SECOND EDITION

Biomedical Photonics Handbook

Volume II
Biomedical Diagnostics

Biomedical Photonics Handbook, Second Edition

Volume I: Fundamentals, Devices, and Techniques

Volume II: Biomedical Diagnostics

Volume III: Therapeutics and Advanced Biophotonics

SECOND EDITION

Biomedical Photonics Handbook

Volume II
Biomedical Diagnostics

Edited by

Tuan Vo-Dinh

Duke University
Durham, North Carolina, USA

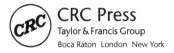

CRC Press
Taylor & Francis Group
Boca Raton London New York

CRC Press is an imprint of the
Taylor & Francis Group, an **informa** business

MATLAB® and Simulink® are trademarks of The MathWorks, Inc. and are used with permission. The MathWorks does not warrant the accuracy of the text or exercises in this book. This book's use or discussion of MATLAB® and Simulink® software or related products does not constitute endorsement or sponsorship by The MathWorks of a particular pedagogical approach or particular use of the MATLAB® and Simulink® software.

CRC Press
Taylor & Francis Group
6000 Broken Sound Parkway NW, Suite 300
Boca Raton, FL 33487-2742

First issued in paperback 2019

© 2015 by Taylor & Francis Group, LLC
CRC Press is an imprint of Taylor & Francis Group, an Informa business

No claim to original U.S. Government works

ISBN-13: 978-1-4200-8514-3 (hbk)
ISBN-13: 978-0-367-37846-2 (pbk)

Library of Congress Cataloging-in-Publication Data

Biomedical photonics handbook / edited by Tuan Vo-Dinh. -- Second edition.
   p. ; cm.
   Includes bibliographical references and indexes.
   Summary: "Biomedical photonics is defined as the science of harnessing light and other forms of radiant energy to address problems in medicine and biology. The field has experienced explosive growth due to the noninvasive or minimally invasive nature and cost-effectiveness of photonic modalities in medical diagnostics and therapy. The first volume of the Biomedical Photonics Handbook, Second Edition focuses on the fundamentals and advanced optical techniques and devices. It is an authoritative reference source for those involved in the research, teaching, learning, and practice of medical technologies"--Provided by publisher.
   ISBN 978-1-4398-0444-5 (set : alk. paper) -- ISBN 978-1-4200-8512-9 (v. 1 : hardcover : alk. paper) -- ISBN 978-1-4200-8514-3 (v. 2 : hardcover : alk. paper) -- ISBN 978-1-4200-8516-7 (v. 3 : hardcover : alk. paper)
   I. Vo-Dinh, Tuan, editor. II. Title: Fundamentals, devices, and techniques. III. Title: Biomedical diagnostics. IV. Title: Therapeutics and advanced biophotonics.
   [DNLM: 1. Diagnostic Imaging--instrumentation. 2. Diagnostic Imaging--methods. 3. Biosensing Techniques--instrumentation. 4. Biosensing Techniques--methods. 5. Photons--diagnostic use. WN 150]

R857.O6
610'.28--dc23
                                                                      2014008504

**Visit the Taylor & Francis Web site at
http://www.taylorandfrancis.com**

**and the CRC Press Web site at
http://www.crcpress.com**

*Inspired by the love and
infinite patience of
my wife, Kim-Chi, and
my daughter, Jade*

*This book is dedicated to the
memory of my parents,
Vo Dinh Kinh and Dang Thi Dinh*

Contents

SECTION I Biomedical Analysis, Sensing, and Imaging

SECTION II   Biomedical Diagnostics and Optical Biopsy

Preface

In the tradition of the *Biomedical Photonics Handbook*, the second edition is intended to serve as an authoritative reference source for a broad audience involved in the research, teaching, learning, and practice of medical technologies. Biomedical photonics is defined as the science that harnesses light and other forms of radiant energy to provide the solution of problems arising in medicine and biology. This research field has recently experienced an explosive growth due to its noninvasive or minimally invasive nature and the cost-effectiveness of photonic modalities in medical diagnostics and therapy.

The field of biomedical photonics did not emerge as a well-defined, single research discipline like chemistry, physics, or biology. Its development and growth have been shaped by the convergence of three scientific and technological revolutions of the twentieth century: the *quantum theory revolution*, the *technology revolution*, and the *genomics revolution*.

The quantum theory of atomic phenomena provides a fundamental framework for molecular biology and genetics because of its unique understanding of electrons, atoms, molecules, and light itself. Out of this new scientific framework emerged the discovery of the structure of DNA, the molecular nature of cell machinery, and the genetic cause of diseases, all of which form the basis of molecular medicine. The formulation of quantum theory not only gave birth to the field of molecular spectroscopy but also led to the development of a powerful set of photonics tools—lasers, scanning tunneling microscopes, and near-field nanoprobes—for exploring nature and understanding the cause of disease at the fundamental level.

Advances in technology also played, and continue to play, an essential role in the development of biomedical photonics. The invention of the laser was an important milestone. Laser is now the light source most widely used to excite tissues for disease diagnosis as well as to irradiate tumors for tissue removal in interventional surgery (*optical scalpels*). The microchip is another important technological development that has significantly accelerated the evolution of biomedical photonics. While the laser has provided a new technology for excitation, the miniaturization and mass production of integrated circuits, sensor devices, and their associated electronic circuitry made possible the development of the microchip, which has radically transformed the ways detection and imaging of molecules, tissues, and organs can be performed in vivo and ex vivo. Recently, nanotechnology, which involves research on materials and species at length scales between 1 and 100 nm, has been revolutionizing important areas in biomedical photonics, especially diagnostics and therapy at the molecular and cellular level. The combination of photonics and nanotechnology has already led to a new generation of devices for probing the cell machinery and elucidating intimate life processes occurring at the molecular level that were heretofore invisible to human inquiry. This will open the possibility of detecting and manipulating atoms and molecules using nanodevices, which have the potential for a wide variety of medical uses at the cellular level. The marriage of electronics, biomaterials, and photonics is expected to revolutionize many areas of medicine in the twenty-first century.

A wide variety of biomedical photonic technologies have already been developed for clinical monitoring of early disease states or physiological parameters such as blood pressure, blood chemistry, pH, temperature, and the presence of pathological organisms or biochemical species of clinical importance. Advanced optical concepts using various spectroscopic modalities (e.g., fluorescence, scattering, reflection, and optical coherence tomography) are emerging in the important area of functional imaging. Many photonic technologies originally developed for other applications (e.g., lasers and sensor systems in defense, energy, and aerospace) have now found important uses in medical applications. From the brain to the sinuses to the abdomen, precision navigation and tracking techniques are critical to position medical instruments precisely within the three-dimensional surgical space. For instance, optical stereotactic systems are being developed for brain surgery, and flexible micronavigation devices are being engineered for medical laser ablation treatments.

With the completion of the sequencing of the human genome, one of the greatest impacts of genomics and proteomics is the establishment of an entirely new approach to biomedical research. With whole-genome sequences and new automated, high-throughput systems, photonic technologies such as biochips and microarrays can address biological and medical problems systematically and on a large scale in a massively parallel manner. They provide the tools to study how tens of thousands of genes and proteins work together in interconnected networks to orchestrate the chemistry of life. Specific genes have been deciphered and linked to numerous diseases and disorders, including breast cancer, muscle disease, deafness, and blindness. Furthermore, advanced biophotonics has contributed dramatically to the field of diagnostics, therapy, and drug discovery in the postgenomic area. Genomics and proteomics present the drug discovery community with a wealth of new potential targets. Biomedical photonics can provide tools capable of identifying specific subsets of genes encoded within the human genome that can cause the development of diseases. Photonic techniques based on molecular probes are being developed to identify the molecular alterations that distinguish a diseased cell from a normal cell. Such technologies will ultimately aid in characterizing and predicting the pathologic behavior of that diseased cell, as well as the cell's responsiveness to drug treatment. Information from the human genome project will one day make personal, molecular medicine an exciting reality.

The second edition of this handbook is intended to present the most recent scientific and technological advances in biomedical photonics, as well as their practical applications, in a single source. The three-volume handbook represents the collective work of over 150 scientists, engineers, and clinicians. It includes many new topics and chapters such as fiber-optics probes design, laser and optical radiation safety, photothermal detection, multidimensional fluorescence imaging, surface plasmon resonance imaging, molecular contrast optical coherence tomography, multiscale photoacoustics, polarized light for medical diagnostics, quantitative diffuse reflectance imaging, interferometric light scattering, nonlinear interferometric vibrational imaging, nanoscintillator-based therapy, SERS molecular sentinel nanoprobes, and plasmonic coupling interference nanoprobes.

The three-volume handbook includes 71 chapters grouped in 8 sections:

1. Volume I: *Biomedical Photonics Handbook*, Second Edition: *Fundamentals, Devices, and Techniques*
2. Volume II: *Biomedical Photonics Handbook*, Second Edition: *Biomedical Diagnostics*
3. Volume III: *Biomedical Photonics Handbook*, Second Edition: *Therapeutics and Advanced Biophotonics*

In Volume I, Section I (Photonics and Tissue Optics) contains introductory chapters on the fundamental optical properties of tissue, light–tissue interactions, and theoretical models for optical imaging. Section II (Basic Photonic Instrumentation and Use) deals with basic instrumentation and hardware systems and contains chapters on lasers and excitation sources, basic optical instrumentation, optical fibers, probe designs, laser use, and optical radiation safety. Section III (Photonic Detection and Imaging Techniques) deals with methodologies and contains chapters on various detection techniques and systems (such as lifetime imaging, microscopy, two-photon detection, photothermal detection, interferometry, Doppler imaging, light scattering, and thermal imaging). Finally, Section IV (Spectroscopic Data) provides a comprehensive compilation of useful information on spectroscopic data of biologically and medically relevant species for over 1000 compounds and systems.

In Volume II, Section I (Biomedical Analysis, Sensing and Imaging) contains chapters describing in vitro diagnostics (e.g., glucose diagnostics, in vitro instrumentation, biosensors, surface plasmon resonance, and flow cytometry) and in vivo diagnostics (optical coherence tomography, polarized light diagnostics, functional imaging and photon migration spectroscopy, and multiscale photoacoustics). Section II (Biomedical Diagnostics and Optical Biopsy) is mainly devoted to novel optical techniques for cancer diagnostics, often referred to as *optical biopsy* (such as fluorescence, scattering, reflectance, interferometric light scattering, optoacoustics, and ultrasonically modulated optical imaging).

In Volume III, Section I (Therapeutic and Interventional Techniques) covers photodynamic therapy as well as various laser-based treatment techniques that are applied to different organs and disease endpoints (dermatology, pulmonology, neurosurgery, ophthalmology, otolaryngology, gastroenterology, and dentistry). There are several chapters dealing with nanotechnology for theranostics, that is, the modality combining diagnostics and therapy. Section II (Advanced Biophotonics and Nanophotonics) is devoted to the most recent advances in methods and instrumentation for biomedical and biotechnology applications. This section contains chapters on emerging photonic technologies (e.g., biochips, nanosensors, quantum dots, molecular probes, molecular beacons, molecular sentinels, plasmonic coupling nanoprobes, bioluminescent reporters, optical tweezers) that are being developed for gene expression research, gene diagnostics, protein profiling, and molecular biology investigations as well as for early diagnostics of disease biomarkers for the *new medicine.*

The goal of the second edition of this handbook is to provide a comprehensive forum that integrates interdisciplinary research and development of interest to scientists, engineers, manufacturers, teachers, students, and clinical providers. Each chapter provides introductory material with an overview of the topic of interest as well as a collection of published data with an extensive list of references for further details. The handbook is designed to present the most recent advances in instrumentation and methods as well as clinical applications in important areas of biomedical photonics. Because light is rapidly becoming an important diagnostic tool and a powerful weapon in the armory of the modern physician, it is our hope that this handbook will stimulate a greater appreciation of the usefulness, efficiency, and potential of photonics in medicine.

Tuan Vo-Dinh
Duke University
Durham, North Carolina

Acknowledgments

The completion of this work has been made possible with the assistance of many friends and colleagues. I wish to express my gratitude to members of the Scientific Advisory Board of the first edition. Their thoughtful suggestions and useful advice in the planning phase of the first edition have been important in achieving the breadth and depth of this handbook. It is a great pleasure for me to acknowledge, with deep gratitude, the contribution of over 150 contributors for the 71 chapters in this handbook. I wish to thank my coworkers at Duke University and the Oak Ridge National Laboratory, and many colleagues in academia, federal laboratories, and industry, for their kind help in reading and commenting on various chapters of the manuscript. My gratitude is extended to all my present and past students, postdoctoral associates, colleagues, and collaborators, who have been traveling with me on this exciting journey of discovery with the ultimate vision of bringing research at the intersection of photonics and medicine to the service of society.

I gratefully acknowledge the support of the US Department of Energy Office of Biological and Environmental Research, the National Institutes of Health, the Defense Advanced Research Projects Agency, the Department of the Army, the Army Medical Research and Materiel Command, the Department of Justice, the Federal Bureau of Investigation, the Office of Naval Research, the Environmental Protection Agency, the Fitzpatrick Foundation, the R. Eugene and Susie E. Goodson Endowment Fund, and the Wallace Coulter Foundation.

The completion of this work has been made possible with the love, encouragement, and inspiration of my wife, Kim-Chi, and my daughter, Jade.

Editor

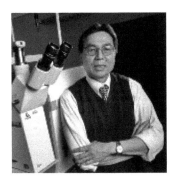

Tuan Vo-Dinh is R. Eugene and Susie E. Goodson Distinguished Professor of Biomedical Engineering, professor of chemistry, and director of the Fitzpatrick Institute for Photonics at Duke University. A native of Vietnam and a naturalized US citizen, he completed high school education in Saigon (now Ho Chi Minh City). He continued his studies in Europe, where he received his BS in physics in 1970 from EPFL (Ecole Polytechnique Federal de Lausanne) in Lausanne and his PhD in physical chemistry in 1975 from ETH (Swiss Federal Institute of Technology) in Zurich, Switzerland. Before joining Duke University in 2006, Dr. Vo-Dinh was director of the Center for Advanced Biomedical Photonics, group leader of Advanced Biomedical Science and Technology Group, and a corporate fellow, one of the highest honors for distinguished scientists at Oak Ridge National Laboratory (ORNL). His research has focused on the development of advanced technologies for the protection of the environment and the improvement of human health. His research activities involve biophotonics, plasmonics, nanobiotechnology, laser spectroscopy, molecular imaging, medical theranostics, cancer detection, nanosensors, chemical sensors, biosensors, and biochips.

Dr. Vo-Dinh has authored over 350 publications in peer-reviewed scientific journals. He is the author of a textbook on spectroscopy and the editor of six books. He holds over 37 US and international patents, 5 of which have been licensed to private companies for commercial development. Dr. Vo-Dinh has presented over 200 invited lectures at international meetings in universities and research institutions. He has chaired over 30 international conferences in his field of research and served on various national and international scientific committees. He also serves the scientific community through his participation in a wide range of governmental and industrial boards and advisory committees.

Dr. Vo-Dinh has received seven R&D 100 Awards for Most Technologically Significant Advance in Research and Development for his pioneering research and inventions of innovative technologies. He has received the Gold Medal Award, Society for Applied Spectroscopy (1988); the Languedoc–Roussillon Award, France (1989); the Scientist of the Year Award, ORNL (1992); the Thomas Jefferson Award, Martin Marietta Corporation (1992); two Awards for Excellence in Technology Transfer, Federal Laboratory Consortium (1995, 1986); the Inventor of the Year Award, Tennessee Inventors Association (1996); the Lockheed Martin Technology Commercialization Award (1998); the Distinguished Inventors Award, UT-Battelle (2003); and the Distinguished Scientist of the Year Award, ORNL (2003). In 1997, he was presented the Exceptional Services Award for distinguished contribution to a healthy citizenry from the US Department of Energy. In 2011, he received the Award for Spectrochemical Analysis from the American Chemical Society (ACS) Division of Analytical Chemistry.

Contributors

Leonardo Allain
Merck & Co., Inc.
Whitehouse Station, New Jersey

Rohit Bhargava
National Institute of Diabetes
and Digestive and Kidney
Diseases
National Institutes of Health
Bethesda, Maryland

Irving J. Bigio
Boston University
Boston, Massachusetts

David A. Boas
Department of Radiology
Harvard Medical School
and
Massachusetts General Hospital
Boston, Massachusetts

and

Athinoula A. Martinos Center
for Biomedical Imaging
Charlestown, Massachusetts

A. Claude Boccara
Institut Langevin
Université Paris VI—Pierre et
Marie Curie
Paris, France

Emmanuel Bossy
Institut Langevin
Université Paris VI—Pierre et
Marie Curie
Paris, France

Michael Canva
Centre National de la Recherche
Scientifique
Université Paris Sud
Palaiseau, France

and

Duke University
Durham, North Carolina

Oscar Carrasco-Zevallos
Department of Biomedical
Engineering
Duke University
Durham, North Carolina

Albert E. Cerussi
Beckman Laser Institute and
Medical Clinic
University of California, Irvine
Irvine, California

Paul Charette
Université de Sherbrooke
Sherbrooke, Québec, Canada

Jean-Pierre Cloarec
Institut des Nanotechnologies
de Lyon
Université de Lyon
Écully, France

and

Centre National de la Recherche
Scientifique
Université de Sherbrooke
Sherbrooke, Québec, Canada

Gerard L. Coté
Department of Biomedical
Engineering
Texas A&M University
College Station, Texas

Brian M. Cullum
Department of Chemistry and
Biochemistry
University of Maryland,
Baltimore County
Baltimore, Maryland

Brian Cummins
Department of Biomedical
Engineering
Texas A&M University
College Station, Texas

Abby E. Deans
University of California,
San Francisco
San Francisco, California

Andrew Fales
Department of Chemistry
Duke University
Durham, North Carolina

S. Douglass Gilman
University of Tennessee
Knoxville, Tennessee

A. Godavarty
Department of Chemistry
and
Department of Chemical
Engineering
Texas A&M University
College Station, Texas

Michel Goossens
Hôpital Henri Mondor
Institut Mondor de Recherche
    Biomédicales
Institut National de la Santé et
    de la Recherche Médicale
Créteil, France

Guy D. Griffin
Department of Biomedical
    Engineering
Duke University
Durham, North Carolina

Michel Gross
Université Montpellier 2
and
Centre National de la Recherche
    Scientifique
Montpellier, France

J.P. Houston
Department of Chemistry
and
Department of Chemical
    Engineering
Texas A&M University
College Station, Texas

Song Hu
Department of Biomedical
    Engineering
Washington University in
    St. Louis
St. Louis, Missouri

Joseph A. Izatt
Department of Biomedical
    Engineering
Duke University
Durham, North Carolina

Steven L. Jacques
Department of Biomedical
    Engineering
and
Department of Dermatology
Oregon Health & Science
    University
Portland, Oregon

E. Kuwana
Department of Chemistry
and
Department of Chemical
    Engineering
Texas A&M University
College Station, Texas

Ira W. Levin
National Institute of Diabetes
    and Digestive and Kidney
    Diseases
National Institutes of Health
Bethesda, Maryland

Hong Liu
Center for Bioengineering
and
Department of Electrical and
    Computer Engineering
University of Oklahoma
Norman, Oklahoma

Anita Mahadevan-Jansen
Vanderbilt University
Nashville, Tennessee

Francis Mandy
Soft Flow Hungary Ltd.
Pécs, Hungary

Roger J. McNichols (Deceased)
BioTex, Inc.
Houston, Texas

Julien Moreau
Centre National de la Recherche
    Scientifique
Université Paris Sud
Palaiseau, France

Judith R. Mourant
Los Alamos National
    Laboratory
Los Alamos, New Mexico

Thomas Nishino
University of Texas Medical
    Branch
Galveston, Texas

Alexander A. Oraevsky
TomoWave Laboratories, Inc.
Houston, Texas

Chetan A. Patil
Vanderbilt University
Nashville, Tennessee

Isaac J. Pence
Vanderbilt University
Nashville, Tennessee

Casey W. Pirnstill
Department of Biomedical
    Engineering
Texas A&M University
College Station, Texas

Nirmala Ramanujam
Department of Biomedical
    Engineering
Duke University
Durham, North Carolina

François Ramaz
Institut Langevin
Université Paris VI—Pierre
    et Marie Curie
Paris, France

**Diether Recktenwald
(Retired)**
BD Biosciences
San Jose, California

Francisco E. Robles
Department of Medical Physics
Duke University
Durham, North Carolina

R. Roy
Department of Chemistry
and
Department of Chemical
    Engineering
Texas A&M University
College Station, Texas

Michael J. Sepaniak
University of Tennessee
Knoxville, Tennessee

E.M. Sevick-Muraca
Department of Chemistry
and
Department of Chemical
    Engineering
Texas A&M University
College Station, Texas

David L. Stokes
EOIR Technologies
Spotsylvania, Virginia

Andrew Taylor
Royal Surrey County Hospital
Surrey, United Kingdom

Neil G. Terry
Department of Biomedical
    Engineering
Duke University
Durham, North Carolina

A.B. Thompson
Department of Chemistry
and
Department of Chemical
    Engineering
Texas A&M University
College Station, Texas

Bruce J. Tromberg
Beckman Laser Institute and
    Medical Clinic
University of California, Irvine
Irvine, California

Joe Trotter
BD Biosciences
San Jose, California

Rudi Varro (Deceased)
BD Biosciences
San Jose, California

Tuan Vo-Dinh
Department of Biomedical
    Engineering
and
Department of Chemistry
Duke University
Durham, North Carolina

Lihong V. Wang
Department of Biomedical
    Engineering
Washington University in
    St. Louis
St. Louis, Missouri

Adam Wax
Department of Biomedical
    Engineering
and
Department of Medical Physics
Duke University
Durham, North Carolina

Molly Donovan Wong
Center for Bioengineering
and
Department of Electrical and
    Computer Engineering
University of Oklahoma
Norman, Oklahoma

Xizeng Wu
Department of Radiology
University of Alabama at
    Birmingham
Birmingham, Alabama

Ming Yan
BD Biosciences
San Jose, California

Arjun G. Yodh
University of Pennsylvania
Philadelphia, Pennsylvania

Bing Yu
Department of Biomedical
    Engineering
University of Akron
Akron, Ohio

Yizheng Zhu
Department of Biomedical
    Engineering
Duke University
Durham, North Carolina

MATLAB Statement

MATLAB® is a registered trademark of The MathWorks, Inc. For product information, please contact:

The MathWorks, Inc.
3 Apple Hill Drive
Natick, MA 01760-2098 USA
Tel: 508-647-7000
Fax: 508-647-7001
E-mail: info@mathworks.com
Web: www.mathworks.com

I

Biomedical Analysis, Sensing, and Imaging

1

1

Biosensors for Medical Applications

Tuan Vo-Dinh
Duke University

Leonardo Allain
Merck & Co., Inc.

Andrew Fales
Duke University

1.1 Introduction

Human beings, along with other mammals, consciously interact with the surrounding world by means of seven sensing mechanisms. In addition to the well-recognized five senses, the abilities to detect temperature and variations in elevation are almost as important. One cannot help being awed by the evolutionary process that brought the development of such senses and by their integration into a brain capable of information processing and storage.

If a better awareness of our surroundings, food supplies, and predators was the main driver for this evolutionary process, a parallel might be drawn with our own human enterprise of creating sensors that help us understand the world we interact with. A sensor can be viewed as the "primary element of a measurement chain, which converts the input variable into a signal suitable for measurement."[1] A sensing scheme is usually based on a transduction principle or mechanism. An input variable is transformed into an output variable through a transduction mechanism. Transduction principles are nothing less than known physical or chemical effects that correlate observations in different domains. For example, the photoelectric effect is used to correlate number of photons with electric current. The piezoelectric effect does the same for stress and electricity, and Biot–Savart's law correlates magnetic field and electric current. In other words, the operating principle of a sensor involves transforming signals between different domains, from a domain we cannot directly access to one we can measure.

A biosensor is a special type of sensor often used in bioanalysis. Humankind has been performing bioanalysis since the dawn of time, using the sensory nerve cells of the nose to detect scents and those of the tongue to taste dissolved substances. As time has progressed, so has our level of understanding about the function of living organisms in detecting trace amounts of biochemicals in complex systems. The abilities of biological organisms to recognize foreign substances are unparalleled and have to some extent been mimicked by researchers in the development of biosensors. Using bioreceptors from biological organisms or receptors that have been patterned after biological systems, scientists have developed a new means of chemical analysis that often has the high selectivity of biological recognition systems. These biorecognition elements in combination with various transduction methods have helped to create the rapidly expanding fields of bioanalysis and related technologies known as biosensors and biochemical sensors.

1.2 Biosensors: Definition and Classification

The two fundamental operating principles of a biosensor are (1) *biological recognition* and (2) *sensing*. Therefore, a biosensor can be generally defined as a device that consists of two basic components connected in series: (1) a biological recognition system, often called a bioreceptor, and (2) a transducer. The basic principle of a biosensor is to detect this molecular recognition and to transform it into another type of signal using a transducer. The main purpose of the recognition system is to provide the sensor with a high degree of selectivity for the analyte to be measured. The interaction of the analyte with the bioreceptor is designed to produce an effect measured by the transducer, which converts the information into a measurable effect, such as an electrical signal. Figure 1.1 illustrates the conceptual principle of the biosensing process.

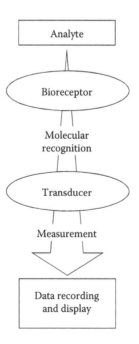

FIGURE 1.1   Conceptual diagram of the biosensing principle.

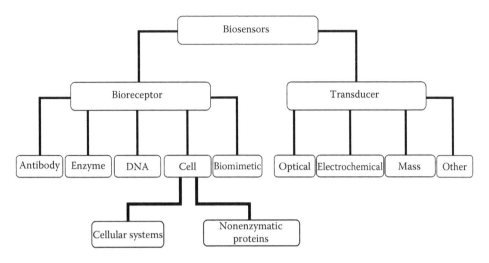

FIGURE 1.2 Biosensor classification schemes.

Biosensors can be classified either by their bioreceptor or by their transducer type (Figure 1.2). A biore-ceptor is a biological molecular species (e.g., an antibody [Ab], an enzyme, a protein, or a nucleic acid) or a living biological system (e.g., cells, tissues, or whole organisms) that utilizes a biochemical mechanism for recognition. The sampling component of a biosensor contains a biosensitive layer. The layer can either contain bioreceptors or be made of bioreceptors covalently attached to the transducer. The most common forms of bioreceptors used in biosensing are based on (a) antibody/antigen (Ag–Ab) interactions, (b) nucleic acid interactions, (c) enzymatic interactions, (d) cellular interactions (i.e., microorganisms, proteins), and (e) interactions using biomimetic materials (i.e., synthetic bioreceptors). For transducer classifica-tion, the previously mentioned techniques (optical, electrochemical, and mass-sensitive) are used.

Bioreceptors are the key to specificity for biosensor technologies. They are responsible for binding the analyte of interest to the sensor for the measurement. These bioreceptors can take many forms, and the different bioreceptors that have been used are as numerous as the different analytes that have been monitored using biosensors. However, bioreceptors can generally be classified into five differ-ent major categories: (1) Ag–Ab, (2) enzymes, (3) nucleic acids/DNA, (4) cellular structures/cells, and (5) biomimetic. Figure 1.3 shows a schematic diagram of two types of bioreceptors: the structure of an immunoglobulin G (IgG) Ab molecule (Figure 1.3a) and DNA and the principle of base pairing in hybridization (Figure 1.3b).

Since the first biosensors were reported in the early 1960s,[2] there has been an accelerated growth of research activities in this area.[3–28] Biosensors have seen a wide variety of applications, primarily in three major areas: biological monitoring, biomedical diagnostics, and environmental sensing applications.

1.3 Transduction Systems

Biosensors can be classified based on the transduction methods they employ. Transduction can be accom-plished through a large variety of methods. Most forms of transduction can be categorized in one of three main classes: (1) optical detection methods, (2) electrochemical detection methods, and (3) mass-based detection methods. Other detection methods include voltaic and magnetic methods. New types of trans-ducers are constantly being developed for use in biosensors. Each of these three main classes contains many different subclasses, creating a large number of possible transduction methods or combination of methods. This section provides a brief overview of the various detection methods used in biosensors. Special emphasis will be placed on the description of optical transducing principles, which is the focus of this chapter.

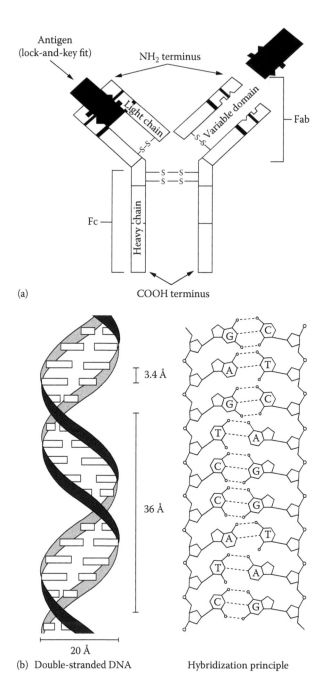

FIGURE 1.3 Schematic diagrams of two types of bioreceptors: (a) IgG Ab and (b) DNA and the hybridization principle.

1.3.1 Optical Detection

Optical detection offers the largest number of possible subcategories of all three of the transducer classes. This is due to the fact that optical biosensors can be used with many different types of spectroscopies (e.g., absorption, fluorescence, phosphorescence, Raman, surface-enhanced Raman scattering [SERS], refraction, dispersion spectrometry) to measure different spectrochemical properties of target species.

These properties include amplitude, energy, polarization, decay time, and/or phase. Amplitude is the most commonly measured parameter of the electromagnetic spectrum, as it can generally be correlated with the concentration of the analyte of interest.

The energy of the electromagnetic radiation measured can often provide information about changes in the local environment surrounding the analyte, its molecular vibrations (i.e., Raman or infrared [IR] absorption spectroscopies), or the formation of new energy levels. Measurement of the interaction of a free molecule with a fixed surface can often be investigated with polarization measurements. Polarization of emitted light is usually random when emitted from a free molecule in solution; however, when a molecule becomes bound to a fixed surface, the emitted light often remains polarized. The decay time of a specific emission signal (i.e., fluorescence or phosphorescence) can also be used to gain information about molecular interactions, since these decay times are highly dependent upon the excited state of the molecules and their local molecular environment. Another property that can be measured is the phase of the emitted radiation. When electromagnetic radiation interacts with a surface, the speed or phase of that radiation is altered, based on the refractive index of the medium (analyte). When the medium changes, via binding of an analyte, the refractive index may change, thus changing the phase of the impinging radiation. This property of electromagnetic radiation has been successfully exploited in commercial applications using surface plasmon resonance (SPR) sensors.

1.3.1.1 Fluorescence

Fluorescence is one of the most sensitive spectroscopic techniques, and its sensitivity makes it uniquely suited for the detection of very low concentrations of bioanalytes. Background information on the photophysical principles of the fluorescence emission process can be found in Chapter 15. When coupled with a high-power light source such as a laser, it can yield very high signal-to-noise (S/N) values. Single-molecule detection using laser-induced fluorescence has been reported in many studies. Because of its inherently high sensitivity, fluorescence has traditionally been the technique of choice for optical detection of trace-level analytes (at the femtomole level or lower). For high-quantum-yield fluorophores, the effective fluorescence cross sections can be as high as 10^{-16} cm²/molecule.

A typical optical setup for a fluorescence biosensor using a laser as the light source is shown in Figure 1.4.[7] The instrument consists of an optical fiber having antibodies immobilized at the sensor tip. Excitation light from a laser is sent through a beam splitter onto the incidence end of the optical fiber. The laser beam is transmitted inside the fiber onto the sensor tip, where it excites the analyte

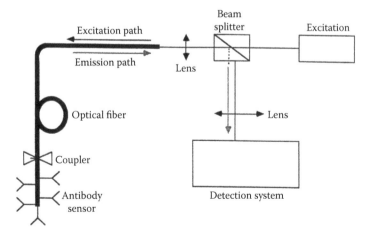

FIGURE 1.4 Schematic diagram of an optical system for an Ab-based biosensor. (From Vo-Dinh, T. et al., *Appl. Spectrosc.*, 41(5), 735, 1987.)

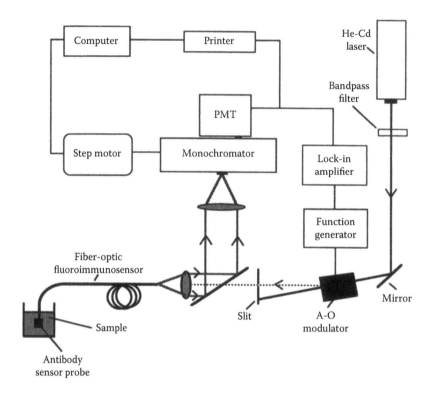

FIGURE 1.5 Schematic diagram of an Ab-based biosensor with phase resolution. (From Vo-Dinh, T. et al., *Appl. Spectrosc.*, 44(1), 128, 1990.)

molecules bound to the antibodies. The excited Ag fluorescence is collected and retransmitted back to the incidence end of the fiber, directed by the beam splitter onto the entrance slit of a monochromator, and recorded by a photomultiplier. This fluoroimmunosensor (FIS) was used to detect the carcinogen benzo[*a*]pyrene (BaP).[7]

Fluorescence detection is also suitable for time- or phase-resolved measurements, yielding additional information from the system of interest. Vo-Dinh and coworkers reported the development of a phase-resolved fiber-optic fluoroimmunosensor (PR-FIS), which can differentiate BaP and its metabolite benzopyrene tetrol (BPT) based on the difference of their fluorescence lifetimes. A diagram for a phase-resolved optical setup is shown in Figure 1.5.[29] The excitation laser beam is modulated with an acousto-optic modulation system. A function generator provides the waveforms to drive the modulator. Laser light is delivered to the sample by an optical fiber, and the fluorescence is collected by the same fiber. The fluorescence from the sensing probe is collimated by appropriate optics and focused onto the entrance slit of a monochromator equipped with a photomultiplier. A lock-in amplifier synchronized with the function generator is used to measure phase-resolved signals. With this setup, BaP and BPT could be detected simultaneously using phase-resolved fluorescence. Their phase-dependent spectrum is shown in Figure 1.6.[29] Figure 1.6a shows the fluorescence of BPT with the use of the optimal phase shift for maximum BPT signal. On the other hand, Figure 1.6b shows the fluorescence of BaP with the use of the optimal phase shift for maximum BaP signal. The results illustrate the capability of the PR-FIS device to reveal the spectrum of 30 fmol of BPT in the presence of much higher amounts of interfering BaP.

Femtomolar sensitivities for fluorescently labeled proteins were reported by Herron and coworkers using a channel-etched thin-film waveguide FIS.[30] A silicon oxynitride thin optical waveguide film was etched to create a channel for small volumes of analyte. Two different types of assays were performed and compared using this biosensor. The first was a direct assay of a fluorescently tagged protein ligand

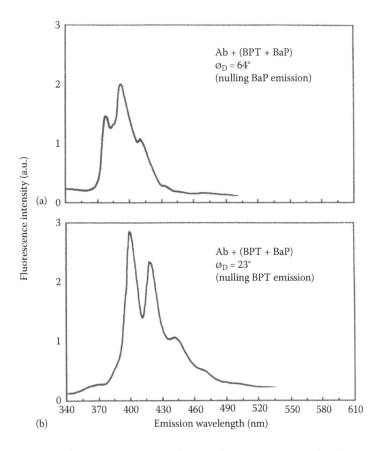

FIGURE 1.6 Phase-resolved fluorescence spectra of BaP and BPT in anti-BPT Ab solution: (a) with detector phase angle at 64° (nulling BaP emission) and (b) with detector phase angle at 23° (nulling BPT emission). (From Vo-Dinh, T. et al., *Appl. Spectrosc.*, 44(1), 128, 1990.)

to a protein receptor that had been immobilized onto the waveguide. The second assay was an indirect sandwich-type assay of a nonfluorescent protein ligand, where the analyte (the protein ligand) binds to a protein bioreceptor that had been immobilized on the waveguide; then a fluorescently tagged secondary receptor was used for measurement purposes. The fluorescent dye used to tag the proteins was Cy5, a red emitting cyanine dye, which reduced the chance of excitation of possible interferents.

An interesting application of fluorescence spectroscopy involves the detection of the lipopolysaccharide endotoxin (LPS), which is the most powerful immune stimulant known and a causative agent in the clinical syndrome known as sepsis. Sepsis is responsible for more than 100,000 deaths annually, in large part due to the lack of a rapid, reliable, and sensitive diagnostic technique. LPS has been detected in *Escherichia coli* at concentrations as low as 10 ng/mL, in 30 s using an evanescent-wave fiber-optic biosensor. Polymyxin B, covalently immobilized onto the surface of the fiber-optic probe, selectively bound fluorescently labeled LPS. The competitive assay format worked in both buffer and plasma with similar sensitivities. This method can be used with other LPS capture molecules such as antibodies, lectins, or antibiotics, to simultaneously detect LPS and determine the LPS serotype. This LPS assay using the fiber-optic biosensor can be applied in both clinical and environmental testing.[31]

1.3.1.2 Surface Plasmon Resonance

Since the first application of the SPR phenomenon for sensing almost two decades ago, this method has made great strides both in terms of instrumentation development and applications.[32] SPR sensor technology has been commercially available, and SPR biosensors have become a useful tool for characterizing and quantifying biomolecular interactions.

SPR makes it possible to monitor the binding process as a function of time by following the increase in refractive index that occurs when one of the interacting partners binds to its ligand immobilized on the surface of an SPR sensor substrate.[33] A technique that does not require that the reactants to be labeled is a major advantage, simplifying the data collection process. Biosensor binding data are also useful for selecting peptides to be used in diagnostic solid-phase immunoassays. Very small changes in binding affinity can be measured with good precision, which is a prerequisite for analyzing the functional effect and thermodynamic implications of limited structural changes in interacting molecules. For example, the on-rate (k_a) and off-rate (k_d) kinetic constants of the interaction between a protein and an Ab can be readily measured and the equilibrium affinity constant, K, can be calculated from the ratio $k_a/k_d = K$.[33]

The transduction principle involved in SPR sensors is based on the arrangement of a dielectric/metal/dielectric sandwich in such way that when light impinges on a metal surface, a wave is excited within the plasma formed by the conduction electrons of the metal.[34,35] A surface plasmon is a surface charge density wave occurring at a metal surface. When a plasmon resonance is induced in the surface of a metal conductor by the impact of light of a critical wavelength and angle, the effect is observed as a minimum in the intensity of the light reflected off the metal surface. The critical angle is naturally very sensitive to the dielectric constant of the medium immediately adjacent to the metal, and it therefore lends itself to exploitation for bioassay. For example, the metal can be deposited as, or on, a grating; upon illumination with a wide band of frequencies, the absence of reflected light at the frequencies at which the resonance matching conditions are met can be observed.

Because of the intrinsic dependence with the index of refraction at the surface, SPR can be used as a sensor transducer to indicate when alterations at the surface happen. The binding event involving Ag–Ab recognition or DNA hybridization at the SPR sensor surface is the most common SPR application. SPR is able to detect small variations of the index of refraction at the metal-coated interface caused by changes in a few monolayers above the surface.

In biosensor devices, the SPR is detected as a very sharp decrease of the light reflectance when the angle of incidence is varied. The resonance angle is very sensitive to variations in the refractive index of the medium just outside the metal film. Since the electric field probes the medium within only a few hundreds of nanometers from the metal surface, the condition for resonance is very sensitive to variations in thin films on this surface. Changes in the refractive index of about 10^{-5} are easily detected.

The surface plasmon wave penetrates in both directions normal to the interface; consequently, the incident angle or frequency at which resonance is observed is dependent on the refractive index of dielectric at the interface. Liedberg and coworkers[34] have shown that SPR can be used as the basis of a genuine reagentless immunosensor if large analytes are to be monitored. The Ab is immobilized on the metal. When a large Ab binds, it displaces solution (having a refractive index of around 1.34) with, for example, protein (having a refractive index of 1.5). The effective refractive index of the dielectric adjacent to the metal is thus changed in proportion to the amount of analyte bound, and the SPR (incident angle or resonance frequency) is shifted accordingly. Flanagan and Pantell have shown that the amount of analyte bound can be directly related to the resonance shift even when the resonance curve is distorted by scattering caused by surface roughness, thus relieving one of the constraints of precise control of metalization, which would be unattractive in the mass production of cheap sensors.

SPR biosensors can provide qualitative information on macromolecular assembly processes under a variety of conditions. Quantitative information, in the form of affinity constants for complex formation, can be obtained in a manner similar to conventional solid-phase assays. The major advantage of SPR biosensors is that the formation and breakdown of complexes can be monitored in real time. This offers the possibility of determining the mechanism and kinetic rate constants associated with a binding event. This information is essential for understanding how biological systems function at the molecular level. However, accurate interpretation of biosensor data is not always straightforward.[36] A few software programs can interpolate SPR data and provide an estimate binding constants. The program CLAMP is a software developed to interpret complex interactions recorded on biosensors.[36] It combines numerical integration and nonlinear global curve-fitting routines. The BIAcore® system is one of the most used among the several commercially available optical biosensors.

For example, the interactions between adenylate kinase (AK) and a monoclonal antibody (MAb) against AK (McAb3D3) were examined with an optical biosensor, and the sensograms were fitted to four models using numerical integration algorithms.[37] The interaction of AK in solution with immobilized McAb3D3 followed a single exponential function and the data fitted well to a pseudo-first-order reaction model.

The application of SPR biosensors in life sciences and pharmaceutical research continues to increase. Several reviews providing a comprehensive analysis of the commercial SPR biosensor literature and highlights of emerging applications are available.[32,38,39] Some general guidelines to help increase confidence in the results reported from biosensor analyses, due to the variability in the quality of published biosensor data, have been compiled as well.[38]

1.3.1.3 Near-Infrared Absorption

Near-infrared (NIR) spectroscopy utilizes wavelengths above 800 nm to excite vibrational overtones and/or low-energy electronic levels of chemical species. Use of NIR usually profits from lower fluorescence background and higher specificity for appropriate dyes. Longer wavelengths also offer better penetration of translucent tissue, another major advantage of NIR for biomedical diagnostics.

A biomolecular probe utilizing NIR for the detection of biological molecules (immunochemical samples) with a semiconductor laser diode (780 nm) has been reported.[40] This probe consists of a modified fiber tip binding site, an NIR dye, and a photodiode detector. Preparation of the NIR biosensor involved the immobilization of anti-IgG Ab to the activated binding site of the fiber, followed by coating with IgG for a sandwich-type probe. The Ab was labeled with the commercially available NIR dye IR-144. The low background signal of the detector allowed the detection of 2.72 ng/mL of IgG in a probe coated with 10 ng/mL Ab at 820 nm.[40]

1.3.1.4 Reflectometric Interference

Gauglitz and coworkers have developed a unique technique based on reflectometric interference spectroscopy (RifS) for detection in biosensors.[41–43] RifS was used for the detection of biomolecular interactions and applied for small-molecule detection by chemical sensor surfaces. The principle of RifS, which does not require the use of labels, is illustrated in Figure 1.7.[41] A thin silica layer on a glass substrate is illuminated from the backside using white light. Light beams are reflected at the different layers and superimposed to form a characteristic interference pattern. Changes in the thickness of the transducer surface caused by biomolecular interactions lead to a shift of the interference pattern, which can be analyzed in real time.

1.3.1.5 Raman

The possibility of using Raman and/or SERS labels as gene probes has been reported.[44–46] The SERS technique has been recently applied to the detection of DNA fragments of the human immunodeficiency virus (HIV)[20,44,45] and of the breast cancer gene.[47] Raman spectroscopy has also proved to be a very useful tool for chemical analysis because it can identify chemical groups. This technique, however, suffers from poor sensitivity, often requiring powerful and expensive laser excitation sources. However, the discovery of the SERS effect,[48–50] which results in increased sensitivities of up to 10^8-fold for some compounds, has renewed interest in this technology for analytical purposes. The feasibility of using surface-enhanced Raman gene (SERGen) probes, which exhibit an extremely narrow small spectral bandwidth, was first demonstrated.[44–46] The ability to use labeled primers extends the utility of the SERGen probes for medical diagnostic purposes.

Because SERGen probes rely on chemical identification rather than emission of radioactivity, they have a significant advantage over radioactive probes. SERGen probes are formed with stable chemicals

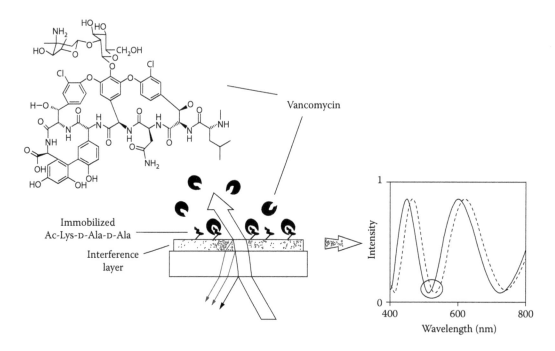

FIGURE 1.7 Principle of reflectometric interference spectrometry. (From Tunnemann, R. et al., *Anal. Chem.*, 73(17), 4313, 2001.)

that do not emit potentially dangerous ionizing radiation. Furthermore, the probes offer the excellent specificity inherent in Raman spectroscopy. While isotope labels are few, many chemicals can be used to label DNA for SERS detection. Potentially, dozens to hundreds of different SERGen probes could be constructed and used to simultaneously probe several DNA sequences of interest (label multiplexing), thus decreasing the time and cost for gene diagnostics and DNA mapping. The multispectral imaging (MSI) system developed in this work, with its rapid wavelength switching of the acousto-optic tunable filter (AOTF) system, could allow very rapid scanning and high-throughput data collection.[44]

For biomedical diagnostics, the SERGen probe could have a wide variety of applications in areas where nucleic acid identification is involved. The SERGen probes may also be used in polymerase chain reaction (PCR) applications for medical diagnostic applications such as for HIV detection. In genomics applications as well as in high-throughput analysis, the SERS gene probe technology could lead to the development of detection methods that minimize the time, expense, and variability of preparing samples by combining the BAC mapping approach with SERS *label multiplex* detection. Large numbers of DNA samples can be simultaneously prepared by automated devices. With the SERGen technique, multiple samples can be separated and directly analyzed using multiple SERGen labels simultaneously (label multiplex scheme). The use of the SERS technique for biomedical application is further described in Chapter 8.

1.3.2 Electrochemical Detection

Electrochemical detection is another possible means of transduction that has been extensively used in biosensors.[51-55] This technique is complementary to optical detection methods such as fluorescence, the most sensitive of the optical techniques. Since many analytes of interest are not strongly fluorescent and tagging a molecule with a fluorescent label is often labor intensive, electrochemical transduction can be very useful. By combining the sensitivity of electrochemical measurements with the selectivity provided by bioreception, detection limits comparable to those of fluorescence biosensors are often achievable.

Electrochemical detection is usually based on the chemical potential of a particular species in solution (the analyte), as measured by comparison to a reference electrode. Therefore, the electrochemical response is dependent on the activity of the analyte species, not their concentration. However, for dilute solutions of low ionic strength, the thermodynamic parameter activity approaches the physical parameter concentration (in molar terms). In comparison, the signal intensity associated with optical detection is usually directly proportional to the number of a specific chromophore within a certain path length and therefore directly dependent on the concentration of the chromophore. The linear relationship between signal intensity and concentration of a species is known as Beer–Lambert's law. The cases in which discrepancies from this linear relationship occur are usually caused by secondary effects such as self-absorbance and equilibrium conditions.

Multiple examples of electrochemical sensors applied to biological systems are known. For example, electrochemical flow-through enzyme-based biosensors for the detection of glucose and lactate have been developed by Cammann and coworkers.[56] Glucose oxidase and lactate oxidase were immobilized in conducting polymers generated from pyrrole, *N*-methylpyrrole, aniline, and *o*-phenylenediamine on platinum surfaces. These various sensor matrices were compared on basis of amperometric measurements of glucose and lactate, and the *o*-phenylenediamine polymer was found to be the most sensitive. This polymer matrix was also deposited on a piece of graphite felt and used as an enzyme reactor as well as a working electrode in an electrochemical detection system. Using this system, a linear dynamic range of 500 µM–10 mM glucose was determined with a detection limit of <500 µM. For lactate, the linear dynamic range covered concentrations from 50 µM to 1 mM with a detection limit of <50 µM.

A biosensor for protein and amino acid estimation has been reported by Turner and Sarkar.[57] A screen-printed biosensor based on a rhodinized carbon-paste working electrode was used in the three-electrode configuration for a two-step detection method. Electrolysis of an acidic potassium bromide electrolyte at the working electrode produced bromine, which was consumed by the proteins and amino acids. The bromine production occurred at one potential while monitoring of the bromine consumption was performed using a lower potential. The method proved very sensitive to almost all of the amino acids, as well as some common proteins, and was even capable of measuring L- and D-proline, which gave no response to enzyme-based biosensors. This sensor has been tested by measuring proteins and amino acids in fruit juice, milk, and urine.

Scheller and coworkers have developed an electrochemical biosensor for the indirect detection of L-phenylalanine via NADH.[58] This sensor is based on a three-step multienzymatic/electrochemical reaction. Three enzymes—L-phenylalanine dehydrogenase, salicylate hydroxylase, and tyrosinase—are immobilized in a carbon-paste electrode. The principle behind this reaction/detection scheme is as follows. First, the L-phenylalanine dehydrogenase, upon binding and reacting with L-phenylalanine, produces NADH. The second enzyme, salicylate hydroxylase, then converts salicylate to catechol in the presence of oxygen and NADH. The tyrosinase then oxidizes the catechol to *o*-quinone, which is detected electrochemically, and reduced back to catechol with an electrode potential of −50 mV vs. a Ag/AgCl reference electrode. This reduction step results in an amplification of signal due to the recycling of catechol from *o*-quinone. Prior to the addition of the L-phenylalanine dehydrogenase to the electrode, it was tested for its sensitivity to NADH, its pH dependence, and its response to possible interferents, urea, and ascorbic acid. From these measurements, it was found that the sensor sensitivity for NADH increased 33-fold by introducing the recycling step over just the salicylate hydroxylase system alone. When this sensor was tested for the detection of L-phenylalanine in human serum, the linear dynamic range was found to cover concentrations ranging from 20 to 150 µM with a detection limit of 5 µM, which is well within the clinical range of 78–206 µM.

1.3.3 Mass-Sensitive Detection

Another form of transduction has also been used in biosensors to measure small changes in mass.[59–61] Mass-based detection is the newest of the three classes of transducers and has already been shown to be capable of sensitive measurements. Mass analysis relies on the use of piezoelectric crystals. These crystals can be made to vibrate at a specific frequency with the application of an electrical signal of a specific frequency. The frequency of oscillation is dependent on the electrical frequency applied to the crystal as well as the crystal's mass. Therefore, when the mass increases due to binding of chemicals, the oscillation frequency of the crystal changes and the resulting change can be measured electrically and be used to determine the mass added to the crystal. In most cases, the added mass consists of antibodies or DNA fragments bound to their biospecific counterparts that have been immobilized on the sensor surface.

Guilbault and coworkers developed a quartz crystal microbalance biosensor for the detection of *Listeria monocytogenes*.[62] Several approaches were tested for the immobilization of *Listeria* onto the quartz crystal through a gold film on the surface. Once bound, the microbalance was then placed in a liquid flow cell, where the Ab and Ag were allowed to form a complex, and measurements were obtained. Calibration of the sensor was accomplished using a displacement assay and was found to have a response range from 2.5×10^5 to 2.5×10^7 cells/crystal. More recently, Guilbault and coworkers have also developed a method for covalently binding antibodies to the surface of piezoelectric crystals via sulfur-based self-assembled monolayers.[63] Prior to Ab binding, the monolayers are activated with 1-ethyl-3-[3-(dimethylamino)propyl] carbodiimide hydrochloride and *N*-hydroxysulfosuccinimide. Using this binding technique, a real-time capture assay based on mouse IgG was performed and results were reported.

The first usage of a horizontally polarized surface acoustic wave biosensor has been reported by Hunklinger and coworkers.[64] This sensor has a dual-path configuration, with one path acting as an analyte-sensitive path and the other path acting as a reference path. A theoretical detection limit of 33 pg was calculated based on these experiments, and a sensitivity of 100 kHz/(ng/mm^2) is reported. In addition, a means of inductively coupling a surface acoustic wave biosensor to its radio-frequency generating circuitry has been reported recently.[65] This technique could greatly reduce problems associated with wire bonding for measurements made in liquids, since the electrodes are coated with a layer of SiO_2.

A relatively new type of mass-based detection system use microcantilevers. Constructed of silicon, these devices are generally shaped like a microsize diving board. Their advantages include their miniature size, high degree of sensitivity, simplicity, low power consumption, low manufacturing cost, and compatibility with array designs.[66] The extremely low mass of the device allows it to sense perturbing forces because of the adsorbed masses at the picogram level, the viscosity of a gas or liquid over several orders of magnitude, and the acoustic and seismic vibrations. Special coatings on the silicon will adapt the cantilever to sense relative humidity, temperature, mercury, lead, ultraviolet (UV) radiation, and IR radiation. By using current micromachining technology, multiple arrays could be used to make multielement or multitarget sensor arrays involving hundreds of cantilevers without significantly increasing the size, complexity, or overall package costs.

1.4 Bioreceptors and Biosensor Systems

1.4.1 Antibody

1.4.1.1 Antibody Bioreceptors

The basis for the specificity of immunoassays is the Ag–Ab binding reaction, which is a key mechanism by which the immune system detects and eliminates foreign matter.[67] The enormous range of potential applications of immunosensors is due, at least in part, to the astonishing diversity possible in one of their key components, Ab molecules. Antibodies are complex biomolecules made up of hundreds of individual amino acids arranged in a highly ordered sequence. The structure of an IgG Ab molecule is schematically illustrated in Figure 1.3a. The antibodies are actually produced by immune system cells (B cells) when such cells are exposed to substances or molecules called Ags. The antibodies called forth following Ag exposure have recognition/binding sites for specific molecular structures (or substructures) of the Ag. The way in which an Ag and an Ag-specific Ab interact may perhaps be understood as analogous to a lock-and-key fit, in which the specific configurations of a unique key enable it to open a lock. In the same way, an Ag-specific Ab fits its unique Ag in a highly specific manner, so that hollows, protrusions, planes, and ridges on the Ag and the Ab molecules (in a word, the total 3D structure) are complementary. Further details of how such complementarity is achieved will be discussed later in this chapter. It is sufficient at this point simply to indicate that, due to this 3D shape fitting and the diversity inherent in individual Ab makeup, it is possible to find an Ab that can recognize and bind to any one of a huge variety of molecular shapes. This unique property of antibodies is the key to their usefulness in immunosensors; this ability to recognize molecular structures allows one to develop antibodies that bind specifically to chemicals, biomolecules, microorganism components, etc. One can then use such antibodies as specific detectors to identify and find an analyte of interest that is present, even in extremely small amounts, in a myriad of other chemical substances. The other Ab property of paramount importance to their analytical role in immunosensors is the strength or avidity/affinity of the Ag–Ab interaction. Because of the variety of interactions that can take place as the Ag–Ab surfaces lie in close proximity one to another, the overall strength of the interaction can be considerable, with correspondingly favorable association and equilibrium constants. What this means in practical terms is that the Ag–Ab interactions can take place very rapidly (for small Ag molecules, almost as rapidly as diffusion processes can bring Ag and Ab together) and that, once formed, the Ag–Ab complex has a reasonable lifetime.

For an immune response to be produced against a particular molecule, a certain molecular size and complexity are necessary: proteins with molecular weights greater than 5000 Da are generally immunogenic. Radioimmunoassay (RIA), which utilizes radioactive labels, has been one of the most widely used immunoassay methods. RIA has been applied to a number of fields, including pharmacology, clinical chemistry, forensic science, environmental monitoring, molecular epidemiology, and agricultural science. The usefulness of RIA, however, is limited by several shortcomings, including the cost of instrumentation, the limited shelf life of radioisotopes, and the potential deleterious biological effects inherent to radioactive materials. For these reasons, there are extensive research efforts aimed at developing simpler, more practical immunochemical techniques and instrumentation, which offer comparable sensitivity and selectivity to RIA. In the 1980s, advances in spectrochemical instrumentation, laser miniaturization, biotechnology, and fiber-optic research provided opportunities for novel approaches to the development of sensors for the detection of chemicals and biological materials of environmental and biomedical interest.

Since the first development of a remote fiber-optic immunosensor for in situ detection of the chemical carcinogen BaP,[7] antibodies have become common bioreceptors used in biosensors today.[8–12,68] The schematics for the optical detection of a bioanalyte is shown in Figure 1.4. In the arrangement shown, a single optical fiber carries both the excitation light source to the sample and the fluorescence signal back to a spectrometer.

Due to fiber-to-fiber differences in fiber-optic biosensors, there is often a great difficulty in normalizing the spectral signal obtained with one fiber to another fiber. Ligler and coworkers reported on a method for calibrating Ab-based biosensors using two different fluorescent dyes.[69] To accomplish this, they labeled the capture antibodies bound to the fiber, with one fluorescent dye and the Ag with a different dye. Both dyes were excited at the same wavelength, and their fluorescence was monitored. The resultant emission spectrum of the fluorescence signal from the capture antibodies was used to normalize the signal from the tagged Ag.

Another example of Ab-based biosensors for bioanalysis is the development of an electrochemical immunoassay for whole blood.[70] This work involved the development of a sandwich-type separationless amperometric immunoassay without any washing steps. The assay is performed on a conducting redox hydrogel on a carbon electrode on which avidin and choline oxidase have been coimmobilized. Biotinylated Ab is then bound to the gel. When the Ag binds to the sensor, another solution of complementary horseradish peroxidase-labeled Ab is bound to the Ag, thus creating an electrical contact between the redox hydrogel and the peroxidase. The hydrogel then acts as an electrocatalyst for the reduction of hydrogen peroxide water.

An important aspect of biosensor fabrication is the binding of the bioreceptor to the sensor solid support or to the transducer. Vogel and coworkers report on a method for the immobilization of histidine-tagged antibodies onto a gold surface for SPR measurements.[71] A synthetic thioalkane chelator is self-assembled on a gold surface. Reversible binding of an antilysozyme Fab fragment with a hexahistidine-modified extension on the C terminal end is then performed. IR spectroscopy was used to determine that the secondary structure of the protein was unaffected by the immobilization process. Retention of Ab functionality upon immobilization was also demonstrated. Due to the reversible binding of such a technique, this could prove a valuable method for regeneration of biosensors for various applications.[71] Enzyme immunoassays can further increase the sensitivity of detection of Ag–Ab interactions by the chemical amplification process, whereby one measures the accumulated products after the enzyme has been allowed to react with excess substrate for a period of time.[72]

With the use of nanotechnology, submicron fiber-optic Ab-based biosensors have been developed by Vo-Dinh and coworkers for the measurements of biochemicals inside a single cell.[73–75] Nanometer-scale fiber-optic biosensors were used for monitoring biomarkers related to human health effects that are associated with exposure to polycyclic aromatic hydrocarbons (PAHs). These sensors use a MAb for benzo[a]pyrene tetrol (BPT), a metabolite of the carcinogen BaP, as the bioreceptor. Excitation light is launched into the fiber and the resulting evanescent field at the tip of the fiber is used to excite any of the BPT molecules that have bound to the Ab. The fluorescent light is then collected via a microscope. Using these Ab-based nanosensors, absolute detection limits for BPT of ca. 300 zmol (10^{-21} mol) have been reported.[73] These nanosensors allow the probing of cellular and subcellular environments in single cells.[19,74,75] The development and applications of optical nanosensors is described in further details in Chapter 23 of *The Biomedical Photonics Handbook: Fundamentals, Devices, and Techniques.*

1.4.1.2 Immunoassay Formats

Biomolecular interactions can be classified into two categories, according to the test format performed (direct or indirect). In a direct format, the immobilized target molecule interacts with a ligand molecule or the immobilized ligand interacts with a target molecule directly. For immunosensors, the simplest situation involves in situ incubation followed by direct measurement of a naturally fluorescent analyte.[7] For nonfluorescent analyte systems, in situ incubation is followed by the development of a fluorophore-labeled second Ab. The resulting Ab sandwich produces a fluorescence signal that is directly proportional to the amount of bound Ag. The sensitivity obtained when using these techniques increases with increasing amounts of immobilized receptor. The indirect format involves competition between fluorophore-labeled and unlabeled Ags.[68] In this case, the unlabeled analyte competes with the labeled analyte for a limited number of receptor binding sites. Assay sensitivity therefore increases with decreasing amounts of immobilized reagent. Figure 1.8 illustrates the principles of (a) a competitive assay, (b) a direct assay, and (c) a sandwich assay.

A sandwich immunoassay using fluorescently labeled tracer antibodies has been developed to detect *cholera* toxin (CT).[76] Using this fluorescence-based biosensor, researchers analyzed six samples simultaneously in 20 min. The biochemical assays utilized a ganglioside-capture format: ganglioside GM1, utilized for capture of the analyte, was immobilized in discrete locations on the surface of the optical waveguide. Binding of CT to the immobilized GM1 was demonstrated with direct assays (using fluorescently labeled CT). The limits of detection for CT were 200 ng/mL in direct assays and 40 ng/mL and 1 μg/mL in sandwich-type assays performed using rabbit and goat tracer antibodies. Binding of CT to other glycolipid capture reagents was also observed. While significant CT binding to loci patterned with GD1b, Gb3, and Gb4 was observed, CT did not bind significantly to immobilized GT1b at the concentrations tested.

A similar planar array, equipped with a charge-coupled device (CCD) as a detector, was used to simultaneously detect three toxic analytes.[16] Wells approximately 2 mm in diameter were formed on

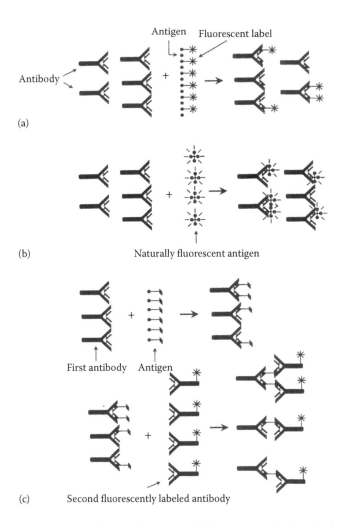

(a)

Naturally fluorescent antigen

(b)

First antibody   Antigen

Second fluorescently labeled antibody

(c)

FIGURE 1.8 Immunoassay formats: (a) competitive assay, (b) direct assay, and (c) sandwich assay.

glass slides using a photoactivated optical adhesive. Antibodies against *staphylococcal* enterotoxin B (SEB), ricin, and *Yersinia pestis* were covalently attached to the bottoms of the circular wells to form the sensing surface. Rectangular wells containing chicken Ig were used as alignment markers and to generate control signals. After the optical adhesive was removed, the slides were mounted over a CCD operating at ambient temperature in inverted (multipin phasing) mode. Cy5-labeled antibodies were used to determine the identity and amount of toxin bound at each location, using quantitative image analysis. Concentrations as low as 25 ng/mL of ricin, 15 ng/mL of *pestis* F1 Ag, and 5 ng/mL of SEB could be routinely measured. A similar assay for ricin, using an immobilized antiricin IgG on an optical fiber surface, was reported.[77] Two immobilization methods were tried: In the first, the Ab was directly coated onto the silanized fiber using a cross-linker; in the second, avidin-coated fibers were incubated with biotinylated antiricin IgG to immobilize the Ab using an avidin–biotin bridge. The assay using the avidin–biotin-linked Ab demonstrated higher sensitivity and wider linear dynamic range than the assay using Ab directly conjugated to the surface. The limits of detection for ricin in buffer solution and river water are 100 pg/mL and 1 ng/mL, respectively.

The use of protein A, an Ig-binding protein, for Ab immobilization on the surface of these fiber probes has been investigated as an alternative immobilization method to the classical avidin–biotin and IgG–anti-IgG interactions.[14] No difference was observed in the binding of fluorescently labeled goat IgG by rabbit anti-goat IgG, regardless of whether the capture Ab was bound to the probe surface via protein A or covalently attached. However, in a sandwich immunoassay for the F1 Ag of *Y. pestis*, probes with rabbit antiplague IgG bound to the surface via protein A generated twice the signal generated by the probes with the Ab covalently attached. Assay regeneration was also examined with protein A probes since Ag–Ab complexes have been successfully eluted from protein A under low pH conditions.

The regeneration of antibodies covalently immobilized to an optical fiber surface is also an important parameter that classifies the usefulness of a biosensor. Ideally, the Ag–Ab complex can be dissociated under mild conditions to regenerate the sensor. In a study by Ligler and coworkers,[78] three different restoring solutions were tested and compared: 0.1 M glycine hydrochloride in 50% (v/v) ethylene glycol, pH 1.75; (b) a basic solution (a) (0.05 M tetraethylamine in 50% [v/v] ethylene glycol, pH 11.0); and (c) 50% (v/v) ethanol in PBS. In this study, optical fibers coated with polyclonal rabbit anti-goat Ab against a large protein retained 70% and 65% of the original signal after five consecutive regenerations with acidic and basic solvent systems, respectively. The fibers coated with monoclonal mouse anti-trinitrobenzene Ab specific for a small organic molecule retained over 90% of the original signal when regenerated with basic and ethanol solutions.

A biosensor based on labeled Cy5 antibodies, using a 635 nm laser diode light source, was used to detect the F1 Ag of *Y. pestis* and the protective Ag of *Bacillus anthracis*. In a blind test containing F1 Ag spiked into 30 of 173 serum samples, this immunosensor was able to achieve 100% detection success for samples with 100 ng/mL or more F1 Ag, with a specificity of 88%.[13]

1.4.1.3 Antibody Probe Regeneration

Removal of Ags bound to antibodies covalently attached to optical fiber surfaces is one of the limiting factors in the development of reusable, inexpensive, and reliable optical fiber immunosensors for environmental and clinical analysis. Chemical reagents were to cleave the binding between Ab and Ag, thus regenerating the biosensor.[79] This chemical procedure is simple but ineffective after multiple regeneration operations (less than five cycles), due to possible denaturation of the Ab. Another approach in the development of regenerable biosensors involves the design of microcapillary systems capable of delivering and removing reagents and Ab-coated microbeads into the sensing chamber without removing the sensor from the sample.[80] Several investigators have searched for fast dissociation protocols that are able to regenerate immobilized antibodies while maintaining their stability for use in routine analysis, commercial immunosorbents,[81] or optical fiber sensors.[78]

Ag–Ab interactions can be classified in three different groups[82]: hydrophobic interactions, electrostatic (or coulombic) interactions, and interactions due to a combination of both forces. Hydrophobic interactions are due to the propensity of nonpolar groups and chains to aggregate when immersed in water. This type of interaction is maximized between the hydrophobic complementary determining regions (CDRs) of the Ab parotopes and the predominantly hydrophilic groups found in the Ag epitope. Electrostatic interactions between Ag and Ab are caused by one or more ionized sites of the epitope and ions of opposite charge on the parotope. After primary binding has occurred through hydrophobic and electrostatic interactions, the epitope and the parotope will be close enough to allow van der Waals and hydrogen bonds to become operative. In order to dissociate the Ag–Ab complexes, the strength of these forces may be reduced by changing the pH, ionic strength, and/or temperature through the addition of dehydrating agents and/or organics. In this sense, strong acids such as HCl or H_2SO_4, mixtures such as glycine HCl, or basic solutions of tetraethylamine, for example, have been used when the primary attractive forces in the bond can be considered as electrostatic interactions.[83]

Lu et al. pointed out that the use of organic solutions such as ethylene glycol could improve the washing efficiency by reducing both the van der Waals and the coulombic forces maintaining the bond.[84] Wijesuriya et al. made a similar observation.[78] Nevertheless, every Ag–Ab pair may differ with respect to the nature of the forces implicated in the binding site. Haga et al. studied the effect of 28 kHz ultrasonic radiation with an intensity of 0.83 W/cm^2 on the dissociation of Ag–Ab complexes immobilized on CH-Sepharose gels.[85] They observed that the percent of dissociation increased with irradiation time and input wattage obtaining a 22% of dissociation after 20 min, whereas the immune reactivity decreased 8% without degradation of the dissolved Ab upon exposure to the ultrasound for times of up to 120 min. Higher-frequency ultrasound (high kHz to low MHz range) is used to remove small (micrometer to submicrometer) particles from the surfaces of silicon wafers.[86,87] This so-called megasonic cleaning process does not damage the surfaces, suggesting that its mode of action does not depend on the strong effects of inertial cavitation that occur with lower-frequency (e.g., 20 kHz) ultrasonic horns and baths. The mechanisms of megasonic cleaning likely involve nonlinear effects such as acoustic streaming and radiation pressure as well as the oscillatory linear forces.[87] Stable cavitation (a less intense process than inertial cavitation) may also play an important role, particularly in enhancing the streaming effects. The success of the gentle but effective megasonic cleaning process suggests that MHz-range ultrasound may have some utility in regeneration of biosensor surfaces.

Vo-Dinh and coworkers described a novel procedure for regenerating antibodies immobilized on a fiber-optic surface with ultrasonic irradiation using a broadband imaging transducer operating near 5 MHz.[22] This type of ultrasound device is commonly used for the detection of flaws in the nondestructive evaluation of engineering materials and measurement of the mechanical properties of various media,[88] including biological tissues.[89] The use of ultrasound for the regeneration of optical fiber immunosensors could be an important advance in the application of these devices for in vivo and in situ measurements since it would no longer be necessary to supply a regeneration solution to the sensor system that could lead to the denaturation of the immobilized Ab.

1.4.2 Enzyme

Enzymes are often used as bioreceptors because of their specific binding capabilities as well as their catalytic activity. In biocatalytic recognition mechanisms, the detection is amplified by a catalytic reaction. This is the basis for the now commonplace enzyme-linked immunosorbent assay (ELISA) technique.

With the exception of a small group of catalytic ribonucleic acid molecules, all enzymes are proteins. Some enzymes require no chemical groups other than their amino acid residues for activity. Others require an additional component called a cofactor, which may be either one or more inorganic ions, such as Fe^{2+}, Mg^{2+}, Mn^{2+}, or Zn^{2+}, or a more complex organic or organometallic molecule called a coenzyme. The catalytic activity provided by enzymes allows for much lower limits of detection than would be obtained with common binding techniques. As expected, the catalytic activity of enzymes depends upon the integrity of their native protein conformation. If an enzyme is denatured, dissociated into its subunits, or broken down into its component amino acids, its catalytic activity is destroyed. Enzyme-coupled receptors can also be used to modify the recognition mechanisms. For instance, the activity of an enzyme can be modulated when a ligand binds at the receptor. This enzymatic activity is often greatly enhanced by an enzyme cascade, which leads to complex reactions in the cell.[90]

Gauglitz and coworkers have immobilized enzymes onto an array of optical fibers for use in the simultaneous detection of penicillin and ampicillin.[91] These biosensors provide an interferometric technique for measuring penicillin and ampicillin based on pH changes during their hydrolysis by penicillinase. Immobilized onto the fibers with the penicillinase is a pH indicator, phenol red. As the enzyme hydrolyzes the two substrates, shifts in the reflectance spectrum of the pH indicator are measured. Various types of data analysis of the spectral information were evaluated using a multivariate calibration method for the sensor array, which consisted of different biosensors.

Rosenzweig and Kopelman described the development and use of a micrometer-sized fiber-optic biosensor for the detection of glucose.[92] These biosensors are 100 times smaller than existing glucose optodes and represent the beginning of a new trend in nanosensor technology.[93] These sensors are based on the enzymatic reaction of glucose oxidase, which catalyzes the oxidation of glucose and oxygen into gluconic acid and hydrogen peroxide. To monitor the reaction, an oxygen indicator, tris(1,10-phenanthroline)ruthenium chloride, is immobilized into an acrylamide polymer with the glucose oxidase, and this polymer is attached to the optical fiber via photopolymerization. A comparison of the response of glucose sensors created on different sizes of fibers found that the micrometer-sized sensors have response times at least 25 times faster (2 s) than the larger fibers. In addition, these sensors are reported to have absolute detection limits of approximately 10^{-15} mol and an absolute sensitivity five to six orders of magnitude greater than current glucose optodes.[93]

A fiber-optic evanescent-wave immunosensor for the detection of lactate dehydrogenase has been developed.[94] Two different assay methods, a one-step and a two-step process, using the sensor based on polyclonal Ab recognition were described. The response of this evanescent-wave immunosensor was then compared to a commercially available SPR-based biosensor for lactate dehydrogenase detection using similar assay techniques, and similar results were obtained. It was also demonstrated that although the same polyclonal Ab can be used for both the one- and the two-step assay techniques, the two-step technique is significantly better when the Ag is large.

1.4.3 Nucleic Acid

1.4.3.1 Nucleic Acid Bioreceptors

Another biorecognition mechanism involves hybridization of DNA or RNA. In the last decade, nucleic acids have received increasing interest as bioreceptors for biosensor and biochip technologies.[93,95–99] The complementarity of the pairing of the nucleotides adenine–thymine (A:T) and cytosine–guanine (C:G) in a DNA ladder (Figure 1.3b) forms the basis for the specificity of biorecognition in DNA biosensors, often referred to as genosensors. If the sequence of bases composing a certain part of the DNA molecule is known, then the complementary sequence, often called a probe, can be synthesized and labeled with an optically detectable compound (e.g., a fluorescent label). By unwinding the double-stranded DNA (dsDNA) into single strands, adding the probe, and then annealing the strands, the labeled probe can be made to hybridize to its complementary sequence on the target molecule.

Grabley and coworkers have reported the use of DNA biosensors for the monitoring of DNA–ligand interactions.[100] SPR was the analytical method used to monitor real-time binding of low-molecular-weight ligands to DNA fragments that were irreversibly bound to the sensor surface via coulombic interactions. The sensor was capable of detecting binding effects between 10 and 400 pg/mm². Binding rates and equilibrium coverages were determined for various ligands by changing the ligand concentration. In addition, affinity constants, association rates, and dissociation rates were also determined for these various ligands.

Sandwich-type biosensors based on liquid-crystalline dispersions formed from DNA–polycation complexes have been described by Yevdokimov and coworkers.[101] These sandwich biosensors have been shown to be useful for the detection of compounds and physical factors that affect the ability of specific DNA cross-linkers, polycationic molecules, to bind between adjacent DNA molecules. The specific case of dispersions from DNA/protamine complexes was investigated, and it was demonstrated that by using this type of sensor with this complex, the hydrolytic enzyme trypsin could be measured down to concentrations of approximately 10^{-14} M.

Karube and coworkers demonstrated another type of biosensor that uses a peptide nucleic acid as the biorecognition element.[96] The peptide nucleic acid is an artificial oligoamide that is capable of binding very strongly to complementary oligonucleotide sequences. By use of an SPR sensor, the direct detection of dsDNA that had been amplified by a PCR has been demonstrated. This technique was capable of monitoring the target DNA over a concentration range of 40–160 nM, corresponding to an absolute detection limit of 7.5 pmol.

Using a unique analytical technique, Vo-Dinh and coworkers have developed a new type of DNA gene probe based on SERS detection.[20,44–46] The SERS probes do not require the use of radioactive labels and have great potential to provide both sensitivity and selectivity via label multiplexing due to the intrinsically narrow bandwidths of Raman peaks. The effectiveness of the new detection scheme is demonstrated using the *gag* gene sequence of the HIV.[20] A SERS-based DNA assay for the breast cancer susceptibility gene (BRCA1) has been also developed. The assay is based on the immobilization of oligonucleotides on a thin silver surface and hybridization with Rhodamine-labeled probes.[21] The silver surface serves as the hybridization support and the means for Raman signal enhancement. The development of a biosensor for DNA diagnostics using visible and NIR dyes has been reported.[23] The system employed a 2D CCD and was used to detect the cancer suppressor *p53* gene.

1.4.3.2 DNA Biosensors

DNA sensors are usually based on hybridization assays and may incorporate simultaneous analytical capability to detect a large number of oligonucleotide fragments. A fiber-optic DNA biosensor microarray for the analysis of gene expression has been reported for the simultaneous analysis of multiple DNA sequences using fluorescent probes.[102]

Fluorescent intercalating and groove-binding dyes that can associate with dsDNA are used for the detection of hybridization in some sensor and biochip designs.[103] It is possible that dye–dye interactions at concentrations relevant to biosensor use can lead to unexpected and undesired emission wavelength shifts and fluorescence quenching interactions. To maximize S/N, many biosensors utilize dye concentrations that are in large excess in comparison to the quantity of immobilized DNA. The linearity of fluorescence intensity response of dyes intercalated to dsDNA may vary with different dye–base pair ratios.[103]

A very common alternative to intercalating fluorescent dyes for the detection of dsDNA are covalently bound dyes. Dyes attached to the terminus of a strand of DNA, through a short hydrocarbon chain (also known as a tether), are continuously available for hybridization and allow the biosensor to be fully reversible.[25]

Another important characteristic of the biosensor assay is the choice of the fluorescent dye, which acts as the signal transducer. Traditionally, ethidium bromide (EB) has been used extensively to detect hybridization of DNA in applications such as electrophoresis, gene chips, and biosensors. A number of dyes with greater quantum efficiency than EB for detection of hybridization have been reported. Furthermore, other practical spectroscopic advantages can be gained in terms of improved S/N by use of dyes with excitation that is redshifted relative to EB. Pyridinium iodide has been shown to be an intercalator of high quantum efficiency and long excitation wavelength.[25]

One type of DNA biosensor utilized the direct synthesis of a single-stranded DNA (ssDNA) sequence directly onto optical fibers, using the well-established solid-phase phosphoramidite methodology. The covalently immobilized oligomers were able to hybridize with available complementary ssDNA, which was introduced into the local environment to form dsDNA. This event was detected by the use of the fluorescent DNA stain EB. The sampling configuration utilized total internal reflection of optical radiation within the fiber, resulting in an intrinsic-mode optical sensor. The nonoptimized procedure used standard hybridization assay techniques to provide a detection limit of 86 ng/mL cDNA and a sensitivity of 83% fluorescence intensity increase per 100 ng/mL of cDNA initially present, with a hybridization analysis time of 46 min. The sensor has been observed to sustain activity after prolonged storage times (3 months) and harsh washing conditions (sonication).[26] A similar sensor fabricated using quartz optical fibers as the support provided very similar results.[104]

A very interesting biosensor capable of detecting triple-helical DNA formation was also based on the direct synthesis of oligonucleotides on the surface of fused silica optical fibers, using a DNA synthesizer. Two sets of oligonucleotides on different fibers were grown in the 3′ to 5′ and 5′ to 3′ directions, respectively. Fluorescence studies of hybridization showed unequivocal hybridization between oligomers immobilized on the fibers and complementary oligonucleotides from the solution phase, as detected by fluorescence from intercalated EB. The complementary origonucleotide, dT(10), which was expected to hybridize when the system was cooled below the duplex melting temperature, provided a fluorescence intensity with a negative temperature coefficient. Upon further cooling, to the point where the pyrimidine motif T*AT triple-helix formation occurred, a fluorescence intensity change with a positive temperature coefficient was observed.[27]

In another study, the same type of sensor, with directly immobilized ssDNA on optical fibers, was used to monitor variation in the melt temperature of dsDNA. Because of the microenvironment conditions, the local ionic strength, the pH, and the dielectric constant at the surface can be substantially different from that in bulk electrolyte solution. The local conditions influence the thermodynamics of hybridization and can be studied by the melt temperature of dsDNA. Fiber-optic biosensors with dT(20) oligonucleotides attached to their surfaces were used to determine the T_m from the dissociation of duplexes of mixtures of fluorescein-labeled and unlabeled dA(20) and d(A(9)GA(10)). Each thermal denaturation of dsDNA at the surface of the optical fibers was accompanied by a two- to threefold reduction in standard enthalpy change relative to values determined for denaturation in bulk solution. The experimental results suggested that the thermodynamic stability of duplexes that are immobilized on a surface is dependent on the density of immobilized DNA. Additionally, the deviation in melt temperature, arising as a result of the presence of a centrally located single base-pair mismatch was significantly larger for thermal denaturation occurring at the surface of the optical fibers ($\Delta T_m = 6°C–10°C$) relative to that observed in bulk solution ($\Delta T_m = 3.8°C–6.1°C$). These results suggest that hybridization at an interface occurs in a significantly different physical environment from hybridization in bulk solution and that surface density can be tuned to design analytical figures of merit.[105] Increased immobilization density resulted in significantly higher sensitivity but reduced dynamic range in all hybridization assays done. Sensitivity and selectivity were functions of temperature; however, the selectivity of hybridization assays done using the sensors could not be predicted by consideration of thermal denaturation temperatures alone.[28]

1.4.4 Cell-Based Systems

Cellular structures and cells comprise a broad category of bioreceptors that have been used in the development of biosensors and biochips.[106–116] These bioreceptors are either based on biorecognition by an entire cell or microorganism or by a specific cellular component that is capable of specific binding to certain species. There are presently three major subclasses of this category: (1) cellular systems, (2) enzymes, and (3) nonenzymatic proteins. Due to the importance and large number of biosensors based on enzymes, these have been given their own classification and were previously discussed in Section 1.4.2. This section deals with cellular systems and nonenzymatic proteins.

1.4.4.1 Cellular Bioreceptors

Microorganisms offer a form of bioreceptor that often allows a whole class of compounds to be monitored. Generally, these microorganism biosensors rely on the uptake of certain chemicals into the microorganism for digestion. Often, a class of chemicals are ingested by a microorganism, therefore allowing a class-specific biosensor to be created. Microorganisms such as bacteria and fungi have been used as indicators of toxicity or for the measurement of specific substances. For example, cell metabolism (e.g., growth inhibition, cell viability, substrate uptake), cell respiration, and bacterial bioluminescence have been used to evaluate the effects of toxic heavy metals. Many cell organelles can be isolated and used as bioreceptors. Since cell organelles are essentially closed systems, they can be used over long periods of time. Whole mammalian tissue slices or in vitro cultured mammalian cells are used as biosensing elements in bioreceptors. Plant tissues are also used in plant-based biosensors; they are effective catalysts because of the enzymatic pathways they possess.[90]

Bilitewski and coworkers have developed a microbial biosensor for the monitoring of short-chain fatty acids in milk.[117] *Arthrobacter nicotianae* microorganisms were immobilized in a calcium alginate gel on an electrode surface. To this gel was added 0.5 mM $CaCl_2$ to help stabilize it. Monitoring the oxygen consumption of the *A. nicotianae* electrochemically allowed its respiratory activity to be monitored, thereby providing an indirect means of monitoring fatty acid consumption. Detection of short-chain fatty acids in milk, ranging from 4 to 12 carbons in length, was accomplished with butyric acid as the major substrate. A linear dynamic range from 9.5 to 165.5 µM was reported, with a response time of 3 min.

1.4.4.2 Nonenzymatic Proteins

Many proteins that are found within cells often serve the purpose of bioreception for intracellular reactions that will take place later or in another part of the cell. These proteins could simply be used for transport of a chemical from one place to another, such as a carrier protein or channel protein on a cellular surface. In any case, these proteins provide a means of molecular recognition through one or another type of mechanism (i.e., active site or potential sensitive site). By attaching these proteins to various types of transducers, many researchers have constructed biosensors based on nonenzymatic protein biorecognition. In one recent application, Cusanovich and coworkers have developed micro- and nanobiosensors for nitric oxide that are free from most potential interferents.[93] These sensors are based on bioreception of nitric oxide by cytochrome *c'*. Two different techniques of immobilization of the cytochrome *c'* to fibers were tested: polymerization in an acrylamide gel and reversible binding using a gold colloid-based attachment. The cytochrome used in this work was labeled with a fluorescent dye that is excited via an energy transfer from the hemoprotein. Response times of faster than 1 s are reported along with a detection limit of 20 μM. Cytochrome *c'* samples from three different species of bacteria were evaluated.

Vogel and coworkers have reported on the use of lipopeptides as bioreceptors for biosensors.[118] A lipopeptide containing an antigenic peptide segment of VP1, a capsid protein of the picornavirus that causes foot-and-mouth diseases in cattle, was evaluated as a technique for monitoring Ag–Ab interactions. The protein was characterized via circular dichroism and IR spectroscopy to verify that upon self-assembly onto a solid surface, it retained the same structure as in its free form. Based on SPR measurements, it was found that the protein was still fully accessible for Ab binding. This technique could provide an effective means of developing biomimetic ligands for binding to cell surfaces.

1.4.5 Biomimetic Receptors

A receptor that is fabricated and designed to mimic a bioreceptor is often termed a *biomimetic receptor*. Several different methods have been developed over the years for the construction of biomimetic receptors.[119–124] These methods include genetically engineered molecules, artificial membrane fabrication, and molecular imprinting. The molecular imprinting technique, which has recently received great interest, consists of mixing analyte molecules with monomers and a large number of cross-linkers. Following polymerization, the hard polymer is ground into a powder, and the analyte molecules are extracted with organic solvents to remove them from the polymer network. As a result, the polymer has molecular holes or binding sites that are complementary to the selected analyte.

Recombinant techniques, which allow for the synthesis or modification of a wide variety of binding sites using chemical means, have provided powerful tools for designing synthetic bioreceptors with desired properties. Hellinga and coworkers reported the development of a genetically engineered single-chain Ab fragment for the monitoring of phosphorylcholine.[125] In this work, protein engineering techniques are used to fuse a peptide sequence that mimics the binding properties of biotin to the carboxy terminus of the phosphorylcholine-binding fragment of IgA. This genetically engineered molecule can be attached to a streptavidin monolayer, and total internal reflection fluorescence was used to monitor the binding of a fluorescently labeled phosphorylcholine analog.

Artificial membranes have been developed for many different bioreception applications. Stevens and coworkers developed an artificial membrane by incorporating gangliosides into a matrix of diacetylenic lipids (5%–10% of which were derivatized with sialic acid).[126] The lipids were allowed to self-assemble into Langmuir–Blodgett layers and were then photopolymerized via UV irradiation into polydiacetylene membranes. When CTs bind to the membrane, its natural blue color changes to red; absorption measurements were used to monitor the toxin concentration. Using these polydiacetylenic lipid membranes coupled with absorption measurements, concentrations of CT as low as 20 μg/mL could be monitored.

Molecular imprinting has been used for the construction of a biosensor based on electrochemical detection of morphine.[127] A molecularly imprinted polymer for the detection of morphine was fabricated on a platinum wire using agarose and a cross-linking process. The resulting imprinted polymer was used to specifically bind morphine to the electrode. Following morphine binding, an electroinactive competitor, codeine, was used to wash the electrode and thus release some of the bound morphine. The freed morphine was then measured by oxidation at the electrode, and concentrations ranging from 0.1 to 10 µg/mL were analyzed, with a reported detection limit of 0.05 µg/mL. One of the major advantages of the molecular imprinting technique is the rugged nature of a polymer relative to a biological sample. The molecularly imprinted polymer can withstand harsh environments such as those experienced in an autoclave or chemicals that would denature a protein.

1.5 Probe Development: Immobilization of Biomolecules

Many of the methods used in biosensor fabrication involve binding of the recognition probe (oligonucleotide strand, Ab, etc.) to a sensor-sensitive surface or to an optically active tag (fluorescent dye). For enzyme-based sensors, immobilization of an enzyme is a critical step and can be accomplished via simple physical adsorption or through more elaborate covalent binding schemes.

Molecules may be either physically immobilized in a solid support through hydrophobic or ionic interactions or covalently immobilized by attachment to activated surface groups.[128] Noncovalent immobilization is effective for many applications and usually requires easier and faster preparation steps.[129-131] In addition, the adsorbed molecules usually preserve their original properties (e.g., wavelength of absorption, excitation, and/or emission, enzymatic activity) because they do not require the structural modification inherent in covalent immobilization to a solid support. However, continuous leaching of the adsorbate from the solid support may reduce the sensor's durability and even render it useless in the worst cases.

Covalent immobilization is often necessary for binding molecules that do not adsorb, adsorb very weakly, or adsorb with improper orientation and conformation to noncovalent surfaces. Covalent immobilization may provide greater stability, reduced nonspecific adsorption, and greater durability.[132-133]

Several synthetic techniques are available for the covalent immobilization of biomolecules or labeling of a sensor probe with a fluorescent dye.[128] Most of these techniques use free amine groups in a polypeptide (enzymes, antibodies, Ags, etc.) or in an amino-labeled DNA strand to react with a carboxylic acid moiety to form amide bonds. As a general rule, a more active intermediate (labile ester) is first formed with the carboxylic acid moiety and in a later stage reacted with the free amine, increasing the coupling yield. A few coupling procedures are described in the following.

1.5.1 Carbodiimide Coupling

Surfaces modified with mercaptoalkyldiols can be activated with 1,1′-carbonyldiimidazole (CDI) to form a carbonylimidazole intermediate. A biomolecule with an available amine group displaces the imidazole to form a carbamate linkage to the alkylthiol tethered to the surface.[134]

1.5.2 *N*-Hydroxysuccinimide and Its Derivatives

Using a succinimide ester intermediate in acylation reactions of 5′-amino-labeled DNA is also a very efficient protocol. The *N*-hydroxysuccinimide (NHS)-activated carboxyl group has a much longer lifetime than the reaction intermediates produced by carbodiimide coupling.[135] NHS can also be used to facilitate amide formation between a carboxylic acid moiety and free amine groups in a polypeptide (enzymes, antibodies, Ags, etc.). NHS reacts almost exclusively with primary amine groups, with the exception of mercaptans. This nucleophilic substitution reaction covalently immobilizes biomolecules via available amine moieties by forming stable amide bonds. Covalent immobilization can be achieved

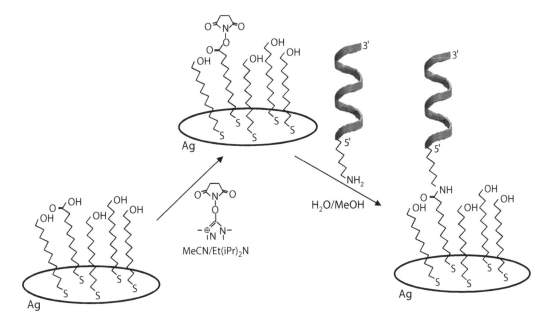

FIGURE 1.9 Binding scheme for biomolecule immobilization.

in as little as 30 min. This surface has been shown to immobilize 5′ amine-modified oligonucleotides, providing an ideal template for hybridization and amplification. Because the DNA is bound at one end rather than at numerous sites along the molecule, the results are high specificity and low background. Since H_2O competes with $-NH_2$ in reactions involving these very labile esters, it is important to consider the hydrolysis kinetics of the esters used in this type of coupling. A derivative of NHS, *O*-(*N*-succinimidyl)-*N,N,N′,N′*-tetramethyluronium tetrafluoroborate, increases the coupling yield by utilizing a leaving group that is converted to urea during the carboxylic acid activation, hence favorably increasing the negative enthalpy of the reaction. The schematic in Figure 1.9 illustrates this approach.

1.5.3 Maleimide

Maleimide can be used to immobilize biomolecules through available –SH moieties. Coupling schemes with maleimide have been proven useful for the site-specific immobilization of antibodies, Fab fragments, peptides, and SH-modified DNA strands. Sample preparation for the maleimide coupling of a protein involves the simple reduction of disulfide bonds between two cysteine residues with a mild reducing agent, such as dithiothreitol, 2-mercaptoethanol, or tris(2-carboxyethyl)phosphine hydrochloride. However, disulfide reduction will usually lead to the protein losing its natural conformation and might impair enzymatic activity or Ab recognition. The modification of primary amine groups with 2-iminothiolane hydrochloride (Traut's reagent) to introduce sulfhydryl groups is an alternative for biomolecules lacking them. Free sulfhydryls are immobilized to the maleimide surface by an addition reaction to unsaturated carbon–carbon bonds.

1.5.4 Hydrazide

Hydrazide is used for the covalent coupling of periodate-activated carbohydrates or glycosylated biomolecules. It can be used for the site-specific immobilization of antibodies, carbohydrates, glycolipids, glycoproteins, and many enzymes. Antibodies are immobilized to the hydrazide surface through the carbohydrate moieties on the Fc region, which allows the Fab regions to be properly oriented (vide Ab probes).

Noncovalent immobilization of biomolecules includes solgel or polymer entrapment of enzymes[136-141] and adsorption of oligonucleotides onto polycationic membranes (polylysine, polymers with quaternarium ammonium groups, etc.).[92,142,143] For solgel or polymeric immobilization, solubility of the biomolecules in the polymerization medium is a major constraint for the use of this technique. In the case of surface adsorption, conformation changes of proteins that might diminish Ab recognition or enzyme activity have to be considered.

A sensor for the nitrate ion based on the encapsulation of an enzyme in a solgel structure is reported to be effective even after a storage period of up to 6 months.[136] The enzyme of choice was the periplasmic nitrate reductase (Nap), extracted from the denitrifying bacterium *Thiosphaera pantotropha*, which reacts specifically with the nitrate (NO^{3-}) anion.

Edmiston and coworkers found evidence that the immobilization of proteins by entrapment in a porous silica matrix prepared by solgel techniques may significantly change the conformation of the proteins. These researchers examined two model proteins, bovine serum albumin (BSA) and horse heart myoglobin (Mb), entrapped in wet solgel glass bulks. They investigated the fluorescence behavior of dissolved and entrapped BSA in the presence of acid, a chemical denaturant, and a collisional quencher. The results show that a large fraction of the BSA added to the sol is entrapped within the gelled glass in a native conformation. However, the reversible conformational transitions that BSA undergoes in solution are sterically restricted in the gel. In contrast, the native properties of Mb are largely lost upon entrapment, as judged by the changes in the visible absorbance spectra of dissolved and entrapped Mb in acidic solutions. Fluorescence studies of dissolved and entrapped apomyoglobin supported this conclusion.[144]

1.6 Biomedical Applications

This section provides an overview of various medical applications of biosensors, especially in the diagnosis of diseases. A large body of work was accomplished using SPR commercial instruments and involves the study of protein and/or DNA interactions relevant for medical applications. Other widely used methods include fluorescence spectroscopy, NIR, and circular dichroism.

1.6.1 Cellular Processes

The staining of cellular organelles is a classic laboratory method that utilizes visible or fluorescent dyes that have high affinity for specific organelles. After staining, visible or UV illumination is used for microscopy identification. Newer techniques explore the same principles to obtain more information on cellular processes as well.

For example, G protein-coupled receptors (GPCRs) represent one of the most important drug targets for medical therapy, and information from genome sequencing and genomic databases has substantially accelerated their discovery.[145] The lack of a systematic approach either to identify the function of a new GPCR or to associate it with a cognate ligand has added to the growing number of orphan receptors. A novel approach to this problem using optical detection of a beta-arrestin2/green fluorescent protein conjugate (beta-arr2–GFP) has been reported. Confocal microscopy demonstrates the translocation of beta-arr2–GFP to more than 15 different ligand-activated GPCRs, providing a real-time and single-cell-based assay to monitor GPCR activation and GPCR–Gr protein-coupled receptor kinase or GPCR–arrestin interactions. The use of beta-arr2–GFP as a biosensor to recognize the activation of pharmacologically distinct GPCRs should accelerate the identification of orphan receptors and permit the optical study of their signal transduction biology, which is intractable to ordinary biochemical methods.[145]

Abscisic acid (ABA) is a plant hormone involved in many developmental and physiological processes, but no ABA receptor has been identified yet.[146] In an attempt to demonstrate that the MAb JIM19 recognizes carbohydrate epitopes of cell surface glycoproteins, researchers have used flow cytometry of rice protoplasts and immunoblotting of purified plasma membranes (PMs).[146] Through use of SPR technology, specific binding of PMs to JIM19 was observed. The interaction was antagonized significantly by ABA but not by the biologically inactive ABA catabolite, phaseic acid. Pretreatment with JIM19 resulted in significant inhibition of ABA-inducible gene expression. Taken together, these data suggest that JIM19 interacts with a functional PM complex involved in ABA signaling.[146]

Another receptor binding study done with optical biosensor technology investigated the affinity and specificity of the putative proximal tubular scavenging receptor for protein reabsorption and the specificity of AGE-modified protein interactions with primary human mesangial cells.[147] An SPR biosensor with a carboxymethyl dextran surface was used for binding competition analysis of five different proteins of the LLCPK cell line (ranging in size and charge). The biosensor data show that there is evidence to support the existence of a single scavenging receptor for all the proteins tested. The proteins competed with each other differing only in their relative binding affinity for the common receptor. This study has also showed that human mesangial cells can bind to AGE-modified human serum albumin (AGE-HSA) immobilized onto the carboxylate surface and that binding can be inhibited by using increasing concentrations of soluble AGE-HSA. However, increasing concentrations of soluble non-AGE-modified HSA can also inhibit binding to a similar extent, which implies that there is relatively little AGE-receptor expression on cultured primary human mesangial cells. The SPR biosensor is a potential tool to explore cellular interactions with renal cells.[147]

1.6.2 Viral Agents

The use of biosensors to detect specific viruses in biological samples offers a great diagnostic tool for medical applications. To date, studies have targeted several viruses, including HIV (discussed separately), measles virus, herpes simplex virus (HSV), rhinoviruses, and foot-and-mouth disease prions. Some of the techniques used in their detection are outlined in the following.

Identifying viruses in clinical materials during the acute phase of infections could give necessary information for the treatment of infections by human immunoglobulin (hIg) or interferon (IF). However, because of a lack of information, most virus infections are not treated. A real-time detection system for viruses in general has been developed using an optical biosensor and a model virus, HSV type 1 (HSV-1). The HSV-1 virus was found to propagate in Vero cells and, when diluted in minimum essential medium (MEM) with 10% fetal bovine serum (FBS), could be detected with an SPR sensor with high sensitivity and a detection limit of 10 infectious units (50% tissue culture infective dose [TCID50] units). When a crude homemade rabbit antiserum was used against measles virus with host cell debris as a ligand, the SPR sensor performed with lower sensitivity, detecting less than 500 infectious (TCID50) units of virus in a 100 μL solution. This real-time viral detection and titration system has sensitivity high enough for clinical purposes.[148]

The herpes virus was also the object of a study of epitope mapping using an SPR optical biosensor. The human herpes virus entry mediator C (HveC), also known as the poliovirus receptor-related protein 1 (PRR1) and as nectin-1, allows the entry of HSV-1 and HSV-2 into mammalian cells. The interaction of the virus envelope glycoprotein D (gD) with such a receptor is an essential step in the process leading to membrane fusion.[149] HveC is a member of the Ig superfamily and contains three Ig-like domains in its extracellular portion. The gD binding site is located within the first Ig-like domain (V domain) of HveC. In a careful study using SPR, 11 MAbs against the ectodomain of HveC were chosen to detect linear or conformational epitopes within the V domain. Besides the biosensor analysis, the HveC was detected by ELISA, Western blotting, and directly on the surface of HeLa cells and human neuroblastoma cell lines, as well as simian Vero cells. A few of the 11 MAbs blocked HSV entry. Competition assays on an optical biosensor showed that CK6 and CK8 (linear epitopes) inhibited the binding of CK41 and R1.302 (conformational epitopes) to HveC and vice versa.[149]

One of the reasons for the traditionally low success for the direct identification of viruses by simple immunological assays is the large variability of their surface epitopes. For example, more than 100 immunologically distinct serotypes of human rhinoviruses (HRV) have been discovered, making detection of surface-exposed capsid Ags impractical. However, the nonstructural protein 3C protease (3Cpro) is essential for viral replication and is relatively highly conserved among serotypes, making it a potential target for diagnostic testing of HRVs. An SPR biosensor having a modified silicon surface with broadly reactive serotype antibodies to 3Cpro has been developed.[150] The in vitro sensitivity, specificity, and multiserotype cross-reactivity of the 3Cpro assay were tested using the SPR sensor in a 28 min, noninstrumented room-temperature test with a visual detection limit of 12 pM of 3Cpro (1000 TCID50 equivalents). Nasal washes from naturally infected individuals were used as test samples. The assay detected 87% (45 of 52) of the HRV serotypes tested but showed no cross-reactivity to common respiratory viruses or bacteria. The SPR assay detected 3Cpro in expelled nasal secretions from a symptomatic individual on the first day of illness. In addition, 82% (9 of 11) concentrated nasal wash specimens from HRV-infected children were positive in the 3Cpro test. Thus, the assay is suitable as a diagnostic test for a point-of-care (POC) setting, where rapid HRV diagnostic test results could contribute to clinical decisions regarding appropriate antibiotic or antiviral therapy.[150]

Another SPR system was applied to the quantitative analysis of the binding of HSV-1 to Vero cells. A commercially available sulfonated hIg preparation was used as the neutralization Ab titer against this virus.[151]

Viruslike particles (VLPs) are multimeric proteins expressed by *Saccharomyces cerevisiae*. These particles are approximately 80 nm in diameter and are used as a framework for a range of biological products, including carriers of viral Ags. An SPR biosensor was developed for the rapid monitoring of purified VLPs. The device can be used for real-time bioprocess monitoring of VLPs. Problems of mass transfer of the analyte were overcome through selection of a planar biosensor surface, instead of the traditional polymer-coated surface. To prolong the surface activity for interaction analysis, a sandwich assay was developed that involved the use of a secondary capture species. It was shown that VLP concentration in pure solution could be determined within 10 min.[152]

An SPR biosensor has been used for the screening of synthetic peptides mimicking the immunodominant region of C-S8c1 foot-and-mouth disease virus (FMDV). The main antigenic site (site A) of the FMDV (strain C-S8c1) may be adequately reproduced by a 15-peptide with the amino acid sequence H-YTASARGDLAHLTTT-NH2 (A15), corresponding to the residues 136–150 of the viral protein VP1.[153] The SPR sensor surface was modified with MAbs raised against antigenic site A. Although these antigenicities have previously been determined from ELISA methods, the SPR-based technique is superior in that it allows a fast and straightforward screening of Ags while simultaneously providing kinetic data for the Ag–Ab interaction.[153]

1.6.3 Human Immunodeficiency Virus

The HIV has been the target of intense research in the past two decades. Some of the research efforts involving optical biosensors are outlined in the following.

The two main proteins on the HIV envelope are glycoproteins gp120 and gp41 (named for their approximate size in kilodaltons). Glycoproteins gp120 and gp41 are associated together noncovalently. Binding of HIV-1 gp120 to T cell receptor CD4 initiates conformational changes in the viral envelope that trigger viral entry into the host cells.[154]

SPR has been used in a number of HIV studies. This technique was applied to observe the conformational changes in gp120 upon binding to certain ligands, to compare the gp120-activation effects of CD4 mimetics, and to examine for CD4 competition and gp120 activation.[155–157] SPR optical biosensors provide a means of looking at the interaction between macromolecules as it occurs in real time, providing information about the kinetics of the interaction, in addition to estimating affinity constants.

SPR optical biosensor assays for the screening of low-molecular-weight compounds, using an immobilized protein target, have been developed. HIV-1 proteinase was immobilized on the sensor surface by direct amine coupling. A large number of inhibitors and noninteracting reference drugs were applied to the sensor surface in a continuous flow of buffer to estimate binding constants. The optimized assay could correctly distinguish HIV-1 inhibitors from other compounds in a randomized series, indicate differences in their interaction kinetics, and reveal artifacts due to nonspecific signals, incomplete regeneration, or carryover.[158]

SPR biosensors have also been used to study the interaction between HIV-1 protease and reversible inhibitors. The steady-state binding level and the time course of association and dissociation could be observed by measuring the binding of inhibitors injected in a continuous flow of buffer to the enzyme immobilized on the biosensor surface. Fourteen low-molecular-weight inhibitors (500–700 Da), including four clinically used HIV-1 protease inhibitors (indinavir, nelfinavir, ritonavir, and saquinavir) were analyzed. Inhibition constants (K_i) were determined by a separate enzyme inhibition assay. Indinavir had the highest affinity (B_{50} = 11 nM) and the fastest dissociation ($t_{1/2}$ = 500 s) among the clinically used inhibitors, while saquinavir had a lower affinity (B_{50} = 25 nM) and the slowest dissociation rate ($t_{1/2}$ = 6500 s). Since these two inhibitors have similar affinities, the differences in dissociation rates reveal important characteristics in the interaction that cannot be obtained by the inhibition studies alone.[159,160] Characterization of another set of HIV-1 protease inhibitors using binding kinetics data from an SPR biosensor-based screen has also been reported.[161]

Fluorescence polarization, circular dichroism, and SPR optical biosensor binding studies were used to investigate the novel virucidal protein cyanovirin-n (cv-n). cv-n binds with equally high affinity to soluble forms of either h9 cell produced or recombinant glycosylated HIV-1 gp120 (sgp120) or gp160 (sgp160). Studies showed that cv-n is also capable of binding to the glycosylated ectodomain of the HIV envelope protein gp41 (sgp41), albeit with considerably lower affinity than the sgp120/cv-n interaction. These optical techniques shed light on the binding of cv-n with both sgp120 and sgp41, providing direct evidence that conformational changes are a consequence of cv-n interactions with both HIV-1 envelope glycoproteins.[162]

1.6.4 Bacterial Pathogens

Several physicochemical instrumental techniques for direct and indirect identification of bacteria—such as IR and fluorescence spectroscopy, flow cytometry, chromatography, and chemiluminescence—have been reviewed as feasible biosensor technologies.[163]

Staphylococcus aureus is a pathogen that commonly causes human infections and intoxication. An evanescent-wave optical sensor was developed for the detection of protein A, a product secreted only by *S. aureus*. A 488 nm laser was used in conjunction with a plastic optical fiber with adsorbed antibodies for protein. A sandwich immunoassay with fluorescein isothiocyanate (FITC) conjugated with anti-(protein A) IgG was used to monitor the Ag–Ab reaction. The detection limit was 1 ng/mL of protein A.[164]

In a different approach, an optical biosensor based on resonant mirrors was used in the detection of whole cells of *S. aureus* (Cowan-1).[165] The bacterium cells, which express protein-A at their surface, were detected through their binding to human IgG, which was immobilized on an aminosilane-derivatized sensor surface at concentrations in the range 8×10^6–8×10^7 cells/mL. A control *S. aureus* strain (Wood-46), which does not express protein-A, produced no significant response. The sensitivity of the technique was increased by three orders of magnitude when a human IgG colloidal gold conjugate (30 nm) was used in a sandwich assay format. *S. aureus* (Cowan-1) cells were detected in spiked milk samples at cell concentrations from 4×10^3 to 1.6×10^6 cells/mL using the sandwich assay.[165]

The same resonant mirror optical biosensor technology was used to characterize *Helicobacter pylori* strains according to their sialic acid binding. In that work, intact bacteria were used in real-time measurements of competition and displacement assays using different glycoconjugates. The authors found that several, but not all, *H. pylori* strains express sialic acid-binding adhesin, specific for α-2,3-sialyllactose. The adhesin, removable from the bacterial surface by water extraction, is not related to other reported *H. pylori* cell surface proteins with binding ability to sialylated compounds such as sialylglycoceramides.[166,167]

A fiber-optic evanescent-wave sensing system that features all-fiber optical design and red semiconductor laser excitation has been developed and tested. A 650 nm laser was used, since biological matrices demonstrate minimal fluorescent background in the red, which helps reduce the background signal of nonessential biomolecules. The fiber directs the fluorescent signal of a sandwich immunoassay to detect *Salmonella* back to a CCD fiber spectrophotometer. The system could detect *Salmonella* with a concentration as low as 10^4 colony-forming units (CFU) per milliliter.[168]

With a similar biodetection approach utilizing laser-induced fluorescence, an optic biosensor was used to detect the fraction 1 (F1) Ag from *Y. pestis*, the etiologic agent of plague.[15] An argon ion laser (514 nm) was used to launch light into a long-clad fiber, and the fluorescence produced by an immunofluorescent complex formed in the evanescent-wave region was measured with a photodiode. Capture antibodies, which bind to F1 Ag, were immobilized on the core surface to form the basis of the sandwich fluoroimmunoassay. The evanescent wave has a limited penetration depth ($<1\lambda$), which restricts detection of the fluorescent complexes bound to the fiber's surface. The direct correlation between the concentration of the F1 Ag and the signal provided an effective method for sample quantitation, and the method was able to detect F1 Ag concentrations from 50 to 400 ng/mL in phosphate-buffered saline, serum, plasma, and whole blood, with a 5 ng/mL detection limit.[15]

A very different detection approach for *Salmonella typhimurium* involved immunomagnetic separation and a subsequent enzyme-linked assay with alkaline phosphatase. The magnetic microbeads coated with anti-*Salmonella* were used to separate *Salmonella* from sample solutions at room temperature for 30 min. A sandwich complex with alkaline phosphatase and the *Salmonella* immobilized on the magnetic beads was formed, separated from the solution by a magnetic filtration, and incubated with a *p*-nitrophenyl phosphate substrate at 37°C for 30 min to produce *p*-nitrophenol by the enzymatic hydrolysis. *Salmonella* was detected by measuring the absorbance of *p*-nitrophenol at 404 nm, with a linear response between 2.2×10^4 and 2.2×10^6 CFU/mL.[169]

1.6.5 Cancer

Optical biosensors have been utilized as tools to aid in the direct diagnosis of carcinogenesis, the identification of genetic markers associated with it, and the quantification of known carcinogens.

Fluorescent detection has become a technique of choice for oligonucleotide hybridization detection. Pairs of high-density oligonucleotide arrays (DNA chips) consisting of more than 96,000 oligonucleotides were designed to screen the entire 5.53 kb coding region of the hereditary breast and ovarian cancer BRCA1 gene for all possible sequence changes in the homozygous and heterozygous states. Fluorescent hybridization signals from targets containing the four natural bases to more than 5592 different, fully complementary 25 mer oligonucleotide probes on the chip varied over two orders of magnitude. To examine the thermodynamic contribution of rU.dA and rA.dT target.probe base pairs to this variability, modified uridine [5-methyluridine and 5-(1-propynyl)-uridine] and modified adenosine (2,6-diaminopurine riboside) 5′-triphosphates were incorporated into BRCA1 targets. Hybridization specificity was assessed based upon hybridization signals from >33,200 probes containing centrally localized single base pair mismatches relative to target sequence. Targets containing 5-methyluridine displayed promising localized enhancements in the hybridization signal, especially in pyrimidine-rich target tracts, while maintaining single-nucleotide mismatch hybridization specificities comparable with those of unmodified targets.[170]

In another study, the breast cancer susceptibility gene BRCA1 was also detected by a relatively new technique based on SERS. A single 24 mer sequence was used as the capture probe and was immobilized on a silver-coated microarray platform for hybridization.[21]

Breast cancer was also the target of a biosensor design to measure the interaction of S100A4 and potential binding partners.[171] Elevated levels of S100A4 induce a metastatic phenotype in benign mammary tumor cells in vivo. In humans, the presence of S100A4 in breast cancer cells correlates strongly with reduced patient survival. There was significant interaction of S100A4 with nonmuscle myosin and *p53* but not with actin, tropomyosin, or tubulin.[171]

A regenerable immunosensor utilizing an Ab against breast cancer Ag has been described. A 65% removal of the Ags bound to the MAb immobilized on the fiber surface is attained after ultrasound regeneration.[22] A multiarray biosensor utilizing DNA probes labeled with visible and NIR dyes has also been developed. The detection system uses a 2D CCD to detect the *p53* cancer gene.[23]

Prostate cancer is the cause of death of many thousands of men worldwide. The screening of men for elevated prostate-specific Ag (PSA) levels is believed to be an important tool for the diagnosis and management of the disease. An assay for measuring PSA in whole blood using the fluorescence capillary fill device has been developed for use in prostate cancer screening programs.[172]

A unique example of the technology being developed is optical nanobiosensors capable of interrogating the contents of a single isolated cell.[173] These submicrometer fiber-optic biosensors have been used to measure carcinogens within single cells. Optical fibers were pulled to a distal-end diameter of 40 nm and were coated with antibodies to selectively bind BPT, a metabolite of BaP, an extremely potent carcinogen. Two different cell lines have been investigated: human mammary carcinoma cells and rat liver epithelial cells. The detection limit of these nanosensors has been determined to be $(0.64 \pm 0.17) \times 10^{-11}$ M for BPT.[74] The development and application of nanosensors are further described in Chapter 23 of *The Biomedical Photonics Handbook: Fundamentals, Devices, and Techniques.*

The carcinogen BaP was itself the target of an Ab-based fiber-optic biosensor.[7] In that biosensor, BaP was the analyte and fluorophore, since it has a large fluorescence cross section. An Ab with high specificity for BaP was immobilized on the tip of an optical fiber. Upon exposure to contaminated samples, the optical fiber was irradiated with a laser and the resulting fluorescence correlated with the BaP concentration.

1.6.6 Parasites

Detection of antibodies specific for the parasite *Leishmania donovani* in human serum samples has been reported. The method is based on an evanescent-wave fluorescence collected by optical fibers that have the purified cell surface protein of *L. donovani* immobilized on their surface. The sensing fibers are incubated with the patient serum for 10 min and then incubated with goat antihuman IgG. Fluorescence was proportional to *L. donovani*–specific antibodies present in the test sera.[174]

1.6.7 Toxins

Ricin, a potently toxic protein, has been detected with an evanescent-wave fiber-optic biosensor with a detection limit of 100 pg/mL and 1 ng/mL for buffer solutions and river water, respectively. This detection was based on a sandwich immunoassay scheme, using an immobilized antiricin IgG on the surface of the optical fiber. Two coupling methods were used. In the first method, the Ab was directly coated to the silanized fiber using a cross-linker, and the second method utilized avidin-coated fibers, which were incubated with biotinylated antiricin IgG to immobilize the Ab using an avidin–biotin bridge. The assay using the avidin–biotin-linked Ab demonstrated higher sensitivity and a wider linear dynamic range than the assay using the Ab directly conjugated to the surface. The linear dynamic range of detection for ricin in buffer using the avidin–biotin chemistry is 100 pg/mL to 250 ng/mL.[77]

The LPS endotoxin is the most powerful immune stimulant known and a causative agent in the clinical syndrome known as sepsis. Sepsis is responsible for more than 100,000 deaths annually, in large part due to the lack of a rapid, reliable, and sensitive diagnostic technique.[18] An evanescent-wave fiber-optic biosensor was developed for the detection of LPS from *E. coli* at concentrations as low as 10 ng/mL, in 30 s.[18] Polymyxin B covalently immobilized onto the surface of the fiber-optic probe was able to selectively bind fluorescently labeled LPS. Unlabeled LPS present in the biological samples was detected in a competitive assay format, by displacing the labeled LPS. The competitive assay format worked in both buffer and plasma with similar sensitivities. This method might also be used with other LPS capture molecules such as antibodies, lectins, or antibiotics, to simultaneously detect LPS and determine the LPS serotype.[18]

An immunoaffinity fluorometric biosensor was developed for the detection of aflatoxins, a family of potent fungi-produced carcinogens commonly found in a variety of agriculture products. The detection system, developed into a fully automated instrument based on immunoassays with fluorescent tags, was able to detect aflatoxins from 0.1 to 50 ppb in 2 min with a 1 mL sample volume.[175]

Parathion was detected with a biosensor based on total internal reflection using a competitive displacement immunoassay. This biosensor utilizes casein–parathion conjugates, immobilized by adsorption on quartz fibers, selectively adsorbed anti-parathion rabbit antibodies raised against BSA–parathion conjugates from polyclonal immune sera. The presence of free parathion inhibited the binding of the rabbit's anti-BSA–parathion. FITC goat anti-rabbit IgG was used to generate the optical signal. It could detect 0.3 ppb of parathion and had a detection limit 100-fold higher for the detection of its oxygen analog, paraoxon.[176] Other biosensor approaches for the detection of parathion include another competition assay that inhibits the alkaline phosphatase generation of a chemiluminescent substance[177] and a direct detection method based on another enzymatic sensor.[178,179]

A very interesting approach for biosensing of toxins involves the integration of multiple transducers with different affinities for a large range of biotoxins. The different transducers are based on membranes made of mixtures of biologically occurring lipids that are deposited on the sensing surface of an SPR optical biosensor. Eight surfaces were prepared, some of which contained various glycolipids as minor components, and one was supplemented with membrane proteins. The researchers analyzed the binding of six protein toxins (CT, CT B subunit, diphtheria toxin, ricin, ricin B subunit, and SEB) and of BSA at pH 7.4 and 5.2 to each of the sensor surfaces.[180] Each of the seven proteins produced a distinct binding pattern to the multitransducer sensor. The same concept had been used earlier for the development of *artificial noses*, which are sensor arrays able to detect a small collection of distinct analytes.

CT has been also detected with a fluorescence-based biosensor using a waveguide platform. The biochemical assay utilized a ganglioside-capture format, where the ganglioside (GM1) that captures the analyte was immobilized in discrete locations on the surface of an optical waveguide. Binding of CT to immobilized GM1 was demonstrated with direct assays (using fluorescently labeled CT) and with *sandwich* immunoassays (using fluorescently labeled tracer antibodies). The detection limits for CT were 200 ng/mL in direct assays and 40 ng/mL and 1 μg/mL in sandwich-type assays performed using rabbit and goat tracer antibodies.[76] A slightly different biosensing approach was also used to detect CT. Instead of direct fluorescence detection, fluorescence quenching was used. The ganglioside GM1 was again used as the recognition unit for CT and was covalently labeled with fluorophores and then incorporated into a biomimetic membrane surface.[122]

In a very nice application of SPR, SPR biosensors have been used to estimate the immunoreactivity of tetanus toxin and *Vipera aspis* venom against new pasteurized preparations of their horse F(ab′)(2) antidotes, in order to investigate immunoreactivity–immunoprotection efficacy relationships. The immunoreactivity data were compared with seroneutralization titers. The association–dissociation rate and affinity constants of the current and the new tetanus toxin-specific F(ab′)(2) preparations were similar, at about 10^4 M^{-1} s^{-1}, 10^{-4} s^{-1}, and 10^8 M^{-1}, respectively.[181]

1.6.8 Blood Factors

SPR was used to determine absolute heparin concentration in human blood plasma. Protamine and polyethyleneimine (PEI) were used to modify the sensor surface and were evaluated for their affinity to heparin. Heparin adsorption onto protamine in blood plasma was specific with a lowest detection limit of 0.2 U/mL and a linear detection range of 0.2–2 U/mL. Although heparin adsorption onto PEI in buffer solution had indicated superior sensitivity to that on protamine, in blood plasma, it was not specific for heparin and adsorbed plasma species to a steady-state equilibrium. By reducing the incubation time and diluting the plasma samples with buffer to 50%, the nonspecific adsorption of plasma could be controlled and a PEI pretreated with blood plasma could be used successfully for heparin determination.

Heparin adsorption in 50% plasma was linear between 0.05 and 1 U/mL so that heparin plasma levels of 0.1–2 U/mL could be determined with a relative error of 11% and an accuracy of 0.05 U/mL.[182]

1.6.9 Congenital Diseases

SPR and biospecific interaction analysis (BIA) have been used to detect the delta F508 mutation (F508del) of the cystic fibrosis transmembrane regulator (CFTR) gene in both homozygous and heterozygous human subjects.[183] The detection method involved the immobilization on a SA5 sensor chip of two biotinylated oligonucleotide probes (one normal, N-508, and the other mutant, F508del) that are able to hybridize to the CFTR gene region involved in F508del mutation. A hybridization step between the oligonucleotide probes immobilized on the sensor chips and (1) wild-type or mutant oligonucleotides, as well as (2) ssDNA allowed for evaluation of the stability of the various DNA/DNA complexes. These nucleic acid samples were obtained using asymmetric PCR, performed using genomic DNA from normal individuals and from F508del heterozygous and F508del homozygous patients. The different stabilities of DNA/DNA molecular complexes generated after hybridization of normal and F508del probes immobilized on the sensor chips were then evaluated. The results strongly suggest that the SPR technology enables a one-step, nonradioactive protocol for the molecular diagnosis of F508del mutation of the CFTR gene. This approach could be of interest in clinical genetics, as the hybridization step is often required to detect microdeletions present within PCR products.[183]

1.7 Recent Applications of Nanotechnology in Biosensor Systems

The use of nanotechnology has brought about great improvements in biosensing techniques over the past few years. This section will highlight a few examples of advances in biosensor technology that have been made possible by nanotechnology. Areas to be discussed include carbon, metal oxide, and plasmonic nanomaterials for biosensor applications.

1.7.1 Carbon Nanomaterials

Carbon nanomaterials, such as carbon nanotubes (CNTs) and graphene, have unique chemical, electrical, mechanical, and thermal properties that make them attractive for biosensor applications. The majority of carbon nanomaterial-based sensing is performed using electrochemical biosensors, as they are relatively inexpensive and offer quick response times with high sensitivity and specificity. In addition to the conventional electrical detection, CNTs have also been used in optical biosensors. An optical immunosensor using individually assembled CNTs coated with a photovoltaic polymer has been developed for the detection of cardiac biomarkers.[184] Chemiluminescent immunoassay was directly performed on the CNT photodetector for an on-chip detection of cardiac troponin T (cTnT) with a detection limit of 12 pg/mL. High sensitivity and reliable selectivity have been achieved through the use of on-chip measurement of chemiluminescent light by the CNT photodetector. As a result, the developed device is envisaged as a new platform for optical immunosensing using the individually self-assembled CNTs for POC clinical diagnostics. A new type of optical biosensor from DNA wrapped semiconductor graphene ribbons (SGRs) has been proposed.[185] In this biosensor design, the single-walled carbon nanotube (SWCNT) is replaced by an SGR. Using a simple theory of exciton in SGRs, transition of DNA secondary structure from the native, right-handed B form to the alternate, left-handed Z form was investigated. This structural phase transition of DNA forms the basis of this optical biosensor at the subcellular level from DNA and SGRs.

Graphene has also been employed in electro-optic devices and shares many of the advantageous electrochemical properties that are observed with CNTs. Among the various graphene forms with lattice-like nanostructure, graphene oxide (GO) exhibits excellent properties for use in a biosensing platform. This material offers good capabilities for direct binding with biomolecules, a heterogeneous chemical and electronic structure, the possibility to be processed in solution, and the capability to be used as an insulator, semiconductor, or semimetal. It is noteworthy that GO exhibits photoluminescence with energy transfer donor/acceptor molecules exposed in a planar surface. This material could be used as an efficient long-range quencher, thus allowing various biosensing schemes. GO has been used in optical biosensing platforms.[186]

1.7.2 Metal Oxide Nanomaterials

Metal oxide nanomaterials (MONs) have also been found to improve the function of optical biosensors. Various metal oxides that have been used in biosensors include titanium, silicon, tin, zirconium, cerium, iron, zinc, vanadium, manganese, copper, and nickel. A highly sensitive biosensor based on nanostructured anodized aluminum oxide (AAO) substrates has been investigated.[187] A gold-deposited AAO substrate exhibits both optical interference and localized SPR (LSPR). A uniform periodic nanopore lattice AAO template by two-step anodizing was fabricated. A layer of C-reactive protein (CRP) Ab on a gold coating was immobilized atop the AAO template. The system was used to detect CRP Ag delivered to the immobilized Ab layer. Detection of a 1fg/mL change in CRP Ag concentration was possible by measuring the LSPR shift caused by a change in refractive index due to membrane thickness upon CRP Ag binding. This method can provide a simple, fast, and sensitive analysis for protein detection in real time.

1.7.3 Plasmonic Nanomaterials

Metal nanomaterials that exhibit LSPR, a collective oscillation of electrons on the surface of the metal that occurs when light is incident on the nanomaterial, are of great interest for use in optical biosensors due to this unique property. Gold and silver nanoparticles are the most studied plasmonic materials, as their LSPRs are in the visible region. The two main optical readout methods used with plasmonic nanoparticles are LSPR sensing and SERS. In LSPR sensing, the extinction spectrum of the nanomaterial is monitored; upon binding of target, a change in the local refractive index around the nanomaterial occurs and redshifts the extinction spectrum. This method is applicable to a wide variety of analytes since gold and silver can be easily modified with the desired bioreceptors. In 1997, Elghanian et al. presented a colorimetric, gold nanoparticle-based sensor for DNA detection.[188] The nanoparticles were functionalized with thiolated ssDNA. Two types of particles were created to bind to a single target strand: one complimentary to the first half of the target DNA and the other complimentary to the second half. When both particles were incubated with the target, the DNA strands hybridized, bringing the two nanoparticles close together. This caused the LSPR to redshift and the color of the solution turned from red (LSPR of single gold nanoparticles) to blue (aggregated particles). This unoptimized system was able to discriminate a single mismatched base and had a detection limit of 10 fmol of oligonucleotides.

The use of SERS in biosensing has only been around for two decades, and is still a rapidly growing area of research. Raman scattering is an inelastic process that occurs when incident light interacts with a molecule and the emitted light is at a higher or lower energy, where this energy difference corresponds to the vibrational states of the molecule. The SERS effect arises from the enhanced electromagnetic field provided by the plasmonic nanostructures, which can increase Raman signals enough to be comparable in intensity to fluorescence. The first demonstration of DNA biosensing using SERS detection was reported in 1994.[44] A study in 2002 reported the use SERS as the readout mechanism in a biosensor.[189] A similar strategy to what is described above was used, but instead of two nanoparticles probes, one of the probe strands was immobilized on a solid support and the other nanoparticle probe included a Raman dye. In the presence of target, the Raman-labeled nanoparticle probes became linked to the substrate and a silver enhancement solution was applied, growing silver nanoparticles around the gold nanoparticle probe and providing the SERS enhancement. By using different probes and Raman dyes, they were able to multiplex the detection of six different oligonucleotides with a detection limit of 20 fM.

Other SERS biosensors have been developed in recent years for a multitude of different analytes. For nucleic acid sensing, there are now one-step homogenous assays, such as the molecular sentinel (MS)[190] and plasmonic coupling interference (PCI) biosensing scheme for nucleic acid targets.[191] The MS probe consists of a DNA strand having a Raman label molecule at one end and a metal nanoparticle at the other end. The plasmonic nanoprobe uses the stem-loop structure to recognize target DNA sequences. Note that hairpin DNA structures have been used in *molecular beacon* systems that are based on fluorescence and electrochemical detection. The sensing principle of MSs, however, is quite different from that of molecular beacons. With MS systems, in the normal configuration (i.e., in the absence of target DNA), the DNA sequence has a hairpin loop, which maintains the Raman label in close proximity of the metal nanoparticle designed to induce an intense SERS signal of the Raman label upon laser excitation. Upon hybridization of a complementary target DNA sequence to the nanoprobe hairpin loop, the Raman label molecule is physically separated from the metal nanoparticle, thus leading to a decreased SERS signal.[190] The PCI method is also a label-free approach using PCI nanoprobes for nucleic acid detection using SERS. To induce a strong plasmonic coupling effect, a nanonetwork of silver nanoparticles having the Raman label located between adjacent nanoparticles is assembled by Raman-labeled DNA-locked nucleic acid (LNA) duplexes. The PCI method then utilizes specific nucleic acid sequences of interest as competitor elements of the Raman-labeled DNA strands to interfere the formation of nanonetworks in a competitive binding process. As a result, the plasmonic coupling effect induced through the formation of the nanonetworks is significantly diminished, resulting in a reduced SERS signal. The PCI technique was used for detecting single-nucleotide polymorphism (SNP) and microRNA sequences involved in breast cancer.[191] Sensing pH in living cells has been performed with nanoparticles[192] and fiber-optic nanoprobes.[193] A SERS-based glucose sensor has even been applied in vivo in a mouse model.[194] The use of SERS in biosensing is still expanding and holds promise for the development of sensors with unrivaled sensitivity and selectivity.

1.8 Conclusion

The past decade has witnessed the rapid development of a wide variety of biosensors for many different analyses and has even seen them begin to advance to clinical and in some cases commercially available technologies, such as SPR biosensors. The increasing interest in the field of optical biosensors has provided a great deal of information about the biochemistry of clinically important ailments and has provided drug discovery research with faster analytical tools to investigate drug–receptor interactions. Optical methods have also been extensively applied to DNA fingerprinting and genotyping, techniques that might find enormous applications in clinical diagnosis in the near future.

As a very positive sign, optical biosensors are reaching a coming-of-age as a bioanalytical tool. A larger number of researchers in different areas now have access to a more user-friendly technology and are able to develop custom applications specific to their research needs, expanding the range of applications for the technology.

For practical medical diagnostic applications, there is a strong need for a truly integrated biosensor system that can be easily operated by relatively unskilled personnel. Some of the currently commercially available technologies have dramatically simplified the data collection operation. While these systems have demonstrated their usefulness in genomic detection, protein interaction analysis, carcinogen monitoring, etc., they are laboratory-oriented and involve relatively expensive equipment and trained, supervised operation.

The outlook is promising for optical biosensor systems, and the near future should bring a larger number of multichannel applications for the simultaneous detection of multiple biotargets, improvements in size and performance, and lower production costs due to a more integrated package. Highly integrated systems lead to a reduction in noise and an increase in signal due to the improved efficiency of sample collection and the reduction of interfaces. The capability of large-scale production using low-cost integrated circuit (IC) technology is an important advantage that cannot be overlooked.

For medical applications, the development of low-cost, disposable biosensor surfaces that can be used for clinical diagnostics at the POC and at home can be a major driving force for the expansion of optical biosensor technologies.

Acknowledgments

This work was sponsored by the US Department of Energy (DOE) Office of Biological and Environmental Research under contract DEAC05-00OR22725 with UT-Battelle, LLC, the National Institutes of Health, the Department of the Army, the Coulter Foundation, and the Defense Advanced Project Research Agency.

References

1. Nauta, J. M., H. vanLeengoed, W. M. Star, J. L. N. Roodenburg, M. J. H. Witjes, and A. Vermey. 1996. Photodynamic therapy of oral cancer—A review of basic mechanisms and clinical applications. *European Journal of Oral Sciences* 104(2):69–81.
2. Clark, L. C. Jr. and C. Lions. 1962. Electrode systems for continuous monitoring in cardiovascular surgery. *Annals of the New York Academy of Sciences* 102:29.
3. Nice, E. C. and B. Catimel. 1999. Instrumental biosensors: New perspectives for the analysis of biomolecular interactions. *Bioessays* 21(4):339–352.
4. Braguglia, C. M. 1998. Biosensors: An outline of general principles and application. *Chemical and Biochemical Engineering Quarterly* 12(4):183–190.
5. Weetall, H. H. 1999. Chemical sensors and biosensors, update, what, where, when and how. *Biosensors & Bioelectronics* 14(2):237–242.
6. Tess, M. E. and J. A. Cox. 1999. Chemical and biochemical sensors based on advances in materials chemistry. *Journal of Pharmaceutical and Biomedical Analysis* 19(1–2):55–68.
7. Vo-Dinh, T., B. J. Tromberg, G. D. Griffin, K. R. Ambrose, M. J. Sepaniak, and E. M. Gardenhire. 1987. Antibody-based fiberoptics biosensor for the carcinogen benzo(a)pyrene. *Applied Spectroscopy* 41(5):735–738.
8. Vo-Dinh, T., J. P. Alarie, R. W. Johnson, M. J. Sepaniak, and R. M. Santella. 1991. Evaluation of the fiberoptic antibody-based fluoroimmunosensor for DNA adducts in human placenta samples. *Clinical Chemistry* 37(4):532–535.
9. Kienle, S., S. Lingler, W. Kraas, A. Offenhausser, W. Knoll, and G. Jung. 1997. Electropolymerization of a phenol-modified peptide for use in receptor–ligand interactions studied by surface plasmon resonance. *Biosensors & Bioelectronics* 12(8):779–786.
10. Pathak, S. S. and H. F. J. Savelkoul. 1997. Biosensors in immunology: The story so far. *Immunology Today* 18(10):464–467.
11. Regnault, V., J. Arvieux, L. Vallar, and T. Lecompte. 1999. Both kinetic data and epitope mapping provide clues for understanding the anti-coagulant effect of five murine monoclonal antibodies to human beta(2)-glycoprotein I. *Immunology* 97(3):400–407.
12. Huber, A., S. Demartis, and D. Neri. 1999. The use of biosensor technology for the engineering of antibodies and enzymes. *Journal of Molecular Recognition* 12(3):198–216.
13. Anderson, G. P., K. A. Breslin, and F. S. Ligler. 1996. Assay development for a portable fiberoptic biosensor. *ASAIO Journal* 42(6):942–946.
14. Anderson, G. P., M. A. Jacoby, F. S. Ligler, and K. D. King. 1997. Effectiveness of protein A for antibody immobilization for a fiber optic biosensor. *Biosensors & Bioelectronics* 12(4):329–336.
15. Cao, L. K., G. P. Anderson, F. S. Ligler, and J. Ezzell. 1995. Detection of *Yersinia-pestis* fraction-1 antigen with a fiber optic biosensor. *Journal of Clinical Microbiology* 33(2):336–341.
16. Wadkins, R. M., J. P. Golden, L. M. Pritsiolas, and F. S. Ligler. 1998. Detection of multiple toxic agents using a planar array immunosensor. *Biosensors & Bioelectronics* 13(3–4):407–415.

17. King, K. D., G. P. Anderson, K. E. Bullock, M. J. Regina, E. W. Saaski, and F. S. Ligler. 1999. Detecting staphylococcal enterotoxin B using an automated fiber optic biosensor. *Biosensors & Bioelectronics* 14(2):163–170.

18. James, E. A., K. Schmeltzer, and F. S. Ligler. 1996. Detection of endotoxin using an evanescent wave fiber-optic biosensor. *Applied Biochemistry and Biotechnology* 60(3):189–202.

19. Cullum, B. M. and T. Vo-Dinh. 2000. The development of optical nanosensors for biological measurements. *Trends in Biotechnology* 18(9):388–393.

20. Isola, N. R., D. L. Stokes, and T. Vo-Dinh. 1998. Surface enhanced Raman gene probe for HIV detection. *Analytical Chemistry* 70(7):1352–1356.

21. Leonardo, R. A. and T. Vo-Dinh. 2002. Surface-enhanced Raman scattering detection of the breast cancer susceptibility gene BRCA1 using a silver-coated microarray platform. *Analytica Chimica Acta* 469(1): 149–154.

22. Moreno-Bondi, M. C., J. Mobley, J. P. Alarie, and T. Vo-Dinh. 2000. Antibody-based biosensor for breast cancer with ultrasonic regeneration. *Journal of Biomedical Optics* 5(3):350–354.

23. Vo-Dinh, T., N. Isola, J. P. Alarie, D. Landis, G. D. Griffin, and S. Allison. 1998. Development of a multiarray biosensor for DNA diagnostics. *Instrumentation Science & Technology* 26(5):503–514.

24. Dremel, B. A. A. and R. D. Schmid. 1992. Optical sensors for bioprocess control. *Chemie Ingenieur Technik* 64(6):510–517.

25. Jakeway, S. C. and U. J. Krull. 1999. Consideration of end effects of DNA hybridization in selection of fluorescent dyes for development of optical biosensors. *Canadian Journal of Chemistry—Revue Canadienne De Chimie* 77(12):2083–2087.

26. Piunno, P. A. E., U. J. Krull, R. H. E. Hudson, M. J. Damha, and H. Cohen. 1994. Fiber optic biosensor for fluorometric detection of DNA hybridization. *Analytica Chimica Acta* 288(3):205–214.

27. Uddin, A. H., P. A. E. Piunno, R. H. E. Hudson, M. J. Damha, and U. J. Krull. 1997. A fiber optic biosensor for fluorimetric detection of triple-helical DNA. *Nucleic Acids Research* 25(20):4139–4146.

28. Watterson, J. H., P. A. E. Piunno, C. C. Wust, and U. J. Krull. 2001. Controlling the density of nucleic acid oligomers on fiber optic sensors for enhancement of selectivity and sensitivity. *Sensors and Actuators B: Chemical* 74(1–3):27–36.

29. Vo-Dinh, T., T. Nolan, Y. F. Cheng, M. J. Sepaniak, and J. P. Alarie. 1990. Phase-resolved fiberoptics fluoroimmunosensor. *Applied Spectroscopy* 44(1):128–132.

30. Plowman, T. E., W. M. Reichert, C. R. Peters, H. K. Wang, D. A. Christensen, and J. N. Herron. 1996. Femtomolar sensitivity using a channel-etched thin film waveguide fluoroimmunosensor. *Biosensors & Bioelectronics* 11(1–2):149–160.

31. Koncki, R. and O. S. Wolfbeis. 1999. Composite films of Prussian blue and N-substituted polypyrroles: Covalent immobilization of enzymes and application to near infrared optical biosensing. *Biosensors & Bioelectronics* 14(1):87–92.

32. Homola, J., S. S. Yee, and G. Gauglitz. 1999. Surface plasmon resonance sensors: Review. *Sensors and Actuators B: Chemical* 54(1–2):3–15.

33. VanRegenmortel, M. H. V., D. Altschuh, and J. Chatellier. 1997. Uses of biosensors in the study of viral antigens. *Immunological Investigations* 26(1–2):67–82.

34. Liedberg, B., C. Nylander, and I. Lundstrom. 1983. Surface plasmon resonance for gas detection and biosensing. *Sensors and Actuators* 4:299.

35. Flanagan, M. T. and R. H. Pantell. 1984. Surface plasmon resonance and immunosensors. *Electronics Letters* 20:968.

36. Morton, T. A. and D. G. Myszka. 1998. Kinetic analysis of macromolecular interactions using surface plasmon resonance biosensors. *Methods in Enzymology* 295:268–294.

37. Luo, J., J. M. Zhou, W. Zou, and P. Shen. 2001. Antibody–antigen interactions measured by surface plasmon resonance: Global fitting of numerical integration algorithms. Production and molecular characterization of clinical phase I anti-melanoma mouse IgG3 monoclonal antibody R24. *Journal of Biochemistry* 130(4):553–559.

38. Rich, R. L. and D. G. Myszka. 2000. Survey of the 1999 surface plasmon resonance biosensor literature. *Journal of Molecular Recognition* 13(6):388–407.

39. Wang, S., S. Boussaad, and N. J. Tao. 2001. Surface plasmon resonance enhanced optical absorption spectroscopy for studying molecular adsorbates. *Review of Scientific Instruments* 72(7):3055–3060.

40. Casay, G. A., M. I. Daneshvar, and G. Patonay. 1994. Development of a fiber optic biomolecular probe instrument using near-infrared dyes and semiconductor-laser diodes. *Instrumentation Science & Technology* 22(4):323–341.

41. Tunnemann, R., M. Mehlmann, R. D. Sussmuth et al. 2001. Optical biosensors. Monitoring studies of glycopeptide antibiotic fermentation using white light interference. *Analytical Chemistry* 73(17):4313–4318.

42. Birkert, O., R. Tunnernann, G. Jung, and G. Gauglitz. 2002. Label-free parallel screening of combinatorial triazine libraries using reflectometric interference spectroscopy. *Analytical Chemistry* 74(4):834–840.

43. Birkert, O., H. M. Haake, A. Schutz et al. 2000. A streptavidin surface on planar glass substrates for the detection of biomolecular interaction. *Analytical Biochemistry* 282(2):200–208.

44. Vo-Dinh, T., K. Houck, and D. L. Stokes. 1994. Surface-enhanced Raman gene probes. *Analytical Chemistry* 66(20):3379–3385.

45. Vo-Dinh, T. 1998. Surface-enhanced Raman spectroscopy using metallic nanostructures. *Trends in Analytical Chemistry* 17(8–9):557–582.

46. Deckert, V., D. Zeisel, R. Zenobi, and T. Vo-Dinh. 1998. Near-field surface enhanced Raman imaging of dye-labeled DNA with 100-nm resolution. *Analytical Chemistry* 70(13):2646–2650.

47. Vo-Dinh, T., L. R. Allain, and D. L. Stokes. 2002. Cancer gene detection using SERS. *Journal of Raman Spectroscopy* 33(7):511–516.

48. Albrecht, M. G. and J. A. Creighton. 1977. Anomalously intense Raman spectra of pyridine at a silver electrode. *Journal of the American Chemical Society* 99:5215.

49. Jeanmaire, D. J. and R. P. Van Dyune. 1977. Surface Raman spectroelectrochemistry: Part I. Heterocyclic, aromatic, and aliphatic amines adsorbed on the anodized silver electrode. *Journal of Electroanalytical Chemistry* 84:1.

50. Fleischchmann, M., P. J. Hendra, and A. J. McQuillan. 1974. Raman spectra of pyridine adsorbed at a silver electrode. *Chemical Physics Letters* 26:63.

51. Gyurcsanyi, R. E., Z. Vagfoldi, K. Toth, and G. Nagy. 1999. Fast response potentiometric acetylcholine biosensor. *Electroanalysis* 11(10–11):712–718.

52. Dobay, R., G. Harsanyi, and C. Visy. 1999. Conducting polymer based electrochemical sensors on thick film substrate. *Electroanalysis* 11(10–11):804–808.

53. Coche-Guerente, L., V. Desprez, J. P. Diard, and P. Labbe. 1999. Amplification of amperometric biosensor responses by electrochemical substrate recycling. Part I. Theoretical treatment of the catechol–polyphenol oxidase system. *Journal of Electroanalytical Chemistry* 470(1):53–60.

54. Dall'Orto, V. C., C. Danilowicz, I. Rezzano, M. Del Carlo, and M. Mascini. 1999. Comparison between three amperometric sensors for phenol determination in olive oil samples. *Analytical Letters* 32(10):1981–1990.

55. Karyakin, A. A., M. Vuki, L. V. Lukachova et al. 1999. Processible polyaniline as an advanced potentiometric pH transducer. Application to biosensors. *Analytical Chemistry* 71(13):2534–2540.

56. Rudel, U., O. Geschke, and K. Cammann. 1996. Entrapment of enzymes in electropolymers for biosensors and graphite felt based flow-through enzyme reactors. *Electroanalysis* 8:1135–1139.

57. Sarkar, P. and A. P. F. Turner. 1999. Application of dual-step potential on single screen-printed modified carbon paste electrodes for detection of amino acids and proteins. *Fresenius Journal of Analytical Chemistry* 364:154–159.

58. Huang, T., A. Warsinke, T. Kuwana, and F. W. Scheller. 1998. Determination of ʟ-phenylalanine based on an NADH-detecting biosensor. *Analytical Chemistry* 70:991–997.

59. Mo, Z. H., X. H. Long, and W. L. Fu. 1999. A new sandwich-type assay of estrogen using piezoelectric biosensor immobilized with estrogen response element. *Analytical Communications* 36(7):281–283.

60. Hengerer, A., C. Kosslinger, J. Decker et al. 1999. Determination of phage antibody affinities to antigen by a microbalance sensor system. *Biotechniques* 26(5):956–960.

61. Wessa, T., M. Rapp, and H. J. Ache. 1999. New immobilization method for SAW-biosensors: Covalent attachment of antibodies via CNBr. *Biosensors & Bioelectronics* 14(1):93–98.

62. Minunni, M., M. Mascini, R. M. Carter, M. B. Jacobs, G. J. Lubrano, and G. C. Guilbault. 1996. A quartz crystal microbalance displacement assay for *Listeria monocytogenes*. *Analytica Chimica Acta* 325:169–174.

63. Vaughan, R. D., C. K. Sullivan, and G. C. Guilbault. 1999. Sulfur based self-assembled monolayers (SAM's) on piezoelectric crystals for immunosensor development. *Fresenius Journal of Analytical Chemistry* 364:54–57.

64. Welsch, W., C. Klein, M. vonSchickfus, and S. Hunklinger. 1996. Development of a surface acoustic wave immunosensor. *Analytical Chemistry* 68:2000–2004.

65. Freudenberg, J., S. Schelle, K. Beck, M. vonSchickfus, and S. Hunklinger. 1999. A contactless surface acoustic wave biosensor. *Biosensors & Bioelectronics* 14:423–425.

66. Ji, H. F. and T. Thundat. 2002. In situ detection of calcium ions with chemically modified microcantilevers. *Biosensors & Bioelectronics* 17(4):337–343.

67. Smith, D. S., M. Hassan, and R. D. Nargessi. 1981. Principles and practice of fluoroimmunoassay procedures. In *Modern Fluorescence Spectroscopy*, Wehry, E.L. (ed.). Springer, New York, pp. 143–191. DOI: 10.1007/978-1-4684-1092-1_4.

68. Tromberg, B. J., M. J. Sepaniak, T. Vo-Dinh, and G. D. Griffin. 1987. Fiberoptic chemical sensors for competitive-binding fluoroimmunoassay. *Analytical Chemistry* 59(8):1226–1230.

69. Wadkins, R. M., J. P. Golden, and F. S. Ligler. 1995. Calibration of biosensor response using simultaneous evanescent-wave excitation of cyanine-labeled capture antibodies and antigens. *Analytical Biochemistry* 232(1):73–78.

70. Campbell, C. N., T. de Lumley-Woodyear, and A. Heller. 1993. Towards immunoassay in whole blood: Separationless sandwich-type electrochemical immunoassay based on in-situ generation of the substrate of the labeling enzyme. *Fresenius Journal of Analytical Chemistry* 364:165–169.

71. Kroger, D., M. Liley, W. Schiweck, A. Skerra, and H. Vogel. 1999. Immobilization of histidine-tagged proteins on gold surfaces using chelator thioalkanes. *Biosensors & Bioelectronics* 14(2):155–161.

72. Vo-Dinh, T., G. D. Griffin, and K. R. Ambrose. 1986. A portable fiberoptic monitor for fluorometric bioassays. *Applied Spectroscopy* 40(5):696–700.

73. Alarie, J. P. and T. Vo-Dinh. 1996. Antibody-based submicron biosensor for benzo[*a*]pyrene DNA adduct. *Polycyclic Aromatic Compounds* 8(1):45–52.

74. Cullum, B. M., G. D. Griffin, G. H. Miller, and T. Vo-Dinh. 2000. Intracellular measurements in mammary carcinoma cells using fiber-optic nanosensors. *Analytical Biochemistry* 277(1):25–32.

75. Vo-Dinh, T., B. Cullum, and G. D. Griffin. 2001. Optical nanosensors for single-cell analysis. *Radiation Research* 156(4):437–438.

76. Rowe-Taitt, C. A., J. J. Cras, C. H. Patterson, J. P. Golden, and F. S. Ligler. 2000. A ganglioside-based assay for cholera toxin using an array biosensor. *Analytical Biochemistry* 281(1):123–133.

77. Narang, U., G. P. Anderson, F. S. Ligler, and J. Burans. 1997. Fiber optic-based biosensor for ricin. *Biosensors & Bioelectronics* 12(9–10):937–945.

78. Wijesuriya, D., K. Breslin, G. Anderson, L. Shriverlake, and F. S. Ligler. 1994. Regeneration of immobilized antibodies on fiber optic probes. *Biosensors & Bioelectronics* 9(8):585–592.

79. Vo-Dinh, T., G. D. Griffin, K. R. Ambrose, M. J. Sepaniak, and B. J. Tromberg. 1988. Fiberoptics immunofluorescence spectroscopy for chemical and biological monitoring. In *Polycyclic Aromatic Hydrocarbons: A Decade of Progress*, M. Cooke and A. J. Dennis (eds.). Battelle Press, Columbus, OH, pp. 885–900.

80. Alarie, J. P., J. R. Bowyer, M. J. Sepaniak, A. M. Hoyt, and T. Vo-Dinh. 1990. Fluorescence monitoring of a benzo[*a*]pyrene metabolite using a regenerable immunochemical-based fiberoptic sensor. *Analytica Chimica Acta* 236(2):237–244.

81. Blanchard, G. C., C. G. Taylor, B. R. Busey, and M. L. Williamson. 1990. Regeneration of immunosorbent surfaces used in clinical, industrial and environmental biosensors—Role of covalent and noncovalent interactions. *Journal of Immunological Methods* 130(2):263–275.

82. Absolom, D. R. and C. J. Vanoss. 1986. The nature of the antigen–antibody bond and the factors affecting its association and dissociation. *CRC Critical Reviews in Immunology* 6(1):1–46.

83. Shriverlake, L. C., K. A. Breslin, P. T. Charles, D. W. Conrad, J. P. Golden, and F. S. Ligler. 1995. Detection of TNT in water using an evanescent-wave fiberoptic biosensor. *Analytical Chemistry* 67(14):2431–2435.

84. Lu, B., C. L. Lu, and Y. Wei. 1992. A planar quartz wave-guide immunosensor based on TIRF principle. *Analytical Letters* 25(1):1–10.

85. Haga, M., T. Shimura, T. Nakamura, Y. Kato, and Y. Suzuki. 1987. Effect of ultrasonic irradiation on the dissociation of antigen–antibody complexes—Application to homogeneous enzyme-immunoassay. *Chemical & Pharmaceutical Bulletin* 35(9):3822–3830.

86. Busnaina, A. A., I. I. Kashkoush, and G. W. Gale. 1995. An experimental-study of megasonic cleaning of silicon-wafers. *Journal of the Electrochemical Society* 142(8):2812–2817.

87. Qi, Q. and G. J. Brereton. 1995. Mechanisms of removal of micron-sized particles by high-frequency ultrasonic-waves. *IEEE Transactions on Ultrasonics Ferroelectrics and Frequency Control* 42(4):619–629.

88. Mobley, J., J. N. Marsh, C. S. Hall, M. S. Hughes, G. H. Brandenburger, and J. G. Miller. 1998. Broadband measurements of phase velocity in Albunex (R) suspensions. *Journal of the Acoustical Society of America* 103(4):2145–2153.

89. Mobley, J., P. M. Kasili, S. N. Norton, and T. Vo-Dinh. 1999. Application of ultrasonic techniques for brain injury diagnostics. In *Biomedical Diagnostics, Guidance and Surgical-Assist Systems*, T. Vo-Dinh, W. S. Grundfest, and D. Benaron (eds.), *Proceedings of the SPIE*, SPIE Publishers, Bellingham, WA, Vol. 3595, pp. 79–90.

90. Diamond, D. (ed.). 1998. *Chemical and Biological Sensors*. Wiley, New York.

91. Polster, J., G. Prestel, M. Wollenweber, G. Kraus, and G. Gauglitz. 1995. Simultaneous determination of penicillin and ampicillin by spectral fibre-optical enzyme optodes and multivariate data analysis based on transient signals obtained by flow injection analysis. *Talanta* 42(12):2065–2072.

92. Rosenzweig, Z. and R. Kopelman. 1996. Analytical properties and sensor size effects of a micrometer-sized optical fiber glucose biosensor. *Analytical Chemistry* 68(8):1408–1413.

93. Barker, S. L. R., R. Kopelman, T. E. Meyer, and M. A. Cusanovich. 1998. Fiber-optic nitric oxide-selective biosensors and nanosensors. *Analytical Chemistry* 70(5):971–976.

94. McCormack, T., G. O'Keeffe, B. D. MacCraith, and R. O'Kennedy. 1997. Optical immunosensing of lactate dehydrogenase (LDH). *Sensors and Actuators B: Chemical* 41:89–96.

95. Vo-Dinh, T. and B. Cullum. 2000. Biosensors and biochips: Advances in biological and medical diagnostics. *Fresenius Journal of Analytical Chemistry* 366(6–7):540–551.

96. Sawata, S., E. Kai, K. Ikebukuro, T. Iida, T. Honda, and I. Karube. 1999. Application of peptide nucleic acid to the direct detection of deoxyribonucleic acid amplified by polymerase chain reaction. *Biosensors & Bioelectronics* 14(4):397–404.

97. Niemeyer, C. M., L. Boldt, B. Ceyhan, and D. Blohm. 1999. DNA-directed immobilization: Efficient, reversible, and site-selective surface binding of proteins by means of covalent DNA–streptavidin conjugates. *Analytical Biochemistry* 268(1):54–63.

98. Marrazza, G., I. Chianella, and M. Mascini. 1999. Disposable DNA electrochemical sensor for hybridization detection. *Biosensors & Bioelectronics* 14(1):43–51.

99. Wang, J., G. Rivas, J. R. Fernandes, J. L. L. Paz, M. Jiang, and R. Waymire. 1998. Indicator-free electrochemical DNA hybridization biosensor. *Analytica Chimica Acta* 375(3):197–203.

100. Piehler, J., A. Brecht, G. Gauglitz et al. 1997. Label-free monitoring of DNA–ligand interactions. *Analytical Biochemistry* 249(1):94–102.

101. Skuridin, S. G., Y. M. Yevdokimov, V. S. Efimov, J. M. Hall, and A. P. F. Turner. 1996. A new approach for creating double-stranded DNA biosensors. *Biosensors & Bioelectronics* 11(9):903–911.

102. Ferguson, J. A., T. C. Boles, C. P. Adams, and D. R. Walt. 1996. A fiber-optic DNA biosensor microarray for the analysis of gene expression. *Nature Biotechnology* 14(13):1681–1684.

103. Hanafi-Bagby, D., P. A. E. Piunno, C. C. Wust, and U. J. Krull. 2000. Concentration dependence of a thiazole orange derivative that is used to determine nucleic acid hybridization by an optical biosensor. *Analytica Chimica Acta* 411(1–2):19–30.

104. Piunno, P. A. E., U. J. Krull, R. H. E. Hudson, M. J. Damha, and H. Cohen. 1995. Fiberoptic DNA sensor for fluorometric nucleic acid determination. *Analytical Chemistry* 67(15):2635–2643.

105. Watterson, J. H., P. A. E. Piunno, C. C. Wust, and U. J. Krull. 2000. Effects of oligonucleotide immobilization density on selectivity of quantitative transduction of hybridization of immobilized DNA. *Langmuir* 16(11):4984–4992.

106. Franchina, J. G., W. M. Lackowski, D. L. Dermody, R. M. Crooks, D. E. Bergbreiter, K. Sirkar, R. J. Russell, and M. V. Pishko. 1999. Electrostatic immobilization of glucose oxidase in a weak acid, polyelectrolyte hyperbranched ultrathin film on gold: Fabrication, characterization, and enzymatic activity. *Analytical Chemistry* 71:3133–3139.

107. Schuler, R., M. WittKampf, and G. C. Chemnitius. 1999. Modified gas-permeable silicone rubber membranes for covalent immobilisation of enzymes and their use in biosensor development. *Analyst* 124:1181–1184.

108. Houshmand, H., G. Froman, and G. Magnusson. 1999. Use of bacteriophage T7 displayed peptides for determination of monoclonal antibody specificity and biosensor analysis of the binding reaction. *Analytical Biochemistry* 268:363–370.

109. Lebron, J. A. and P. J. Bjorkman. 1999. The transferrin receptor binding site on HFE, the class I MHC-related protein mutated in hereditary hemochromatosis. *Journal of Molecular Biology* 289:1109–1118.

110. Kim, H. J., M. S. Hyun, I. S. Chang, and B. H. Kim. 1999. A microbial fuel cell type lactate biosensor using a metal-reducing bacterium, *Shewanella putrefaciens*. *Journal of Microbiology and Biotechnology* 9:365–367.

111. Nelson, R. W., J. W. Jarvik, B. E. Taillon, and K. A. Tubbs. 1999. BIA/MS of epitope-tagged peptides directly from *E. coli* lysate: Multiplex detection and protein identification at low-femtomole to subfemtomole levels. *Analytical Chemistry* 71:2858–2865.

112. Hara-Kuge, S., T. Ohkura, A. Seko, and K. Yamashita. 1999. Vesicular-integral membrane protein, VIP36, recognizes high-mannose type glycans containing $\alpha 1 \rightarrow 2$ mannosyl residues in MDCK cells. *Glycobiology* 9:833–839.

113. Pemberton, R. M., J. P. Hart, P. Stoddard, and J. A. Foulkes. 1999. A comparison of 1-naphthyl phosphate and 4 aminophenyl phosphate as enzyme substrates for use with a screen-printed amperometric immunosensor for progesterone in cows' milk. *Biosensors & Bioelectronics* 14:493–503.

114. Blake, R. C., A. R. Pavlov, and D. A. Blake. 1999. Automated kinetic exclusion assays to quantify protein binding interactions in homogeneous solution. *Analytical Biochemistry* 272:123–124.

115. Patolsky, F., M. Zayats, E. Katz, and I. Willner. 1999. Precipitation of an insoluble product on enzyme monolayer electrodes for biosensor applications: Characterization by Faradaic impedance spectroscopy, cyclic voltammetry, and microgravimetric quartz crystal microbalance analyses. *Analytical Biochemistry* 71:3171–3180.

116. Barker, S. L. R., Y. D. Zhao, M. A. Marletta, and R. Kopelman. 1999. Cellular applications of a sensitive and selective fiber optic nitric oxide biosensor based on a dye-labeled heme domain of soluble guanylate cyclase. *Analytical Chemistry* 71(11):2071–2075.

117. Schmidt, A., C. StandfussGabisch, and U. Bilitewski. 1996. Microbial biosensor for free fatty acids using an oxygen electrode based on thick film technology. *Biosensors & Bioelectronics* 11(11):1139–1145.

118. Boncheva, M., C. Duschl, W. Beck, G. Jung, and H. Vogel. 1996. Formation and characterization of lipopeptide layers at interfaces for the molecular recognition of antibodies. *Langmuir* 12(23):5636–5642.

119. Cornell, B. A., V. L. B. Braach-Maksvytis, L. G. King, P. D. J. Osman, B. Raguse, L. Wieczorek, and R. J. Pace. 1997. A biosensor that uses ion-channel switches. *Nature* 387:580–583.

120. Wollenberger, U., B. Neumann, and F. W. Scheller. 1999. Development of a biomimetic alkane sensor. *Electrochimica Acta* 43:3581–3585.

121. Ramsden, J. J. 1999. Biomimetic protein immobilization using lipid bilayers. *Biosensors & Bioelectronics* 13:593–598.

122. Song, X. D. and B. I. Swanson. 1999. Direct, ultrasensitive, and selective optical detection of protein toxins using multivalent interactions. *Analytical Chemistry* 71(11):2097–2107.

123. Cotton, G. J., B. Ayers, R. Xu, and T. W. Muir. 1999. Insertion of a synthetic peptide into a recombinant protein framework: A protein biosensor. *Journal of the American Chemical Society* 121:1100–1101.

124. Zhang, W. T., G. Canziani, C. Plugariu, R. Wyatt, J. Sodroski, R. Sweet, P. Kwong, W. Hendrickson, and L. Chaiken. 1999. Conformational changes of gp120 in epitopes near the CCR5 binding site are induced by CD4 and a CD4 miniprotein mimetic. *Biochemistry* 38:9405–9416.

125. Piervincenzi, R. T., W. M. Reichert, and H. W. Hellinga. 1998. Genetic engineering of a single-chain antibody fragment for surface immobilization in an optical biosensor. *Biosensors & Bioelectronics* 13(3–4):305–312.

126. Charych, D., Q. Cheng, A. Reichert et al. 1996. A "litmus test" for molecular recognition using artificial membranes. *Chemistry & Biology* 3(2):113–120.

127. Kriz, D. and K. Mosbach. 1995. Competitive amperometric morphine sensor-based on an agarose immobilized molecularly imprinted polymer. *Analytica Chimica Acta* 300(1–3):71–75.

128. Veilleux, J. K. and L. W. Duran. March 1996. Covalent immobilization of bio-molecules to preactivated surfaces. *IVD Technology Magazine* 2:26–31.

129. Allain, L. R., K. Sorasaenee, and Z. L. Xue. 1997. Doped thin-film sensors via a sol-gel process for high acidity determination. *Analytical Chemistry* 69(15):3076–3080.

130. Allain, L. R. and Z. L. Xue. 2000. Optical sensors for the determination of concentrated hydroxide. *Analytical Chemistry* 72(5):1078–1083.

131. Yost, T. L., B. C. Fagan, L. R. Allain et al. 2000. Crown ether-doped sol-gel materials for strontium(II) separation. *Analytical Chemistry* 72(21):5516–5519.

132. Rasmussen, S. R., M. R. Larsen, and S. E. Rasmussen. 1991. Covalent immobilization of DNA onto polystyrene microwells: The molecules are only bound at the 5′ end. *Analytical Biochemistry* 198:138–142.

133. Larsson, P. H., S. G. O. Johansson, A. Hult et al. 1987. Covalent binding of proteins to grafted plastic surfaces suitable for immunoassays. I. Binding capacity and characteristics of grafted polymers. *Journal of Immunological Methods* 98:129–135.

134. Potyrailo, R. A., R. C. Conrad, A. D. Ellington, and G. M. Hiefje. 1998. Adapting selected nucleic acid ligands (aptamers) to biosensors. *Analytical Chemistry* 70:3419–3425.

135. Yoo, S. K., M. Yoon, U. J. Park, H. S. Han, J. H. Kim, and H. J. Hwang. 1999. A radioimmunoassay method for detection of DNA based on chemical immobilization of anti-DNA antibody. *Experimental and Molecular Medicine* 31(3):122–125.

136. Aylott, J. W., D. J. Richardson, and D. A. Russell. 1997. Optical biosensing of nitrate ions using a sol-gel immobilized nitrate reductase. *Analyst* 122(1):77–80.

137. Blyth, D. J., S. J. Poynter, and D. A. Russell. 1996. Calcium biosensing with a sol-gel immobilized photoprotein. *Analyst* 121(12):1975–1978.

138. Blyth, D. J., J. W. Aylott, D. J. Richardson, and D. A. Russell. 1995. Sol-gel encapsulation of metalloproteins for the development of optical biosensors for nitrogen-monoxide and carbon-monoxide. *Analyst* 120(11):2725–2730.

139. Doong, R. A. and H. C. Tsai. 2001. Immobilization and characterization of sol-gel-encapsulated acetylcholinesterase fiber-optic biosensor. *Analytica Chimica Acta* 434(2):239–246.

140. Li, J., K. M. Wang, X. H. Yang, and D. Xiao. 1999. Sol-gel horseradish peroxidase biosensor for the chemiluminescent flow determination of hydrogen peroxide. *Analytical Communications* 36(5):195–197.

141. Lin, J. and C. W. Brown. 1997. Sol-gel glass as a matrix for chemical and biochemical sensing. *Trends in Analytical Chemistry* 16(4):200–211.

142. Situmorang, M., J. J. Gooding, and D. B. Hibbert. 1999. Immobilisation of enzyme throughout a polytyramine matrix: A versatile procedure for fabricating biosensors. *Analytica Chimica Acta* 394(2–3):211–223.

143. Lee, Y. C. and M. H. Huh. 1999. Development of a biosensor with immobilized L-amino acid oxidase for determination of L-amino acids. *Journal of Food Biochemistry* 23(2):173–185.

144. Edmiston, P. L., C. L. Wambolt, M. K. Smith, and S. S. Saavedra. 1994. Spectroscopic characterization of albumin and myoglobin entrapped in bulk sol-gel glasses. *Journal of Colloid and Interface Science* 163(2):395–406.

145. Barak, L. S., S. S. G. Ferguson, J. Zhang, and M. G. Caron. 1997. A beta-arrestin green fluorescent protein biosensor for detecting G protein-coupled receptor activation. *Journal of Biological Chemistry* 272(44):27497–27500.

146. Desikan, R., D. Hagenbeek, S. J. Neill, and C. D. Rock. 1999. Flow cytometry and surface plasmon resonance analyses demonstrate that the monoclonal antibody JIM19 interacts with a rice cell surface component involved in abscisic acid signalling in protoplasts. *FEBS Letters* 456(2):257–262.

147. Newman, D. J., H. Thakkar, M. K. Lam-Po-Tang, and J. T. C. Kwan. 1999. The use of optical sensors to understand cellular interactions with renal cells. *Renal Failure* 21(3–4):349–357.

148. Inoue, K., T. Arai, and M. Aoyagi. 1999. Sensitivity of real time viral detection by an optical biosensor system using a crude home-made antiserum against measles virus as a ligand. *Biological & Pharmaceutical Bulletin* 22(2):210–213.

149. Krummenacher, C., I. Baribaud, M. P. de Leon et al. 2000. Localization of a binding site for herpes simplex virus glycoprotein D on herpesvirus entry mediator C by using antireceptor monoclonal antibodies. *Journal of Virology* 74(23):10863–10872.

150. Ostroff, R., A. Ettinger, H. La et al. 2001. Rapid multiserotype detection of human rhinoviruses on optically coated silicon surfaces. *Journal of Clinical Virology* 21(2):105–117.

151. Inoue, K., T. Arai, and M. Aoyagi. 1997. Real time observation of binding of herpes simplex virus type 1 (HSV-1) to Vero cells and neutralization of HSV-1 by sulfonated human immunoglobulin. *Journal of Biochemistry* 121(4):633–636.

152. Tsoka, S., A. Gill, J. L. Brookman, and M. Hoare. 1998. Rapid monitoring of virus-like particles using an optical biosensor: A feasibility study. *Journal of Biotechnology* 63(2):147–153.

153. Gomes, P., E. Giralt, and D. Andreu. 1999. Surface plasmon resonance screening of synthetic peptides mimicking the immunodominant region of C-S8c1 foot-and-mouth disease virus. *Vaccine* 18(3–4):362–370.

154. Li, C., C. S. Dowd, W. Zhang, and I. M. Chaiken. 2001. Phage randomization in a charybdotoxin scaffold leads to CD4-mimetic recognition motifs that bind HIV-1 envelope through non-aromatic sequences. *Journal of Peptide Research* 57(6):507–518.

155. Hoffman, T. L., G. Canziani, L. Jia, J. Rucker, and R. W. Doms. 2000. A biosensor assay for studying ligand-membrane receptor interactions: Binding of antibodies and HIV-1 Env to chemokine receptors. *Proceedings of the National Academy of Sciences of the United States of America* 97(21):11215–11220.

156. Dowd, C. S., W. T. Zhang, C. Z. Li, and I. M. Chaiken. 2001. From receptor recognition mechanisms to bioinspired mimetic antagonists in HIV-1/cell docking. *Journal of Chromatography B* 753(2):327–335.

157. Zeng, X. X., Y. Nakaaki, T. Murata, and T. Usui. 2000. Chemoenzymatic synthesis of glyco-polypeptides carrying alpha-Neu5Ac-(2 → 3)-beta-D-Gal-(1 → 3)-alpha-D-GalNAc, beta-D-Gal-(1 → 3)-alpha-D-GalNAc, and related compounds and analysis of their specific interactions with lectins. *Archives of Biochemistry and Biophysics* 383(1):28–37.

158. Markgren, P. O., M. Hamalainen, and U. H. Danielson. 1998. Screening of compounds inter-acting with HIV-1 proteinase using optical biosensor technology. *Analytical Biochemistry* 265(2):340–350.

159. Markgren, P. O., M. Hamalainen, and U. H. Danielson. 2000. Kinetic analysis of the interaction between HIV-1 protease and inhibitors using optical biosensor technology. *Analytical Biochemistry* 279(1):71–78.

160. Markgren, P. O., M. T. Lindgren, K. Gertow, R. Karlsson, M. Hamalainen, and U. H. Danielson. 2001. Determination of interaction kinetic constants for HIV-1 protease inhibitors using optical biosensor technology. *Analytical Biochemistry* 291(2):207–218.

161. Hamalainen, M. D., P. O. Markgren, W. Schaal et al. 2000. Characterization of a set of HIV-1 pro-tease inhibitors using binding kinetics data from a biosensor-based screen. *Journal of Biomolecular Screening* 5(5):353–359.

162. O'Keefe, B. R., S. R. Shenoy, D. Xie et al. 2000. Analysis of the interaction between the HIV-inactivating protein cyanovirin-N and soluble forms of the envelope glycoproteins gp120 and gp41. *Molecular Pharmacology* 58(5):982–992.

163. Ivnitski, D., I. Abdel-Hamid, P. Atanasov, and E. Wilkins. 1999. Biosensors for detection of patho-genic bacteria. *Biosensors & Bioelectronics* 14(7):599–624.

164. Chang, Y. H., T. C. Chang, E. F. Kao, and C. Chou. 1996. Detection of protein a produced by *Staphylococcus aureus* with a fiber-optic-based biosensor. *Bioscience Biotechnology and Biochemistry* 60(10):1571–1574.

165. Watts, H. J., C. R. Lowe, and D. V. Pollardknight. 1994. Optical biosensor for monitoring microbial-cells. *Analytical Chemistry* 66(15):2465–2470.

166. Hirmo, S., E. Artursson, G. Puu, T. Wadstrom, and B. Nilsson. 1998. Characterization of *Helicobacter pylori* interactions with sialylglycoconjugates using a resonant mirror biosensor. *Analytical Biochemistry* 257(1):63–66.

167. Hirmo, S., E. Artursson, G. Puu, T. Wadstrom, and B. Nilsson. 1999. *Helicobacter pylori* interac-tions with human gastric mucin studied with a resonant mirror biosensor. *Journal of Microbiological Methods* 37(2):177–182.

168. Zhou, C. H., P. Pivarnik, S. Auger, A. Rand, and S. Letcher. 1997. A compact fiber-optic immu-nosensor for *Salmonella* based on evanescent wave excitation. *Sensors and Actuators B: Chemical* 42(3):169–175.

169. Liu, Y. C., Y. H. Che, and Y. B. Li. 2001. Rapid detection of *Salmonella typhimurium* using immu-nomagnetic separation and immune-optical sensing method. *Sensors and Actuators B: Chemical* 72(3):214–218.

170. Hacia, J. G., S. A. Woski, J. Fidanza et al. 1998. Enhanced high density oligonucleotide array-based sequence analysis using modified nucleoside triphosphates. *Nucleic Acids Research* 26(21):4975–4982.

171. Chen, H. L., D. G. Fernig, P. S. Rudland, A. Sparks, M. C. Wilkinson, and R. Barraclough. 2001. Binding to intracellular targets of the metastasis-inducing protein, S100A4 (p9Ka). *Biochemical and Biophysical Research Communications* 286(5):1212–1217.

172. Oneill, P. M., J. E. Fletcher, C. G. Stafford, P. B. Daniels, and T. Bacaresehamilton. 1995. Use of an optical biosensor to measure prostate-specific antigen in whole-blood. *Sensors and Actuators B: Chemical* 29(1–3):79–83.

173. Vo-Dinh, T., J. P. Alarie, B. M. Cullum, and G. D. Griffin. 2000. Antibody-based nanoprobe for measurement of a fluorescent analyte in a single cell. *Nature Biotechnology* 18(7):764–767.

174. Nath, N., S. R. Jain, and S. Anand. 1997. Evanescent wave fibre optic sensor for detection of *L. donovani* specific antibodies in sera of kala azar patients. *Biosensors & Bioelectronics* 12(6):491–498.

175. Carlson, M. A., C. B. Bargeron, R. C. Benson et al. 2000. An automated, handheld biosensor for aflatoxin. *Biosensors & Bioelectronics* 14(10–11):841–848.

176. Anis, N. A., J. Wright, K. R. Rogers, R. G. Thompson, J. J. Valdes, and M. E. Eldefrawi. 1992. A fiber-optic immunosensor for detecting parathion. *Analytical Letters* 25(4):627–635.

177. Ayyagari, M. S., S. Kamtekar, R. Pande et al. 1995. Chemiluminescence-based inhibition-kinetics of alkaline-phosphatase in the development of a pesticide biosensor. *Biotechnology Progress* 11(6):699–703.

178. Mulchandani, A., S. T. Pan, and W. Chen. 1999. Fiber-optic enzyme biosensor for direct determination of organophosphate nerve agents. *Biotechnology Progress* 15(1):130–134.

179. Mulchandani, A., I. Kaneva, and W. Chen. 1998. Biosensor for direct determination of organophosphate nerve agents using recombinant *Escherichia coli* with surface-expressed organophosphorus hydrolase. 2. Fiber optic microbial biosensor. *Analytical Chemistry* 70(23):5042–5046.

180. Puu, G. 2001. An approach for analysis of protein toxins based on thin films of lipid mixtures in an optical biosensor. *Analytical Chemistry* 73(1):72–79.

181. PepinCovatta, S., C. Lutsch, M. Grandgeorge, and J. M. Scherrmann. 1997. Immunoreactivity of a new generation of horse F(ab′)(2) preparations against European viper venoms and the tetanus toxin. *Toxicon* 35(3):411–422.

182. Gaus, K. and E. A. H. Hall. 1998. Surface plasmon resonance sensor for heparin measurements in blood plasma. *Biosensors & Bioelectronics* 13(12):1307–1315.

183. Feriotto, G., M. Lucci, N. Bianchi, C. Mischiati, and R. Gambari. 1999. Detection of the Delta F508 (F508del) mutation of the cystic fibrosis gene by surface plasmon resonance and biosensor technology. *Human Mutation* 13(5):390–400.

184. Shim, J. S. and C. H. Ahn. 2012. Optical immunosensor using carbon nanotubes coated with a photovoltaic polymer. *Biosensors & Bioelectronics* 34:208–214.

185. Phan, A. D. and N. A. Viet. 2012. A new type of optical biosensor from DNA wrapped semiconductor graphene ribbons. *Journal of Applied Physics* 111:114703–114708.

186. Morales-Narváez, E. and A. Arben Merkoçi. 2012. Graphene oxide as an optical biosensing platform. *Advanced Materials* 24:3298–3308.

187. Yeom, S.-H., O.-G. Kim, B.-H. Kang, K.-J. Kim, H. Yuan, D.-H. Kwon, H.-R. Kim, and S.-W. Kang. 2011. Highly sensitive nano-porous lattice biosensor based on localized surface plasmon resonance and interference. *Optics Express* 19:22882–22891.

188. Elghanian, R., J. J. Storhoff, R. C. Mucic, R. L. Letsinger, and C. A. Mirkin. 1997. Selective colorimetric detection of polynucleotides based on the distance-dependent optical properties of gold nanoparticles. *Science* 277(5329):1078–1081.

189. Cao, Y. C., R. Jin, and C. A. Mirkin. 2002. Nanoparticles with Raman spectroscopic fingerprints for DNA and RNA detection. *Science* 297(5586):1536–1540.

190. Wabuyele, M. B. and T. Vo-Dinh. 2005. Detection of human immunodeficiency virus type 1 DNA sequence using plasmonics nanoprobes. *Analytical Chemistry* 77(23):7810–7815.

191. Wang, H. N. and T. Vo-Dinh. 2011. Plasmonic coupling interference (PCI) nanoprobes for nucleic acid detection. *Small* 7(21):3067–3074.

192. Talley, C. E., L. Jusinski, C. W. Hollars, S. M. Lane, and T. Huser. 2004. Intracellular pH sensors based on surface-enhanced Raman scattering. *Analytical Chemistry* 76(23):7064–7068.

193. Scaffidi, J. P., M. K. Gregas, V. Seewaldt, and T. Vo-Dinh. 2009. SERS-based plasmonic nanobiosensing in single living cells. *Analytical and Bioanalytical Chemistry* 393(4):1135–1141.

194. Stuart, D. A., J. M. Yuen, N. Shah et al. 2006. In vivo glucose measurement by surface-enhanced Raman spectroscopy. *Analytical Chemistry* 78(20):7211–7215.

$$2$$

Glucose Monitoring

Casey W. Pirnstill
Texas A&M University

Brian Cummins
Texas A&M University

Gerard L. Coté
Texas A&M University

Roger J. McNichols
BioTex, Inc.

2.1 Introduction

Glucose is one of the most important carbohydrate nutrient sources and is fundamental to almost all biological processes. Quantification of glucose concentration is important in the monitoring and analysis of agricultural products, control and regulation of cell culture, and diagnosis and control of human diseases including diabetes. A wide range of parameters including glucose concentration levels, volume of glucose solution available, and required accuracy exist across these applications. For instance, the sugar concentration in many agricultural products (e.g., fruit juices) is hundreds of grams per liter, while the glucose concentration for an online cell culture system may be in the milligrams per deciliter range. Additionally, the volume, or more importantly for optical approaches the available optical path length, for online process control and agricultural applications can be tens of centimeters, while *in vivo*, these are typically millimeters to centimeters. Consequently, the glucose monitor sensitivity *in vivo* needs to be orders of magnitude better than in the agricultural industry. Finally, the challenges associated with the *in vivo* environment make monitoring more difficult than typical industrial applications because of a range of potential confounders that cannot be controlled. These include temperature and pH variations, confounding chemical species, pressure changes, and correlated physiological changes.

For biotechnological processes such as cell culture, measurements of analytes such as glucose are currently obtained using off-line methods that require sample extraction from the process or bioreactor. The off-line measurements may cause cell contamination, can be time-consuming and expensive, and may not reflect the real-time status of the cells. In order to overcome many of these limitations, nondestructive optical methods have been proposed as a solution.

A significant role for physiological glucose monitoring is in the diagnosis and management of diabetes. Diabetes mellitus is a metabolic disease that presents as a complex group of syndromes related in large part to problems with insulin production and/or utilization. Because insulin is the primary hormone responsible for glucose regulation in the body, the blood glucose levels in people with diabetes may fluctuate between 40 and 400 mg/dL. Normally, these values are maintained between 90 and 120 mg/dL. Over time, elevated glucose levels may damage the kidneys, eyes, nerves, and heart, and severely low glucose levels may cause a patient to go into shock or even die. Therefore, a goal of diabetes management is tight maintenance of blood glucose levels via insulin injection, modified diet, exercise, or a combination of these, and in order to guide this therapy, regular measurement of blood glucose levels (up to five or more times per day) is recommended [1]. Because current glucose-monitoring methods require a painful and inconvenient puncture of the skin to obtain a blood sample for analysis, optically based noninvasive and implantable glucose meters have been and continue to be investigated [2–6]. The techniques include direct light transmission or reflection through blood-containing body parts including the earlobe, the finger, and the forearm or optical interrogation of non-blood-containing compartments that correlate to blood glucose such as the aqueous humor of the eye or interstitial fluid of the dermis. The invasive approaches have the advantage of direct contact with the media of interest and thereby enhanced specificity, but they often suffer from biocompatibility issues. The noninvasive approaches do not suffer from the biocompatibility issues but are less specific and must account for the fact that they simultaneously probe multiple volumes including interstitial fluid, blood, and intracellular fluid.

2.2 History of Diabetes Monitoring

The disease *diabetes mellitus* is a condition marked by the body's inability to control blood glucose levels. Diabetes affects millions of people worldwide, with these numbers steadily increasing and expected to continue over the next several years with the increase in obesity and an increase in an aging population. Elevated glucose concentrations give rise to increased passing of glucose in urine and excessive urination. It is from this symptom that the disease gets its name diabetes mellitus where *diabetes* in Greek means *a siphon* and *mellitus* originates from the Greek and Latin word for honey. The increased passing of glucose in urine also later became the first method for diagnosing the condition.

The Ebers papyrus (1550 BC) appears to be the earliest and most comprehensive reference to diabetes as it covers one of the principal associated symptoms, excessive urination. It was not until the second century AD that the condition was described in more detail by Aretaeus of Cappadocia. The word diabetes was first used to describe the condition by Aretaeus, and his description of the disease focused on increased urination, weight loss, degradation of tissue, and unquenchable thirst. The first known method of diagnosing diabetes mellitus occurred in the second millennium AD, where *water tasters* tasted a patient's urine to determine if it had a sweet taste. It was suggested in 1776 by Mathew Dobson, a British physician and chemist, the sweetness in both the blood serum and urine was due to sugar [6–8]. This led to urine tasting as an indicator of diabetes throughout the seventeenth and eighteenth centuries [6,8]. Then in 1778, an Englishman by the name of Thomas Cowley was successful in separating saccharine matter from urine in a free state [9]. In the early 1800s, attention toward diabetes began considering the condition as a metabolic disease and resulted in the conclusion that the development of analytical devices and techniques would allow for reliable glucose monitoring. Initial research into analytical methods for determining glucose measurements can be greatly attributed to work of Cowley, Bernard, Bouchardat, Priestly, Lavoisier, Chevreul, Wöhler, and Benedict [7–9]. As noted by prominent French physiologist Claude Bernard in his lecture at the College de France in the late 1800s, the three prominent methods used during that time for the detection of glucose included polarimetry, reduction of Cu(II)–Cu(I) by the reduction of sugars, and the development of CO_2 from the fermentation of a glucose-containing solution [6]. Although it was known at the time that the reduction of Cu(II) is not specific to glucose, it was this method involving the reduction of Cu(II)–Cu(I) by reducing sugars through the use of Fehling's solution or the closely related Benedict's solution that became the dominant method for analyzing glucose over the next 100 years until the early 1940s.

In 1941, the Ames Division of Miles Laboratories (now known as Bayer) developed a tablet known as the Clinitest®, essentially the Benedict's reagent in the form of a tablet, which could be combined with a few drops of a glucose-containing sample such as urine to produce an exothermic reaction resulting in color change [6,10]. This color change could then be compared to a reference sheet for an estimate of the approximate level of glucose within the sample. Then in 1956, Bayer developed a dip-and-read test for glucose in urine known as Clinistix®, which represented the first technology to use glucose oxidase

(GOx) and peroxidase as opposed to the previous reagents to detect the presence of glucose. Although urine-based test strips for determining glucose still exist today, it has been shown that the glucose present in urine is a poor index for blood glucose concentrations [8]. Some of the current handheld meters used to date still employ the use of GOx and peroxidase as discussed later in this chapter. It was this technique that led to the development of the first test strip used for measuring blood glucose by the name Dextrostix®, named after dextrose, developed at Ames by Anton (Tom) Clemens in 1964. The Dextrostix was designed to be read using a reflectance meter, which was called the Ames Reflectance Meter, a departure from previous techniques that relied on the individual to use their eyes to assess a comparison of color change on the test strip to a color scale chart. Due to the expensive price of the device for that time period ($400), it was primarily meant for use in a doctor's office but was used by a limited number of patients. Another significant development in 1979 by Ames was the first fingerpick lancet device for simplifying blood sampling in patients called the Ames Autolet®.

2.3 Current Commercial Blood Glucose Monitoring Technologies for Diabetes

Many of the home blood glucose monitors currently in use rely on the so-called electroenzymatic and colorimetric approach to glucose monitoring. The colorimetric method consists of three basic steps: (1) the invasive withdrawal of a small blood sample, (2) the application of the blood sample to a specially formulated *test strip*, and (3) the automated reading of the test strip results via an electrical or optical meter.

Glucose monitor test strips are available from a number of manufacturers and in several varieties. However, all commercially available glucose monitor test strips (be they electroenzymatic or colorimetric) rely on the quantification of reaction of glucose with the naturally occurring enzyme GOx. While a number of redox reaction–based methods for determining the concentration of reducing sugars exist, the specificity afforded by GOx makes it the standard practiced assay. GOx is a protein approximately 160,000 daltons (Da) in size and is composed of two identical 80 kDa subunits linked by disulfide bonds. Each subunit contains 1 mol of Fe and 1 mol of flavin adenine dinucleotide (FAD). During the oxidation of glucose, the FAD groups become temporarily reduced; thus, GOx is one of the family of flavoenzymes. The reaction, which is catalyzed by GOx, is shown in Figure 2.1. In the presence of oxygen, reduced GOx further reacts to drive the reaction to the right. The reaction, which results in the production of hydrogen peroxide (H_2O_2), is shown in Figure 2.2.

Commercially available colorimetric sensors employ a peroxidase enzyme (commonly horseradish peroxidase) and a redox-coupled dye pair to generate chromophore concentrations, which are proportional to the amount of H_2O_2 produced. One such dye pair is the oxygen acceptor 3-methyl-2-benzothiazolinone hydrazone plus 3-(dimethylamino)benzoic acid (MBTH–DMAB), which has an absorption peak at 635 nm. Production of hydrogen peroxide by oxidation of glucose and reduction of oxygen

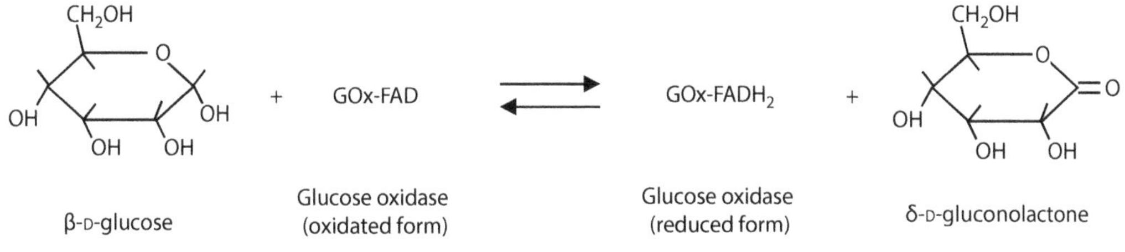

FIGURE 2.1 Oxidation of glucose to gluconolactone by the flavoenzyme GOx.

$$GOx\text{-}FADH_2 \quad + \quad O_2 \quad \longrightarrow \quad GOx\text{-}FAD \quad + \quad H_2O_2$$

FIGURE 2.2 Production of hydrogen peroxide by reduced GOx in the presence of oxygen.

drives the peroxidase-catalyzed production of active MBTH–DMAB chromophore, thus, resulting in a measurable increase in absorbance of light at 635 nm. Oxygen acceptor dyes that can also be used include *o*-dianisidine, benzidine, and 4-aminoantipyrene and chromotropic acid (AAP–CTA), among others [11].

Optical measurement of the dye product (and hence glucose concentration) is based on the Beer's law increase in absorbance of the dye product. In practice, this increase in absorbance is usually quantified by measuring the attendant decrease in reflectance of the active site on a test strip. The relationship between absorbance and reflectance is described by the Kubelka–Munk equation (see, e.g., [12]), $K/S = (1 - R)^2/2R$, where K is the concentration-dependent absorbance, S is a constant related to the scattering coefficient, and R is the measured reflectance.

Practical colorimetric measurement systems typically employ a multiwavelength detection scheme to increase accuracy and account for variables like the background absorbance of blood, the oxygenation state of blood, and the hematocrit of the blood under test. For the case of the MBTH–DMAB dye pair, the absorbance peak at 635 nm is fairly sharp and absorbance by the dye at 700 nm is negligible. Therefore, a second reflectance measurement at 700 nm affords a correction factor, which is used to account for background and sample variations. Since the GOx reaction is progressive, the timing of measurements is also extremely important. Early measurement systems required that a timer be started when blood was placed on the strip and that a reading be taken after a specific period of time (typically 15–60 s). Modern systems overcome this inconvenience by taking continuous reflectance measurements as soon as a new test strip is inserted into the meter. When a drop of blood is placed on the meter, an immediate change in the reflectance signals the start of the reaction, and multiple reflectance readings may be taken during the reaction to further increase accuracy or dynamic range of the sensor.

Findings released by the National Institute of Health (NIH) have shown that improved glycemic control can significantly reduce the risk of many secondary associated complications such as kidney failure, blindness, heart disease, and gangrene [1,13]. Current commercial methods of monitoring are invasive, requiring a finger or forearm stick to draw blood each time a reading is needed or by using an implanted sensor for continuous glucose monitoring (CGM). Although it has been shown that proper education and self-management of the disease can significantly improve health outcomes and the quality of life in people with diabetes [1,13], current approaches are painful, cumbersome, can be embarrassing and raise concerns about blood-borne pathogens. CGMs also require calibration with the finger stick devices one or more times daily. Thus, it is oftentimes difficult to obtain the appropriate motivation and dedication on the part of the patients to commit to an intensive blood sugar monitoring regiment.

2.4 Optical Approaches for Glucose Monitoring

In an effort to overcome several of the concerns with current glucose monitoring technology, over the past 30 years, there has been significant research conducted toward the development of optical methods for the determination of blood glucose. The primary optical approaches applied toward glucose monitoring continue to be optical absorption and scatter spectroscopy [14–18] including Raman spectroscopy (inelastic scatter) [19–21], fluorescence spectroscopy [22,23], and polarimetry [24–38]. In addition, there have been a few other optical approaches that have been suggested but are less prevalent in the literature such as optical coherence tomography (OCT) [39–41] and photoacoustic spectroscopy [42,43] that we will mention briefly. Note that in this chapter, we cover primarily the application of each of these optical approaches as they relate to glucose monitoring. Some of the details of the physics behind each approach have been skipped as they are covered in other chapters in this book.

2.4.1 Polarimetric Measurements of Aqueous Glucose

Polarimetry is a sensitive, nondestructive technique for measuring the optical activity exhibited by inorganic and organic compounds. A compound is considered to be chiral if it has at least one center about which no structural symmetry exists. Such molecules are said to be optically active since linearly polarized light is rotated when passing through them. The amount of optical rotation is determined by the molecular structure of the molecule, the concentration of chiral molecules in the substance, and the pathlength the light traverses through the sample. Each optically active substance has its own specific rotation as defined by Biot's law:

$$[\alpha]_{\lambda,\mathrm{pH}}^{T} = \frac{\alpha}{LC} \tag{2.1}$$

where
  L is the layer thickness in decimeters
  C is the concentration of solute in grams per mL of solution
  α is the observed rotation in degrees

In Equation 2.1, the specific rotation $[\alpha]_{\lambda,\mathrm{pH}}^{T}$ of a molecule is dependent upon temperature, T; wavelength, λ; and the pH of the solvent. The specific rotation is given in degrees/(dm g/mL).

This observation of optical rotation is commonly done using a setup as depicted in Figure 2.3. It is common for light to exist in the unpolarized state. The unpolarized light can then be passed through a device known as a linear polarizer, as depicted in Figure 2.3, which only allows the transmission of light in a single plane, and the output is known as plane-polarized light. Another polarizer, often referred to as an analyzer and typically oriented with its transmission axis 90° from the initial polarizer, can be used to block out the light that was transmitted through the initial polarizer. However, when an optically active sample is placed between the initial polarizer and analyzer, the plane of polarization is rotated by some amount as described by Equation 2.1. Because of this wavelength dependent rotation caused by the optically active sample, some light will pass through the analyzer, which can be measured with an optical detector.

This simply described polarimetric method has been employed in quality and process control in addition to research in the pharmaceutical, chemical, essential oil, flavor, and food industries. It is so well established that the US Pharmacopeia and the Food and Drug Administration (FDA) include polarimetric specifications for numerous substances [44]. Since the late 1800s, one of the earliest applications of polarimetry has been the development of benchtop polarimeters, known as saccharimeters, designed solely for the estimation of starch and/or sugar in food and beverage manufacturing in addition to the sugar industry [45]. For these agricultural industrial applications, in which the concentrations and pathlengths are high, commercial benchtop units similar to the system depicted in Figure 2.3 are adequate. However, for evaluating low glucose concentrations found in cell culture systems and *in vivo*, more sophisticated polarimetry systems are required to monitor the glucose.

For polarimetry to be used as a noninvasive technique for blood glucose monitoring, the polarized light signal must be able to pass from the source, through the body (sample), and to a detector without

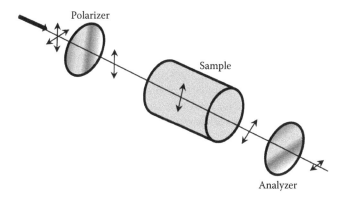

FIGURE 2.3 Illustration of optical rotation of plane-polarized light.

total depolarization of the input signal. Since most tissues possess high scattering coefficients, maintaining polarization information in a beam passing through a thick piece of tissue (i.e., 1 cm), which includes skin, is not feasible. Even polarized examination in tissue of thicknesses less than 4 mm incur 95% depolarization of the light due to scattering occurring within the tissue. In addition, in these highly scattering surfaces, there are a large amount of proteins and other chiral substances that have a much stronger rotation than that due to glucose making it very difficult to measure the millidegree rotations required for physiological glucose monitoring. Thus, due to the lack of scatter, the aqueous humor (AH) of the eye as a site for detection of *in vivo* glucose concentrations has been suggested as an alternative to transmitting light through skin [24–38]. For polarimetric approaches exploring the eye as a sensing location, the cornea and fluid contained in the anterior chamber (AC), the AH, not only provide a low scattering window into the body, but also a highly specific medium for physiologic glucose monitoring since the AH is virtually devoid of proteins leaving glucose as the primary optically chiral molecule present.

Unlike online processing systems that measure relatively high sugar concentrations (grams) and allow for longer pathlengths (10 cm), the *in vivo* glucose concentration is smaller, and if the eye is to be used as the sensing site, the pathlength in an adult human eye measures between 1 and 1.2 cm with a volume of approximately 250 μL [46]. Advances in polarimetric instrumentation have only recently made it possible to measure the small rotations due to glucose at physiological levels. For example, at a wavelength of 670 nm (red), glucose will rotate the linear polarization of a light beam by approximately 0.4 mdeg per 10 mg/dL for a 1 cm sample pathlength. In order to measure such small rotations, a very sensitive and stable polarimeter must be employed. Throughout the past few decades, many researchers have investigated techniques that are capable in the development of such sensitive devices [26–38]. The primary approaches being investigated today include at a minimum the following components: a light source (typically low powered lasers), a means of modulating the plane of polarization (photoelastic modulator, Faraday rotator, etc...), and a means of detecting and demodulating the signal. Detection and demodulation of the signal is performed typically by using a lock-in amplifier or some means of heterodyne detection.

The eye as a sensing site for polarimetric glucose monitoring, however, is not without its share of problems that need to be overcome, prior to the approach demonstrating a viable monitoring device for diabetes in human subjects. Although the eye is great at coupling light into the body for the purpose of vision, it provides a couple of challenges when it is desired to couple the light into and back out of the AC of the eye, as required for glucose monitoring. In particular, for polarimetric monitoring, the light must travel across the AC of the eye, but due to its curvature and change in the refractive index (RI), the eye naturally tries to focus all the light impinging on it toward the retina. In addition, the cornea is birefringent, meaning it is capable of producing changes in the state of polarization of the light (i.e., somewhat like a quartz crystal). The birefringent change that occurs in the polarized signal due to the corneal surfaces is often time-varying in the presence of eye motion, which can confound the polarization signal due to glucose. Through the use of a lock-in amplifier, the amplitude of the second harmonic or twice the modulation frequency of the signal can be monitored continuously over the course of an experiment. In an ideal situation (i.e., no motion is present) the value observed should be constant represented in the form of a straight line. However, Figure 2.4 shows the spectral components of *in vivo* rabbit data corresponding to the time-varying motion-induced signal. The two dominant components appear at 1.4 and 3.4 Hz, which corresponds to the respiration and cardiac cycles in a rabbit. Therefore, the key issues that need to be addressed for a polarimetric approach to be feasible in monitoring glucose include building an instrument that can accommodate for the large birefringence of the cornea, particularly in the presence of motion artifact, in addition to developing an instrument that can safely and simply couple the light source across the AC of the eye.

Over the past decade, research in polarimetric glucose monitoring has focused primarily on methods toward overcoming motion-induced time-varying corneal birefringence and briefly the coupling of light across the anterior chamber of the eye [29–32,48]. Primarily two techniques have been presented to account for motion artifact, which include the use of a phase-sensitive element to compensate for

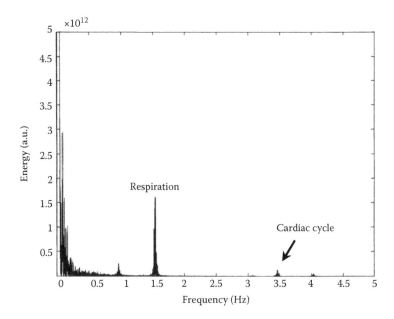

FIGURE 2.4 Frequency analysis indicating the common sources of motion artifact caused by the cardiac (3.4 Hz) and respiratory (1.6 Hz) cycles. (Reproduced from Cameron, B.D., The application of polarized light to biomedical diagnostics and monitoring, in *Biomedical Engineering*, Texas A&M, 2000. With permission.)

the corneal birefringence [49] and/or the use of a dual-wavelength polarimetric system, which, coupled with a multiple linear regression (MLR) signal processing approach, can account for time-varying birefringence [29–31,48]. To couple light through the AC of the eye in the evaluation of these polarized approaches during *in vivo* studies with New Zealand white rabbits, an index-matched coupling device has been used [32,33,37,38,50]. Although index matching to allow coupling of light across the cornea is useful for experimental testing of polarimetric systems in animals and could potentially be done using a scleral lens in humans, solutions for coupling light through the AC (e.g., light incidence at a grazing angle) are also currently being investigated [30,51].

2.4.2 Fluorescence Spectroscopy

Fluorescence spectroscopy is an analytical method that monitors the fluorescence intensity and/or lifetime of a sample to collect information regarding the local environment of the fluorophores. Interaction between the interrogated fluorophores and their immediate environment (neighboring fluorophores, analytes, etc.) can change the optical properties of the fluorophore and be detected as a change in the fluorescence at the macroscale. Fluorescence is an extremely sensitive technique that causes minimal damage to the host system. Glucose, however, is not fluorescent, and there are no known endogenous fluorescent molecules that respond sufficiently to monitor glucose concentrations *in vivo*. Therefore, exogenous reagents have been used to engineer assays that induce a fluorescent response according to the amount of glucose within the sample. These assays implement a recognition (binding) scheme using a certain receptor to make it selective to glucose and transduce that binding event by tracking some change in the local environment with fluorescence. For *in vivo* purposes, these assays can be packaged into deliverable constructs, embedded into the interstitial space, and interrogated using light. For a full review, there are many thorough and detailed discussions on the subject [5,6,22,23,52]. This section is an introduction to the key fluorescence sensing assay strategies that have been engineered to monitor the concentration of glucose *in vivo* according to their recognition scheme.

2.4.2.1 Enzymatic Sensors

2.4.2.1.1 Glucose Oxidase via By-Products

One of the first and most successful optical assays for glucose monitoring has used the enzymatic reaction catalyzed by GOx, as shown in Equation 2.2. Typically synthesized from fermentative production using *Aspergillus niger*, GOx is an enzyme that is highly specific for β-D-glucose, having a very low affinity to other saccharides (including the α-anomer of glucose) [53]. Several groups have used the fluorescence from the enzyme (intrinsic and exogenous) to directly track glucose binding and enzymatic activity [54,55]. However, the primary optical method in which GOx is used for CGM tracks glucose indirectly by monitoring the concentration of the products and reactants of the catalyzed reaction. Assays use fluorescent probes that are sensitive to oxygen, hydrogen peroxide, and/or pH [56,57].

$$\beta\text{-}D\text{-glucose} + O_2 \rightarrow D\text{-glucono-1,5-lactone} + H_2O_2$$
$$D\text{-glucono-1,5-lactone} + H_2O_2 \rightarrow \text{gluconate} + H^+ \tag{2.2}$$

2.4.2.1.2 Oxygen

Many groups have tracked the fluorescence intensity and lifetime of an oxygen-sensitive fluorophore to follow the dynamics of the previously described enzymatic reaction. Given an appropriate concentration of active GOx and molecular oxygen, an increase in the glucose concentration can increase the rate of consumption of the products. This would decrease the concentration of the quencher (oxygen) and increase the fluorescence of the oxygen-sensitive label. Fluorophores such as ruthenium, platinum porphyrin, palladium porphyrin, or decacyclene have been used due to their ability to be dynamically quenched with molecular oxygen and relatively long lifetimes [56,58,59]. A disadvantage of this simple approach is that a decrease in local oxygen content may not be distinguished from a rise in glucose concentration. Li and Walt have attempted to solve this problem by creating a dual-channel sensor with a ruthenium–GOx channel and a second ruthenium-only channel [60]. Thus, the second O_2-sensitive channel can be used to correct for changes in the local oxygen tension. Development of GOx-based optic sensors is currently ongoing, and more elaborate sensors have been described [61,62]. These assays are also being encapsulated into microspheres that can be delivered in the dermal layers of the tissue, and there have been studies done to determine the appropriate diffusion conditions to achieve the required kinetics [63,64].

2.4.2.1.3 Hydrogen Peroxide

Hydrogen peroxide offers an attractive alternative to oxygen levels since the naturally occurring levels in the body are very low. Therefore, monitoring the formation of hydrogen peroxide produced in the enzymatic reaction has a low, steady background *in vivo* [65]. To form a measurable product, GOx is coupled with peroxidase to oxidize the hydrogen peroxide with a nonfluorescent substrate. The addition of glucose causes the enzymatic reaction to proceed, resulting in the substrate being oxidized and increasing its ability to fluoresce [53,66]. However, many of these fluorescent probes are irreversible and useless for continuous monitoring applications [67]. Wu et al. displayed the first example of a functional continuous glucose sensor based on hydrogen peroxide by using europium(III) tetracycline (EuTc) [68]. EuTc is weakly fluorescent until complexed with hydrogen peroxide. In addition, this probe has a decay time on the order of microseconds, enabling the time-resolved measurement of fluorescence [68].

2.4.2.1.4 pH

As the reaction shown in Equation 2.1 progresses forward, the product gluconolactone increases and is converted into gluconic acid. This increase in the gluconic acid concentration decreases the pH of the immediate environment and can be directly monitored by using a pH-sensitive fluorophore [57,69]. In addition, a hydrogel can be synthesized that changes its swelling ratios depending on its pH. Stable, fluorescent dyes can be embedded within the hydrogel network cross-linked to the tip of an optical fiber. The fluorescence collected from excited fluorophores correlates to the swelling of the hydrogel that is induced by the pH of the local environment. Concerns with this approach center around the response time to reach steady-state swelling of the hydrogel [70]. Overall, researchers monitoring glucose concentrations by tracking the local pH changes induced by GOx have struggled to overcome the problems associated with an unknown initial pH and an unknown buffering capacity of the sample [6].

2.4.2.1.5 Hexokinase

Hexokinase catalyzes the phosphorylation reaction shown in Equation 2.2. However, in the absence of ATP, this reaction is nonconsuming and the enzyme can be used as a binding protein similar to those used in affinity sensors [71,72]. Yeast hexokinase is a protein that exists as a dimer; each subunit consists of two lobes with a cleft. The binding of glucose induces a large conformational change where the protein rearranges itself and completely surrounds the glucose molecule. Upon binding, the N-terminal of the protein rotates by 12° relative to the C-terminal domain [73]. This induced conformational change upon binding to glucose has been shown to be tracked via intrinsic fluorescence upon addition of glucose [74,75]. The tryptophan fluorescence intensity has been shown to decrease 30% upon addition of 12 mM glucose [76]. It has also been used with an environmentally sensitive dye that is translated from hydrophobic portions of the protein prior to binding to the hydrophilic environment found at the exterior of the protein [77].

2.4.2.2 Affinity Sensors

Opposed to the consuming nature of enzymatic glucose sensors, affinity sensors provide a receptor (protein or synthetic) that simply binds to the sugar due to its binding affinity for glucose. Affinity sensors may involve a detectable change in the receptor upon glucose binding, or they may employ a competitive binding approach wherein a glucose analog is competitively displaced from the receptor according to the glucose concentration. In either case, such sensors have the distinct feature that their signals are based on an eventual equilibrium at a particular glucose concentration and are unaffected by factors like mass transport and local oxygen tension, which may affect response sensitivity. In addition, affinity-based sensors do not produce reaction by-products like H_2O_2, which may be locally cytotoxic.

2.4.2.2.1 Glucose-Binding Protein

Several researchers have used a protein commonly found in the periplasmic space of the Gram-negative bacteria, *Escherichia coli* (*E. coli*). These glucose-binding proteins (GBPs) are ellipsoidal and possess a single binding site for glucose. Upon binding to the analyte, the protein undergoes a large conformational change in which the glucose is buried within the cleft [78,79]. This change in conformation can be monitored optically by attaching environmentally sensitive fluorophores in locations that would be transferred from a hydrophobic environment to a hydrophilic environment upon binding [80]. This binding event can also be tracked by incorporating Forster resonance energy transfer (FRET) dye pairs that are conjugated to specific sites on each of the two domains [81,82].

The high affinity of native GBP for glucose ($K_d \sim 0.2\ \mu M$) does not allow it to be an effective receptor for CGM systems at physiological levels [80]. However, induced mutations to the protein have decreased its affinity to glucose, and this mutated GBP has been shown to be a functional sensor to physiological concentrations of glucose. The GBP binds to glucose via hydrogen-bonding and the stacking forces by aromatic amino acid residues in the cleft. Fehr et al. introduced a mutation of GBP's phenylalanine-16 into alanine to decrease those stacking forces. This decreased the affinity (increased the dissociation constant) from a K_d of 0.2 μM to 0.6 mM, allowing the system to improve the dynamic range to have an upward limit of 10 mM [83]. Thomas et al. have since engineered a mutated GBP with cysteine mutations for optimal fluorophore attachment that also decreased the affinity further to a K_d of 12 mM [84].

2.4.2.2.2 Boronic Acid

Boronic acids have been used in glucose monitoring due to their ability to rapidly and reversibly form cyclic esters with 1,2-diols and 1,3-diols in aqueous media. They act as weak Lewis bases and react with water to convert from the neutral trigonal form into the anionic tetrahedral form [85]. When a cyclic ester is formed with a diol of a saccharide, the electrophilicity of the boronic acid group intensifies and reduces its pK_a value from ~9 to ~6. In that pH range, the boronic acid receptor is in a trigonal form. Upon addition of saccharides and subsequent binding, the boronic acid converts to the anionic tetrahedral form, changing the fluorescent emission of any conjugated fluorophore [86]. Due to the synthetic nature of the receptor, the selectivity of the sensor is oftentimes the greatest concern. However, for the same reasons, it is more highly resistant to denaturation and would be a good candidate for long-term continuous glucose monitoring in that regard.

The first fluorescent saccharide sensor using boronic acid as the recognition element was reported in 1992 by Yoon and Czarnik. Due to the chelation-enhanced quenching effect, it showed a ~30% quenching effect to the fluorescence intensity upon the addition of fructose, and the receptor appeared to have a much higher affinity for fructose than glucose [87]. A system developed by Shinkai in 1993 implemented a spacer with a tertiary amine between the anthracene fluorophore and the boronic acid to lower the pK_a of the boronic acid and increase the binding strength. When unbound to a saccharide, the lone pair electrons on the nitrogen of the amine quench the fluorescence of the anthracene through photoinduced electron transfer (PET). When the glucose was bound, it eliminated this quenching effect [88]. This fluorophore–spacer–receptor design, shown in Figure 2.5, continues to be used to engineer PET fluorescent modular receptors for glucose and other analytes [89]. In 1994, a receptor was engineered to display a higher binding affinity for glucose when compared to other saccharides by Shinkai's group upon adding a second benzylic amine

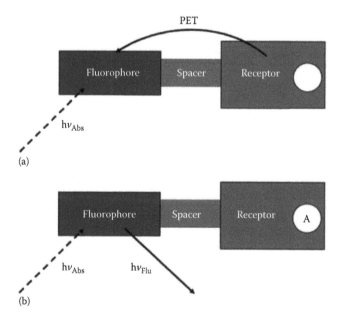

FIGURE 2.5 A schematic representation of a modular PET sensor with a receptor, spacer, and fluorophore. In (a), the excited fluorophore does not emit due to the energy transfer from the free receptor. In (b), the receptor has bound an analyte, preventing energy transfer to the excited fluorophore. This increases the fluorescence intensity of the sample. (From Springsteen, G. and Wang, B., A detailed examination of boronic acid–diol complexation, *Tetrahedron*, 58(26), 5291–5300, 2002. Reproduced by permission of The Royal Society of Chemistry.)

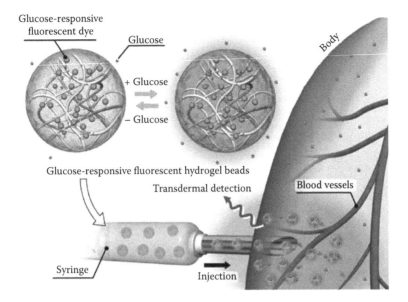

FIGURE 2.6 Schematic representation of implantable glucose-responsive fluorescent microspheres based on a modular boronic acid sensing scheme. (From Shibata, H. et al., Injectable hydrogel microbeads for fluorescence-based *in vivo* continuous glucose monitoring, *Proceedings of the National Academy of Sciences of the United States of America*, 107(42), 17894–17898, 2010. Reproduced by permission of The Proceedings of the National Academy of Sciences of the United States of America.)

group. It has since been determined that a diboronic acid receptor can be used to achieve selectivity for monosaccharides [88,90].

Shibata et al. have recently synthesized injectable hydrogel microbeads based on this recognition scheme, displayed in Figure 2.6. They have generated a glucose-responsive fluorescent monomer using the fluorophore–spacer–receptor design using anthracene, a tertiary amine, and a diboronic acid. They conjugated the monomer to the polyacrylamide hydrogel with flexible linkers in an attempt to immobilize the receptor without significantly decreasing the mobility of the receptor. They show ~400% increase in signal to 1000 mg/dL glucose in vitro [91]. They later implanted hydrogel fibers with the same glucose-responsive monomer and displayed a fluorescent response to glucose concentration changes for up to 140 days [92].

2.4.2.2.3 Concanavalin A

Concanavalin A (Con A) is a glucose-binding lectin that is derived from the jack bean. It is a tetrameric C-type protein at physiological pH (pH 7.4) that has a single binding site for glucose at each monomer. Below pH 5, the protein exists primarily as a dimer. It is possible to alter the protein through succinylation and permanently dimerize the protein at all pH. Con A is not a highly selective receptor, as it binds to fructose, mannose, and sucrose in addition to glucose. However, the typical *in vivo* concentrations of other sugars are low enough as to not interfere with the recognition process of glucose. Unlike the aforementioned affinity-based systems, Con A does not undergo a significant conformational change upon binding. It is instead used as the receptor of a competitive binding system, which is made possible due to its low selectivity for specific saccharides [15,93].

One of the first non–oxygen-based fluorescence assays investigated for glucose monitoring *in vivo* used an indwelling fiber-optic approach. A dialysis membrane was attached to the optical fiber, and competitive binding chemistry was held within. The receptor, Con A, was attached to the inner surface of the membrane and fluorescent dextran was in free solution. In the absence of glucose, the dextran

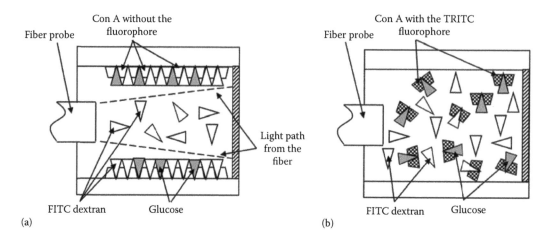

FIGURE 2.7 Characterization of a fiber optic fluorescence assay using (a) a single fluorescent molecule bound to dextran. Note that the light path is critical in this configuration since it is necessary to measure fluorescence only from the free dextran and not from that bound to Con A on the walls of the sensor. (b) A FRET approach that uses two fluorescent molecules (FITC and TRITC), one bound to Con A and the other to dextran. Note that the FITC is quenched when placed in close proximity to the TRITC, as would be the case in the absence of glucose. The beam alignment is no longer critical.

bound to the Con A at the surface of the fiber, decreasing the fluorescence that was collected by the fiber (Figure 2.7a). Upon addition of sufficient levels of glucose, this dextran is displaced from the receptor, and the collected fluorescence increases. Since the approach only used a single fluorophore, the probe was sensitive to alignment and had to be made to insure the beam did not shine on the walls of the membrane [94,95].

Another approach used FRET to transduce the displacement of a similar competitive binding system according to glucose concentrations. This system was now independent of the beam path into the fiber [96,97]. In this case, fluorescein isothiocyanate (FITC) was bound to dextran and tetramethylrhodamine isothiocyanate (TRITC) was bound to Con A (Figure 2.7b). This donor/acceptor FRET pair has a Forster radius of ~50 Å, allowing the competitive binding of Con A to dextran in response to glucose to be tracked by the level of energy transfer. Using this approach, glucose concentrations can be measured by monitoring the intensity of the FITC fluorescence peak. Another potential means of monitoring the change with glucose is based on phase-modulation fluorimetry, which is a technique that measures fluorescent lifetimes [98].

Assays have been synthesized in an attempt to engineer it appropriately for *in vivo* applications by increasing the sensitivity and using fluorophores with excitation/emission profiles that are minimally attenuated in physiological tissue [99,100]. Additional improvements include stabilization of the Con A protein within a polysaccharide matrix and inclusion of longer-wavelength more dyes, which exhibit greatly improved long-term stability [101–103]. An illustration of a prototype of this sensor that was evaluated in human subjects with diabetes [103] is shown in Figure 2.8.

In addition, as an alternative to fiber optic–based sensing, it has been proposed that fully implantable fluorescence-based glucose assays could be used [104–106]. An example of a porated microsphere loaded with competitive binding chemistry based on Con A and its associated response is shown in Figure 2.9. In order for this type of implantable device to be useful, it must be biocompatible, must not exhibit acute reagent consumption or degradation, and must provide a means of communicating the sensor output to the physician or patient. Also, once injected, the implant will not be exposed to blood but will rather be exposed to interstitial fluid. The fluorescent assay itself has the potential problem of limited chemical and photochemical stability over the long term, and fluorophores that are resistant to photobleaching are ideal.

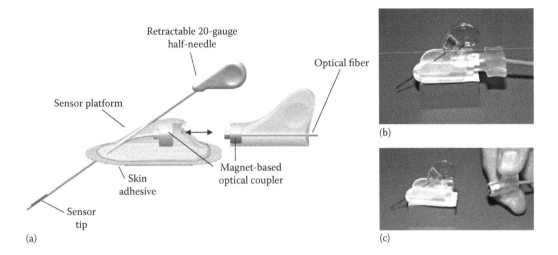

FIGURE 2.8 Illustration of a prototype sensor that has been evaluated in human diabetic subjects. (a) The right figure shows an illustration of a prototype of a sensor that was evaluated in human diabetic subjects. The individual components of the sensor are listed with arrows indicating their position in the overall sensor design. (b) A picture of the actual sensor configured similar to the illustration shown in (a). (c) A picture of the prototype sensor in a different configuration with the optical source fiber being held apart from the rest of the sensor.

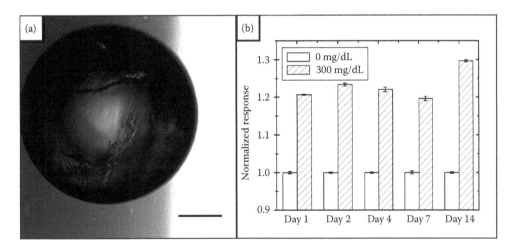

FIGURE 2.9 (a) The right figure shows a hybrid confocal fluorescence/brightfield image of a porated microsphere with competitive binding chemistry based on Con A embedded inside. (b) The fluorescent response to 300 mg/dL glucose consistently increased ~20% over the course of 2 weeks. (Reproduced from Cummins, B.M. et al., *Biomed. Opt. Express*, 2(5), 1243, 2011. With permission.)

2.4.3 Absorption and Scattering Spectroscopy

Infrared (IR) and near-infrared (NIR) absorption spectroscopy techniques have long been mainstays of nondestructive chemometric analysis and are therefore thought to hold great potential for the development of noninvasive blood glucose measurement techniques. The NIR methods are attractive because, in theory, a beam of nonionizing radiation may be directed through an aqueous mixture or solution and the exiting light analyzed to determine the content of glucose or other molecules of interest. In the IR region and more specifically the mid-infrared (MIR) region (from about 5 to 50 μm), the so-called fingerprint spectrum can be found. Absorption bands in this region are due to fundamental resonances of specific functional groups and bonds contained within the molecule, and they tend to be rather sharp. The fingerprint spectrum, therefore, offers highly specific information about the molecular makeup of the compound or mixture under study. In contrast, absorption bands in the NIR are composed of complex overtone or combination bands and tend to be broad, overlapping, and much less specific. Figure 2.10a and b shows, respectively, portions of the MIR and NIR absorption spectra for glucose.

Despite the specificity offered by IR absorption spectroscopy, its application to quantitative blood glucose measurement is limited. A strong background absorption by water and other components including blood and tissue severely limits the pathlength that may be used for transmission spectroscopy to roughly 100 μm or less. Further, the magnitude of the absorption peaks themselves and

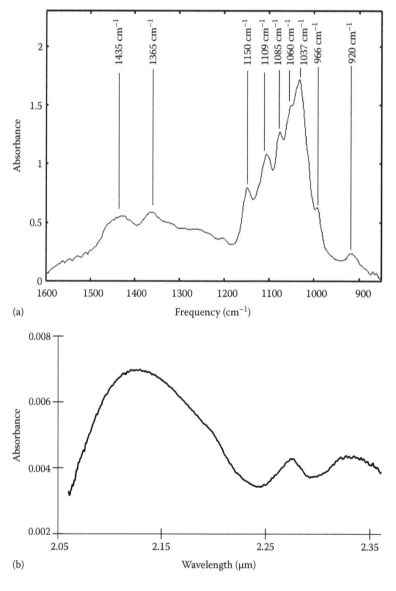

FIGURE 2.10 Optical absorption spectra for glucose. (a) MIR region extending from 1600 to 900 cm⁻¹ or 6.25 to 11 μm and showing absorption peak assignments. (b) NIR region extending from 2.0 to 2.5 μm or 5000 to 4000 cm⁻¹. Note that the magnitude of the three absorbance peaks in the NIR region is much smaller.

the dynamic range required to record them makes quantitation based on these sharp peaks difficult. Nonetheless, attempts have been made to quantify blood glucose using IR absorption spectroscopy both in vitro and *in vivo* [107–111].

2.4.3.1 NIR Absorption and Scattering

In contrast to the IR and MIR spectrum, the NIR spectrum passes relatively easily through water and body tissues allowing moderate pathlengths in the millimeter to centimeter range to be used for measurements. The NIR region of the optical spectrum extends from 700 to 2500 nm (0.7 to 2.5 µm) and can be used for quantitative measurement of organic functional groups, especially C—H, O—H, N—H, and C=O. Absorption bands in the NIR are composed primarily of overtone and combination bands of stretching and vibrational modes of organic molecules. These bands tend to be rather broad and overlap considerably; thus, the NIR region is not particularly well suited for qualitative analysis.

Both NIR transmission spectroscopy and diffuse reflectance spectroscopy have been investigated for online glucose monitoring and process control [14,112–125]. NIR spectroscopy has been developed extensively in the agricultural and food industries for more than thirty years. Although challenging for use in qualitative analysis, an advancement that has enabled NIRS as an analytical tool has been the development of sophisticated multivariate data analysis or chemometric techniques for quantitative analysis. The use of NIR spectroscopy for glucose monitoring in industrial and agricultural applications has been well described in several other sources [12,126–128]. NIR spectroscopy has also been applied to online measurement of glucose concentration in bioreactors and cell cultures. These applications represent a more challenging application of NIR glucose measurement since the media involved are more complex and the analyte concentrations involved are significantly lower than those found in current industrial applications. Specifically, cell culture applications require careful maintenance of a number of factors including pH, temperature, and more importantly, glucose concentration. The automated control of glucose concentration via online continuous monitoring could result in improved culture productivity and efficiency, but optical NIR measurement of glucose is further complicated by the complex nature of cell culture media itself, which contain proteins, amino acids, salts, and other small carbohydrates and nutrients including glucose. A typical NIR spectrum of GTSF-2 cell culture medium in the 2–2.5 µm range with respect to an air background is shown in Figure 2.11. When one compares this to the NIR spectrum for aqueous glucose

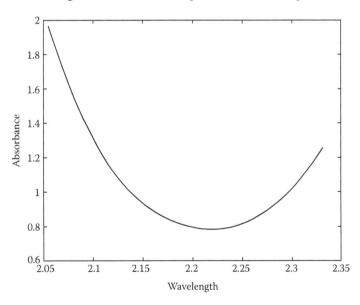

FIGURE 2.11 NIR absorbance spectrum of cell culture media with air as the background. Note that absorption amplitude is orders of magnitude larger than the glucose absorption shown in Figure 2.10b.

at a concentration of 500 mg/dL (27.5 mM), with the background removed (shown in Figure 2.10b), it is important to note the magnitude of the absorbance units on the *y*-axis. Specifically, the absorbance by water and proteins is at least three orders of magnitude greater than that of glucose. Thus, the stability and signal-to-noise ratio of a NIR instrument must be very good if it is to be used to distinguish changes in the glucose concentration. Further, the temperature of the sample must also be very tightly controlled since, with even a slight change in temperature, the absorbance of the background water spectrum will shift, severely impacting measurement of the glucose signal. Figure 2.12 demonstrates the effect of varying temperature on the NIR spectrum of cell culture medium. Techniques such as digital filtering combined with high-order multivariate statistics have been used to compensate for and model such variations.

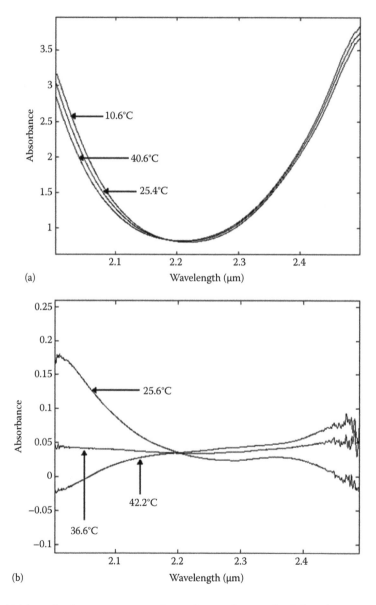

FIGURE 2.12 (a) Water absorbance spectrum, referenced to air, showing the shift in the water peaks with temperature. (b) Glucose (500 mg/dL) absorbance spectrum taken at different temperatures, referenced to a water background taken at one temperature showing the baseline water peak shifts.

Additionally, cell culture applications typically exhibit well-controlled temperature and are amenable to inclusion of a fixed pathlength for optical measurements making online NIR glucose monitoring in cell culture promising. Detailed discussion of specific NIR spectroscopic studies of glucose measurement in cell culture media may be found in the referenced literature [116,125,128].

Though all optical glucose-monitoring methodologies require the use of a prediction model relating optical measurements to glucose concentration, the broad overlapping peaks and complicated nature of multicomponent NIR spectra make single- or dual-wavelength models inadequate. As with cell culture, NIR absorption bands for *in vivo* glucose detection may be significantly influenced by factors such as temperature, pH, the degree of hydrogen bonding present, and the unknown influence of background spectra. The changes in pressure and different glucose-containing compartments in the body (interstitial, blood, and intercellular) further complicate the problem. For this reason, research toward quantitative NIR spectroscopy for *in vivo* glucose monitoring has long relied on the development of very high-order multivariate prediction models and empirical calibration techniques. A brief analysis of the signal variation due to glucose in a typical sample should serve to illustrate the problem at hand.

The physiological range of glucose values seen in the normal human body may range from 80 to 120 mg/dL and should ideally remain around 100 mg/dL (5.5 mM). In people suffering from diabetes, blood sugar may rise as high as 500 mg/dL. The generally accepted figure of merit for required sensitivity of a useful glucose meter is 10 mg/dL (0.55 mM). For the most identifiable NIR glucose peak at approximately 2.27 μm, molar absorptivity is roughly 0.23 M^{-1} cm^{-1}. That of water at the same wavelength is 0.41 M^{-1} cm^{-1}, and the concentration of the water in typical body tissues is approximately 39 M. Consider a transmission measurement made through 1 mm of body tissue. The background absorbance due to water will be about 1.6 and that due to glucose will be about 1.26×10^{-4}. To meet the accuracy requirement, we must further be able to discern an absorbance change of about 1.26×10^{-5} on a background of 1.6, and it is evident that even a change in tissue hydration of 1/1000th of a percent would result in a larger signal change than would a 10 mg/dL change in glucose concentration. For this reason, high-order multivariate models that incorporate analysis of entire spectra must be used to extract NIR glucose information. A number of excellent and authoritative sources on such methods are available [127,129–131], and these methods will not be discussed here other than to introduce some of the terminology associated with their formulation, use, and practice.

Multivariate calibration techniques focus on finding a response matrix, which is suitable to describe spectral observations obtained when analyzing a solution containing particular concentrations of a number of analytes. Once this response matrix has been found, it may then be inverted in order to relate analyte concentrations to observed spectral readings. The most direct method is the classical least squares method in which spectral observations are made of a number of samples with known analyte concentrations. The problem can be written mathematically as $\mathbf{A} = \mathbf{KC}$ where $\mathbf{A}$ is the matrix containing spectral observations for each sample, $\mathbf{K}$ is the response matrix, and $\mathbf{C}$ is the concentration matrix containing analyte concentrations for each known sample. In the classical least squares solution, $\mathbf{K}$ is computed from $\mathbf{A}$ and $\mathbf{C}$ as $\mathbf{K} = \mathbf{AC}^{\mathrm{T}}(\mathbf{CC}^{\mathrm{T}})^{-1}$, and estimates of the concentration of analytes in subsequent samples may be determined from the spectral observations $\mathbf{a}$ as $\mathbf{c} = (\mathbf{K}^{\mathrm{T}}\mathbf{K})^{-1}\mathbf{K}^{\mathrm{T}}\mathbf{a}$. This approach assumes that all measurement errors occur in the spectral observations and that the concentration matrix $\mathbf{C}$ is known exactly. This is often not the case, and alternate formulations for the least squares calibration model solution have been proposed including inverse least squares and partial least squares (PLS). The latter has become overwhelmingly popular due to its robust ability to model complex data interactions and to formulate powerful prediction models. The PLS technique employs an iterative singular value decomposition of the $\mathbf{A}$ matrix to extricate spectral changes most strongly correlated to analyte concentration changes and thereby creates a number of model *factors* that may be linear combinations of many of the observations in $\mathbf{A}$. In the practical application of PLS, data observations are typically split into two groups, one of which is used for formulation of the model (calibration) and the other which is used for validation of the model (prediction). Two common statistics are the standard error of calibration (SEC), which is the root mean square (RMS) prediction error of the model compared to the calibration data set, and standard error of prediction (SEP), which is the RMS prediction error of the model when applied to the validation set. A problem that can arise in PLS modeling is *overfitting* of the data in which noise or spurious trends evident in the calibration data may actually be factored into the model if chance correlation to analyte concentrations exists. The separation of calibration and validation data sets is one technique which is used to detect potential overfitting.

For the purposes of discussion of the literature, it is useful to break the NIR region into the very NIR region (from 700 to 1300 nm) and the NIR region (from 2.0 to 5.0 μm). The attraction to the very NIR region is that optical detectors and sources in this region are particularly easy to come by, transmission through tissue is rather good, and transmissive fiber optics may be employed to facilitate probe design. However, glucose absorption bands are particularly weak in this region, and it is maybe difficult to acquire signals with substantial signal to noise to allow robust measurement. Examples of very NIR studies of glucose determination include [15,18,132–134].

Longer in the NIR spectrum, a relative dip in the water absorbance spectrum opens a unique window in the 2.0–2.5 μm wavelength region. This window, saddled between two large water absorbance peaks, allows pathlengths or penetration depths on the order of millimeters and contains specific glucose peaks at 2.13, 2.27, and 2.34 μm. So far, this region has offered the most promising results for quantifiable glucose measurement using NIR spectroscopy. The instrumentation required for spectral measurements in this region is somewhat more expensive. Typically, FTIR spectrometers with InSb, HgCdTe, or extended InGaAs are required to obtain spectra with sufficient signal to noise. A further challenge is that fiber optic materials appropriate for this spectral region are not as readily available. Chalcogenide fibers have typically high refractive indices leading to large Fresnel losses during coupling. They also exhibit sharp bands in transmission, which may be bend dependent. Very low-OH glass fibers provide partial transmission out to about 2.3 μm but fall off very rapidly in this region. Sapphire fibers are transmissive in this region and offer promise; however, they are quite expensive and typically more brittle and less flexible than glass fibers. Investigations of glucose determination using this spectral region include [135–138].

In addition to the NIR absorption, in the very near infrared, the scatter and the RI of a material can be used to determine sugar concentrations in syrups, honey, molasses, tomato products, and jams for which the glucose concentration is very high. The RI of a solution of carbohydrate such as glucose increases with increasing concentration and so can be used to measure the amount of carbohydrate present. The RI of a liquid can easily be determined by optically measuring the angle of refraction at a boundary between the liquid and a solid of known RI. The RI is also temperature and wavelength dependent and so measurements are usually made at a specific temperature (20°C) and wavelength (589.3 nm). This method is quick and simple to carry out and can be performed with simple handheld instruments.

Since the change in RI is also directly related to a change in the elastic scatter of a molecule, the measurement of light scatter in the NIR region has been investigated for potentially quantifying glucose noninvasively both in vitro and *in vivo* [139–142]. This is much more challenging than for the agricultural measurement because *in vivo* blood glucose, as opposed to in vitro sugars such as that found in syrup, has very small concentrations. In addition, the specificity is potentially problematic since other physiologic effects, unrelated to glucose concentration, could produce similar variations of the reduced scattering coefficient with time. The measurement precision of the reduced scattering coefficient and separation of scatter and absorption changes is another potential problem with this approach. Tissue scattering is caused by a variety of substances and organelles (membranes, mitochondria, nucleus, etc...), and all of them have different refractive indices; thus, this approach also needs to take into account the different refractive indices of tissue. Lastly, there is a need to account for factors that might change the reduced scattering coefficient such as variations in temperature, red-blood-cell concentration, electrolyte levels, and movements of extracellular and intracellular water.

2.4.3.2 Raman Spectroscopy

In addition to NIR absorption and elastic scatter, the optical method known as Raman spectroscopy is an inelastic scattering technique that has been investigated as a method for potentially rapid, precise,

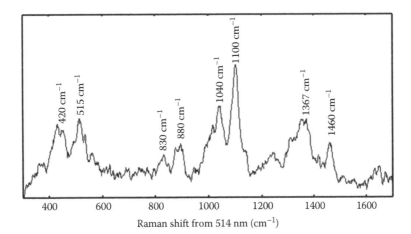

FIGURE 2.13 Baseline-corrected Raman spectra of glucose showing the narrow peaks that can be obtained when compared with the NIR spectra of Figure 2.10b.

and accurate analysis of glucose concentration and biochemical composition [143]. Raman spectroscopy provides information about the inelastic scattering that occurs when vibrational or rotational energy is exchanged with incident probe radiation. When monochromatic radiation is incident upon Raman-active media, most of the incident light of frequency v_o is elastically scattered at the same frequency (Rayleigh scattering), but a very small portion of the light undergoes Raman scattering and exhibits frequency shifts of $\pm v_m$, which are associated with transitions between the rotational and vibrational levels [144,145]. Energy decreases ($v_o - v_m$) are referred to as Stokes shifts, and energy increases ($v_o + v_m$) are referred to as anti-Stokes shifts. Since Stokes shifts are much more prevalent, most studies utilize the Stokes type of scattering bands. Therefore, the Raman bands of interest are shifted to longer wavelengths relative to the excitation wavelength. As with IR spectroscopic techniques, Raman spectra can be utilized to identify molecules such as glucose since these spectra are characteristic of variations in the molecular polarizability and dipole moments. However, in contrast to IR and NIR spectroscopy, Raman spectroscopy has a spectral signature that is less influenced by water. In addition, as shown in Figure 2.13, Raman spectral bands are considerably narrower than those produced in NIR spectral experiments. Raman also has the ability to permit the simultaneous estimation of multiple analytes, requires minimum sample preparation, and would allow for direct sample analysis (i.e., would be online), and since different bonds scatter different wavelengths of EM radiation, this method gives quantitative information about the total biochemical composition of a sample, without its destruction.

The fundamental instrumentation required to produce a Raman spectrum includes a monochromatic light source such as a laser, a wavelength separation system such as a dispersive monochromator or nondispersive Fourier transform (FT) spectrometer, and a detection system such as a charge-coupled device (CCD) array for the dispersive case or point detector for the FT Raman case. In either system, it is very important to eliminate the elastically scattered light, which is roughly 10^5 times greater in intensity and occurs at the same wavelength. Many typical optical filters are not adequate to remove enough of this elastically scattered light, and therefore holographic notch filters or very sharp high-pass filters are typically required. One application of dispersive Raman spectroscopy is the noninvasive, online determination of the biotransformation by yeast of glucose to ethanol [146]. Using a diode-laser exciting at 780 nm and a CCD detector along with PLS multivariate analysis, both glucose and ethanol could be measured to within 5%.

Although these early attempts to employ Raman techniques to directly measure glucose concentration online and in aqueous solutions, serum, and plasma have been met with some success in vitro [147–151], efforts to utilize these techniques *in vivo* for transcutaneous measurement of whole blood glucose levels have met with considerable difficulty [151,152]. This is partly because whole blood and most tissue are highly absorptive. In addition, most tissues contain many fluorescent and Raman-active confounders [152]. As a surrogate to blood glucose measurement, several investigators have suggested using Raman spectroscopy to obtain the glucose signal from the aqueous humor of the eye [152–154]. The glucose content of the aqueous humor reflects an age-dependent steady-state value of approximately 70% of that found in blood, and the time lag between aqueous humor and blood glucose has been shown to be on the order of minutes. For Raman sensing, the aqueous humor of the eye is relatively nonabsorptive and contains much fewer Raman-active molecules than whole blood. However, even though only four or five Raman-active constituents are present in significant concentrations in the AH, it is still necessary to use both linear and nonlinear multifactor analytical techniques to obtain accurate estimates of glucose concentrations from the total Raman spectrum [152]. In addition, as with other tissues, when excited in the NIR region (700–1300 nm), Raman spectra encounter less fluorescence background. However, although the background fluorescence falls off when excitation is moved to the NIR region, the Raman signal also falls off to the fourth power with wavelength. Thus, unlike the polarization approach through the eye, Raman requires higher power and it remains to be seen if it could be measured at laser intensities that can be used safely in the eye. Due to the power required and the associated safety concerns related to the use of Raman for glucose monitoring in the eye, this technique has been extended to alternative sensing locations. Because of the low signal to noise associated with traditional Raman techniques *in vivo*, multivariate analyses have been employed that are similar to those used in glucose-related NIR spectroscopic approaches [19,155,156].

Alternatively, the Raman spectra acquired for a sample can be greatly enhanced (by some 10^6–10^8-fold) if the molecules of interest are sufficiently close to a suitably roughened metal surface (i.e., Cu, Ag, or Au) [157]. This method, called surface-enhanced Raman scattering (SERS) [158,159], has received much attention within biomedicine [159] and genomics [160]. Since the development of reproducible SERS on a silver-coated alumina substrate by Vo-Dinh [161], this technology has emerged as a very powerful biochemical detection method. It is noteworthy as well that the fluorescence background typically observed in many online samples using dispersive Raman may potentially be reduced by using SERS. Recently, an approach utilizing surface-enhanced spatially offset Raman spectroscopy (SESORS) was used for *in vivo* monitoring of glucose in rats as shown in Figure 2.14 [20,21]. Spatially

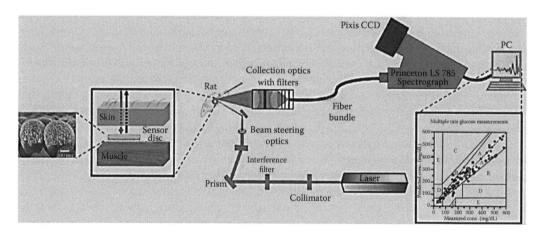

FIGURE 2.14 Optical setup illustrating the design of a surface-enhanced spatially offset Raman spectroscopy (SESORS) system used for transcutaneous glucose sensing *in vivo* in rats. Image on the far left represents an image of the coated surface for glucose detection and on the far right at the bottom of the figure is a result of the predicted versus actual glucose concentration in multiple rats for greater than 17 days plotted on a Clarke error grid. (Reprinted with permission from Ma, K. et al., *In vivo*, transcutaneous glucose sensing using surface-enhanced spatially offset Raman spectroscopy: Multiple rats, improved hypoglycemic accuracy, low incident power, and continuous monitoring for greater than 17 days, *Anal. Chem.*, 83(23), 2011, 9146–9152. Copyright 2011 American Chemical Society.)

offset Raman spectroscopy (SORS) is used to increase the sensing depth of SERS techniques for *in vivo* applications [162,163]. This work used silica nanoparticles covered with a silver film, termed silver or Ag film over nanoparticles (AgFONs), which have displayed enhancement factors of up to 10^7 [6]. These films were then functionalized with a self-assembled monolayer to increase the number of glucose molecules probed, allowing CGM *in vivo* up to 17 days without the need for multiple calibrations [20,21].

2.4.4 Other Optical Glucose Diagnostic Approaches

2.4.4.1 Photoacoustic Spectroscopy

Photoacoustic spectroscopy (PAS) can be used to noninvasively acquire absorption spectra from samples including biological ones. The photoacoustic signal is obtained by probing the sample with a monochromatic radiation that is modulated or pulsed. Absorption of probe radiation by the sample results in localized short-duration heating. Thermal expansion then gives rise to a pressure wave, which can be detected with a suitable transducer. An absorption spectrum for the sample can be obtained by recording the amplitude of generated pressure waves as a function of probe beam wavelength. Because high signal-to-noise measurements require reasonable penetration of the sample by the probe radiation, the NIR region holds the same attraction in PAS techniques as described above for more conventional NIR spectroscopy approaches. A purported advantage of PAS, however, is that the signal recorded is a direct result of absorption alone with the absence of scatter or dispersion producing change in the acquired signal.

PAS techniques using the NIR region face many of the same challenges attendant to other NIR spectroscopic methods, namely, that complicated and empirical calibration models must be created in order to account for the broad overlapping spectral bands associated with the NIR spectrum, temperature changes, pressure changes, and varied glucose compartments. Further, the technique requires expensive instrumentation and the measurements are particularly sensitive to variables including temperature, transducer pressure, and sample morphology. Some examples of PAS techniques applied to glucose monitoring include [164–169].

2.4.4.2 Optical Coherence Tomography

OCT provides a means for measuring the optical properties of turbid media including scatter and RI. OCT is an optical ranging technique in which a very short coherence length source is coupled to an interferometer with a sample in one arm and a reference reflector in the other. As the reference reflector is scanned, depth-resolved interference fringes are produced with amplitude dependent on the amplitude of backscattered radiation. Since the scattering coefficient of tissue is dependent on the bulk index of refraction, an increase in RI and a decrease in scatter can be detected as a change in the slope of falloff of the depth-resolved OCT amplitude. As the glucose concentration present in interstitial fluid rises, a change in the RI occurs. Using OCT, the delay in backscattered light is compared to light that is reflected by the reference arm. Like similar scatter and RI approaches described previously in this chapter, it has yet to be shown that OCT can overcome specificity and other limitations when applied *in vivo*. In addition, OCT techniques also suffer from large signal fluctuations due to motion artifact along with other environmental and physiological conditions [3,39]. Several groups have explored the use of OCT based systems for measurement of glucose *in vivo* [6,39–41,170–176]. To enhance specificity, an additional variation on OCT-based glucose monitoring has also been proposed in which the bulk RI and scattering change of a suspension of small polysaccharide beads and cross-linked dextran molecules were mediated by the competitive binding of both glucose and dextran to Con A (see Section 2.4.2.2) bound to the beads. Encapsulated within a dialysis membrane, this sensor displayed varying optical turbidity with glucose that was discernible by OCT [177].

References

1. The Diabetes Control and Complications Trial Research Group, The effect of intensive treatment of diabetes on the development and progression of long-term complications in insulin-dependent diabetes mellitus. *The New England Journal of Medicine*, 1993. 329(14): 977–986.
2. McNichols, R.J. and G.L. Cote, Optical glucose sensing in biological fluids: An overview. *Journal of Biomedical Optics*, 2000. 5(1): 5–16.
3. Tura, A., A. Maran, and G. Pacini, Non-invasive glucose monitoring: Assessment of technologies and devices according to quantitative criteria. *Diabetes Research and Clinical Practice*, 2007. 77(1): 16–40.
4. Oliver, N.S. et al., Glucose sensors: A review of current and emerging technology. *Diabetic Medicine*, 2009. 26(3): 197–210.
5. Tuchin, V.V., ed., *Handbook of Optical Glucose in Biological Fluids and Tissues*. 2009, Boca Raton, FL: Taylor & Francis Group.
6. Cunningham, D.D. and J.A. Stenken, eds., *In Vivo Glucose Sensing*. 2010, Hoboken, NJ: John Wiley & Sons.
7. Papaspyros, N.S., *The History of Diabetes Mellitus*, 2nd edn. 1964, Stuttgart, Germany: Georg Thieme Verlag.
8. Bilous, R. and R. Donnelly, *Handbook of Diabetes*, 4th edn. 2010, Chichester, U.K.: John Wiley & Sons.
9. Morgan, W., *Diabetes Mellitus: Its History, Chemistry, Anatomy, Pathology, Physiology, and Treatment*, 1st edn. 1877, London, U.K.: The Homeopathic Publishing Company.
10. Smith, J.L., *The Pursuit of Noninvasive Glucose: "Hunting the Deceitful Turkey"*, 2nd edn. 2011.
11. Phillips, R., G. McGarraugh, F.A. Jurik, and R.D. Underwood, U.S. patent 5,563,042, Whole blood glucose test strip. October 8, 1996.
12. Osbourne, B.G. and T. Fearn, *Near Infrared Spectroscopy in Food Analysis*. 1986, Harlow, Essex, England: Longman Scientific and Technical.
13. Nathan, D.M. et al., Intensive diabetes treatment and cardiovascular disease in patients with type 1 diabetes. *New England Journal of Medicine*, 2005. 353(25): 2643–2653.
14. Suzuki, Y. et al., Preliminary evaluation of optical glucose sensing in red cell concentrations using near-infrared diffuse-reflectance spectroscopy. *Journal of Biomedical Optics*, 2012. 17(1): 017004–017008.
15. Huang, Z.-H. et al., *Noninvasive Blood Glucose Sensing on Human Body with Near-Infrared Reflection Spectroscopy*. 2011, Beijing, China: SPIE.
16. Burmeister, J.J., M.A. Arnold, and G.W. Small, Noninvasive blood glucose measurements by near-infrared transmission spectroscopy across human tongues. *Diabetes Technology & Therapeutics*, 2000. 2(1): 5–16.
17. Marquardt, L.A., M.A. Arnold, and G.W. Small, Near-infrared spectroscopic measurement of glucose in a protein matrix. *Analytical Chemistry*, 1993. 65: 3279–3289.
18. Robinson, M.R. et al., Noninvasive glucose monitoring in diabetic patients: A preliminary evaluation. *Clinical Chemistry*, 1992. 38(9): 1618–1622.
19. Dingari, N.C. et al., Investigation of the specificity of Raman spectroscopy in non-invasive blood glucose measurements. *Analytical and Bioanalytical Chemistry*, 2011. 400(9): 2871–2880.
20. Ma, K. et al., In vivo, transcutaneous glucose sensing using surface-enhanced spatially offset raman spectroscopy: Multiple rats, improved hypoglycemic accuracy, low incident power, and continuous monitoring for greater than 17 days. *Analytical Chemistry*, 2011. 83(23): 9146–9152.
21. Yuen, J.M. et al., Transcutaneous glucose sensing by surface-enhanced spatially offset Raman spectroscopy in a rat model. *Analytical Chemistry*, 2010. 82(20): 8382–8385.
22. Pickup, J.C. et al., Fluorescence-based glucose sensors. *Biosensors and Bioelectronics*, 2005. 20(12): 2555–2565.
23. Moschou, E.A. et al., Fluorescence glucose detection: Advances toward the ideal in vivo biosensor. *Journal of Fluorescence*, 2004. 14(5): 535–547.

24. March, W.F., B. Rabinovitch, and R.L. Adams, Noninvasive glucose monitoring of the aqueous humor of the eye: Part II. Animal studies and the scleral lens. *Diabetes Care*, 1982. 5(3): 259–265.

25. Rabinovitch, B., W.F. March, and R.L. Adams, Noninvasive glucose monitoring of the aqueous humor of the eye: Part I. Measurement of very small optical rotations. *Diabetes Care*, 1982. 5(3): 254–258.

26. Cameron, B.D. et al., The use of polarized laser light through the eye for noninvasive glucose monitoring. *Diabetes Technology & Therapeutics*, 1999. 1(2): 135–143.

27. King, T.W. et al., Multispectral polarimetric glucose detection using a single Pockels cell. *Optical Engineering*, 1994. 33(8): 2746–1753.

28. Knighton, R.W., X.R. Huang, and L.A. Cavuoto, Corneal birefringence mapped by scanning laser polarimetry. *Optics Express*, 2008. 16(18): 13738–13751.

29. Malik, B.H. and G.L. Coté, Real-time, closed-loop dual-wavelength optical polarimetry for glucose monitoring. *Journal of Biomedical Optics*, 2010. 15(1): 017002.

30. Pirnstill, C.W. and G.L. Coté, Modeling the Optical Coupling across the Anterior Chamber of the Eye towards Polarimetric Glucose Sensing. *In SPIE Photonics West BIOS*, 2014, San Francisco, CA: SPIE.

31. Malik, B.H., C.W. Pirnstill, and G.L. Coté, Dual wavelength polarimetric glucose sensing in the presence of birefringence and motion artifact using anterior chamber of the eye phantoms. *Journal of Biomedical Optics*, 2013. 18(1): 017007–017007.

32. Purvinis, G., B.D. Cameron, and D.M. Altrogge, Noninvasive polarimetric-based glucose monitoring: An in vivo study. *Journal of Diabetes Science and Technology*, 2011. 5(2): 380–387.

33. Pirnstill, C.W., B.H. Malik, V.C. Gresham, and G.L. Coté, *In vivo* glucose monitoring using dual-wavelength polarimetry to overcome corneal birefringence in the presence of motion. *Diabetes Technology & Therapeutics*, 2012. 14(9): 819–827.

34. Cote, G.L., M.D. Fox, and R.B. Northrop, Noninvasive optical polarimetric glucose sensing using a true phase measurement technique. *IEEE Transactions on Biomedical Engineering*, 1992. 39(7): 752–756.

35. Cameron, B.D. and G.L. Cote, Noninvasive glucose sensing utilizing a digital closed-loop polarimetric approach. *IEEE Transactions on Biomedical Engineering*, 1997. 44(12): 1221–1227.

36. Chou, C. et al., Noninvasive glucose monitoring in vivo with an optical heterodyne polarimeter. *Applied Optics*, 1998. 37(16): 3553–3557.

37. Cameron, B.D., J.S. Baba, and G.L. Coté, Measurement of the glucose transport time delay between the blood and aqueous humor of the eye for the eventual development of a noninvasive glucose sensor. *Diabetes Technology & Therapeutics*, 2001. 3(2): 201–207.

38. Webb, A.J. and B.D. Cameron, *The Use of Optical Polarimetry as a Noninvasive In Vivo Physiological Glucose Monitor*. 2011, San Francisco, CA: SPIE.

39. Sudheendran, N. et al., Assessment of tissue optical clearing as a function of glucose concentration using optical coherence tomography. *Journal of Innovative Optical Health Sciences*, 2010. 3(3): 169–176.

40. Larin, K. et al., Potential application of optical coherence tomography for non-invasive monitoring of glucose concentration. *Proceedings of SPIE*, 2001. 4263: 83–90.

41. Larin, K.V. et al., Noninvasive blood glucose monitoring with optical coherence tomography. *Diabetes Care*, 2002. 25(12): 2263–2267.

42. Weiss, R. et al., Noninvasive continuous glucose monitoring using photoacoustic technology—Results from the first 62 subjects. *Diabetes Technology & Therapeutics*, 2007. 9(1): 68–74.

43. Zeng, L. et al., Design of a portable noninvasive photoacoustic glucose monitoring system integrated laser diode excitation with annular array detection. *Proceedings of SPIE, Seventh International Conference on Photonics and Imaging in Biology and Medicine*, 2009. 7280: 72802F-1–72802F-8.

44. Analytical, R.R., Polarimetry definitions [Web page]. Available from: http://www.rudolphresearch.com/polarimetry.htm, cited April 2, 2012.

45. Browne, C.A. and F.W. Zerban, *Physical and Chemical Methods of Sugar Analysis*, 3rd edn. 1941, New York: John Wiley & Sons.

46. Krachmer, J.H., M.J. Mannis, and E.J. Holland, eds., *Fundamentals, Diagnosis, and Management*, 3rd edn. *Cornea*, Vol. 1. 2011, Philadelphia, PA: Mosby Elsevier.

47. Cameron, B.D., The application of polarized light to biomedical diagnostics and monitoring. Dissertation, 2000, College Station, TX: Texas A&M University.

48. Malik, B.H. and G.L. Coté, Modeling the corneal birefringence of the eye toward the development of a polarimetric glucose sensor. *Journal of Biomedical Optics*, 2010. 15(3): 037012.

49. Cameron, B.D. and H. Anumula, Development of a real-time corneal birefringence compensated glucose sensing polarimeter. *Diabetes Technology & Therapeutics*, 2006. 8(2): 156–164.

50. Baba, J.S. et al., Effect of temperature, pH, and corneal birefringence on polarimetric glucose monitoring in the eye. *Journal of Biomedical Optics*, 2002. 7(3): 321.

51. Malik, B.H. and G.L. Coté, Characterizing dual wavelength polarimetry through the eye for monitoring glucose. *Biomedical Optics Express*, 2010. 1(5): 1247–1258.

52. Steiner, M.S., A. Duerkop, and O.S. Wolfbeis, Optical methods for sensing glucose. *Chemical Society Reviews*, 2011. 40(9): 4805–4839.

53. Bankar, S.B. et al., Glucose oxidase—An overview. *Biotechnology Advances*, 2009. 27(4): 489–501.

54. Sanz, V. et al., Fluorometric sensors based on chemically modified enzymes glucose determination in drinks. *Talanta*, 2003. 60(2–3): 415–423.

55. Sierra, J.F., J. Galbán, and J.R. Castillo, Determination of glucose in blood based on the intrinsic fluorescence of glucose oxidase. *Analytical Chemistry*, 1997. 69(8): 1471–1476.

56. Dremel, B.A.A., S.Y. Li, and R.D. Schmid, On-line determination of glucose and lactate concentrations in animal cell culture based on fibre optic detection of oxygen in flow-injection analysis. *Biosensors and Bioelectronics*, 1992. 7(2): 133–139.

57. Ertekin, K. et al., Glucose sensing employing fluorescent pH indicator: 4-[(*p-N,N*-dimethylamino) benzylidene]-2-phenyloxazole-5-one. *Dyes and Pigments*, 2005. 67(2): 133–138.

58. Papkovsky, D.B., Luminescent porphyrins as probes for optical (bio)sensors. *Sensors and Actuators B: Chemical*, 1993. 11(1–3): 293–300.

59. Rosenzweig, Z. and R. Kopelman, Analytical properties and sensor size effects of a micrometer-sized optical fiber glucose biosensor. *Analytical Chemistry*, 1996. 68(8): 1408–1413.

60. Li, L. and D.R. Walt, Dual-analyte fiber-optic sensor for the simultaneous and continuous measurement of glucose and oxygen. *Analytical Chemistry*, 1995. 67(20): 3746–3752.

61. Gunasilgham, H., C.H. Tan, and J.K.L. Seow, Fiber-optic glucose sensor with electrochemical generation of indicator reagent. *Analytical Chemistry*, 1990. 62(7): 755–759.

62. Abdel-Latif, M.S. and G.G. Guilbault, Fiber-optic sensor for the determination of glucose using micellar enhanced chemiluminescence of the peroxyoxalate reaction. *Analytical Chemistry*, 1988. 60(24): 2671–2674.

63. Brown, J.Q. and M.J. McShane, Modeling of spherical fluorescent glucose microsensor systems: Design of enzymatic smart tattoos. *Biosensors and Bioelectronics*, 2006. 21(9): 1760–1769.

64. Brown, J.Q., R. Srivastava, and M.J. McShane, Encapsulation of glucose oxidase and an oxygen-quenched fluorophore in polyelectrolyte-coated calcium alginate microspheres as optical glucose sensor systems. *Biosensors and Bioelectronics*, 2005. 21(1): 212–216.

65. Wolfbeis, O.S. et al., A europium-ion-based luminescent sensing probe for hydrogen peroxide. *Angewandte Chemie—International Edition*, 2002. 41(23): 4495–4498.

66. Koncki, R. and O.S. Wolfbeis, Composite films of Prussian blue and N-substituted polypyrroles: Covalent immobilization of enzymes and application to near infrared optical biosensing. *Biosensors and Bioelectronics*, 1999. 14(1): 87–92.

67. Schaeferling, M., D.B.M. Groegel, and S. Schreml, Luminescent probes and nanoparticles for detection and imaging of hydrogen peroxide. *Microchimica Acta*, 2011. 174: 1–18.

68. Wu, M. et al., Time-resolved enzymatic determination of glucose using a fluorescent europium probe for hydrogen peroxide. *Analytical and Bioanalytical Chemistry*, 2004. 380(4): 619–626.

69. Piletsky, S.A. et al., Polyaniline-coated microtiter plates for use in longwave optical bioassays. *Fresenius' Journal of Analytical Chemistry*, 2000. 366(8): 807–810.

70. McCurley, M.F., An optical biosensor using a fluorescent, swelling sensing element. *Biosensors and Bioelectronics*, 1994. 9(7): 527–533.

71. Steitz, T.A. et al., High resolution crystal structures of yeast hexokinase complexes with substrates, activators, and inhibitors. Evidence for an allosteric control site. *Journal of Biological Chemistry*, 1977. 252(13): 4494–4500.

72. D'Auria, S. et al., A novel fluorescence competitive assay for glucose determinations by using a thermostable glucokinase from the thermophilic microorganism *Bacillus stearothermophilus*. *Analytical Biochemistry*, 2002. 303(2): 138–144.

73. Kramp, D.C. and I. Feldman, Tryptophan distribution in yeast hexokinase isoenzyme B. *Biochimica et Biophysica Acta*, 1978. 537(2): 406–416.

74. Woolfitt, A.R., G.L. Kellett, and J.G. Hoggett, The binding of glucose and nucleotides to hexokinase from *Saccharomyces cerevisiae*. *Biochimica et Biophysica Acta (BBA)/Protein Structure and Molecular*, 1988. 952(C): 238–243.

75. Hussain, F., D.J.S. Birch, and J.C. Pickup, Glucose sensing based on the intrinsic fluorescence of sol–gel immobilized yeast hexokinase. *Analytical Biochemistry*, 2005. 339(1): 137–143.

76. Maity, H., N.C. Maiti, and G.K. Jarori, Time-resolved fluorescence of tryptophans in yeast hexokinase-PI: Effect of subunit dimerization and ligand binding. *Journal of Photochemistry and Photobiology B: Biology*, 2000. 55(1): 20–26.

77. Maity, H. and S.R. Kasturi, Interaction of bis(1-anilino-8-naphthalenesulfonate) with yeast hexokinase: A steady-state fluorescence study. *Journal of Photochemistry and Photobiology B: Biology*, 1998. 47(2–3): 190–196.

78. Sack, J.S., M.A. Saper, and F.A. Quiocho, Periplasmic binding protein structure and function: Refined X-ray structures of the leucine/isoleucine/valine-binding protein and its complex with leucine. *Journal of Molecular Biology*, 1989. 206(1): 171–191.

79. Vyas, N.K., M.N. Vyas, and F.A. Quiocho, Sugar and signal-transducer binding sites of the *Escherichia coli* galactose chemoreceptor protein. *Science*, 1988. 242(4883): 1290–1295.

80. Tolosa, L. et al., Glucose sensor for low-cost lifetime-based sensing using a genetically engineered protein. *Analytical Biochemistry*, 1999. 267(1): 114–120.

81. Garrett, J.R. et al., pH-insensitive glucose indicators. *Biotechnology Progress*, 2008. 24(5): 1085–1089.

82. Ye, K. and J.S. Schultz, Genetic engineering of an allosterically based glucose indicator protein for continuous glucose monitoring by fluorescence resonance energy transfer. *Analytical Chemistry*, 2003. 75(14): 3451–3459.

83. Fehr, M. et al., In vivo imaging of the dynamics of glucose uptake in the cytosol of COS-7 cells by fluorescent nanosensors. *Journal of Biological Chemistry*, 2003. 278(21): 19127–19133.

84. Thomas, J. et al., Synthesis and biosensor performance of a near-IR thiol-reactive fluorophore based on benzothiazolium squaraine. *Bioconjugate Chemistry*, 2007. 18(6): 1841–1846.

85. Springsteen, G. and B. Wang, A detailed examination of boronic acid–diol complexation. *Tetrahedron*, 2002. 58(26): 5291–5300.

86. Mader, H.S. and O.S. Wolfbeis, Boronic acid based probes for microdetermination of saccharides and glycosylated biomolecules. *Microchimica Acta*, 2008. 162(1–2): 1–34.

87. Yoon, J. and A.W. Czarnik, Fluorescent chemosensors of carbohydrates. A means of chemically communicating the binding of polyols in water based on chelation-enhanced quenching. *Journal of the American Chemical Society*, 1992. 114: 5874–5875.

88. James, T.D. et al., Novel saccharide-photoinduced electron transfer sensors based on the interaction of boronic acid and amine. *Journal of the American Chemical Society*, 1995. 117(35): 8982–8987.

89. de Silva, A.P., T.S. Moody, and G.D. Wright, Fluorescent PET (Photoinduced Electron Transfer) sensors as potent analytical tools. *Analyst*, 2009. 134(12): 2385–2393.

90. James, T.D., K.R.A. Samankumara Sandanayake, and S. Shinkai, A glucose-selective molecular fluorescence sensor. *Angewandte Chemie (International Edition in English)*, 1994. 33(21): 2207–2209.

91. Shibata, H. et al., Injectable hydrogel microbeads for fluorescence-based in vivo continuous glucose monitoring. *Proceedings of the National Academy of Sciences of the United States of America*, 2010. 107(42): 17894–17898.

92. Heo, Y.J. et al., Long-term in vivo glucose monitoring using fluorescent hydrogel fibers. *Proceedings of the National Academy of Sciences of the United States of America*, 2011. 108(33): 13399–13403.

93. Huet, C. et al., Temperature effects on the concanavalin A molecule and on concanavalin A binding. *Biochimica et Biophysica Acta*, 1974. 365(1): 28–39.

94. Mansouri, S. and J.S. Schultz, A miniature optical glucose sensor based on affinity binding. *Biotechnology*, 1984. 2(10): 885–890.

95. Schultz, J.S., S. Mansouri, and I.J. Goldstein, Affinity sensor: A new technique for developing implantable sensors for glucose and other metabolites. *Diabetes Care*, 1982. 5(3): 245–253.

96. Meadows, D. and J.S. Schultz, Fiber-optic biosensors based on fluorescence energy transfer. *Talanta*, 1988. 35(2): 145–150.

97. Meadows, D.L. and J.S. Schultz, Design, manufacture and characterization of an optical fiber glucose affinity sensor based on an homogeneous fluorescence energy transfer assay system. *Analytica Chimica Acta*, 1993. 280(1): 21–30.

98. Lakowicz, J.R. and B. Maliwal, Optical sensing of glucose using phase-modulation fluorimetry. *Analytica Chimica Acta*, 1993. 271(1): 155–164.

99. Ibey, B.L. et al., Competitive binding assay for glucose based on glycodendrimer-fluorophore conjugates. *Analytical Chemistry*, 2005. 77(21): 7039–7046.

100. Ballerstadt, R. et al., In vivo performance evaluation of a transdermal near-infrared fluorescence resonance energy transfer affinity sensor for continuous glucose monitoring. *Diabetes Technology & Therapeutics*, 2006. 8(3): 296–311.

101. Ralph Ballerstadt, C.E., A. Gowda, and R. McNichols, In vivo performance evaluation of a transdermal near-infrared fluorescence resonance energy transfer affinity sensor for continuous glucose monitoring. *Diabetes Technology & Therapeutics*, 2006. 8(3): 296–311.

102. Ballerstadt, R. et al., Fiber-coupled fluorescence affinity sensor for 3-day in vivo glucose sensing. *Journal of Diabetes Science and Technology*, 2007. 1(3): 384–393.

103. Ballerstadt, R. et al., A human pilot study of the fluorescence affinity sensor for continuous glucose monitoring in diabetes. *Journal of Diabetes Science and Technology*, 2012. 6(2): 362–370.

104. Russell, R.J. et al., A fluorescence-based glucose biosensor using concanavalin A and dextran encapsulated in a poly(ethylene glycol) hydrogel. *Analytical Chemistry*, 1999. 71(15): 3126–3132.

105. Ballerstadt, R. and J.S. Schultz, A fluorescence affinity hollow fiber sensor for continuous transdermal glucose monitoring. *Analytical Chemistry*, 2000. 72(17): 4185–4192.

106. Cummins, B.M. et al., Encapsulation of a concanavalin A/dendrimer glucose sensing assay within microporated poly (ethylene glycol) microspheres. *Biomedical Optics Express*, 2011. 2(5): 1243–1257.

107. Zeller, H., P. Novak, and R. Landgraf, Blood glucose measurement by infrared spectroscopy. *International Journal of Artificial Organs*, 1989. 12(2): 129–135.

108. Heise, H.M. et al., Multivariate determination of glucose in whole blood by attenuated total reflection infrared spectroscopy. *Analytical Chemistry*, 1989. 61(18): 2009–2015.

109. Robinson, K., Blood analysis: Noninvasive methods hover on horizon. *Biophotonics International*, 1998. 5(3): 48–52.

110. Bhandare, P. et al., Glucose determination in simulated plasma solutions using infrared spectrophotometry. In *1992 14th Annual International Conference of the IEEE Engineering in Medicine and Biology Society*, Paris, France, 1992.

111. Bhandare, P. et al., Multivariate determination of glucose in whole blood using partial least-squares and artificial neural networks based on mid-infrared spectroscopy. *Applied Spectroscopy*, 1993. 47(8): 1214–1221.

112. Schügerl, K., Progress in monitoring, modeling and control of bioprocesses during the last 20 years. *Journal of Biotechnology*, 2001. 85(2): 149–173.

113. Fayolle, P., D. Picque, and G. Corrieu, On-line monitoring of fermentation processes by a new remote dispersive middle-infrared spectrometer. *Food Control*, 2000. 11(4): 291–296.

114. Ducommun, P. et al., On-line determination of animal cell concentration. *Biotechnology and Bioengineering*, 2001. 72(5): 515–522.

115. Heise, H.M., A. Bittner, and R. Marbach, Near-infrared reflectance spectroscopy for noninvasive monitoring of metabolites. *Clinical Chemistry and Laboratory Medicine*, 2000. 38(2): 137–145.

116. Lewis, C.B. et al., Investigation of near-infrared spectroscopy for periodic determination of glucose in cell culture media in situ. *Applied Spectroscopy*, 2000. 54(10): 1453–1457.

117. Hazen, K.H., M.A. Arnold, and G.W. Small, Measurement of glucose and other analytes in undiluted human serum with near-infrared transmission spectroscopy. *Analytica Chimica Acta*, 1998. 371(2–3): 255–267.

118. Riley, M.R. et al., Simultaneous measurement of glucose and glutamine in insect cell culture media by near infrared spectroscopy. *Biotechnology and Bioengineering*, 1997. 55(1): 11–15.

119. Rileys, M.R. et al., Adaptive calibration scheme for quantification of nutrients and byproducts in insect cell bioreactors by near-infrared spectroscopy. *Biotechnology Progress*, 1998. 14(3): 527–533.

120. Yeung, K.S.Y. et al., Near-infrared spectroscopy for bioprocess monitoring and control. *Biotechnology and Bioengineering*, 1999. 63(6): 684–693.

121. Fayolle, P., D. Picque, and G. Corrieu, Monitoring of fermentation processes producing lactic acid bacteria by mid-infrared spectroscopy. *Vibrational Spectroscopy*, 1997. 14(2): 247–252.

122. Li, Y. et al., Non-invasive fermentation analysis using an artificial neural network algorithm for processing near infrared spectra. *Journal of Near Infrared Spectroscopy*, 1999. 7(2): 101–108.

123. Cavinato, A.G. et al., Noninvasive method for monitoring ethanol in fermentation processes using fiber-optic near-infrared spectroscopy. *Analytical Chemistry*, 1990. 62(18): 1977–1982.

124. Vaccari, G. et al., A near-infrared spectroscopy technique for the control of fermentation processes: An application to lactic acid fermentation. *Biotechnology and Bioengineering*, 1994. 43(10): 913–917.

125. McShane, M.J. and G.L. Coté, Near-infrared spectroscopy for determination of glucose, lactate, and ammonia in cell culture media. *Applied Spectroscopy*, 1998. 52(8): 1073–1078.

126. Burns, D.A. and E.W. Ciurczak, *Handbook of Near-Infrared Analysis*. 1992, New York: Marcel Dekker.

127. McClure, G.L., *Computerized Quantitative Infrared Analysis*. 1987, Philadelphia, PA: American Society of Testing and Materials.

128. Mattu, M.J., G.W. Small, and M.A. Arnold, Application of multivariate calibration techniques to quantitative analysis of bandpass-filtered Fourier transform infrared interferogram data. *Applied Spectroscopy*, 1997. 51(9): 1369–1376.

129. Haaland, D.M. and E.V. Thomas, Partial least-squares methods for spectral analyses. 1. Relation to other quantitative calibration methods and the extraction of qualitative information. *Analytical Chemistry*, 1988. 60(11): 1193–1202.

130. Martens, H. and T. Naes, *Multivariate Calibration*. 1989, New York: John Wiley & Sons.

131. Pan, T., G.Q. Jiang, and J.M. Chen, Waveband selection of NIR spectroscopy analysis for glucose aqueous solution based on Savitzky–Golay smoothing. *Advanced Materials Research*, 2011. 181–182: 712–716.

132. Amato, I., Race quickens for non-stick blood monitoring technology. *Science*, 1992. 258(5084): 892–893.

133. Rosenthal, R.D., L.N. Paynter, and L.H. Mackie, Non-invasive measurement of blood glucose, U.S. patent 5,028,787, 1991.

134. Samann, A. et al., Non-invasive blood glucose monitoring by means of near infrared spectroscopy: Investigation of long-term accuracy and stability. *Experimental and Clinical Endocrinology and Diabetes*, 2000. 108(6): 406–413.

135. Chung, H. et al., Simultaneous measurements of glucose, glutamine, ammonia, lactate, and glutamate in aqueous solutions by near-infrared spectroscopy. *Applied Spectroscopy*, 1996. 50(2): 270–276.

136. Haaland, D.M. et al., Reagentless near-infrared determination of glucose in whole blood using multivariate calibration. *Applied Spectroscopy*, 1992. 46(10): 1575–1578.

137. Marbach, R. et al., Noninvasive blood glucose assay by near-infrared diffuse reflectance spectroscopy of the human inner lip. *Applied Spectroscopy*, 1993. 47(7): 875–881.

138. Pan, S. et al., Near-infrared spectroscopic measurement of physiological glucose levels in variable matrices of protein and triglycerides. *Analytical Chemistry*, 1996. 68(7): 1124–1135.

139. Kohl, M. et al., Influence of glucose concentration on light scattering in tissue-simulating phantoms. *Optics Letters*, 1994. 19(24): 2170–2172.

140. Maier, J.S. et al., Possible correlations between blood glucose concentration and the reduced scattering coefficient of tissues in the near infrared. *Optics Letters*, 1994. 19(24): 2062–2064.

141. Bruulsema, J.T. et al., Correlation between blood glucose concentration in diabetics and noninvasively measured tissue optical scattering coefficient. *Optics Letters*, 1997. 22(3): 190–192.

142. Kessoku, S. et al., Influence of blood glucose level on the scattering coefficient of the skin in near-infrared spectroscopy. In *ASME/JSME 8th Thermal Engineering Joint Conference Proceedings*, 2011, Honolulu, Hawaii: ASME. 38921: T10007-1–T10007-7.

143. Harrigan, G.G. and R. Goodacre, eds., *Metabolic Profiling: Its Role in Biomarker Discovery and Gene Function Analysis*. 2003, Boston, MA: Kluwer Academic Publishers.

144. Berger, A.J., Introduction to concepts in laser technology for glucose monitoring. *Diabetes Technology & Therapeutics*, 1999. 1(2): 121–128.

145. Long, D.A., *Raman Spectroscopy*. 1977, New York: McGraw-Hill.

146. Shaw, A.D. et al., Noninvasive, on-line monitoring of the biotransformation by yeast of glucose to ethanol using dispersive Raman spectroscopy and chemometrics. *Applied Spectroscopy*, 1999. 53(11): 1419–1428.

147. Wang, S.Y. et al., Analysis of metabolites in aqueous solutions by using laser Raman spectroscopy. *Applied Optics*, 1993. 32(6): 925–929.

148. Goetz Jr., M.J. et al., Application of a multivariate technique to Raman spectra for quantification of body chemicals. *IEEE Transactions on Biomedical Engineering*, 1995. 42(7): 728–731.

149. Dou, X. et al., Biological applications of anti-Stokes Raman spectroscopy: Quantitative analysis of glucose in plasma and serum by a highly sensitive multichannel Raman spectrometer. *Applied Spectroscopy*, 1996. 50(10): 1301–1306.

150. Berger, A.J., I. Itzkan, and M.S. Feld, Feasibility of measuring blood glucose concentration by near-infrared Raman spectroscopy. *Spectrochimica Acta—Part A: Molecular Spectroscopy*, 1997. 53(2): 287–292.

151. Koo, T.W. et al., Reagentless blood analysis by near-infrared Raman spectroscopy. *Diabetes Technology & Therapeutics*, 1999. 1(2): 153–157.

152. Borchert, M.S., M.C. Storrie-Lombardi, and J.L. Lambert, A noninvasive glucose monitor: Preliminary results in rabbits. *Diabetes Technology & Therapeutics*, 1999. 1(2): 145–151.

153. Tarr, R.V. and P.G. Steffes, Non-invasive blood glucose measurement system and method using stimulated Raman spectroscopy, U.S. patent 5,243,983, Sept. 14, 1993.

154. Wicksted, J.P. et al., Raman spectroscopy studies of metabolic concentrations in aqueous solutions and aqueous humor specimens. *Applied Spectroscopy*, 1995. 49(7): 987–993.

155. Dingari, N.C. et al., Wavelength selection-based nonlinear calibration for transcutaneous blood glucose sensing using Raman spectroscopy. *Journal of Biomedical Optics*, 2011. 16(8): 087009–087010.

156. Shim, B. et al., *An Investigation of the Effect of In Vivo Interferences on Raman Glucose Measurements*. 2011, San Francisco, CA: SPIE.

157. Moskovits, M., Surface-enhanced spectroscopy. *Reviews of Modern Physics*, 1985. 57(3): 783–826.

158. Chang, R.K. and T.E. Furtak, *Surface Enhanced Raman Scattering*. 1982, New York: Plenum Press.

159. Kneipp, K. et al., Surface-enhanced Raman scattering: A new tool for biomedical spectroscopy. *Current Science*, 1999. 77(7): 915–924.

160. Vo-Dinh, T. et al., Surface-enhanced Raman Scattering (SERS) method and instrumentation for genomics and biomedical analysis. *Journal of Raman Spectroscopy*, 1999. 30(9): 785–793.

161. Vo-Dinh, T., Surface-enhanced Raman spectroscopy using metallic nanostructures. *TrAC—Trends in Analytical Chemistry*, 1998. 17(8–9): 557–582.

162. Matousek, P. et al., Subsurface probing in diffusely scattering media using spatially offset Raman spectroscopy. *Applied Spectroscopy*, 2005. 59(4): 393–400.

163. Matousek, P. et al., Numerical simulations of subsurface probing in diffusely scattering media using spatially offset Raman spectroscopy. *Applied Spectroscopy*, 2005. 59(12): 1485–1492.

164. Christison, G.B. and H.A. MacKenzie, Laser photoacoustic determination of physiological glucose concentrations in human whole blood. *Medical and Biological Engineering and Computing*, 1993. 31(3): 284–290.

165. Quan, K.M. et al., Glucose determination by a pulsed photoacoustic technique: An experimental study using a gelatin-based tissue phantom. *Physics in Medicine and Biology*, 1993. 38(12): 1911–1922.

166. Pleitez, M., H. von Lilienfeld-Toal, and W. Mäntele, Infrared spectroscopic analysis of human interstitial fluid in vitro and in vivo using FT-IR spectroscopy and pulsed quantum cascade lasers (QCL): Establishing a new approach to non invasive glucose measurement. *Spectrochimica Acta: Part A: Molecular and Biomolecular Spectroscopy*, 2012. 85(1): 61–65.

167. von Lilienfeld-Toal, H. et al., A novel approach to non-invasive glucose measurement by mid-infrared spectroscopy: The combination of quantum cascade lasers (QCL) and photoacoustic detection. *Vibrational Spectroscopy*, 2005. 38(1–2): 209–215.

168. Camou, S., Y. Ueno, and E. Tamechika, Towards non-invasive and continuous monitoring of blood glucose level based on CW photoacoustics: New concept for selective and sensitive measurements of aqueous glucose. In *2011 Fifth International Conference on Sensing Technology (ICST)*, Palmerston North, New Zealand, 2011.

169. Kottmann, J. et al., Glucose sensing in human epidermis using mid-infrared photoacoustic detection. *Biomedical Optics Express*, 2012. 3(4): 667–680.

170. Solanki, J. et al., Cyclic correlation of diffuse reflected signal with glucose concentration and scatterer size. *Journal of Modern Physics*, 2012. 3: 64–68.

171. Larin, K.V. et al., Specificity of noninvasive blood glucose sensing using optical coherence tomography technique: A pilot study. *Physics in Medicine and Biology*, 2003. 48: 1371–1390.

172. Guo, X. et al., In vivo quantification of propylene glycol, glucose and glycerol diffusion in human skin with optical coherence tomography. *Laser Physics*, 2010. 20(9): 1849–1855.

173. Popov, A. et al., Glucose sensing in flowing blood and intralipid by laser pulse time-of-flight and optical coherence tomography techniques. *IEEE Journal of Selected Topics in Quantum Electronics*, 2011. 1(1): 99.

174. Li, Z. et al., Feasibility of glucose monitoring based on Brownian dynamics in time-domain optical coherence tomography. *Laser Physics*, 2011. 21(11): 1995–1998.

175. Ullah, H. et al., Can temporal analysis of optical coherence tomography statistics report on dextrorotatory-glucose levels in blood? *Laser Physics*, 2011. 21(11): 1962–1971.

176. Larin, K.V. et al., Noninvasive functional imaging of tissue abnormalities using optical coherence tomography. In *2010 IEEE Sensors*, Waikoloa, HI, 2010.

177. Ballerstadt, R. et al., Affinity-based turbidity sensor for glucose monitoring by optical coherence tomography: Toward the development of an implantable sensor. *Analytical Chemistry*, 2007. 79(18): 6965–6974.

3

Biochips and Microarrays: Tools for New Medicine

Tuan Vo-Dinh
Duke University

Guy D. Griffin
Duke University

3.1 Introduction

Biochips and microarrays are technologies that benefit directly from the research advances in micro-manufacturing, nanotechnology, and the postsequencing era in genomics. Experimental genomics in combination with the growing body of sequence information promise to revolutionize the way cells and cellular processes are studied and diseases diagnosed and treated. Information on genomic sequence can be used experimentally with high-density DNA arrays that allow complex mixtures of RNA and DNA to be interrogated in a parallel and quantitative fashion. DNA arrays can be used for many different purposes, especially to measure levels of gene expression (messenger RNA [mRNA] abundance) for tens of thousands of genes simultaneously.[1-4] On the other hand, portable, self-contained biochips with integrated detection microchip systems have great potential for use by the physician at the point of care.[5–11]

As a result, there has been an explosion of interest in the development and applications of biochips and microarrays.[1–5,7,11–29] Biochips are integrated microdevices designed to rapidly and inexpensively perform biochemical procedures for biomedical applications. Because of their miniaturization, low cost, and potential for large-scale automation, biochips can perform more efficiently than currently available laboratory equipment. Biochips with high- and medium-density arrays of oligonucleotides, complementary DNAs (cDNAs), proteins, and antibodies are among the most powerful and versatile tools in genomics and proteomics for taking full advantage of the large and rapidly increasing body of information on gene structure and function. One of the greatest impacts of microarray and biochip technologies in conjunction with bioinformatics is in enabling an entirely new approach to biological and biomedical research. In the past, researchers studied one or a few genes at a time. With whole-genome sequences and new automated, high-throughput microarray and biochip technologies, they can investigate a medical problem systematically and on a large scale. They can study all the genes in a genome or all the gene products in a particular tissue, tumor, or organ. Furthermore, they can investigate how tens of thousands of genes and proteins work together in interconnected networks in a living system. Such knowledge will have a profound impact on the way disorders are diagnosed, treated, and prevented and will bring about revolutionary changes in biomedical research and clinical practice.

This chapter describes the development and applications of biochip and microarray technology in biological research and medical applications.

3.2 Biochips and Microarrays: Definition and Classification

3.2.1 Biochips and Microarrays: A Definition

The terms *biochip* and *microarray* have been often used indiscriminately. However, these two systems are different in design and concept. The term *biochip* was coined in analogy to the phrase *computer chip*, which of course refers to the silicon-based substrate used in the fabrication of miniaturized electronic circuits. Therefore, in the generic sense, the term *biochip* involves the concept of an integrated circuit (IC). However, the term has taken on a variety of meanings over the years. A biochip is often referred to as a material or a substrate that has an array of probes for biochemical assays. In general, any device or component incorporating a 2D array of reaction sites having biological materials on a solid substrate has been referred to as a biochip. Biochips involve both miniaturization, usually in microarray formats, and the possibility of low-cost mass production. In the literature, various terms have been used to describe this new technology: if the probes are nucleic acids, the devices are called DNA biochips, DNA chips, genome chips, DNA microarrays, gene arrays, and genosensor arrays. GeneChip is a registered trademark of Affymetrix, Inc., which uses this term to refer to its high-density, oligonucleotide-based DNA arrays. If the probes consist of antibodies or proteins, the devices are referred to as protein chips or protein biochips. A recently developed system with both DNA and antibody probes on the same platform is referred to as multifunctional biochip (MFB).[7–9,11]

We define the term *biochip* in the same way that the International Union of Pure and Applied Chemistry (IUPAC) defines *biosensor*.[30] According to IUPAC, a biosensor is "a self-contained integrated device, which is capable of providing specific quantitative or semi-quantitative analytical information using a biological recognition element (biochemical receptor), which is retained in direct spatial contact with a transduction element." The interaction of the analyte with the bioreceptor is designed to produce an effect measured by the transducer, which converts the information into a measurable effect, such as an electrical signal. Figure 3.1 illustrates the conceptual principle of the biosens-

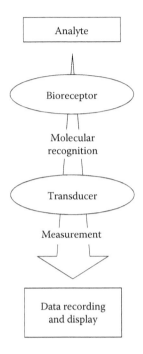

FIGURE 3.1 Principle of the biosensing process.

ing process. Biochips can be considered an array of individual biosensors that can be individually monitored and generally are used for the analysis of multiple analytes.

We group microarrays and biochips into two general classes:

- Microarray systems, which consist of arrays of probes on a substrate (chip)
- Integrated biochips, which also include detector-array microchips

Microarrays (often called *chips*) consist only of arrays of probes (in a chip format) but do not include sensor microchips integrated into the system.[10] Microarrays usually have separate, relatively large detection systems that are suitable for laboratory-based research applications (Figure 3.2). They can have large numbers of probes (tens of thousands) that could be used to identify multiple biotargets with very high speed and high throughput by matching with different types of probes via hybridization. Therefore, array plates are very useful for gene discovery and drug discovery applications, which often require tens of thousands of assays on a single plate.

On the other hand, integrated biochips include an IC microsensor, which makes these devices very portable and inexpensive (Figure 3.3). These devices generally have medium-density probe arrays (10–100 probes) and are most appropriate for medical diagnostics at the physician's office or at the point of care in the field. The characteristic features of microarrays and biochips are summarized in Table 3.1.

3.2.2 Biochip Classification

Both microarrays and biochips use probes that consist of biological recognition systems, often called bioreceptors. Biochips can be classified either by the nature of their bioreceptors or by the type of transducer used (Figure 3.4). A detailed description of various types of bioreceptors and transducers is provided in Chapter 1 in this handbook. A bioreceptor is a biological molecular species (e.g., an antibody, an enzyme, a protein, or a nucleic acid) or a living biological system (e.g., cells, tissue, or whole

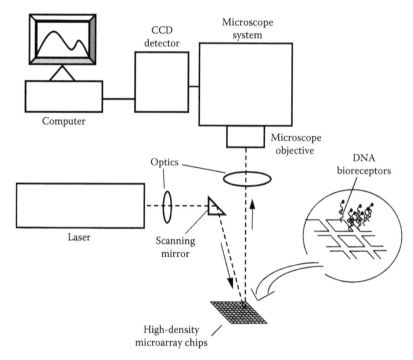

FIGURE 3.2 Schematic diagram of a microarray system. Microarrays (often called *chips*) consist of high-density arrays of probes (in a chip format) but do not include sensor microchips integrated into the system. These microarrays usually have separate detection systems that are relatively large and are suitable for laboratory-based research applications.

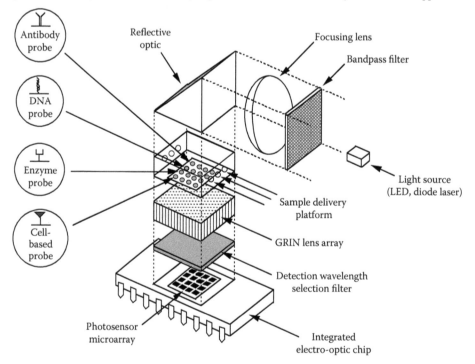

FIGURE 3.3 Schematic diagram of an integrated biochip. Integrated biochips also include an IC microsensor, which make these devices very portable and inexpensive. These devices generally have medium-density probe arrays (10–100 probes) and are most appropriate for medical diagnostics at the physician's office or at the point of care in the field.

TABLE 3.1   Characteristic Features of Microarrays and Biochips

Systems	Bioreceptor	Format	Probe Density	Detection System	Applications
Microarrays	DNA Antibody Proteins Cells, etc.	Array	High density $(10^3–10^5)$	Separate system (laboratory system)	Research tools
Biochip	DNA Antibody Proteins Cells, etc.	Array	Low–medium density $(10–10^2)$	Integrated system (portable)	Physicians tool (field monitor)

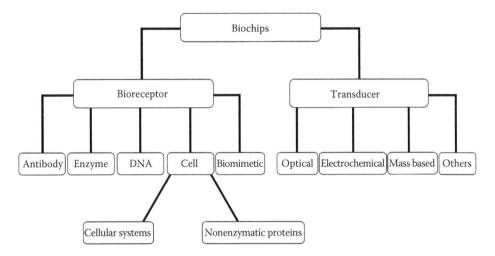

FIGURE 3.4   Biochip classification schemes.

organisms) that uses a biochemical mechanism for recognition. Bioreceptors are the key to specificity for biochip technologies, responsible for binding the analyte of interest to the sensor for the measurement. Bioreceptors can take many forms and are as numerous as the different analytes that have been monitored using biosensors. Bioreceptors can generally be classified into five major categories: (1) antibody/antigen, (2) enzymes, (3) nucleic acids/DNA, (4) cellular structures/cells, and (5) biomimetic probes (synthetic probes that mimic receptors of living systems).

Biochips can also be classified by the type of transducers used. The conventional transducer techniques are (1) optical measurements (luminescence, absorption, surface plasmon resonance [SPR], etc.), (2) electrochemical measurements, and (3) mass-sensitive measurements (surface acoustic wave, microbalance, etc.).

3.3 Microarray Systems

3.3.1 Basic Principles

Nucleic acids have been widely used as bioreceptors for microarray and biochip technologies.[31–38] The complementarity of adenine/thymine (A/T) and cytosine/guanine (C/G) pairing in DNA forms the basis for the specificity of biorecognition in DNA biochips. If the sequence of bases composing a certain part of the DNA molecule is known, then the complementary sequence can be synthesized and labeled with an optically detectable compound (e.g., a radioactive label or a fluorescent label). When unknown fragments of single-stranded (ss) DNA samples, called the target, react (or hybridize) with the probes on the chip, double-stranded (ds) DNA fragments are formed only when the target and the probe are complementary according to the base-pairing rule. When the targets contain more than one type of sample, each is labeled with its specific tag.

The microarrays of probes serve as reaction sites, each reaction site containing single strands of a specific sequence of a DNA fragment. The DNA fragments can either be short oligonucleotides—for example, 20- to 100-nucleotide (nt) sequences—or longer strands of cDNA. The relatively large nucleic acid components—those longer than 100 nt—are often used in RNA expression analysis,[1] and those with short nucleic acids—with oligonucleotides up to 25 nt—can be used for both RNA expression[39] and sequence analysis.

Probes based on a synthetic biorecognition element, peptide nucleic acid (PNA), have been developed.[34] PNA is an artificial oligoamide that is capable of binding very strongly to complementary oligonucleotide sequences. An SPR sensor has been used to directly detect dsDNA that had been amplified by a polymerase chain reaction (PCR).

Synthetic antibody-like probes produced by molecular imprint methods are often used as biomimetic probes. Another type of biomimetic probes are aptamers, which are artificial nucleic acid ligands that can be produced against amino acids, proteins, and other molecules.

3.3.2 Microarray Fabrication

DNA arrays, often called DNA chips, can be fabricated using high-speed robotics on a variety of substrates. The substrates can be thin plates made of silicon, glass, gel, gold, or a polymeric material such as plastic or nylon or may even be composed of beads at the ends of fiber-optic bundles.[40] Oligonucleotide microarrays are fabricated either by in situ light-directed combinatorial synthesis that uses photographic masks for each chip[41] or by conventional synthesis followed by immobilization on glass substrates.[1,2,12]

Arrays with more than 250,000 different oligonucleotide probes or 10,000 different cDNAs per cm^2 have been produced.[42] Sequence information is used directly to design high-density, 2D arrays of synthetic oligonucleotides. The probe arrays, made using spatially patterned, light-directed combinatorial chemical synthesis, contain up to hundreds of thousands of different oligonucleotides on a small glass surface. The arrays have been designed and used for quantitative and highly parallel measurements of gene expression, to discover polymorphic loci, and to detect the presence of thousands of alternative alleles.

A maskless fabrication method of light-directed oligonucleotide microarrays replaces the chrome mask with virtual computer-generated masks. These virtual masks are relayed to a digital micromirror array capable of synthesizing microarrays containing more than 76,000 features measuring 16 m^2. A reflective imaging system forms an ultraviolet image of the virtual mask on the active surface of the glass substrate, which is mounted in a flow cell reaction chamber connected to a DNA synthesizer. Programmed chemical coupling cycles follow light exposure, and steps are repeated to achieve the desired pattern.[43]

Modified chemistries should allow for other types of arrays to be manufactured using photolithography. Alternative processes, such as ink-jet[44] and spotting techniques, can also be used.[13,14] One method for constructing these arrays using light-directed DNA synthesis with photoactivatable monomers can currently achieve densities on the order of 10^6 sequences/cm^2. One of the challenges facing the developers of this technology is to further increase the volume, complexity, and density of sequence information encoded in these arrays. An approach for synthesizing DNA probe arrays that combines standard solid-phase oligonucleotide synthesis with polymeric photoresist films serving as the photoimageable component opens the way to exploiting high-resolution imaging materials and processes from the microelectronics industry for the fabrication of DNA probe arrays with substantially higher densities.[44]

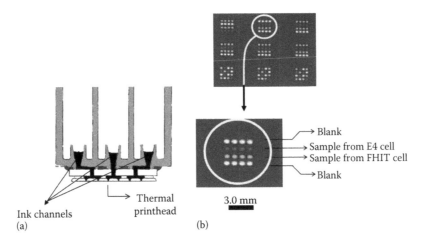

FIGURE 3.5 **(See color insert.)** (a) Schematic diagram of a generic bubble-jet cartridge illustrating the connection of ink channels to the printhead. (b) Membrane printed with biological materials using the bubble-jet technology. For purposes of better visualization of the spotting, different fluorescent dyes were added for the preparation of this sample. (From Allain, L.R. et al., *Fresenius J. Anal. Chem.*, 371(2), 146, 2001.)

Activated DNA has been immobilized in aldehyde-containing polyacrylamide gel for use in manufacturing microarrays.[13] In this process, abasic sites were generated in DNA by partial acidic depurination. Amino groups were then introduced into the abasic sites by reaction with ethylenediamine and reduction of the aldimine bonds formed. It was found that DNA could be fragmented at the site of amino group incorporation or preserved mostly unfragmented. In similar reactions, both amino-DNA and amino-oligonucleotides were attached through their amines to polyacrylamide gel derivatized with aldehyde groups. ssDNA and dsDNA of 40–972 nt or base pairs (bp's) were immobilized on the gel pads to manufacture DNA microarrays.[13]

Microarrays containing PCR-amplified genomic DNA extracts from mice tumors on a Zeta-Probe® membrane have been fabricated using a modified thermal ink-jet printer.[45] This method, using a modified bubble-jet printing system, is a simple and cost-effective procedure for the fabrication of microarrays containing biological samples. Figure 3.5 shows a cross-section view of a generic bubble-jet cartridge illustrating the connection of ink channels to the printhead (Figure 3.5a) and a membrane printed with biological materials extracted from mice tumors—cell with fragile histidine triad (FHIT) gene—and control cells (cells labeled as E4). For purposes of better visualization of the spotting, different fluorescent dyes were added for the preparation of this figure.[45] Because of their mass-produced design, ink-jet printers are a much cheaper alternative to conventional spotting techniques.

3.3.3 Assay Detection

Because of its inherently sensitive detection capability, fluorescence is the most commonly used technique in DNA hybridization assays. Fluorescent labels can be inserted during the PCR process; subsequently, the sample is tested for hybridization to the microarray. In general, microarray systems are based on fiber-optic probes. Glass and silica plates are used as the probe substrates and are externally connected to a photosensing system, which generally consists of a conventional detection device, such as a photomultiplier or a charge-coupled device (CCD). Although the probes on the sampling platform are small, the entire device—containing excitation laser sources and detection systems (often a confocal microscope system)—is relatively large, for example, tabletop size. The high density of the array and the small size of the probes often require powerful excitation source and high-precision scanning systems, which are also relatively large. These systems have demonstrated their usefulness in genomics research and analysis, but they are laboratory oriented and involve relatively expensive equipment.

Other optical techniques, such as SPR, have also been used to monitor real-time binding of low-molecular-weight ligands to DNA fragments that were irreversibly bound to the sensor surface via Coulombic interactions. Ellipsometry confirmed that the DNA layer remained stable over a period of several days. Binding rates and equilibrium coverages were determined for various ligands by changing the ligand concentration. In addition, affinity constants and association and dissociation rates were also determined for these various ligands. A label-free optical technique, based on reflectometric interference spectroscopy, has also been used in characterization of low-molecular-weight ligand–DNA interaction.[46]

Ellipsometric and interferometric detection methods have also been used for characterization of DNA probes immobilized on a combinatorial arrays.[47] The hybridization reaction may be solution based, or it may be driven by an electric field.[48] This technology has been successfully applied to the simultaneous assay of expression of many thousands of genes and to large-scale gene discovery, as well as to polymorphism screening and mapping of genomic DNA.

Several researchers have investigated sensing system-based sandwich-type biosensors formed from liquid-crystalline dispersions formed from DNA–polycation complexes.[49] These sandwich biosensors have been used to detect compounds and physical factors that affect the ability of specific DNA cross-linkers, polycationic molecules, to bind between adjacent DNA molecules.

The application of the principles of atomic force microscopy (AFM) for the use of supported lipid bilayers for anchoring subcellular to the submolecular biomolecules such as DNA, enzymes, and crystalline protein arrays has been studied.[50] Chemical force microscopy (CFM) has also been used to probe the mechanics of molecular recognition between surfaces. The technique uses DNA-modified probes to scan the interactions between short segments of ssDNA containing complementary sequences. These substrates consisted of micron-scale patterned arrays of one or more distinct oligonucleotides.[51]

Raman spectroscopy has recently been used as a detection technique for gene assays. For this method, researchers developed a new type of spectral label for DNA probes based on surface-enhanced Raman scattering (SERS) detection.[29,52-55] The SERS probes have great potential to provide both sensitivity and selectivity via label multiplexing because of the intrinsically narrow bandwidths of Raman peaks. The effectiveness of the new detection scheme was demonstrated using the *gag* gene sequence of the human immunodeficiency (HIV) virus.[55] The development of a multiarray system for DNA diagnostics using visible and near-infrared (NIR) dyes has been reported.[28]

3.3.4 Target Sample Amplification

An important step in DNA microarray assay involves efficient and reproducible mRNA and DNA amplification methods. Various amplification technologies are described in detail in Chapter 16 in Book 3 of this handbook. This section briefly discusses two main approaches: (1) a PCR-based approach that has been used to make single-cell cDNA libraries[56,57] and (2) a method that uses multiple rounds of linear amplification based on cDNA synthesis and a template-directed in vitro transcription (IVT) reaction. Although the PCR technique is most widely used, the IVT method shows significant promise. Labeled material can be sufficiently produced through multiple-round cDNA/IVT amplification. The IVT technique is highly reproducible and introduces less quantitative bias than PCR-based amplification.[58,59] mRNA from single live neurons has been characterized using the IVT method.[60,61]

The need for only minute amounts of starting material is a significant advantage of the microarray and biochip technologies. This feature in conjunction with the capability of laser-capture microdissection technology to provide pure samples has greatly enhanced the reliability and the value of the DNA chip technology as a sophisticated genetic testing technique.[62,63] The combination of microarrays generated with DNA, or RNA extracted from pure cell populations within the tissue, and powerful amplification strategies promises to be especially important for studies that involve human biopsy material from inhomogeneous tissue, as well as for research in developmental biology, immunology, and neurobiology.

3.3.5 DNA Sequence Analysis

Microarray-based sequence analyses are generally performed using arrays designed to evaluate specific sequences. There are several approaches for analyzing a DNA sequence of interest for all possible changes. The first approach uses probes complementary to a significant subset of sequence changes (such as those described for the cystic fibrosis transmembrane regulator[64]) and measures gain of hybridization signal to these probes relative to reference samples. The approach allows for a partial scan of a DNA segment for all possible sequence variations. Probes are designed such that the location of the interrogated target base is in the centermost position of the potential target/probe duplex and thus provides the best discrimination for hybridization specificity. The probe arrays are made using spatially patterned, light-directed combinatorial chemical synthesis and contain up to hundreds of thousands of different oligonucleotides on a small glass surface. The arrays have been designed and used for quantitative and highly parallel measurements of gene expression, to discover polymorphic loci, and to detect the presence of thousands of alternative alleles.[42] In another study, the entire 297 bp HIV-1 protease gene coding sequence from 167 viral isolates was screened for all single-nucleotide changes using this gain-of-signal approach. The DNA sequence of US HIV-1 clade B proteases was found to be extremely variable, with 47% of the 99 amino acid positions varied.[65] Naturally occurring mutations in HIV-1-infected patients have important implications for therapy and the outcome of clinical studies.

The second approach for scanning DNA analyses involves the selective loss of hybridization signal to perfect-match probes, which are complementary to wild-type sequence in a manner analogous to comparative genomic hybridization (CGH) studies.[66,67] In the loss-of-signal approach, sequence variations are scored by quantifying relative losses of hybridization signal to perfect-match oligonucleotide probes relative to wild-type reference targets. Loss-of-signal analysis allows for a practical screen to be set up for virtually any sequence variation. A disadvantage of loss-of-signal analysis is that the mutation cannot be discerned; the identity of the sequence change must be established by subsequent dideoxysequencing of the region surrounding the loss-of-signal signature. This approach has been further improved by using internal standards using two-color assays. In this scheme, reference targets with a known sequence can be cohybridized to the arrays along with the test target. Labeling each target with a different fluorophore allows a direct comparison of hybridization signals from the two targets to be made. High-density arrays consisting of over 96,600 oligonucleotides 20 nt in length screen for a wide range of heterozygous mutations in the 3.45 kilobases (kb) exon 11 of the hereditary breast and ovarian cancer gene *BRCA1*.[67] Reference and test samples were cohybridized to these arrays and differences in hybridization patterns quantified by two-color analysis. The ability to scan a large gene rapidly and accurately for all possible heterozygous mutations in large numbers of patient samples will be critical for the future of medicine. DNA minisequencing assays couple target hybridization with enzymatic primer extension reactions to provide a powerful means of scanning for all possible sequence variations.[22,68,69]

Representational difference analysis (RDA), which compares the results for two tissue samples, is another analysis method used for DNA microarrays and biochips. Subtraction of one set of results from the other shows which genes are active in one sample but less active or completely inactive in the other. The comparison is usually performed between normal and cancer cells or between metastatic and nonmetastatic cancers. In this way, the evaluation may pinpoint an abnormal cellular process occurring mainly (or even exclusively) in diseased cells. The evaluation may thus serve not only as a diagnostic tool but also as a means to identify therapeutic targets. RDA of cDNA was used for a comparison of the global transcript level of tumor of the larynx and the corresponding normal epithelial tissue for detecting differentially expressed genes. Overall, some 130 gene fragments were identified.[70] After further analysis, these genes could be put in functional groups such as genes whose overexpression was a result of tumor growth or dedifferentiation, genes that played major roles in signal transduction pathways, and apoptosis, oncogenes, or tumor suppressor genes, in addition to new, entirely unknown genes.

3.3.6 Protein Microarrays

Recently, antibodies have received increasing interest as bioreceptors for research in proteomics. When microarray probes consist of antibodies or proteins, the microarrays are sometimes called protein chips or protein biochips.[45,71-79] The basis for the specificity of immunoassays is the antigen–antibody (Ag–Ab) binding reaction, which is a key mechanism by which the immune system detects and eliminates foreign matter.[80-82] The way in which an antigen and an antigen-specific antibody interact may perhaps be understood as analogous to a lock-and-key fit, in which the specific configurations of a unique key enable it to open a lock. In the same way, an antigen-specific antibody fits its unique antigen in a highly specific manner, so that hollows, protrusions, planes, and ridges on the antigen and the antibody molecules (in a word, the total 3D structure) are complementary. How such complementarity is achieved will be discussed later in this chapter. It is sufficient at this point simply to indicate that, due to this 3D shape fitting and the diversity inherent in individual antibody makeup, it is possible to find an antibody that can recognize and bind to any one of a huge variety of molecular shapes. This unique property of antibodies is the key to their usefulness in immunosensors, since this ability to *recognize* molecular structures allows researchers to develop antibodies that bind specifically to chemicals, biomolecules, microorganism components, etc. Such antibodies can then be used as specific detectors to identify and find an analyte of interest that is present, even in extremely small amounts, in a myriad of other chemical substances.

Protein microarrays have received great interest because it is not sufficient just to know the genes involved and their DNA sequences.[71] Proteins formed as a result of the activity of certain genes induce the symptoms of illnesses. To understand and manage disease, it is important to investigate those proteins in the body that are responsible for all the biological processes (growth, metabolism, disease, etc.). The number of these proteins is estimated at several hundred thousands. For this reason, it is expected that microarray and biochip technologies will play an important role in the investigation of proteomics.[83]

Proteomics research has two main objectives: (1) quantification of all the proteins expressed in a cell and (2) the functional study of thousands of protein in parallel. The standard methods for identification and quantification are 2D gel separation and mass spectrometry. Microarray-based assays are being used to study protein–protein and protein–ligand interactions because the rapid development of this technology has shortened the analysis process and made it more reliable.[84]

3.4 Biochips

3.4.1 Integrated Biochip Concept

Biochips that integrate conventional biotechnology with semiconductor processing, microelectromechanical systems (MEMS), optoelectronics, and digital signal and image acquisition and processing have received a great deal of interest. There is a strong need for a truly integrated biochip system that comprises probes, samplers, and detectors as well as amplifier and logic circuitry on board. Such a system will be useful in physicians' offices and can be used by relatively unskilled personnel.

An integrated biochip using bioreceptor probes and a detection system into a self-contained microdevice has been developed.[5,7-9,11] As illustrated schematically in Figure 3.3, the biochip concept involves the combination of IC elements, an electro-optic excitation/detection system, and bioreceptor probes in a self-contained and integrated microdevice. A basic biochip includes (1) an excitation light source with related optics, (2) a bioprobe, (3) a sampling platform and delivery system, (4) an optical detector with associated optics and dispersive device, and (5) a signal amplification/treatment system.

Construction of a biochip involves the integration of several basic elements of very different natures. The basic steps are (1) the selection or development of the bioreceptor, (2) the selection of the excitation source, (3) the selection or development of the transducer, and (4) the integration of the excitation source–bioreceptor–transducer system. The development of the biochip comprises three major elements. The first element involves the development of a bioreceptor probe system: a microarray of bioreceptor probes on a multiarray sampling platform. The second element involves the development of nonradioactive methods for optical detection: the fluorescence technique. The third element involves the development of an integrated electro-optic IC system on a single chip for biosensing: a photodiode–amplifier microchip using complementary metal oxide semiconductor (CMOS) technology.

3.4.2 Integrated Circuit Fabrication

Most microarray detection systems are very large when the excitation source and detector are considered, making them impractical for anything but laboratory usage. For biochips, however, the sensors, amplifiers, discriminators, and logic circuitry are all built onto the chip. The integrated biochip involves integrated electro-optic sensing photodetectors. Highly integrated biosensors are possible partly because multiple optical sensing elements and microelectronics can be fabricated on a single IC. The biochips include a large-area, n-well integrated amplifier–photodiode array that has been designed as a single, custom IC fabricated for the biochip. This IC device is coupled to the multiarray sampling platform and is designed for monitoring very low light levels. The individual photodiodes have 900 μm^2 sizes and are arrayed on a 1 mm spacing grid. The photodiodes and the accompanying electronic circuitry were fabricated using a standard 1.2 μm n-well CMOS process. The use of this standard process allows for the production of photodiodes and phototransistors as well as other numerous types of analog and digital circuitry in a single IC chip. This feature is the main advantage of the CMOS technology as compared to other detector technologies such as CCDs or charge-injection devices. The photodiodes themselves are produced using the n-well structure that is generally used to make resistors or as the body material for transistors. Since the anode of the diode is the p-type substrate material, which is common to every circuit on the IC chip, only the cathode is available for monitoring the photocurrent, and the photodiode is constrained to operate with a reverse bias. Figure 3.6 shows a 16 (4 × 4)-array microchip fabricated for the DNA biochip.

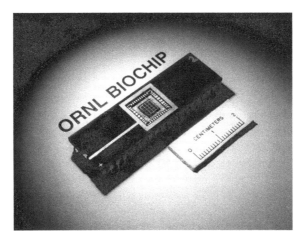

FIGURE 3.6 (See color insert.) Photograph of an IC microchip for a biochip with 4 × 4 sensor array. (From Vo-Dinh, T., *Sens. Actuat. B*, 51, 52, 1998.)

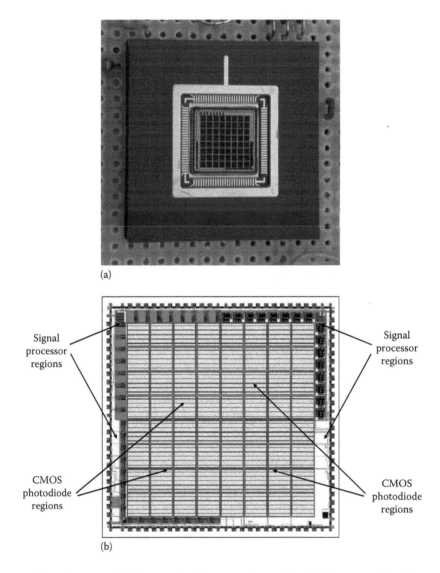

FIGURE 3.7 **(See color insert.)** (a) Photograph of the 8 × 8 IC microchip. (b) Schematic of the electronic design of the 8 × 8 microchip with CMOS photodiode regions and signal processor regions.

An analog multiplexer was designed to allow any of the elements in the array to be connected to an amplifier. The multiplexer is made from 16 cells for the 4 × 4 array device. Each cell has a CMOS switch controlled by the output of the address decoder cell. The switch is open, connecting the addressed diode to an amplifier. This arrangement allows connecting a 4 × 4 (8 × 8 or 10 × 10) array of light sources (e.g., different fluorescent probes) to the photodiode array and reading out the signal levels sequentially.

Figure 3.7a shows a photograph of 64 (8 × 8)-array IC microchips. Figure 3.7b shows the design of the different CMOS photodiode regions and signal processor regions of the 8 × 8 microchip. The CMOS technology makes possible highly integrated biosensors, partly through the capability of fabricating multiple optical sensing elements and microelectronics on a single IC. A 2D array of optical detector amplifiers was integrated on a single IC chip.

3.4.3 Multifunctional Biochip: A Hybrid Chip for Genomics and Proteomics

The development of the first integrated DNA biochip having a phototransistor IC microchip was reported by Vo-Dinh and coworkers.[5–7,85] This work involved the integration of 4 × 4 optical biosensor arrays onto an IC. The usefulness and potential of this DNA biochip were illustrated by the detection of gene fragments of the HIV system.[5]

Nucleic acids are not, however, the only possible substances of interest in medical diagnosis. For example, proteins also need to be analyzed using biochips having antibody probes. These antibody-based biochips are often referred to as protein chips. In general, biochips employ only one type of bioreceptor as probes—that is, either nucleic acid or antibody probes. A novel integrated biochip system that uses multiple bioreceptors with different functionalities on the same biochip, allowing simultaneous detection of several types of biotargets on a single platform, has been developed.[8,9] This device is referred to as the MFB. The integrated electro-optic microchip system developed for this work involved integrated electro-optic sensing photodetectors for the biosensor microchips.

The MFB allows simultaneous detection of several disease end points using different bioreceptors, such as DNA and antibodies on a single biochip system. The multifunctional capability of the MFB device is illustrated by measurements of different types of bioreceptors using DNA probes specific to gene fragments of the *Mycobacterium tuberculosis* (TB) system and antibody probes targeted to the cancer-related tumor suppressor gene *p53* on a single biochip platform (Figure 3.8).

3.5 Applications in Biology and Medicine

3.5.1 Genomics Research

Microarray and biochip technologies provide powerful tools to identify all the genes as well as to understand their functions and how these components work together to coordinate the functions of cells and organisms.[21] Two important applications for the high-density DNA microarray technology involve

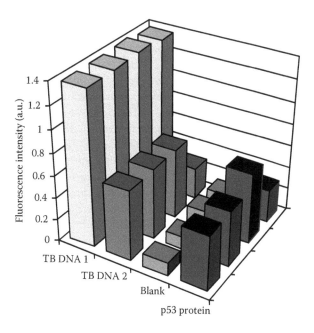

FIGURE 3.8 (**See color insert.**) MFB used for simultaneous detection of the p53 protein (antibody probe) and the *M. tuberculosis* gene (DNA probe).

identification of sequence (gene mutation) and determination and monitoring of expression level—for example, mRNA abundance—of genes (gene expression).

DNA microarray and biochip technologies for genome-scale screening and the availability of genome information will enable rapid mapping and identification of disease-related genes, which can then be analyzed in more detail. Until recently, functional studies of genes were carried out in the one gene—one protein at a time approach. High-density microarray technology can simultaneously analyze the expression of all genes in a given organism containing thousands of different genes.

The collection of genes that are expressed or transcribed from genomic DNA (the expression profile) is a major determinant of cellular phenotype and function that changes rapidly and dramatically in response to various stimulations and during normal cellular events. Microarray hybridization has been applied for a genome-wide transcriptional analysis of cellular mitotic process.[86] A comprehensive identification of cell-cycle-regulated genes of the yeast *Saccharomyces cerevisiae* has been accomplished.[87] Transcription alterations in DNA replication genes, genes involved with cell-cycle control and chromosomes, and a large collection of genes involved with smooth muscle function, apoptosis, intercellular adhesion, and cell motility have been measured.[88]

With the human genome sequencing phase now completed, the postgenomics phase of research involves information analysis and experimental activities initiated as the results of genome information. For instance, the information from open reading frames (ORFs), which indicate the particular parts within the genome encoded for proteins, allows functional assignment of the given genes. Functional assignment is performed using several methods: systematic disruption of the gene to observe the effects of the absence of the functional genes, expression of the genes in transgenic animals, and expression of recombinant proteins.

3.5.1.1 Application of Human Expressed Sequence Tags and cDNA Microarrays

Human expressed sequence tags (ESTs) in combination with high-density cDNA microarray techniques have been used to map the genome, to explore genes, and to profile downstream gene changes in a host of experiments. EST is a short strand of DNA that is a part of a cDNA molecule and can act as the identifier of a gene. ESTs represent sequences expressed in an organism under particular conditions that are often used in locating and mapping genes. For instance, in lung cancer, the effects of overexpression of a tumor suppressor—the phosphatase and tensin homology deleted on chromosome 10 (phosphatase and tensin homology [PTEN])—has been studied.[89] In prostate cancer, ESTs have been used for identification of several potential markers for prostate cancer.[90] Prostate cancer tends to become transformed to androgen-independent disease over time when treated by androgen-deprivation therapy. In one study, two variants of the human prostate cancer cell line LNCaP were used to study gene expression differences during prostate cancer progression to androgen-independent disease.[90]

The cDNA microarray technique is a unique tool that exploits this wealth of information for the analysis of gene expression. In this method, DNA probes representing cDNA clones are arrayed on a glass slide and interrogated with fluorescently labeled cDNA targets. The power of the DNA biochip technology is the ability to perform a genome-wide expression profile of thousands of genes in one experiment. In a study of breast cancer, cell lines have been used for rapid identification and comparison of the differential pattern of gene expression.[91] In an alternative approach for selecting tissue-appropriate cDNAs that can be used to examine the expression profiles of developmental processes and diseases, ESTs were employed to identify 21 neural crest-derived melanocytes in a library of 198 cDNA for microarray analysis.[92]

3.5.1.2 Single-Nucleotide Polymorphism

Single-nucleotide polymorphisms (SNPs) are the most frequent type of variation in the human genome. Although more than 99% of human DNA sequences are the same across the population, variations in DNA sequence can have a major impact on how humans respond to disease; to such environmental insults as bacteria, viruses, toxins, and chemicals; and to drugs and other therapies. Methods are being developed to detect different types of variation, particularly SNPs, which occur about once every 100–300 bases. SNPs provide powerful tools for a variety of medical genetic studies. It is believed that SNP maps will help researchers identify the multiple genes associated with such complex diseases as cancer, diabetes, vascular disease, and some forms of mental illness. These associations are difficult to establish with conventional gene-hunting methods because a single altered gene may make only a small contribution to disease risk. Detection of the presence of particular mutations or polymorphisms using oligonucleotide array-based analysis of known genomic DNA sequence was first reported in 1989.[93] Genotype was determined nonradioactively by the binding of streptavidin–horseradish peroxidase (HRP) to the biotinylated DNA in a colorimetric assay that detected the signal intensity produced by each allele-specific probe.

In a large-scale survey for SNPs employing a combination of gel-based sequencing and high-density microarray DNA chips, 2.3 megabases of human genomic DNA were examined by a combination of gel-based sequencing and high-density-variation detection DNA chips. The study identified a total of over 3000 candidate SNPs. A genetic map was constructed showing the location of over 2000 of these SNPs. Prototype genotyping chips were developed that allow simultaneous genotyping of 500 SNPs. The study provides a characterization of human diversity at the nucleotide level and demonstrates the possibility of large-scale identification of human SNPs.[22]

Most human cancers are characterized by genomic instability, the accumulation of multiple genetic alterations, and allelic imbalance throughout the genome. Loss of heterozygosity (LOH) is a common form of allelic imbalance, and the detection of LOH has been used to identify genomic regions that harbor tumor suppressor genes and to characterize tumor stages and progression. Researchers have used high-density oligonucleotide arrays for genome-wide scans for LOH and allelic imbalance in human tumors.[94] The detection of LOH and other chromosomal changes using large numbers of SNP markers should enable identification of patterns of allelic imbalance, with potential prognostic and diagnostic utility. Prototype genotyping chips have been produced to detect 400, 600, and 3000 of these SNPs.[95] Methods have been developed for rapid genotyping of these SNPs using oligonucleotide arrays.[96,97] Each allele of an SNP marker is represented on the array by a set of perfect-match and mismatch probes. High-density DNA-chip-based analysis has also been used to determine the distant history of SNPs, polymorphism detection, and genotyping in current human populations. The studies demonstrate that microarray-based assays allow rapid comparative sequence analysis of intra- and interspecies genetic variation.[96,97]

3.5.1.3 Gene Expression Studies

DNA microarrays and biochips can also be used to probe gene expression patterns throughout a genome. For this purpose, the probes are selected not to cover the length of an individual gene but to have sequence characteristic of different genes (so-called partial sequence tags). When a gene is expressed (active), its code is transcribed into ss mRNAs, through which the gene transmits its instructions for cellular biosynthesis of a specific protein. Hence, a cell's cytoplasm contains a variety of messengers, depending on which genes are expressed. The messengers' hybridizations with one or another partial sequence tag on a biochip can serve to reveal the patterns of genes being expressed. Microarray analyses have been successfully applied to identify amplified and overexpressed genes in chromosomal region 17q23, which is known to be augmented in up to 20% of primary breast cancers.[98]

An important objective of current cancer research is to develop a detailed molecular characterization of gene expression in tumor cells and tissues that is linked to clinical information. One study used differential display to identify approximately one-quarter of all genes that were aberrantly expressed in a breast cancer cell line.[99] Two clusters of genes, represented by *p53* and maspin, had expression patterns strongly associated with estrogen receptor status. A third cluster that included HSP-90 tended to be associated with the clinical tumor stage, whereas a fourth cluster that included keratin 14 tended to be associated with tumor size. The expression levels of these clinically relevant gene clusters allowed breast tumors to be grouped into distinct categories. Gene expression fingerprints that include these four gene clusters could improve prognostic accuracy and therapeutic outcomes for breast cancer patients.[99]

High-density oligonucleotide arrays were used to measure mRNA levels and to evaluate the transcriptional profiles of fibroblast cultures taken from different age donors. mRNA levels were measured in actively dividing fibroblasts isolated from young, middle-aged, and old humans and from humans with progeria, a rare genetic disorder characterized by accelerated aging. The study identified genes whose expression is associated with age-related phenotypes and diseases. The data suggest that an underlying mechanism of the aging process involves increasing errors in the mitotic machinery of dividing cells in the postreproductive stage of life. Results indicated that a central underlying process of aging involves errors in the mitotic machinery that lead to chromosomal pathologies and ultimately to misregulation of essential structural, signaling, and metabolic genes.[100]

Complex changes in patterns of gene expression that accompany the development and progression of cancer and the experimental reversal of tumorigenicity can be investigated by microarray and biochip technologies. The tumorigenic properties of human melanoma cell line can be suppressed by introduction of a normal human chromosome 6. The introduction of this chromosome results in a reduced growth rate, restored contact inhibition, and suppressed soft agar clonogenicity and tumorigenicity in nude mice. A high-density microarray of 1161 DNA elements was used to search for differences in gene expression associated with tumor suppression in this system. Fluorescent probes for hybridization from two sources of cellular mRNA were labeled with different fluorophores to provide a direct and internally controlled comparison of the mRNA levels corresponding to each arrayed gene. The fluorescence signals representing hybridization to each arrayed gene were analyzed to determine the relative abundance in the two samples of mRNAs corresponding to each gene.[3]

High-density cDNA arrays have been used to detect tumorigenesis- and angiogenesis-related alterations in gene transcript expression profiles in ovarian cancer.[101] In the ovary, an abundance of specific tumor markers, increased macrophage recruitment mediators, a late-stage angiogenesis profile, and the presence of chemoresistance-related markers distinguished normal and advanced ovarian cancer tissue samples. The detection of such parallel changes in pathway- and tissue-specific markers may prove a potential approach ready for application in reproductive disease diagnostic and therapeutic developments.[101]

Similarly, investigators have applied general approaches to cancer classification based on gene expression profiles monitored by DNA microarrays to a systematic characterization of gene expression in B cell malignancies.[102] The molecular classification of tumors on the basis of gene expression can be used to identify previously undetected and clinically significant subtypes of cancer.[102]

A damaging change during cancer progression is the switch from a locally growing tumor to a metastatic killer. This switch is believed to involve numerous alterations that allow tumor cells to complete the complex series of events needed for metastasis. DNA microarrays were used to investigate this metastasis process where a defined pattern of gene expression that correlates with progression from a locally growing tumor to a metastatic phenotype had been discerned.[103] The results demonstrated an enhanced expression of several genes involved in extracellular matrix assembly and of a second set of genes that regulate the actin-based cytoskeleton.[103]

Many genes and signaling pathways controlling cell proliferation, death and differentiation, and genomic integrity are involved in cancer development. Identification of prognostic markers and prognostic parameters for renal cell carcinoma has been performed using cDNA microarray and biochip technologies.[104] Finally, DNA microarray technologies have been applied in genomic analysis and monitoring of the expression profiles of a host of cancerous organs including glioma,[105] ovary,[101] breast,[106] blood,[107] liver,[108] nasopharyngeal,[109] and lung.[110]

3.5.2 Gene Profile Analysis

High-density DNA microarrays allow massively parallel genomics profiling and gene discovery studies and could provide researchers with information on tens of thousands of genes simultaneously. These arrays can be used to test an individual gene throughout all or part of its length for single-base variations from the gene's usual sequence. DNA chips, available from various commercial sources such as Affymetrix, Inc., can be used to detect single-base variations in the human genes *BRCA1* and *BRCA2* (breast cancer related), *p53* (a tumor suppressor gene mutated in many forms of cancer), and *P450* (coding for a key liver enzyme system that metabolizes drugs). Other Affymetrix's GeneChips™ analyze the HIV genome for variations within the code for the viral protease and reverse transcriptase. Predicting the drug resistance of a given patient's viral strain is a possible application for these chips.

Measurements of the expression of thousands of genes in a single experiment, revealing many new, potentially important cancer genes, have become possible with techniques such as serial analysis of gene expression and cDNA microarrays. These genome screening tools are capable of analyzing one tumor at a time. However, there is often a need to have techniques to survey hundreds of specimens from patients in different stages of disease in order to establish the diagnostic, prognostic, and therapeutic importance of each of the emerging cancer gene candidates. To facilitate rapid screening for molecular alterations in many different malignancies, a tissue microarray consisting of samples from 17 different tumor types was generated. Altogether, 397 individual tumors—such as breast, colon, kidney, lung, ovary, bladder, colon, stomach, testis, head and neck, and endometrial cancer, as well as in melanoma—were arrayed in a single paraffin block. The results confirmed and even extend existing data in the literature for the amplification of three extensively studied oncogenes, CCND1, CMYC, and ERBB2.[111]

A high-throughput microarray technique that facilitates gene expression and copy-number surveys of very large numbers of tumors has been developed.[15] This technique can analyze as many as 1000 cylindrical tissue biopsies from individual tumors distributed in a single tumor tissue microarray. Sections of the microarray provide targets for parallel in situ detection of DNA, RNA, and protein targets in each specimen on the array, and consecutive sections allow the rapid analysis of hundreds of molecular markers in the same set of specimens. Detection of six gene amplifications as well as *p53* and estrogen receptor expression in breast cancer demonstrates the usefulness and potential of this method for identifying new subgroups of tumors.

Gene amplifications and deletions have often been associated with pathogenetic roles in cancer. Thirty thousand radiation-hybrid-mapped cDNAs provide a genomic resource to map these lesions with high resolution. Researchers report the development of a multiplex assay to detect small deletions and insertions by using a modified PCR to evenly amplify each amplicon (PCR/PCR), followed by ligase detection reaction (LDR).[112] This study demonstrates that microarray analysis of PCR/PCR/LDR2 products permits rapid identification of small insertion and deletion mutations in the context of both clinical diagnosis and population studies.

Another group of researchers have developed a cDNA microarray-based comparative genomic hybridization (CGH) method for analyzing DNA copy-number changes across thousands of genes simultaneously.[26] With this procedure, DNA copy-number alterations of twofold or less could be reliably detected. The researchers have mapped regions of DNA copy-number variation at high resolution in breast cancer cell lines, revealing previously unrecognized genomic amplifications and deletions and new complexities of amplicon structure. They have also identified recurrent regions of DNA amplification, which may harbor novel oncogenes, and performed comparison and correlations of alterations of DNA copy number and gene expression in parallel analyses. For breast tumors, DNA copy-number information is being compared and correlated with data already collected on *p53* status, microarray gene expression profiles, and treatment response and clinical outcome. Genome-wide DNA copy-number information on a set of 9 breast cancer cell lines and over 35 primary breast tumors has been collected in the study.

3.5.3 Pharmacogenomics and Drug Discovery

High-throughput microarray and biochip technologies have generated increasing interest in the field of pharmacogenomics, which is aimed at finding correlations between therapeutic responses to drugs and the genetic profiles of patients. It is hoped that the discovery of genetic variances that affect drug action will lead to the development of new diagnostic procedures and therapeutic products that enable drugs to be prescribed selectively to patients for whom they will be effective and safe. Many people die each year from adverse responses to medications that are beneficial to others. Others experience serious reactions or fail to respond at all. DNA variants in genes involved in drug metabolism, particularly the cyto-chrome *P450* multigene family, are the focus of much current research in this area. Enzymes encoded by these genes are responsible for metabolizing most drugs, and their function affects patients' responses to both the drug and the dose. Within the next decade, researchers will begin to correlate DNA variants with individual responses to medical treatments, identify particular subgroups of patients, and develop drugs customized for those populations. This *customized medicine* approach has now come to be recognized as a significant commercial opportunity for genomics.[17]

A number of attempts are ongoing to treat cystic fibrosis, a lethal recessive disease affecting children in the United States and Europe, either by gene therapy or pharmacotherapy. Recently, cDNA array technology was used in a cystic fibrosis study of human cells concerned with global gene expression and drug effects.[113] The results provided useful pharmacogenomic information with significant relevance to both gene and pharmacological therapy. The functional similarity and specificity of different purine analogues have been determined by comparing the expression profiles of their genome-wide effects on treated yeast, murine, and human cells. Purine libraries have also been shown to be useful tools for analyzing a variety of signaling and regulatory pathways and may lead to the development of new therapeutics.[114]

A method for drug target validation and identification of secondary drug target effects based on genome-wide gene expression patterns using DNA biochip microarrays has been demonstrated in several experiments, which included treatment of mutant yeast strains defective in calcineurin, immunophilins, or other genes with the immunosuppressants cyclosporin A or FK506.[115] The described method permits the direct confirmation of drug targets and recognition of drug-dependent changes in gene expression that are modulated through pathways distinct from the drug's intended target. Such a method may prove useful in improving the efficiency of drug development programs.

The molecular mechanisms underlying the progression of prostate cancer during hormonal therapy have remained poorly understood. A study of hormone therapy for prostate cancer developed a new strategy, using of a combination of cDNA and tissue microarray technologies, for the identification of differentially expressed genes in hormone-refractory human prostate cancer.[116]

Microarray and biochip technologies in conjunction with genomic data and bioinformatics are expected to make drug development faster, cheaper, and more effective. Most drugs today are based on about 500 molecular targets; genomic research on the genes involved in diseases, disease pathways, and drug-response sites will lead to the discovery of thousands of new targets.

3.5.4 Toxicogenomics

The availability of genome-scale DNA sequence information and reagents has led to the development of a new scientific subdiscipline combining the fields of toxicology and genomics.[23] This subdiscipline, often referred to as toxicogenomics, involves the study of how genomes respond to environmental stressors or toxicants.[117] Toxicogenomics combines genome-wide mRNA expression profiling with protein expression patterns using bioinformatics to understand the role of gene–environment interactions in disease and dysfunction. The goal of toxicogenomics is to find correlations between toxic responses to toxicants and changes in the genetic profiles of the objects exposed to such toxicants. For these applications, DNA microarray and biochip technologies, which allow the monitoring of the expression levels of thousands of genes simultaneously, provide an important analytical tool.[27] A general method by which gene expression, as measured by cDNA microarrays, can be used as a highly sensitive and informative marker for toxicity has been described.[23]

Arrays containing ESTs for xenobiotic metabolizing enzymes, proteins associated with glutathione regulation, DNA repair enzymes, heat shock proteins, and housekeeping genes were used to examine gene expression in response to β-naphthoflavone (β-NF) with results comparable to those of northern blotting analysis.[118]

3.5.5 Genetic Screening of Diseases

An important area of DNA biochip application involves screening genetic diseases. Gene tests can be used to diagnose disease, confirm a diagnosis, provide prognostic information about the course of disease, confirm the existence of a disease, and, potentially, predict the risk of future disease in healthy individuals or their progeny. Currently, several hundred genetic tests are in clinical use, with many more under development. Most current tests detect mutations associated with rare genetic disorders that follow Mendelian inheritance patterns. These diseases include myotonic and Duchenne muscular dystrophies, cystic fibrosis, neurofibromatosis type 1, sickle cell anemia, and Huntington's disease.

These screening procedures are often performed prenatally. DNA biochip technology could be a sensitive tool for the prenatal detection of genetic disorders. Newborn blood cards provide high-quality DNA samples that can reliably support highly multiplexed PCRs. In a single assay, a DNA microarray facilitates the codetection of amplification products diagnostic for several genetic diseases. Initial data utilizing the model systems of sickle cell disease, an autosomal recessive condition caused by a single amino acid substitution in the β-globin protein, have been reported.[119]

Genetic alterations and abnormalities could lead to uncontrolled cell division and metastasis, resulting ultimately in cancer. Genetic studies have identified a number of genes that must mutate in order to induce cancer or promote the growth of malignant cells. For example, mutations in *BRCA1*, a gene on chromosome 17, have been found to be related to breast cancer. A high percentage of women with a mutated *BRCA1* gene will develop breast cancer or have an increase in ovarian cancer. A second breast cancer gene, *BRCA2*, is located in chromosome 13. Another important gene associated with cancer is the *p53* gene, which encodes a nuclear protein that serves as a transcription factor. The *p53* gene is a tumor suppressor gene that regulates passage of the cell from the G1 into the S phase in the cell cycle. Mutations of *p53* have been associated with a wide variety of cancers, including colon, lung, breast, and bladder cancers. DNA biochips are available for the analysis of human genes, including *BRCA1*, *BRCA2*, *p53*, and *P450*.

Information on genetic abnormalities that are characteristic of certain tumor types or stages of tumor progression is provided by the rapidly expanding database of CGH publications, which already covers about 1500 tumors. CGH data have led to the discovery of six new gene amplifications, as well as a locus for a cancer-predisposition syndrome. The approach based on CGH has now been established as a first-line screening procedure for cancer researchers and will serve as a basis for ongoing efforts to develop the next-generation genome scanning techniques, such as high-resolution microarray technology.[120] Recent microarray studies have involved identification of genes involved in the development or progression of ovarian cancer,[121,122] prostate cancer,[90,123,124] breast cancer,[125] renal cell carcinoma,[104] and urinary bladder cancer.[126]

With the availability of sequence data on the human genome, it is expected that biochips will soon be used for a wide variety of other genetic tests. The use of DNA microarrays has been suggested for evaluating renal function and disease,[127] analysis of gene expression in multiple sclerosis lesions,[128] and quantitative histological analysis of Alzheimer's disease.[129]

3.5.6 Pathogen Detection

Another important application of miniaturized biochip devices involves the detection of biological pathogens (e.g., bacteria and viruses) present in the environment, at occupational sites such as hospitals and offices or in public places. To achieve the required level of sensitivity and specificity in detection, it is often necessary to use a device that is capable of identifying and differentiating a large number of biochemical constituents in complex environmental samples. DNA biochip technologies could offer a unique combination of performance capabilities and analytical features of merit not available in any other current bioanalytical system. Biochip devices that combine automated sample collection systems and multichannel sensing capability will allow simultaneous detection of multiple pathogens present in complex environmental samples. In this application, the biochip technology could provide an important tool to warn off exposure to pathogenic agents for use in human health protection and disease prevention.

The list of expected biochip applications could include biochips for diagnosis of infectious diseases such as HIV. Nucleic acid arrays have been constructed for many different organisms and have been successfully employed in a host of different experiments.[130–134] In an investigation to obtain a more comprehensive view of the global effects of HIV infection of CD4-positive T cells at the mRNA level, cDNA microarray analysis was performed on approximately 1500 cellular cDNAs at 2 and 3 days postinfection (p.i.) with HIV-1. Host cell gene expression changed little at 2 days p.i., but at 3 days p.i., 20 cellular genes were identified as differentially expressed. Genes involved in T cell signaling, subcellular trafficking, and transcriptional regulation, as well as several uncharacterized genes, were among those whose mRNAs were differentially regulated.[135]

Current applications of microarray research involve complete profiling of the genomic sequences of microbial pathogens and hosts. Such studies will ultimately lead to sophisticated new strategies for studying host–pathogen interactions.[136] One such study looked at *Pseudomonas aeruginosa*, an opportunistic pathogen that plays a major role in lung function deterioration in cystic fibrosis patients. To identify critical host responses during infection, the investigators used high-density DNA microarrays, consisting of 1506 human cDNA clones, to monitor gene expression in the *A549* lung pneumocyte cell line during exposure to *P. aeruginosa*. Identification of differentially regulated genes was analyzed by expression microarray analysis of human cDNAs.[137]

Bacillus Calmette–Guerin (BCG) vaccines are live attenuated strains of *Mycobacterium bovis* administered to prevent tuberculosis. To provide for rational approaches to the design of improved diagnostics and vaccines and better understand the differences between *M. tuberculosis*, *M. bovis*, and the various BCG daughter strains, researchers studied their genomic compositions by performing comparative hybridization experiments on a DNA microarray.[138]

3.5.7 Rapid Clinical Diagnosis

In general, because high-density microarray technologies involve relatively expensive and bulky detection systems, they are useful for laboratory applications but are not appropriate for clinical use in the physician's office. On the other hand, integrated biochip systems, having medium-density arrays (10–100 probes) and a miniaturized detection microchip, are most appropriate for medical diagnostics at the point of care, that is, the physician's office. Recently, an integrated biochip device with a 16-photodiode array was developed and evaluated for the detection of HIV-1 gene fragments.[5,6] This integrated, portable system, described in Section 3.4, is an illustration of the usefulness of the DNA biochip for detection of a specific HIV gene sequence. Actual detection of HIV viruses will require simultaneous detection of multiple gene sequence regions of the viruses. It has been observed that progression of the AIDS disease causes an increase in the genotype diversity in HIV viruses. HIV viruses appear to defeat the immune system by producing and accumulating these gene mutations as the disease progresses. In this study, a specific DNA sequence fragment was used as the model system for a feasibility demonstration. Other sequence fragments of HIV viruses or other pathogens of medical interest, such as the *M. tuberculosis* bacterium or the *p53* cancer gene, have been used on the same biochip.[5–8]

As noted earlier, biosensors and biochips usually employ only one type of bioreceptor as probes, that is, either nucleic acid or antibody probes. Biochips with DNA probes are often called gene chips, and biochips with antibody probes are often called protein chips. An integrated DNA biochip that uses multiple bioreceptors with different functionalities on the same biochip, allowing simultaneous detection of several types of biotargets on a single platform, has been developed.[9–11] This device is referred to as the MFB.

The unique feature of the MFB is its capability to perform different types of bioassay on a single platform using DNA and antibody probes simultaneously. Figure 3.9 illustrates the detection of

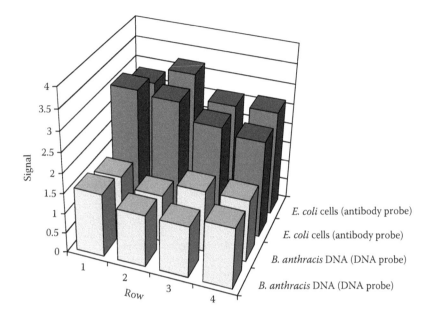

FIGURE 3.9 Detection of *E. coli* and *B. anthracis* using the MFB system. Two rows of the biochip were used for the detection of 1×10^6 *E. coli* cells via Cy5-labeled antibody probes, while the other two rows were used for the detection of the 41.2 pmol *B. anthracis* using Cy5-labeled DNA probes.

Escherichia coli and *Bacillus anthracis* with the MFB system. Each signal bar of the graph represents the signal acquired with an individual detection element of the 4×4 photosensor array.[9] Sensing arrays on half the biochip show the detection of 1×10^6 *E. coli* cells via Cy5-labeled antibody probes, while the other half detected the 41.2 pmol *B. anthracis* gene fragment via Cy5-labeled DNA probes. Hybridization of a nucleic acid probe to DNA biotargets (e.g., gene sequences, bacteria, viral DNA) offers a very high degree of accuracy for identifying DNA sequences complementary to that of the probe. In addition, the MFB's antibody probes take advantage of the specificity of immunological recognition. Figures 3.10 and 3.11 demonstrate the quantitative capability of the biochip in monitoring the immobilization of various biomolecules of medical and environmental interest. Figure 3.10 shows a calibration curve for the detection of a segment of the Bac 816 gene of *B. anthracis* through

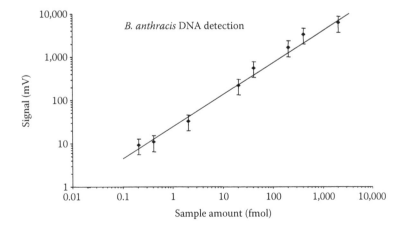

FIGURE 3.10 Calibration curve for the detection of *B. anthracis* using DNA probes.

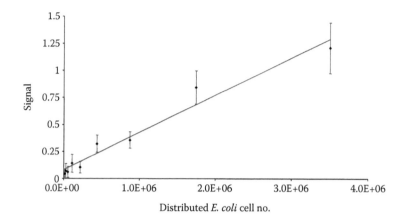

FIGURE 3.11   Calibration curve for the detection of *E. coli* using antibody probes.

hybridization of a Cy5-labeled DNA probe. Figure 3.11 shows a calibration curve for the detection of immobilized *E. coli* 157:H7. In contrast to the *B. anthracis* study described earlier, this screening method involved antibody/antigen interaction, analogous to the western blot assay. This study demonstrates the feasibility of the MFB for the detection of multiple biotargets of different functionality (DNA, proteins, etc.) on a single biochip platform.

3.5.8 Microparticle/Nanoparticle Applications for Biochips

The recent developments in production and utilization of particles with micro- and nanoscale dimensions have resulted in interesting applications of such materials to biochips. Use of these micro-/nano-sized particles can produce large increases in surface area available for biomolecule loading, powerful increases in detection capability (e.g., quantum dot labeling, plasmonics-based nanoprobes), and novel applications of synthetic nanoparticles for biobased assay development. We provide some representative developments in this section.

Sung et al.[139] discuss the use of polystyrene nanobeads to coat a cyclic olefin copolymer (COC) plastic surface. The use of these beads increases dramatically the surface area available for immobilization of capture antibodies, thus enhancing sensitivity of immunoassays on solid surfaces, such as biochips. Importantly, the authors first coat the cyclic olefin substrate with an amphiphilic copolymer consisting of benzyl, polyethylene glycol (PEG), and reactive ester moieties, to produce a hydrophilic surface on the hydrophobic olefin solid surface to which the nanobeads are attached. Benefits of the large increase in capture antibody surface density included a wide dynamic range for analyte detection, high specificity, and a 100-fold increase in sensitivity compared to a conventional enzyme-linked immunosorbent assay (ELISA). Sung et al. pointed out that the use of PEG in the copolymer layer results in less nonspecific protein absorption and hence helps alleviate biofouling. Also of interest, these workers found that the nanobeads formed multilayers on the copolymer surface, instead of a monolayer, which was initially expected.

Roh et al.[140] applied quantum dot-labeled RNA oligonucleotides to the detection of a hepatitis C-associated viral protein using a biochip. This assay would presumably be a diagnostic for hepatitis C virus (HCV) infection. Currently, HCV infection is diagnosed by the detection of anti-HCV antibodies using an ELISA immunoassay. The ELISA sometimes generates false positives or false negatives and does not detect HCV infection at early stages, before antibody production in response to infection occurs. In the experiments described in Roh et al., an HCV nonstructural protein 5B, which is a viral RNA-dependent RNA polymerase, is immobilized on the surface of the biochip, and RNA oligonucleotides, conjugated to the surface of quantum dots, are then allowed to interact with the protein-coated surface. The immobilized protein recognizes and binds the RNA oligonucleotide, and in turn, the quantum dot is immobilized, producing the detection signal. The authors note a linear relationship between protein concentration and range from 1 μg/mL to 1 ng/mL, with a detection limit of 1 ng/mL.

A technology involving magnetic nanoparticles and using a magnetoresistive biochip that carries out biorecognition assays by detection of magnetically labeled targets is described by Germano et al.[141] and applied for the detection of nucleic acids.[142] The magnetoresistive biochips appeared to offer higher sensitivity, increased portability, and lower costs compared to biochips using standard florescence detection techniques. The experimental procedure is applicable to both nucleic acids and cells (bacteria). In the example used by Germano et al., a DNA oligonucleotide, serving as a capture probe, is immobilized on a biochip surface. The target DNA analyte, previously labeled with magnetic particles (MP; nanoparticles of 250 nm diameter), is then microfluidically added and binds to the immobilized capture probe because of base complementarity. Upon application of an external magnetic field, the fringe field produced by the immobilized magnetic particles is detected by a sensor and the electrical resistance observed is related to the number of biomolecules captured by the capture probes. The system was able to detect the 250 nm magnetic particles at a concentration of 41 fM.

Martins et al.[142] used the same magnetoresistive sensing system but did work to optimize biofunctionalization of the biochip, as well as reducing nonspecific absorption of magnetic particles to the sensing surface. A thiol–gold surface chemistry was used to attach the capture DNA oligonucleotide probes to the cleaned gold surface of the biochip. A blocking solution of PEG-SH of 3 kDa was found to be more effective than bovine serum albumin (BSA), in terms of reducing nonspecific binding of magnetic particles. The protocol for assay involved incubation of the biotinylated target probe with the immobilized capture probe to allow hybridization, followed by incubation with streptavidin-labeled magnetic particles, washing, and subsequent readout. Limit of detection was found to be around 1 pM with a working concentration range between 10 nM to low pM levels. Additional improvements to the functional biochip involved fine-tuning of the microfluidic system and use of a magnetic focusing system. There is a need to label the target DNA with biotin, so as to allow capture of the streptavidin-labeled MP. The system was only tested using analyte prepared in buffer solutions; the efficiency of analysis in physiologic solutions is thus not known.

Huang et al.[143] devised a scheme for detecting bacteria (*Salmonella* or *E. coli*) using gold nanospheres (25–35 nm diameter) that were coated with specific antibodies for the bacteria to capture the bacteria from samples. Following capture, the nanosphere-conjugated bacteria could be collected by dielectrophoretic forces and enumerated by impedance measurements on a biochip substrate that contained interlaced comb-like electrodes. The device described is not a self-contained system as microfluidics is not integrated into the detection platform. Quantification is demonstrated using several different concentrations of bacteria.

3.5.9 Cell-Based Biochips

Several investigators have extrapolated the concept of immobilization of biomolecules on biochips for medical diagnostics, etc., to the actual use of whole cells immobilized on a biochip-like surface. Advantages associated with use of whole cells include the vastly more complex biochemistry of the intact cell, thus providing a *snapshot* of potentially the whole organism's response to medicinal drugs, toxins, and pollutants, as well as an integrating aspect to each analyte being tested. Disadvantages include difficulty in interpreting results from whole cell assays, as such results could reflect cascades of signaling and metabolic activities within the cell, making deductions about cause and effect difficult to perform. An even more immediate problem is the issue of culturing cells, that is, keeping them viable and metabolically stable on the biochip platform. Nevertheless, it seems in the future that whole cells will command more and more attention as possible detection elements in specific biochip applications.

Hu et al.[144] presented a mammalian whole cell-based biosensor for in vitro drug analysis, which uses a light-addressable potentiometric sensor (LAPS) and an electrical cell-substrate impedance sensor (ECIS) to monitor cell growth status and cell energy metabolism status in real time. The cell growth status is monitored by ECIS, which provides data corresponding to cell number, adhesion, and morphology, while the LAPS monitors extracellular pH, thus providing evidence of cell metabolic status. Neonatal SD rat renal cells were used in the described experiments. The cell-based sensor's use is demonstrated with the anticancer drug doxorubicin. Regarding the control of medium flow to the cellular sensor, the authors indicated that a low buffer capacity in the culture medium was required so that the sensor system could be enabled to detect small pH changes.

Baxter[145] discussed the use of an interactive, cell-based microfluidic biochip called a Hurel™, which is designed to have living cells segregated into discrete compartments, so that a more realistic mimic of the in vivo situation can be attained, compared to usual in vitro cell culture. As an example, Baxter shows a four-organ component device, in which liver cells metabolize xenobiotics, lung cells (for example) provide a target tissue, adipocytes provide a site for bioaccumulation of hydrophobic chemicals, and an *other tissue* compartment assists in mimicking the whole organism. All cell/organ compartments are connected by the microfluidic system, which mimics the blood circulation. Baxter presents experimental results in which, by use of a chemotherapy drug (tegafur) requiring metabolic activation, the Hurel device provides metabolic activation (by liver cells) and detects subsequent cytotoxicity to target cells. On the other hand, if the target cells are cultured in static culture outside the Hurel device with the prodrug, no cytotoxic effect is observed. The Hurel device thus performs a dynamic assessment of potential toxicity, metabolism, and bioavailability of candidate chemicals. Other results are reported.

Curtis et al.[146] described a cell-based biosensor for field testing of drinking water samples, to evaluate the samples for presence of possible toxicants. In this device, which is already commercialized, long-term (9 days to more than a month) culture of mammalian cells on a biochip surface is accomplished by use of a compact self-contained media circulation and disposal system. Toxic effects on the cells in the biochip are assessed by the use of an electric detection system, that is, cell-substrate impedance sensing technology. Impedance measurements are compared between microchannels containing cells immersed in only media versus microchannels where cells are exposed to water samples. Endothelial cells are used as the cellular sensors, because they organize in vitro to form a restrictive barrier under normal conditions. Thus, electrical resistance of endothelial cell monolayers can provide quantitative information regarding changes in cell morphology, cell movements, and changes in cell function. Results are shown where various toxicants are spiked into water samples.

One approach to using in vitro cell cultures to simulate, at least in some sense, the complex interactions of in vivo systems is to use different types of cells in culture to mimic metabolic activity of differing cell types upon an analyte, such as the Hurel device (Baxter[145]) discussed earlier. Another approach, probably more direct, is to use actual tissue slices, composed of differing cell types, to metabolize analytes in a more or less exact replica of the same tissue in the whole organism. Tissue slices, however, present a whole set of complications, probably chiefly with respect to insuring that the cells in the slices are adequately perfused to maintain viability. Van Midwoud et al.[147] addressed this issue by developing a microfluidic biochip that was designed to provide a highly controlled environment in which rat liver slices could be kept fully functional for at least 24 h. Liver slices were chosen because the liver is the organ directly involved in initial metabolism of various drugs and environmental toxicants. Precision-cut liver slices were incubated in 25 µL microchambers, under conditions of constant medium flow (10 µL/min). There was complete change of the medium every 2.5 min in the microchamber using the microfluidic system. The suffusion of the liver slices by the medium is termed *perifusion*, rather than perfusion, since the medium flows around the tissue slice, rather than through it. Studies of leakage of lactate dehydrogenase (LDH) from the cells in the slice indicated a low percentage of leakage, indicating good cell viability. Tests with a model compound, 7-ethoxycoumarin, showed that metabolism of this compound by liver slices correlated well with the in vivo situation. Although the design of the liver slice biochip was rather complex, this approach does offer the potential for drug and toxicant kinetic studies that are likely to provide data of direct relevance to intact liver function.

The previous studies discussed in this section used mammalian cells (sometimes human cells) as the detector organisms in biochip assay devices. Kwon et al.[148] demonstrate a very novel microorganism manipulation technique, which is targeted to such microbes as viruses, bacteria, and fungi. These micro-organisms could also be used in biochip applications, to assess concentration and biological activity of various chemicals or bioactive molecules. The emphasis in the article by Kwon et al. is, however, on the development of methods for aggregating, patterning, translation (i.e., directed movement), and size-based separation of populations of single or mixed microorganisms. The basis of the technique, which is called rapid electrokinetic patterning (REP), is to rapidly and dynamically move and assemble microparticles onto an electrode surface by applying laser illumination to the electrode surface biased also with a uniform AC electric field. The theory of this technique is discussed in the article. Kwon et al. demonstrate that REP can be used to manipulate microorganisms and that the technique is also biocompatible. Microorganisms used in the demonstration included *Shewanella oneidensis* MR-1, *Sa. cerevisiae*, and *Staphylococcus aureus*. The authors demonstrate aggregation and translation of *Sh. oneidensis* MR-1 by the REP technique, and no evidence of cell death was seen. REP was also applied to showing size-based separation of microorganisms. In this case, *S. aureus* and *Sa. cerevisiae* were successfully separated by changing the AC frequency, although the separation was not 100% efficient.

3.5.10 New Advances in Biochip Techniques and Applications

Zhu et al.[149] developed a biochip device that can be used for rapid (6 h analysis time) identification of mycobacterial species from either sputum samples or culture isolates. Not only is accurate and sensitive identification of mycobacterial species of importance for tuberculosis diagnosis, but the incidence of opportunistic infections by nontuberculous mycobacteria has shown a gradual increase. Furthermore, the slow growth of mycobacteria can result in ambiguous results standard diagnostic methods, which can take 4–8 weeks to complete. The biochip identified 17 common mycobacterial strains simultaneously by assessing differences in the diagnostic sequences of 16S ribosomal RNA of the different species. The complete system included the biochip itself, sample preparation apparatus, hybridization device, chip washing machine, and laser confocal scanner. However, this total instrumentation appeared to be assembled from individual components and was not a fully integrated one-use dedicated device. Oligonucleotide probes specific for the various species were immobilized on the glass surface of the biochip. PCR was used to amplify and fluorescently label the diagnostic sequences of each of the strains to be assayed. Hybridization was carried out on-chip. Limits of detection, reproducibility studies, and specificity studies were carried out. The concordance rate between the biochip assay results and species diagnosis by direct DNA sequencing was 100%.

Javanmard et al.[150] describe an interesting system that could be eventually used for high-throughput, multiplex analysis and that does not use a standard 2D array common to many biochip schemes. In their case, the heart of the detection system is a protein-functionalized microchannel with integrated electrodes. Microspheres (of comparable size to the microchannel geometry) decorated with receptors that specifically bind analyte molecules are first reacted with the analyte of interest, and the microspheres are then introduced into the microchannel, which has, immobilized upon its surface, other receptors also specific for the analyte. The functionalized area of the microchannel is bounded by two electrodes. The microspheres immobilized, via specific binding of analyte/receptor, to the surface of the microchannel produce a change in resistance of the solution in the microchannel as current is passed between the two electrodes, and this resistance change is proportional to the concentration of the analyte. Javanmard et al. demonstrated the functionality of this approach using antibodies as receptors to detect the presence of anti–human chorionic gonadotropin (hCG) antibody in PBS. The anti-hCG antibody was from rabbits, and therefore, the antibody bound to the 10 μm microspheres was anti–rabbit IgG. Anti–rabbit IgG was also used to coat the microchannel surface, and unreacted sites on the microchannel surface were blocked with BSA. The microspheres were incubated with the anti-hCG antibody for 45 min and subsequently introduced into the microchannel. Specific binding of the microspheres to the microchannel was found to occur in less than 1 min, and after washing with buffer, the electrical impedance was measured. Results with this system indicated a detection limit, for the anti-hCG antibody, of 1 ng/mL, with a dynamic range of three orders of magnitude, and an analysis time of less than 1 h. Anti-hCG antibody is a biomarker useful in diagnosing infertility in women if present in the serum at concentrations higher than 35 ng/mL, so the assay as described could have clinical relevance, although the authors point out that the protein chosen was for demonstration purposes, and the technique has general relevance.

Pernagallo et al.[151] described a biochip platform, which takes advantage of two previously developed technologies. One technology is a silicon-based microelectromechanical system developed by STMicroelectronics as part of their *In-Check* platform. This device provides microfluidic handling, miniaturized PCR reactor, and a nucleic acid microarray detection module, all in a compact benchtop footprint. The second technology is called Chem-NAT, which has been commercialized by DestiNA Genomics. This technology uses what the developers call dynamic chemistry to essentially produce probes that recognize specific nucleic acid sequences and also contain an *abasic* position, which can be filled with a fluorescently labeled aldehyde-modified nucleobase. One claimed advantage of the Chem-NAT system is that false positives are almost impossible to obtain, as the nucleobase incorporation can only take place in the presence of target templating strands. The authors tested the hybrid system by detecting a small RNA based on micro-RNA 122 or a small fragment of the mengo virus RNA. The DestiNA probe is configured such that it can be tethered to the lab-on-a-chip platform via amino-terminated PEGylated spacer. The other end of the probe has a complementary sequence to the target nucleic acid, but with one *blank* site in the sequence. Upon hybridization of the probe and target strands, this so-called chemical pocket is filled by reaction with a fluorescein-labeled aldehyde nucleoside, which is subsequently detected. Importantly, this incorporation of the labeled base can take place only when the probe and target strands form a perfect complementary duplex. The silicon-based platform was blocked with dimethylamine, to prevent nonspecific binding of the fluorophore-tagged base. Results indicated low background, with specificity shown toward the appropriate targets.

Kraus et al.[152] described the construction and application of a biochip designed to detect quantitatively the presence of HCV antibodies in human blood or serum. In this device, HCV core protein is immobilized on the microfluidic chip, which serves to capture HCV antibodies, if present, in the serum of patients suspected of having HCV infection. An ELISA antibody sandwich assay is carried out, with enzymatic amplification of the detection event, and the readout employs gold electrode arrays. Good sensitivity was found, and assay time was 20 min. The analysis could be done in whole blood, with no increase in background or loss of sensitivity.

Marcy et al.[153] developed a device, called a live hybridization machine (LHM), which integrates a real-time fluorescence reader with a hybridization/washing station equipped with highly efficient mixing and precise temperature controls. The current generation of microarray devices can detect thousands of DNA sequences immobilized on a small surface area but depends for this detection upon the end point of hybridization. There is no reliable predictor of on-chip hybridization efficiency, because predictions based upon solution-phase hybridizations are not relevant to the solid phase. Therefore, the ability to monitor these hybridization events in real time under adjustable temperature would allow one to quickly optimize conditions for effective hybridization. Using SNPs as a model system, Marcy et al. demonstrated the utility of the LHM to perform experiments, which would not be possible with standard microarrays.

Seefeld et al.[154] discussed the development of a microfluidic biochip to detect DNA and proteins in very small microliter volumes using the technique of SPR imaging. The 4 × 3 microarray of the biochip is constituted of 12 thin film gold spots each in an individually addressable 0.5 μL microchannel. The SPR imaging technique allows the detection of surface absorption events on the gold surface, due to a change in reflectivity upon binding events occurring. Either nucleic acids or proteins can be detected, if suitable capture molecules preattached to the surface are used. In the case of Seefeld et al., ssDNA or ssRNA was attached to the surface of the biochip, allowing the detection of complementary nucleic acids. Protein binding was detected by attaching an aptamer to the biochip surface, which recognized thrombin. Detection of either nucleic acid or protein was extremely fast, on the order of tens of seconds.

Limits of detection were in the range of nM (or fmol absolute amounts, given the small size of the microchannels) for both nucleic acid and protein. With the clever use of an enzymatic amplification step involving RNase H, the investigators were able to detect ssDNA at extremely low levels, that is, with a detection limit of 10 fM or 30 zmol absolute. Incredibly, this highly sensitive assay could be carried out in the neighborhood of 200 s, since the enzymatic amplification detection technique is not limited by diffusion of DNA. The amplification technique basically involves introducing a solution of target ssDNA and RNase H to the microarray, which has immobilized upon it ssRNA molecules with sequence complementary to the target DNA. When the target DNA hybridizes to the immobilized RNA, RNase H hydrolyzes the heteroduplex, thus releasing the RNA from the surface. Also, continued hydrolysis results in digestion of the RNA leaving the target DNA now free to react with another immobilized RNA molecule. Therefore, a very small number of DNA molecules can remove a large percentage of the immobilized RNA, which can be detected by SPR reflectivity.

A novel device for cell lysis and DNA purification prior to PCR amplification of genomic material is presented by Chen et al.[155] Integration of a microfluidic component that features a carefully designed mixing chamber for blending blood and lysing reagent, along with a porous silicon matrix for efficient extraction of released DNA, is featured in the completed device. Two mixing models were compared for efficiency of cell lysis, one a T-type mixing model and the other a sandwich-type mixing model. The sandwich-type mixing module featuring a coiled channel was found to be the better choice. Cell lysis and purification of DNA to a PCR-amplifiable stage can be done in 20 min. Measurements of amount of genomic DNA extracted from 1 µL of whole blood were in the range of 40 ng, considerably higher than could be extracted using a commercial kit. The authors proposed that combining their device with PCR might result in a fully integrated analysis system for genomic studies.

Kim et al.[156] used immobilized aptamers on a glass biochip surface as a device to specifically and sensitively capture tumor cells that express certain marker proteins on their cell surfaces. The aptamers were evolved to specifically bind to human epidermal growth factor receptor 2 (HER2) or prostate-specific membrane antigen (PSMA), and the biochips were tested against cell lines that expressed these proteins to various levels. The aptamers were found to be equivalent or superior to antibodies in terms of specificity and sensitivity. The detection limit for the PSMA sensor was found to be $\sim10^3$ cells, for the human prostate cancer cell line, LNCaP. One of the more unique aspects of this work is the fact that the biochip could be denatured and reused many times, although the regeneration process did involve reestablishing the chemistry binding the aptamer to the biochip surface.

Fang et al.[157] presented an interesting concept for an integrated biochip in which electrochemistry is used for detection of isothermal DNA amplification. The authors stated that isothermal DNA amplification has greater amplification efficiency and gives higher DNA yields, because of the uninterrupted and sustained amplifying enzyme activity. Among the advantages of their design are the facts that only a simple heater is needed (no thermal cycling), there is no immobilization of capture DNA molecules on the electrode surfaces, and the use of interdigitated electrodes increases the sensitivity of the assay substantially. In their system, microwells between the interdigitated electrodes are filled with analyte solution, which has target DNA strands, enzymes, and deoxynucleotide triphosphates (dNTPs), all of which contribute to the capacitance of the solution. During amplification, accumulation of DNA strands and particularly depletion of the dNTPs lead to changes of the conductance of the solution, which is the parameter measured. Using this concept, there is no need for probe labeling or immobilization of capture biomolecules. The authors used strand displacement amplification and rolling circle amplification for isothermal amplification techniques. The target DNA used in demonstrating the use of the described biochip was a segment (nesda T) of the epidermal growth factor gene, but the size of this fragment was not given. In the case of strand displacement amplification, starting concentrations of DNA of 1 or 10 nM could be distinguished from a negative control, while for rolling circle amplification, the concentration of the DNA detected was not given. The authors pointed out that a further advantage of their system is the potential for real-time detection, as the change in impedance can be detected in less than 15 min for the 1 nM DNA sample.

Wen et al.[158] presented a biochip system that uses plastic biochips and colorimetric detection. The advantages of such a system in terms of point-of-care diagnostics are low cost, disposability, and ease of fabrication and modification. Wen et al. used polycarbonate sheets (from CDs) as the substrate, and the assay format is a typical sandwich assay, in which capture probes bind the analyte, and in turn, reporter probes bind to the analyte. In this scheme, the reporter probes are biotinylated, and subsequent to the reporter binding event, gold nanoparticle-labeled streptavidin reacts with the reporter, and finally, the immobilized complex is stained with silver staining solution. The colorimetric readout of the assay can be imaged on a conventional flatbed scanner. The authors found that operating in the transmission mode was best for imaging the biochip. The procedure is demonstrated for both an immunoassay (IgG) and a DNA oligonucleotide. The detection limit for the DNA analyte was stated to be 10 nM, while the detection limit for IgG was ≤0.1 μg/mL if the silver staining time was prolonged. Wen et al. contrasted optical imaging outputs using their assay technique with an enzyme-catalyzed reaction giving a colored precipitate and with a fluorescence labeling technique. In each case, the assay was carried out in the immunoassay procedure, using human IgG as the target antigen, and all assays were carried out on the plastic biochip. The results demonstrated greater sensitivity for the silver staining procedure than for the other two detection techniques.

Some recent studies that assayed for a variety of analytes have used as their basis the *Evidence Investigator* analyzer (Randox Laboratories, Crumlin, United Kingdom), a high-throughput automated analyzer that employs a biochip array as the substrate upon which analysis takes place. The integrated system is described in some detail in the article by Fitzgerald et al.[159] In this article, Fitzgerald and coauthors discuss, in considerable detail, the issue of optimizing immobilization of ligands on a biochip surface and the related issue of denaturation of antibodies immobilized upon such a surface. The solid substrate chosen by these investigators is aluminum oxide, which is then treated with a silanation process prior to additional reactions with a bifunctional linker. A variety of surface chemistry modifications are described, and the resulting surfaces were analyzed by x-ray photoelectron spectroscopy and secondary ion mass spectrometry. Contact-angle measurements of water droplets on the biochip surface were done to assess the hydrophobicity of the various surfaces produced. Details can be found in Fitzgerald et al. The most hydrophobic surface was produced by treating the substrate with a proprietary polymer, as assessed by contact-angle measurements, while the most hydrophilic surface was the aluminum oxide substrate itself, and the second most hydrophilic was obtained by treatment with only 3-glycidoxypropyltrimethoxysilane (GOPTS). The authors assessed the effects of various surface activation techniques using two differing assay systems. In one, a typical immunoassay sandwich technique was used, in which capture antibody was immobilized on the activated surface, and various cytokines served as the analytes, which were detected by binding of a detector antibody with attached horse radish peroxidase (HRP), which was coupled to a chemiluminescence detection scheme. The other assay involved a competitive assay for drugs of abuse, in which unlabeled drug and HRP-labeled drug competed for immobilized antibody sites. Interestingly, the results obtained indicated that the proprietary polymer (the most hydrophobic activated surface) was optimal for the cytokine sandwich assay, while the GOPTS surface was better for the competitive assay for drugs of abuse. The authors point out that surface chemistry is obviously of great importance for ligand attachment, analyte binding, and final assay output for biochip systems. Fitzgerald et al. also discuss the mechanics of the automated device and provide validation numbers for assay performance using the integrated system.

Bunger et al.[160] used the same basic *Evidence Investigator* analyzer to apply biochip technology to colon cancer screening, using sandwich-based immunoassay procedures. Nine protein targets were assayed in blood samples of colorectal cancer patients and controls, and results were analyzed. They were able to show that a panel of serum protein markers (CEA + IL-8 and CEA + CRP; CEA = carcino-embryonic antigen, IL-8 = interleukin 8, CRP = C-reactive protein) had the best screening performance, for colon cancer, with 47% sensitivity; for early carcinomas, with 33% sensitivity; and for adenomas, with 18% sensitivity, at an overall specificity of 86%. In another article using this same biochip system, Porter et al.[161] assayed for the presence of more than 20 anthelmintic drugs in milk and food animal tissue. Anthelmintic drugs are used in veterinary practice to treat for infections caused by parasitic worms. If they are extensively used in food-producing animals, residues of the drugs can be present in animal tissues used for food. Thus, for protection of the consumer, it is important to screen for anthelmintic residues, to be sure they are within acceptable levels. The assay in this case was a competitive immunoassay as described earlier in Fitzgerald et al.[159] The limits of detection found using this biochip assay system were below levels usually set for maximum residue limits, and the advantages of multiplex screening for this many analytes were discussed.

Many researchers have demonstrated successful operation of biochip devices. Very few, however, have shown experimental results where the analyte of interest was successfully detected at relevant concentrations from actual physiological fluids (i.e., blood, in the most common case). The issues of biofouling and nonspecific binding of biomolecules to sensor surfaces can quickly degrade the active surface areas of microsensing chips. In the case of biomarkers for various disease states, the biomarkers are often present in very low levels, at least in the early stages of the disease, when it might be most important to make a definitive diagnosis. Thus, the analyst would ideally like a biochip system that is highly sensitive and able to deal effectively with samples in whole blood. In addition, the oft-invoked requirement for labeling (usually with fluorescent dyes) adds additional complication and time to the assay procedure. Label-free sensing technologies could be added to the *wish list* for ideal biomolecule detection.

Stern et al.[162] propose an ingenious solution to the dilemmas presented earlier. In their system, a two-stage approach is implemented to provide a purification of the desired analytes from whole blood, using a microfluidic purification chip (MPC), which is consecutively followed by specific sensing with a silicon nanoribbon detector. The MPC depends upon the specificity of antigen/antibody reaction to capture the analyte from whole blood, but the capture antibody is bound to the surface via a specific DNA oligonucleotide (a 19 mer), which is, in turn, linked to the actual chip surface with a photolabile cross-linker. After capture of the analyte from whole blood, the resulting sample can be washed extensively, to remove extraneous components, followed by UV irradiation to cleave the cross-linker and release the analyte–antibody complex. This complex then is transferred by microfluidics to the detector nanowire surface, where there are other antibodies that are also specific for the analyte/biomarkers of interest. Thus, the specificity of the assay is greatly increased, as two separate antibodies, recognizing different epitopes, are required to complete a successful detection. A modified ELISA completes the sensing scheme. Here, a biotinylated 19-mer DNA complementary to the DNA oligonucleotide in the purification complex is hybridized to this primary DNA, and streptavidin complexed with HRP is added, to provide enzyme amplification to the positive signal. The authors provide data for two biomarkers, prostate-specific antigen (PSA) and carbohydrate antigen 15.3 (CA15.3, a marker for breast cancer). Studies of the purification efficiency of the MPC indicated a monotonic relationship between the amount of biomarker spiked into the blood samples and the amount released into the pure sensing buffer going to the sensing chip. The yield of purified biomarker from the MPC was in agreement with modeling studies (although data presented in the paper did not show a particularly high yield, the authors point out that capture conditions can be adjusted to significantly increase the capture efficiency). The authors demonstrate detection of PSA at both 2.5 and 2.0 ng/mL (with discrimination between the two concentrations) as well as detection of CA15.3 at 30 and 15 U/mL.

Pedrero et al.[163] provided a fairly recent review of the status of biochip-like devices for detection/identification of foodborne pathogens. The issue of contamination of foods by microbial pathogens is an important public health concern, and the development of rapid, reliable, specific, sensitive, and low-cost methods for detection will be a significant achievement. Biochip development for this purpose is discussed in this article, with focus particularly on electrochemical sensors that use microarray and other types of platforms. The usual methods of detection involve either antibody–antigen (immunochemistry) or DNA hybridization interactions, but other approaches such as the monitoring of oxygen consumption are also discussed.

Nasedkina et al.[164] discussed the use of diagnostic biochips and microarrays in hematologic oncology in a review article. Hematologic malignancies are complex diseases, which involve a variety of genomic alterations, among them, changes in gene expression, chromosomal aberrations, and gene mutations. The authors discuss the use of gene expression profiling using microarrays and applications to malignant lymphoma and leukemias. Also discussed are the use of array-based CGH and the applications of SNP arrays in the diagnosis and study of various hematologic cancers. The authors devote most of the review, however, to a discussion of application of gel-based biochips to clinical uses in hematologic oncology. In the gel-based biochip technology, an array of semispherical gel drops is spotted onto a hydrophobic surface. The gel drops provide a discrete localization for immobilized oligonucleotide probes within the droplets, as well as providing a nanoliter-sized reaction vessel in which such steps as hybridization, PCR amplification, and ligation can take place. The gel monomer is methylacrylamide, which polymerizes into a porous gel. The size of the gel drops can vary from 50 to 600 μm. The immobilized probes (immobilized via an amino group on one end of the probe) are distributed uniformly throughout the gel. Detection of reactions between probe and target is visualized apparently by fluorescence. The authors discussed use of this technology for such applications as (1) analysis of rearranged T cell receptor loci in T lymphocyte populations, of relevance to T cell lymphomas, and (2) polymorphism analysis of drug metabolizing enzymes, which can aid in designing appropriate chemotherapies for individual patients.

3.5.11 Nanomaterial Applications to Biochips

Various investigators have used nanomaterials for biochips, particularly for structural elements that may have certain advantages for either bioassays or in regard to specific detection schemes. In regard to the latter case, some investigators have developed specially structured nanosurfaces that allow the use of surface-enhanced Raman spectroscopy (SERS) for optical detection.[29,52–55]

Wang et al.[165] developed a unique *molecular sentinel-on-chip* (MSC) technology for biosensing using SERS detection. This approach uses the unique *molecular sentinel* (MS) biosensing scheme,[166,167] a label-free detection of the nucleic acid molecules on chips developed on a wafer scale having controlled nanostructures exhibiting plasmonic-active properties. The MS probe consists of a DNA sequence having a middle section (probe section) and two arms, with SERS-active molecule attached to the end of one arm and a metallic nanoparticle attached to the end of the other arm. The middle section contains a sequence complementary to the target sequence to be detected, and two arms have complementary sequences so they can hybridize to form a hairpin loop configuration under normal conditions. In the normal configuration and in the absence of target DNA, the hairpin loop maintains the Raman label in close proximity of the metal nanostructured chip (nanochip) surface, which induces an intense SERS effect producing a strong Raman signal upon laser excitation. The metal nanostructure is used as a signal-enhancing platform for the SERS signal associated with the label. The enhancement is due to the SERS effect from the nanostructured metal surface scattering process (nanoenhancers), which increases the intrinsically weak normal Raman scattering. Upon hybridization of a complementary target DNA sequence to the nanoprobe hairpin DNA, the Raman label is physically separated from the metal nanochip, thus quenching the SERS signal. Wang et al. employed a combination of deep UV lithography, atomic layer deposition, and metal deposition to develop a plasmonic-active substrate based on triangular-shaped nanowire (TNW) arrays having controlled sub-10 nm gap nanostructures over an entire 6 in. wafer. The detection of a nucleic acid sequence of the *Ki-67* gene, a critical breast cancer biomarker, illustrates the usefulness and potential of the MSC technology as a novel biosensing platform on chip substrates.

Yi et al.[168] have developed procedures for fabricating vertically aligned silicon nanowire (SiNW) arrays that are decorated with silver nanoparticles. ssDNA oligonucleotide probes are then immobilized on the silver surface via sulfhydryl groups. Hybridization to cDNA (the analyte) results in a ds structure, which is then discriminated from the ssDNA probe by some differences in the SERS spectra. SEM and TEM images show the successful growth of the vertically aligned arrays, with the silver nanoparticles tending to be more concentrated at the tips of the SiWNs. The SERS spectra were of sufficient quality to allow the differentiation of perfectly matched DNA sequences from partially mismatched sequences.

The approach of these investigators could provide possible solutions to the difficult problem of producing SERS-active substrates, which are highly reproducible. Also, the apparent enhancement factor for the SiNW substrate is reported by the authors to be 10^8–10^{10}.

Strelau et al.[169] developed a chip-based system combined with a microfluidic platform for the detection of specific sequences of DNA using SERS as the detection technology. In this demonstration, capture DNAs (30 bp oligonucleotides) were immobilized to the chip surface, in defined locations, and following washing, the target oligonucleotide, labeled with a SERS-active dye, was washed into the chip using the microfluidic system. Hybridization was facilitated by an embedded thermal management system in the chip, which allowed adjustment of the hybridization temperature. Following hybridization, the active surface of the chip was coated with a solution of silver colloid, which produced, under their experimental conditions, an aggregate of silver nanoparticles. This provided the conditions for SERS enhancement. Results obtained showed that labeled target DNA complementary to the capture DNA produced a strong SERS signal, when the hybridization spot was interrogated by a laser. On the other hand, noncomplementary capture DNA spots did not give a signal distinguishable from areas of the chip where no modifications were made. It is noteworthy that Isola et al.[55] have previously reported a similar SERS-based assay where SERS-labeled oligonucleotides can be used as primers for PCR amplification of target sequences. The capture probe sequences bound onto N-oxysuccinimide-derivatized probes readily hybridize to the amplified product, and the SERS signals can be readily detected by deposition of a silver layer over the hybridized samples.

Bhuvana and Kulkarni[170] describe the conceptualization of nanocrystalline Pd films into a biochip format to which biomolecules could be attached and detected by SERS. The enhancement factor of ~10^5 described by these authors is probably not large enough for sensitive applications, however. Only SERS spectra of various biomolecules on the Pd nanocrystals are presented, and no actual analysis is discussed.

Ali et al.[171] discussed the development of a microfluidic biochip that uses nanostructured nickel oxide to electrochemically detect cholesterol. The NiO sensors are fabricated as nanorods, of approximate dimensions of 5–10 nm diameter and 30–50 nm length. They are embedded in a microchannel of 200 μm width × height, through which the analyte solution flows. Cholesterol esterase and cholesterol oxidase are immobilized on the NiO nanorods and serve as the working electrode. Detection of cholesterol at clinically relevant concentrations was obtained, although the detection was from buffered solutions of cholesterol, not blood samples.

Hong et al.[172] developed a biochip designed to sensitively measure the concentration of the anesthetic propofol using molecularly imprinted nanocavities produced in polymer films. Accurately determining the depth of anesthesia is an important goal in surgical procedures. To detect the concentration of anesthetics such as propofol in blood of patients undergoing surgery is therefore valuable, but to date, analytical techniques such as HPLC or GC-MS in general do not deliver real-time detection. This fact motivated Hong et al. to develop a biochip detection scheme for propofol. Using propofol to imprint the nanocavities formed during the polymerization process, the authors investigated various aspects of the imprinting process. It was found that smaller nanocavities (10–14 nm) had more specificity and sensitivity for detection of the analyte than larger nanocavities. A microfluidic system flowed analyte-containing samples past the molecularly imprinted polymer, and the nanocavities trapped the analyte. Following washing, a color reagent was run through the flow system, which reacted with the analyte, and the resulting color was optically detected and related to concentration. The experimental device developed was designed to monitor propofol concentrations in real time. Sensitivity of the optimal imprinted polymer appeared to be around 1 ppm of propofol.

Birnbaumer et al.[173] also used molecularly imprinted polymers to detect viruses. They developed a micrototal analysis system that was capable of continuous monitoring for viral contamination with high sensitivity and selectivity, using a copolymer of vinylpyrrolidone and methacrylic acid upon which a virus stamp (in this case tobacco mosaic virus [TMV]) was pressed before polymerization. The TMV stamp was fabricated by depositing a TMV solution onto a glass substrate and allowing virus particle assembly to proceed for 30 min. The virus particles on the stamp, pressed into the surface of the monomers before polymerization, produced microcavities upon polymerization that mirrored the viral shapes. Detection of virus particles using the imprinted polymers was carried out using contactless bioimpedance spectroscopy, optimized for certain frequencies. Basically, intrinsic dielectric differences in the polymer used to fabricate the imprinted chip and the virus particles were the parameters detected. Birnbaumer et al. used a poly (methacrylic acid-co-vinylpyrrolidone) polymer that was not imprinted as a negative control surface, to take into account nonspecific binding. Results obtained with native polymer versus imprinted polymer indicated that the dielectric spectroscopy was able to distinguish intrinsic structural differences in the two polymers. The authors showed that they were able to detect TMV in solutions containing 4 μg/mL of TMV using polymers imprinted for TMV, while no viral signal was detected in the native polymer. The impedance signal from the imprinted polymer chamber increased for 90 min and then remained steady, although the perfusion was continued for 12 h, indicating that the virally imprinted sites were saturated. Selectivity of the molecularly imprinted polymer was also studied, using imprinted polymers with TMV cavities. If human rhinovirus, serotype 2 (HRV2), was flowed through this biochip, no impedance signal above background was detected, while with TMV, there was a significant signal increase. The authors note that specific recognition of TMV by the imprinted polymer can be ascribed to inherent shape differences between the two viruses tested, since the rod-shaped cavities in the imprinted polymer were 18 nm in diameter and 300 nm long, while the HRV2 virus particles are larger, that is, about 30 nm in diameter.

Zhang et al.[174] described a biosensor for optical detection of DNA, which is based on a porous silicon microcavity (PSM) on a silicon-on-insulator wafer. Although the device as demonstrated is not a biochip, the potential exists for integration of this technology into a multicomponent sensor. Porous silicon has recently attracted interest as the substrate for optical biosensors because of favorable properties, such as low-cost manufacture and the fact that the very large internal surface area permits immobilization of more probe molecules, which increases the probability of capturing lower amounts of analyte from test solutions. Zhang et al. produced a PSM on a silicon-on-insulator wafer using electrochemical etching, which was then used for detection of DNA at 1555 nm. The basic principle involved in the detection is that when DNA molecules are captured by hybridization to immobilized DNA in the PSM, there is a red shift in the reflectance spectrum of the detecting light, due to a change in the optical thickness of the silicon wall plus biomolecules. The preparation of the PSM is rather complex and is described in detail in Zhang et al.[174] Also, there is considerable wet chemistry that must be performed to prepare the PSM for use, including oxidation, silanization, and immobilization steps. The nanoscale structure of the PSM is shown by SEM in Zhang et al. The PSM structure consists of alternating layers of high and low porosity (each high-porosity layer is about 240 nm, while each low-porosity layer is about 190 nm). The total thickness of the PSM layer on the silicon-on-insulator wafer is approximately 7.3 μm. The average diameter of the pores is ~20 nm. To demonstrate DNA detection, a 19-mer oligonucleotide is immobilized on the PSM, and complementary or noncomplementary target oligonucleotides are exposed under hybridization conditions. With cDNA, there was a red shift in the reflectance spectrum of 41 nm, while with the non-cDNA, no shift is seen. Since the extent of the red shift in the reflectance is dependent on analyte concentration, Zhang et al. showed a calibration curve for the oligonucleotide target used and found a limit of detection of about 44 nM.

3.5.12 Applications of Biochips to Basic Biological Systems

A number of recent articles have taken advantage of advances in technology of microfabrication, modification of surfaces, and micro-/nanomachining, to develop devices that can be used to study basic aspects of biological interactions. For example, Zhang et al.[175] have developed a microfluidic device that permits analysis of pathogen–host interaction at the single-cell level. Understanding the association dynamics between bacteria and host cells is important in understanding mechanisms of pathogenesis. Polydimethylsiloxane (PDMS) biochips with 900 microwells were fabricated and were loaded with single cells using one-step vacuum-driven microfluidics. The single cell/well was established by using a very dilute cell suspension, such that the probability favored one cell/well. Host (human) cells were incubated with bacteria (*P. aeruginosa*) prior to introduction to the microwells. Using real-time PCR targeted to the test bacteria, the investigators were able to quantify the number of adhering bacteria per well, with a single bacterium sensitivity of detection.

In another example, Ma et al.[176] used laser-patterned biochips to define contact modes for stem cells interacting with cardiomyocytes. The object of this study was to develop a system in which the contact mode of the two cell types could be rigorously defined and the cellular interactions could be studied at the single-cell level. The long-term research objective was to understand how stem cells interact with cardiomyocytes, since cell-based therapies might restore cardiomyocyte loss as a consequence of cardiac diseases or myocardial infarction. Ingeniously, the investigators prepared two types of microwells, one contact promoting and one contact preventing. In the promoting microwell, the shape was rectangular (50 μm long and 25 μm wide), while the preventative microwell was dumbbell shaped, with two circles (30 μm diameter) connected by a channel of 30 μm long and 15 μm wide. In the case of the promoting microwell, the two cells (stem cell and myocyte) could engage in unrestricted physical contact, while in the case of the preventative microwell, the cells were inhibited from interaction and remained in separate parts of the microwell. Single cells of both types were moved to specific locations in the microwells by laser-guided micropatterning. Cell interactions were then studied as the cells were incubated in the biochips for a number of days. This biochip device could allow study of specific cellular interactions, such as electrical coupling, mechanical coupling, and mitochondria transfer.

Marhefka and Abbud-Antali[177] described the development of a first-generation test cancer biochip. This concept uses microwells to hold cancer cells in soft agar, and also, the soft agar contains various silencing RNAs (siRNAs). The effect of the various siRNAs on growth of the cancer cells in a 3D matrix can thus be studied, and this effect, as monitored in soft agar, is postulated to be of special relevance to cancer biology because anchorage-independent growth assays are considered to be the gold standard for chemosensitivity assessment. siRNAs, which specifically affect 3D growth of cancer cells, can be uniquely detected in this assay, and this knowledge may help to identify clinically relevant breast cancer targets.

3.5.13 Biochip Surfaces, Biomolecule Immobilization

COCs have found recent favor as substrates for biochip applications, due to a range of favorable properties, such as heat resistance, ease of embossability, and superior optical transparency as well as low autofluorescence. Nevertheless, the COC polymers demonstrate undesirable characteristics such as nonspecific protein absorption and cell adhesion. Jena and Yue[178] demonstrated that surface modification of COC by the use of a 2-methacryloylethyl phosphorylcholine (MPC) moiety reduced significantly the tendency of the COC to absorb protein and capture cells.

Bearinger et al.[179] discussed the use of photocatalytic lithography (PCL) as a technique to produce patterned substrates in an inexpensive, fast, and robust manner. They described the use of porphyrin-based PCL for patterning poly (propylene sulfide) block copolymer films on gold substrates, with both micron- and submicron-scale precision. In this article, they demonstrated biomolecular patterning results with fluorescently labeled proteins and protein-linked beads.

Sollier et al.[180] presented the use of a *print-n-shrink* technology for fabrication of microfluidic biochips. In this procedure, a microfluidic design is screen printed onto PolyShrink™ polystyrene sheets. The print is subsequently shrunk by heating to 163°C for 30 s. The shrinking results in an isotropic reduction in size in the x–y plane, but a size increase in the z plane. Various microfluidic designs can be easily prepared by this method. Interestingly, the authors also deposit proteins on the print surface before printing. Surprisingly, the thermal conditions of shrinking seem to leave a significant proportion of the deposited proteins in native form (not denatured), as demonstrated by immunochemical reactions carried out on the shrunken sheet. Thus, antibodies spotted upon the sheet before shrinking still recognize and bind their appropriate antigens. The authors also demonstrate that the shrunken polysty-rene sheets can be used as satisfactory surfaces for culture of mammalian cells, provided materials such as fibronectin or collagen were deposited on the polystyrene before shrinking.

Chakra et al.[181] described the use of microcontact printing in fabricating biochip surfaces with precise positioning of biomolecules in specified locations. The authors built a microprinting device that allowed them to consecutively and selectively print patterns of antibodies at the bottom of a glass microchannel. Among the innovations of this microprinter was ultrafine control of the stamp's compression during the contact process. Chakra et al. demonstrated the application of this device by using it to lay down patterns of antibody placement in a glass microchannel and performing an immunoassay, with fluores-cence detection. The authors indicated that microcontact printing has the capability of producing bio-molecule patterns from several mm down to 50 nm, but their actual experiments involved imprinting of 30×250 μm spots in a 70 μm flow channel.

3.5.14 Miniaturized Systems for In Vivo Applications and Implantable Biochips

Although many analytical applications have been developed for biochips, most involve analyzing for specific biomolecules in, at best, a hospital, a clinical laboratory setting, or a physician's office. Many of the biochip analyses so far described in the literature have not even been advanced to this level, but remain research laboratory demonstrations. Miniaturized light sources and detectors are important components for the development of implantable biosensing platforms. Vertical cavity surface-emitting lasers (VCSELs) are useful elements of many integrated biosensors and biochips. Harris and coworkers developed integrated biosensor VCSELs and monolithically integrated optical sensors for in vivo molec-ular monitoring in small animals.[182] A major barrier to implantable monitors that can function over any reasonable period of time in vivo is the response of the body itself to this essentially foreign object. To mitigate the issues of biofouling and foreign body response is therefore a major research problem to be overcome in terms of implantable biochips. In this section, we provide only a brief overview of recent work, and that mainly directed to attempts to broach this biocompatibility barrier.

Guiseppi-Elie[183] discussed an implantable biochip design, whose ultimate goal is to develop an implantable, integrated glucose and lactate biosensor and communicating biochip that can monitor these compounds as an indicator of physiologic status during hemorrhage and for intensive care unit stays. The author provides much discussion for the clinical value of such monitoring during cases of treatment of severe trauma-induced hemorrhage. Suffice it to say that glucose and lactate both expe-rience widely fluctuating levels as a result of hemorrhage, and ability to monitor these metabolites continuously over an extended time in the in vivo compartment would be of great benefit to thera-peutic intervention. Guiseppi-Elie proposes a dual responsive, amperometric biotransducer, which uses a microdisc electrode format upon which are immobilized glucose oxidase and lactate oxidase in discrete areas. Glucose and lactate levels are related to current output, which is reported telemetri-cally to a remote receiver. Much of the article is concerned with the preparation of electroconduc-tive hydrogels, which are coated with a bioactive hydrogel layer that has phosphorylcholine and PEG pendant moieties, to promote indwelling biocompatibility. To evaluate the biocompatibility of the electroconductive hydrogel outer layer (i.e., the hydrogel in contact with in vivo tissue), cells (either rat pheochromocytomas [PC12] or human muscle fibroblasts [RMS13]) were seeded and cultured on various prepared hydrogel surfaces. Growth was compared with a positive control, which were cells grown on standard plastic culture dishes. Cell viability was assessed by trypan blue staining and cell morphology was evaluated using fluorescent stains on fixed cells. Also, human aortic vascular smooth muscle (HA-VSMC) was cultured on hydrogels, to evaluate biomaterial cytotoxicity. Finally, to test in vivo biocompatibility, the bioactive hydrogels, which would form the outer layer of the device, were implanted into the trapezius muscle of rats, and the sites of implantation were evaluated histologically after a certain time period.

Among the results reported were that hydrogels with increasing MPC (monomer) content also showed an increase in the percent hydration. The in vitro cell studies found that all hydrogel formulations produced >80% viability when HA-VSMC cells were cultured with the hydrogels. Interestingly, it was found that RMS13 cells were retained inside the hydrogel matrix and the degree of retention was strongly dependent on both the PEG and MPC content of the hydrogel. Implantation in the rat model for 2 weeks showed that the base hydrogel elicited significant encapsulation of the implant and accumulation of foreign body material, while the modified hydrogel with 1 mol% of MPC only showed a thin band of encapsulation and much reduced residual inflammation. It therefore appeared that the inclusion of the phosphorylcholine in the hydrogel, in some manner, conferred an outer cell membrane similarity to the hydrogel surface. When the functional implant was surgically introduced into the rat trapezius muscle, and hemorrhage was simulated, it was found that the lactate levels recorded by the implanted sensor were not concordant with lactate levels as measured by conventional means, using an ABL 705 blood gas and metabolite analyzer during the hemorrhage simulation. The implanted sensor showed a more rapid rise of lactate levels early in the hemorrhage process. Further experimentation is needed to resolve and understand these discrepancies.

A review article by Carrara et al.[184] provides details regarding various aspects of biochip platforms for implantable biosensing. As opposed to single metabolite biosensing, the focus of this article is definitely on multianalyte sensing, using a biochip platform. This article focuses exclusively on electrochemical sensing, as the detection technology. Although the benefits of this technology for in vivo sensing are, in some sense, obvious, it is not clear that this is the only viable detection technology for biosensor implants. The review by Carrara et al. provides thorough coverage of most aspects relevant to the development of implantable sensors. Thus, there is discussion of the use of nanomaterials to enhance sensor performance, discussion of most common proteins used as sensing moieties, and integration of nano- and biomaterials onto silicon platforms. Further topics covered include issues involving microelectronics for the biosensing component as well as remote powering. Also, the major problem of biocompatibility is discussed. Finally, the concerns regarding security and privacy attendant upon wireless transmission of data are discussed and the review ends with a section on future developments.

As indicated earlier, this article by Carrara et al. is focused on implantable biochip platforms. As the authors point out, new diagnostic and monitoring technologies are needed in all healthcare systems, but particularly in low- and middle-income countries. Here, particularly, the requirements for low-power, low-cost, and robust operation become important, and remote telemetry monitoring of health status becomes almost a necessity. Glucose and lactate monitoring with commercially available devices is already possible, but sensor lifetime in vivo is still an issue. The fact that the sensor operates in the in vivo environment presents unique challenges with regard to calibration, the foreign body response, and signaling. In the following section, we make brief comments about some aspects discussed in greater detail by Carrara et al.

Nanomaterials as biosensor elements are discussed in some detail in Carrara et al., particularly carbon nanotubes and carbon nanotube-hybrid materials. Also, the use of nanoparticles, nanowires, and conductive polymers/nanocomposites is discussed. All of these materials have advantages for sensing surfaces, related to their electrical properties and their large surface area, allowing immobilization of more biomolecules. Immobilization of the biomolecule sensing element onto the electroconducting surface in such a fashion that bioactivity is retained is an important consideration. Techniques such as adsorption, covalent attachment, bioaffinity immobilization (e.g., lectins, biotin), and physical entrapment in conductive polymers are discussed. The authors particularly make the point that biomolecules can be entrapped in the polymers not only through physical adsorption but cross-linking with glutaraldehyde, covalent attachment, and, perhaps most efficiently, by electrochemical polymerization. By this latter process, the enzyme (or other biomolecules) is incorporated in a homogeneous manner into the polymer, as polymerization takes place. Other techniques, such as self-assembled monolayers, Langmuir–Blodgett films, and layer-by-layer processes, are also discussed.

Integration of biomolecules and nanomaterials on multielectrode platforms is discussed in some detail, particularly with regard to attachment processes involved. Thus, direct growth of nanomaterials onto the biochip surface (i.e., particularly with regard to carbon nanotubes), covalent attachment of nanomaterials onto electrode surfaces (i.e., carbon nanotubes onto gold electrodes), and microspotting of nanomaterials onto microelectrodes are all possible options.

There are two sections in this article dealing with electrical issues associated with these implantable biochips. One section concerns the front-end electronics, which must be integrated and miniaturized into a single chip. The other involves remote powering. The front-end electronics involve both a readout circuit and a voltage generator/potentiostat. CMOS designs for chips are discussed as is the issue of electrical noise. Remote powering seems, naively, to be no problem, given the battery developments of recent years, but when it is recognized that implantable sensors need to minimize device size, battery power on board the sensor may not be so attractive. Possibilities for remote powering are therefore discussed.

Biocompatibility of the implanted biochip is perhaps the most crucial issue to be dealt with regarding all such implantable sensors; if biocompatibility is ignored, severe inflammation and necrosis of tissue can occur in the short term, with potentially even more severe effects in the long term (e.g., cancer). If there is a severe mismatch between the implant and surrounding local tissue, a strong foreign body response will occur, in which the implant is walled off by fibrotic tissue 3–4 weeks after implantation. At this point, little contact between the sensor and body fluids is possible. An additional point to be considered is biostability. If body fluids corrode and disable the operating components of the sensor, there is little point to implanting it. The authors list three important factors that need to be carefully evaluated for achieving success of implanted biochips: grafting factors, implant fabrication factors, and sensor biofouling factors. Solutions to the problem of the implant as graft include procedures to improve cell adhesion, promote vascularization, and reduce the inflammatory response. Thus, the implant material's morphology, porosity, and mechanical properties can all influence cell response to the implant. Porous coatings like poly-L-lactic acid or hydrogels seem to enhance blood vessel formation and reduce fibrosis. Inclusion of a drug that can be released from the implant coating may reduce the risk of biofilm formation by bacteria. In terms of implant fabrication, the implant, by definition, has some nonbiocompatible materials (e.g., batteries). One does not want diffusion of subcomponents of such nonbiocompatible materials (e.g., metal ions from batteries) into the body tissue nor is penetration of body fluids into the active implant desirable, since corrosion of the sensor may occur, with further deleterious consequences, such as leaching of toxic components into the body. Devices such as pacemakers solve these problems by enclosing the whole device in a titanium box, with ceramic/polymer feedthrough for the leads. Unfortunately, this box design is limited in how miniature it can be made, and its rigidity is also quite foreign to most tissue in which it is implanted. Thus, ceramic or polymer films have properties that may be advantageous for implant use. Biofouling is the accumulation of biomaterial on the surface of the device; this accumulation of cells, macromolecules, and small molecules has been found to be detrimental for effective biosensor functioning. Hydrogel overlays or Nafion coatings have been employed to reduce biofouling. Careful choice of all components/raw materials for the implanted sensor is important, and clearly, refinement of biocompatibility issues will benefit from further research. Following discussion of privacy issues and future perspectives for implantable sensors, the authors concluded with the prediction that in a 5–10-year time frame, they anticipated that reliable technology will be developed for remote sensing/telemetry of various metabolic products.

3.6 Conclusion and Future Perspectives

Rapid, simple, cost-effective medical devices for screening multiple diseases and infectious pathogens are essential for early diagnosis and, thus, timely and improved treatments of many illnesses. An important factor in medical diagnostics is rapid, selective, and sensitive detection of biochemical substances, biomarkers, or biological pathogens at ultratrace levels in biological samples (tissues, blood, and other bodily fluids).

In research laboratories, microarray technology enables massive parallel mining of biological data, with biological chips providing hybridization-based expression monitoring, polymorphism detection, and genotyping on a genomic scale. High-density microarray biochips containing sequences representative of many human genes may soon permit the expression analysis of the entire human genome in a single reaction. These *genome chips* will provide unprecedented access to key areas of human health, including disease prognosis and diagnosis, drug discovery, toxicology, aging, and mental illness.

At the physician's office, integrated biochip systems offer several advantages in size, performance, analysis capabilities, and cost because of their integrated optical sensing microchip. The small probes (microliter to nanoliter in size) minimize sample treatment and reduce reagent requirements and waste. Highly integrated systems reduce noise and increase signal due to the improved efficiency of sample collection and the reduction of interfaces. The IC technology used in the systems will allow large-scale production and, therefore, low cost. The assembly of the various components of the system is made simple by the integration of multiple elements on a single chip. For medical applications, this cost advantage will allow the development of extremely low-cost, disposable biochips that can be used for in-home medical diagnostics of diseases without the need to send samples to a laboratory for analysis.

It is apparent, from the survey of recent work reviewed for this chapter, that much has been accomplished to date. Novel techniques of detection, promising greater sensitivity, have been developed and are being explored. New materials, notably nano-based in nature, will likely bring unique capabilities to biochip fabrication and detection technologies. Yet, in spite of the advances, there are big challenges to overcome in the area of practical biochip applications.

Integration of components, such as microfluidics, biosensing surfaces, and detection technology into a seamless system, which is truly a *lab on a chip*, still remains an urgent goal, rather than an accomplished fact. An integrated biochip analysis system, where a clinical (or other) sample is injected into one port and the output is automatically read out (at some subsequent point in time), is by no means the norm, but is relatively uncommon. A related issue, of great importance, is the complex nature of many clinical samples, such as blood. Without a preparatory purification step, the large number of components in blood can limit the effectiveness of almost any assay envisioned. Thus, seamless integration of microseparation systems with detection technology may be important for practical analysis under field conditions or at the point of care. For example, nucleic acid analysis for such applications as evaluating samples for bacterial pathogens will require effective lysis procedures and some degree of sample purification before detection, with or without amplification, takes place.

Coupled with the issue of integration is the question of time to complete sample analysis. If many preliminary steps must be accomplished off-chip, before the readout of the detection system occurs, the process can hardly be called integrated, and the total time of analysis could become a concern. For clinical usefulness, as well as for environmental or contamination monitoring, one of the points in favor of analysis using a biochip is hopefully a significant savings in time of analysis.

It is apparent, also, that advances in micromachining and microfabrication, while of great significance in development of more effective lab-on-a-chip systems, also raise some unique problems, such as the issue of effective mixing of sample and analysis components in microchannels, as well as the associated problem of efficiently moving microliter volumes (or less) of fluids. Nanostructured materials, be they particles, surfaces, wires, etc., also present challenges as well as opportunities. Nanosurfaces present much greater surface area for immobilization of bioprobes but also present this same increased surface area as a site for nonspecific binding.

Many of the articles reviewed for this updated chapter use electrochemical detection due to the relative simplicity of electronic circuitry. The benefits of this technology are many, but there are analysis issues with conductivity changes and electrode corrosion due to various components in samples and in buffers. Optical detection has certain advantages in analysis, especially with current advances in miniaturization of optical systems (nanolasers, detectors on a chip).

Sensitivity and specificity are twin problems with almost all biochip systems. Much beneficial work has been done to address both issues. The problem of protein and biological probe denaturation (e.g., antibodies) continues to be a potential problem, if proteins are involved as the biosensing probe or bioreceptor. The potential of imprinted polymers to provide a stable sensing surface may offer a robust biomimetic probe for sensors, but the issue of specificity still must be addressed in a thorough manner. Nucleic acids may be more stable than proteins in a thermodynamic sense, but are still susceptible to degradation by enzymes in the sample (such as RNases in blood samples).

Finally, there is the ultimate goal of biochip applications, a truly implantable sensor that can provide a reliable and real-time snapshot of in vivo health status over a reasonably long period of time. In many ways, this will be the greatest challenge to overcome. Much modern technology can be brought to bear to deal with issues of biocompatibility, remote detection wireless telemetry, and miniaturization for subcutaneous (or other sites) implantation. It is clear, however, that a number of investigators are vigorously addressing these formidable challenges using biomimicry, novel chemistry, ultrasensitive detection, system miniaturization, and nanoengineering of surfaces in order to minimize the foreign body response and enhance sensitivity and specificity as well as improve the lifetime of the biosensing system.

Acknowledgments

The authors acknowledge the contributions of their coworkers A.L. Wintenberg, N. Ericson, M. Askari, D.L. Stokes, J. Mobley, B. Cullum, R. Maples, G.H. Miller, and H.N. Wang. The authors acknowledge the sponsorship of the US Department of Energy (DOE) Office of Biological and Environmental Research, the DOE Chemical and Biological Nonproliferation Program, the Department of Navy, the National Institutes of Health, the US Army Research, the Wallace Coulter Foundation, and the Defense Advanced Research Project Agency (DARPA).

References

1. Schena, M., Shalon, D., Davis, R. W., and Brown, P. O., Quantitative monitoring of gene-expression patterns with a complementary-DNA microarray, *Science* 270(5235), 467–470, 1995.
2. Blanchard, A. P. and Hood, L., Sequence to array: Probing the genome's secrets, *Nature Biotechnology* 14(13), 1649, 1996.
3. DeRisi, J., Penland, L., Brown, P. O., Bittner, M. L., Meltzer, P. S., Ray, M., Chen, Y. D., Su, Y. A., and Trent, J. M., Use of a cDNA microarray to analyse gene expression patterns in human cancer, *Nature Genetics* 14(4), 457–460, 1996.
4. Wallace, R. W., DNA on a chip: Serving up the genome for diagnostics and research, *Molecular Medicine Today* 3(9), 384–389, 1997.
5. Vo-Dinh, T., Alarie, J. P., Isola, N., Landis, D., Wintenberg, A. L., and Ericson, M. N., DNA biochip using a phototransistor integrated circuit, *Analytical Chemistry* 71(2), 358–363, 1999.
6. Vo-Dinh, T., Development of a DNA biochip: Principles and applications, *Sensors and Actuators B* 51, 52–59, 1998.
7. Vo-Dinh, T. and Cullum, B., Biosensors and biochips: Advances in biological and medical diagnostics, *Fresenius Journal of Analytical Chemistry* 366(6–7), 540–551, 2000.
8. Vo-Dinh, T., The multi-functional biochip, in *Sixth Annual Biochip Technologies: Chips for Hits'99*, Cambridge Health Institute, Berkeley, CA, 1999.
9. Vo-Dinh, T., Griffin, G. D., Stokes, D. L., and Wintenberg, A. L., A multi-functional biochip for biomedical diagnostics and pathogen detection, *Sensors and Actuators* 90(1–3), 104–111, 1999.
10. Vo-Dinh, T. and Askari, M., Micro arrays and biochips: Applications and potential in genomics and proteomics, *Current Genomics* 2, 399–415, 2001.
11. Vo-Dinh, T., Cullum, B. M., and Stokes, D. L., Nanosensors and biochips: Frontiers in biomolecular diagnostics, *Sensors and Actuators B: Chemical* 74(1–3), 2–11, 2001.

12. Blanchard, G. C., Taylor, C. G., Busey, B. R., and Williamson, M. L., Regeneration of immunosorbent surfaces used in clinical, industrial and environmental biosensors—Role of covalent and noncovalent interactions, *Journal of Immunological Methods* 130(2), 263–275, 1990.

13. Proudnikov, D., Timofeev, E., and Mirzabekov, A., Immobilization of DNA in polyacrylamide gel for the manufacture of DNA and DNA-oligonucleotide microchips, *Analytical Biochemistry* 259(1), 34–41, 1998.

14. Blanchard, A. P., Kaiser, R. J., and Hood, L. E., High-density oligonucleotide arrays, *Biosensors & Bioelectronics* 11(6–7), 687–690, 1996.

15. Kononen, J., Bubendorf, L., Kallioniemi, A., Barlund, M., Schraml, P., Leighton, S., Torhorst, J., Mihatsch, M. J., Sauter, G., and Kallioniemi, O. P., Tissue microarrays for high-throughput molecular profiling of tumor specimens, *Nature Medicine* 4(7), 844–847, 1998.

16. Marshall, A. and Hodgson, J., DNA chips: An array of possibilities, *Nature Biotechnology* 16(1), 27–31, 1998.

17. Housman, D. and Ledley, F. D., Why pharmacogenomics? Why now? *Nature Biotechnology* 16(6), 492–493, 1998.

18. Kricka, L. J., Revolution on a square centimeter, *Nature Biotechnology* 16(6), 513–514, 1998.

19. Service, R. F., Microchip arrays put DNA on the spot, *Science* 282(5388), 396–399, 1998.

20. Service, R. F., Future chips—Labs on a chip—Coming soon: The pocket DNA sequencer, *Science* 282(5388), 399–401, 1998.

21. Schena, M., Heller, R. A., Theriault, T. P., Konrad, K., Lachenmeier, E., and Davis, R. W., Microarrays: Biotechnology's discovery platform for functional genomics, *Trends in Biotechnology* 16(7), 301–306, 1998.

22. Wang, D. G., Fan, J. B., Siao, C. J., Berno, A., Young, P., Sapolsky, R., Ghandour, G. et al., Large-scale identification, mapping, and genotyping of single-nucleotide polymorphisms in the human genome, *Science* 280(5366), 1077–1082, 1998.

23. Nuwaysir, E. F., Bittner, M., Trent, J., Barrett, J. C., and Afshari, C. A., Microarrays and toxicology: The advent of toxicogenomics, *Molecular Carcinogenesis* 24(3), 153–159, 1999.

24. Ekins, R. and Chu, F. W., Microarrays: Their origins and applications, *Trends in Biotechnology* 17(6), 217–218, 1999.

25. Khan, J., Saal, L. H., Bittner, M. L., Chen, Y. D., Trent, J. M., and Meltzer, P. S., Expression profiling in cancer using cDNA microarrays, *Electrophoresis* 20(2), 223–229, 1999.

26. Pollack, J. R., Perou, C. M., Alizadeh, A. A., Eisen, M. B., Pergamenschikov, A., Williams, C. F., Jeffrey, S. S., Botstein, D., and Brown, P. O., Genome-wide analysis of DNA copy-number changes using cDNA microarrays, *Nature Genetics* 23(1), 41–46, 1999.

27. Afshari, C. A., Nuwaysir, E. F., and Barrett, J. C., Application of complementary DNA microarray technology to carcinogen identification, toxicology, and drug safety evaluation, *Cancer Research* 59(19), 4759–4760, 1999.

28. Vo-Dinh, T., Isola, N., Alarie, J. P., Landis, D., Griffin, G. D., and Allison, S., Development of a multiarray biosensor for DNA diagnostics, *Instrumentation Science & Technology* 26(5), 503–514, 1998.

29. Vo-Dinh, T., Allain, L. R., and Stokes, D. L., Cancer gene detection using SERS, *Journal of Raman Spectroscopy* 33(7), 511–516, 2002.

30. Thevenot, D. R., Toth, K., Durst, R. A., and Wilson, G. S., Electrochemical biosensors: Recommended definitions and classification (technical report), *Pure and Applied Chemistry* 71(12), 2333–2348, 1999.

31. Wang, J., Rivas, G., Fernandes, J. R., Paz, J. L. L., Jiang, M., and Waymire, R., Indicator-free electrochemical DNA hybridization biosensor, *Analytica Chimica Acta* 375(3), 197–203, 1998.

32. Barker, S. L. R., Kopelman, R., Meyer, T. E., and Cusanovich, M. A., Fiber-optic nitric oxide-selective biosensors and nanosensors, *Analytical Chemistry* 70(5), 971–976, 1998.

33. Erdem, A., Kerman, K., Meric, B., Akarca, U. S., and Ozsoz, M., DNA electrochemical biosensor for the detection of short DNA sequences related to the hepatitis B virus, *Electroanalysis* 11(8), 586–588, 1999.

34. Sawata, S., Kai, E., Ikebukuro, K., Iida, T., Honda, T., and Karube, I., Application of peptide nucleic acid to the direct detection of deoxyribonucleic acid amplified by polymerase chain reaction, *Biosensors & Bioelectronics* 14(4), 397–404, 1999.

35. Niemeyer, C. M., Boldt, L., Ceyhan, B., and Blohm, D., DNA-directed immobilization: Efficient, reversible, and site-selective surface binding of proteins by means of covalent DNA-streptavidin conjugates, *Analytical Biochemistry* 268(1), 54–63, 1999.

36. Niemeyer, C. M., Ceyhan, B., and Blohm, D., Functionalization of covalent DNA-streptavidin conjugates by means of biotinylated modulator components, *Bioconjugate Chemistry* 10(5), 708–719, 1999.

37. Marrazza, G., Chianella, I., and Mascini, M., Disposable DNA electrochemical sensor for hybridization detection, *Biosensors & Bioelectronics* 14(1), 43–51, 1999.

38. Bardea, A., Patolsky, F., Dagan, A., and Willner, I., Sensing and amplification of oligonucleotide-DNA interactions by means of impedance spectroscopy: A route to a Tay-Sachs sensor, *Chemical Communications*, 21–22, 1999.

39. Lockhart, D. J., Dong, H. L., Byrne, M. C., Follettie, M. T., Gallo, M. V., Chee, M. S., Mittmann, M. et al., Expression monitoring by hybridization to high-density oligonucleotide arrays, *Nature Biotechnology* 14(13), 1675–1680, 1996.

40. Walt, D. R., Biological warfare detection, *Analytical Chemistry* 72(23), 738A–746A, 2000.

41. Hacia, J. G., Woski, S. A., Fidanza, J., Edgemon, K., Hunt, N., McGall, G., Fodor, S. P. A., and Collins, F. S., Enhanced high density oligonucleotide array-based sequence analysis using modified nucleoside triphosphates, *Nucleic Acids Research* 26(21), 4975–4982, 1998.

42. Lipshutz, R. J., Fodor, S. P. A., Gingeras, T. R., and Lockhart, D. J., High density synthetic oligonucleotide arrays, *Nature Genetics* 21, 20–24, 1999.

43. Singh-Gasson, S., Green, R. D., Yue, Y. J., Nelson, C., Blattner, F., Sussman, M. R., and Cerrina, F., Maskless fabrication of light-directed oligonucleotide microarrays using a digital micromirror array, *Nature Biotechnology* 17(10), 974–978, 1999.

44. McGall, G., Labadie, J., Brock, P., Wallraff, G., Nguyen, T., and Hinsberg, W., Light-directed synthesis of high-density oligonucleotide arrays using semiconductor photoresists, *Proceedings of the National Academy of Sciences of the United States of America* 93(24), 13555–13560, 1996.

45. Allain, L. R., Askari, M., Stokes, D. L., and Vo-Dinh, T., Microarray sampling-platform fabrication using bubble-jet technology for a biochip system, *Fresenius Journal of Analytical Chemistry* 371(2), 146–150, 2001.

46. Piehler, J., Brecht, A., Gauglitz, G., Maul, C., Grabley, S., and Zerlin, M., Specific binding of low molecular weight ligands with direct optical detection, *Biosensors & Bioelectronics* 12(6), 531–538, 1997.

47. Gray, D. E., CaseGreen, S. C., Fell, T. S., Dobson, P. J., and Southern, E. M., Ellipsometric and interferometric characterization of DNA probes immobilized on a combinatorial array, *Langmuir* 13(10), 2833–2842, 1997.

48. Edman, C. F., Raymond, D. E., Wu, D. J., Tu, E. G., Sosnowski, R. G., Butler, W. F., Nerenberg, M., and Heller, M. J., Electric field directed nucleic acid hybridization on microchips, *Nucleic Acids Research* 25(24), 4907–4914, 1997.

49. Skuridin, S. G., Yevdokimov, Y. M., Efimov, V. S., Hall, J. M., and Turner, A. P. F., A new approach for creating double-stranded DNA biosensors, *Biosensors & Bioelectronics* 11(9), 903–911, 1996.

50. Czajkowsky, D. M., Iwamoto, H., and Shao, Z. F., Atomic force microscopy in structural biology: From the subcellular to the submolecular, *Journal of Electron Microscopy* 49(3), 395–406, 2000.

51. Mazzola, L. T., Frank, C. W., Fodor, S. P. A., Mosher, C., Lartius, R., and Henderson, E., Discrimination of DNA hybridization using chemical force microscopy, *Biophysical Journal* 76(6), 2922–2933, 1999.

52. Vo-Dinh, T., Houck, K., and Stokes, D. L., Surface-enhanced Raman gene probes, *Analytical Chemistry* 66(20), 3379–3383, 1994.

53. Vo-Dinh, T., Surface-enhanced Raman spectroscopy using metallic nanostructures, *Trends in Analytical Chemistry* 17(8–9), 557–582, 1998.

54. Vo-Dinh, T., Stokes, D. L., Griffin, G. D., Volkan, M., Kim, U. J., and Simon, M. I., Surface-enhanced Raman scattering (SERS) method and instrumentation for genomics and biomedical analysis, *Journal of Raman Spectroscopy* 30(9), 785–793, 1999.

55. Isola, N. R., Stokes, D. L., and Vo-Dinh, T., Surface enhanced Raman gene probe for HIV detection, *Analytical Chemistry* 70(7), 1352–1356, 1998.

56. Jena, P. K., Liu, A. H., Smith, D. S., and Wysocki, L. J., Amplification of genes, single transcripts and cDNA libraries from one cell and direct sequence analysis of amplified products derived from one molecule, *Journal of Immunological Methods* 190(2), 199–213, 1996.

57. Wang, A. M., Doyle, M. V., and Mark, D. F., Quantitation of messenger-RNA by the polymerase chain-reaction, *Proceedings of the National Academy of Sciences of the United States of America* 86(24), 9717–9721, 1989.

58. Kwoh, D. Y., Davis, G. R., Whitfield, K. M., Chappelle, H. L., Dimichele, L. J., and Gingeras, T. R., Transcription-based amplification system and detection of amplified human immunodeficiency virus type-1 with a bead-based sandwich hybridization format, *Proceedings of the National Academy of Sciences of the United States of America* 86(4), 1173–1177, 1989.

59. Guatelli, J. C., Whitfield, K. M., Kwoh, D. Y., Barringer, K. J., Richman, D. D., and Gingeras, T. R., Isothermal, in vitro amplification of nucleic-acids by a multienzyme reaction modeled after retroviral replication, *Proceedings of the National Academy of Sciences of the United States of America* 87(5), 1874–1878, 1990.

60. Luo, L., Salunga, R. C., Guo, H. Q., Bittner, A., Joy, K. C., Galindo, J. E., Xiao, H. N. et al., Gene expression profiles of laser-captured adjacent neuronal subtypes, *Nature Medicine* 5(1), 117–122, 1999.

61. Eberwine, J., Yeh, H., Miyashiro, K., Cao, Y. X., Nair, S., Finnell, R., Zettel, M., and Coleman, P., Analysis of gene-expression in single live neurons, *Proceedings of the National Academy of Sciences of the United States of America* 89(7), 3010–3014, 1992.

62. Bonner, R. F., EmmertBuck, M., Cole, K., Pohida, T., Chuaqui, R., Goldstein, S., and Liotta, L. A., Cell sampling—Laser capture microdissection: Molecular analysis of tissue, *Science* 278(5342), 1481–1483, 1997.

63. Ohyama, H., Zhang, X., Kohno, Y., Alevizos, I., Posner, M., Wong, D. T., and Todd, R., Laser capture microdissection-generated target sample for high-density oligonucleotide array hybridization, *Biotechniques* 29(3), 530–536, 2000.

64. Cronin, M. T., Fucini, R. V., Kim, S. M., Masino, R. S., Wespi, R. M., and Miyada, C. G., Cystic fibrosis mutation detection by hybridization to light-generated DNA probe arrays, *Human Mutation* 7(3), 244–255, 1996.

65. Kozal, M. J., Shah, N., Shen, N. P., Yang, R., Fucini, R., Merigan, T. C., Richman, D. D. et al., Extensive polymorphisms observed in HIV-1 clade B protease gene using high-density oligonucleotide arrays, *Nature Medicine* 2(7), 753–759, 1996.

66. Chee, M., Yang, R., Hubbell, E., Berno, A., Huang, X. C., Stern, D., Winkler, J., Lockhart, D. J., Morris, M. S., and Fodor, S. P. A., Accessing genetic information with high-density DNA arrays, *Science* 274(5287), 610–614, 1996.

67. Hacia, J. G., Brody, L. C., Chee, M. S., Fodor, S. P. A., and Collins, F. S., Detection of heterozygous mutations in BRCA1 using high density oligonucleotide arrays and two-colour fluorescence analysis, *Nature Genetics* 14(4), 441–447, 1996.

68. Nikiforov, T. T., Rendle, R. B., Goelet, P., Rogers, Y. H., Kotewicz, M. L., Anderson, S., Trainor, G. L., and Knapp, M. R., Genetic bit analysis—A solid-phase method for typing single nucleotide polymorphisms, *Nucleic Acids Research* 22(20), 4167–4175, 1994.

69. Pastinen, T., Kurg, A., Metspalu, A., Peltonen, L., and Syvanen, A. C., Minisequencing: A specific tool for DNA analysis and diagnostics on oligonucleotide arrays, *Genome Research* 7(6), 606–614, 1997.

70. Frohme, M., Scharm, B., Delius, H., Knecht, R., and Hoheisel, J. D., Use of representational difference analysis and cDNA arrays for transcriptional profiling of tumor tissue, in *Colorectal Cancer: New Aspects of Molecular Biology and Immunology and Their Clinical Applications*, Hanski, C., Mann, B., and Scherübl, H., eds. New York Academy of Science, New York, 2000, pp. 85–105.

71. Askari, M., Alarie, J. P., Moreno-Bondi, M., and Vo-Dinh, T., Application of an antibody biochip for p53 detection and cancer diagnosis, *Biotechnology Progress* 17(3), 543–552, 2001.

72. Hancock, W. S., Wu, S. L., and Shieh, P., The challenges of developing a sound proteomics strategy, *Proteomics* 2(4), 352–359, 2002.

73. Volinia, S., Francioso, F., Venturoli, L., Tosi, L., Marastoni, M., Carinci, P., Carella, M., Stanziale, P., and Evangelisti, R., Use of peptide microarrays for assaying phospho-dependent protein interactions, *Minerva Biotecnologica* 13(4), 281–285, 2001.

74. Service, R. F., Protein chips—Searching for recipes for protein chips, *Science* 294(5549), 2080–2082, 2001.

75. Zhu, H., Klemic, J., Bilgin, M., Hall, D., Bertone, P., Gerstein, M., Reed, M., and Snyder, M., Analysis of yeast proteins using protein chips, *Yeast* 18, S108, 2001.

76. Borrebaeck, C. A. K., Ekstrom, S., Hager, A. C. M., Nilsson, J., Laurell, T., and Marko-Varga, G., Protein chips based on recombinant antibody fragments: A highly sensitive approach as detected by mass spectrometry, *Biotechniques* 30(5), 1126–1130, 2001.

77. Voss, D., Protein chips—New microarrays show how proteins interact, *Technology Review* 104(4), 35, 2001.

78. Zhu, H., Klemic, J. F., Chang, S., Bertone, P., Casamayor, A., Klemic, K. G., Smith, D., Gerstein, M., Reed, M. A., and Snyder, M., Analysis of yeast protein kinases using protein chips, *Nature Genetics* 26(3), 283–289, 2000.

79. Borrebaeck, C. A. K., Antibodies in diagnostics—From immunoassays to protein chips, *Immunology Today* 21(8), 379–382, 2000.

80. Vo-Dinh, T., Tromberg, B. J., Griffin, G. D., Ambrose, K. R., Sepaniak, M. J., and Gardenhire, E. M., Antibody-based fiberoptics biosensor for the carcinogen benzo(a)pyrene, *Applied Spectroscopy* 41(5), 735–738, 1987.

81. Vo-Dinh, T., Nolan, T., Cheng, Y. F., Sepaniak, M. J., and Alarie, J. P., Phase-resolved fiberoptics fluoroimmunosensor, *Applied Spectroscopy* 44(1), 128–132, 1990.

82. Vo-Dinh, T., Alarie, J. P., Cullum, B. M., and Griffin, G. D., Antibody-based nanoprobe for measurement of a fluorescent analyte in a single cell, *Nature Biotechnology* 18(7), 764–767, 2000.

83. Ziebolz, B., Proteomics: The treasure hunt for diagnosis and treatment, *PharmaChem* 3, 5–7, 2002.

84. Seeskin, E., Chemical array: The drug discovery superhighway, *Drug Discovery World*, Spring 43–47, 2002.

85. Vo-Dinh, T., A hetero-functional biochip for environmental monitoring, *Abstracts of Papers of the American Chemical Society* 221, 57-AGRO, 2001.

86. Cho, R. J., Campbell, M. J., Winzeler, E. A., Steinmetz, L., Conway, A., Wodicka, L., Wolfsberg, T. G. et al., A genome-wide transcriptional analysis of the mitotic cell cycle, *Molecular Cell* 2(1), 65–73, 1998.

87. Spellman, P. T., Sherlock, G., Zhang, M. Q., Iyer, V. R., Anders, K., Eisen, M. B., Brown, P. O., Botstein, D., and Futcher, B., Comprehensive identification of cell cycle-regulated genes of the yeast *Saccharomyces cerevisiae* by microarray hybridization, *Molecular Biology of the Cell* 9(12), 3273–3297, 1998.

88. Lockhart, D. J. and Winzeler, E. A., Genomics, gene expression and DNA arrays, *Nature* 405(6788), 827–836, 2000.

89. Hong, T. M., Yang, P. C., Peck, K., Chen, J. J. W., Yang, S. C., Chen, Y. C., and Wu, C. W., Profiling the downstream genes of tumor suppressor PTEN in lung cancer cells by complementary DNA microarray, *American Journal of Respiratory Cell and Molecular Biology* 23(3), 355–363, 2000.

90. Vaarala, M. H., Porvari, K., Kyllonen, A., and Vihko, P., Differentially expressed genes in two LNCaP prostate cancer cell lines reflecting changes during prostate cancer progression, *Laboratory Investigation* 80(8), 1259–1268, 2000.

91. Yang, G. P., Ross, D. T., Kuang, W. W., Brown, P. O., and Weigel, R. J., Combining SSH and cDNA microarrays for rapid identification of differentially expressed genes, *Nucleic Acids Research* 27(6), 1517–1523, 1999.

92. Loftus, S. E., Chen, Y., Gooden, G., Ryan, J. F., Birznieks, G., Hilliard, M., Baxevanis, A. D. et al., Informatic selection of a neural crest-melanocyte cDNA set for microarray analysis, *Proceedings of the National Academy of Sciences of the United States of America* 96(16), 9277–9280, 1999.

93. Saiki, R. K., Walsh, P. S., Levenson, C. H., and Erlich, H. A., Genetic-analysis of amplified DNA with immobilized sequence-specific oligonucleotide probes, *Proceedings of the National Academy of Sciences of the United States of America* 86(16), 6230–6234, 1989.

94. Mei, R., Galipeau, P. C., Prass, C., Berno, A., Ghandour, G., Patil, N., Wolff, R. K., Chee, M. S., Reid, B. J., and Lockhart, D. J., Genome-wide detection of allelic imbalance using human SNPs and high-density DNA arrays, *Genome Research* 10(8), 1126–1137, 2000.

95. Sapolsky, R. J., Hsie, L., Berno, A., Ghandour, G., Mittmann, M., and Fan, J. B., High-throughput polymorphism screening and genotyping with high-density oligonucleotide arrays, *Genetic Analysis: Biomolecular Engineering* 14(5–6), 187–192, 1999.

96. Rose, N. R., Bigazzi, P. E., and Rapid, T.-A., *Methods in Immunodiagnosis*, Wiley, New York, 1999.

97. Hacia, J. G., Fan, J. B., Ryder, O., Jin, L., Edgemon, K., Ghandour, G., Mayer, R. A. et al., Determination of ancestral alleles for human single-nucleotide polymorphisms using high-density oligonucleotide arrays, *Nature Genetics* 22(2), 164–167, 1999.

98. Barlund, M., Forozan, F., Kononen, J., Bubendorf, L., Chen, Y. D., Bittner, M. L., Torhorst, J. et al., Detecting activation of ribosomal protein S6 kinase by complementary DNA and tissue microarray analysis, *Journal of the National Cancer Institute* 92(15), 1252–1259, 2000.

99. Martin, K., Kritzman, D. M., Price, L. M., Koh, B., Kwan, C. P., Zhang, X. H., Mackay, A. et al., Linking gene expression patterns to therapeutic groups in breast cancer, *Cancer Research* 60(8), 2232–2238, 2000.

100. Ly, D. H., Lockhart, D. J., Lerner, R. A., and Schultz, P. G., Mitotic misregulation and human aging, *Science* 287(5462), 2486–2492, 2000.

101. Martoglio, A. M., Tom, B. D. M., Starkey, M., Corps, A. N., Charnock-Jones, D. S., and Smith, S. K., Changes in tumorigenesis- and angiogenesis-related gene transcript abundance profiles in ovarian cancer detected by tailored high density cDNA arrays, *Molecular Medicine* 6(9), 750–765, 2000.

102. Alizadeh, A. A., Eisen, M. B., Davis, R. E., Ma, C., Lossos, I. S., Rosenwald, A., Boldrick, J. G. et al., Distinct types of diffuse large B-cell lymphoma identified by gene expression profiling, *Nature* 403(6769), 503–511, 2000.

103. Clark, E. A., Golub, T. R., Lander, E. S., and Hynes, R. O., Genomic analysis of metastasis reveals an essential role for RhoC, *Nature* 406(6795), 532–535, 2000.

104. Moch, H., Schraml, P., Bubendorf, L., Mirlacher, M., Kononen, J., Gasser, T., Mihatsch, M. J., Kallioniemi, O. P., and Sauter, G., High-throughput tissue microarray analysis to evaluate genes uncovered by cDNA microarray screening in renal cell carcinoma, *American Journal of Pathology* 154(4), 981–986, 1999.

105. Galloway, A. M. and Allalunis-Turner, J., cDNA expression array analysis of DNA repair genes in human glioma cells that lack or express DNA-PK, *Radiation Research* 154(6), 609–615, 2000.

106. Perou, C. M., Sorlie, T., Eisen, M. B., van de Rijn, M., Jeffrey, S. S., Rees, C. A., Pollack, J. R. et al., Molecular portraits of human breast tumours, *Nature* 406(6797), 747–752, 2000.

107. Liu, T. X., Zhang, J. W., Tao, J., Zhang, R. B., Zhang, Q. H., Zhao, C. J., Tong, J. H. et al., Gene expression networks underlying retinoic acid-induced differentiation of acute promyelocytic leukemia cells, *Blood* 96(4), 1496–1504, 2000.

108. Saurin, J. C., Joly-Pharaboz, M. O., Pernas, P., Henry, L., Ponchon, T., and Madjar, J. J., Detection of Ki-ras gene point mutations in bile specimens for the differential diagnosis of malignant and benign biliary strictures, *Gut* 47(3), 357–361, 2000.

109. Fung, L. F., Lo, A. K. F., Yuen, P. W., Liu, Y., Wang, X. H., and Tsao, S. W., Differential gene expression in nasopharyngeal carcinoma cells, *Life Sciences* 67(8), 923–936, 2000.

110. Lindblad-Toh, K., Tanenbaum, D. M., Daly, M. J., Winchester, E., Lui, W. O., Villapakkam, A., Stanton, S. E. et al., Loss-of-heterozygosity analysis of small-cell lung carcinomas using single-nucleotide polymorphism arrays, *Nature Biotechnology* 18(9), 1001–1005, 2000.

111. Schraml, P., Kononen, J., Bubendorf, L., Moch, H., Bissig, H., Nocito, A., Mihatsch, M. J., Kallioniemi, O. P., and Sauter, G., Tissue microarrays for gene amplification surveys in many different tumor types, *Clinical Cancer Research* 5(8), 1966–1975, 1999.

112. Favis, R., Day, J. P., Gerry, N. P., Phelan, C., Narod, S., and Barany, F., Universal DNA array detection of small insertions and deletions in BRCA1 and BRCA2, *Nature Biotechnology* 18(5), 561–564, 2000.

113. Srivastava, M., Eidelman, O., and Pollard, H. B., Pharmacogenomics of the cystic fibrosis transmembrane conductance regulator (CFTR) and the cystic fibrosis drug CPX using genome microarray analysis, *Molecular Medicine* 5(11), 753–767, 1999.

114. Gray, N. S., Wodicka, L., Thunnissen, A., Norman, T. C., Kwon, S. J., Espinoza, F. H., Morgan, D. O. et al., Exploiting chemical libraries, structure, and genomics in the search for kinase inhibitors, *Science* 281(5376), 533–538, 1998.

115. Marton, M. J., DeRisi, J. L., Bennett, H. A., Iyer, V. R., Meyer, M. R., Roberts, C. J., Stoughton, R. et al., Drug target validation and identification of secondary drug target effects using DNA microarrays, *Nature Medicine* 4(11), 1293–1301, 1998.

116. Bubendorf, L., Kolmer, M., Kononen, J., Koivisto, P., Mousses, S., Chen, Y. D., Mahlamaki, E. et al., Hormone therapy failure in human prostate cancer: Analysis by complementary DNA and issue microarrays, *Journal of the National Cancer Institute* 91(20), 1758–1764, 1999.

117. Medlin, J. F., Timely toxicology, *Environmental Health Perspectives* 107(5), A256–A258, 1999.

118. Bartosiewicz, M., Trounstine, M., Barker, D., Johnston, R., and Buckpitt, A., Development of a toxicological gene array and quantitative assessment of this technology, *Archives of Biochemistry and Biophysics* 376(1), 66–73, 2000.

119. Dobrowolski, S. F., Banas, R. A., Naylor, E. W., Powdrill, T., and Thakkar, D., DNA microarray technology for neonatal screening, *Acta Paediatrica* 88, 61–64, 1999.

120. Forozan, F., Karhu, R., Kononen, J., Kallioniemi, A., and Kallioniemi, O. P., Genome screening by comparative genomic hybridization, *Trends in Genetics* 13(10), 405–409, 1997.

121. Wang, K., Gan, L., Jeffery, E., Gayle, M., Gown, A. M., Skelly, M., Nelson, P. S. et al., Monitoring gene expression profile changes in ovarian carcinomas using cDNA microarray, *Gene* 229(1–2), 101–108, 1999.

122. Ono, K., Tanaka, T., Tsunoda, T., Kitahara, O., Kihara, C., Okamoto, A., Ochiai, K., Takagi, T., and Nakamura, Y., Identification by cDNA microarray of genes involved in ovarian carcinogenesis, *Cancer Research* 60(18), 5007–5011, 2000.

123. Xu, J. C., Stolk, J. A., Zhang, X. Q., Silva, S. J., Houghton, R. L., Matsumura, M., Vedvick, T. S. et al., Identification of differentially expressed genes in human prostate cancer using subtraction and microarray, *Cancer Research* 60(6), 1677–1682, 2000.

124. Elek, J., Park, K. H., and Narayanan, R., Microarray-based expression profiling in prostate tumors, *In Vivo* 14(1), 173–182, 2000.

125. Sgroi, D. C., Teng, S., Robinson, G., LeVangie, R., Hudson, J. R., and Elkahloun, A. G., In vivo gene expression profile analysis of human breast cancer progression, *Cancer Research* 59(22), 5656–5661, 1999.

126. Richter, J., Wagner, U., Kononen, J., Fijan, A., Bruderer, J., Schmid, U., Ackermann, D. et al., High-throughput tissue microarray analysis of cyclin E gene amplification and overexpression in urinary bladder cancer, *American Journal of Pathology* 157(3), 787–794, 2000.

127. Hsiao, L. L., Stears, R. L., Hong, R. L., and Gullans, S. R., Prospective use of DNA microarrays for evaluating renal function and disease, *Current Opinion in Nephrology and Hypertension* 9(3), 253–258, 2000.

128. Whitney, L. W., Becker, K. G., Tresser, N. J., Caballero-Ramos, C. I., Munson, P. J., Prabhu, V. V., Trent, J. M., McFarland, H. F., and Biddison, W. E., Analysis of gene expression in multiple sclerosis lesions using cDNA microarrays, *Annals of Neurology* 46(3), 425–428, 1999.

129. Hanzel, D. K., Trojanowski, J. Q., Johnston, R. F., and Loring, J. F., High-throughput quantitative histological analysis of Alzheimer's disease pathology using a confocal digital microscanner, *Nature Biotechnology* 17(1), 53–57, 1999.

130. DeRisi, J. L., Iyer, V. R., and Brown, P. O., Exploring the metabolic and genetic control of gene expression on a genomic scale, *Science* 278(5338), 680–686, 1997.

131. Wodicka, L., Dong, H. L., Mittmann, M., Ho, M. H., and Lockhart, D. J., Genome-wide expression monitoring in *Saccharomyces cerevisiae*, *Nature Biotechnology* 15(13), 1359–1367, 1997.

132. White, K. P., Rifkin, S. A., Hurban, P., and Hogness, D. S., Microarray analysis of *Drosophila* development during metamorphosis, *Science* 286(5447), 2179–2184, 1999.

133. Chambers, J., Angulo, A., Amaratunga, D., Guo, H. Q., Jiang, Y., Wan, J. S., Bittner, A. et al., DNA microarrays of the complex human cytomegalovirus genome: Profiling kinetic class with drug sensitivity of viral gene expression, *Journal of Virology* 73(7), 5757–5766, 1999.

134. Gingeras, T. R., Ghandour, G., Wang, E. G., Berno, A., Small, P. M., Drobniewski, F., Alland, D., Desmond, E., Holodniy, M., and Drenkow, J., Simultaneous genotyping and species identification using hybridization pattern recognition analysis of generic *Mycobacterium* DNA arrays, *Genome Research* 8(5), 435–448, 1998.

135. Geiss, G. K., Bumgarner, R. E., An, M. C., Agy, M. B., van't Wout, A. B., Hammersmark, E., Carter, V. S., Upchurch, D., Mullins, J. I., and Katze, M. G., Large-scale monitoring of host cell gene expression during HIV-1 infection using cDNA microarrays, *Virology* 266(1), 8–16, 2000.

136. Cummings, C. A. and Relman, D. A., Using DNA microarrays to study host-microbe interactions, *Emerging Infectious Diseases* 6(5), 513–525, 2000.

137. Ichikawa, J. K., Norris, A., Bangera, M. G., Geiss, G. K., van't Wout, A. B., Bumgarner, R. E., and Lory, S., Interaction of *Pseudomonas aeruginosa* with epithelial cells: Identification of differentially regulated genes by expression microarray analysis of human cDNAs, *Proceedings of the National Academy of Sciences of the United States of America* 97(17), 9659–9664, 2000.

138. Behr, M. A., Wilson, M. A., Gill, W. P., Salamon, H., Schoolnik, G. K., Rane, S., and Small, P. M., Comparative genomics of BCG vaccines by whole-genome DNA microarray, *Science* 284(5419), 1520–1523, 1999.

139. Sung, D., Yang, S., Park, J. W., and Jon, S., High-density immobilization of antibodies onto nanobead-coated cyclic olefin copolymer plastic surfaces for application as a sensitive immunoassay chip, *Biomedical Microdevices* 15(4), 691–698, 2013. doi 10.1007/s10544-012-9732-x (published online: December 29, 2012).

140. Roh, C., Lee, H.-Y., Kim, S.-E., and Jo, S.-K., A highly sensitive and selective protein detection method based on RNA oligonucleotide nanoparticle, *International Journal of Nanomedicine* 5, 323–329, 2010.

141. Germano, J., Martins, V. C., Cardosa, F. A., Almeida, T. M., Sousa, L., Freitas, P. P., and Piedade, M. S., A portable and autonomous magnetic detection platform for biosensing, *Sensors* 9, 4119–4437, 2009.

142. Martins, V. C., Cardosa, F. A., Freitas, P. P., and Fonseca, L. P., Picomolar detection limit on a magnetoresistive biochip after optimization of a thiol–gold based surface chemistry, *Journal of Nanoscience and Nanotechnology* 10, 5994–6002, 2010.

143. Huang, J.-T., Hou, S.-Y., Fang, S.-B., Yu, H.-W., Lee, H.-C., and Yang, C.-Z., Development of a biochip using antibody-coated gold nanoparticles to detect specific bioparticles, *Journal of Industrial Microbiology and Biotechnology* 35, 1377–1385, 2008.

144. Hu, N., Zhou, J., Su, K., Zhang, D., Xiao, L., Wang, T., and Wang, P., An integrated label-free cell-based biosensor for simultaneously monitoring of cellular physiology multiparameter *in vitro*, *Biomedical Microdevices* 15(3), 473–480, 2013.

145. Baxter, G., Hurel™—An in vivo-surrogate assay platform for cell-based studies, *Alternatives to Laboratory Animals* 37(Supplement 1), 11–18, 2009.

146. Curtis, T. M., Widder, M. W., Brennan, L. M., Schwager, S. J., van der Schalie, W. H., Fey, J., and Salazar, N., A portable cell-based impedance sensor for toxicity testing of drinking water, *Lab on a Chip* 9, 2176–2183, 2009.

147. Van Midwoud, P. M., Groothuis, G. M. M., Merema, M. T., and Verpoorte, E., Microfluidic biochip or the perifusion of precision-cut rat liver slices for metabolism and toxicology studies, *Biotechnology and Bioengineering* 105(1), 184–194, 2010.

148. Kwon, J.-S., Ravindranath, S. P., Kumar, A., Irudayara, J., and Wereley, S. T., Opto-electrokinetic manipulation for high-performance on-chip bioassays, *Lab on a Chip* 12, 4955–4959, 2012.

149. Zhu, L., Jiang, G., Wang, S., Wang, C., Li, Q., Yu, H., Zhou, Y. et al., Biochip system for rapid and accurate identification of mycobacterial species from isolates and sputum, *Journal of Clinical Microbiology* 48(10), 3654–3660, 2010.

150. Javanmard, M., Talasaz, A. H., Nemat-Gorgoni, M., Pease, F., Ronaghi, M., and Davis, R. W., Electrical detection of protein biomarkers using bioactivated microfluidic channels, *Lab on a Chip* 9(10), 1429–1434, 2009.

151. Pernagallo, S., Ventimiglia, G., Cavalluzo, C., Alessi, E., Ilyine, H., Bradley, M., and Diaz-Mochon, J. J., Novel biochip platform for nucleic acid analysis, *Sensors* 12, 8100–8111, 2012.

152. Kraus, S., Kleines, M., Albers, J., Blohm, L., Piechotta, G., Puttmann, C., Barth, S., Nahring, J., and Nebling, E., Quantitative measurement of human anti-HCV core immunoglobulins on an electrical biochip platform, *Biosensors & Bioelectronics* 26, 1895–1901, 2011.

153. Marcy, Y., Cousin, P.-Y., Rattier, M., Cerovic, G., Escalier, G., Bena, G., Gueron, M. et al., Innovative integrated system for real-time measurement of hybridization and melting on standard format microarrays, *Biotechniques* 44(7), 913–920, 2008.

154. Seefeld, T. H., Zhou, W.-J., and Corn, R. M., Rapid microarray detection of DNA and proteins in microliter volumes with SPR imaging measurements, *Langmuir* 27(10), 6534–6540, 2011.

155. Chen, X., Cui, D. F., and Liu, C. C., On-line cell lysis and DNA extraction on a microfluidic biochip fabricated by microelectromechanical system technology, *Electrophoresis* 29, 1844–1851, 2008.

156. Kim, J., Lee, G.-H., Jung, W., and Hah, S. S., Selective and quantitative cell detection based on aptamers and the conventional cell-staining methods, *Biosensors & Bioelectronics* 43, 362–365, 2013.

157. Fang, X., Jin, Q., Jing, F., Zhang, H., Zhang, F., Mao, H., Xu, B., and Zhao, J., Integrated biochip for label-free and real-time detection of DNA amplification by contactless impedance measurements based on interdigitated electrodes, *Biosensors & Bioelectronics* 44, 241–247, 2013.

158. Wen, J., Shi, X., He, Y., Zhou, J., and Li, Y., Novel plastic biochips for colorimetric detection of biomolecules, *Analytical and Bioanalytical Chemistry* 404, 1935–1944, 2012.

159. Fitzgerald, S. P., Lamont, J. V., McConnell, R. I., and Benchikh, E. O., Development of a high-throughput automated analyzer using biochip array technology, *Clinical Chemistry* 51(7), 1165–1176, 2005.

160. Bunger, S., Haug, U., Kelly, M., Posorski, N., Klempt-Giessing, K., Cartwright, A., Fitzgerald, S. P. et al., A novel multiplex-protein array for serum diagnostics of colon cancer: A case-control study, *BMC Cancer* 12, 393, 2012.

161. Porter, J., O'Loan, N., Bell, B., Mahoney, J., McGarrity, M., McConnell, R. I., and Fitzgerald, S. P., Development of an evidence biochip array kit for the multiplex screening of more than 20 anthelmintic drugs, *Analytical and Bioanalytical Chemistry* 403, 3051–3056, 2012.

162. Stern, E., Vacic, A., Rajan, N. K., Criscione, J. M., Park, J., Ilic, B. J., Mooney, D. J., Reed, M. A., and Fahmy, T. M., Label-free biomarker detection from whole blood, *Nature Nanotechnology* 5(2), 138–142, 2010.

163. Pedrero, M., Campuzano, S., and Pingarron, J. M., Electroanalytical sensors and devices for multiplexed detection of foodborne pathogen microorganisms, *Sensors* 9, 5503–5520, 2009.

164. Nasedkina, T. V., Guseva, N. A., Gra, O. A., Mityaeva, O. N., Chudinov, A., and Zasedatelev, A. S., Diagnostic microarrays in hematologic oncology, *Molecular Diagnosis and Therapy* 13(2), 91–102, 2009.

165. Wang, H. N., Dhawan, A., Du, Y., Batchelor, D., Leonard, D. N., Misra, V., and Vo-Dinh, T., Molecular sentinel-on-chip for SERS-based biosensing, *Physical Chemistry Chemical Physics* 15(16), 6008–6015, April 28, 2013. doi: 10.1039/c3cp00076a.

166. Wabuyele, M. and Vo-Dinh, T., Detection of HIV type 1 DNA sequence using plasmonics nanoprobes, *Analytical Chemistry* 77, 7810–7815, 2005.

167. Wang, H.-N. and Vo-Dinh, T., Multiplex detection of breast cancer biomarkers using plasmonic molecular sentinel nanoprobes, *Nanotechnology* 20, 065101-1–065101-6, 2009.

168. Yi, C., Li, C.-W., Fu, H., Zhang, M., Qi, S., Wong, N.-B., Lee, S.-T., and Yang, M., Patterned growth of vertically aligned silicon nanowire arrays for label-free DNA detection using surface-enhanced Raman spectroscopy, *Analytical and Bioanalytical Chemistry* 397, 3143–3150, 2010.

169. Strelau, K. K., Kretschmer, R., Moller, R., Fritzsche, W., and Popp, J., SERS as tool for the analysis of DNA-chips in a microfluidic platform, *Analytical and Bioanalytical Chemistry* 396, 1381–1384, 2010.

170. Bhuvana, T. and Kulkarni, G. U., A SERS-active nanocrystalline Pd substrate and its nanopatterning leading to a biochip fabrication, *Small* 4(5), 670–676, 2008.

171. Ali, M. A., Solanki, P. R., Patel, M. K., Dhayani, H., Agrawal, V. V., John, R., and Malhotra, B. D., A highly efficient microfluidic nano biochip based on nanostructured nickel oxide, *Nanoscale* 5, 2883–2891, 2013.

172. Hong, C.-C., Lin, C.-C., Hong, C.-L., and Chang, P.-H., Enhanced anesthetic propofol biochips by modifying molecularly imprinted nanocavities of biosensors, *Biomedical Microdevices* 14, 435–441, 2012.

173. Birnbaumer, G. M., Lieberzeit, P. A., Richter, L., Schirhagl, R., Milnera, M., Dickert, F. L., Bailey, A., and Ertl, P., Detection of viruses with molecularly imprinted polymers integrated on a microfluidic biochip using contact-less dielectric microsensors, *Lab on a Chip* 9, 3549–3556, 2009.

174. Zhang, H., Jia, Z., Lv, X., Zhou, J., Chen, L., Liu, R., and Ma, J., Porous silicon optical microcavity biosensor on silicon-on-insulator wafer for sensitive DNA detection, *Biosensors & Bioelectronics* 44, 89–94, 2013.

175. Zhang, R., Gong, H.-Q., Zeng, X. D., and Sze, C. C., A high-throughput microfluidic biochip to quantify bacterial adhesion to single host cells by real-time PCR assay, *Analytical and Bioanalytical Chemistry* 405(12), 4277–4282, 2013.

176. Ma, Z., Yang, H., Liu, H., Xu, M., Runyon, R. B., Eisenberg, C. A., Markwald, R. R., Borg, T. K., and Gao, B. K., Mesenchymal stem cell–cardiomyocytes interactions under defined contact modes on laser-patterned biochips, *PLoS ONE* 8(2), e56554, 2013.

177. Marhefka, J. N. and Abbud-Antali, R. A., Validation of the cancer BioChip system as a 3D siRNA screening tool for breast cancer targets, *PLoS ONE* 7(9), e46086, 2012.

178. Jena, R. K. and Yue, C. Y., Cyclic olefin copolymer based microfluidic devices of biochip applications: Ultraviolet surface grafting using 2-methacryloyloxyethyl phosphorylcholine, *Biomicrofluidics* 6, 012822-1–012822-12, 2012.

179. Bearinger, J. P., Stone, G., Hiddessen, A. L., Dugan, L. C., Wu, L., Hailey, P., Conway, J. W., Kuenzler, T., Feller, L., Cerritelli, S., and Hubbell, J. A., Photocatalytic lithograph of poly(propylene sulfide) block copolymers: Towards high throughput nanolithography for biomolecular arraying applications, *Langmuir* 25(2), 1238–1244, 2009.

180. Sollier, K., Mandon, C. A., Heyries, K. A., Blum, L. J., and Marquette, C. A., "Print-n-Shrink" technology for the rapid production of microfluidic chips an d protein microarrays, *Lab on a Chip* 9, 3489–3494, 2009.

181. Chakra, E. B., Hannes, B., Veillard, J., Mansfield, C. D., Mazurczyk, R., Bouchard, A., Potempa, J., Krawczyk, S., and Cabrera, M., Grafting of antibodies inside integrated microfluidic-microoptic devices by means of automated microcontact printing, *Sensors and Actuators B: Chemical* 140(1), 278–286, 2009.
182. O'Sullivan, T. D., Munro, E., Parashurama, N., Conca, C., Harris, J. S., Gambhir, S. S., and Levi, O., Implantable semiconductor biosensor for continuous in vivo sensing of far-red fluorescent molecules, *Optics Express* 18, 12513–12525, 2010.
183. Guiseppi-Elie, A., An implantable biochip to influence patient outcomes following trauma-induced hemorrhage, *Analytical and Bioanalytical Chemistry* 399, 403–419, 2011.
184. Carrara, S., Ghoreishizadeh, S., Olivo, J., Taurino, I., Baj-Rossi, C., Cavallini, A., de Beeck, M. O. et al., Fully integrated biochip platforms for advanced healthcare, *Sensors* 12, 11013–11060, 2012.

4

Atomic Spectrometry in Clinical and Biological Analysis

Andrew Taylor
*Royal Surrey County
Hospital*

4.1 Introduction

Within biological systems, elements may be classified as those essential to the well-being of the organism and those that have no known or demonstrable function and are therefore regarded as nonessential.[1,2] On the basis of the usual concentrations within tissues and body fluids, they may also be classified as major or trace elements, trace elements being defined as those that individually contribute no more than 0.01% of the dry body mass.[3] All the major elements and a limited number of trace elements are essential (Table 4.1); all others that may be detected are nonessential. Essential elements are required for various biological functions,[1] for example,

- Enzyme structure and function
- Hormone structure and function
- Vitamin structure and function (e.g., B_{12})
- Transport of oxygen
- Structure of macromolecules

When any are present in less than optimal concentrations, symptoms of morbidity will be evident—indeed, the severity of deficiency may be such that death is the eventual outcome (Figure 4.1). At the same time, all elements, whether essential or nonessential, are toxic if they accumulate in tissues to sufficiently large concentrations.[3]

Therefore, it is important that accurate measurements in biological and clinical specimens may be obtained for fundamental research involving mechanistic aspects of trace element biology and so that deficiencies or excess may be detected in various situations.[1,4] In addition to these concepts of essentiality

TABLE 4.1   Major Elements and Essential Trace Elements in Clinical and Biological Samples

	Minerals	Nonminerals
Major elements	Calcium, iron, magnesium, potassium, sodium	Carbon, chlorine, hydrogen, nitrogen, oxygen, phosphorus, sulfur
Essential elements (not all proven to have essential roles in man)	Chromium, cobalt, copper, iron, manganese, molybdenum, nickel, selenium, silicon, vanadium, zinc	Fluorine, iodine

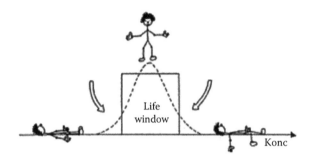

FIGURE 4.1   Representation of the relationship between essential elements and well-being.

and nonessentiality and deficiency and toxicity, elements are also used therapeutically and concentrations in body fluids may be required to monitor the effectiveness and safety of the treatment.[3]

The analytical techniques used must afford the sensitivity necessary to measure concentrations below 1 ppm, often low ppb levels, in specimens of just a few microliters or milligrams with almost total specificity and relatively few interferences. These demands are met by the atomic spectrometry techniques described in this chapter.

Put very simply, spectroscopy is concerned with the study of interactions between electromagnetic radiation and matter, while spectrometry is the exploitation of these interactions to gain analytical (quantitative or qualitative) information. As indicated by the terminology, the interactions studied in atomic spectrometry involve atoms (rather than molecules) and the purpose is to determine the concentration or, more rarely, simply the presence of an element within a sample. The appropriate energy required to interact with atoms is that derived from the UV–visible section, and by high-energy particles, of the electromagnetic spectrum. In practice, atomic spectrometry involves the emission, absorption, or fluorescence of such energy. Thus, this chapter describes atomic emission spectrometry (AES), atomic absorption spectrometry (AAS), atomic fluorescence spectrometry (AFS), and x-ray fluorescence spectrometry (XRF). Although these procedures are used extensively, elements may also be determined by a number of other techniques; of particular relevance to biological and clinical specimens are those involving inorganic mass spectrometry, activation analysis, and anodic stripping voltammetry.[5] Recognizing the importance of these techniques, brief reference will be included, particularly where features overlap with the more conventional atomic spectrometry.

4.2 Principles

Analytical AES, AAS, and AFS are quantitative techniques that exploit interactions between UV–visible light and the outer shell electrons of free, gaseous, uncharged atoms. In XRF and related techniques, high-energy particles interact with inner shell electrons to initiate further electron transitions within the atom that conclude with the emission of x-ray photons.

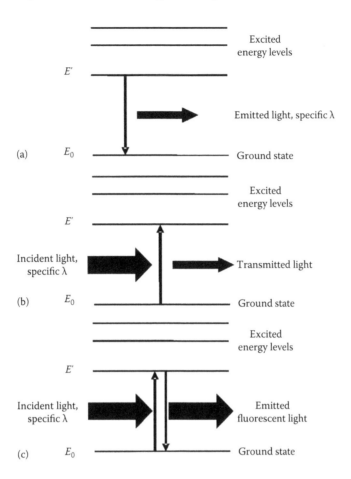

FIGURE 4.2 Energy transitions associated with (a) atomic emission, (b) absorption, and (c) fluorescence.

Each element has a characteristic atomic structure with a positively charged nucleus surrounded by electrons in orbital shells to provide neutrality. These electrons occupy discrete energy levels, but it is possible for an electron to be moved from one level to another within the atom by the introduction of energy (Figure 4.2). This energy may be supplied by collisions with other atoms, that is, heating (for AES), as photons of light (for AAS and AFS), or as high-energy particles (for XRF). Such transitions occur only if the available energy is equal to the difference between two levels (ΔE). Uncharged atoms may exist at the lowest energy level or ground state (E_0), or at any one of a series of excited states (E_n) depending on how certain electrons have been moved to higher energy levels, although it is usual to consider just the first transition. Energy levels and the ΔEs associated with electron transitions are unique for each element.

The ΔE for movements of outer shell electrons in most elements correspond to the energy equivalent to UV–visible radiation and these transitions are used for AES, AAS, and AFS. The energy of a photon (E) is characterized by

$$E = h\nu \tag{4.1}$$

where
    h is Planck's constant
    ν is the frequency of the waveform corresponding to that photon

Furthermore, frequency and wavelength are related as

$$v = \frac{c}{\lambda} \tag{4.2}$$

where
   c is the velocity of light
   λ is the wavelength

Therefore,

$$E = \frac{hc}{\lambda} \tag{4.3}$$

and it follows that a specific transition, ΔE, is associated with a unique wavelength.[6]

Under appropriate conditions, outer shell electrons of vaporized atoms may be excited by thermal energy (i.e., collisions with other atoms). As these electrons return to the more stable ground state, energy is lost. As Figure 4.2 shows, some of this energy will be in the form of emitted light, which can be measured with a detector; this is AES. When light (radiant energy) of a characteristic wavelength enters an analytical system, outer shell electrons of the corresponding atoms will be excited as energy is absorbed. Consequently, the amount of light transmitted from the system to the detector will be attenuated; this is understood as AAS. Finally, some of the radiant energy absorbed by ground-state atoms can be emitted as light as the atom returns to the ground state, that is, AFS.

When high-energy photons, electrons, or protons strike a solid sample, an electron from the inner shells (K, L, or M) of a constituent atom may be displaced (i.e., ionization). The structure of this atom is then unstable and the resulting orbital vacancy is filled by an outer shell electron *falling* into the hole. This movement releases energy, as emission of an x-ray photon, the energy being equal to the difference between the energy levels involved. This emission is known as XRF. The energy of the emission, that is, the wavelength, is characteristic of the atom (element) from which it originated, while the intensity of the emission is related to the concentration of the atoms in the sample. The transitions are given names that describe the movement of electrons: L to K is Kα, M to K is Kβ, and M to L is Lα (Figure 4.3).

Depending on the principle of the spectrometer employed to measure the emission, XRF is divided into wavelength dispersive XRF (WDXRF) or energy dispersive XRF (EDXRF). Total reflection XRF (TXRF) is usually described as a separate technique although it may be seen as a modification of

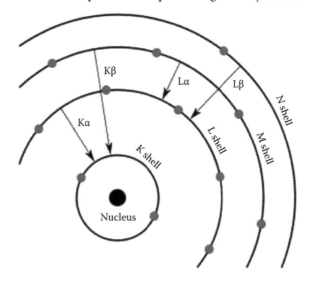

FIGURE 4.3   XRF electronic transitions in a calcium atom.

EDXRF. High-energy hydrogen or helium ions may also be used as incident radiation to displace an electron from a K or L shell with an emission of characteristic x-rays. This is known as particle-induced x-ray emission (PIXE). In addition to being an independent analytical technique, PIXE can be used with electron microscopy to provide elemental analysis of visualized specimens.

Analogous to XRF and PIXE, when an atom is bombarded with charged particles, a radioactive nuclide may be formed. Gamma radiation then emitted is characteristic of the nuclide and the intensity of the emission is proportional to the analyte concentration. Neutrons are most often used for excitation and the technique is then called neutron activation analysis. This multielement technique requires specialized facilities and is not widely available.[5]

The high-temperature inductively coupled plasma (ICP) (see Section 4.3.4) is an effective ion source for a mass spectrometer; the technique of ICP-mass spectrometry (ICP-MS) is extensively used for measurements of trace elements in clinical and biological materials. It affords very sensitive multielement analysis and also provides for the determination of stable isotopes.[7,8]

Anodic stripping voltammetry is an electrochemical procedure that offers exceptional sensitivity for some applications. It is ideally suited for large sample volumes such as water specimens, but it is widely applied to the measurement of lead in blood,[5] particularly in North America.

It follows from Equations 4.1 through 4.3 that the wavelengths of the absorbed and emitted energies are unique to a given element. It is this that makes atomic spectrometric techniques specific, so that one element can be determined even in the presence of an enormous excess of a chemically similar element.[6]

4.3 Instrumentation

Formation of the atomic vapor, that is, atomization, is central to emission, absorption, and fluorescence by atoms. Atomizers and the devices for sample introduction are the heart of the instrumentation, with an associated spectrometer for wavelength separation and detection of light. Atomization involves the following steps: removal of solvent (drying), separation from anion or other components of the matrix, and reduction of ions to the ground-state atom. Energy necessary to accomplish these steps is supplied as heat. The proportion of an atom population within the vapor, as the excited- or the ground-state atoms, is influenced by the temperature and the atomic structure of the element. At the temperatures of flame and electrothermal atomizers, around 2–3000 K, the ratio is at least 10^{-6}:1 for most elements and AAS affords superior sensitivity to AES. With the much higher temperatures provided by an ICP atomizer, the proportion changes and AES may be favored.

An essential requirement for atomic absorption is a highly intense source of radiant energy. Hollow cathode lamps (HCLs) or electrodeless discharge lamps (EDLs) are traditionally used, which have the additional feature of transmitting light of a very narrow and specific wavelength. Consequently, AAS is essentially a single-element technique so that if more than one element is to be determined, the lamp has to be changed for each analysis and the samples remeasured.

Multielement analytical systems, with continuum light sources to give radiation over a wide spectral range, have been constructed in the past but performance was rarely as good as with HCL or EDL. Interest has been revived following technical developments, and high-resolution continuum source AAS instrumentation employing a high-intensity xenon short-arc lamp as the continuum radiation source, a high-resolution double-echelle monochromator, and a CCD array detector, providing a resolution of ~2 pm per pixel, is now commercially available. The potential advantages of this development were described in detail by Welz et al.,[9] and several examples of application to real analytical problems have since been published.[10]

4.3.1 Flame Atomizers

The flame provides for simple, rapid measurements with few interferences and is preferred wherever the analyte concentration is suitable. The typical pneumatic nebulizer for sample introduction is inefficient

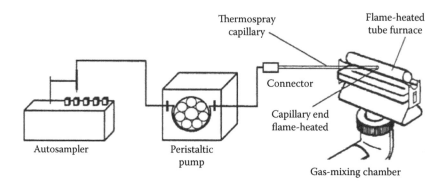

FIGURE 4.4　Flame furnace atomizer.

and although elements such as Na and K may be measured in biological specimens by flame AES, flame atomization is more usually suited to AAS and AFS. With AAS, measurements are possible with specimens where concentrations are around 1 μg/mL or more. Devices have been developed that overcome the limitations of the pneumatic nebulizer by bypassing the nebulizer so that 100% of the sample is atomized; they also introduce the sample as a single, rapid pulse rather than by continuous flow. These approaches are also features of electrothermal atomization and vapor generation procedures (see Sections 4.3.3 and 4.5.4). Lower detection limits are obtained with AFS but various constraints restrict this technique, with a few exceptions, to the hydride-forming elements (see Section 4.5.4).[11]

4.3.2　Flame Furnace

The sensitivity of flame AAS (FAAS) can be improved by employing flame furnace AAS (FFAAS) in which the sample is directly injected into a Ni tube positioned in the flame (Figure 4.4). This provides for 100% of sample being atomized and detection limits can be improved by up to at least 30-fold with little degradation of precision. Different techniques for introducing the sample have been used but the most effective is to create a thermospray so that the liquid sample disperses at the point of entry.[12] A recent development involves a double atomizer, with a Ti tube inside a Ni tube.[13]

4.3.3　Electrothermal Atomizers

Most systems use an electrically heated graphite tube, a technique often called graphite furnace atomization, although other materials are sometimes employed.[11,14] With a programmed temperature sequence, the test solution (10–50 μL) is dried, organic material destroyed, and the analyte ions dissociated from anions for reduction to ground-state atoms. The temperatures achieved by this technique can be up to 3000 K so that refractory elements such as aluminum and chromium will form an atomic vapor. Because all of the sample is atomized and retained within the small volume of the furnace, a dense atom population is produced. The technique is, therefore, very sensitive and allows measurement of μg/L concentrations. Although the technique is widely used for AAS, electrothermal atomization is also suitable for AES and for sample introduction into an ICP.[11,15]

4.3.4　Inductively Coupled Plasmas

As stated previously, high-temperature atomizers are required to provide useful numbers of excited atoms for AES. Historical sources include arcs and sparks but modern instruments use argon, or some other inert gas, in the form of a plasma. The plasma is formed when gas atoms are ionized, $Ar + e^- \leftrightarrow Ar^+ + 2e^-$—a process generated by seeding from a high-voltage spark—and is sustained with energy from an induction

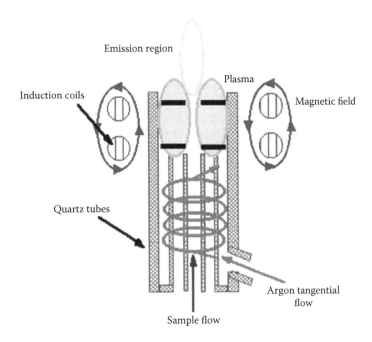

FIGURE 4.5 (**See color insert.**) ICP torch.

coil connected to a radio-frequency generator. This is known as an ICP; other plasmas (direct coupled, glow discharge) have been described but are not widely employed. Plasmas exist at temperatures of up to 10,000 K and in the instrument have the appearance of a torch (Figure 4.5). Samples can be introduced via a nebulizer, by vapor generation procedures, by vaporization from a graphite atomizer, or by laser ablation of solid specimens.

The main feature of AES is that it permits multielement analysis. Optical systems direct the emitted light via a monochromator to a single detector or to an array of monochromators and detectors positioned around the plasma. With the first arrangement, a sequential series of readings are made with the monochromator driven to give each of the wavelengths of interest in turn. Simultaneous readings can be made with the second arrangement. For most elements, the analytical sensitivity for ICP-AES is similar to that obtained with flame AAS at the part per million level although with recent developments in instrumentation, performance may rival that seen with electrothermal AAS.[16]

4.3.5 X-Ray Fluorescence

XRF requires that specimens be irradiated by high-energy photons. In most instruments, the source is the polychromatic primary beam from x-ray tubes. Of interest to biological applications, however, is the use of radioactive isotopes as sources. Isotopes such as [244]Cm, [241]Am, [55]Fe, and [109]Cd are used.[10,17] The latter is particularly important as the source in portable instruments developed for in vivo XRF (see Section 4.5.5). A growing number of publications refer to the use of synchrotron radiation that acts as a high-resolution highly energetic source.[17]

Because sample matrix contributes considerably to signal intensity, calibration can be difficult, usually requiring the use of different reference materials or internal standardization. Fewer problems are encountered with samples prepared as very thin films and in TXRF. Together with the effect of the matrix, sensitivity is also influenced by wavelength, such that lighter elements present a difficult analytical challenge.

In WDXRF, high-intensity x-rays (e.g., from a 3 kW x-ray tube) are used to induce the fluorescence emission, which is dispersed into individual spectral lines by reflection at an analyzer crystal.

The diffracted beams are collimated and directed onto a photon detector. As with ICP-AES, spectrometers may operate sequentially, with a number of interchangeable crystals, to permit the measurement of the full range of elements, or in a multichannel (simultaneous) mode usually preset for specific analytes. Detection limits for light elements are 10–100 times lower than with EDXRF. Resolution is good, although less so at shorter wavelengths. Sequential instruments require long analysis times to measure several elements compared with the more expensive simultaneous instruments or EDXRF technology.

For EDXRF, x-rays emitted from the sample are directed together into a crystal detector. A pulse of current is generated with a height proportional to the energy of the x-ray photon. The different energies associated with the various atoms (elements) in the sample are sorted electronically. Lower energy sources (a low-power x-ray tube or an isotopic source) are used. The detector must be maintained at a very low temperature and in a clean vacuum. Analysis times are 10–30 times longer than with WDXRF but, as a truly multielement technique, the total time is not necessarily any greater.

When a collimated beam of x-rays is directed against an optically flat surface at an angle of around 5′, total reflection will occur. This is the principle of TXRF in which the sample is exposed to primary and total reflected beams and is excited to fluoresce. Emitted radiation is resolved and measured as an ED spectrum. There is effectively no absorption by the matrix, so measurement and calibration are much simpler and sensitivities are greater than with other x-ray techniques.

4.4 Sample Preparation

While there are some exceptions, most analytical systems for measuring metals require samples to be in a liquid form. The objectives for preparation of biomedical specimens are to ensure the specimen is in a suitable form for introduction to the analytical instrument, to remove interfering components from the matrix, and to adjust the concentration of analyte to facilitate the actual measurement. These objectives may be realized by a number of approaches (Table 4.2).

Methods for destruction of the organic matrix by simple heating or by acid digestion have been used extensively and are thoroughly validated. Microwave heating is now well established for this purpose, with specifically constructed apparatus to avoid dangers of excessive pressure within reaction vessels. Although the number of specimens that can be processed is not large, microwave heating affords rapid digestion and low reagent blanks. More recent developments include continuous flow systems for automated digestion linked directly to the instrument for measurement of the analytes.

Preconcentration by liquid–liquid partitioning is a widely used procedure. Analyte atoms in a large volume of aqueous specimen are complexed with an appropriate agent and then extracted into a smaller volume of organic solvent. This leads to enhancement of concentration and also removes the analyte from potential or real interferences in the original matrix. It is used to measure lead in blood and metals in urine and for other applications. Trapping onto solid-phase media represents the area where much of the recent interest in FAAS has been focused.[10,18] The original work involved adsorption onto material such as charcoal or alumina but newer phases include ion-exchange resins and novel support systems to which functional groups are added to confer increased selectivity and capacity.[19]

TABLE 4.2   Approaches to Sample Preparation

Procedure	Remarks
Dilution, protein precipitation	Using simple offline arrangements or flow-injection manifold
Dry ashing	Using a muffle furnace or a low-temperature asher
Acid digestion	1. In open vessels with convection or microwave heating
	2. In sealed vessels to increase the reaction pressure
Base dissolution	Using quaternary ammonium hydroxides
Chelation and solvent extraction	For analyte enhancement and removal of interferences
Trapping onto solid-phase media	For analyte enhancement and removal of interferences

Trapping of analyte from dilute sample and elution into a small volume of release solution may be accomplished offline; however, developments in flow-injection analysis provide for the assembly of simple online manifolds so that complete measurements may be carried through automatically.[10,20] Developments in these applications involving a wide range of biological and clinical sample types and elements are regularly published.

Vapor generation procedures were referred to in earlier sections. These permit the rapid introduction of 100% of the sample into the atomizer and are used for AAS, AFS, ICP-AES, and ICP-MS.[11] Certain elements such as arsenic, selenium, and bismuth readily form gaseous hydrides, for example, arsine (AsH_3), that are transferred by a flow of inert gas to a heated silica tube positioned in the light path. The tube is heated by the air–acetylene flame or by an electric current and the temperature is sufficient to cause dissociation of the hydride and atomization of the analyte. Thus, there is no loss of specimen, all the atoms enter the light path within a few seconds and they are trapped within the silica tube, which retards their dispersion. Hydride generation AAS allows the detection of a few nanograms of analyte from whatever sample volume is placed into the reaction flask.

Mercury forms a vapor at ambient temperatures and this property is the basis for cold vapor generation. A reducing agent is added to the sample solution to convert Hg^{2+} to the elemental mercury. Agitation or bubbling of gas through the solution causes rapid vaporization of the atomic mercury, which is then transferred to a flow-through cell placed in the light path. As with hydride generation, the detection limit is a few nanograms and common instrumentation to accomplish both procedures has been developed by some manufacturers.

Appreciation of the importance of determining not just the total concentration of an element in a specimen but also something of its distribution is now well established. This concept of speciation is applied to associations with different molecules such as proteins, to different organometallic compounds, and to different valence states.[21] A number of preparative procedures are available to separate or speciate the analyte,[22] but much innovation is directed to chromatographic and electrophoretic techniques that are coupled directly to the atomic spectrometric equipment to form an integrated analytical arrangement. Examples are presented in the following section. Contrasting with measurement of total concentration, in which destruction of the sample matrix facilitates the analysis, the intrinsic structures and forms of the analytes must be maintained prior to measurement. Therefore, more subtle preparative techniques are required to extract analyte species. Methods used include ultrasonic-assisted extraction, pressure extraction, and lytic enzymes.[10]

4.5 Recent Developments and Applications

Measurements of major and trace elements in biological and clinical specimens are required in many situations.

Work to determine mechanisms of action within biological systems at cellular and biochemical levels, of essentiality and of toxicity, involves knowing concentrations within the experimental systems.

Determining trace element and mineral physiology, routes of absorption, tissue distribution, and concentrations in normal subjects and in patients with inborn errors involves these processes, for example, copper and Wilson's disease.

Nutritional studies investigate possible deficiencies of essential elements, for example, in subjects with poor diets or patients receiving long-term total parenteral feeding (where protocols for regular monitoring are generally recommended).[1] In addition to measuring trace elements in blood and urine, such work may include analysis of foods and special investigations to assess intestinal absorption.

Investigation of undue exposure to elements[4]: Increased exposure to minerals and trace elements can cause morbidity and some are carcinogenic. While the function of many organs may be perturbed by accumulation of metals, the kidney, liver, nervous, intestinal, and hemopoietic systems are more likely to be involved. Accidental (or even deliberate suicidal or homicidal) exposures to trace elements feature in the differential diagnosis when considering signs and symptoms involving these sites. Increased exposure may be consequent on sources within the environment or in the home, associated with hobbies or from unusual cosmetics and remedies. In an occupational setting, biological monitoring is important in the implementation of health and safety regulations.[23]

In other situations, iatrogenic poisoning can occur. Profound toxicity has been observed for many elements including aluminum, bismuth, and manganese.[4]

4.5.1 Atomic Emission Spectrometry

Sodium, potassium, and lithium are usually measured by flame AES or with ion-selective electrodes although they can also be determined by flame AAS. At the temperature of the flame, there is no useful emission of other biologically important elements. However, with the greater energy of the ICP, lower detection limits are obtained and many elements may be determined simultaneously in solutions prepared from biological tissues. Furthermore, a few elements, such as boron, phosphorus, and sulfur, cannot be measured by AAS but are determined by ICP-AES.

Developments with the optical systems and array detectors have led to improvements in sensitivity and data collection. In consequence, elements such as copper, zinc, and aluminum may be measured in blood plasma,[24–26] while the expanded information caught by detectors is making it possible for powerful chemometric manipulation of individual signals to be undertaken. ICP-AES now has an established role for monitoring patients with possible compromised nutritional status[24] and those who receive hemodialysis to treat chronic renal failure and are at risk of developing aluminum toxicity.[25] With the multielement feature of the technique, ICP-AES is widely used for analysis of foodstuffs and tissues samples.[10] The convenience of this approach has, however, encouraged the dubious *diagnostic practice* of hair analysis among some laboratories.[27] Vapor generation techniques for sample introduction (see Section 4.5.4) are possible.

4.5.2 Atomic Absorption Spectrometry

Measurement of calcium in serum was the first analysis to which AAS was applied and is an obvious example of how the technique is useful for biomedical analysis. Elements present in biological fluids at a sufficiently high concentration to be measured by flame AAS are lithium and gold, when used to treat depression and rheumatoid arthritis, respectively, and calcium, magnesium, iron, copper, and zinc. Flame AAS is used by the large majority of laboratories needing to measure these elements. It fulfills an important role in the investigation of patients with possible nutritional problems, genetic disorders, or other relevant clinical challenges. Other elements are present in fluids at too low a concentration to be measured by conventional FAAS with pneumatic nebulization. With more exotic fluids, for example, seminal plasma or cerebrospinal fluid, analysis may just be possible for a very few elements.

The concentrations of many metals in plant, animal, or human tissues are usually much higher than in biological fluids and very often the weight of an available specimen is such that a relatively large mass of analyte is recovered into a small volume of solution, thus enhancing the concentration still further. For the analysis of tissues (including specimens such as hair and the cellular fractions of blood) following sample dissolution steps, FAAS is suitable for measurement of many of the biologically important elements.[10]

The flame furnace and various accessories for atom trapping such as the slotted quartz tube increase the sensitivity associated with FAAS for more volatile elements[28]; sporadic reports appear of their use in simplified methods for analysis of biological fluids. However, if concentrations are low, it is more usual to take advantage of the lower limits of detection provided by electrothermal AAS.

Virtually all the trace elements of biological interest may be determined by electrothermal AAS. Although it is relatively slow, a single-element technique, and subject to various interferences, it is extensively used throughout the world for clinical investigations and for monitoring occupational exposures, as well as in the other settings mentioned earlier. The design and construction of furnaces are subject to continuous development to improve detection limits and to reduce interferences.[11,18] Devices to measure nonatomic absorption, for example, Zeeman-effect background correction, are essential. Commercial furnaces are made from electrographite, electrographite with a pyrolytic coating, or total pyrolytic graphite, although publications showing the advantages of other materials as coatings or for the furnace itself regularly appear.[14] Typically, these refer to analysis of elements that form extremely refractory carbides in graphite furnaces, for example, molybdenum.

Design developments are introduced with the objective of separating the appearance of the atomic vapor from components that cause an interference with the atomization signal. These innovations include graphite platforms and probes but, as with automobiles, there are continuous refinements to the overall shape and dimensions to effect improvements in performance. An authoritative review of materials suitable for use in furnace construction and of recent developments in design has been prepared by Frech.[14] Several research groups have designed very novel atomizers with the purpose of separating the analyte from interfering species, to permit simple atomic absorption.[29-31] Although some appear to be effective, none are commercially available.

It was shown some years ago that a 150 W tungsten filament from a light bulb could be used as an electrothermal atomizer. More recently, this concept has been used to develop very small portable instruments for on-site measurement of lead in blood.[32] Excellent results have been reported but a commercial model is still awaited.

In addition, effective analysis of most biological samples requires the addition of reagents that modify the behavior of the specimen during the heating program so as to reduce interferences.[10] The chemical modifiers most commonly employed with biological specimens are given in Table 4.3. Triton X-100 is used at a concentration of around 0.1% w/v and is included with the sample diluent. Gaseous oxygen or air is an effective ashing aid but will cause rapid deterioration of the graphite furnace unless a desorption step is included before the temperature is increased for atomization. Other modifier solutions can be included with the sample diluent or separately added by the autosampler to the specimen inside the furnace. The choice of modifier often depends on the availability of a source material that is free from contamination.

4.5.3 Atomic Fluorescence Spectrometry

Recent innovations in AFS follow almost entirely from the development of commercial instruments specifically designed for use with vapor generation applications; the particular applications of interest will be considered in the next section. For various reasons, earlier attempts to exploit the inherent sensitivity of AFS using flame systems were never fully realized. However, with improvements in light source technology and other instrumentation, this niche area has progressed rapidly in recent years.[10,11]

TABLE 4.3 Chemical Modifiers Used in the Analysis of Biomedical Specimens by ETAAS

Modifier	Purpose
Triton X-100	To promote drying of protein-rich specimens, avoid a dried crust around a liquid core
Gaseous oxygen or air	To promote destruction of organic matrix, reduce smoke formation and particulates that give nonatomic absorption
Ni, Cu, Pd	To stabilize volatile elements, for example, Se, As, during the dry and ash phases
Potassium dichromate	Stabilizes Hg up to a temperature of 200°C
HNO_3 or NH_4NO_3	To stabilize analyte atoms by removal of halides as HCl or NH_4Cl during the ash phase
$Mg(NO_3)_2$	Becomes reduced to MgO, which traps the metals to reduce volatilization losses, delays atomization, and separates the analyte signal from the background absorption
$NH_3H_2PO_4$ or $(NH_3)_2HPO_4$	Usually used with $Mg(NO_3)_2$, reduces volatilization losses and delays atomization to separate the analyte signal from the background absorption

4.5.4 Vapor Generation Procedures

Depending on the nature of the exposure to mercury—inorganic salts, organomercury compounds, and the metal or its vapor—it may be necessary to analyze specimens of urine, blood or tissues, and foods. Mercury is used extensively in industry and occupational monitoring continues to be relevant. There is now considerable interest in two particular environmental sources of exposure, that is, from dental amalgam and from the diet, especially fish. Although no good evidence exists for mercury leaching from amalgam fillings in amounts that can cause toxicity, many members of the public believe that their health is affected and seek to have the mercury removed, even after analysis of blood or urine has failed to show increased concentrations of the metal.[33] Concern has been raised that undue exposure to methylmercury may occur from eating large amounts of seafoods. Those at risk are young children in utero and during early childhood. Long-term studies are in progress within communities where basic foods contain mercury and maternal hair concentrations of it are high. Mercury intakes and neurological development are being monitored within the target groups.[34]

Considerable interest in methods to measure arsenic and other hydride-forming elements has been evident in recent years. The basic procedure involves careful digestion of the specimens to convert all the different species to a single valency form, reduction with BH_4^-, and vaporization to the hydride, which is then transferred by a stream of inert gas to a quartz tube heated in an air–acetylene flame or with electrical thermal wire. Atomization is then achieved by the high temperature. Some work has been reported in which the hydride is transferred into a cold graphite furnace where it is trapped onto the surface. Atomization takes place as the furnace is rapidly heated and, as with conventional electrothermal AAS, improved sensitivity is observed due to the high atom density within the small volume of the furnace.

Trapping is more efficient when the graphite is coated with a metal salt, for example, Ag, Pd, and Ir.[35,36] The chemical hydride reaction is impaired by other hydride-forming elements and by transition metals so that careful calibration is essential. An emerging development involves an electrolytic process in which nascent hydrogen is produced as an alternative to chemical hydride generation. With this arrangement, the interferences are much less and the reagents employed introduce less contamination.[37]

The biological and clinical importance of selenium receives much current interest; more attention is focused on measurement of this element than on any other. The stimuli to this flurry of activity are (1) the association between selenium status and cardiovascular disease coupled to the demonstration that dietary intakes are low in some regions and are declining in others[38] and (2) epidemiological data suggesting a relationship between selenium status and the incidence of certain carcinomas.[39] Measurements of selenium in foods, biological fluids, and tissues, using vapor generation techniques, electrothermal AAS, or ICP-MS, are integral to many large-scale studies now in progress or recently completed.

There is also much interest in the determination of arsenic. This element is important within the microelectronics industry and in other occupations, but extensive environmental exposure is also associated with naturally high concentrations in drinking water. Arsenic in drinking water is a problem in several areas of the world; however, the situation that now exists in Bangladesh and West Bengal, India, is extraordinary, with millions of people consuming highly toxic and carcinogenic water.[40] Measurement of total arsenic is not always entirely helpful. Fish contain large amounts of organoarsenic species that are absorbed and excreted without further metabolism and with no adverse health effects. These species will be included in a total arsenic determination and can mask attempts to measure toxic As^{3+} and metabolites. Thus, methods to measure the individual species or related groups of compounds in urine or other samples provide more meaningful results. These methods include separation by chromatography or solvent extraction and pretreatment steps that transform only the species of interest into the reducible form.

As this speciation work has become more refined, additional arsenic-containing compounds have been demonstrated and, very recently, some of these have been identified as methylated As species containing As[III]. It is well known that methylated species with As[V] are found in blood and urine following exposure to inorganic arsenic and believed to represent steps in the detoxification pathway. Methylarsenic[III] species are potent enzyme inhibitors and cytotoxins and their formation may be involved in the mechanism of arsenic toxicity. In one study,[41] biliary and urinary arsenic species were determined in rats exposed to As^{III} and As^V. MonomethylAsIIIarsonate (MMA^{III}) was present in bile but not in urine; the authors hypothesized that MMA^{III} was subsequently oxidized to MMA^V and excreted in urine. In a separate investigation, arsenic species were measured in water, urine, and cultured cells, and methylarsenic^{III} species were identified in the urine of individuals who had consumed water contaminated with inorganic As.[42]

Other elements that form gaseous hydrides, such as antimony, bismuth, and tellurium, are also relevant to investigations in clinical and biological specimens.

4.5.5 X-Ray Fluorescence Spectrometry

XRF and other x-ray techniques offer no particular advantage over the many other procedures for simple quantitative measurement of minerals and trace elements in clinical and biochemical specimens. Alternative methods are widely available, well established, and relatively simple. Nevertheless, a few interesting applications have been reported with recent examples of Fe, Cu, and Zn in placenta tissues.[43] In certain applications involving clinical and biochemical specimens, however, XRF does have a specific role. These include elemental mapping[44] and in vivo analyses.

By virtue of the very narrow x-ray beam (100 μm or less), it is possible to take repeat measurements over a very small surface and develop a map of the distribution of elements within a structure. This approach is regularly applied to solid materials including hairs, teeth, and other calcareous materials. Results have also been reported in which single cells have been investigated, for example, in a study to compare iron and other elements within neuromelanin aggregates in neuronal cells of patients with Parkinson's disease and their controls.[45]

Developments involving in vivo XRF have flourished in the last few years although the majority of the many publications originate from just a few centers. Most of the work is concerned with measurement of lead in bone by ^{109}Cd-based XRF. Analytically, recent improvements refer to detection systems to reduce detection limits to low part per million levels and to the methods for calibration. Phantoms (often plaster of Paris) containing known amounts of Pb are generally used. Recent alternative materials that are reported to behave more like bone are a synthetic apatite matrix and a material with polyurethane and CaCO$_3$. It has been shown that the measurement location, that is, proximal–distal sites, influences the measured XRF intensity and its uncertainty. Considerable differences in mean bone Pb concentrations between the left and right legs of the same individual (0.8 and 2.0 μg/g bone mineral) have also been demonstrated.[46] Using this technique, cumulative exposures to lead at work have been assessed and results compared with other markers such as blood and urine lead concentrations.[47] Blood and bone lead concentrations were determined and related to the development of hypertension. A positive association was found between the baseline bone Pb level and the incidence of hypertension but no association was found with blood Pb level.[48] Bone lead has also been shown to be released into the circulation during pregnancy, with an implied risk to the fetus if the mother has a history of previous lead absorption.

There are reports of the determination of other elements by in vivo XRF. Skin iron concentrations correlated strongly with iron in the internal organs of rats injected with iron dextran, and it was concluded that this technique had great potential in the diagnosis and treatment of hereditary hemochromatosis and β-thalassemia.[49] A method for measuring platinum in kidneys of patients receiving Pt-based chemotherapy drugs has been developed.[50] These few examples illustrate that the potential for in vivo elemental analysis is hugely exciting.

4.6 Quality Assurance

Apart from the actual analysis, adventitious contamination, which can occur during collection and storage of specimens, the preparative procedure, and the spectrometric measurement, has the greatest impact on the quality of results. Data from proficiency testing schemes indicate that specialist trace element centers tend to maintain the highest standards of analytical performance. This observation reflects the continuing application of practices that minimize contamination and the expertise and experience to ensure optimal functioning of equipment. Because of the stability of inorganic analytes and the purity with which standard materials can be prepared, there are reasonable numbers of reference materials available for use to validate methods and for internal and external quality control.[51] Proficiency testing schemes relating to occupational and environmental laboratory medicine are organized in most countries and all laboratories involved in this work should have access to an appropriate scheme to demonstrate the reliability of their analytical data.[52]

References

1. Taylor, A., Detection and monitoring of disorders of essential trace elements, *Ann. Clin. Biochem.*, 33, 486, 1996.
2. Taylor, A., ed., *SAS Trace Element Laboratories. Clinical and Analytical Handbook*, 4th edn., Royal Surrey County Hospital, Guildford, Surrey, U.K., 2006. www.SAS-centre.org.
3. Taylor, A., ed., *Trace Elements in Human Disease. Clinics in Endocrinology and Metabolism*, W.B. Saunders, Eastbourne, U.K., 1985.
4. Baldwin, D.R. and Marshall, W.J., Heavy metal poisoning and its laboratory investigation, *Ann. Clin. Biochem.*, 36, 267, 1999.
5. Flanagan, R.J., Taylor, A., Watson, I.D. et al., *Fundamentals of Analytical Toxicology*, Wiley, Chichester, U.K., 2008.
6. Lajunen, L.H.J. and Peramaki, P., *Spectrochemical Analysis by Atomic Absorption and Emission*, Royal Society of Chemistry, London, U.K., 2005.
7. Holland, J.G. and Tanner, S.D., *Plasma Source Mass Spectrometry: The New Millenium*, Royal Society of Chemistry, Cambridge, U.K., 2001.
8. Giessman, U. and Greb, U., High resolution ICP-MS—A new concept for elemental mass spectrometry, *Fresenius J. Anal. Chem.*, 50, 186, 1994.
9. Welz, B., Becker-Ross, H., Stefan Florek, S. et al., High-resolution continuum-source atomic absorption spectrometry—What can we expect? *Braz. Chem. Soc.*, 14, 220, 2003.
10. Taylor, A., Branch, S., Day, M.P. et al., Atomic spectrometry update. Clinical and biological materials, foods and beverages, *J. Anal. At. Spectrom.*, 25, 453, 2010 (Updated annually).
11. Evans, E.H., Day, J.A., Palmer, C. et al., Advances in atomic spectrometry and related techniques, *J. Anal. At. Spectrom.*, 25, 760, 2010 (Updated annually).
12. Berndt, H. and Pulvermacher, E., A recent development involves a double atomizer, with a Ti tube inside a Ni tube, *Anal. Bioanal. Chem.*, 382(8), 1826–1834, 2005.
13. Gomes, M.D. and Pereira, E.R., Ti and Ni tubes combined in thermospray flame furnace atomic absorption spectrometry (TS-FF-AAS) for the determination of copper in biological samples, *Microchem. J.*, 93(1), 93–98, 2009.
14. Frech, W., Recent developments in atomizers for electrothermal atomic absorption spectrometry, *Fresenius J. Anal. Chem.*, 355, 475, 1996.
15. Turner, J., Hill, S.J., Evans, E.H. et al., Accurate analysis of selenium in water and serum using ETV-ICP-MS with isotope dilution, *J. Anal. At. Spectrom.*, 15, 743, 2000.
16. Rahil-Khazen, R., Henriksen, H., Bolann, B. et al., Validation of ICP-AES for multi-element analysis of trace elements in human serum, *Scand. J. Clin. Lab. Invest.*, 60, 677, 2000.
17. West, M., Ellis, A.T., Potts, P.J. et al., Atomic spectrometry update. X-ray fluorescence spectrometry, *J. Anal. At. Spectrom.*, 24, 1289, 2009 (Updated annually).
18. Taylor, A., Applications of recent developments for trace element analysis, *J. Trace Elem. Med. Biol.*, 11, 185, 1997.
19. Pacheco, P.H., Olsina, R.A., Smichowski, P. et al., On-line preconcentration and speciation analysis of inorganic vanadium in urine using L-methionine immobilised on controlled pore glass, *Talanta*, 74, 593, 2008.

20. Suleiman, J.S., Hu, B., Huang, C.Z. et al., Determination of Cd, Co, Ni and Pb in biological samples by microcolumn packed with black stone (Pierre noire) online coupled with ICP-OES, *J. Hazard. Mater.*, 157, 410, 2008.

21. Harrington, C.F., Clough, R.A., Hansen, H.R. et al., Atomic spectrometry update. Elemental speciation, *J. Anal. At. Spectrom.*, 25, 1185, 2010 (Updated annually).

22. Szpunar, J., Bio-inorganic speciation analysis by hyphenated techniques, *Analyst*, 125, 963, 2000.

23. European Union, Council Directive 98/24/EC of April 7, 1998 on the protection of the health and safety of workers from the risks related to chemical agents at work (fourteenth individual Directive within the meaning of Article 16(1) of Directive 89/391/EEC), *Official J.*, 131, 11, 1998.

24. Chappuis, P., Poupon, J., and Rousselet, F., A sequential and simple determination of zinc, copper and aluminium in blood samples by ICP-AES, *Clin. Chim. Acta*, 206, 155, 1992.

25. Lyon, T.D., Cunningham, C., Halls, D.J. et al., Determination of aluminium in serum, dialysate fluid and water by ICP-OES, *Ann. Clin. Biochem.*, 32, 160, 1995.

26. Norman, P.T., Joffe, P., Martinsen, I. et al., Quantification of gadodiamide as Gd in serum, peritoneal dialysate and faeces by inductively coupled plasma atomic emission spectroscopy and comparative analysis by high-performance liquid chromatography, *J. Pharm. Biomed. Anal.*, 22, 939, 2000.

27. Taylor, A., Usefulness of measurements of trace elements in hair, *Ann. Clin. Biochem.*, 23, 364, 1986.

28. Brown, A.A. and Taylor, A., Determination of copper and zinc in serum and urine by use of a slotted quartz tube and flame atomic absorption spectrometry, *Analyst*, 109, 1455, 1984.

29. Smith, C.M.M. and Harnley, J.M., Characterization of a modified two-step furnace for atomic absorption spectrometry for selective volatilization of iron species in hemin, *J. Anal. At. Spectrom.*, 11, 1055, 1996.

30. Kitagawa, K., Ohta, M., Kaneko, T. et al., Packed glassy carbon tube atomizer for direct determinations by atomic absorption spectrometry free of background absorption, *J. Anal. At. Spectrom.*, 9, 1273, 1994.

31. Ohta, K., Koike, Y., and Mizuno, T., Determination of zinc in biological materials by sequential metal vapor elution analysis with atomic absorption detection, *Anal. Chim. Acta*, 329, 191, 1996.

32. Zhou, Y., Parsons, P.J., Aldous, K.M. et al., Atomization of lead from whole blood using novel tungsten filaments in electrothermal atomic absorption spectrometry, *J. Anal. At. Spectrom.*, 16, 82, 2001.

33. Bailer, J., Rist, F., Rudolf, A. et al., Adverse health effects related to mercury exposure from dental amalgam fillings: Toxicological or psychological causes? *Psych. Med.*, 31, 255, 2001.

34. Myers, G.J., Davidson, P.W., Cox, C. et al., Prenatal methylmercury exposure from ocean fish consumption in the Seychelles child development study, *The Lancet*, 361, 1686, 2003.

35. Zhe-Ming, N., Bin, H., and Heng-Bin, H., In situ concentration of selenium and tellurium hydrides in a silver-coated graphite atomizer, *J. Anal. At. Spectrom.*, 8, 995, 1993.

36. Tsalev, D.L., D'ulivo, A., Lampugnani, L. et al., Thermally stabilized iridium on an integrated, carbide-coated platform as a permanent modifier for hydride-forming elements in electrothermal atomic absorption spectrometry, *J. Anal. At. Spectrom.*, 11, 979, 1996.

37. Schickling, C., Yang, J., and Broekaert, J., The optimization of electrochemical hydride generation coupled to microwave induced plasma atomic emission spectrometry for the determination of arsenic and its use for the analysis of biological tissue samples, *J. Anal. At. Spectrom.*, 11, 739, 1996.

38. Rayman, M., Dietary selenium: Time to act, *Br. Med. J.*, 314, 387, 1997.

39. Clark, L.C., Coombs, G., Jr., Turnbull, B.W. et al., Effects of selenium supplementation for cancer prevention in patients with carcinoma of the skin, *J. Am. Med. Assoc.*, 276, 1957, 1996.

40. Chatterjee, A., Das, D., Mandal, B.K. et al., Arsenic in groundwater in six districts of West Bengal, India: the biggest arsenic calamity in the world, *Analyst*, 120, 643, 1995.

41. Gregus, Z., Gyurasics, A., and Csanaky, I., Monomethylarsonous acid as a major biliary metabolite in rats, *Toxicol. Sci.*, 56, 18, 2000.

42. Del Razo, L.M., Stybo, M., Cullen, W.R. et al., Determination of trivalent methylated arsenicals in biological matrices, *Toxicol. Appl. Pharmacol.*, 174, 282, 2001.

43. Ozdemir, Y., Borekci, B., Levet, A. et al., Assessment of trace element concentration distribution in human placenta by wavelength dispersive X-ray fluorescence: Effect of neonate weight and maternal age, *Appl. Radiat. Isotopes*, 67, 1790, 2009.

44. Durak, R., Gulen, Y., Kurudirek, M. et al., Determination of trace element levels in human blood serum from patients with type II diabetes using WDXRF technique: A comparative study, *J. X-Ray Sci. Technol.*, 18, 111, 2010.

45. Ektessabi, A., Yoshida, S., and Takada, K., Distribution of iron in a single neuron of patients with Parkinson's disease, *X-Ray Spectrom.*, 28, 456, 1999.

46. Hoppin, J.A., Aro, A., Hu, H. et al., Measurement variability associated with KXRF bone lead measurement in young adults, *Environ. Health Perspect.*, 108, 239, 2000.

47. Britto, J., McNeil, F., Chettle, D. et al., Study of the relationships between bone lead levels and its variation with time and the cumulative blood lead index, in a repeated bone lead survey, *J. Environ. Monit.*, 2, 271, 2000.

48. Cheng, Y.W., Schwartz, D., Sparrow, A. et al., Bone lead and blood lead levels in relation to baseline blood pressure and the prospective development of hypertension—The Normative Aging Study, *Am. J. Epidemiol.*, 153, 164, 2001.

49. Farquharson, M.J., Bagshaw, A.P., Porter, J. et al., The use of skin Fe levels as a surrogate marker for organ Fe levels, to monitor treatment in cases of iron overload, *Phys. Med. Biol.*, 45, 1387, 2000.

50. Kadhim, R., Al-Hussany, A., Ali, P.A. et al., In vivo measurement of platinum in the kidneys using X-ray fluorescence, *In Vivo Body Comp. Stud.*, 90, 263, 2000.

51. Roelandts, I., Biological and environmental reference materials: Update 1996, *Spectrochim. Acta*, 52B, 1073, 1997.

52. Arnaud, J., Weber J.-P., Weykamp, C. et al., Quality specifications for the determination of copper, zinc, and selenium in human serum or plasma: Evaluation of an approach based on biological and analytical variation, *Clin. Chem.*, 54, 1892, 2008.

5

Flow Cytometry

Francis Mandy
Soft Flow Hungary Ltd.

Joe Trotter
BD Biosciences

Rudi Varro
BD Biosciences

Ming Yan
BD Biosciences

Diether Recktenwald
BD Biosciences

5.1 Introduction

Flow cytometry allows the analysis and sorting of particles of biological interest at rates of more than 10^4 s^{-1}, based on the analysis of light scatter and fluorescence. It also permits the quantitative analysis of many cellular constituents based on fluorescence measurements. Measurements at the single-molecule level have been reported. Based on the versatility and richness of information of flow cytometry, it is used in biological and biomedical research and for clinical data collection. This chapter provides an overview of flow cytometry and its biomedical and clinical applications. For readers interested in further details, we provide references to additional reviews of subtopics. A comprehensive account of flow cytometry, covering all aspects until 2003, can be found in *Practical Flow Cytometry* (Shapiro 2003).

5.2 Hardware

Flow cytometers measure multiple optical properties of particles generally without spatial resolution from about 20 μm down to submicroscopic size at rates of several thousand per second. A typical flow cytometer consists of a fluidics system, the optical components, and analog and/or digital electronics for data processing, storage, and evaluation (Figure 5.1). Special cytometers also sort particles into different fractions, based on optical particle properties. Several sorting mechanisms have been used as described in the following.

5.3 Fluidics

In the fluidics system of a cytometer, a particle suspension from a tube or well of a microtiter plate is injected into a second fluid stream of aqueous sheath fluid—mostly saline—to create a very narrow, quasi 1D file of particles for intersection with a light beam for optical measurements. Typical stream velocities are 10 m/s. The ratio of sheath fluid volume to sample volume with the size of the observation cuvette determines the diameter of the sample stream and influences the precision of the optical measurements. Typical total stream diameters are on the order of 100 μm and sample streams on the order of 10 μm. The sample stream diameter can be controlled by the differential pressure between the sheath and sample fluid (Peters et al. 1985). The sample stream diameter usually relates to the sample flow rate. The low flow rate corresponds to the small sample stream diameter. Coefficients of variation (CV) better than 2% are quite common for measurements of the DNA content of cell nuclei. Typically, the better CV is achieved by low sample flow rate due to uniform light beam illumination on the entire sample core stream.

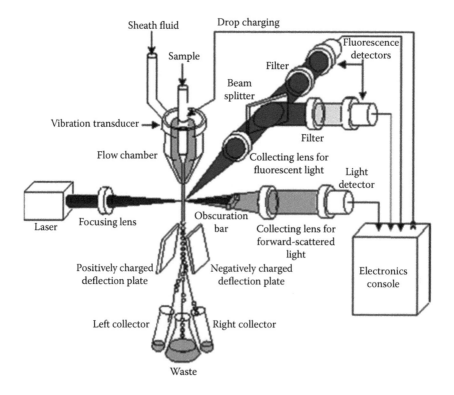

FIGURE 5.1 Components of a typical flow cytometer with droplet cell sorting feature.

5.4 Optics

To perform optical measurements on the particle stream in a cytometer, a light beam, commonly from a laser, is focused on the center of the fluid stream either in a cuvette or a free flowing stream in air for most cell sorters. Figure 5.2 shows a typical optical diagram for a three-laser sorter. Mercury arc lamps and LEDs are also used as excitation light sources. Cylindrical lenses are used frequently to achieve a better uniformity of light intensity for the particle illumination with a typical beam height of about 10–20 μm. Research flow cytometers are capable of measuring several light scatter and fluorescence emission intensities. Many fluorescence measurements on biological systems require a very low limit of detection. Therefore, high numerical aperture lenses are used for the collection of emitted light. Dichroic filters separate scattered and fluorescent light into separate wavelength bands. Photomultipliers (PMTs) measure the light intensities in the different wavelength bands. With an optimized instrument, photon-noise-limited measurements can be performed, and less than 100 molecules per particle (approx. 10^{-21} mol) of some fluorescent dyes can be detected. Some newer specialized systems use avalanche photodiodes in place of PMTs; light scatter can be detected with photodiodes. The number of detectors has increased significantly due to multiple color assay development. The numerous designs of detector arrays have been deployed for better compact design and low loss performance. Figure 5.3 shows a fiber optic–linked PMT detector array design (Oostman et al. 2006). High-end research systems offer multiple

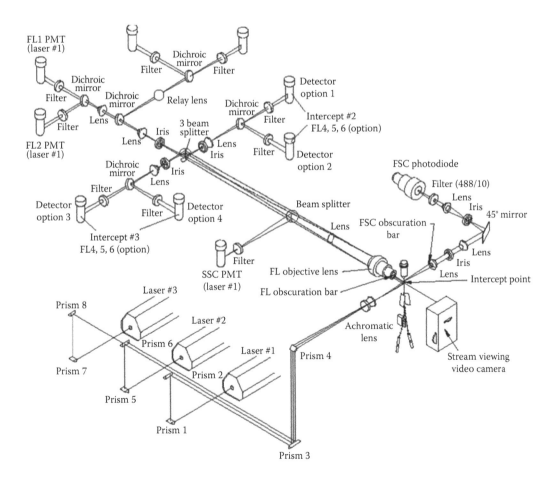

FIGURE 5.2 Optical diagram of a three-laser flow cytometer with droplet sorting feature.

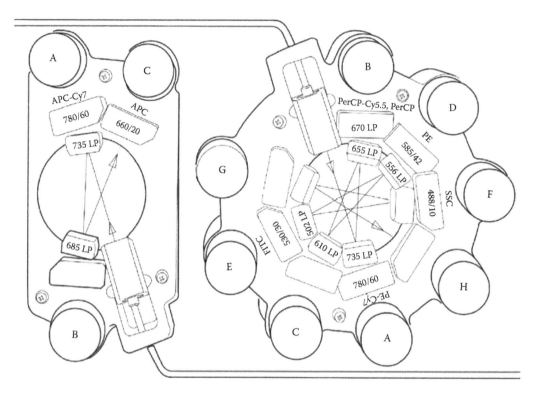

FIGURE 5.3 Schematic design PMT detector array for large number of fluorochrome detection. When light arrives at an array, a longpass mirror (filter) transmits the highest wavelength to the first PMT in the series and reflects lower wavelengths to the next PMT. Similarly, the next PMT's longpass mirror transmits the next highest wavelengths and reflects lower wavelengths and so on around the array. A bandpass filter (or additional longpass mirror) in front of each PMT further screens unwanted light.

excitation light sources, either in a colinear arrangement or for more flexibility for the resolution of multiple fluorophores with completely separate spatial optical paths and temporal synchronization.

5.5 Electronics

Signals from the light detectors are amplified. To allow the measurement of small and large signal intensity ranges, linear and logarithmic (typically four decades) ranges are provided on most instruments. Signal subtraction circuitry, linking adjacent spectral fluorescence emission bands, allows for the correction for spectral overlap between fluorescent dyes to express the intensity measurements in relative units of dye concentration rather than light intensities. After baseline subtraction, an analog pulse height or pulse area and a calculated pulse width are provided to an analog-to-digital converter (ADC). The ADC is triggered by a pulse height threshold, based on a Boolean combination of the measurement parameters, and after digitization, all of the particle measurements including those from separate light beams—after temporal synchronization—are stored as a record for the particle in the data matrix. Approaches for the extraction of population information from this data matrix are described in Section 5.7.

Recently, digital electronics has been used to derive the particle measurements from a continuous digitization of detector output through high-speed ADCs. All of the signal calculations on the pulses, including height, area, width, logarithms, and spectral overlap correction, are performed with high-speed digital signal processors. Calculations of signal parameters are performed with higher accuracy than by analog approximation, and the approach also provides more flexibility for future applications of modern signal signature analysis for flow cytometry.

5.6 Cell Sorting with Cloning

As mentioned earlier, several approaches have been used to sort particles in essentially real time, based on the measurements of a flow cytometer. Cell sorting has been reviewed in detail in a book chapter (Hoffman and Houck 1998). The most common method for flow cytometric cell sorting uses a piezoelectric actuator, which breaks the stream containing the particles under analysis into droplets. Charging the droplets at the right time with a charge pulse, triggered by the results of the optical analysis, allows the electrostatic deflection into typically four positions, where a collection tube can be placed. Sorting rates of higher than $10^4\,s^{-1}$ can be achieved for the purification of millions of purified particles (cells) with specific properties in under an hour.

In another setup, the particles of interest are deflected into a multiwell plate (typically 96 wells in an 8×12 well arrangement) or onto a plate with cell nutrient under xy control. For cloning, single cells can be deposited there to achieve a cultured cell population, which can be traced back to an individual cell.

5.7 Data Analysis

As mentioned earlier, data from flow cytometric measurements are stored in a data matrix, where each row contains the measurement for an individual particle with a column for each of the measurement parameters. One of the measurement parameters can be a time tag for kinetic data evaluation. For most analyses, information on at least 5000 particles is stored, in many cases substantially more. At least 1 byte of data is stored for each of the parameters; in many cases, the resolution is higher. Newer digital instruments store data as high-resolution floating point numbers. This kind of data file is called a listmode file. This designation comes from the times when data storage was very expensive. To economize on usage of memory, data were also stored as histogram data (see below).

The listmode data matrix is the basis for all subsequent data analysis, but by itself cannot be evaluated easily without computer-based data transformation.

A simple analysis of the data consists of calculating a histogram of the number of particles at each parameter value for all of the parameters. In the most simple implementation, the digital parameter value for each of the particles in the matrix is used as an address for an array (1024 elements long for a 10-bit parameter resolution), and the content of the corresponding array element is incremented by 1, every time the respective value is observed. Data histograms (Figure 5.4a) provide a view of intensity distribution for the subpopulations in a particle ensemble; however, information about the correlation between parameters is lost.

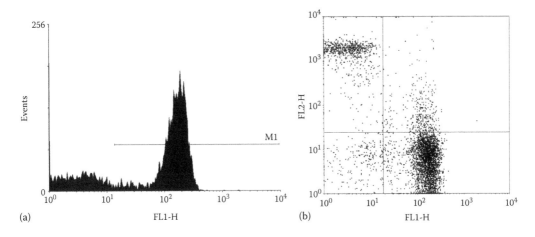

FIGURE 5.4 Histogram (a) and dot plot (b) from a two-color immunofluorescence measurement of mammalian lymphocytes.

A so-called dot plot (Figure 5.4b) shows the intensity distribution with pairs of two measurement parameters. In a 2D plot, dots are displayed for each particle at xy coordinates corresponding to two parameter values. This plot shows population locations and widths with some relative frequency information from the dot density. Quantitative frequency information is lost, because overlapping dots show only as one.

Density and contour plots show quantitative population frequency information with two parameters. Both are based on 2D histograms. A density plot uses a gray scale or colors to represent the z-axis (frequency information), whereas a contour plot uses different contour levels to show histogram height or probability contours show population frequency.

All the data representations earlier show only up to two parameters correlated simultaneously. The listmode data matrix may contain many parameters, for most measurements at least four. Therefore, the problem remains to look at subpopulations of the particle ensemble in multidimensional space. A process called gating uses 1D or 2D dot plot displays to select parameter value sets to include or exclude from additional data displays. In this way, properties of particle subpopulations can be determined for all measured parameters. A special case of novel multiparameter *gating* is detailed in Bierre and Thiel (1998). Several software packages offer additional features for multiparameter data analysis. Paint-A-Gate™ (Conrad et al. 1989) uses color to highlight populations selected in one display in five more 2D displays in real time. For automated multiparameter analysis, density-based or nearest neighbor cluster algorithms have been used among others. Further details on data analysis methods for flow cytometry have been discussed elsewhere (Watson 1992).

5.8 Flow Cytometry Measurements

A flow cytometric measurement characterizes one or more populations of a particle suspension with a count value and several optical parameter intensities and their distributions. From the partial count, particle concentrations can be calculated, if the sample volume is known. Regardless of the capabilities of the instrumentation to record sample volumes, a known concentration of a reference particle with scatter and fluorescence properties different from the particles of the sample can be added to obtain concentrations of all of the particle populations. However, many applications of flow cytometry only report the relative frequency of a sample particle subset as fraction of a subset in a superset of the particle sample, that is, T cells as a percentage of lymphocytes.

The optical parameter intensities are used to derive physical properties of the particles in a sample. Light scatter intensities are related to the size and index of refraction of particles; fluorescence intensities are related to the mass of fluorophores per particle. With calibration of the system, absolute masses of analyte per particle can be determined from fluorescence intensities. However, for most application, relative quantities are reported. Limits of detection for fluorescence measurements with commercial systems are on the order of 100 fluorescent molecules per particle (Coventry et al. 1994); with specialized instrumentation, single-molecule detection has been achieved (Harding and Keller 1992).

5.9 Flow Cytometer Characterization and Setup

Measurement of instrument characteristics and its correlation to assay performance provides quantitative criteria for quality assurance and quality control. One simple measure of sensitivity is the difference in fluorescence intensity of a specific positive cell and unstained population divided by twice the standard deviation of the unstained population. This normalized signal-to-background approach is best used to either compare sensitivity for a specific reagent among cytometers or to determine which dye color might be optimal for any specific marker when planning multicolor reagent panels. However, it does not directly address the underlying contributions that ultimately determine the fluorescence sensitivity of the cytometer itself, that is, optics, fluidics, and electronics. In a multicolor assay, the ability to accurately detect spectral spillover from other fluorescence dyes is also an important factor. The cytometer performance can be simplified as instrument performance factor Q (detection efficiency), B (background), standard deviation of electronic noise (SDen), and linearity (Chase and Hoffman 1998; Gaucher et al. 1988). The dye-embedded polystyrene bead exhibits broad fluorescence spectrum that enables us to measure the performance from a cytometer for at least 18 different colors commonly used simultaneously. A bead set consisting of different fluorescence intensity levels allows users to assess the cytometer performance including laser alignment, Q, B, SDen, and linearity within the dynamic range typically used for immunofluorescence. The instrument performance Q and B are usually normalized to a fluorescence intensity standard. The molecules of equivalent soluble fluorochromes (MESF) is a commonly used standard (Henderson et al. 1998; Lenkei et al. 1998a) with only a few fluorochromes available. Equivalent reference fluorescence (ERF) was proposed as an alternative (Wang et al. 2008) method to cross-calibrate various fluorescence standards, usually traceable from lot to lot by bead manufacturers. Large fluorescence intensity variation of different antibody-linked fluorochromes requires the assay-specific instrument setup. Typically, a fluorochrome-labeled bead or dye-embedded bead is used for instrument setup prior to running biological samples. Proper setup provides the consistency for the assay from sample to sample. The fluorescence cross talk from the detectors measured from multiple fluorochromes, called spillover, is usually required to know before performing an assay. The spillover is due to fluorescence spectral overlap and can be compensated mathematically during data processing. Measured fluorescence intensity distributions can be described as the combination of Q, B, and electronic noise in a multicolor cytometer. Along with the background light from the spillover of other fluorescence channels, the experimental results from a multicolor assay on an instrument with known and varied combinations of these factors are compared to theoretical predictions (Hoffman and Woods 2007). The ability to predict assay performance based on measured instrument characteristics is the critical factor for quality assurance of cytometer-based assays.

5.10 New Approaches to Data Transformation and Analysis

5.10.1 Data Transformation

In flow cytometry, the need often arises to measure signal changes over a significantly large dynamic range. Immunologists measure a wide range of expression levels for specific cell surface markers, and this has for many years largely been solved by employing a simple logarithmic transformation to span the dynamic range requirements, either by the use of a logarithmic amplifier in hardware or by displaying high-resolution linear data on a log scale. In many cases, the simultaneous display of a negative cell population (essentially unstained) and a positive (stained) population on the same scale necessitates two to four or more decades of dynamic range; only the standard logarithmic transformation does a poor job of handling populations with low medians and high variances and cannot handle data values less than or equal to zero. Several alternatives to the logarithmic transformation have been proposed and implemented in software that mitigate issues intrinsic to the log scale by allowing the lower end of the scale to be nearly linear, yet become and remain logarithmic for the upper decades, and allow for the display of values less than or equal to zero (Bagwell 2005; Parks et al. 2006; Trotter 2007). After immunofluorescence data are properly compensated, and various positive population medians are translocated to be orthogonal to unstained populations in other dye dimensions, their higher variance due to photoelectron statistics results in what most investigators term *spread* in the data. As a result, properly compensated data sets frequently contain populations with large variances and low medians, and the data often extend far below zero. Since zero and negative values remain undefined within the log transformation, that approach only satisfies the dynamic range requirement for immunofluorescence data visualization and seriously confounds the proper display of dimly stained and unstained cell populations. Figure 5.5 shows an example data set using both the log and logicle transformations to demonstrate the usefulness of an other than log transformation for immunofluorescence data that spans several decades' dynamic range.

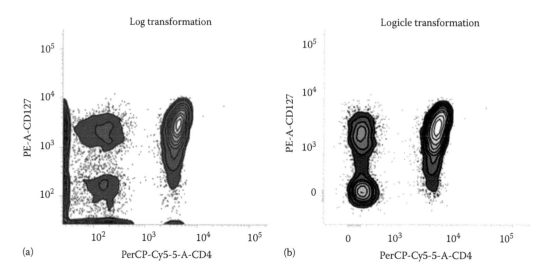

FIGURE 5.5 Shows the same data set plotted (a) using the log transformation and (b) using the logicle transformation. Note the ambiguity in the log display as to the nature and extents of CD4-negative populations in the CD127 dimension, where log artifacts obfuscate the expression levels of CD127. The logicle transformation mitigates this through its variance-normalizing approach and properly displaying the cell populations of interest.

5.10.2 Analysis

Promising new approaches have been proposed for the analysis and display of high-dimensional flow data to satisfy the need to simultaneously deconvolve and display events in k dimensions. The traditional multiple 1D and 2D plots using subjective gating can often ignore key interactions between parameters within a single multivariate data file. Flow fingerprinting (Rogers et al. 2009) extends probability binning (Roederer et al. 2001) to help deconvolve complex data sets by representing the multivariate probability density function as a fingerprint and is an unbiased, model-free representation of multivariate density that is complimentary to flowClust (http://www.bioconductor.org/packages/release/bioc/html/flowClust.html), a model-based clustering package, and more recently flowType and RchyOptimyx (Aghaeepour et al. 2012, O'Neill et al. 2014), also available in Bioconductor (R) flow cytometry package (http://www.bioconductor.org/packages/release/bioc/html/flowCore.html).

Probability State Modeling (http://www.vsh.com/publication/inokumaISAC2010Poster.pdf) is a different approach whereby the events in a flow cytometry data file are classified using their probability state rather than traditional, often subjective, graphical gates to classify the data. The probability state algorithms use fitting routines to classify cells into their most probable states based on the characteristics defined for each parameter and allow n-dimensional data to be deconvolved based on a progression among all the exhibited states. As a modeling system, it allows for both characterization and assessing whether an unknown sample fits any given accepted model, such as *normal* for a set of parameters.

5.11 Biological Applications

5.11.1 Cell Cycle/Proliferation Analysis

DNA content (including assessment of aneuploidy and S phase) can be measured with propidium iodide (PI), the Hoechst dyes, or other compounds. PI intercalates in the DNA helix and fluoresces strongly orange red. It has the advantage that it is excited by 488 nm light and can be used on most common flow cytometers. The Hoechst dyes bind AT pairs in the DNA and enter viable cells without the need for fixation. These dyes are UV excited and so cannot be used on many benchtop flow cytometers. However, they may allow dye combinations that are not possible with PI (van den Engh et al. 1986).

Bromodeoxyuridine (BrdU) incorporation for specific cell proliferation can also be measured by immunofluorescence. This is often done along with DNA staining. Cell cycle and synchronization analysis can be performed allowing quantitative analysis of cell cycle phases. This can be used with or without antibody staining to characterize the transition between cell cycle phases in terms of expression of control proteins (Jensen et al. 1994).

5.11.2 Ca Flux

Ca^{2+} is the most common signal transduction element in cells, and it is involved in diverse cellular processes. Flow cytometry can be used to measure calcium flux (Vandenberghe and Ceuppens 1990). The calcium flux assay can be combined with immunofluorescent stain and identify cell subpopulations by immunofluorescence and measure calcium flux in response to an activating signal.

5.11.3 Cellular Antigen Quantitation

Antigens per cell can be quantitated by standardized fluorescent measurements (Davis et al. 1998). Quantitative measurements can be used to characterize receptor expression and cellular activation. A number of bead-based methods are available to calibrate flow cytometers and provide quantitative results on density of antigen on cells (Lenkei et al. 1998b).

5.12 Clinical Flow Cytometry Applications

5.12.1 T Cell Subset Analysis and the Management of HIV Disease

In the late twentieth century, flow cytometry was catapulted into clinical utility because of a global viral pandemic. A worldwide infectious disease threat was identified. It was the sudden appearance of the acquired immunodeficiency syndrome (AIDS). As the syndrome could be rapidly detected with the aid of a flow cytometer, this situation accelerated the availability of clinical flow cytometers. This section of the chapter offers a brief introduction to the evolution of a clinical instrument development. In the early 1980s, it was a direct implementation-oriented response to demands for translational medicine for a clinical diagnostic technology. It was developed for long-term monitoring and eventual management of an incurable infectious viral disease.

Contrary to expectations back in the late twentieth century, it was AIDS, not the management of lymphoma and leukemia, that was responsible for the massive and rapid worldwide mobilization of flow cytometers into clinical immunology and hematopathology laboratories. In 1981, reports appeared from various parts of the United States involving young men who had an unusual immune suppression linked with opportunistic infections (Gottlieb et al. 1981; Siegal et al. 1981). Soon, it was discovered that the hallmark of this new epidemic, AIDS, was a dramatic decrease of CD4 T cells (helper cells) in peripheral blood (Ammann et al. 1983). In subsequent years, the causative viral agent was discovered, the human immunodeficiency virus (HIV) (Barre-Sinoussi et al. 1983; Gallo et al. 1984). It was determined that the T helper cell in the presence of a coreceptor is the primary target for HIV, and the CD4 epitopes on cell surface are the primary means for viral entry and the subsequent massive viral replication (McDougal et al. 1986). The current generation of antiretroviral drug cocktails can suppress viral replications for decades, but none of the available therapies can completely eliminate HIV from the host. Hence, lifelong monitoring of HIV-positive patients is required. T cell subsets are followed throughout the course of the disease as they remain the best surrogate marker for immune status monitoring (Stein et al. 1992). Normal T helper cell levels are about 1000 cells/μL of blood (with a range from 600 to 1400); generally, levels below 500 cells/μL indicate that the virus has already damaged the immune system (Fahey et al. 1990). Usually, the overall level of T cells remains relatively constant until the late symptomatic phase of the disease (Nicholson and Mandy 2000). Throughout the disease, the CD8 T cell numbers proportionally increase as CD4 T cell population declines (Giorgi et al. 1987). A definition for AIDS was established based on a CD4 T cell count of less than 200 cells/µL (CDC 1993). This CD4 T cell level is associated with the early manifestation of acquired immunosuppression symptoms. Accurate and reproducible measurement of T cell subsets is an important part of lifelong clinical management of HIV-infected patients (Bergeron et al. 1998). In the past decade, therapies have improved; the intervention point with antiretroviral therapy (ART) has shifted from 200 to 350 CD4 T cell counts per µL. Following intervention with ART, the T helper cell population will usually rise (Koot et al. 1993). However, the CD4 T cell reset point always occurs below the preinfection level. Current therapies usually extend life for years adding productive quality life for individuals living with HIV; however, the virus is almost never completely eliminated. Eventually, death occurs resulting from long-term drug toxicity combined with viral drug resistance and various complications associated with opportunistic infections.

While epifluorescent microscopy was the initial technology, most frequently, the analysis of T cell subsets from peripheral whole blood is achieved with flow cytometry–based immunophenotyping. Fresh whole blood with anticoagulant is the usual requirement for immunophenotyping. In industrialized countries, to evaluate effective therapy, both viral load and T cell subset assays are performed at regular intervals. Clinical flow cytometers handle minimum 5 or 6 distinct parameters: forward scatter (FS), side scatter (SS), and three or more fluorescence light (FL) signals, FL1, FL2, FL3, and more, respectively. The two light scatters are intrinsic parameters that define morphological features of leukocytes, such as size and granularity. The FL parameters measure extrinsic attributes, such as identification of surface antigens, via fluorescence emission from excited fluorochrome-labeled monoclonal antibodies (MAbs) (Shapiro 1994). Fluorescein isothiocyanate (FITC) and R-phycoerythrin (PE) are the most frequently used fluorochromes. Both dyes can be simultaneously excited using 488 nm air-cooled laser. As third and fourth dyes, both natural and man-made tandem dyes are utilized. Peridinin chlorophyll protein (PerCP) was the first directly conjugated commercially available natural tandem dye. Other frequently used dyes are energy-coupled dye (ECD), R-phycoerythrin–CyChrome 5 (PE-Cy5), allophycocyanin (APC), CyChrome 5 (Cy5), and allophycocyanin–CyChrome 7 (APC-Cy7). Currently, in resource-rich regions, the simultaneous four-color immunophenotyping protocol is the most frequently used method. Such polychromatic application is accomplished either by adding a fourth PMT for the detection in the far red or by using an additional red laser to accommodate the fourth PMT. Most frequently, an additional red diode laser is installed that excites at 635 nm; APC is often the choice as the fourth fluorochrome; see Table 5.1. For HIV immunophenotyping, both single- and dual-laser instruments produce similar results (Mandy et al. 1997; O'Gorman and Nicholson 2000). In most clinical instruments, samples are incubated with fluorochrome-labeled monoclonal antibodies (MAbs) followed by

TABLE 5.1 Available MAb–Fluorochrome Conjugates for Single- and Dual-Laser Immunophenotyping

Dye	Excitation with 488 nm 1st Laser	Excitation with 635 nm 2nd Laser	Emission (nm)	Extinction Coefficient (cm^{-1} M^{-1})	Quantum Yield	Molecular Weight (Da)
FITC	x		519	67,000	0.71	389
PE	x		578	1,960,000	0.68	240,000
PerCP	x		675	na	1	35,000
ECD	x		613	na	na	250,000
PE-Cy5	x		675	1,960,000	na	241,000
APC		x	660	700,000	0.68	104,000
Cy5		x	670	250,000	0.28	792
APC-Cy7		x	767	700,000	na	105,000

Notes: This table includes typical fluorochromes that are commercially available already conjugated to MAbs for immunophenotyping T cell subsets. Under the column of excitation, the first laser refers to the conventional argon ion source installed on most clinical instruments. The second laser is available as an option on most modern flow cytometers. A comprehensive list of fluorochromes can be found at http://flowcyt.salk.edu/fluo.html.

na, not available.

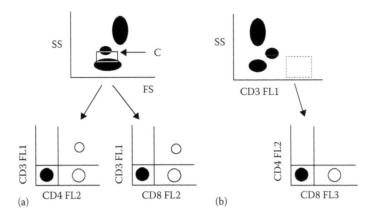

FIGURE 5.6 Gating strategies based on intrinsic and extrinsic cell attributes. Illustrations of homogeneous (Panel a) and heterogeneous (Panel b) gating strategies as they are applied to simultaneous three-color immunophenotyping. Panel (a) is an example of the traditional homogeneous approach to gating, where the two parameters are both intrinsic attributes based on cellular morphology. The three regions in the upper part of Panel (a) in descending order are granulocytes, monocytes, and lymphocytes, respectively. Arrow C points to an interface between lymphocytes and monocytes. It is focusing on a common dilemma: how to resolve, where does the monocyte gate ends, and where the lymphocyte gate begins? Panel (b) illustrates the advantage of the heterogeneous gating strategy. An extrinsic attribute is harnessed (CD3 FL1) in combination with an intrinsic one (SS).

red blood cell lysing (Hoffman et al. 1980). Leukocyte subsets are then identified with a combination of intrinsic and extrinsic cell surface markers (Graedel and McGill 1982). Resulting graphic presentation provides not only the relative location of lymphocytes in a dual-parameter dot plot but also the clustering of monocyte and granulocyte populations. Thus, a three-part differential of leukocytes is obtained.

Initially, there was an inherent problem with immunophenotyping displays based on intrinsic cell attributes alone. While the three cell populations were easy to locate, the light scatter gating protocol did not resolve the interface between the populations. For example, there was usually a zone between lymphocytes and monocytes where it was possible to find both types of cells; see Figure 5.6. The operator often had to set a lymphocyte gate that either included all the lymphocytes but not only lymphocytes or it included only lymphocytes but not all of them. This type of gating strategy predisposed the assay to compromise in purity and or recovery of lymphocytes. By the end of the twentieth century, more practical implementation of lineage and function-specific cell markers coupled with more effective gating software eliminated much of the data acquisition challenges. For example, a T gating protocol for simultaneous three-color application was developed in Mandy et al. (1992). With this method, T cells (CD3) are identified with a bivariate dot plot using heterogeneous parameters, SS (an intrinsic parameter), and CD3 fluorescence (an extrinsic parameter) (Figure 5.1). From the T gate, either CD4- or CD8-positive cells can be identified by conventional dual-color bivariate quadrant analysis. Such heterogeneous protocols can easily be modified for absolute cell counting. The most frequently used heterogeneous parameter combination is a single-tube assay containing CD45, CD3, CD4, and CD8 (Nicholson et al. 1993). In this case, the heterogeneous gating strategy combines SS and bright CD45 fluorescence. CD45 is an epitope variably expressed on leukocytes in combination with SS; it allows for the identification of lymphocytes. This innovative use of heterogeneous gating protocol significantly improved diagnostic capacity (Mandy et al. 1995).

Originally, most clinical flow cytometers were designed to analyze distribution of positive cells within a gated region. Therefore, traditionally, CD4 and CD8 T cells were reported as percentage of the lymphocyte gate. However, most guidelines for CD4 T cell immunophenotyping recommend reporting absolute cell numbers (Calvelli et al. 1993; CDCP 1997). Absolute cell count (cell concentration) per unit volume can be acquired on these clinical instruments by using the single platform technology (SPT). When the absolute count is generated exclusively with a flow cytometer, the counting process is referred to as SPT. An additional reagent, microfluorospheres, is added to each specimen to produce an internal

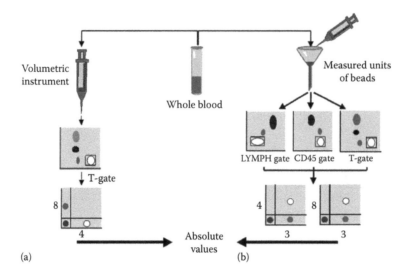

FIGURE 5.7 Various SPT for T cell subset enumeration. Two SPT approaches are presented for T cell subset enumeration. They are depicted in Panels (a) and (b). Panel (a) represents a dedicated volumetric instrument where a measured unit of blood is analyzed. Panel (b) illustrates a situation where a known concentration of fluorospheres is added to a known volume of blood. The volume of the mixture is calculated. With the added fluorosphere unit, an accurate T cell subset count per volume is possible. Three gating options are illustrated in the middle of Panel (b). One homogeneous and two heterogeneous gating strategies are illustrated.

control for absolute T cell subset count without a need for additional data from a hematology instrument (Mandy and Brando 2000). Currently, in industrialized countries, SPT is the default protocol for T cell subset determination (see Figure 5.7). For most clinical instruments, known concentrations of microfluorospheres are added to the whole blood, and automatic calculations are made of the ratio between microfluorospheres and the volume of sample analyzed. Relatively robust and reliable absolute counts can be achieved with SPT (Nicholson et al. 1997).

Natural killer (NK) cells (CD16) decrease with HIV infection, particularly in the later phase of the disease (Hardy 1992; Lucia et al. 1995). Additional uses of flow cytometry in the detection of HIV infection include evaluation of cell functions such as activation, in vitro proliferation, cytotoxic T lymphocyte responses, detection of various cytokine-producing cells, study of the role of coreceptors at time of viral fusion, and measurement of in situ HIV antigens. These research-oriented applications are frequently used during drug and vaccine development. For routine evaluation of drug efficacy for HIV disease in some resource-poor regions with extremely limited infrastructure, T cell subset is used as the essential surrogate marker for the individual's immune status (Gilks et al. 2009). There is one large-scale clinical application of an activation marker for HIV disease monitoring in South Africa. In the Glencross flow cytometry laboratory in Johannesburg, CD8/CD38 expression is routinely monitored as a surrogate marker for ART efficacy (Glencross et al. 2008a).

To support global implementation of ART, there is an enormous need for affordable robust technology that can withstand hostile rural environments. In response to the relentless international demand to treat millions more of HIV-infected individuals in regions such as sub-Saharan Africa, there is an ongoing significant progress in instrument development. While the choice for robust *time-tested* instruments is still very limited, the number of innovative solutions to format enhanced instrument capacity suitable for remote applications is astonishing. Most of the quintessential features associated with a traditional flow cytometry have been discarded on many of the new affordable instruments (see Table 5.2). Eliminated features include color compensation for dual-color assays, hydrodynamic focusing, laser as monochromatic light source, fluorescent-tagged MAbs, sheath fluid, refrigerated reagents,

TABLE 5.2 Over Time: Alternative and Innovative Solutions Are Emerging

Required Function	Traditional Solution	Innovative Solution	System
Aligning cells for optical interrogation	Hydrodynamic focusing	Microcapillary flow system Acoustic focusing system	Guava PCA Attune
Labeled MAbs to identify cell surface receptors	Fluorescent dye conjugated to MAb	Colloidal metal conjugated to MAb	PointCare
Dual-color immunophenotyping	Compensate for spectral spillover	Observe two colors in Cartesian space as is	FACSCount[a]
Absolute cell counting	Add known con. of microfluorospheres	Install intrinsic volumetric feature	Partec[a] CyFlow
Stable source of monochromatic light	Air-cooled laser	Low-power LED	PointCare[a]
Specimen handling	Manual/automated open system	Cap piercing fully closed system	PointCare[a]
Fluid propulsion method	Sheath fluid under pressure	Peristaltic pump-driven system	Accuri[a]
Red cell interference	Use lysing reagent	Trigger on fluorescent signal, no lysing	FACSCount[a]

[a] The first and not necessarily the only system to introduce this feature.

reagent-dependent SPT, manual specimen manipulation step postphlebotomy, and lysing reagent. Some of these ingenious innovative solutions will have impact on how all portable flow cytometers will be constructed in the future. The three significant challenges that require addressing when designing systems for remote rural application are (1) minimal human resource requirement, (2) cost that includes supply chain and sustainability issues, and (3) reduced environment/energy requirements (Mandy et al. 2008). Earlier in the twenty-first century, Keating and Cambrosio recognized clinical flow cytometry as a biomedical platform that is redefining our understanding of normal and pathological conditions (Keating and Cambrosio 2003). Most clinical instruments are compatible with Internet-based rigorous internal and external quality management options. Such data management features are now harvested by some of the international external quality assessment schemes (Bergeron et al. 2010). The South African National Health Laboratory Services (NHLS) has invested in a sophisticated internal and external CD4 T cell enumeration quality management monitoring system (Glencross et al. 2008b). Intensive data management practices avail opportunities to evaluate new methodologies and protocols at critical intervention points. In a recent publication, Stevens et al. introduced a method assessment strategy that incorporates upward and downward misclassification probabilities for CD4 T cell enumeration methods at critical clinical intervention points (Stevens et al. 2008). Because of the persistent and consistent global efforts to deal with HIV disease, it is possible for major leaps in clinical assessment of the limits of reliability of specific models of a flow cytometer. In the quest to eradicate the AIDS pandemic, the development of rapid and reproducible CD4 T cell immunophenotyping has made an invaluable contribution. Flow cytometry has been an exemplary technology to demonstrate how to generate a response to a demand from translational medicine (Janossy and Mandy 2010). Unfortunately, universal implementation has been slow. Nevertheless, persistent demand driven by resource-restricted regions of humanity for affordable quality instrumentation is making steady progress; on the long run, both economic divides will profit from the pressures of continuous and ingenious innovation.

5.12.2 Blood Banking

Flow cytometry interrogates the properties of every cell, which moves by the laser beam. This feature is exploited in characterizing therapeutic blood products, either to count an enriched cell population or to validate the effectiveness of the removal of unwanted cells.

An example for the first type of application is the enumeration of hematopoietic stem cells by flow cytometry (To et al. 1997). Transplantation of hematopoietic progenitor cells is used increasingly in the treatment of blood disorders, malignancies, and genetic abnormalities. A cell surface molecule, CD34, is present on immature hematopoietic cells and all hematopoietic colony-forming cells (Civin et al. 1989). The relative frequency of the CD34+ cell population is 1%–4% of the mononuclear cells in normal bone marrow and less than 0.1% in normal peripheral blood (Loken et al. 1988).

An accurate measure of the CD34 cell count is necessary for defining the dose of transplanted stem cells. Cell surface markers (CD34, CD45) and DNA binding dyes are useful to identify stem cells, while the absolute count of CD34 cells is determined by their proportion to a known number of fluorescent beads (McNiece et al. 1998).

The second category of flow assays identifies the presence of unwanted cells in a purified blood concentrate. Platelet and red blood cell concentrates are regularly used in patient care. Leukocytes could cause graft-versus-host disease, alloimmunization, and other transfusion-related adverse reactions. Flow cytometry provides a rapid and sensitive method of enumerating *residual* white blood cells in leukoreduced blood products. White blood cells are detected by their binding of a DNA dye. A fluorescent counting bead in the same tube is used as an internal concentration standard (Barclay et al. 1998).

Flow cytometry is a sensitive and rapid research tool for the study of platelet disorders. Quantitation of surface receptors and secreted platelet proteins (CD62P, CD63, thrombospondin, fibrinogen) is possible with flow cytometry (Michelson 1996). Conformational changes in platelet glycoproteins, especially GPIIb–IIIa, can be measured using MAbs (Shattil et al. 1987). These antibodies and multicolor testing strategies are useful to monitor effects of drugs to inhibit platelet activation (Coller et al. 1995).

5.12.3 Cancer

Another clinical area, where flow cytometry has contributed to the understanding of the disease, is in cancer diagnosis. Cells from leukemias differ in their molecular, genetic, and immunologic characteristics. Different leukemias have different prognoses and require different therapies. Multiparameter flow cytometry with fluorochrome-labeled MAbs has improved the diagnosis and classification of the diseases substantially, as reviewed in detail by Weir and Borowitz (2001) and Karthick et al. (2010). In leukemias and other cell proliferation diseases, the analysis of the cellular DNA content (DNA ploidy) has been used to differentiate between healthy and disease-associated cells. High-resolution DNA analysis with a precision of close to 1% in DNA content provides information on abnormal DNA content, based on chromosome losses or additions, and on the fraction of actively dividing cells (S phase cells), which is a measure for the growth rate of the tumor. More detail on S phase and ploidy measurements in human cancer tissues can be found in the literature (D'Urso et al. 2009).

5.12.4 Clinical Microbiology

Flow cytometry has been demonstrated in many clinical infectious disease applications. Nucleic acid dyes like ethidium bromide have been used to detect bacteria in blood after lysis of blood cells. Identification of bacteria can be performed by immunofluorescence followed by flow cytometric detection. Fungi and parasites can also be measured by flow cytometry. Other microbiological applications are the detection and quantitation of viral antigens and nucleic acids and testing of antimicrobial agents and especially susceptibility to antibiotics. More detail on these and other applications in clinical microbiology are found in a recent review with 347 references by Alvarez-Barrientos et al. (2000). Another reference covers the measurement of microbial susceptibility measurements by flow cytometry (Braga et al. 2003).

5.13 Biological and Medical Research

5.13.1 Antigen-Specific T Cells/Immune Function in Infectious Diseases

Quantitative and qualitative measurement of antigen-specific T cells is possible by flow methods. It offers effective monitoring of immune status during disease and in assessing vaccine efficacy. Single-cell flow assays of antigen-specific T cells include MHC–peptide tetramer staining (Savage et al. 1999) and intracellular cytokine assays (Suni et al. 1998). Each of these assays can provide truly quantitative readouts since they enumerate antigen-specific cells.

Tetrameric complexes of HLA molecules can be used to stain antigen-specific T cells in FACS analysis. The enumeration and phenotypical analysis of antigen-specific cellular immune responses against viral, tumor, or transplantation antigens has applications in various experimental and clinical settings.

A typical intracellular cytokine assay utilizes a three-color combination of fluorochrome-labeled anticytokine, CD69, and CD4 antibodies. CD69 is an early activation antigen whose expression is induced during in vitro antigen stimulation. The T cells respond to stimulation by cytokine expression, and the secretion of the cytokines is arrested by secretion inhibitors, such as Brefeldin A inside the cells. The cells are fixed and permeabilized, and the frequency of the T cells, which respond to specific stimulation, is determined by the ratio of the cytokine-expressing T cells to the total T cell population. This technique allows the detection of functional populations of memory T cells that respond to specific soluble antigens in short-term restimulation assays.

Similar assays are described for detecting antigen-specific CD8 T cells, using overlapping peptides as stimulants (Maecker et al. 2001). These functional assays assist in delineating the cellular immune response to natural infections or to vaccines.

5.13.2 Measurement of Soluble Analytes Using Multiplex Bead Assays

Flow cytometry may be used as readout for immunoassays. Bead-based single analyte flow immunoassays were described for α-fetoprotein assay (Frengen et al. 1993), β_2-microglobulin (Bishop and Davis 1997), and for immune complexes (McHugh 1994). The single assay principle was expanded to the detection of multiple analytes from a single sample, using bead technology.

Beads of different size or color are used for multiplexed immunoassays. Fulwyler et al. (1988) and McHugh (1994) used beads of different sizes as carriers for antigens or antibodies. The beads were differentiated by their scatter characteristics, and the immunoassay signal was generated through the binding of fluorescent conjugates.

Collins et al. (1998) used a single bead to measure three different analytes. Three antibodies were coated to the same bead, and the corresponding antigens were detected through binding of MAbs, each carrying a different fluorochrome. The three different fluorescent signals were simultaneously detected by three-color flow cytometry.

Beads can be also identified by one type of fluorescence, while the signal is generated by conjugates carrying a second type of fluorescent signal (Camilla et al. 1998). This concept is useful to create low-complexity bead sets (Chen et al. 1999). Experience with biological applications of multiplex assays was summarized in Morgan et al. (2004).

Mixing two different fluorescent dyes for the identification of bead populations creates a larger set of distinguishable beads. An example of a 2D bead set is shown in Figure 5.8.

The immunoassay signal is generated by conjugates, coupled to a third type of fluorescent dye. Fulton et al. (1997) described this system, which could differentiate 64 unique bead populations by indexing their position in 2D fluorescent space. This strategy was further expanded by inclusion of a third fluorescent dye into the beads, thus creating a 3D indexing system. This expansion created the potential to include several hundred simultaneous assays in a single sample well.

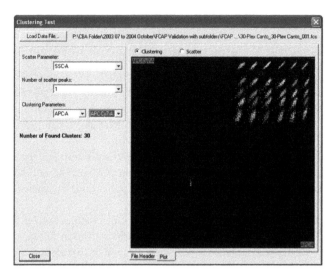

FIGURE 5.8 Dual stained Flex-set bead clusters for multiplex immunoassays. Thirty bead populations with varying levels of a red and infrared dye are detected on a BD™ FACSCanto II instrument. Analysis software is FCAP Array from Soft Flow.

Multiplex beads simplify panel assays. Only a single sample is needed to detect and quantify a number of analytes, an advantage when the sample volume is limited (e.g., pediatric samples, clinical studies, experiments in animal models). The multiple independent measurements within each bead population assure good precision. The wide detection range (at least three orders of magnitude) for fluorescent signal is another advantage.

An interesting application for the bead assays was demonstrated by van Dongen and collaborators (2009). One of the characteristics of several blood cancers is the presence of a fusion protein, which is the product of chromosome translocations. While multiple translocations occur within one family of malignant diseases, the resulting fusion proteins share the N-terminal and C-terminal sequences. This feature allowed the formulation of a simple immunobead assay for fusion proteins like BCR–ABL, PML–RARA, and others. Using MAbs against the shared N-terminal and C-terminal portion of the individual fusion protein, one of the antibodies served as capture reagent, coupled to beads, while the other antibody, coupled with a fluorescent molecule, functioned as detector.

Bead assays are well suited to monitor antibody responses against a panel of antigens from infectious agents. McHugh et al. (1997) presented a prototype hepatitis C virus antibody assay for potential use in the blood bank.

Detection and quantitation of cytokines are a natural area for flow multiplex assays. Figure 5.9 shows a multiplex assay with six cytokines. Oliver et al. (1998), Camilla et al. (1998), Chen et al. (1999), and others have described multiplex methods to measure panels of secreted cytokines in serum. Carson and Vignali (1999) demonstrated a multiplex bead assay for simultaneous quantitation of 15 cytokines, using the FlowMetrix™ system.

Pei et al. (1999) developed a multiplex bead method to detect antibodies against HLA Class I and Class II antigens. Pierangeli et al. (1999) described a flow multiplex assay for the simultaneous detection of IgG and IgM antibodies to cardiolipin and phosphatidylserine (PS). Lund-Johansen et al. (2000) applied a bead multiplex assay to assess the level of phosphorylation of different proteins. MAbs were coupled to latex beads, which in turn bound protein kinase substrate proteins. Phosphorylation of the captured proteins was detected with PE-labeled antiphosphotyrosine antibody.

Clinical applications were developed utilizing the multiplex bead assays. These include autoimmune disease diagnostic assays from multiple companies, allergy testing, and HLA typing. Rules-Based Medicine, an Austin-based company, has further developed the multiplex assay strategy as a centralized

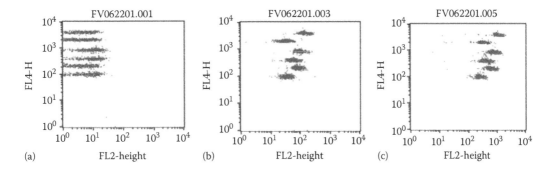

FIGURE 5.9 Multiplex bead immunoassay of six human cytokines. Three levels [(a) 0, (b) 80, and (c) 625 pg/mL] of each of the six cytokines] from a standard curve are shown. The order of the cytokines from top down: IL2, IL4, IL5, IL10, interferon-γ, and tumor necrosis factor-α. (From Chen, R. and Varro, R., Unpublished data, R&D, BD Biosciences.)

comprehensive laboratory service provider. They offer exclusive panels for various pharmaceutical studies, such as renal function assays to support drug toxicity studies as part of drug development.

5.13.3 Immunoglobulin Isotyping

Stall et al. (1998) constructed a single-tube immunoassay for isotyping of MAbs. Seven beads of different red fluorescence intensities were coated with mouse heavy-chain-specific antibodies. A mixture of FITC-labeled anti-κ and PE-labeled anti-λ antibodies subsequently identified the heavy- and light-chain isotypes of the captured MAb.

5.14 Polymerase Chain Reaction, Strand Displacement Amplification and Organon Technica and MSI

Molecular biology techniques are compatible with bead assays. Different amplification strategies were used to demonstrate flow methods to measure HIV viral load (Mehrpouyan et al. 1997; Van Cleve et al. 1998).

Defoort et al. (1998) and Fert (1999) developed a flow cytometric reverse transcriptase–polymerase chain reaction (RT-PCR) bead assay to quantitate HIV-1 mRNA.

5.14.1 SNP Detection, Gene Defects

The multiplex bead method is also compatible with nucleic acid hybridization. Iannone et al. (2000) describe a multiplex bead method to detect single nucleotide polymorphisms (SNPs). The SNP sites were identified by oligonucleotide ligation (OLA) and subsequent bead capture. Nine SNP markers were simultaneously tested by this method. Armstrong et al. (2000) used direct hybridization to determine the genotypes of eight polymorphic genes in a 32-plex flow assay.

Cai and collaborators have developed a sensitive and rapid flow cytometry-based assay for the multiplexed analysis of SNPs based on polymerase-mediated primer extension, or minisequencing, using microspheres as solid supports (Cai et al. 2000).

Horejsh developed a molecular beacon-based bead assay (Horejsh et al. 2005) and demonstrated that synthetic nucleic acid control sequences could be specifically detected for three respiratory pathogens, including the SARS coronavirus. This method was further expanded to monitor mRNA levels during fermentation (Dong et al. 2010) and to detect viral pathogens (Marshall et al. 2007).

Another bead-based molecular biology assay format was developed by Tm Biosciences for population-based screening for cystic fibrosis (Strom et al. 2006).

5.14.2 Other Cell Function Assays (Phagocytosis, Oxidative Burst, Basophils)

Flow cytometry is very useful for tracking apoptotic responses. Cellular viability (cytoplasmic membrane permeability) can be monitored using antitubulin antibody (O'Brien and Bolton 1995).

In the early phase of apoptosis, the cells lose the asymmetry of their membrane phospholipids. PS, a negatively charged phospholipid located in the inner leaflet of the plasma membrane, becomes exposed at the cell surface. Annexin V, a calcium and phospholipid-binding protein, binds preferentially to PS, with high affinity. Apoptotic cells are stained by annexin V before the dying cell changes its morphology and hydrolyzes its DNA (Koopman et al. 1994).

Other apoptosis assays include detection of Fas, FasL, caspase enzymes, and other biomolecules (Labroille et al. 2000).

Whole blood flow assays are adaptable for cell function testing. The phagocytic function of granulocytes and monocytes may be measured by detection of ingested fluorescent, opsonized bacteria (Sawyer et al. 1989). One can determine the overall percentage of monocytes and granulocytes showing phagocytosis in general (ingestion of one or more bacteria per cell) and the individual cellular phagocytic activity (number of bacteria per cell).

A variation of this method is used to evaluate the oxidative burst of leukocytes. Unlabeled opsonized bacteria are incubated with heparinized whole blood, and the generated reactive oxidants are detected by a fluorogenic substrate. Phagocytosis by polymorphonuclear neutrophils and monocytes constitutes an essential arm of host defense against bacterial or fungal infections; reduced oxidative burst may signal inborn defects (Donadebian 1989; Smith and Curnutte 1991).

Flow cytometry is an effective method to detect expression levels of receptors on cell surfaces. An example of this type of application is the quantitative determination of low-density lipoprotein (LDL) receptor expression on human monocytes. This method is suitable to identify people with the genetically inherited familial hypercholesterolemia (FH) disorder (Goldstein and Brown 1979). Individuals, homozygous for FH, carry mutant forms of the LDL receptor (frequency, one in 1,000,000) and have a high risk for atherosclerosis and coronary heart disease. Isolated peripheral blood mononuclear cells (lymphocytes and monocytes) are cultured, and the amount of LDL receptors is determined by flow cytometry after staining the cells with a MAb against the LDL receptor. This method is useful to identify the genetic defect.

Human basophils represent a very small portion of circulating leukocytes. They are hypersensitive effector cells of the immune system and play an important role in host defense mechanisms and allergic reactions. The binding of allergens to specific IgE fixed on the basophil membrane via the FceRI receptor triggers cellular activation, degranulation, and the release of potent mediators, including histamine and leukotriene C_4 (Dembo and Goldstein 1978; Kurimoto et al. 1991). Multicolor whole blood flow cytometric assays were constructed to detect the degranulation of basophils upon allergen exposure. These assays utilize the appearance of CD63, a member of the tetraspanin superfamily on activated basophils, as a marker for basophil degranulation (Sainte-Laudy et al. 1996). In Figure 5.10, such an assay is shown. In this case, the basophil phenotype is defined as HLA-DR-negative, CD123-positive cell population, and the degranulation is detected by the expression of CD63. A negative and a positive control are shown together with the effect of a specific allergen challenge.

The cytotoxic activity of human NK cells may be detected by flow cytometry. Fluorescently labeled K562 target cells are incubated with whole blood samples, and the killed target cells are identified by a DNA stain, which penetrates the dead cells and specifically stains their nuclei. This method can detect altered NK function found in various disorders (Rosenberg and Fauci 1989; Sibbitt and Bankhurst 1985) and can also be used to evaluate the effects of drugs on NK activity (Henney et al. 1981).

5.14.3 Thermodynamic and Kinetic Analysis of Binding Phenomena

Flow cytometry is increasingly used for rapid analysis in drug screening (Nolan et al. 1999). When combined with autosampler, pumps, and microwell plates, the potential throughput can reach 100,000 samples or more per day (Kuckuck et al. 2001). Sample valve systems allow pressure-free

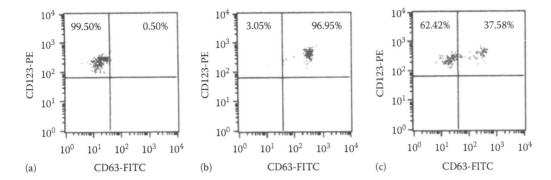

FIGURE 5.10 Basophil degranulation is detected by the rapid appearance of a CD63+ population in the upper right quadrant: (a) a negative control, (b) pollen mixture stimulated, and (c) fMLP stimulated. (From Chen, C.-H. and Varro, R., Unpublished data.)

introduction of very small samples, creating a *plug flow* instrument for rapid sequential flow cytometric sample analysis (Edwards et al. 1999).

Flow cytometry is uniquely capable of making sensitive and quantitative measurements of molecular interactions. These measurements can be made in real time with subsecond kinetic resolution using purified biomolecules or living cells (Nolan and Sklar 1998). The role of ligand/receptor binding in signal transduction may be studied in real time using bead bound receptors (Sklar et al. 2000) or by studying cell surface receptor interactions and signaling pathways in engineered cells, which contain fusion proteins, carrying fluorescent signals. The use of variants of the green fluorescent protein (GFP) provides valuable in vivo methods to explore protein binding, transduction pathways, and binding reactions, exploiting the fluorescence resonance energy transfer (FRET) phenomenon (Chan et al. 2001).

Live cell assays may be combined with methodology, which provide information on the longitudinal changes of assay parameters through subsequent generations of cells. Carboxyfluorescein succinimidyl ester (CFSE) binds to cell membranes and then equally distributes into daughter cells during cell division. After a few days in culture, the amount of cell division may be measured by the decreasing amount of fluorescence of each progeny population. CFSE staining can be combined with calcium flux, mitochondrial activity, pH, and free radical production to measure live cell populations in real time (Lyons and Parish 1994).

Technologies are also available to enhance the detection of antigens, expressed at low levels. A signal enhancement method, based on localized DNA amplification, was demonstrated by Gusev et al. (2001). The method substantially improved staining sensitivity of cellular antigens.

Enzyme-based amplification of the fluorescent staining is another way to increase signal intensities (Kaplan and Smith 2000).

5.15 Molecular and Cellular Biology Research: Genomics and Proteomics

High-speed sorting of chromosomes, especially at the US National Laboratories in Livermore (Gray et al. 1987) and Los Alamos (Cram 1990), provided the early material for the human genome project. Chromosomes were prepared from cell division metaphase stages, when they are condensed and stable. After staining with fluorescent or fluorogenic dyes, different chromosomes were separated, based on fluorescence intensity. The nucleic acid base sequence of the chromosomes was determined mostly by restriction enzyme digestion and electrophoresis-based sequencing. Based on the ability of specialized flow cytometers to detect single molecules (Habbersett and Jett 2004), it has been proposed to sequence long single nucleic acid strands by identifying bases, released by an enzyme cleaving off terminal bases. Even though this proposal has not been implemented yet, a nucleic acid analyzer based on the analysis of single fragment molecules from a restriction enzyme digestion of RNAs has been described (Nguyen et al. 1987). Other applications of flow cytometry in genomics are the identification of specific nucleic acid sequences in single cells by fluorescence in situ hybridization and the fluorescence-based detection of the transfection of cells with genetic material in combination with some marker gene like an enzyme (Fiering et al. 1991) or a fluorescent protein (Mateus and Avery 2000). One of the earliest applications of flow cytometry is based on MAb technology. In the past 20 years, thousands of antibodies have been developed against cellular structures. The reaction of fluorophore-labeled antibodies with cell suspensions followed by a flow cytometric analysis measures cell subsets carrying the structures identified by the antibodies. To date, 247 cell surface structures of white blood cells have been characterized with this method and are tabulated by an international organization as numbered cluster designations (http://www.uniprot.org/docs/cdlist) (Zola et al. 2005, Schlossman et al. 2005).

As mentioned in the section on medical applications of this chapter, these surface markers have helped in our understanding of diseases like AIDS. The characterization of these molecules has also contributed substantially to the knowledge in cell biology. Combined with high-speed cell sorting, these markers provide the basis for the large-scale isolation of specific cell subsets, which can be further characterized by 2D gel electrophoresis and mass spectrometry for identifying the complete proteome of different cell types or organelles (Godfrey et al. 2005).

5.16 Industrial and Environmental Cytometry

Flow cytometry has found applications in several industrial settings for quality control and process monitoring. Examples are the monitoring of industrial cell culture (Zhao et al. 1999), clone improvement by sorting and recloning highly productive single cells (Borth et al. 1999), and the sorting of transfectants based on expression of coexpressed fluorescent proteins (Van Tendeloo et al. 2000).

In agriculture, flow cytometry is used for sperm counting (Eustache et al. 2001) and sorting (Johnson 2000). Methods for counting microbes in foods like milk have been described (Gunasekera et al. 2000). For environmental testing, the technique has been proposed for water quality monitoring (Vesey et al. 1994) and for measuring bioburden in air (Hairston et al. 1997). Marine biologists are using it to count bacteria and viruses in seawater (Li and Dickie 2001).

Acknowledgment

The authors thank Hailey Tipton for help with the preparation of the manuscript.

References

Aghaeepour N, Jalali A, O'Neill K, Chattopadhyay PK, Roederer M, Hoos HH, Brinkman RR. 2012. RchyOptimyx: Cellular hierarchy optimization for flow cytometry. *Cytometry A*, 12:1022–1030.

Alvarez-Barrientos A, Arroyo J, Canton R, Nombela C, Sanchez-Perez M. April 2000. Applications of flow cytometry to clinical microbiology. *Clin. Microbiol. Rev.*, 13(2), 167–195.

Ammann AJ, Abrams D, Conant M, Chudwin D, Cowan M, Volberding P. 1983. Acquired immune dysfunction in homosexual men: Immunologic profiles. *Clin. Immunol. Immunopathol.*, 27, 315.

Armstrong B, Stewart M, Mazumder A. 2000. Suspension arrays for high throughput, multiplexed single nucleotide polymorphism genotyping. *Cytometry*, 40, 102–108.

Bagwell CB. 2005. Hyperlog—A flexible log-like transform for negative, zero, and positive valued data. *Cytometry A*, 64(1), 34–42.

Barclay R, Walker B, Allan R, Reid C, Duffin E, Kane E, Turner M. 1998. Flow cytometric determination of residual leucocytes in filter-depleted blood products: An evaluation of Becton–Dickinson's LeucoCOUNT system. *Transf. Sci.*, 19, 399–403.

Barre-Sinoussi R, Chermann JC, Rey F et al. 1983. Isolation of a T-lymphotropic retrovirus from a patient at risk for acquired immune deficiency syndrome (AIDS). *Science*, 220, 868.

Bergeron M, Ding T, Houle G et al. 2010. QASI, an international quality management system for CD4 T-cell enumeration focused to make a global difference. *Clin. Cytom. B*, 78(1), 41–48.

Bergeron M, Faucher S, Minkus T, Lacroix F, Ding T, Phaneuf S, Somorjai R, Summers R, Mandy F. 1998. Impact of unified procedures as implemented in the Canadian Quality Assurance Program for T lymphocyte subset enumeration. Participating Flow Cytometry Laboratories of the Canadian Clinical Trials Network for HIV/AIDS Therapies. *Cytometry*, 33(2), 146.

Bierre P, Thiel DE. 1998. Algorithmic engine for automated N-dimensional subset analysis. United States Patent 5,739,000. April 14, 1998.

Bishop JE, Davis KA. 1997. A flow cytometric immunoassay for β_2-microglobulin in whole blood. *J. Immunol. Methods*, 210, 79–87.

Borth N, Strutzenberger K, Kunert R, Steinfellner W, Katinger H. 1999. Analysis of changes during subclone development and ageing of human antibody-producing heterohybridoma cells by northern blot and flow cytometry. *J. Biotechnol.*, 67(1), 57–66.

Braga PC, Bovio C, Calicic M, Dal Sasso M. 2003. Flow cytometric assessment of susceptibilities of *Streptococcus pyogenes* to erythromycin and rokitamycin. *Antimicrob. Agents Chemother.*, 47, 408–412.

Cai H, White PS, Torney D, Deshpande A, Wang Z, Keller RA, Marrone B, Nolan JP. 2000. Flow cytometry-based minisequencing: A new platform for high-throughput single-nucleotide polymorphism scoring. *Genomics*, 66, 135–143.

Calvelli T, Denny TN, Paxton H, Gelman R, Kagan J. 1993. Guidelines for flow cytometric immunophenotyping: A report from the National Institutes of Allergy and Infectious Diseases, Division of AIDS. *Cytometry*, 14, 702.

Camilla C, Defoort JP, Delaage M, Auer R. Quintana J, Lary T, Hamelik R, Prato S, Casano B, Martin M, Fert V. 1998. A new flow cytometry-based multi-assay system. 1. Application to cytokine immunoassays. *Cytometry*, 8(Suppl.), 132 (Abstract).

Carson RT, Vignali DA. 1999. Simultaneous quantitation of fifteen cytokines using a multiplexed flow cytometric assay. *J. Immunol. Methods*, 227, 41–45.

Centers for Disease Control (CDC). 1993. Revised classification system for HIV infection and expanded surveillance case definition for AIDS among adolescents and adults. *Morbid. Mortal. Wkly. Rep.*, 41, 1.

Centers for Disease Control and Prevention (CDCP). 1997. Revised guidelines for performing CD4+ T-cell determinations in persons infected with human immunodeficiency virus (HIV). *Morbid. Mortal. Wkly. Rep.*, 46, 1.

Chan FK, Siegel RM, Zacharias D, Swofford R, Holmes KL, Tsien RY, Lenardo MJ. 2001. Fluorescence resonance energy transfers analysis of cell surface receptor interactions and signaling using spectral variants of the green fluorescent protein. *Cytometry*, 44, 361–368.

Chase ES, Hoffman RA. 1998. Resolution of dimly fluorescent particles: A practical measure of fluorescence sensitivity. *Cytometry*, 33, 267–269.

Chen R, Lowe L, Wilson JD, Crowther E, Tzeggai K, Bishop JE, Varro R. 1999. Simultaneous quantification of six human cytokines in a single sample using microparticle-based flow cytometric technology. *Clin. Chem.*, 9, 1693–1694.

Civin CI, Trischman TW, Fackler MJ et al. 1989. Report on the CD34 cluster workshop. In: Knapp W, Dorken B, Gilks WR et al. (eds.), *Leucocyte Typing IV: White Cell Differentiation Antigens*. Oxford University Press, Oxford, U.K., pp. 818–829.

Coller BS, Anderson K, Weisman HF. 1995. New antiplatelet agents: Platelets GpIIb/IIIa antagonists. *Thromb. Haemost.*, 74, 302–308.

Collins DP, Luebering BJ, Shaut DM. 1998. T-lymphocyte functionality assessed by analysis of cytokine receptor expression, intracellular cytokine expression, and femtomolar detection of cytokine secretion by quantitative flow cytometry. *Cytometry*, 33, 249–255.

Conrad MP, Reichert TA, Bezdek JC. 1989. Method of displaying multi-parameter data sets to aid in the analysis of data characteristics. United States Patent 4,845,653. July 4, 1989.

Coventry BJ, Neoh SH, Mantzioris BX, Skinner JM, Zola H, Bradley J. August 1994. A comparison of the sensitivity of immunoperoxidase staining methods with high-sensitivity fluorescence flow cytometry-antibody quantitation on the cell surface. *J. Histochem. Cytochem.*, 42(8), 1143–1147.

Cram LS. 1990. Flow cytogenetics and chromosome sorting. *Hum. Cell*, 3(2), 99–106 (Review).

Davis KA, Abrams B, Iyer SB, Hoffman RA, Bishop JE. 1998. Determination of CD4 antigen density on cells: Role of antibody valency, avidity, clones, and conjugation. *Cytometry*, 33, 197–205.

Defoort JP, Camilla C, Delaage M et al. 1998. A new flow cytometry-based multi-assay system. 2. Application to HIV1 mRNA quantification. *Cytometry*, 8(Suppl.), 132 (Abstract).

Dembo M, Goldstein B. 1978. Theory of equilibrium bridging of symmetric bivalent haptens to cell surface antibody. Application to histamine release from basophils. *J. Immunol.*, 121, 345–352.

Donadebian HD. 1989. Congenital and acquired neutrophil abnormalities. In: Klempner MS et al. (eds.), *Phagocytes and Disease*. Kluwer, Dordrecht, the Netherlands, pp. 103–118.

Dong D, Pang Y, Gao Q, Huang X, Xu Y, Li R. 2010. Rapid monitoring of mRNA levels with a molecular beacon during microbial fermentation. *J. Biotechnol.*, 145(3), 310–316

Edwards BS, Kuckuck F, Sklar LA. 1999. Plug flow cytometry: An automated coupling device for rapid sequential flow cytometric sample analysis. *Cytometry*, 37, 156–159.

Eustache F, Jouannet P, Auger J. 2001. Evaluation of flow cytometric methods to measure human sperm concentration. *J. Androl.*, 22(4), 558–567.

Fahey JL, Taylor JMG, Detels R, Hofmann B, Melmed R, Nishanian P, Giorgi JV. 1990. The prognostic value of cellular and serologic markers in infection with human immunodeficiency virus type 1. *N. Engl. J. Med.*, 322, 166.

Fert V. 1999. Simultaneous immuno- and nucleic acid probe assays on flow cytometer, critical parameters for assay design and applications as a screening tool for understanding immune disease. *Cytometry*, 38, 94.

Fiering SN, Roederer M, Nolan GP, Micklem DR, Parks DR, Herzenberg LA. 1991. Improved FACS-Gal: Flow cytometric analysis and sorting of viable eukaryotic cells expressing reporter gene constructs. *Cytometry*, 12(4), 291–301.

Frengen J, Schmid R, Kierulf B, Nustad K, Paus E, Berge A, Lindmo T. 1993. Homogeneous immunofluorometric assays for α-fetoprotein with macroporous monosized particles and flow cytometry. *Clin. Chem.*, 39, 2174–2181.

Fulton RJ, McDade RL, Smith PL, Kienker LJ, Kettman JR. 1997. Advanced multiplexed analysis with the FlowMetrix system. *Clin. Chem.*, 43, 1749.

Fulwyler MJ, McHugh TM, Schwadron R, Scillian JJ, Lau D, Busch MP, Roy S, Vyas GN. 1988. Immunoreactive bead (IRB) assay for the quantitative and simultaneous flow cytometric detection of multiple soluble analytes. *Cytometry*, 2(Suppl.), 19 (Abstract).

Gallo RC, Salahuddin SZ, Popovic M, Shearer GM, Kaplan M, Haynes BF, Palker TJ, Redfield R, Oleske J, Safai B. 1984. Frequent detection and isolation of cytopathic retroviruses (HTLV-III) from patients with AIDS and at risk for AIDS. *Science*, 224, 500.

Gaucher JC, Grunwald D, Frelat G. 1988. Fluorescence response and sensitivity determination for the ATC 3000 flow cytometer. *Cytometry*, 9(6), 557–565.

Gilks CF, Mugyenyi P, Hakim J, Reid A, Bray D, Darbishire LH, Gibb DM, Babiker AG. 2009. Routine versus clinically driven laboratory monitoring of HIV antiretroviral therapy in Africa (DART): A randomized non-inferiority trial. *Lancet*, 375, 123.

Giorgi JV, Fahey JL, Smith DC, Hultin LE, Cheng H, Mitsuyasu RT. 1987. Early effects of HIV on CD4 lymphocytes in vivo. *J. Immunol.*, 138, 3725.

Glencross DK, Aggett HM, Stevens WS, Mandy F. 2008a. African regional external quality assessment for CD4 T-cell enumeration: Development, outcomes, and performance of laboratories. *Clin. Cytom. B*, 74(1), S69–S79.

Glencross DK, Janossy G, Coetzee LM, Lawrie D, Scott LE, Sanne I, McIntyre JA, Stevens W. 2008b. CD8/CD38 activation yields important clinical information of effective antiretroviral therapy: Findings from the first year of the CIPRA-SA cohort. *Cytometry B: Clin. Cytom.*, 74(Suppl. 1), S131–S140.

Godfrey WL, Rudd CJ, Iyer S, Recktenwald D. 2005. Purification of cellular and organelle populations by fluorescence-activated cell sorting for proteome analysis. In: Walker JM (ed.), *The Proteomics Protocols Handbook*. Springer, New York, pp. 67–78.

Goldstein JL, Brown MS. 1979. The LDL receptor locus and the genetics of familial hypercholesterolemia. *Ann. Rev. Genet.*, 13, 259–289.

Gottlieb MS, Schroff R, Schanker HM, Weisman JD, Fan PT, Wolf RA, Saxon A. 1981. *Pneumocystis carinii* pneumonia and mucosal candidiasis in previously healthy homosexual men. *N. Engl. J. Med.*, 305, 1426.

Graedel TE, McGill R. 1982. Graphical presentation of results from scientific computer models. *Science*, 215, 1191.

Gray JW, Dean PN, Fuscoe JC, Peters DC, Trask BJ, van den Engh GJ, Van Dilla MA. 1987. High-speed chromosome sorting. *Science*, 238(4825), 323–329 (Review).

Gunasekera TS, Attfield PV, Veal DA. 2000. A flow cytometry method for rapid detection and enumeration of total bacteria in milk. *Appl. Environ. Microbiol.*, 66(3), 1228–1232.

Gusev Y, Sparkowski J, Raghunathan A et al. 2001. Rolling circle amplification: A new approach to increase sensitivity for immunohistochemistry and flow cytometry. *Am. J. Pathol.*, 159, 63–69.

Habbersett RC, Jett JA. 2004. An analytical system based on a compact flow cytometer for DNA fragment sizing and single-molecule detection. *Cytometry A*, 60(2), 125–134.

Hairston PP, Ho J, Quant FR. April 1997. Design of an instrument for real-time detection of bioaerosols using simultaneous measurement of particle aerodynamic size and intrinsic fluorescence. *J. Aerosol. Sci.*, 28(3), 471–482.

Harding JD, Keller RA. 1992. Single-molecule detection as an approach to rapid DNA sequencing. *Trends Biotechnol.*, 10(1–2), 55–57.

Hardy NM. 1992. Lymphocyte subset changes in persons infected with human immunodeficiency virus. *Ann. Clin. Lab. Sci.*, 22, 286.

Henderson LO, Marti GE, Gaigalas AK, Hannon WH, Vogt RF. 1998. Terminology and nomenclature for standardization in quantitative fluorescence cytometry. *Cytometry*, 33, 97–105.

Henney CS, Kuribayashi K, Kern DE, Gillis S. 1981. Interleukin-2 augments natural killer cell activity. *Nature*, 291, 335.

Hoffman RA, Houck DW. 1998. Cell separation using flow cytometric cell sorting. In: Recktenwald D, Radbruch A (eds.), *Cell Separation Methods and Applications*. Marcel Dekker, New York, Chapter 11, pp. 237–269.

Hoffman RA, Kung PC, Hansen WP, Goldstein G. 1980. Simple and rapid measurement of human T lymphocytes and their subclasses in peripheral blood. *Proc. Natl. Acad. Sci. USA*, 77, 4914.

Hoffman RA, Wood JCS. 2007. Characterization of flow cytometer instrument sensitivity. *Current Protocols in Cytometry*. John Wiley & Sons, New York, pp. 1.20.1–1.20.18.2.

Horejsh D, Martini F, Poccia F, Ippolito G, Di Caro A, Capobianchi MR. 2005 A molecular beacon, bead-based assay for the detection of nucleic acids by flow cytometry. *Nucleic Acids Res.*, 33(2), e13.

Iannone MA, Taylor JD, Chen J, Li MS, Rivers P, Slentz-Kesler KA, Weiner MP. 2000. Multiplexed single nucleotide polymorphism genotyping by oligonucleotide ligation and flow cytometry. *Cytometry*, 39, 131–140.

Janossy G, Mandy F. 2010. Translational medicine as implementation science in the field of monitoring HIV and TB, new concepts emanating from resource poor countries. *Cytometry Part B*, 78, 183–187.

Jensen PO, Larsen JK, Christensen IJ, van Erp PE. 1994. Discrimination of bromodeoxyuridine labeled and unlabelled mitotic cells in flow cytometric bromodeoxyuridine/DNA analysis. *Cytometry*, 15, 154–161.

Johnson LA. 2000. Sexing mammalian sperm for production of offspring: The state-of-the-art. *Anim. Reprod. Sci.*, 60–61, 93–107 (Review).

Kaplan D, Smith D. 2000. Enzymatic amplification staining for flow cytometric analysis of cell surface molecules. *Cytometry*, 40, 81–85.

Karthick RMR, Kovarova L, Jajek R. 2010. Review of phenotypic markers used in flow cytometric analysis of MGUS and MM and applicability of flow cytometry in other plasma cell disorders. *Brit. J. Haematol.*, 149, 334–351.

Keating P, Cambrosio A. 2003. *Biomedical Platform—Realigning the Normal and the Pathological in the Late-Twentieth-Century Medicine*. MIT, London, U.K.

Koopman G, Reutelingsperger CPM, Kuijten GAM, Keehnen RMJ, Pals ST, Nan Oers, MHJ. 1994. Annexin V for flow cytometric detection of phosphatidylserine expression on B cells undergoing apoptosis. *Blood*, 84, 1415–1420.

Koot M, Schellekens PTA, Mulder JW, Lange JMA, Roos MTL, Coutinho RA, Tersmette M, Miedema F. 1993. Viral phenotype and T cell reactivity in human immunodeficiency virus type 1-infected asymptomatic men treated with zidovudine. *J. Infect. Dis.*, 168, 733.

Kuckuck FW, Edwards BS, Sklar LA. 2001. High throughput flow cytometry. *Cytometry*, 44, 83–90.

Kurimoto YA, de Week AL, Dahinden CA. 1991. The effect of interleukin-3 upon IgE-dependent and IgE-independent basophil degranulation and leukotriene generation. *Eur. J. Immunol.*, 21, 361–368.

Labroille G, Dumain P, Lacombe F, Belloc F. 2000. Flow cytometric evaluation of fas expression in relation to response and resistance to anthracyclines in leukemic cells. *Cytometry*, 39, 195–202.

Lenkei R, Gratama JW, Rothe G, Schmitz G, D'hautcourt JL, Arekrans A, Mandy F, Marti G. 1998a. Performance of calibration standards for antigen quantitation with flow cytometry. *Cytometry*, 33, 188–196.

Lenkei R, Mandy F, Marti G, Vogt R (eds.). 1998b. Quantitative fluorescence cytometry: An emerging consensus. *Cytometry*, 33, 1–287.

Li WK, Dickie PM. 2001. Monitoring phytoplankton, bacterioplankton, and virioplankton in a coastal inlet (Bedford Basin) by flow cytometry. *Cytometry*, 44(3), 236–246.

Loken MR, Shah VO, Hollander Z, Civin CI. 1988. Flow cytometric analysis of normal B lymphoid development. *Pathol. Immunopathol. Res.*, 7, 357–370.

Lucia B, Jennings C, Cauda R, Ortona L, Landay AL. 1995. Evidence of a selective depletion of a CD16+ CD56+ CD8+ natural killer cell subset during HIV infection. *Cytometry*, 22, 10.

Lund-Johansen F, Davis K, Bishop J, de Waal Malefyt R. 2000. Flow cytometric analysis of immunoprecipitates: High-throughput analysis of protein phosphorylation and protein–protein interactions. *Cytometry*, 39, 250–259.

Lyons AB, Parish CR. 1994. Determination of lymphocyte division by flow cytometry. *J. Immunol. Methods*, 171, 131–137.

Maecker HT, Dunn HS, Suni MA et al. 2001. Use of overlapping peptide mixtures as antigens for cytokine flow cytometry. *J. Immunol. Methods*, 255(1–2), 27–40.

Mandy F, Brando B. 2000. Enumeration of absolute cell counts using immunophenotyping techniques. *Curr. Protoc. Cytom.*, Unit 6.8.

Mandy F, Janossy G, Bergeron M, Pilon R, Faucher S. 2008. Affordable CD4 T-cell enumeration for resource-limited regions: A status report for 2008. *Cytometry B: Clin. Cytom.*, 74(Suppl. 1), S27–S39.

Mandy FF, Bergeron M, Minkus T. 1995. Principles of flow cytometry. *Transf. Sci.*, 16, 303.

Mandy FF, Bergeron M, Minkus T. 1997. Evolution of leukocyte immunophenotyping as influenced by the HIV/AIDS pandemic: A short history of the development of gating strategies for CD4 T-cell enumeration. *Cytometry*, 30, 157.

Mandy FF, Bergeron M, Recktenwald D, Izaguirre CA. 1992. A simultaneous three-color T cell subsets analysis with single laser flow cytometers using T cell gating protocol. *J. Immunol. Methods*, 156, 151.

Marshall DJ, Reisdorf E, Harms G, Beaty E, Moser MJ, Lee W-M, Gern JE, Nolte FS, Shult P, Prudent JR. 2007. Evaluation of a multiplexed PCR assay for detection of respiratory viral pathogens in a public health laboratory setting. *J. Clin. Microbiol.*, 8(12), 3875–3882.

Mateus C, Avery SV. 2000. Destabilized green fluorescent protein for monitoring dynamic changes in yeast gene expression with flow cytometry. *Yeast*, 16(14), 1313–1323.

McDougal JS, Kennedy MS, Sligh JM, Cort SP, Mawle A, Nicholson JKA. 1986. Binding of HTLV-III/LAV to CD4+ T cells by a complex of the 100 K viral protein and the T4 molecule. *Science*, 231, 382.

McHugh TM. 1994. Flow microsphere immunoassay for the quantitative and simultaneous detection of multiple soluble analytes. *Methods Cell Biol.*, 42, 575–595.

McHugh TM, Viele MK, Chase ES, Recktenwald DJ. 1997. The sensitive detection and quantitation of antibody to HCV using a microsphere-based immunoassay and flow cytometry. *Cytometry*, 29, 106–112.

McNiece I, Kern B, Zilm K, Brunaud C, Dziem G, Briddell R. 1998. Minimization of CD34+ cell enumeration variability using the ProCOUNT standardized methodology. *J. Hematother.*, 7, 499–504.

Mehrpouyan M, Bishop JE, Ostrerova N, Van Cleve M, Lohman KL. 1997. A rapid and sensitive method for non-isotopic quantitation of HIV-1 RNA using thermophilic SDA and flow cytometry. *Mol. Cell. Probes*, 11, 337–347.

Michelson AD. 1996. Flow cytometry: A clinical test of platelet function. *Blood*, 87, 4925–4936.

Morgan E, Varro R, Sepulveda H et al. 2004. Cytometric bead array: A multiplexed assay platform with applications in various areas of biology. *Clin. Immunol.*, 110(3), 252–266.

Nguyen DC, Keller RA, Jett JH, Martin JC. 1987. Detection of single molecules of phycoerythrin in hydrodynamically focused flows by laser-induced fluorescence. *Anal. Chem.*, 59(17), 2158–2161.

Nicholson JKA, Jones BM, Hubbard M. 1993. CD4 T-lymphocyte determinations on whole blood specimens using a single-tube three-color assay. *Cytometry*, 14, 685.

Nicholson JKA, Mandy FF. 2000. Immunophenotyping in HIV infection. In: Stewart CC, Nicholson JKA (eds.), *Immunophenotyping*. Wiley-Liss, New York, Chapter 1, pp. 267–268.

Nicholson JKA, Stein D, Mui T, Mack R, Hubbard M, Denny T. 1997. Evaluation of a method for counting absolute numbers of cells with a flow cytometer. *Clin. Diag. Lab. Immunol.*, 4, 309.

Nolan JP, Lauer S, Prossnitz ER, Sklar LA. 1999. Flow cytometry: A versatile tool for all phases of drug discovery. *Drug Discov. Today*, 4, 173–180.

Nolan JP, Sklar LA. 1998. The emergence of flow cytometry for sensitive, real-time measurements of molecular interactions. *Nat. Biotechnol.*, 16, 633–638.

O'Brien MC, Bolton WE. 1995. Comparison of cell viability probes compatible with fixation and permeabilization for combined surface and intracellular staining in flow cytometry. *Cytometry*, 19, 243–255.

O'Gorman MRG, Nicholson JKA. 2000. Adoption of single-platform technologies for enumeration of absolute T-lymphocyte subsets in peripheral blood. *Clin. Diag. Lab. Immunol.*, 7, 333.

Oliver KG, Kettman JR, Fulton RJ. 1998. Multiplexed analysis of human cytokines by use of the FlowMetrix system. *Clin. Chem.*, 44, 2057–2060.

O'Neill K, Jalali A, Aghaeepour N, Hoos H, Brinkman RR. 2014. Enhanced flowType/RchyOptimyx: A bioconductor pipeline for discovery in high-dimensional cytometry data. *Bioinformatics* [Epub ahead of print].

Oostman Jr CA, Blasenheim BJ. 2006. Fluorescence detection instrument with reflective transfer legs for color decimation. United States Patent 7,129,505. October 31, 2006.

Parks DR, Roederer M, Moore WA. 2006. A new "logicle" display method avoids deceptive effects of logarithmic scaling for low signals and compensated data. *Cytometry A*, 69(6), 541–551.

Pei R, Lee J, Chen T, Rojo S, Terasaki PI. 1999. Flow cytometric detection of HLA antibodies using a spectrum of microbeads. *Hum. Immunol.*, 60, 1293–1302.

Peters D, Branscomb E, Dean P, Merrill T, Pinkel D, Van Dilla M, Grayref JW. 1985. The LLNL high-speed sorter: Design features, operational characteristics, and biological utility. *Cytometry*, 6, 290–301.

Pierangeli SS, Silva LK, Harris EN. 1999. A flow cytometric assay for the detection of antiphospholipid antibodies. *Am. Clin. Lab.*, 18, 18–19.

Roederer M, Moore W, Treister A, Hardy RR, Herzenberg LA. 2001. Probability binning comparison: A metric for quantitating multivariate distribution differences. *Cytometry*, 45, 47–55.

Rogers WT, Moser AR, Holyst HA. 2009. FlowFP: A bioconductor package for fingerprinting flow cytometric data. *Adv. Bioinform.*, Article ID 193947, 11p., doi:10.1155/2009/193947.

Rosenberg ZF, Fauci AS. 1989. The immunopathogenesis of HIV infection. *Adv. Immunol.*, 47, 377–431.

Sainte-Laudy J, Vallon C, Guerin JC. 1996. Diagnosis of latex allergy: Comparison of histamine release and flow cytometric analysis of basophil activation. *Inflamm. Res.*, 45(Suppl. 1), S35–S36.

Savage PA, Boniface JJ, Davis MM. 1999. A kinetic basis for T cell receptor repertoire selection during an immune response. *Immunity*, 10, 485–492.

Sawyer DW, Donowitz GR, Mandell GL. 1989. Polymorphonuclear neutrophils: An effective antimicrobial force. *Rev. Infect. Dis.*, 11, S1532–S1544.

Schlossman SF, Schwartz-Albiez R, Simmons P, Tedder TF, Uguccioni M, Warren H. 2005. CD molecules 2005: Human cell differentiation molecules. *Blood*, 106(9), 3123–3126.

Shapiro HM. 2003. *Practical Flow Cytometry*. Wiley-Liss Inc., New York.

Shapiro HN. 1994. Parameters and probes. In: Shapiro A. (ed.), *Practical Flow Cytometry*. Wiley-Liss Inc., New York, Chapter 7.2, pp. 243–248.

Shattil SJ, Cunningham M, Hoxie JA. 1987. Detection of activated platelets in whole blood using activation-dependent monoclonal antibodies and flow cytometry. *Blood*, 70, 307–315.

Sibbitt WL, Bankhurst AD. 1985. Natural killer cells in connective tissue disorders. *Clin. Rheum. Dis.*, 11, 507.

Siegal FP, Lopez C, Hammer GS et al. 1981. Severe acquired immunodeficiency in male homosexuals, manifested by chronic perianal ulcerative herpes simplex lesions. *N. Engl. J. Med.*, 305, 1439.

Sklar LA, Vilven J, Lynam E, Neldon D, Bennett TA, Prossnitz E. 2000. Solubilization and display of G protein-coupled receptors on beads for real-time fluorescence and flow cytometric analysis. *Biotechniques*, 28, 976–980.

Smith RM, Curnutte JT. 1991. Molecular basis of chronic granulomatous disease. *Blood*, 77, 673–686.

Stall A, Sun Q, Varro R, Lowe L, Crowther E, Abrams B, Bishop J, Davis K. 1998. A single tube flow cytometric multibead assay for isotyping mouse monoclonal antibodies. Abstract 1877, *Experimental Biology Meeting*, San Francisco, CA.

Stein DS, Korvick JA, Vermund SH. 1992. CD4+ lymphocyte cell enumeration for prediction of clinical course of human immuno-deficiency virus disease: A review. *J. Infect. Dis.*, 165, 352.

Stevens W, Gelman R, Glencross DK, Scott LE, Crowe SM, Spira T. 2008. Evaluating new CD4 enumeration technologies for resource-constrained countries. *Nat. Rev. Microbiol.*, 6, 529–537.

Strom CM, Janeszco M, Quan F, Wang S-B, Buller A, McGinnis M, Sun W. 2006. Technical validation of a Tm biosciences luminex-based multiplex assay for detecting the American College of Medical Genetics recommended cystic fibrosis mutation panel. *J. Mol. Diagn.*, 8(3), 371–375.

Suni MA, Picker LJ, Maino VC. 1998. Detection of antigen-specific T cell cytokine expression in whole blood by flow cytometry. *J. Immunol. Methods*, 212, 89–98.

To LB, Haylock DN, Simmons PJ, Juttner CA. 1997. The biological and clinical uses of blood stem cells. *Blood*, 89, 2233–2258.

Trotter J. 2007. Alternatives to log-scale data display. *Curr. Protocols Cytom.*, 42, 10.16.1–10.16.11.

Van Cleve M, Ostrerova N, Tietgen K, Cao W, Chang C, Collins ML, Kolberg J, Urdea M, Lohman K. 1998. Direct quantitation of HIV by flow cytometry using branched DNA signal amplification. *Mol. Cell. Probes*, 12, 243–247.

Vandenberghe PA, Ceuppens JL. 1990. Flow cytometric measurement of cytoplasmic free calcium in human peripheral blood T lymphocytes with Fluo-3, a new fluorescent calcium indicator. *J. Immunol. Methods*, 127, 197–205.

van den Engh GJ, Trask BJ, Gray JW. 1986. The binding kinetics and interaction of DNA fluorochromes used in the analysis of nuclei and chromosomes by flow cytometry. *Histochemistry*, 84, 501–508.

Van Tendeloo VF, Ponsaerts P, Van Broeckhoven C, Berneman ZN, Van Bockstaele DR. 2000. Efficient generation of stably electrotransfected human hematopoietic cell lines without drug selection by consecutive FACsorting. *Cytometry*, 41(1), 31–35.

Vesey G, Hutton P, Champion A, Ashbolt N, Williams KL, Warton A, Veal D. 1994. Application of flow cytometric methods for the routine detection of Cryptosporidium and Giardia in water. *Cytometry*, 16(1), 1–6.

Vittorio D, Angelo C, Eliseo M, Antonio G, Luigi B. 2009. Cytometry and DNA ploidy: Clinical uses and molecular perspective in gastric and lung cancer. *J. Cell. Physiol.*, 222(3), 532–539.

Wang L, Gaigalas AK, Marti G, Abbasi F, Hoffman RA. 2008. Toward quantitative fluorescence measurements with multicolor flow cytometry. *Cytometry A*, 73, 279–288.

Watson JV. 1992. *Flow Cytometry Data Analysis*. Cambridge University Press, Cambridge, U.K.

Weerkamp F, Dekking E, Ng YY et al. 2009. Flow cytometric immunobead assay for the detection of BCR–ABL fusion proteins in leukemia patients. *Leukemia*, 23, 1106–1117.

Weir EG, Borowitz MJ. April 2001. Flow cytometry in the diagnosis of acute leukemia. *Semin. Hematol.*, 38(2), 124–138.

Zhao R, Natarajan A, Srienc F. 1999. A flow injection flow cytometry system for on-line monitoring of bioreactors. *Biotechnol. Bioeng.*, 62(5), 609–617.

Zola H, Swart B, Nicholson I et al. 2005. CD molecules 2005: Human cell differentiation molecules. *Blood*, 106(9), 3123–3126.

6

Capillary Electrophoresis Techniques in Biomedical Analysis

S. Douglass Gilman
University of Tennessee

Michael J. Sepaniak
University of Tennessee

6.1 Overview

Capillary electrophoresis (CE) is a microscale analytical separation technique that has matured rapidly over the past 20 years since the groundbreaking publications of Jorgenson and Lukacs.[1,2] Biomedical applications of CE are a leading factor driving the development of what has now evolved into a broad family of related separation techniques. Certainly the most prominent biomedical application of CE is the sequencing of the human genome.[3] The accelerated achievement of this goal depended on CE separations.[3-5] From 1981 through the writing of this text, more than 14,000 papers were published that included CE and related techniques. A survey of this literature over the past 12 months indicates that more than 70% of these reports include bioanalytical applications of CE.

Clearly, a comprehensive review of biomedical applications of CE is well beyond the scope of a single book chapter. This chapter first reviews basic CE separations; readers are directed to review articles for in-depth coverage of related CE separation methods. Next, the role of photonics in CE, primarily for detection purposes, is discussed. Finally, the chapter reviews specific examples of biomedical applications of CE that feature photonics, to provide the reader with a view of the possibilities of this approach for biomedical analysis.

Capillary electrophoresis typically is performed in 25–75 μm internal diameter (ID), fused-silica capillaries (15–100 cm in length) filled with aqueous, buffered solutions. Each end of the capillary is immersed in a buffer reservoir, and a potential of 10–30 kV is applied across the capillary using Pt electrodes in each reservoir. In its simplest form, capillary zone electrophoresis (CZE), different charged compounds in an injected sample zone are separated based on their relative electrophoretic migration rates. For newcomers to this technique, an intuitive feel for this separation method can perhaps best be developed by comparing and contrasting CE with two more familiar and related separation techniques: high pressure liquid chromatography (HPLC) and slab gel electrophoresis.

Like HPLC, CE is a column-based separation technique. Sample plugs are injected into the CE column. Compounds separate as they pass through the column, and separated compound zones are detected as they elute past a fixed point. One obvious difference between the two separation techniques is scale. Typical internal diameters for CE are 25–75 μm compared to 1–5 mm for HPLC. A 50 μm ID CE column 1 m in length has a total column volume of only 2 μλ. Typical CE injection volumes are only a few nanoliters; column flow rates are ordinarily a few hundred nanoliters per minute, although linear flow velocities are generally greater than in HPLC. One consequence of the scale of CE is that it is well suited for analysis of small-volume samples such as single cells.[6,7] In addition, insignificant volumes of solvent waste are generated compared to HPLC. Due to its small scale, CE is primarily an analytical technique, and is not as practical as HPLC for preparative work. Analyte detection is also more challenging at smaller scales, as discussed later in this chapter.

Capillary electrophoretic separations typically exhibit higher separation efficiencies (narrower peaks) and are rapid compared to HPLC. Typically, a CE separation will generate 10–100 times more theoretical plates than an HPLC separation for the same compounds and separation time. High separation efficiencies are primarily due to the plug-shaped electroosmotic flow profile and the electrophoretic separation mechanism of CZE. Peaks for HPLC are typically broader due to the parabolic flow profile of pressure-driven flow, effects of the particles used to pack stationary phases for HPLC, and resistance to mass transfer between the mobile phase and separation phase in HPLC. This last source of peak broadening for HPLC underscores the primary difference between the two techniques, which is separation mechanism. HPLC is a chromatographic technique where separation depends on the relative partitioning of different compounds between a mobile phase and a stationary phase. Separation in CZE is based on electrophoretic migration rates in free solution. Related CE techniques that include partitioning as part of the separation also have been developed and will be discussed later in this chapter.

The most common forms of slab gel electrophoresis, SDS–PAGE for proteins and PAGE for DNA analysis, separate molecules based on sieving behavior through a polymer gel while the separation mechanism for CZE is electrophoretic migration in free solution. Gel-free electrophoretic separations are possible with CE due to the small scale of the technique compared to slab gel electrophoresis. The reduced scale of CE results in lower electrophoretic currents and higher surface-to-volume ratios. The small electrophoretic current in CE generates relatively low joule heating, and the heat that is produced is dissipated more effectively. Capillary separations are much more rapid than slab gel separations, in part because much higher potential fields can be applied (hundreds of volts per centimeter) due to reduced electrophoretic currents and increased heat dissipation.

For slab gel electrophoresis, the gel is required to dissipate heat and reduce zone broadening due to convective flow in addition to providing a sieving medium. Like HPLC, slab gel electrophoresis is superior to CE for preparative work. Capillary electrophoresis, however, is better suited to volume-limited samples. In addition, slab gels are ideally suited for parallel separations and two-dimensional separations. Capillary array electrophoresis has been developed for parallel separations,[4,5] and CE has been used for two-dimensional separations,[8] but in both cases sophisticated instrumentation had to be developed to realize the advantages of these separation strategies with CE.

6.2 Capillary Electrophoresis Basics

6.2.1 Capillary Zone Electrophoresis

6.2.1.1 Fundamentals

Capillary zone electrophoresis separations are based on differences in electrophoretic migration of ionic species in solution. For practical reasons, which will be explained later, a positive potential is normally applied at the injection end of the capillary, and the opposite end of the capillary is held at a relatively negative potential. Figure 6.1 illustrates a basic CZE instrument and separations with and without fluid flow.

Consider a sample zone at the injection end of a capillary column containing a mixture of cationic, anionic, and neutral compounds when a separation potential is applied (Figure 6.1b). In the absence of fluid flow, cationic compounds will migrate down the column toward the detector. Anionic compounds will immediately exit the column at the injection end. Neutral compounds (not shown) will be unaffected by the separation potential. The following relation describes electrophoretic migration of ionic species in free solution:

$$v_{ep} = u_{ep}E \tag{6.1}$$

where
v_{ep} is the electrophoretic velocity of a charged compound
u_{ep} is the electrophoretic mobility
E is the applied field strength (V/cm)

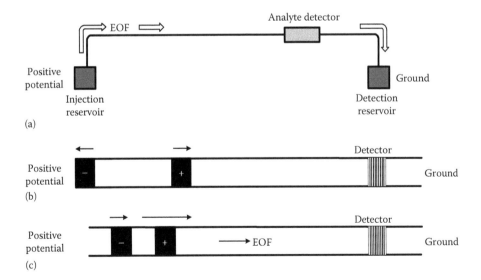

FIGURE 6.1 (a) Capillary electrophoresis instrument. A potential is applied through Pt electrodes (not shown) in the injection and detection reservoirs. (b) Migration of anions and cations in the absence of EOF (fluid flow). (c) Migration of anions and cations in the presence of strong EOF.

The electrophoretic mobility, u_{ep} is defined as

$$u_{ep} = \frac{q}{6\pi\eta r} \tag{6.2}$$

where

  q is the charge of the compound
  η is the viscosity of the solution
  r is the compound's hydrodynamic radius

In the absence of fluid flow, only cationic species can be separated with the experimental setup illustrated in Figure 6.1a. Anionic species could be separated by reversing the polarity of the applied potential.

In practice, CZE experiments typically include bulk fluid flow in the capillary due to electroosmosis.[9] Electroosmotic flow (EOF) is generated at the capillary surface in the presence of an applied potential by electrophoretic migration of solvated ions near the capillary surface. If the capillary surface includes charged functional groups (e.g., Si–O$^-$ for fused silica), a double-layer structure is formed in solution at the surface (typically nanometer in scale), which contains an excess of ions opposite in charge to the bound surface charge on the capillary inner wall. In the presence of an applied potential, these solvated counter ions in the diffuse part of the double layer will migrate toward one electrode, generating a bulk fluid flow. In effect, the entire capillary inner surface acts as a fluid pump for CE. For the experimental arrangement shown in Figure 6.1 with a fused-silica capillary filled with an aqueous solution near neutral pH, EOF is in the direction from the injection end of the capillary (positive polarity) to the detection end of the capillary (negative polarity) and is proportional to the applied potential:

$$v_{eof} = u_{eof} E \tag{6.3}$$

where

  v_{eof} is the EOF velocity
  u_{eof} is the electroosmotic mobility
  E is the applied field strength

The electroosmotic mobility is described by

$$u_{eof} = \frac{\varepsilon\zeta}{4\pi\eta} \tag{6.4}$$

The structure of the double layer defines the zeta potential, ζ and ε is the dielectric constant of the buffer filling the capillary. Electroosmosis is typically greater in magnitude than electrophoretic migration of charged species so cationic and anionic compounds will have a net migration toward the detection end of the capillary (Figure 6.1c). This is a critical point because strong EOF allows the simultaneous separation of cationic and anionic species. Neutral molecules (not shown) migrate at the EOF rate and are not separated from each other by CZE. Other CE techniques for separations of neutrals will be discussed later in this chapter. The net electrophoretic migration of ionic species in the presence of EOF is described by

$$v_{net} = u_{net} E = (u_{ep} + u_{eof})E \tag{6.5}$$

where

  v_{net} is the net velocity of a compound due to electrophoresis and EOF
  u_{net} is the net electrophoretic mobility

The resolving ability of CE is the primary reason for the technique's rapid development and widespread application. The resolution, R, for two compounds (1 and 2) by CE is

$$R = \frac{0.177(u_{ep,1} - u_{ep,2})V^{1/2}}{\sqrt{(u_{avg} + u_{eof})D}}$$ (6.6)

where
  u_{avg} is the average electrophoretic mobility of the two compounds
  D is the diffusion coefficient of the compounds
  V is the applied potential (volts)

High separation efficiency is the primary reason that CE provides good resolution compared to other separation techniques. The number of theoretical plates for a CZE separation is given by:

$$N = \frac{(u_{ep} + u_{eof})V}{2D}$$ (6.7)

This equation shows that, ideally, CZE peaks are only broadened by axial diffusion. There is no stationary phase in a CZE separation, and, therefore, no mass transfer terms or particle packing terms are in Equation 6.7. Furthermore, EOF has a very flat, plug-shaped flow profile, so resistance to mass transfer in the mobile phase (running buffer) does not contribute to peak broadening. Separations with 10^5 theoretical plates are common and plate counts over 10^6 have been reported. Other factors can degrade separations for CE, however. Unwanted adsorption to the capillary surface is frequently encountered. Temperature changes due to excessive joule heating can cause peak broadening. Sample injection and detection can degrade separation efficiencies in some cases. Zone broadening for CE has been reviewed.[10,11]

6.2.1.2 Practical Considerations

Basic CE instruments are straightforward to construct in the laboratory, and much of the research in this field has relied on laboratory-constructed instrumentation. Commercial instrumentation for CE is widely available, however, and these instruments offer many advantages for new users of CE and experienced researchers who also use laboratory-constructed instruments. The most common instrument is a single-capillary device with a UV/VIS absorbance detector. Laser-induced fluorescence (LIF) detectors, electrochemical detectors, and instruments designed to interface with mass spectrometers are also available. Most complete CE systems include autoinjectors (pressure and electrokinetic) and capillary thermostats. Capillary array instruments are also available for applications requiring high throughput.

Most CE experiments are performed in bare fused-silica capillaries filled with buffered, aqueous solutions (running buffer) near neutral pH. Applied potentials typically range from 10 to 30 kV, and Pt electrodes are commonly used in the two buffer reservoirs for this purpose. One of the main advantages of CE is that selectivity can be changed substantially by simply altering the separation buffer. The simplest and most effective means to control selectivity is to change the running buffer pH to alter the net charge of analytes. The running buffer pH also influences EOF; as seen in Equation 6.6, this can have subtle to dramatic effects on resolution. Altering the buffer composition and ionic strength can also affect separation selectivity and EOF, but the effects of these changes are subtle and not as easy to predict as with a pH change. As described in following sections, compounds can be added to the buffer to alter the separation mechanism. Water-miscible organic solvents are often added to CE buffers, and nonaqueous CE has been studied extensively.[12]

Sample injections typically are performed by placing the injection end of the capillary into the sample container and applying pressure or an electrical potential. Both methods can be automated, and the precision for pressure injection can be as much as a factor of 2 better than for electrokinetic injection.[13,14] Electrokinetic injection suffers from injection bias for charged species due to differences in electrophoretic mobilities between sample components. Theoretical descriptions of these injection techniques, which include equations for calculating injection volumes, are available in the literature.[14] Sample stacking describes a family of related methods used to preconcentrate samples electrophoretically in the capillary column at the start of a CE separation. A number of variations of this technique have been developed to achieve sample preconcentration factors ranging from 10 to 1000 for charged analytes, and related methods have been developed to preconcentrate neutral analytes.[15,16] Preconcentration methods using solid phase supports also have been developed for CE.[16] Preconcentration is particularly important for CE methods due to the difficulty in detecting analytes at low concentrations with this separation method.

A typical CE capillary is 15–100 cm in length and has an ID from 25 to 75 μm. Capillaries made from materials other than fused silica are rarely used. One reason for this is the superior properties of fused-silica capillaries for on-column optical detection. The inner surface of the capillary is commonly modified, however. One goal of capillary surface modification is to reduce band broadening and sample loss due to adsorption of analytes to the capillary surface, which can be especially problematic for protein analysis. A second goal is to suppress EOF. Because EOF is sensitive to the solution composition and the surface chemistry at the capillary surface, it can be irreproducible or unstable, leading to poor analytical reproducibility. Coating the capillary surface can reduce these problems. Covalently bound coatings, adsorbed coatings, and separation buffer additives are used to modify the capillary surface.[17–20]

6.2.2 Biomedically Significant Variations on the Capillary Electrophoresis Theme

The facile addition of a wide variety of reagents to the CE running buffer to influence migration behavior and enhance separations is a major advantage of the technique. Among the additives that have been used are chelating agents such as crown ethers, surfactants above and below the critical micelle concentration (CMC), macrocyclic reagents such as cyclodextrins, antibiotics, and calixarenes, and sieving media such as soluble polymers.[17,21,22] In some cases, these reagents have served sufficiently unique and valuable purposes that specialized variants of the CE have been dubbed. We will cover the basic principles of a few of those variations on the CE theme.

A disadvantage of the conventional CZE technique is that neutral species migrate with EOF and co-elute at or very near the void time of the system. Given the preponderance of neutral compounds of biological and medical significance, this limitation is significant. Neutral compounds can be separated, however, if they acquire different effective electrophoretic mobilities due to differential association with charged running buffer additives. The most commonly used approach involves the addition of surfactant at concentrations above its CMC to form charged aggregates of surfactant molecules (micelles).

This technique, micellar electrokinetic capillary chromatography (MEKC), was first introduced by Terabe and co-workers.[23] Instrumental and operational aspects of MEKC are virtually indistinguishable from CZE; however, MEKC also shares many of the features of HPLC. The running buffer assumes the role of the mobile phase and is transported at the EOF rate, while the micellar phase constitutes a secondary (albeit not stationary) phase that migrates at a different velocity (usually slower than EOF as negatively charged micelles attempt to migrate in opposition to EOF). The technique differs from HPLC in that movement of the secondary phase creates a distinct elution window, bound by the void time of the capillary (t_0) and the effective migration time of a micelle (t_{mic}), within which neutral species elute. In a typical experiment the ratio of t_0 to t_{mic} might take a value of 0.3. Efficiencies are generally not as high as in CZE because resistance to mass transfer between the running buffer and micellar

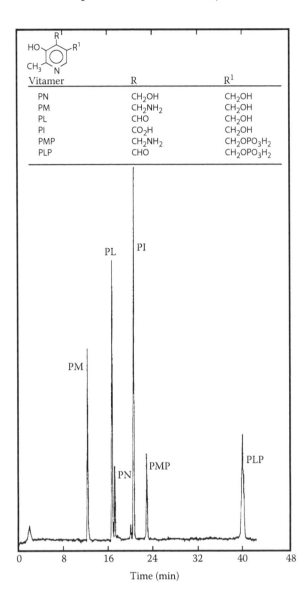

FIGURE 6.2 Separation of vitamin B6 and its metabolites by MEKC using a running buffer containing 0.05 M sodium dodecyl sulfate.

phases is involved.[23,24] Efficiencies are much higher in MEKC than in HPLC, however. As with HPLC, resolution in MEKC depends on efficiency, selectivity, and system retention as seen in Equation 6.8:

$$R = \frac{\sqrt{N}}{4} \cdot \frac{\alpha-1}{\alpha} \cdot \frac{k_2'}{1+k_2'} \cdot \frac{1-(t_0/t_{mic})}{1+(t_0/t_{mic})k_1'} \tag{6.8}$$

where
k_1' and k_2' are the capacity factors of the two analytes
α is the selectivity factor defined as k_2'/k_1'

A unique aspect of having micelles present in the running buffer is that biomedical samples containing charged and neutral species can be efficiently separated. Figure 6.2 is a separation of vitamin B6 (pyridoxine) and several of its metabolites using MEKC (sodium dodecyl sulfate as the surfactant) with LIF detection.[25] This group of metabolites contains both acidic and basic functionalities, and, as such, charged and neutral species are present at any pH.

There are two significant limitations of the MEKC technique. First, hydrophobic solutes associate very strongly with the micellar phase and tend to bunch up near t_{mic}. A ramification of the elution window is that R (see Equation 6.8) tends to show an optimum at k' values <5.[23] The use of mixed aqueous-organic running buffers expands the elution window and reduces the capacity factors of hydrophobic solutes.[26] Unfortunately, organic solvents at greater than about 25% v/v seriously inhibit micelle formation. A second limitation of MEKC is that control over selectivity is rather limited. A good number of surfactants are available, but many are not applicable to the MEKC technique, and when combining different types of surfactants, mixed micelles are formed with unpredictable selectivity effects.

These limitations have led to the use of other running buffer additives to address the separation of neutral solutes. The cyclodextrins (CD) are particularly useful reagents for this purpose. Native CDs are neutral, cylindrically shaped macrocyclic sugar molecules that possess a hydrophobic cavity and a hydrophilic exterior.[27] The size of the cavity depends on the number of sugar units in the structure ($\alpha = 6$, $\beta = 7$, and $\gamma = 8$ are most common). Inclusion complex formation between a solute and the cavity of the CD is very selective, and, given that native CDs can be derivatized with a wide variety of neutral and ionizable functional groups, the possibilities to tune selectivity are extensive.

CD-modified MEKC has been shown to be useful for separating hydrophobic compounds.[28] Alternately, systems comprising strictly CDs can be created with a technique referred to as cyclodextrin distribution capillary electrochromatography (CDCE).[29,30] With CDCE, running buffer-CD "cocktails" containing combinations of charged and neutral CDs are created that exhibit the correct selectivity for a given application. Figure 6.3 shows the process of a solute distributing between CD phases and a typical CDCE separation showing high efficiency and selectivity.

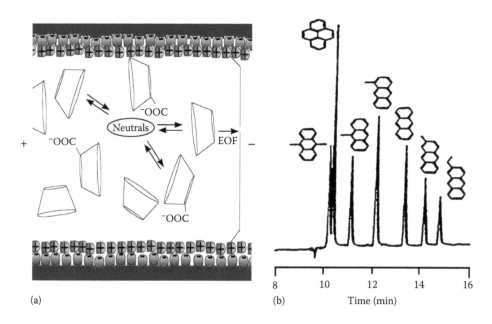

(a)   (b)   Time (min)

FIGURE 6.3 (a) Depiction of the CDCE process. The neutral CDs migrate with EOF and the negative CDs migrate more slowly toward the cathode. Neutral compounds migrate at an intermediate rate that depends on their distribution between the CDs. (b) Separation of alkyl anthracene compounds using a running buffer with β-CD and carboxymethyl-β-CD.

Cyclodextrins are also used as a secondary phase to carry out chiral CE separations. Because cyclodextrins are enantiomeric molecules, they can differentially bind pairs of small-molecule enantiomers such as amino acids or small molecules of pharmaceutical importance. This approach for chiral separations has been reviewed extensively.[21,31] A broad range of additional chiral molecules have been used to form secondary phases for chiral CE separations. These include proteins, crown ethers, linear polysaccharides, macrocyclic antibiotics, and chiral surfactants.[21,31]

Analytical methodologies involving DNA and proteins are widely used in the life sciences, and a comparison of slab gel electrophoresis and CE approaches to DNA analysis was made earlier in this chapter. DNA fragments possess a charge and, hence, an electrophoretic mobility. Unfortunately, differences in migration rates for differently sized fragments are extremely small because they possess similar charge-to-mass ratios.[32,33] In order to separate DNA fragments, discrimination must be based on differences in size and is accomplished using sieving media.

One approach is to add a soluble polymer such as methylcellulose to the running buffer at concentrations above the entanglement threshold of the polymer. This creates a dynamic mesh in the capillary with a characteristic mesh size that can be varied by adjusting polymer concentration or molecular weight.[34] In practice, the size-selective capillary electrophoresis (SSCE) technique usually employs a surface-modified capillary that does not have appreciable EOF. Detection of the negatively charged DNA fragments, in order of increasing base pair number, is accomplished at the anodic side of the capillary. Because SSCE separations involve large biopolymers migrating through very dense media, axial diffusion is extremely slow and efficiencies numbering millions of theoretical plates are routinely achieved.[34] Figure 6.4a illustrates high efficiency in a temporal study of the digestion of a DNA sample,[35] and Figure 6.4b illustrates the ability to study biomedically significant protein–DNA interactions using

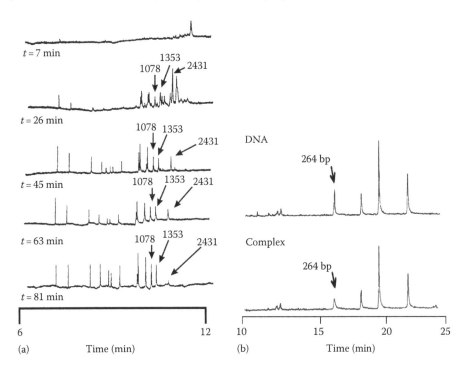

FIGURE 6.4 (a) The use of SSCE for a temporal study of the digestion of φX-174 DNA with *HaeIII* restriction enzyme. The intermediate fragment at 2431 base pairs is digesting to the 1078 and 1353 fragments. On-column labeling with EB is employed. (b) The interaction of digested pBKH26 plasmid DNA with *trp* repressor protein. LIF detection is employed: top, prior to exposure of the digested plasmid to *trp* repressor protein and, bottom, after post-column EB labeling within a sheath flow cell.

this technique.[36] In both instances, fluorescence labeling protocols and photonics-based detection played a critical role (see below). Moreover, the development of SSCE separations with polymer solutions paved the way for the practical development of large capillary array electrophoresis instruments and their application to sequencing the human genome.[3–5,22]

6.2.3 Additional Capillary Electrophoresis Separation Modes

During the active development of CE in the 1980s, most separations were based on CZE or on MEKC. Over the next decade, a number of additional separation modes were developed, and several of these have found widespread application (e.g., see preceding discussion). All of the CE-based separation methods currently being developed and applied cannot be discussed adequately in a single chapter; the reader is directed to detailed reviews of these CE-based separation methods. Isotachophoresis and isoelectric focusing have been used with CE technology.[37,38] Capillary electrochromatography is similar to reverse-phase HPLC, except that electrophoretic migration and EOF are used to propel analytes through a packed capillary chromatographic column.[39,40]

6.3 Applications of Photonics to Capillary Electrophoresis

The most prominent role played by photonics in CE is detection of separated analytes. Many of the advantages offered by CE as a separation technique are a result of its small scale, which is a significant limitation for detection of analyte bands. The most common detection method used for liquid-phase separation methods is UV/VIS absorption, and it best illustrates the detection challenges for CE. Beer's law describes absorbance detection, $A = \varepsilon bc$. Here A is the absorbance, ε is the molar absorptivity, b is the detection cell pathlength, and c is the analyte concentration.

The pathlength for a standard cuvette used for absorption measurements is 1 cm. Optical detection for CE is most often carried out on-column using the fused-silica capillary as an optical cell. The pathlength for a 50 μm ID capillary is, therefore, only about 50 μm. An absorbance measurement of a compound in a capillary will produce an absorbance that is only 5×10^{-3} that of the absorbance measured in a 1 cm cuvette. A 5 mm pathlength cell for an HPLC detection system will provide an absorbance reading 100× that for a typical CE capillary. Due to the short pathlength provided by a typical CE column and extremely small sample volumes, concentration detection limits are a critical issue when considering detection methods for CE.

6.3.1 Detection of Native Analytes

Ideally, all separated components in a CE separation would be detected sensitively and selectively in their native chemical form by a single detector. Of course, this ideal has not been realized in practice, and a wide range of detection strategies are used for CE separations. Although many of these detection methods require chemical modification of an analyte in order to detect it sensitively, a number of detection methods are able to detect compounds in their native state. Detection of an analyte in its native form is preferred if sufficient sensitivity and selectivity for the application at hand can be achieved. Native detection simplifies the overall analytical method and typically results in better measurement precision and accuracy by reducing the total number of steps required for analysis.

6.3.1.1 UV/VIS Absorbance

Despite the aforementioned sensitivity limitations due to short optical pathlengths, the most common detection method used for commercial and laboratory-constructed CE instruments is UV/VIS absorbance. The primary reasons for the popularity of UV/VIS absorbance detection are that it is a relatively general detection technique and can be used to detect a broad range of molecules in their native state with moderate sensitivity and selectivity. Single-wavelength UV/VIS absorbance detectors and

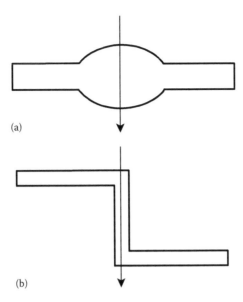

(a)

(b)

FIGURE 6.5 (a) Bubble capillary to increase the optical pathlength through the capillary column (only the capillary bore is shown). (b) Z cell to increase the detection pathlength through the capillary. The arrows indicate the light path from the source.

diode-array based instruments capable of collecting spectra are commercially available. It is possible to use detection wavelengths near 200 nm when using aqueous solution with inorganic buffers, which do not absorb at these wavelengths. Peptides and proteins can be detected at these wavelengths regardless of sequence. Detection selectivity can be obtained by adjusting the detection wavelength using a variable, single- or dual-wavelength absorbance detector. Absorbance spectra can be used to help confirm peak identity or purity if a diode array-based detector is used.

A number of approaches have been used in an attempt to overcome the pathlength limitation of UV/VIS absorbance detection for CE. Most of these methods are based on increasing the optical pathlength by changing the capillary geometry in the region where on-column detection is performed.[41] Figure 6.5 illustrates two common approaches: the Z cell and the bubble cell. These methods have been used to reduce detection limits for CE; however, there is a limit to the usefulness of this approach. As the pathlength is increased using either of the approaches shown in Figure 6.5, eventually a point will be reached where separation efficiency will be compromised due to the increased volume in the detection zone. Other interesting approaches for reducing detection limits for UV/VIS absorbance detection have been reported, such as on-column signal averaging using diode array detectors[42] and thermal lens methods.[43] These approaches, however, are not commercially available and have not been widely used.

6.3.1.2 Native Fluorescence

Laser-induced fluorescence is clearly the most sensitive detection method available for CE.[44] Single molecule detection has been demonstrated for CE.[45–47] Unfortunately, most molecules are not highly fluorescent in their native state. In cases where a molecule can be detected by native fluorescence and by UV/VIS absorbance, native fluorescence typically provides detection limits that are orders of magnitude lower.[48,49] Most proteins and some small peptides can be detected in their native state due to the fluorescence of tryptophan, tyrosine, and phenylalanine. Proteins have been detected after CE separation at low pM concentrations by native fluorescence.[50] Some nucleotides are also natively fluorescent, as well as catecholamine neurotransmitters.[51,52] NADH and NADPH are fluorescent; this property has been exploited to follow on-column enzyme reactions by CE.[53] These examples of native fluorescence all require excitation at UV wavelengths. Although NADH and NADPH can be excited effectively with

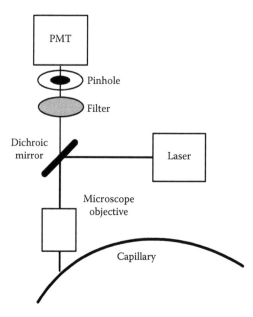

FIGURE 6.6 Schematic of an LIF detector for CE. The same microscope objective is used to focus the laser beam on the capillary and to collect emitted fluorescence for detection at the PMT (photomultiplier tube).

a modestly priced He–Cd laser at 325 nm, native fluorescence of peptides, catecholamines, and nucleotides requires excitation at wavelengths below 300 nm. At these wavelengths, special UV optics are necessary and lasers are relatively expensive. Although these technological barriers will be overcome eventually, at present they still limit the widespread use of native fluorescence of peptides, proteins, and nucleotides with CE. Some compounds of biological interest, such as green fluorescent protein and porphyrins, are fluorescent at visible wavelengths, but this is relatively rare.[54,55]

Concentration detection limits for LIF are less affected by the short optical pathlength of CE because the fluorescence signal can be increased by increasing the laser power until substantial photobleaching begins to dominate.[56] With a small CE capillary, this typically requires a beam of only a few milliwatts focused to the dimensions of the capillary bore. Figure 6.6 shows a common design for LIF detection with a 180° geometry. This optical design is essentially the same as a fluorescence microscope. Detection at 90° with separate objective lenses for focusing the laser beam and collecting fluorescence is also common. Although LIF detection is commercially available, it is less common than absorbance detection, and LIF detectors are substantially more expensive. In addition, it is often necessary to use different lasers for different applications. Most LIF detectors for CE are simple filter fluorometers. Laser-induced fluorescence detectors with CCD detection, which can rapidly collect emission spectra, have been developed, and have been applied to native fluorescence detection.[57,58] Recently, LIF detection with multiphoton excitation has been developed for CE and applied to study natively fluorescent species.[59]

6.3.1.3 Additional Detection Methods

Refractive index (RI) detection is common for HPLC but has rarely been used with CE. This technique has the advantage of being universal. Unfortunately, RI detection is less selective and less sensitive than UV/VIS absorbance detection. Furthermore, miniaturizing RI detection for CE has proven to be challenging. Recently, Bornhop and co-workers have reported a simple but effective method for performing RI detection for CE.[60,61] This technique uses interference fringes from light backscattered through the capillary bore to detect RI changes. Instrumentally simple and inexpensive, it produces detection limits close to those obtained by UV/VIS absorbance for CE. One challenge is that it is necessary to thermostat the CE capillary carefully to obtain low detection limits because the RI detector response is extremely sensitive to temperature.

Electrochemical techniques are important for detection of native analytes separated by CE. These detection methods are not optical, however, and will not be discussed in detail in this chapter. Amperometry, voltammetry, potentiometry, and conductivity detection have all been used with CE, and detailed reviews about electrochemical detection are available in the literature.[62,63]

6.3.2 Detection Involving Reactions and Indirect Methods

In many instances the photonic responses of the analytes of interest are weak or nonexistent. However, such responses can be elicited via chemical reactions between the analyte and carefully tailored chromophoric reagents. Alternately, the analytes can be made to modulate a running buffer additive's photonic response in order to measure the analyte indirectly.

6.3.2.1 Derivatization (Fluorescence Labeling) in LIF

The low detection limits and selectivity that can be obtained with LIF provide strong motivation to extend the use of this detection method beyond the relatively few compounds that exhibit modest to high fluorescence quantum efficiencies (QE). This can be accomplished by derivatizing the analytes with suitable reagents. The derivatization can involve the formation of covalent bonds between the analyte and reagent or noncovalent association between these species. The reagent may be a natural fluorophore or it may fluoresce strongly only when associated with the analyte. The timing of the derivatization process relative to the CE separation is a critical factor; preseparation, on-column, or post-separation derivatization all have positive and negative characteristics.[64] These characteristics are much the same as in HPLC but are sometimes exacerbated by the small volumes and high efficiencies inherent to CE.

In some cases, preseparation derivatization does not involve specific reagents but, rather, a transformation of the analytes to fluorescent products. For example, the antibiotic ampicillin can be degraded preseparation to a fluorescent species.[65] In most cases, however, covalent interactions between functional groups on the analyte and on the derivatization reagent are involved. Examples of reagents commonly used for CE include *o*-phthalaldehyde (OPA), dansyl-Cl, and fluorescein isothiocyanate (FITC).[64] All of these reagents react to form fluorescent products with many amines, including those found in free amino acids, proteins, and many drugs. A recent review indicates that most covalent derivatization reagents used with CE react with amine groups, although a few reports include derivatization of thiols, carboxylic acids, carbonyls, hydroxyls, and the reducing end of saccharides.[64] A general review citing reagents that are specific for carboxylic acids has been published.[66] Guttman reported the use of 8-aminopyrene-3,6,8-trisulfonate to label sugar moieties and produce low femtomole quantification levels in CE–LIF.[67]

Relatively few compounds are natively fluorescent in the near-infrared (NIR) and, therefore, derivatization to produce molecules that fluoresce in the NIR offers high sensitivity with reduced interference from other compounds in a sample. McWhorter and Soper recently reviewed the use of NIR detection in CE–LIF.[68] Using a variety of newly developed derivatization dyes many measurements of biological samples have been performed. For example, subattomole limits of detection were achieved for amino acids derivatized preseparation with pyronin succinimidyl ester.[69] Another significant advantage of the NIR–LIF approach is that inexpensive diode lasers can be used for excitation.

Certain reagents form sufficiently strong noncovalent associations with analytes such that preseparation labeling can be performed and the separation and LIF detection can be conducted without dissociation of the label–analyte complex. For example, the cationic dye DTTCI was used to label proteins prior to CE separation[70] and certain cyanine intercalation dyes are used in this manner for DNA analysis.[71] Noncovalent labeling of proteins for CE–LIF has been reviewed by Colyer.[72]

The literature is replete with other examples of preseparation labeling.[64] Nevertheless, the preseparation derivatization technique is not always the approach of choice—it can be time consuming and often produces chemical by-products that complicate the sample. It is also possible to form multiple derivatization products when more than one functional group is available for reaction on the analyte.

Swaile and Sepaniak compared native fluorescence and preseparation FITC labeling of proteins in terms of detection and of separation performance.[73] The 514 nm output of an Ar+ laser was used for excitation in the FITC case, and native fluorescence of the protein was excited via frequency doubling of the Ar+ laser output. In the case of conalbumin, which has over 100 side chain amine groups, the native fluorescence approach was less sensitive but produced a single high-efficiency peak, while the FITC labeling approach produced multiple unresolved peaks resulting from the creation of multiple products (differing labeling ratios) that spanned a range of electrophoretic mobilities.

Ultrahigh CE–LIF sensitivity is possible for analytes derivatized with strongly fluorescing reagents. For example, Dovichi and co-workers demonstrated single molecule detection for a highly fluorescent macromolecule, β-phycoerythin.[46] β-Phycoerythin has been used as a preseparation label.[74] It is important to note that derivatization is prohibitively slow in ultra-dilute solutions, and often the reported ultrahigh sensitivity involves dilution of samples that are derivatized at much higher concentrations. Nevertheless, it is still possible for derivatization at high concentration, when coupled with ultrahigh sensitivity, to provide unique analytical capabilities. For instance, Yeung and co-workers performed "single-molecule electrophoresis" to measure antibody bound and unbound β-phycoerythrin-digoxigenin.[74] The unique single-molecule electrophoresis technique is a direct product of advances in photonic detection. This technique truly takes advantage of the ability to detect single molecules for an analysis application. A relatively large number of migrating molecules are imaged individually and their mobilities measured simultaneously. Differences in the mobilities of the bound and unbound single molecules facilitated determination of the ratio of these species in the digoxigenin assay.[74]

On-column derivatization is a dynamic labeling process wherein a reagent is added to the running buffer that associates reversibly with analyte migrating in the capillary. Because the mobilities of the labeled and unlabeled analyte will usually differ, fast association–dissociation exchange is required to maintain efficiency. Thus, association constants generally are relatively modest in magnitude. It is essential that the spectral properties of the running buffer reagents be altered upon association. Swaile and Sepaniak investigated this mode of CE–LIF to measure metals in blood serum.[75] The reagent employed at low mM concentrations, 8-hydroxy-quinoline-5-sulfonic acid, is a nonfluorescent, bidentate ligand that forms fluorescent complexes with many metals.[76] Excitation of the complexes is conveniently supplied with the 325 nm output of an He–Cd laser. The same authors demonstrated the on-column dynamic labeling of proteins using hydrophobic probes such as 1-anilinonaohthalene-8-sulfonate.[73] This compound intercalates into the hydrophobic regions of proteins with association constants in the 10^{-4}–10^{-6} range and experiences a considerable increase in fluorescence QE upon binding. Limits of detection using He–Cd (325 nm) excitation were not as low as with the preseparation labeling approach using FITC, partly because of an appreciable fluorescence background; however, the aforementioned multiple-labeling problem was not encountered.

The most significant use of on-column labeling involves the intercalation of dyes such as ethidium bromide (EB) or newer classes of monomeric and dimeric cyanine dyes into the structure of double-stranded DNA.[71,77–79] The combination of SSCE and on-column labeling provides a powerful tool for DNA analysis. The cyanine dyes generally outperform the more traditionally used EB in terms of sensitivity. However, EB is extremely reliable and always yields high separation efficiency. Upon intercalation, EB experiences roughly a 20-fold increase in fluorescence QE (less than is observed with the cyanine dyes) and also a bathochromic shift in the lowest energy absorption band convenient for excitation using the 543 nm output of an He–Ne "greenie" laser. Using low μM concentrations of EB in the running buffer, it is relatively easy to achieve subattomole limits of detection for injections of modest-sized DNA fragments.[80] The separation shown in Figure 6.4a was obtained using SSCE–LIF with a running buffer containing 2.5 μM EB.

Several types of reactors have been used for post-separation derivatization in CE–LIF; one of the most successful approaches involves sheath flow cells.[36,81,82] In this approach, a sheathing capillary or tube surrounds the end of the separation capillary and a coaxial flow is maintained. The sheathing flow serves to focus the effluent from the capillary hydrodynamically to minimize post-capillary band dispersion. It

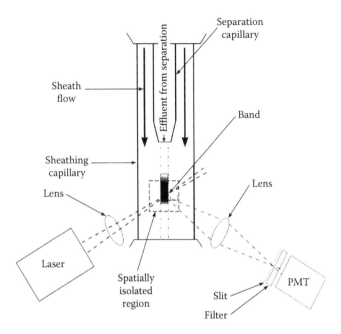

FIGURE 6.7 Depiction of the sheath flow cell used for the experiment shown in Figure 6.4b. The sheathing fluid contained 2.5 μM EB.

also has photonics-related advantages, such as reduced background due to Rayleigh scattering from the capillary (as compared to on-column detection). When used as a post-separation derivatization reactor, the reagents involved in the reaction are added to the sheathing fluid. To minimize post-separation band dispersion and maximize signal levels, it is critical that the derivatization reaction is rapid. The experiment shown in Figure 6.4b was performed using a sheath flow cell such as that depicted in Figure 6.7.[36]

Discerning the specifics of protein–DNA interactions is very important in genomic–proteomic studies. Unfortunately, preseparation labeling is problematic when dealing with biopolymers (see above). Similarly, on-column labeling with an intercalator can interfere with interactions between the biopolymers. *Try* repressor protein is responsible for the regulation of L-trytophan in *Escherichia coli*. When the amino acid concentration is low, *trp* operon is expressed. The separation in Figure 6.4b demonstrates that the correct (operand-containing) DNA fragment in a digested plasmid can be identified via SSCE–LIF. In this case EB in the sheathing fluid is used to label the separated DNA fragments as they exit the capillary. When EB is used in the normal manner (on-column labeling) in the running buffer, the protein–DNA interaction is suppressed (not shown).

6.3.2.2 Indirect Detection

Indirect detection involves the addition of a background electrolyte (BE) to the running buffer to create a relatively large optical background. The technique relies on the displacement of the BE from analyte bands by various mechanisms; the most efficient mechanism being charge displacement. A vacancy zone of BE within the analyte band results in a negative response peak as the band passes the point of detection. An obvious advantage of this technique is that detected analytes need not exhibit the measured optical property. A broad range of analytes have been detected using indirect absorbance and fluorescence, and many of these are of biological significance.[83] Typical BEs include creatine and chromate for indirect absorbance detection, and salicylate and quinine sulfate for indirect LIF.

Unfortunately, several problems are associated with indirect detection. The large BE background signal can be noisy, and baseline disturbances due to nonanalyte displacement of the BE can occur. The addition of a fairly large concentration of BE can also result in distorted (fronted or tailed) peaks due to field inhomogeneity in the analyte band.[84] This problem is exacerbated when the mobilities of the BE and analyte differ greatly. The linear dynamic range (dynamic reserve) for indirect detection is determined by the ratio of the background signal to the noise in that signal and can be small.

The inherent instability of laser sources translates into background fluctuations and results in far less sensitivity than with direct LIF. In early work in this area, Yeung and Kuhr achieved 10^{-7} M limits of detection for amino acids, but this required them to go to some length to reduce noise from the laser source.[85] More generally, the limits of detection for indirect LIF detection are in the 10^{-5}–10^{-6} M range. This is about the same as for indirect absorbance detection where conventional light sources are employed. These sources exhibit better stability than laser sources.[83] Newer diode lasers have been reported to provide detection limits similar to those reported previously by Kuhr and Yeung due to their improved stability.[86] A technique that is somewhat similar to indirect fluorescence involves quenching the background emission of a phosphorescent running buffer system by analytes.[87] Limits of detection in the 10^{-7}–10^{-8} M range were achieved with this technique.

6.3.2.3 Chemiluminescence Detection

Chemiluminescence (CL) is an increasingly common detection method for CE and has been reviewed by several authors.[88–90] Chemiluminescence involves the excitation of an emitting species via a chemical reaction and can be classified as a direct or as a sensitized detection technique. In the direct case the reaction leaves the emitting analyte species in an excited state. In sensitized CL the reaction generates an excited state species that transfers its energy to a fluorescent analyte. An example of the latter is the peroxyoxalate system.[88–90] The obvious advantage of CL is that a light source is not needed, and the background is extremely low. However, a major challenge in implementing CL detection is executing the necessary reactions without degrading the separation. The efficiency of CL depends on the local chemical environment; hence, running buffer conditions such as pH are important.

A few basic configurations are used to implement CL detection in CE at the exit of the separation capillary. In many cases a coaxial design is used in which the separation capillary is slipped through a tee and also through a reaction capillary with an ID greater than the OD of the separation capillary.[82,88–90] The CL reagents flow in the reaction capillary and convectively mix with the effluent at the end of the CE capillary. Convectional mixing reduces problems with slow mixing kinetics but tends to degrade separation efficiency to values of 10^4 theoretical plates or less. In one example, Ruberto and Grayeski employed a system wherein acridinium ester is oxidized by hydrogen peroxide to an excited state derivative of acridine.[91] This system is amenable to analytes tagged with an acridinium moiety or those that affect peroxide concentration.

A very simple approach employed by Zare and co-workers for CL detection that involves placing the reagents in a relatively large reservoir at the end of the CE capillary has been used with luminol CL and firefly luciferase bioluminescence systems.[92] Limits of detection were 2×10^{-8} M for luminol, but separation efficiencies were still limited to less than 2×10^4 theoretical plates with this approach. This approach would be problematic with sensitized CL because the background level would increase over time as fluorescent species collect in the reservoir.

Dovichi and co-workers utilized a coaxial approach in a sheath flow cell to mix CL reagents contained in the sheathing fluid with CE effluent.[93] Since mixing is based on diffusion, sensitivity can be reduced due to slow mixing kinetics. The authors demonstrated that signals increased moving away from the end of the capillary up to a distance of about 4 mm and then diminished sharply. Absolute limits of detection in the subfemtomole level were quoted for the isoluminol thiocarbamyl derivative of valine. More importantly, the reported separation efficiencies were approximately 10^5 theoretical plates.

6.3.3 Information-Rich Photonic Detection

Despite the qualitative analysis advantages afforded by the excellent resolving power of CE, keen interest in mating electrophoretic separations with information-rich (sometimes referred to as "hyphenated") detection techniques remains. Information-rich techniques provide unambiguous analyte identification, structural elucidation, and high selectivity for those cases where adequate resolution is not achieved. In addition, problems associated with poor EOF reproducibility that have inhibited widespread acceptance of CE by the research community are mitigated, to a degree, when one can track eluted analytes with certainty based on distinctive spectra. Nuclear magnetic resonance (NMR) spectrometry provides unmatched structural information and has been employed for detection in capillaries and in CE using microcoils directly surrounding the measurement capillary.[94] Unfortunately, the inherent insensitivity of the technique makes its implementation in CE detection very challenging.

Conversely, significant progress has been made in hyphenating mass spectrometry (MS) with CE.[95,96] Mass spectrometry has been interfaced with CE primarily using electrospray ionization (ESI). Interfacing CE to ESI–MS also poses some challenges. A compromise must be made between a buffer solution ideal for the CE separation and one optimal for ESI. The electrical interface between the CE capillary and the ESI capillary has proven to be a significant challenge. The coupling of CE to MS has been successful in that amol mass detection limits have been obtained for many analytes, and mass spectrometry can provide unambiguous identification of an analyte peak.

Although MS has been used with CE rather extensively, the expense and complications associated with CE–MS provide motivation to develop complementary photonic approaches to performing information-rich detection in CE. Fourier transform infrared (FTIR) spectrometry has been employed in conjunction with separations.[97] However, complications arise from short optical pathlengths and the absorption of IR radiation by running buffers and capillaries when FTIR is employed with CE. One fluorescence-based technique used in CE is fluorescence line narrowing spectrometry (FLNS). FLNS is a very low-temperature spectral technique that does not exhibit inhomogeneous broadening contributions to vibronic bands. Thus, distinctive, sharp line spectra are obtained. FLNS detection has been employed on-line in CE,[98] an approach that involves jacketing a portion of the CE capillary near its outlet to permit submersion in liquid helium. In operation, the CE flow is stopped and the capillary and its contents rapidly frozen prior to acquiring spectra. The obvious limitations of this approach are the stop flow aspect and the fact that it is limited to natural fluorophores.

The advantages of Raman spectroscopy, relative to FTIR, in accommodating glass sample cells and aqueous solvents are realized when the technique is applied to CE. Raman vibrational bands are distinctive and can be used to determine chemical structure and provide selectivity. Lasers operating in the visible to NIR spectral regions are generally used for excitation. Normal Raman spectroscopy suffers from poor sensitivity. Raman scattering cross sections are often 10 orders of magnitude smaller than for more efficient photonic processes such as absorbance or fluorescence. Batchelder and co-workers recently reported an efficient hyperhemispherical detector configuration that provided mid- to low-millimolar detectability in CE.[99] Morris and colleagues have made effective and impressive use of CE preconcentration (sample stacking) and zone-sharpening effects of capillary isotachophoresis to perform normal Raman detection.[100–102] In this approach, sub- to low-micromolar concentrations of analytes such as ribonucleotides, herbicides, and oxyanions are concentrated to detectable levels; distinctive spectra have been obtained, as shown in Figure 6.8.

The inherent inefficiency of normal Raman scattering has been overcome with remarkable success using resonance- and surface-enhanced techniques. Surface-enhanced Raman scattering (SERS) occurs when analytes are adsorbed onto or very near the nanofeatured surfaces of certain metals.[103–105] SERS active media range from simple silver colloidal solutions and silver island films on glass to sophisticated nanolithographically prepared planar substrates.[103–105] In some instances, extreme sensitivity reaching the single molecule level with enhancement factors greater than 10^{12} has been achieved by resonance-enhanced SERS.[106]

There have been a few reports of SERS detection in CE.[107–109] Sepaniak and co-workers have employed on-column and postseparation approaches. The on-column approach is simple and involves adding

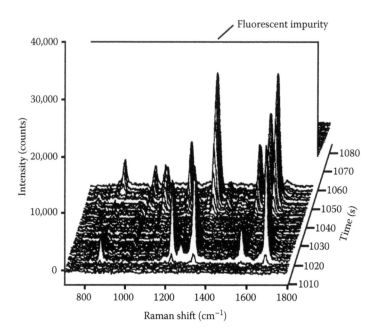

FIGURE 6.8   On-column normal Raman spectra of 1.5×10^{-5} M paraquat and diquat acquired in conjunction with a capillary isotachophoresis separation. (From Walker, P.A., III et al., *Appl. Spectrosc.*, 51, 1394, 1997. With permission.)

silver colloidal solution to the CE running buffer.[109] Spectra are acquired on the fly by positioning the microscope objective of a commercial Raman spectrometer directly above the CE capillary in a confocal optical arrangement. Figure 6.9 shows very good CE–SERS sensitivity with this approach, although a strong-to-modest resonance enhancement is also occurring with these analytes. Unfortunately, in many cases the running buffer conditions needed for detection, e.g., silver colloid and electrolytes, degrade separation performance and shorten capillary life. However, the postseparation approach allows independent control over separation and detection conditions.

In one case, the effluent of the CE capillary is efficiently transferred to a moving, planar SERS substrate via a modification of the ESI sampling technique that is used extensively in MS.[108] In this case, the substrate was a frosted microscope slide onto which silver colloid had been deposited. The separation is deposited as a track of bands on the moving substrate, which acts as a semipermanent record of the separation and is available for performing manipulations (e.g., rinsing or derivatization) without the time constraints imposed by on-column detection. Spectra were demonstrated for low- to submicromolar concentrations of pharmaceutically significant analytes.[108] Moreover, the CE separation was transferred to the substrate with only a minor loss in separation efficiency. In the future, advances in SERS substrate design will probably improve this approach to performing information-rich photonic detection in CE.

6.3.4 Optically Gated Injection

Optically gated injection represents an unusual application of optical methods to CE, which has been applied to study research problems of biomedical interest. Monnig and Jorgenson first developed optically gated injection in order to perform extremely rapid CE separations (less than 2 s).[110] To perform an optically gated injection, a sample containing fluorescent analytes is continually introduced into a

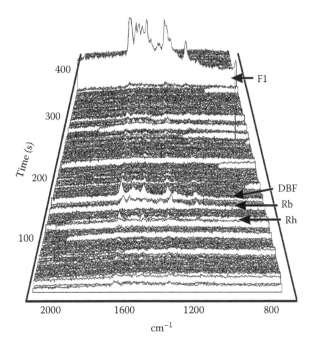

FIGURE 6.9 SERS spectra obtained for the CE separation of rhodamine 6G (Rh), riboflavin (Rb), dibenzofluorescein (DBF), and fluorescein (Fl). The running buffer contained ~0.5% by weight Ag nanoparticles. Excitation was provided by an Ar^+ laser (515 nm, 5 mW). The weak Rh spectrum corresponds to the injection of 10^{-8} M.

capillary by electrophoresis. The gating beam is a high-intensity laser beam, which almost completely photobleaches the fluorescent analytes. To perform an injection, the gating beam is briefly blocked, allowing a small plug of fluorescent analytes to pass through the gating beam area. The compounds in this plug are separated before they are detected by an LIF detector as shown in Figure 6.10. Optically gated injections have been used for a number of bioanalytical applications.[111] This technique has been used with fast CE separations as the second step of two-dimensional separation methods, as well as applied to perform injections for on-line analysis of microdialysis samples.[8,111] Moore and Jorgenson applied optically

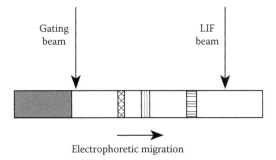

FIGURE 6.10 Optically gated injection for CE. The gating beam bleaches the fluorescent sample migrating from the left. When the beam is briefly blocked, a fluorescent sample plug is injected. The schematic shows three analyte zones that have separated but not yet reached the LIF detector.

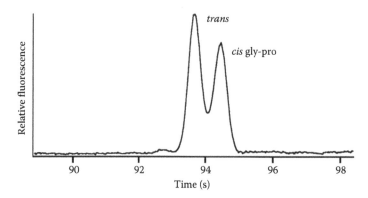

FIGURE 6.11   Separation of fluorescein-labeled *trans* and *cis* gly-pro with optically gated injection (100 ms). The separation distance was 13.7 cm, and the applied field was 508 V/cm. (From Moore, A.W., Jr. and Jorgenson, J.W., *Anal. Chem.*, 67, 3464, 1995. With permission.)

gated injections to perform rapid separations of *cis* and *trans* isomers of proline-containing peptides.[112] Figure 6.11 shows an example of a separation of *cis* and *trans* glycyl proline from this work.

6.4 Biomedical Applications

Much of the development of CE has been undertaken with biochemical applications in mind, and CE techniques have been applied to a wide range of biomedical problems. The chemical contents of single cells have been analyzed by CE, taking advantage of the technique's small-volume sampling capabilities.[6,7] Capillary electrophoresis has been applied extensively to the analysis of nucleic acids,[3–5,113] and applications to study protein conformational changes and protein folding have emerged in recent years.[114,115] Affinity CE has been developed to study the binding interactions of biological molecules with other chemical species by measuring shifts in electrophoretic mobilities when zones of interacting analytes electrophorese through each other.[116,117] Capillary electrophoresis methods have been applied to analyze and characterize enzymes and to quantify enzyme substrates.[118–120] Capillary electrophoresis is emerging as an important tool for clinical analysis.[121–123] Two specific examples of the application of CE to address biomedical problems are discussed in this section.

6.4.1 Analysis of Substance P Metabolites in Microdialysis Samples

Capillary electrophoresis was used by Lunte and co-workers to separate and detect metabolites of substance P from microdialysis samples collected from rat brains.[124] Substance P is an 11 amino acid neuropeptide, and it is metabolized in the brain by several cytosolic and membrane-bound peptidases. Microdialysis samples were collected from the rat striatum over 15 min intervals throughout the experiments. Substance P (100 μM) was perfused through the microdialysis probe for the first 6 h of the experiments, and microdialysis samples were collected for an additional 5.5 h after substance P was removed from the perfusing solution. Figure 6.12b shows an electropherogram from a microdialysis sample collected at 120 min during the perfusion of substance P. The peak labels identify the corresponding fragment sequences. The peaks were identified based on co-elution with standard samples.

This application of CE takes advantage of the technique's strengths in the areas of separation and sampling and exposes its primary weakness—detection sensitivity. Resolution of the substance P fragments as shown in Figure 6.12b was accomplished using CD-modified MEKC. A very challenging separation was accomplished by simply adding a cyclodextrin (sulfobutyl ether(IV) β-cyclodextrin) and a surfactant (sodium cholate) to a simple aqueous buffer. The microdialysis samples were collected every 15 min at a flow rate of 0.2 μL/min, resulting in 3 μL sample volumes. Fast sampling rates and low probe flow rates

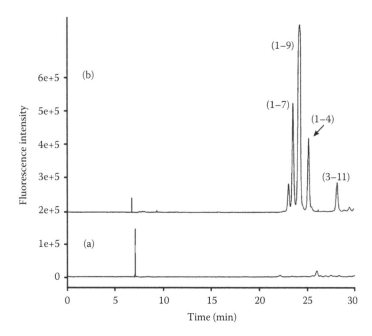

FIGURE 6.12 (a) Blank microdialysis sample prior to introduction of substance P. (b) Brain microdialysis sample 120 min after substance P introduction. (From Freed, A.L. et al., *J. Neurosci. Methods*, 109, 23, 2001. With permission.)

are desirable for microdialysis, but they are limited by the sample volume requirements of the analytical methods used to analyze the samples. In principle, hundreds of nanoliters-volume CE injections could be made from a 3 μL sample. In practice, the minimum sample volume required here was limited by the requirements for the derivatization reaction used to enhance analyte detection and by the volume required to immerse one end of the CE capillary in the sample for injection. Nonetheless, the low sample volume requirements of CE allow researchers to use lower flow rates and to collect samples over shorter time intervals compared to experiments using other analysis methods.[125,126] In addition, multiple injections can be made from a single sample to improve accuracy and reproducibility. Because CE typically uses buffered, aqueous solutions, microdialysates can be injected directly with minimal sample preparation.

Achieving adequate detection sensitivity for these experiments was challenging, however. Detection limits for the substance P fragments ranged from 2.5 to 26 nM, and several enhancement strategies were used to achieve these results. The substance P metabolites were detected by LIF, but these peptides are either nonfluorescent or weakly fluorescent in their native state. The microdialysis samples were derivatized prior to CE analysis with naphthalene-2,3-dicarboxaldehyde and CN^- to form highly fluorescent compounds (λ_{ex} = 442 nm, λ_{em} = 488 nm). A short reaction time was used (2 min) so that the reagent derivatized the amine groups on lysine side chains but did not react extensively with terminal amine groups. This resulted in less interference from other compounds in the dialysate, but it also limited the substance P metabolites detected to those fragments containing the lysine at position 3. In addition, sample stacking by injection of a plug of water preceding the analyte plug was used to lower detection limits. Finally, it was found that the cyclodextrin and sodium cholate added to the buffer enhanced the fluorescence of the labeled analytes by a factor of 2–3.

6.4.2 Capillary Electrophoretic Enzyme Inhibition Assays

Whisnant and co-workers have developed an on-column CE method for studying enzyme inhibition.[127,128] Figure 6.13 illustrates the basic technique. The capillary is filled with a substrate for the enzyme under

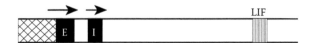

FIGURE 6.13 CEEI assay. The enzyme–substrate zone (E) migrates faster than the inhibitor zone (I) and will overtake it in the capillary later in the experiment. The hashed region behind the enzyme–substrate zone is product formed by the enzyme-catalyzed reaction, which will be detected later by LIF.

study. A zone of inhibitor is first injected into the capillary and an electrophoretic potential is applied for a few seconds. Then a zone of enzyme is injected into the capillary and an electrophoretic potential is applied again. A high concentration of substrate is used to ensure that the enzyme is saturated, and the enzyme zone is actually a zone of enzyme–substrate complex. Because the enzyme–substrate complex has a greater migration rate than the inhibitor zone, the two zones will merge in the capillary, and the enzyme-catalyzed reaction will be inhibited. The two zones will separate again as the experiment continues. The enzyme-catalyzed reaction rate is monitored throughout the experiment based on detection of the reaction product when it migrates past the CE detector. Saevels and co-workers have used a related approach to study the inhibition of adenosine deaminase by erythro-9-(2-hydroxyl-3-nonyl) adenine.[129] In their work the capillary was filled with inhibitor and zones of enzyme and substrate were electrophoretically mixed in the capillary.

Figure 6.14 shows a capillary electrophoretic enzyme inhibition (CEEI) electropherogram for the inhibition of alkaline phosphatase by sodium arsenate.[128] Sodium arsenate is a reversible, competitive inhibitor for this enzyme. A commercial, fluorogenic substrate for alkaline phosphatase, AttoPhos, was used to determine alkaline phosphatase activity. The concentration of fluorescent reaction product detected by LIF indicates the reaction rate for the enzyme-catalyzed reaction as the enzyme traveled down the capillary. The negative peak at 4.05 min indicates inhibition when the zone of 125 µM sodium arsenate overlaps with the zone of enzyme–substrate complex. When the inhibitor is not injected, the electropherogram appears as a flat plateau formed as the enzyme migrates from the injection end of the capillary to the LIF detector. A flat plateau indicates a constant reaction rate throughout the experiment. The enzyme concentration was 0.18 nM; only 1.9 amol of enzyme were injected.

The shape of the electropherogram in Figure 6.14 indicates that sodium arsenate is a reversible inhibitor. The enzyme returns to its original activity when the zones of enzyme–substrate complex and inhibitors separate again after mixing. Figure 6.15 shows a CEEI electropherogram for an irreversible inhibitor of alkaline phosphatase, EDTA, at 4 mM. In this case, the enzyme activity does not recover after the two zones mix, indicating irreversible inhibition. Note that the electropherogram is "reversed"

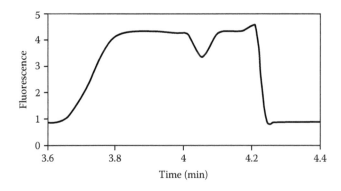

FIGURE 6.14 CEEI assay showing the reversible inhibition of alkaline phosphatase (0.18 nM) by sodium arsenate (125 µM). The sodium arsenate zone was injected first, and then the enzyme was injected after 60 s of electrophoresis. The fluorescence signal is due to product from the enzyme-catalyzed reaction of AttoPhos (0.1 mM).

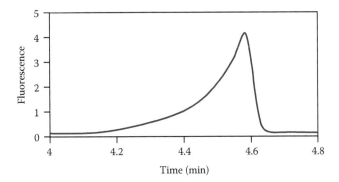

FIGURE 6.15 CEEI assay showing the irreversible inhibition of alkaline phosphatase (0.18 nM) by EDTA (4 mM). The EDTA zone was injected first, and then the enzyme was injected after 180 s of electrophoresis.

compared to what one might expect. This is a result of the enzyme–substrate complex having a greater migration rate than the reaction product.[127,130] This CEEI technique also showed that EDTA unexpectedly activated alkaline phosphatase at concentrations from 20 to 400 μM.[128]

Quantitative analysis of sodium arsenate and sodium vanadate, also a competitive reversible inhibitor of alkaline phosphatase, has been demonstrated using CEEI assays.[128] The CEEI data for a range of inhibitor concentrations was analyzed using a Michaelis–Menten-based treatment of competitive enzyme inhibition kinetics to construct a calibration curve for the inhibitors. The K_i values calculated based on this analysis were consistent with values obtained using traditional methods for studying enzyme inhibition kinetics.[128] Theophylline, a noncompetitive, reversible inhibitor was quantified using a similar approach.[127,128]

References

1. Jorgenson, J.W. and Lukacs, K.D., Zone electrophoresis in open-tubular capillaries, *Anal. Chem.*, 53, 1298, 1981.
2. Jorgenson, J.W. and Lukacs, K.D., Capillary zone electrophoresis, *Science*, 222, 266, 1983.
3. Venter, J.C. et al., The sequence of the human genome, *Science*, 291, 1304, 2001.
4. Kheterpal, I. and Mathies, R.A., Capillary array electrophoresis DNA sequencing, *Anal. Chem.*, 71, 31A, 1999.
5. Dovichi, N.J. and Zhang, J., How capillary electrophoresis sequenced the human genome, *Angew. Chem. Int. Ed.*, 39, 4463, 2000.
6. Shaner, L.M. and Brown, P.R., Single cell analysis using capillary electrophoresis, *J. Liq. Chromatogr. Relat. Technol.*, 23, 975, 2000.
7. Zabzdyr, J.L. and Lillard, S.J., New approaches to single-cell analysis by capillary electrophoresis, *Trends Anal. Chem.*, 20, 467, 2001.
8. Liu, Z. and Lee, M.L., Comprehensive two-dimensional separations using microcolumns, *J. Microcolumn Sep.*, 12, 241, 2000.
9. Rice, C.L. and Whitehead, R., Electrokinetic flow in a narrow cylindrical capillary, *J. Phys. Chem.*, 69, 4017, 1965.
10. Gas, B. and Kenndler, E., Dispersive phenomena in electromigration separation methods, *Electrophoresis*, 21, 3888, 2000.
11. Huang, X., Coleman, W.F., and Zare, R.N., Analysis of factors causing peak broadening in capillary zone electrophoresis, *J. Chromatogr.*, 480, 95, 1989.
12. Riekkola, M.-L., Jussila, M., Porras, S.P., and Valko, I.E., Non-aqueous capillary electrophoresis, *J. Chromatogr. A*, 892, 155, 2000.

13. Schaeper, J.P. and Sepaniak, M.J., Parameters affecting reproducibility in capillary electrophoresis, *Electrophoresis*, 21, 1421, 2000.

14. Rose, D.J., Jr. and Jorgenson, J.W., Characterization and automation of sample introduction methods for capillary zone electrophoresis, *Anal. Chem.*, 60, 642, 1988.

15. Quirino, J.P. and Terabe, S., Sample stacking of cationic and anionic analytes in capillary electrophoresis, *J. Chromatogr. A*, 902, 119, 2000.

16. Stroink, T., Paarlberg, E., Waterval, J.C.M., Bult, A., and Underberg, W.J.M., On-line sample preconcentration in capillary electrophoresis, focused on the determination of proteins and peptides, *Electrophoresis*, 22, 2374, 2001.

17. Corradini, D., Buffer additives other than the surfactant sodium dodecyl sulfate for protein separations by capillary electrophoresis, *J. Chromatogr. B*, 699, 221, 1997.

18. Horvath, J. and Dolnik, V., Polymer wall coatings for capillary electrophoresis, *Electrophoresis*, 22, 644, 2001.

19. Liu, C.-Y., Stationary phases for capillary electrophoresis and capillary electrochromatography, *Electrophoresis*, 22, 612, 2001.

20. Righetti, P.G., Gelfi, C., Verzola, B., and Castelletti, L., The state of the art of dynamic coatings, *Electrophoresis*, 22, 603, 2001.

21. Vespalec, R. and Bocek, P., Chiral separations in capillary electrophoresis, *Chem. Rev.*, 100, 3715, 2000.

22. Quesada, M.A. and Menchen, S., Replaceable polymers for DNA sequencing by capillary electrophoresis, in *Capillary Electrophoresis of Nucleic Acids*, Vol. I, Mitchelson, K.R. and Cheng, J., eds., Humana Press, Totowa, NJ, 2001, p. 139.

23. Terabe, S., Otsuka, K., and Ando, T., Electrokinetic chromatography with micellar solution and open-tubular capillary, *Anal. Chem.*, 57, 834, 1985.

24. Sepaniak, M.J. and Cole, R.O., Column efficiency in micellar electrokinetic capillary chromatography, *Anal. Chem.*, 59, 472, 1987.

25. Burton, D.E., Sepaniak, M.J., and Maskarinec, M.P., Analysis of B6 vitamers by micellar electrokinetic capillary chromatography with laser-excited fluorescence detection, *J. Chromatogr. Sci.*, 24, 347, 1986.

26. Balchunas, A.T. and Sepaniak, M.J., Extension of elution range in micellar electrokinetic capillary chromatography, *Anal. Chem.*, 59, 1466, 1987.

27. Culha, M., Fox, S., and Sepaniak, M., Selectivity in capillary electrochromatography using native and single isomer anionic cyclodextrin reagents, *Anal. Chem.*, 72, 88, 2000.

28. Copper, C.L. and Sepaniak, M.J., Cyclodextrin-modified micellar electrokinetic capillary chromatography separations of benzopyrene isomers: Correlation with computationally derived host–guest energies, *Anal. Chem.*, 66, 147, 1994.

29. Lurie, I.S., Klein, R.F.X., Dal Cason, T.A., LeBelle, M.J., Brenneisen, R., and Weinberger, R.E., Chiral resolution of cationic drugs of forensic interest by capillary electrophoresis with mixtures of neutral and anionic cyclodextrins, *Anal. Chem.*, 66, 4019, 1994.

30. Sepaniak, M.J., Copper, C.L., Whitaker, K.W., and Anigbogu, V.C., Evaluation of a dual-cyclodextrin phase variant of capillary electrokinetic chromatography for separations of nonionizable solutes, *Anal. Chem.*, 67, 2037, 1995.

31. Rizzi, A., Fundamental aspects of chiral separations by capillary electrophoresis, *Electrophoresis*, 22, 3079, 2001.

32. Dolnik, V. and Novotny, M., Capillary electrophoresis of DNA fragments in entangled polymer solutions: A study of separation variables, *J. Microcolumn Sep.*, 4, 515, 1993.

33. Grossman, P.D. and Soane, D.S., Experimental and theoretical studies of DNA separations by capillary electrophoresis in entangled polymer solutions, *Biopolymers*, 31, 1221, 1991.

34. Clark, B.K., Nickles, C.L., Morton, K.C., Kovac, J., and Sepaniak, M.J., Rapid separation of DNA restriction digests using size selective capillary electrophoresis with application to DNA fingerprinting, *J. Microcolumn Sep.*, 6, 503, 1994.

35. Stebbins, M.A., Schar, C.R., Peterson, C.B., and Sepaniak, M.J., Temporal analysis of DNA restriction digests by capillary electrophoresis, *J. Chromatogr. B*, 697, 181, 1997.

36. Nirode, W.F., Staller, T.D., Cole, R.O., and Sepaniak, M.J., Evaluation of a sheath flow cuvette for postcolumn fluorescence derivatization of DNA fragments separated by capillary electrophoresis, *Anal. Chem.*, 70, 182, 1998.

37. Rodriguez-Diaz, R., Wehr, T., and Zhu, M., Capillary isoelectric focusing, *Electrophoresis*, 18, 2134, 1997.

38. Gebauer, P. and Bocek, P., Recent progress in capillary isotachophoresis, *Electrophoresis*, 21, 3898, 2000.

39. Colon, L.A., Burgos, G., Maloney, T.D., Cintron, J.M., and Rodriguez, R.L., Recent progress in capillary electrochromatography, *Electrophoresis*, 21, 3965, 2000.

40. Unger, K.K., Huber, M., Walhagen, K., Hennessy, T.P., and Hearn, M.T.W., A critical appraisal of capillary electrochromatography, *Anal. Chem.*, 74, 200A, 2002.

41. Albin, M., Grossman, P.D., and Moring, S.E., Sensitivity enhancement for capillary electrophoresis, *Anal. Chem.*, 65, 489A, 1993.

42. Culbertson, C.T. and Jorgenson, J.W., Lowering the UV absorbance detection limit and increasing the sensitivity of capillary electrophoresis using a dual linear photodiode array detector and signal averaging, *J. Microcolumn Sep.*, 11, 652, 1999.

43. Seidel, B.S. and Faubel, W., Fiber optic modified thermal lens detector system for the determination of amino acids, *J. Chromatogr. A*, 817, 223, 1998.

44. Li, T. and Kennedy, R.T., Laser-induced fluorescence detection in microcolumn separations, *Trends Anal. Chem.*, 17, 484, 1998.

45. Haab, B.B. and Mathies, R.A., Single molecule fluorescence burst detection of DNA fragments separated by capillary electrophoresis, *Anal. Chem.*, 67, 3253, 1995.

46. Chen, D.Y. and Dovichi, N.J., Single-molecule detection in capillary electrophoresis: Molecular shot noise as a fundamental limit to chemical analysis, *Anal. Chem.*, 68, 690, 1996.

47. Shortreed, M.R., Li, H., Huang, W.-H., and Yeung, E.S., High-throughput single-molecule DNA screening based on electrophoresis, *Anal. Chem.*, 72, 2879, 2000.

48. Yeung, E.S., Study of single cells by using capillary electrophoresis and native fluorescence detection, *J. Chromatogr. A*, 830, 243, 1999.

49. Gooijer, C., Kok, S.J., and Ariese, F., Capillary electrophoresis with laser-induced fluorescence detection for natively fluorescent analytes, *Analysis*, 28, 679, 2000.

50. Lee, T.T. and Yeung, E.S., High-sensitivity laser-induced fluorescence detection of native proteins in capillary electrophoresis, *J. Chromatogr.*, 595, 319, 1992.

51. Milofsky, R.E. and Yeung, E.S., Native fluorescence detection of nucleic acids and DNA restriction fragments in capillary electrophoresis, *Anal. Chem.*, 65, 153, 1993.

52. Chang, H.-T. and Yeung, E.S., Determination of catecholamines in single adrenal medullary cells by capillary electrophoresis and laser-induced native fluorescence, *Anal. Chem.*, 67, 1079, 1995.

53. Xue, Q. and Yeung, E.S., Variability of intracellular lactate dehydrogenase isoenzymes in single human erythrocytes, *Anal. Chem.*, 66, 1175, 1994.

54. Wu, N., Li, B., and Sweedler, J.V., Recent developments in porphyrin separations using capillary electrophoresis with native fluorescence detection, *J. Liq. Chromatogr.*, 17, 1917, 1994.

55. Korf, G.M., Landers, J.P., and O'Kane, D.J., Capillary electrophoresis with laser-induced fluorescence detection for the analysis of free and immune-complexed green fluorescent protein, *Anal. Biochem.*, 251, 210, 1997.

56. Mathies, R.A., Peck, K., and Stryer, L., Optimization of high-sensitivity fluorescence detection, *Anal. Chem.*, 62, 1786, 1990.

57. Timperman, A.T., Oldenburg, K.E., and Sweedler, J.V., Native fluorescence detection and spectral differentiation of peptides containing tryptophan and tyrosine in capillary electrophoresis, *Anal. Chem.*, 67, 3421, 1995.

58. Park, Y.H., Zhang, X., Rubakhin, S.S., and Sweedler, J.V., Independent optimization of capillary electrophoresis separation and native fluorescence detection conditions for indolamine and catecholamine measurements, *Anal. Chem.*, 71, 4997, 1999.

59. Shear, J.B., Multiphoton-excited fluorescence in bioanalytical chemistry, *Anal. Chem.*, 71, 598A, 1999.

60. Swinney, K., Markov, D., and Bornhop, D.J., Ultrasmall volume refractive index detection using microinterferometry, *Rev. Sci. Instrum.*, 71, 2684, 2000.

61. Swinney, K.A. and Bornhop, D.J., Universal detection for capillary electrophoresis using microinterferometric backscatter detection, *J. Microcolumn Sep.*, 11, 596, 1999.

62. Zemann, A.J., Conductivity detection in capillary electrophoresis, *Trends Anal. Chem.*, 20, 346, 2001.

63. Baldwin, R.P., Recent advances in electrochemical detection in capillary electrophoresis, *Electrophoresis*, 21, 4017, 2000.

64. Waterval, J.C.M., Lingeman, H., Bult, A., and Underberg, W.J.M., Derivatization trends in capillary electrophoresis, *Electrophoresis*, 21, 4029, 2000.

65. Miyazaki, K., Ohtani, K., Sunada, K., and Arita, T., Determination of ampicillin, amoxicillin, cephalexin, and cephradine in plasma by high-performance liquid chromatography using fluorometric detection, *J. Chromatogr.*, 276, 478, 1983.

66. Mukherjee, P.S. and Karnes, H.T., Ultraviolet and fluorescence derivatization reagents for carboxylic acids suitable for high performance liquid chromatography: A review, *Biomed. Chromatogr.*, 10, 193, 1996.

67. Guttman, A., Capillary gel electrophoresis of 8-aminopyrene-3,6,8-trisulfonate-labeled oligosaccharides, in *Techniques in Glycobiology*, Townsend, R.R. and Hotchkiss, A.T., Jr., eds., Marcel Dekker, New York, 1997, p. 377.

68. McWhorter, S. and Soper, S.A., Near-infrared laser-induced fluorescence detection in capillary electrophoresis, *Electrophoresis*, 21, 1267, 2000.

69. Fuchigami, T., Imasaka, T., and Shiga, M., Subattomole detection of amino acids by capillary electrophoresis based on semiconductor laser fluorescence detection, *Anal. Chim. Acta*, 282, 209, 1993.

70. Legendre, B.L., Jr. and Soper, S.A., Binding properties of near-IR dyes to proteins and separation of the dye/protein complexes using capillary electrophoresis with laser-induced fluorescence detection, *Appl. Spectrosc.*, 50, 1196, 1996.

71. Gibson, T.J. and Sepaniak, M.J., Examination of cyanine intercalation dyes for rapid and sensitive detection of DNA fragments by capillary electrophoresis, *J. Cap. Electrophor.*, 5, 73, 1998.

72. Colyer, C., Noncovalent labeling of proteins in capillary electrophoresis with laser-induced fluorescence detection, *Cell Biochem. Biophys.*, 33, 323, 2000.

73. Swaile, D.F. and Sepaniak, M.J., Laser-based fluorometric detection schemes for the analysis of proteins by capillary zone electrophoresis, *J. Liq. Chromatogr.*, 14, 869, 1991.

74. Ma, Y., Shortreed, M.R., Li, H., Huang, W., and Yeung, E.S., Single-molecule immunoassay and DNA diagnosis, *Electrophoresis*, 22, 421, 2001.

75. Swaile, D.F. and Sepaniak, M.J., Determination of metal ions by capillary zone electrophoresis with on-column chelation using 8-hydroxyquinoline-5-sulfonic acid, *Anal. Chem.*, 63, 179, 1991.

76. Soroka, K., Vithanage, R.S., Phillips, D.A., Walker, B., and Dasgupta, P.K., Fluorescence properties of metal complexes of 8-hydroxyquinoline-5-sulfonic acid and chromatographic applications, *Anal. Chem.*, 59, 629, 1987.

77. Clark, S.M. and Mathies, R.A., Multiplex dsDNA fragment sizing using dimeric intercalation dyes and capillary array electrophoresis: Ionic effects on the stability and electrophoretic mobility of DNA-dye complexes, *Anal. Chem.*, 69, 1355, 1997.

78. Glazer, A.N. and Rye, H.S., Stable dye-DNA intercalation complexes as reagents for high-sensitivity fluorescence detection, *Nature*, 359, 859, 1992.

79. Rye, H.S., Yue, S., Wemmer, D.E., Quesada, M.A., Haugland, R.P., Mathies, R.A., and Glazer, A.N., Stable fluorescent complexes of double-stranded DNA with bis-intercalating asymmetric cyanine dyes: Properties and applications, *Nucl. Acids Res.*, 20, 2803, 1992.

80. Clark, B.K. and Sepaniak, M.J., Evaluation of on-column labeling with intercalating dyes for fluorescence detection of DNA fragments separated by capillary electrophoresis, *J. Microcolumn Sep.*, 5, 275, 1993.

81. Oldenburg, K.E., Xi, X., and Sweedler, J.V., Simple sheath flow reactor for post-column fluorescence derivatization in capillary electrophoresis, *Analyst*, 122, 1581, 1997.

82. Zhu, R. and Kok, W.T., Post-column derivatization for fluorescence and chemiluminescence detection in capillary electrophoresis, *J. Pharm. Biomed. Anal.*, 17, 985, 1998.

83. Doble, P. and Haddad, P.R., Indirect photometric detection of anions in capillary electrophoresis, *J. Chromatogr. A*, 834, 189, 1999.

84. Colburn, B.A., Starnes, S.D., Hinton, E.R., and Sepaniak, M.J., Quantitative aspects of rare earth metal determinations using capillary electrophoresis with indirect absorbance detection, *Sep. Sci. Technol.*, 30, 1511, 1995.

85. Yeung, E.S. and Kuhr, W.G., Indirect detection methods for capillary separations, *Anal. Chem.*, 63, 275A, 1991.

86. Melanson, J.E., Boulet, C.A., and Lucy, C.A., Indirect laser-induced fluorescence detection for capillary electrophoresis using a violet diode laser, *Anal. Chem.*, 73, 1809, 2001.

87. Kuijt, J., Brinkman, U.A.T., and Gooijer, C., Quenched phosphorescence, a new detection method in capillary electrophoresis, *Electrophoresis*, 21, 1305, 2000.

88. Staller, T.D. and Sepaniak, M.J., Chemiluminescence detection in capillary electrophoresis, *Electrophoresis*, 18, 2291, 1997.

89. Kuyper, C. and Milofsky, R., Recent developments in chemiluminescence and photochemical reaction detection for capillary electrophoresis, *Trends Anal. Chem.*, 20, 232, 2001.

90. Huang, X.-J. and Fang, Z.-L., Chemiluminescence detection in capillary electrophoresis, *Anal. Chim. Acta*, 414, 1, 2000.

91. Ruberto, M.A. and Grayeski, M.L. Investigation of acridinium labeling for chemiluminescence detection of peptides separated by capillary electrophoresis, *J. Microcolumn Sep.*, 6, 545, 1994.

92. Dadoo, R., Seto, A.G., Colon, L.A., and Zare, R.N., End-column chemiluminescence detector for capillary electrophoresis, *Anal. Chem.*, 66, 303, 1994.

93. Zhao, J.-Y., Labbe, J., and Dovichi, N.J., Use of a sheath flow cuvette for chemiluminescence detection of isoluminol thiocarbamyl-amino acids separated by capillary electrophoresis, *J. Microcolumn Sep.*, 5, 331, 1993.

94. Olson, D.L., Lacey, M.E., and Sweedler, J.V., The nanoliter niche, *Anal. Chem.*, 70, 257A, 1998.

95. von Brocke, A., Nicholson, G., and Bayer, E., Recent advances in capillary electrophoresis/electrospray–mass spectrometry, *Electrophoresis*, 22, 1251, 2001.

96. Naylor, S. and Tomlinson, A.J., Capillary electrophoresis–mass spectrometry of biologically active peptides and proteins, in *Clinical and Forensic Applications of Capillary Electrophoresis*, Petersen, J.R. and Mohammad, A.A., eds., Humana Press, Totowa, NJ, 2001.

97. Somsen, G.W., Hooijschuur, E.W.J., Gooijer, C., Brinkman, U.A.Th., Velthorst, N.H., and Visser, T., Coupling of reversed-phase liquid column chromatography and Fourier transform infrared spectrometry using postcolumn on-line extraction and solvent elimination, *Anal. Chem.*, 68, 746, 1996.

98. Jankowiak, R., Roberts, K.P., and Small, G.J., Fluorescence line-narrowing detection in chromatography and electrophoresis, *Electrophoresis*, 21, 1251, 2000.

99. Ruddick, A., Batchelder, D.N., Bartle, K.D., Gilby, A.C., and Pitt, G.D., Development of a Raman detector for capillary electrophoresis, *Appl. Spectrosc.*, 54, 1857, 2000.

100. Kowalchyk, W.K., Walker, P.A., III, and Morris, M.D., Rapid normal Raman spectroscopy of sub-ppm oxy-anion solutions: The role of electrophoretic preconcentration, *Appl. Spectrosc.*, 49, 1183, 1995.

101. Walker, P.A., III, Shaver, J.M., and Morris, M.D., Identification of cationic herbicides in deionized water, municipal tap water, and river water by capillary isotachophoresis/on-line Raman spectroscopy, *Appl. Spectrosc.*, 51, 1394, 1997.

102. Walker, P.A., III and Morris, M.D., Capillary isotachophoresis with fiber-optic Raman spectroscopic detection. Performance and application to ribonucleotides, *J. Chromatogr. A*, 805, 269, 1998.

103. Vo-Dinh, T., Surface-enhanced Raman spectroscopy using metallic nanostructures, *Trends Anal. Chem.*, 17, 557, 1998.

104. Weaver, M.J., Zou, S., and Chan, H.Y.H., The new interfacial ubiquity of surface-enhanced Raman spectroscopy, *Anal. Chem.*, 72, 38A, 2000.

105. Campion, A. and Kambhampati, P., Surface-enhanced Raman scattering, *Chem. Soc. Rev.*, 27, 241, 1998.

106. Nie, S. and Emory, S.R., Probing single molecules and single nanoparticles by surface-enhanced Raman scattering, *Science*, 275, 1102, 1997.

107. He, L., Natan, M.J., and Keating, C.D., Surface-enhanced Raman scattering: A structure-specific detection method for capillary electrophoresis, *Anal. Chem.*, 72, 5348, 2000.

108. DeVault, G.L. and Sepaniak, M.J., Spatially focused deposition of capillary electrophoresis effluent onto surface-enhanced Raman-active substrates for off-column spectroscopy, *Electrophoresis*, 22, 2303, 2001.

109. Nirode, W.F., Devault, G.L., Sepaniak, M.J., and Cole, R.O., On-column surface-enhanced Raman spectroscopy detection in capillary electrophoresis using running buffers containing silver colloidal solutions, *Anal. Chem.*, 72, 1866, 2000.

110. Monnig, C.A. and Jorgenson, J.W., On-column sample gating for high-speed capillary zone electrophoresis, *Anal. Chem.*, 63, 802, 1991.

111. Kennedy, R.T., Bioanalytical applications of fast capillary electrophoresis, *Anal. Chim. Acta*, 400, 163, 1999.

112. Moore, A.W., Jr. and Jorgenson, J.W., Resolution of *cis* and *trans* isomers of peptides containing proline using capillary zone electrophoresis, *Anal. Chem.*, 67, 3464, 1995.

113. Mitchelson, K.R. and Cheng, J., eds., *Capillary Electrophoresis of Nucleic Acids*, Vols. I and II, Humana Press, Totowa, NJ, 2001.

114. Righetti, P.G. and Verzola, B., Folding/unfolding/refolding of proteins: Present methodologies in comparison with capillary zone electrophoresis, *Electrophoresis*, 22, 2359, 2001.

115. Rochu, D. and Masson, P., Mulitple advantages of capillary zone electrophoresis for exploring protein conformational stability, *Electrophoresis*, 23, 189, 2002.

116. Heegaard, N.H.H., Nissen, M.H., and Chen, D.D.Y., Applications of on-line weak affinity interactions in free solution capillary electrophoresis, *Electrophoresis*, 23, 815, 2002.

117. Duijn, R.M.G.-V., Frank, J., Dedem, G.W.K.V., and Baltussen, E., Recent advances in affinity capillary electrophoresis, *Electrophoresis*, 21, 3905, 2000.

118. Bao, J.J., Fujima, J.M., and Danielson, N.D., Determination of minute enzymatic activities by means of capillary electrophoretic techniques, *J. Chromatogr. B*, 699, 481, 1997.

119. Schultz, N.M., Tao, L., Rose, D.J., Jr., and Kennedy, R.T., Immunoassays and enzyme assays using capillary electrophoresis, in *Handbook of Capillary Electrophoresis*, 2nd edn., Landers, J.P., ed., CRC Press, Boca Raton, FL, 1997, p. 611.

120. Harmon, B.J. and Regnier, F.E., Electrophoretically mediated microanalysis, *Chem. Anal.*, 146, 925, 1998.

121. Jenkins, M.A., Clinical applications of capillary electrophoresis: Status at the new millennium, *Mol. Biotechnol.*, 15, 201, 2000.

122. Harvey, M.D., Paquette, D.M., and Banks, P.R., Clinical applications of CE, *J. Liq. Chromatogr. Relat. Technol.*, 24, 1871, 2001.

123. Petersen, J.R. and Mohammad, A.A., eds., *Clinical and Forensic Applications of Capillary Electrophoresis*, Humana Press, Totowa, NJ, 2001.

124. Freed, A.L., Cooper, J.D., Davies, M.I., and Lunte, S.M., Investigation of the metabolism of substance P in rat striatum by microdialysis sampling and capillary electrophoresis with laser-induced fluorescence detection, *J. Neurosci. Methods*, 109, 23, 2001.

125. Dawson, L.A., Capillary electrophoresis and microdialysis: Current technology and applications, *J. Chromatogr. B*, 697, 89, 1997.
126. Denoroy, L., Bert, L., Parrot, S., Robert, F., and Renaud, B., Assessment of pharmacodynamic and pharmacokinetic characteristics of drugs using microdialysis sampling and capillary electrophoresis, *Electrophoresis*, 19, 2841, 1998.
127. Whisnant, A.R., Johnston, S.E., and Gilman, S.D., Capillary electrophoretic analysis of alkaline phosphatase inhibition by theophylline, *Electrophoresis*, 21, 1341, 2000.
128. Whisnant, A.R. and Gilman, S.D., Studies of reversible inhibition, irreversible inhibition and activation of alkaline phosphatase by capillary electrophoresis, *Anal. Biochem.*, 307, 266, 2002.
129. Saevels, J., Van den Steen, K., Schepdael, A.V., and Hoogmartens, J., Study of competitive inhibition of adenosine deaminase by erythro-9-(2-hydroxy-3-nonyl)adenine using capillary zone electrophoresis, *J. Chromatogr. A*, 745, 293, 1996.
130. Bao, J. and Regnier, F.E., Ultramicro enzyme assays in a capillary electrophoretic system, *J. Chromatogr.*, 608, 217, 1992.

7

Surface Plasmon Resonance Imaging Sensors: Principle, Development, and Biomedical Applications—Example of Genotyping

Julien Moreau
Université Paris Sud

Jean-Pierre Cloarec
Université de Lyon
and
Université de Sherbrooke

Paul Charette
Université de Sherbrooke

Michel Goossens
Institut National de la Santé
et de la Recherche Médicale

Michael Canva
Université Paris Sud
and
Duke University

Tuan Vo-Dinh
Duke University

7.1 Introduction

Chemical sensing and biosensing are playing an increasingly important part in many smart systems by providing important information that enable making the right decisions at reasonable cost. This is especially true and of primary importance in the biomedical field, both in developing countries that face many illnesses and limited health-care resources and in developed countries facing rapid aging of society and increasing demand for higher-quality health services.

High-throughput detection of biomolecular interactions between probe and target molecules on a sensing surface is a challenge that has been met in numerous ways. Direct detection schemes without any labeling of the probe or target molecules have the advantages of simplicity and reliability as labels can structurally and functionally alter an assay. Toward these goals, many integrated systems have been developed recently, some reaching the level of *lab on a chip* (LOC) as they are now referred to. Mostly, these methods rely on micro- or nanoelectromechanical sensors [1], photonic microresonators [2], electrical measurement systems such as conductance in silicon nanowire arrays [3], or electrochemical detection devices [4]. However, these devices are quite difficult to apply to multiplex systems as the complexity of the detection scheme increases exponentially with the number of molecular interactions one wishes to simultaneously monitor.

Photonics is one of the major players in this field, and numerous examples discussed in this book underline this point. Within the field of photonics lie plasmonics, which deals with special electromagnetic modes that are confined in the immediate vicinity of metal–dielectric interfaces. Because such optical modes can be very sensitive to minute changes in the dielectric material, this plasmonic field also offers many opportunities for biomedical sensing applications as illustrated in several chapters of this book. As will be shown in this specific chapter, one can image a large surface, of the order of cm^2, with lateral spatial resolution in the range of a few microns and subnanometer resolution in thickness. This allows parallel monitoring of numerous biomolecular binding events onto a so-called biochip format. Plasmonic sensing has been successfully implemented in the detection of a large number of different types of molecular interactions, as illustrated by the few following examples: DNA and RNA and peptides [5–11], immunoassays [12], proteins [13–15], and cell studies [16].

Figure 7.1 shows bibliographic data reflecting the rapidly growing field related to plasmonic sensing. In particular, DNA-related work is very prominent, accounting for about 20% of published work. Plasmonic sensing in an imaging format, with applications such as biochip microarrays, is also a major area of focus.

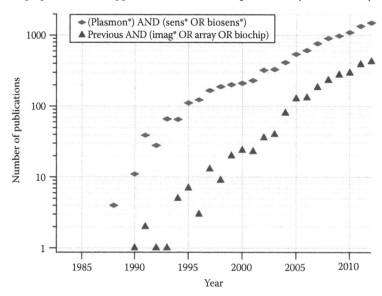

FIGURE 7.1 Illustration of bibliographic data extracted from ISI Web of Science in March 2011 using the following keywords: (1) ([plasmon*] AND [biosens* OR sens*]) and (2) adding (imag* OR array* OR biochip*).

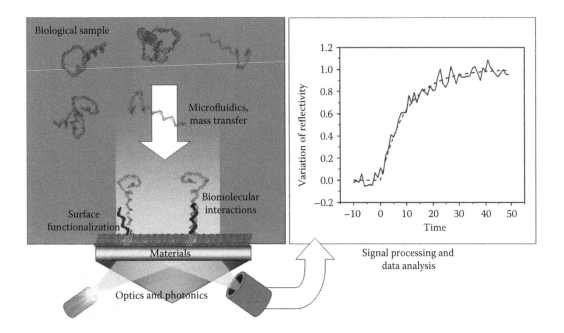

FIGURE 7.2 Sketch of an optical biochip/bioarray plasmonic sensor showing the complementary expertise needed for quantitative and reproducible results in biosensing experiments.

Many complementary areas of expertise are required to design, develop, and operate a plasmonic biochip system. As schematically illustrated in Figure 7.2, these include photonics, plasmonics, surface (bio)functionalization, biomolecular interactions, microfluidics, electrooptics, data processing, and analysis.

In this chapter, we will start by describing the surface plasmon resonance (SPR) phenomenon, described in detail on how it can be used to accurately monitor surface biomolecular interaction kinetics in an imaging format. We will then describe how the sensing surface can be functionalized, structured, and organized into an array, capable of parallel monitoring of biomolecular surface interactions. To be adequately characterized, such surface interactions must occur in controlled microfluidic conditions, which we will detail. We will then describe how raw data must be processed to provide information, both qualitatively and quantitatively. We will also discuss the challenges of genetic diagnostics in the important case of cystic fibrosis (CF), as a model study of DNA–DNA interactions, and provide experimental data issued from such an SPR imaging (SPRI) biochip system. Finally, we will briefly describe other biomedical applications before the conclusion.

7.2 Plasmonic Biochip Reader System

7.2.1 Surface Plasmon Resonance Imaging

7.2.1.1 Surface Plasmon Resonance Effect

Metallic surfaces at visible wavelengths have a high reflectivity, above 80% for gold, silver, or aluminum. However, if monochromatic transverse magnetic (TM)-polarized light is irradiated upon a very thin metallic layer (~50 nm) through a glass substrate, reflectivity will drop to almost zero for a very specific incidence angle. At this resonance angle, most of the light energy is absorbed by the free electrons at the surface of the metallic layer, creating an evanescent surface wave, which propagates along the metal/dielectric interface (see Figure 7.3). Away from this resonance angle, a high reflectivity is observed like with any thick metallic layer. This sharp drop in the angular reflectivity is called SPR and is observed for visible and near-infrared (IR) wavelengths in metals such as gold, silver, and aluminum. Note that light–plasmon coupling is only possible if the light momentum is first increased since plasmon excitation by light impinging directly on

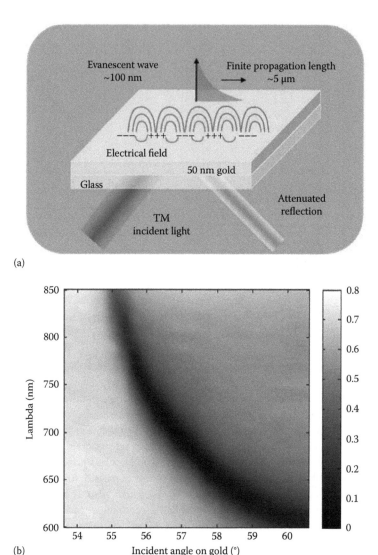

(a)

(b)

FIGURE 7.3 **(See color insert.)** (a) Diagram of the SPR effect where TM monochromatic light is reflected from a 50 nm gold layer through a glass substrate. At the resonance angle, an evanescent surface wave is created and a drop in reflectivity is observed; (b) experimentally measured reflectivity, as a function of the incidence angle and wavelength, for a typical SPR biochip made of a 50 nm gold layer on a SF10 glass substrate. The SPR resonance appears as a valley of almost zero reflectivity.

a metal–dielectric interface is not possible: details of the underlying mechanisms involved in SPR can be found in previous review articles [17] or [18]. The most useful feature of SPR in biosensing is its sensitivity to minute changes in the dielectric refractive index in the vicinity of the metallic surface.

With a gold or a silver layer, resonance can be observed at any wavelength above 500 nm to the near IR, where the specific resonance angle corresponding to a particular wavelength will always be above the total internal reflection angle of the glass/dielectric interface. As mentioned earlier, the thickness, t, of the metallic layer is critical in this matter. If the metallic layer is too thick, the entire incident light is absorbed before reaching the upper surface of the metal; if it is too thin, not enough energy is absorbed by the free electrons and the SPR effect is negligible. Optimum thickness is around 50 nm for a gold or silver layer across most of the visible and near-IR ranges. The intensity of a surface plasmon wave, generated at a given point on the surface, will decrease due to the metal absorption as it propagates along the surface, with a propagation length, L, which strongly depends on the incident excitation wavelength: as short as 2 μm for a Ag layer excited at 500 nm and reaching almost 40 μm at 900 nm. This propagation length limits the spatial resolution that can be obtained in imaging and has practical consequences for SPR biochips as will be discussed later in this chapter. The spatial extension of the plasmon evanescent field above the metallic layer is extremely limited. The typical penetration depth, L_z, in the medium above the surface, usually water, is typically less than 300 nm. This is a key parameter for biochip applications, which ensures that SPR will only sense refractive index changes in the immediate vicinity of the surface.

When such a refractive index perturbation occurs, in particular when a molecular layer binds to the surface, the coupling conditions between the incident light and surface plasmons change. This leads to a shift in the resonance curve. The idea of using SPR for sensing begins in the 1980s [19], with the first commercial systems appearing in the 1990s. Figure 7.4a shows a typical angular reflectivity measurement curve for a 50 nm gold layer covered with water, deposited on a SF10 glass substrate, at an incident wavelength of 633 nm (corresponding to a He–Ne laser), and the subsequent shift due to the binding of

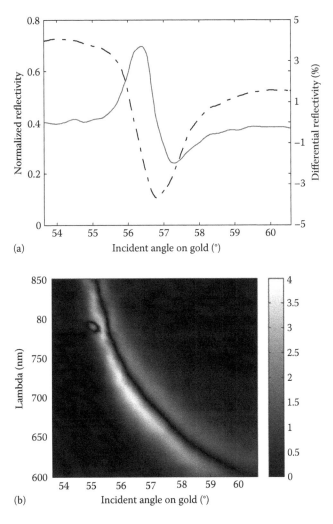

FIGURE 7.4 **(See color insert.)** (a) Solid line, angular reflectivity curve for an incident wavelength of 633 nm extracted from Figure 7.1; dashed line, variation of reflectivity due to the binding of BSA on the gold surface; (b) map of the reflectivity variation due to the BSA-binding, experimental data.

bovine serum albumin (BSA) on gold. The plasmon resonance is angularly shifted and a 3% variation in maximum reflectivity is observed. Not surprisingly, this maximum in reflectivity variation is measured at the incidence angle where the reflectivity slope is the greatest. Figure 7.4b shows the complete shift measurement of resonance after the BSA binding for incident wavelengths between 600 and 800 nm. All TM reflectivity measurements are normalized by the transverse electric (TE) reflectivity measurements. Such an example shows how the sensitivity of plasmon resonance to refractive index changes close to the gold surface can be used as a transducer to convert a chemical or biological event, here the binding of BSA, to an optical signal.

Compared to more conventional fluorescence detection, SPR detection is significantly different in the sense that the signal is related to a change in the refractive index, which in turn is related to the change in mass density of the molecular layer binding to the sensing surface. A high surface coverage of small target molecules, such as short oligonucleotides, will give a signal similar to a low surface concentration of large target molecules, such as proteins, because of steric hindrance. In fluorescence detection, the signal will only depend on the number of fluorescent molecules in the detection zone and not on the size or the mass of the molecule of interest to which the fluorescent tag is attached. SPR techniques, therefore, are not suitable for the detection of small target molecules at very low surface concentration.

Tables 7.1 and 7.2 show two measures of theoretical sensitivity as a function of reflectivity change, as well as the characteristic lengths of SPs for gold and silver sensing layers, respectively. The first expression, $\delta R/\delta n$, is the maximum rate of change in reflectivity, R, as a function of bulk refractive index change, δn, in the dielectric above the metal layer. The second expression, $\delta R/\delta e$, is the maximum rate of change of reflectivity as a function of biological layer thickness change, δe, atop the metal layer (assuming an index of refraction equal to 1.45 for the biological layer). These quantities are calculated considering an ideal system with optimized parameters, angular divergence of the incident beam, and spectral width of the source not being considered. Adhesion layers, typically chromium or titanium, are also not taken into account. Experimental data have shown that actual measurements are very close to these results.

The first observation that can be made from these results is that, as the incident wavelength increases from 500 to 900 nm, the penetration depth of the surface plasmon (SP) in the dielectric medium increases. This in turn leads to an improvement in the sensitivity in terms of $\delta R/\delta n$ by a similar factor. The $\delta R/\delta e$ sensitivity to the binding of a molecular layer to a gold or silver sensing surface is, however, much less dependent on penetration depth. A first-order calculation, detailed in Section 7.2.1.3, shows that

$$\frac{\delta R}{\delta e} \propto \frac{\delta R}{\delta n} \frac{1}{L_z} \tag{7.1}$$

TABLE 7.1 Key Parameters for a Gold Layer on a SF10 Glass Substrate

λ (nm)	t (nm)	$\delta R/\delta n$ (%/RIU)	$\delta R/\delta e$ (%/nm)	L (μm)	L_z (nm)
500	—	—	—	—	—
650	52	3,300	6.3	3	83
750	47	9,100	12.5	12.7	148
900	42	15,100	15.6	28.6	238

The numerical calculations are done with an optimum thickness, t, defined by a minimum of the SP resonance. Indices of refraction are from [25]. $\delta R/\delta n$ and $\delta R/\delta e$ are calculated at the maximum slope of the angular reflectivity curves. No significant SP coupling in gold is possible below 500 nm.

TABLE 7.2 Key Parameters for a Silver Layer on a SF10 Glass Substrate

λ (nm)	t (nm)	$\delta R/\delta n$ (%/RIU)	$\delta R/\delta e$ (%/nm)	L (μm)	L_z (nm)
500	44	3,300	7.6	2.3	58
650	47	8,300	12.0	9.4	114
750	47	12,700	14.5	18.3	159
900	46	20,200	16.2	37.1	240

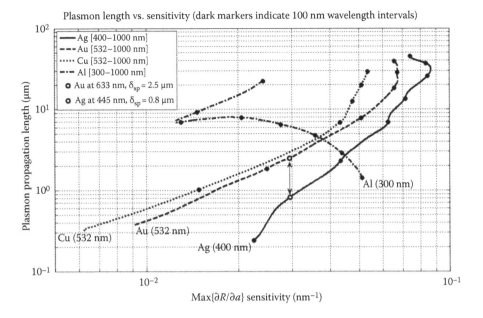

FIGURE 7.5 Plasmon propagation length as a function of sensitivity for Au, Ag, Al, and Cu at optimal film thicknesses for each metal, across a range of wavelengths (black markers on the curves). The combination of highest sensitivity and shortest propagation length is in the lower right-hand corner of the graph. The vertical arrow in the figure indicates that the sensitivity for Ag at 450 nm is roughly equivalent to that of Au at 633 nm.

One must not conclude, however, that working at a longer wavelength is always preferable for biochip applications. For a given metal/dielectric interface, there is an unavoidable trade-off between plasmon length (L) and SPR sensitivity ($\delta R/\delta e$): if conditions are adjusted to reduce the plasmon length in order to increase imaging spatial resolution, the sensitivity decreases correspondingly in most cases. Indeed, the propagation length dramatically increases at higher wavelengths. For gold, between 650 and 900 nm, a 10-fold increase in the propagation length is observed, which in turn will reduce the spatial resolution by the same amount as discussed in Section 7.2.1.3. Also, the increase in penetration depth with increasing wavelength will degrade the rejection of bulk disturbances, emanating, for example, from temperature variations. Several authors have investigated the sensitivity/resolution compromise using a variety of metals at different wavelengths, such as gold, silver, aluminum, and copper [20–24].

Figure 7.5 illustrates the sensitivity/resolution compromise for a model chip structure consisting of an SF10 glass substrate, a 3 nm chromium (Cr) adhesion layer, a plasmon-guiding metal film (Ag, Au, Cu, Al), a 5 nm biofilm (index of 1.5, typical of DNA), and a semi-infinite bulk water volume. Dispersion data from the literature for the metals were used in all calculations [25]. The dispersion data for the glass were approximated using the Sellmeier model. The combination of highest sensitivity and shortest propagation length is in the lower right-hand corner of the graph. The vertical arrow in the figure indicates that the sensitivity for Ag at 450 nm is roughly equivalent to that of Au at 633 nm, a classic SPR configuration having excellent sensitivity. However, Ag at 450 nm has a plasmon propagation length of 0.8 µm, that is, 1/3 that of Au at 633 nm.

An interesting approach to the sensitivity/resolution compromise, first proposed by [26] and refined by [27], makes use of the interference between coherent surface plasmons to confine the SPR response to a diffraction-limited spot. In this way, submicron imaging resolution can be achieved using a microscope objective of sufficiently high numerical aperture. However, scanning is required to build up an image, as with a confocal microscope, so that spatial resolution improvement comes at the expense of temporal resolution.

Finally, a change in the resonance curve, $R(\alpha, \lambda, x, y, T)$, can be detected in many different ways as the reflectivity of the metal sensing surface depends on at least five parameters: the incidence angle α, the excitation wavelength λ, the position (x, y) on the sensing surface, and time T. As such, the measured variable can be an angular shift in the minimum measured at a fixed excitation wavelength λ_0, a spectral shift at a fixed incidence angle α_0, or a variation of reflectivity at a given angular–spectral (α_0, λ_0) working point.

7.2.1.2 SPR Imaging Systems

Figure 7.6 shows a typical SPRI system [28,29]. The light source, collimated and linearly polarized, is reflected from a rotating mirror to control the incidence angle. Two afocal systems conjugate the mirrors with the gold biochip and the charge-coupled device (CCD) camera. A prism is used to enable plasmon resonance at the metal/water interface (light momentum increase). The metal layer can be deposited directly on the prism, but a better and less costly solution is to deposit the metal on a glass coverslip with the same index of refraction as the prism. Index-matching oil is then required to minimize secondary reflections between the prism and the glass coverslip.

Using a prism, however, distorts the images seen by the camera through the second afocal system. The index of refraction of the glass prism and the prism angle must be chosen so that the plasmon resonance is obtained with incident (and reflected) light at an angle close to the normal to the prism face in order to minimize these aberrations. Figure 7.7 shows the combination of prism material (index of refraction) and prism geometry (summit angle, A), which ensures working in such an optimized configuration. Calculations were performed for a 50 nm gold layer covered with water at 650 nm. Also, because of the compression of the images in the y direction (x being parallel to the prism face) due to the oblique incidence, it is also preferable to use a prism with the highest possible summit angle, as the compression factor is equal to $\sin(A/2)$. Working with high-index prisms is not always possible in practice as oils with indices of refraction higher than 1.8 usually contain arsenic that makes them toxic and difficult to use.

To inject different solutions containing target molecules, the metal sensing surface is covered by a microfluidic cell. The simplest configuration is a cylindrical vessel with single input and output points. For a cylindrical vessel 1 cm in diameter and 100 μm in depth, the total volume is 10 μL. A detailed discussion on microfluidic aspects is given in Section 7.2.3. The temperature of the cell should be controlled as temperature drifts of 0.01°C or greater could affect the detection limit of the system.

The possible choices for the light source are limited by the fact that though a highly collimated and quasi-monochromatic source such as a laser is desirable for imaging purposes, the speckle effect strongly degrades image quality. Various solutions to this problem in optics have been previously reported in the literature and have been applied in the case of SPRI [30] with some success. Still, LED is the simplest light source that can be used with negligible interference effects and high brightness. Of course, the

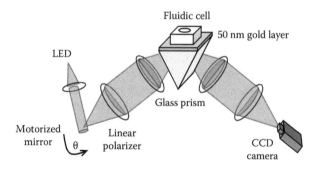

FIGURE 7.6 Typical SPRI setup. A LED light source is collimated and TM polarized. A motorized rotating mirror is used to adjust the incidence angle on the gold sensing layer, through a prism. The gold surface is covered with a fluidic cell. Afocal systems conjugate the mirrors with the gold surface and the CCD camera.

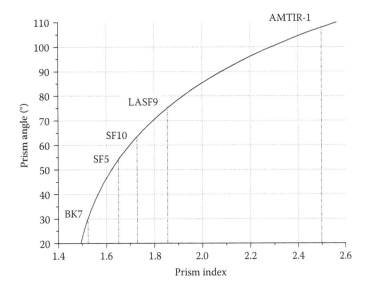

FIGURE 7.7 Graph of prism summit angle versus prism index of refraction required for an optimized imaging configuration (SP resonance obtained for incident and reflected light beams normal to the prism faces).

spectral width and the larger angular divergence of an LED compared to a laser both have an impact on the overall performance of the SPRI setup, but the effect on the sensitivity is small (less than 10%). The incident light must be TM polarized in order to observe the SP effect. Some more complex polarization setups can also be used to enhance the sensitivity by working in a dark field configuration [31]. Finally, the choice of the wavelength involves a trade-off between sensitivity and spatial resolution as discussed in Tables 7.1 and 7.2.

7.2.1.3 SPR System Performance

7.2.1.3.1 Detection Limit

In many probe–target detection applications, chemical and biological related drift is usually the limiting factor in the sensitivity of the sensor. Temperature, if not carefully controlled, can also be an important source of a noise, especially for low-concentration detection or weakly interacting species where the incubation time can be in order of hours. Finally, shot noise, being a fundamental limit in optics, will always be the ultimate limiting factor in the minimum refractive index change detectable by an SPR sensor. It is interesting to estimate the detection limit imposed by shot noise as it is easy to calculate and does not depend on the exact nature of the optical system, keeping in mind that it is not always possible to reach this limit in actual applications.

In optics, if an ideal light source emits n photons per unit time, then the noise as measured by an ideal detector will be proportional to $\sqrt{n}$. Thus, we can write the relative noise of a reflectivity measurement on a given area of the sensing surface as

$$\text{Noise }(\%) = \frac{100}{\sqrt{R \times N_e \times N_{\text{acc}} \times n_{\text{px}}}} \tag{7.2}$$

where
    R is the mean reflectivity of the measured area
    N_e is the full-well capacity of camera pixel
    N_{acc} is the number of accumulated images
    n_{px} is the number of pixels averaged over the measurement area

Note that as shot noise is white, Equation 7.2 does not directly depend on the acquisition speed of the detector or any other temporal parameter: it only depends on the total number of photoelectrons acquired, limited by the capacity of the detector and the spatial or temporal averaging.

The typical full-well capacity of a megapixel CCD camera is around 20,000 e⁻ (N_e is proportional to the pixel size, which means that cameras with a high number of pixels will have lower performance in terms of shot noise of individual pixels). The number of images averaged, N_{acc}, must be chosen according to the time resolution needed for a given experiment. As an example, a camera with an acquisition speed of 10 images/s ($N_{acc} = 10$) with $R = 30\%$ at the working angle results in an individual pixel shot noise of 0.4%. Averaging the signal over an area of 10×10 pixels will further reduce the shot noise to 0.04%. This is equivalent to a change in the refractive index of the water above the gold layer of 1.2×10^{-5} (at 650 nm), which in turn is what can be expected from a temperature variation in the fluidic cell of ~0.01°C at 20°C.

For the study of molecular interactions, it is useful to express the detection limit of a SPRI system not in terms of reflectivity variation but in terms of surface coverage, Γ (mass/volume), of the target molecules on the sensing surface. The relationship between the measured reflectivity, R, and the variation of the index of refraction, Δn, above the metallic layer is given to a first-order approximation by

$$R = R_0 + \frac{\delta R}{\delta n} \Delta n \qquad (7.3)$$

If we consider a thin molecular layer on the sensing surface with a thickness e and a concentration C, a first-order development of the index of refraction of the layer, n_{layer}, can be written as

$$n_{layer} = n_0 + \frac{\delta n}{\delta C} C \qquad (7.4)$$

where
    n_0 is the index of the dielectric medium, usually water, and the rate of change of refractive index with respect to concentration
    $\delta n/\delta C$ depends on the nature of the target molecules

As the SP has a penetration depth L_z of a few hundred nanometers and will extend far above the molecular layer, only a small part of the evanescent wave will *see* the molecular layer. If we consider that the target molecular layer thickness is much smaller than L_z, then the variation of refraction index seen by the SP due to the binding of the molecular layer will be equal to

$$\Delta n = \frac{e}{L_z}(n_{layer} - n_0) = C \frac{\delta n}{\delta C} \frac{e}{L_z} \qquad (7.5)$$

We can therefore write that the reflectivity variation, ΔR, measured with an SPRI system will be related to the molecular layer parameters by

$$\Delta R = C \frac{\delta n}{\delta C} \frac{\delta R}{\delta n} \frac{e}{L_z} \qquad (7.6)$$

where $\delta R/\delta n$ is the sensitivity of the system to a bulk index of refraction variation, as defined in Section 2.1.1. From Equation 7.6, neglecting all second-order terms, a simple proportionality relationship between the major parameters of SPR biochips can be also obtained:

$$\frac{\delta R}{\delta e} \propto \frac{\delta R}{\delta n} \frac{1}{L_z} \qquad (7.7)$$

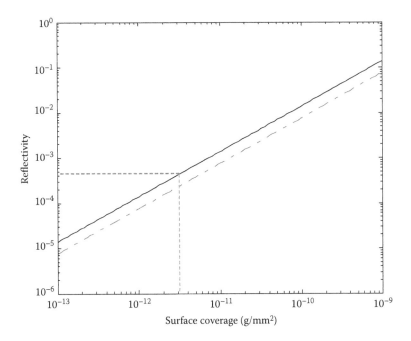

FIGURE 7.8 Sensitivity, in terms of reflectivity variations of gold (dashed line) and silver (solid line) SPR biochips as a function of the surface coverage of a molecular layer for an incident wavelength of 650 nm ($\delta n/\delta C = 0.19$ mL/g).

This helps to understand some of the results obtained in Tables 7.1 and 7.2, in particular the small increase in $\delta R/\delta e$ sensitivity and the large increase in $\delta R/\delta n$ sensitivity with increasing wavelength. In terms of surface coverage, using the fact that $\Gamma = C \times e$, we finally find the following:

$$\Delta R = \Gamma \frac{\delta n}{\delta C} \frac{\delta R}{\delta n} \frac{1}{L_z} \qquad (7.8)$$

Figure 7.8 shows the TM reflectivity variation as a function of the surface coverage, for gold and silver layers at 650 nm, using the parameters of Tables 7.1 and 7.2. Since refractive index characteristics across different proteins are fairly similar [32], we have chosen a representative value $\delta n/\delta C = 0.19$ mL/g. With a noise level of 0.04%, the minimum surface coverage detectable is therefore a few pg/mm². This threshold can also be expressed as a minimum surface concentration of target molecules, ranging from around 50 amol/mm² for large molecules, such as streptavidin protein with a mass of 52,800 Da, to 0.5 fmol/mm² for very small molecules such as 20-base single-stranded DNA (ssDNA) with a mass of 6,200 Da.

7.2.1.3.2 Spatial Resolution

In a conventional optical imaging system, the spatial resolution will be limited by the size and the number of pixels of the image sensor, the aberrations of the optics, and the diffraction limit. Features on the metallic surface, such as different areas functionalized with different molecular probes, can only be distinguishable if their separation is greater than the SP propagation length, L. This is true only in the direction of propagation, given by the projected direction of the incident beam of light on the metallic surface. In the perpendicular direction, the spatial resolution is limited by the optics and diffraction like in any classical optical system. SPRI images will therefore exhibit strong resolution anisotropy, particularly at long wavelengths, as L increases with the excitation wavelength. This effect is distinct from the geometrical compression of the image due to the oblique incidence of the illumination beam through the prism.

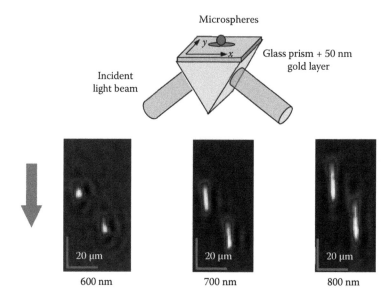

FIGURE 7.9 SPR reflectivity images taken at different wavelengths of microspheres deposited on a gold surface. For each wavelength, the incidence angle is chosen in order to be at the SPR angle. The arrow shows the direction of propagation of the surface plasmons.

Figure 7.9 shows an experiment to illustrate the anisotropic spatial resolution in SPRI: 10 μm diameter polystyrene microspheres were deposited onto a gold film biochip substrate, and the fluidic cell was filled with water. Due to evanescent nature of SP, only the fraction of the sphere directly in contact with the gold surface falls within the range of the evanescent field. A simple calculation shows that for a penetration depth of 100 nm, the 10 μm diameter microspheres appear as 1 μm diameter circular objects. As the spatial resolution of the setup is ~6 μm, limited by the numerical aperture of the imaging system, the spheres can be considered as point objects. Using a thermal white light source and a monochromator, SPR reflectivity images were taken at various wavelengths. At each wavelength, the incident angle was tuned in order to be at the SPR angle of the gold/water interface. The microspheres, having a high index of refraction compared to the surrounding medium, appear as bright objects on a dark background in the SPR images. At 600 nm, the spatial resolution is more or less isotropic. As the wavelength increases, the SPR images of the microspheres are more and more elongated in the direction of SP propagation, but the spatial resolution in the perpendicular direction remains constant. The plasmonic reflectivity profiles of the microspheres at different wavelengths are given in Figure 7.10.

7.2.1.4 Dynamic Measurement (Kinetics)

A typical SPRI experiment will begin with the choice of the working incidence angle. Usually this is done by measuring the mean reflectivity over the whole biochip as a function of the incidence angle around the expected SP resonance angle as shown in Figure 7.11a. The highest sensitivity will be achieved by choosing a working angle where the slope is the greatest. When the incidence angle is chosen, reflectivity images are acquired at video rates, while different solutions are injected in the fluidic cell.

Figure 7.11b shows the mean reflectivity variation during the injection of calibrated refractive index solutions using a peristaltic pump connected to the fluidic cell. Changes in the refractive index, from water to phosphate buffer solutions (PBSs), change the angular position of the SP resonance and lead to a variation in reflectivity. Figure 7.11c shows a series of images obtained during kinetics measurements with an SPRI setup, in this example when water is replaced by a PBS 0.1× solution. A reflectivity variation of about 0.75% is observed, shown in false color. Note that the total refractive index variation in this case is around 10^{-4}.

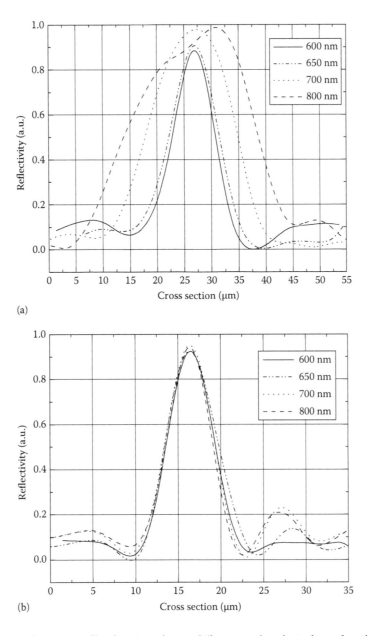

FIGURE 7.10 TM reflectivity profile of a microsphere at different wavelengths in the surface plasmon propagation direction (a) and perpendicular direction (b).

The intrinsic temporal resolution of an SPRI instrument is mostly useful when biomolecular interactions are studied as a dynamical measurement (kinetics of biomolecular interactions). First, the association and dissociation rates between the probe and the target molecule can be extracted from the data, in addition to the final surface concentration of the target, after the washing phase, obtained with a single end-point measurement. This allows studies of the influence of external parameters such as temperature or salt condition on the probe–target duplex interaction. Kinetics data also increase the range of interaction strengths that can be detected. A very weak binding duplex will not be seen with an end-point measurement as most of the duplex will dissociate during rinsing, whereas it can be detected in the kinetics SPR signal. Figure 7.12 illustrates such advantages brought about by dynamical measurements.

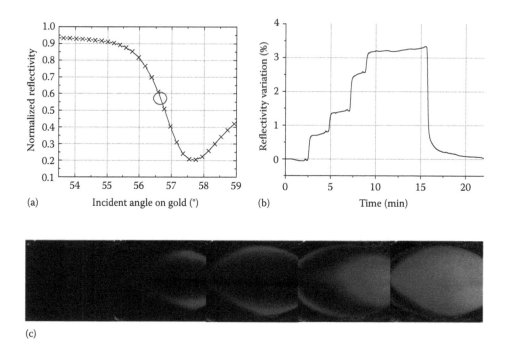

(a)   Incident angle on gold (°)   (b)   Time (min)

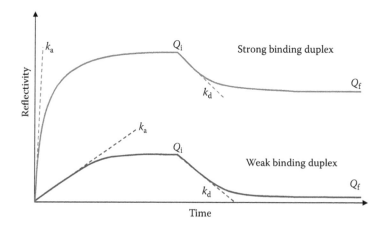

(c)

FIGURE 7.11 (a) TM/TE reflectivity around the resonant angle for a 50 nm gold layer deposited on a SF10 glass substrate and covered with water. The circle indicates the maximum slope, which must be chosen as the operating point. (b) Mean reflectivity of the gold biochip, as a function of time. Solutions injected successively are water, PBS 0.1×, PBS 0.2×, PBS 0.3×, and PBS 0.5×. (c) SPR images taken during the solution change between water and PBS 0.1×. Reflectivity variation is shown in false color. The diameter of the fluidic cell is 1 cm.

FIGURE 7.12 Schematic of a dynamical reflectivity measurement of a probe–target duplex in weak interaction (lower curve) and strong interactions (upper curve). In both cases, association and dissociation rates (k_a, k_d) can be measured as well as the reflectivity level before and after (Q_i, Q_f) rising, these last two quantities being proportional to the surface concentration of the target on the biochip at the time. Q_f can be very small and even undetectable if the duplex interaction is weak. However, using the dynamical information, the study of the interaction is still possible with the measurement of k_a and k_d.

7.2.2 Biochips for SPRI

SPRI biochips exhibit specific characteristics, compared to more conventional biochips using fluorescence measurements. In this section, we describe the specificities of biochips for SPRI, emphasizing the importance of surface functionalization on the efficiency of the SPRI signals. We then describe several functionalization strategies involving alkanethiols, a class of coupling agents commonly used for grafting biomolecular probes on gold supports. Our goal is to show the diversity of probes that can be grafted and the related chemical reactions used to bind them. We finally discuss two strategies in more details, involving dextran and cysteamine, as examples to illustrate mechanisms of gold chemical and biomolecular functionalization.

7.2.2.1 Specificities of Plasmonic Label-Free Biochip Surfaces

As pointed out in the precedent section, SPRI biochip systems exhibit two main characteristics, namely, label-free detection and kinetics analysis, presenting advantages as well as limitations compared to fluorescence biochips, as summarized in Table 7.3.

Indeed, the first interest of SPRI biochips lies in their ability to perform real-time detection of *nonlabeled* species. Labeling of biomolecules, that is, by fluorophores, classically involves costly reagents, additional time for labeling reaction, and loss of biomolecular targets due to purification following the labeling reaction. Moreover, in some cases, the recognition behavior of labeled biomolecules may be modified by the incorporated labels. SPRI biochips thus provide a way to avoid these limitations.

By comparison, fluorescence-based biochips involve end-point measurements and labeled targets. End-point measurements are of course simpler to analyze than kinetics data, but they also produce

TABLE 7.3 Comparison of SPRI and Fluorescence Biochips

Bioanalytical Tool	Characteristics	Advantages	Drawbacks
SPRI biochips	Label-free detection	No labeling step Biomolecular recognition not influenced by labels	Need for a close-to-perfect surface functionalization for correctly interpreting measurements
			Poor limit of detection compared to fluorescence
	Kinetics analysis	Access to dissociation and association rate constants	Needs a correct mixing during biomolecular recognition
		Real-time monitoring of biomolecular recognition	
Fluorescence biochips	Fluorescent labeling	Better inferior limit of detection than SPR Possibility to combine information from different labels (e.g., double-channel fluorescence for transcriptome analysis)	Fluorescent labels may modify biomolecular recognition Additional cost and time; loss of biological material due to final purification step
	End-point measurement	Access to dissociation constants using several concentrations of probes and targets (therefore needing more complex spotting)	No access to kinetic behavior No way to monitor if equilibrium is reached during the molecular recognition Depending on the implementation (e.g., single- or dual-channel fluorescence biochip), may need for correct mixing

far less information and do not give access easily to affinity constants between probes and targets [33–35]. Labeling targets, though involving drawbacks already cited, offer the possibility to combine several different labels. This allows to use internal reference during competitive assay, for instance, for transcriptome analysis biochips.

7.2.2.1.1 Importance of Surface Functionalization

Using nonlabeled species imposes an important constraint on SPRI systems: any molecule binding to the sensor surface may cause a variation in the measured ΔR output signal. Obtaining reflectivity variations accounting only for binding of targeted biomolecules implies to modify the metal surface in order to (1) maximize the binding of target molecules to the sensor surface and (2) prevent binding of any other molecules present in the biological sample to be analyzed (interfering molecules). This modification is usually performed in two steps named chemical and biological functionalizations.

Modifying the surface of the metal basically involves a change of the metallic chemical functions. This first operation, referred to as *chemical functionalization*, does not affect the bulk of the metal but only its surface. Chemical functionalization allows further modifications, usually aimed at grafting on the support biomolecules, that is, the biorecognition probes. The probes are chosen for their ability to specifically (as much as possible) bind the biomolecules to be detected, that is, analytes or targets. The so-called probe layer therefore consists of a layer of bioreceptors, which depending on applications can be such diverse as DNA and antibody and are deposited at operational, as defined later, concentrations.

Thus, SPR biosensors, like other classical affinity biosensors, are made of a bioreceptor layer aimed at specifically bound targets and a transducer converting the binding events into a physical signal.

7.2.2.1.2 Functionalized Surfaces and Nonspecific Adsorption

Figure 7.13 illustrates several key challenges associated with surface chemistry for biosensors.

Case a corresponds to an ideal situation, in which all the immobilized probes are available for binding targets. Furthermore, the biofunctionalized surface is fully covered by the probe, thus exhibiting no other site susceptible to cause nonspecific binding of interfering molecules from the biological sample. In this case, target molecules can be captured, while other biomolecules are repelled.

Case b introduces a probe layer including two types of probes: probes presenting a correct structure, which can bind the targets, and probes exhibiting some modification in their geometrical structure. These modifications lower the ability of the probes to correctly bind the targets, thus decreasing their biomolecular affinity (sometimes named *biological activity*). These defects can be caused by the steps involved in the chemical and/or biological functionalization. It can also be caused by interactions between the immobilized probes and the support. These defects can be either permanent or transient. This type of problem usually depends on the nature of the biomolecular probes. Nucleic acids are usually considered as robust and not easily degraded after immobilization—provided their anchorage is stable. On the contrary, proteins are commonly considered as fragile, being easily denatured. Among proteins, antibodies are certainly the most robust, while globular proteins' (e.g., enzymes) biological activity is easily degraded after immobilization on a support.

Case c corresponds to a loss of activity of the bioreceptor film, due to an incorrect orientation of some of the probes. This is directly related to the method used for immobilizing the probes. This case illustrates the compromise in choosing between the efficiency and the complexity of the immobilization method. The final balance has to be related to the specific biological application. For instance, if the target concentration of the biological samples is routinely particularly low compared to the limit of detection of the transducer, it is better to optimize the immobilization method, which of course involves additional complex steps. On the contrary, when inferior limit of detection is not a problem, because the targets are concentrated enough compared to the inferior limit of detection of the transducer, the immobilization steps can be simplified.

Case d illustrates a common case in which the sensor surface can either capture targets with probes through specific (i.e., expected) probe/target interactions or adsorb both targets and interfering molecules

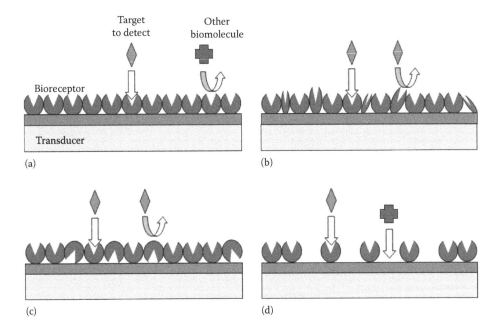

FIGURE 7.13 Four typical configurations for surface functionalization: (a) ideal case, the bioreceptor layer is highly specific (only the target can bind to it, while other biomolecules are repelled); all the probes are biologically active and they fully cover the transducer surface. (b) Because of the immobilization method and/or because of interactions with their direct environment, some molecular probes of the bioreceptor are not biologically active and cannot capture targets. (c) Some probes of the bioreceptor are not correctly oriented and are not available for capturing targets. (d) The surface exhibits both active probes and nonspecific binding sites.

on other sites, through nonexpected (thus named *nonspecific*) interactions. This decreases the specificity of the detection [36] and causes false-positive signals. In the case of biomolecules commonly encountered in affinity biosensors, nonspecific interactions between the surface and the molecules are related to physical bonds and the phenomenon of physical adsorption [37–39] and involve van der Waals forces (Table 7.4).

Specific biomolecular recognition may involve more various types of interactions [39–41] such as hydrophobic interactions (protein–target, for instance, antibody–antigen or protein–carbohydrates), π–π stacking (nucleic acids), and hydrogen bonding (nucleic acids; proteins). Cases b, c, and d may usually be de facto combined and yield surfaces with nonexplicit behavior.

TABLE 7.4 Different Types of Physical Interactions between Two Chemical or Biochemical Species

Interaction Type	Distance Dependence of Potential Energy	Typical Bond Energy (kJ/mol)
Ion–ion	$1/r$	250
Ion–dipole	$1/r^2$	15
Dipole–dipole	$1/r^{3a}$	2
	$1/r^{6b}$	0.6
	$1/r^{6c}$	2
Hydrogen bond	Contact	10–40

Source: After Atkins, P. and De Paula, J.D., eds., *Physical Chemistry*, W.H. Freeman and Co., New York, 2009, p. 630.

[a] Interactions between stationary dipoles.

[b] Interaction between rotating polar molecules.

[c] Interaction between all types of molecules.

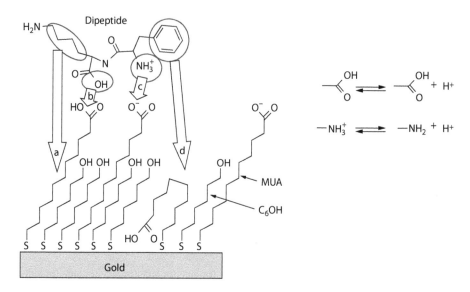

FIGURE 7.14 Diversity of physical interactions coexisting between a surface and a biomolecule. In this example, a dipeptide interacts with a gold support modified with MUA and C_6OH thiols, such as used in [45]. (a) van der Waals interactions between alkyl ($-CH_2-$) chains; (b) hydrogen bonding; (c) electrostatic bonding; (d) hydrophobic interaction. Depending on the pH of the medium, $-COOH$ and $-NH_2$ moieties can be protonated or deprotonated.

7.2.2.1.3 Nonspecific Adsorption Can Arise from Various Physical Interactions

The goal of surface functionalization is to provide a surface in which the interactions between probe and target are significantly more stable than nonspecific interactions. A difficulty arises from the fact that biomolecular targets usually bear a large diversity of functional groups, some being polar, apolar, charged, or neutral. Figure 7.14 shows an example of chemical bonds potentially involved between a dipeptide target (a molecule formed of two amino acids, constituents of proteins) and a gold support functionalized with a classical self-assembled monolayer (SAM) made of 1-mercapto-11-undecanoic acid (MUA) and 1-mercapto-6-hexanol (C6OH) [42–45].

In the given example, the mixed SAM is imperfect, since one MUA makes a hairpin. Considering that the dipeptide is in a solution buffered at pH 7, $-NH_2$ groups and $-COOH$ groups of the system are statistically charged. Some $-NH_2$ (pK_a #8.5) are protonated in their form NH_3^+, while some $-COOH$ (pK_a #4.7) are deprotonated in their form $-COO^-$. Additionally, the dipeptide exhibits functional groups susceptible to establish hydrophobic interactions and van der Waals interactions. Considering Table 7.4, one can see that the influence of each type of possible bond depends on its distance to the SAM groups. Nonspecific bindings of the dipeptide to the surface also depend on the temperature, since each type of bond involves a typical average energy. The more energetic a bond is, the more stable it stands at a given temperature. Hydrogen bonds are thus more stable than van der Waals forces, but less stable than electrostatic ion–ion interactions. Finally, one should not forget the fact that counterions present in the buffer solution have a screening effect on the biomolecule functional groups.

The presence of defects in a chemical layer can thus influence nonspecific binding of biomolecular species present in the solution to analyze with SPR.

7.2.2.1.4 Effects of Surface Functionalization on SPRI Measurements

Figure 7.15 shows three typical chronograms related to surface functionalization, in the simple case of the detection of one single type of target. In each chronogram, the black curve corresponds to the global signal measured versus time; the green curve corresponds to the contribution of binding targets; and the red curve corresponds to the contribution of other interfering biomolecules. In this

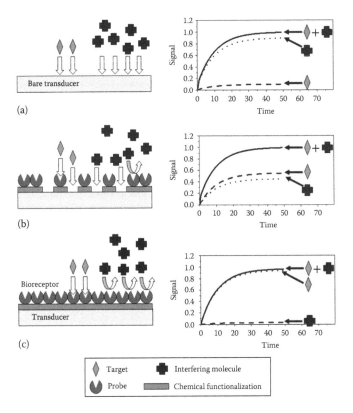

FIGURE 7.15 Influence of surface functionalization on the SPR biosensor signals. Right: chronograms give output signal versus time. Continuous lines: actual global output signal resulting from specific + non specific interactions. Dot lines: contribution of non specific binding to the signal. Dashed lines: contribution of specific binding to the signal. Left: corresponding typical bioreceptor structures. (a) bare gold, no surface functionalization; (b) intermediate case; and (c) most efficient surface functionalization.

example, the mass of each individual interfering biomolecule is considered as equivalent to the mass of a target molecule.

Figure 7.15 illustrates three different cases. (a) In the case of a transducer bearing no surface functionalization, any biomolecule (either the targets or other interfering species) binding to the surface causes a signal change. The sensor is fully nonspecific: each individual target and interfering molecule both yield equal contribution to the measured signal. Since interfering biomolecules are classically more concentrated than targets in the biological sample to be analyzed, the global signal mainly corresponds to false-positive contributions, that is, contribution which is actually not related to the target to be detected. (b) The sensor exhibits a bioreceptor layer that is not fully efficient. In this precise example, the metal layer is only partially covered by the chemical functionalization layer. Other defects may be involved. For instance, even if the metal layer is fully covered by the chemical functionalization layer, the bioreceptor layer coverage could be partial. Although probes can capture targets, some sites of the surface are available for nonspecific adsorption of both targets and interfering biomolecules. The overall signal, therefore, also includes a nonspecific contribution that prevents from a correct interpretation of the chronogram. (c) An ideal surface functionalization allows avoiding nonspecific binding of interfering species. The output signal thus corresponds only to the contribution of the binding targets. The biosensor is thus fully specific.

In SPRI biochips, different bioreceptor zones (each zone being composed of one type of probe) are implemented on the metal surface, in order to analyze in the same run different targets (Figure 7.16).

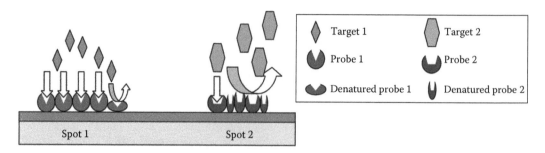

FIGURE 7.16   Heterogeneity of probes on a same support for SPRI. Spot 1 is composed of protein probes ("probe 1") mainly biologically active (i.e., not denatured). Protein targets can thus correctly bind to probes 1. On the contrary, spot 2 is made of probes 2 that are mainly denatured. Spot 2 thus exhibits a poor affinity toward the target 2. In a SPRI experiment, spot 1 will yield a signal change much higher than spot 2, even if targets 1 and 2 are present with the same concentration. In order to compare correctly the chronograms, it would be advantageous to evaluate relative densities of active probes of each spot.

In this case, an additional difficulty is to ensure that the behavior of each spot can actually be compared with the other spot behaviors. When working with nucleic acids, one can commonly use the same type of surface chemistry for all the probes. On the contrary, proteins exhibit various structures and do not behave equally on a given surface [33–35]. Protein probe behaviors thus need to be assessed before comparing output raw biosensor signals between spots.

Before detailing some specifics about the surface biofunctionalization, it is worth pointing out that, as a general comment, such biofunctionalization request is one of the toughest parts to master especially in a homogeneous manner across the biochip. Indeed, it is in our view the main cause of data dispersion. When great precision is needed, we have suggested and demonstrated the use of especially designed probes in order to be able to quantify and take into account the spatial ineluctable inhomogeneities [46]. The bases for such self-calibration method, detailed later in this chapter, are based on the use of multifunctional probes based on two *sensing* parts, one as explained before and the *extra* one, referred as calibration probe part, common to all probes. The use of a unique calibration target therefore allows quantifying the active probe concentration all over the biochip surface. As demonstrated in the genotyping section, this brings huge gain in spot-to-spot comparison precision and therefore releases some of the constraint of the biofunctionalization.

7.2.2.2 Surface Functionalization with Alkanethiols: Classical Steps and Bottlenecks

This section describes gold functionalization using alkanethiols, a widely used approach for modifying gold supports. Other approaches, for instance, polypyrrole functionalization, are also well known and would deserve more specific explanations [15,47–56]. Figure 7.17 summarizes indicative successive steps for gold functionalization using alkanethiols [57–64].

The implementation of a functionalized support using alkanethiol monolayer involves the following common steps: metal coating and reorganization, alkanethiol monolayer formation, optionally grafting of additional linkers/intermediate biomolecules, probe grafting, and capping/blocking of the surface.

7.2.2.2.1 Metal Coating and Reorganization

After a first washing step, a glass slide (a) is coated with an anchoring layer, followed by evaporation of a thin metal film, commonly gold (b). The anchoring layer is classically chromium or titanium dioxide. Mercaptosilanes can also be used [65]. The anchoring layer is aimed at optimizing adhesion of gold on the support. After evaporation, gold is immediately coated by carbonated particles or aerosol present in the atmosphere. It is nearly impossible to obtain a gold surface absolutely free from organic contamination, even in vacuum. The obtained gold support is amorphous, exhibiting a globular geometry that is not adapted for forming a correct and regular SAM. Gold surface can be reorganized in order to form

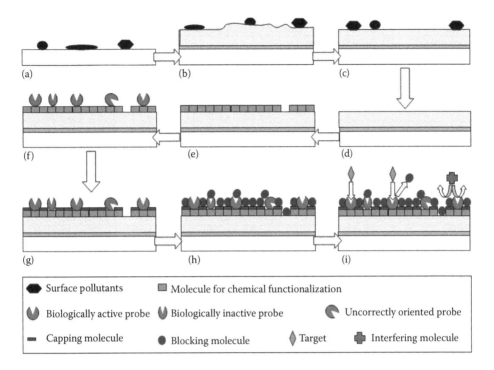

FIGURE 7.17 Common successive steps for implementing a SPRI biochip (a) glass support. (b) Anchoring layer (usually chromium) + gold thin film. (c) Metallic surface reorganization (e.g., by flaming). (d) Washing prior to functionalization. (e) Chemical functionalization. (f) Immobilization of probes. It should be followed by a washing prior to capping, in order to remove unbound probes. (g) Capping of chemical sites unreacted with probes. (h) Blocking by physisorption. (i) Biomolecular recognition with targets. Capping and blocking are critical steps for obtaining the best affinity behavior.

larger $\langle 100 \rangle$ crystallites terraces, more adapted for further surface functionalization (c) [45,57,66–75]. Annealing, electrochemical reorganization, and chemical treatments [57] are different ways to equalize the gold topography. However, these approaches are more adapted for 200 nm thickness gold films than for classical 48 nm thin films used for SPR, and they may damage SPR supports.

7.2.2.2.2 Alkanethiol Monolayer Formation

A washing step has to be performed to remove organic surface pollutants before chemical functionalization. Piranha solution ($H_2O_2 + H_2SO_4$) is classically used [57], although it may be too strong for some supports, depending on the adhesion of gold on the anchoring layer. UV/ozone may also be used for degrading organic pollutions. An alkanethiol monolayer can then be formed by self-assembly (e). The monolayer can be either pure or mixed that is composed of two alkanethiols. In this case, one, the alkanethiol, is used for further probe grafting (typically mercaptoundecanoic acid), while the other is chosen for limiting nonspecific adsorption (typically 1-mercaptohexanol) [45,57,76]. The quality of the metallic coating and the conditions of self-assembly can greatly influence the SAM compacity and coverage [57]. The interest of alkanethiols lies in the diversity of available functional groups. The choice of functional groups has to be made depending on the biomolecular probes to immobilize, as described in Table 7.5 [77–79].

7.2.2.2.3 Additional Linker or Intermediate Biomolecules

The alkanethiol monolayer can be modified following different pathways, depending on the biomolecular probes to be bound and the expected performances. When surface functional groups are carboxylic acids (a classical moiety), they have to be activated prior to probe grafting. A classical activation procedure is the

TABLE 7.5 General Examples of Typical Functional Groups Used to Bind Biomolecules onto Solid Supports

Surface Functional Group	Probe Functional Group	Notes	References
(a) –NH₂ Primary amine	HO—⟩=O—Protein Carboxylic acid	–NH₂ can be used for on-chip peptide and oligonucleotide direct synthesis. Carboxylic acid requires chemical activation. Amine can also bind isothiocyanate and aldehyde groups.	Boujday et al. [61–63], Calevro et al. [36], Haddour [144], and Spadavecchia et al. [91]
(b) –NH₃⁺ Protonated primary amine	⁻O—⟩=O—Protein Deprotonated carboxylic acid	Electrostatic interactions. Protonation/deprotonation depends on pH. –NH₃⁺ surface groups can also be used for binding nucleic acids or negatively charged polymers.	Bassil et al. [6] (protein) and Balladur et al. [145] (nucleic acids)
(c) O=⟨–OH Carboxylic acid	H₂N—protein Primary amine	Carboxylic acid –COOH requires chemical activation. It can be reacted with linkers containing –NH₂ groups. –NH₂ can also be incorporated into synthetic oligonucleotides (*amine linker*).	Bessueille et al. [94], Bras [146], Bres [147], Calevro [148], Dugas et al. [82], El Khoury et al. [86], Haddour [144], Li et al. [44], Wang et al. [150], Löfås and Johnsson [80], Manelli et al. [29], Mazurczyk et al. [95], Mosquet [151], Soultani-Vigneron et al. [81], and Tombelli et al. [99]
(d) Biotin	Streptavidin, neutravidin, extravidin	Very stable complex useful for binding probes in various configurations (nucleic acids, proteins, carbohydrates).	Bassil et al. [6], Cosnier et al. [152], Haddour [153], Hou et al. [101], Maalouf et al. [76], Manelli et al. [29], and Vidic [154]
(e) –OH Alcohol	Dilution function for nonspecific adsorption	Used as dilution function to lower nonspecific adsorption of proteins or nucleic acids. Also used for on-chip oligonucleotide synthesis.	Briand et al. [45], Briand [155], and Tielens et al. [64]
(f) –O⌒OH Ethylene glycol	Dilution function for nonspecific adsorption	Used as dilution function to lower nonspecific adsorption of proteins or nucleic acids. Also used for on-chip oligonucleotide synthesis.	Bres et al. [147], Cloarec et al. [77], and Li et al. [44]

Cited articles refer to either gold supports modified with alkanethiols, gold electrodes modified by pyrrole copolymerization, glass/silica supports modified with organosilanes, or carboxylatex dispersed supports. Once the first chemical functionalization has been performed, biological functionalization presented in these articles can be employed on gold supports for SPRI. Further details on reaction schemes are given in Löfås [78] and Hermanson [79].

NHS/EDC reaction [79–82]. Activated surfaces can then be used for direct probe grafting (f). Alternatively, surface groups such as primary amine or alcohol can be used for direct synthesis of oligomers [83–90]. This type of approach is more difficult to implement, but more versatile [77]. Instead of immobilizing probes, surface functional groups can first be modified by an additional linker. This linker both provides more degrees of freedom to the immobilized probes and allows adjusting surface properties in order to lower nonspecific adsorption. The linker can either be bifunctional (1,4-phenylenediisothyocyanate [PDC] [91], polyethyleneglycol [88–90,92], amino-polyethyleneglycol [93,94], Jeffamine [81,85,95], glutaraldehyde [63,96]) or polymeric (polyethylenimine [PEI] [6,96], dextran [29,80,97–99], MAMVE [86]). This linker is then used for binding the probe itself or an additional molecule itself used for binding the probe (avidin [63,91,98,100–102], protein A [63,96,103]). Table 7.5 summarizes some typical surface groups and chemical moieties available on proteins and nucleic acids. Further information is presented in [78,79]. Probes in excess have to be washed after the grafting step, in order to obtain a stable bioreceptor film [104].

7.2.2.2.4 Capping and Blocking

After probe immobilization, the surface has to be treated in order to prevent coupling of undesired molecules and to lower nonspecific adsorption. Two complementary processes, named herein *capping* and *blocking*, can be performed to modify the surface properties. We call *capping* a chemical deactivation of unreacted sites after probe grafting [45,77,80,84,85,98,105] (g). A capping reagent is usually a small molecule; it is used in excess compared to the surface groups, in order to ensure a high yield of deactivation. Ethanolamine is, for instance, a classical capping reagent for MUA-functionalized supports. Its amine reacts with activated ester of MUA, while its hydrophilic alcohol function tends to bind water and prevent protein adsorption.

We call herein *blocking* a preventive physisorption of biomolecular species, prior to analysis of samples containing the targets. These blocking molecules are used for binding to every site that may still interact with biomolecules through physical interactions. BSA, milk proteins, IgG, and Denhardt's reagent [36,77,101] are classical blocking molecules. BSA exhibits both hydrophobic and polar sites and is able to bind to a large diversity of supports (oxides, metals). It usually forms a monolayer that repels other proteins. The blocking reagent does not prevent probes to bind targets, because specific probe/ target interactions are usually far stronger than other nonspecific interactions.

Capping and blocking are key complementary steps that affect drastically the final behavior of the functionalized surface.

7.2.2.2.5 Examples of Surface Functionalization Pathways

We present herein examples of surface functionalization adapted for SPRI (Table 7.6 and Figure 7.18). The chosen examples illustrate the diversity of the possible functionalization strategies, for binding probes such as proteins, nucleic acids, and living cells. The methods are compared in terms of chemical functionalization time and needs for specific experimental setup. Three types of bioprobes are indicated: antibodies, living cells, and oligodeoxyribonucleotides (ODNs).

The most complex method of Table 7.6 uses dextran hydrogel. This functionalization takes at least 89 h and involves various chemical reactions. The protocol is long and complex but considerably lowers nonspecific adsorption for protein detection [105]. Moreover, this approach is compatible with another approach

TABLE 7.6 Examples of Functionalization Strategies

Surface Functionalization Strategy	Indicative Duration Time		Specific Experimental Setup for SPRI Biochip Manufacturing	References
	Initial Surface Functionalization	Probe Grafting		
(a) Alkanethiol SAM + dextran + antibodies	89 h	Spotting time	Surface chemistry setup; spotter	Löfås and Johnsson [80], Manelli et al. [29], and Tombelli et al. [99]
(b) Alkanethiol SAM + thiols + protein A + antibodies	26.5 h	1 h	Surface chemistry setup; spotter	Boujday et al. [61,63], Lu et al. [156], Babacan et al. [96], and Grubor et al. [103]
(c) Poly-lysine + cells	35 min	Cell culture	Surface chemistry setup; cell culture	Chabot et al. [16]
(d) Cysteamine + neutravidin + ODN	36 h	Spotting time	Surface chemistry setup; spotter	Spadavecchia et al. [91]
(e) Polypyrrole + ODN	10 min	Spotting time	Organic chemistry setup; surface chemistry setup; electrospotter	Livache et al. [51] and Descamps et al. [48]

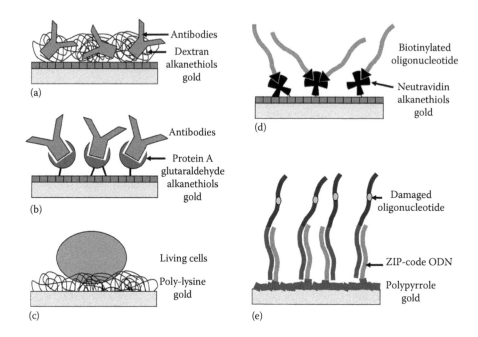

FIGURE 7.18 Examples of functionalization strategies. See Table 7.6 for details.

for binding antibodies using protein A [63]. This protein has the ability to bind Fc part of IgG and has been used in immunosensors. This approach requires less time and less complex implementation process.

More details about carboxydextran and cysteamine reaction pathways are given in the following, as described by [80,91].

7.2.2.2.6 Dextran Reaction Pathway

The described dextran pathway is used to immobilize proteins (such as antibodies), molecules rich in primary amines $-NH_2$. In the dextran functionalization approach proposed by Löfås and Johnsson [80], gold is firstly modified with 16-mercaptohexadecan-1-ol, forming a SAM making the surface hydrophilic (Figure 7.19A, left column). The alcohol moieties (–OH) react with the chloride groups –Cl of epichloro-hydrin molecules, in a mixture of sodium hydroxide and diglyme during 4 h at 25°C (Figure 7.19B). The epoxy functional group of epichlorohydrin can then react with a basic dextran solution (dextran T500) in sodium hydroxide during 20 h at 25°C. The dextran must then be converted to carboxymethyl-dextran by reaction with bromoacetic acid. Another possibility is to directly use a carboxymethyl-dextran for reacting with epoxy, as described in Figure 7.19c. Carboxy groups (–COOH) are intrinsically poorly reactive but can be activated using a N-ethyl-N'-(3-dimethylaminopropyl)carbodiimide hydrochloride (EDC) and N-hydroxysuccinimide (NHS) in water (Figure 7.19D). Activated esters can then react with primary amines ($-NH_2$) present in proteins such as antibodies (Figure 7.19E), forming amide groups (–CO–NH), for instance, in acetate buffer at pH 5. The nonreactive activated esters must be deactivated, for instance, by using ethanolamine hydrochloride at pH 8.5. The surface, implemented in about 90 h, is highly stable and can stand acidic and basic conditions.

7.2.2.2.7 Cysteamine Reaction Pathway

The cysteamine functionalization pathway proposed by Spadavecchia et al. [91] is described for immo-bilizing biotinylated oligonucleotide probes. The gold support is cleaned in a boiling aqueous H_2O_2/NH_3 solution, before being immersed in an unstirred 10 mM ethanolic solution of β-mercaptoethanolamine during 6 h (Figure 7.19A, right column). After washings, the support is treated with PDC in pyridine/dimethylformamide solution for 2 h (Figure 7.19B). PDC is a bifunctional linker reacting with primary

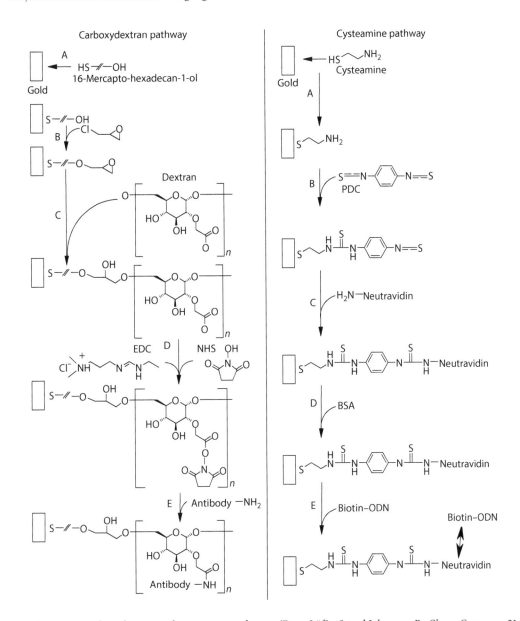

FIGURE 7.19 Carboxydextran and cysteamine pathways. (From Löfås, S. and Johnsson, B., *Chem. Commun.*, 21, 1526, 1990; Löfas, S. and Mcwhirter, A., The art of immobilization for SPR biosensors, *Surface Plasmon Resonance Based Biosensors*, Springer Series on Chemical Sensors and Biosensors 2006, vol. 4, Springer, Berlin, Germany, pp. 117–151, 2006; Spadavecchia, J. et al., *Sens. Actuat. B Chem.*, 143(1), 139, 2009.)

amines. Neutravidin, a globular protein bearing primary amines on its external envelop, is then reacted during 40 min with PDC available isothiocyanate groups (Figure 7.19C). Since primary amines exhibit a pK_a of approximately 8.5 in aqueous solution, it is adapted to perform the reaction at a pH above 8.5 to ensure that neutravidin $-NH_2$ groups are not protonated. The nonreacted isothiocyanate groups are then reacted with BSA (Figure 7.19D). This blocks the surface, preventing any chemical reaction or physical adsorption of the targets on the surface. Biotinylated probes can then interact with the neutravidin surface (Figure 7.19E) in PBS (pH 7.2). Since the interaction between biotin and neutravidin is particularly strong, BSA molecules potentially adsorbed on neutravidins cannot prevent the neutravidin/biotin interaction.

Alternatively, the cysteamine pathway can be modified for binding NH_2-containing molecules, for instance, proteins or oligonucleotides bearing a terminal $-NH_2$ group (aminolink); the other $-NH_2$ groups of nucleotides are less accessible because, for instance, of steric hindrance. Binding proteins or aminolink-modified oligonucleotides only require replacing the neutravidins with the desired $-NH_2$-rich molecule in step C. Blocking step D is then performed, while step E is discarded.

The cysteamine approach requires 36 h for binding probes, which is approximately 3 times shorter than the dextran approach. It yields a surface standing easily basic solutions (e.g., 0.5 mM NaOH solution), but not acidic media.

7.2.2.2.8 SPRI Biochip Conclusion

SPRI biochips have to be chemically and biologically functionalized in order to ensure a specific and efficient capture of biomolecular targets yielding change of reflectivity of the SPRI transducer. Surface functionalization relies on chemical modification (covalent binding) and physical interactions (physisorption). The blocking step is important to reduce nonspecific interactions between probes and interfering species present in the medium to be analyzed. Duration, complexity, and performances of some protocols have been described to show that a wide variety of protocols can be adapted to different system needs and applications.

7.2.3 Microfluidics

To design reliable miniaturized biosensors, it is critical to understand certain fundamental concepts in surface chemistry kinetics and microfluidics. In this section, we discuss basic, but highly useful models of kinetics and key concepts in fluid flow and molecular diffusion, which are unfortunately too often overlooked. The reader is strongly encouraged to consult review articles from [106] on microfluidics and the series of papers by Rich and Myszka such as [107] on good practices in biosensing experimental design and measurement, from which this section is heavily inspired.

7.2.3.1 Binding Kinetics

7.2.3.1.1 Single Probe/Target Binding Kinetics

In the simplest case of probe/target binding kinetics, there is a single species of target in solution and a single probe species immobilized on a flat surface with homogeneous surface coverage (Figure 7.20). Each target molecule is either free in solution or bound to a single probe molecule on the surface, in a *target + probe* complex.

Once binding has occurred, the target + probe complexes remain bound for a certain amount of time before dissociating. In such single probe/target binding kinetics, the following two parameters can be defined, where the square brackets "[]" indicate bulk concentration in the case of the targets and surface density in the case of the probes and probe–target complexes (see Table 7.7 for model parameter units):

The *rate of association* of target + probe complexes is equal to [target] × [probe] × k_a, where k_a is the *association rate* constant (note that "[probe]" indicates the *unbound* probe surface density).

The *rate of dissociation* of the target + probe complexes is equal to [target + probe] × k_d, where k_d is the *dissociation rate* constant.

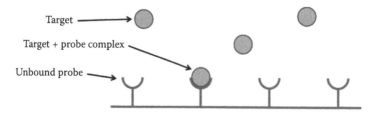

FIGURE 7.20   Single probe/target binding kinetics.

TABLE 7.7 Single Probe/Target Binding Kinetics Model Parameters

Name	Symbol	Units
Association rate constant	k_a	$M^{-1} s^{-1}$
Dissociation rate constant	k_d	s^{-1}
Equilibrium dissociation constant	K_D	M

Equilibrium is reached when the rate at which new target + probe complexes are formed equals the rate at which existing complexes dissociate. At equilibrium, therefore,

$$[\text{Target}] \times [\text{Probe}] \times k_a = [\text{Target} + \text{Probe}] \times k_d$$

Rearranging, the *equilibrium dissociation constant*, K_D, is defined as

$$\frac{[\text{Probe}][\text{Target}]}{[\text{Probe} + \text{Target}]} = \frac{k_d}{k_a} = K_D \tag{7.9}$$

K_D has a clear physical meaning. By setting [target] equal to K_D in (7.9), the K_D terms cancel out and we are left with [probe] = [target + probe], that is, the surface densities of bound and unbound probes are *equal*. In other words, when the bulk concentration of targets in solution equals K_D, half the probes on the surface will be occupied at equilibrium.

If the probe has a *high* affinity for the target, K_D will be *low*, as it will take a low concentration of targets to bind to half the probes. Table 7.8 shows the fractional probe occupancy (percentage of probes bound to targets) as a function of target concentration, expressed in multiples of K_D.

7.2.3.1.2 Langmuir Isotherm

The aforementioned relationships are best expressed mathematically, using the following variable definitions:

$B(t)$ = surface density of *bound* probes
R_T = total surface density of probes (bound + unbound)
C_0 = bulk concentration of (unbound) targets in solution

The following equations express the kinetics of single probe/target binding:
Rate of association of probes:

$$\frac{dB(t)}{dt} = k_a(R_T - B(t))C_0 \tag{7.10}$$

TABLE 7.8 Fractional Probe Occupancy as a Function of Target Concentration

Target	Fractional Probe Occupancy (%)
0	0
$0.01\ K_D$	1
$0.1\ K_D$	9
$0.5\ K_D$	33
K_D	50
$4\ K_D$	80
$9\ K_D$	90
$99\ K_D$	99

Rate of dissociation of probes:

$$\frac{dB(t)}{dt} = k_d B(t) \tag{7.11}$$

Rate of change of bound probe surface density:

$$\frac{dB(t)}{dt} = k_a (R_T - B(t))C_0 - k_d B(t) \tag{7.12}$$

Solving (7.12) with null initial conditions ($B = 0$ at time $t = 0$) yields the *Langmuir isotherm* kinetics model in the three unknowns, R_T, k_a, and k_d:

$$\frac{B(t)}{R_T} = \frac{k_a C_0}{k_a C_0 + k_d}[1 - e^{-(k_a C_0 + k_d)t}] \tag{7.13}$$

By considering the limiting behavior of the model at key points, the dynamics of the model are revealed. In the case of association (adsorption), by replacing the exponential with the first two terms of a Taylor series expansion of the exponential about 0 ($e^x \sim 1 + x$), the behavior at $t = 0^+$ reduces to the following linear relationship:

$$\left.\frac{B(t)}{R_T}\right|_{t=0+} = (k_a C_0)t \tag{7.14}$$

Similarly, the behavior at $t = \infty$ tends asymptotically toward a constant plateau:

$$\left.\frac{B(t)}{R_T}\right|_{t=\infty} = \frac{k_a C_0}{k_a C_0 + k_d} \tag{7.15}$$

Equations 7.14 and 7.15 are shown graphically in Figure 7.21.

In the case of dissociation (desorption) following rising with the buffer solution ($C_0 = 0$), the limiting behavior is also linear and can be deduced by solving (7.11) with the appropriate initial conditions (7.15), followed with a Taylor approximation for the exponential about $t = t_a$ (see Figure 7.21):

$$\left.\frac{B(t)}{R_T}\right|_{t=t_a+} \approx \left(\frac{k_a c_0}{k_a C_0 + k_d}\right)\{1 - k_d(t - t_a)\} \tag{7.16}$$

7.2.3.1.3 Fitting Reaction-Limited Kinetics to the Langmuir Model

The Langmuir model assumes that the bulk concentration of targets in solution, C_0, is constant, that is, there is an infinite supply of targets in solution and they reach the probes on the surface infinitely fast—this is referred to as *reaction-limited* kinetics. In most practical situations, however, chemical reactions are sufficiently fast to consume targets more rapidly that they can be replenished locally by diffusion—this situation is referred to as *mass-transport-limited* kinetics and will be detailed further, emphasizing the importance of the actual microfluidic conditions in a dynamical biochip system.

In the Langmuir model, the unknown parameters (probe density, R_T, and parameters, k_a, k_d) can be determined from a numerical fit to a set of kinetic-response curves (association/dissociation)

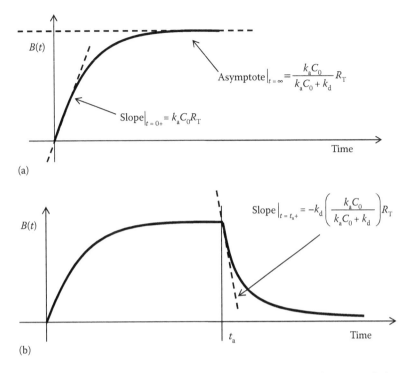

(a)

(b)

FIGURE 7.21 (a) Limiting behavior of the Langmuir isotherm for association (adsorption); (b) limiting behavior of the Langmuir isotherm for dissociation (desorption).

measured on the same sample. The association curves in a set are measured at different target concentrations ($C_{01}...C_{05}$ in Figure 7.22 interspaced by dissociation curves resulting from a rinse with buffer solution). Figure 7.22 shows two sets of association/dissociation curves, where the respective measurements at the different target concentrations are overlaid, having been aligned to the same starting point in time.

In a reaction-limited situation, kinetics are *independent of probe surface density.* Hence, once normalized to their respective maximum asymptote values (the plateaus at equilibrium for the C_{05} curves in sets

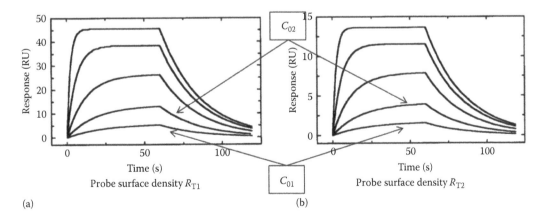

(a)

(b)

FIGURE 7.22 Langmuir model fits to reaction-limited kinetics measured with SPR. The individual curves at corresponding target concentrations in sets a and b have a one-to-one correspondence between them at the two different probe surface densities, R_{T1} and R_{T2}. (From Myszka, D.G. et al., *Biophys. J.*, 75(2), 583, 1998.)

a and b), curves taken at a particular target concentration are *identical* across different probe surface coverage densities (R_{T1} and R_{T2} in Figure 7.22).

The Langmuir model assumes the following conditions:

- All probes are equally accessible to targets.
- Probes are either free or bound to targets. The model does not allow for more than one affinity state or states of partial binding.
- Binding does not alter the target or probe.
- The bulk concentration of targets in solution, C_0, is constant.

BUT: The last condition is rarely fulfilled in practice, unless the reaction is sufficiently slow and the bulk target concentration and diffusion speed are sufficiently high to ensure reaction-limited kinetics. As stated earlier, if $C_0 \neq$ constant, the system is mass-transport-limited and *the kinetics do not follow the Langmuir model.*

7.2.3.1.4 Mass-Limited Transport: The Two-Compartment Model

The *two-compartment* model takes into account the effect of the finite diffusion speed of target molecules in the fluid. The following discussion describing the two-compartment model is heavily inspired by [108]—the reader is referred to this publication for additional details.

In the two-compartment model, the fluid volume is split into an (large) outer compartment with *constant* target concentration, C_T, and an (thin) inner compartment with *variable* target concentration, $C(t)$; see Figure 7.23. The two-compartment model includes a third parameter, k_M, which is the transport coefficient describing the diffusive movement of targets between the two compartments.

The two-compartment model is governed by the following two equations, where h_i is the height of the inner compartment:

$$\frac{dC(t)}{dt} = \{-k_a C(t)(R_T - B(t)) + k_d B(t) + k_M (C_T - C(t))\}\frac{1}{h_i} \tag{7.17}$$

$$\frac{dB(t)}{dt} = k_a (R_T - B(t))C(t) - k_d B(t) \tag{7.18}$$

Equation 7.18 is identical to the Langmuir model (7.12), except that the target concentration above the sensor, $C(t)$, is *variable* in time and given by Equation 7.17. If conditions are such that binding occurs over periods longer than a few seconds, it can be shown that, after a brief transient, the target concentration in the inner compartment, C, can effectively be considered constant [108]. In the steady-state approximation ($dC/dt = 0$), (7.17) yields an expression for $B(t)$ that is independent of the height of the inner compartment, h_i. Inserting this expression for $B(t)$ into (7.18), Equation 7.19 is obtained, where

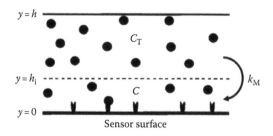

FIGURE 7.23 The two-compartment model. (From Myszka, D.G. et al., *Biophys. J.*, 75(2), 583, 1998.)

the rate constants, k_a and k_d, of the Langmuir model have been replaced with the effective rate constants, k_a' and k_d' [109]. The following must be solved numerically:

$$\frac{dB(t)}{dt} = k_a'(R_T - B(t))C_T - k_d'B(t) \tag{7.19}$$

where,

$$k_a' = \frac{k_M k_a}{k_M + k_a(R_T - B(t))} \quad \text{and} \quad k_d' = \frac{k_M k_d}{k_M + k_a(R_T - B(t))}$$

Note that in the case where the forward reaction rate $(k_a R_T)$ is slow compared to the rate of diffusive movement of analytes between the compartments, that is, $(k_a R_T) \ll k_M$, the effective rate constants, k_a' and k_d', reduce to the true rate constants, k_a and k_d, and (7.19) simplifies to the Langmuir model (7.12).

7.2.3.1.5 Model Fitting to Mass-Transport-Limited Kinetics

SPR measurements from two mass-transport-limited experiments are shown in Figure 7.24. As seen in (a) and (b), the Langmuir model (red lines) fits mass-transport-limited data (black lines) poorly, whereas the two-compartment model shows a good fit to the data from the two experiments (c) and (d). Furthermore, under mass-transport-limited conditions, kinetics are not independent of probe surface coverage density. Hence, normalized kinetic curve sets taken at identical target concentrations change with probe surface coverage density, that is, though the individual curves in sets (c) and (d) have a one-to-one correspondence in terms of target concentration, their shapes are different. This property is an *excellent test to ascertain whether the data are mass-transport-limited or not.*

In the following sections, the phenomena in fluid mechanics that are particularly relevant to microfluidics in relation to surface-based biosensing are discussed. In particular, the importance of certain key dimensionless numbers used in fluid mechanics to describe physical behavior independently of scale is described.

7.2.3.2 Fluidic Regimes

7.2.3.2.1 Reynolds Number (Re): Inertial versus Viscous Forces in Flow

An important dimensionless parameter in microfluidics is the *Reynolds number*, which expresses the relative importance of viscous forces to inertial forces in fluid flow.

> *If inertial forces dominate*: The motion of individual particles is governed by their mass and speed—past history, that is, conservation of momentum, plays a dominant role in determining individual particle motion at a given time. Flow is more chaotic.
> *If viscous forces dominate*: Instantaneous particle motion is governed by the relationship to the immediate surroundings (drag, *stickiness* to neighbors and surfaces)—the past history of individual particles plays a much lesser role. Flow is smoother.

The Reynolds number, *Re*, is defined as

$$Re = \frac{\text{Inertial forces}}{\text{Viscous forces}} = \frac{\text{Length scale} \times \text{Density} \times \text{Speed}}{\text{Viscosity}} \tag{7.20}$$

The flow is considered

- *Laminar* when $Re < 2300$ (viscous forces dominate)
- *Transient* when $2300 < Re < 4000$
- *Turbulent* when $4000 < Re$ (inertial forces dominate)

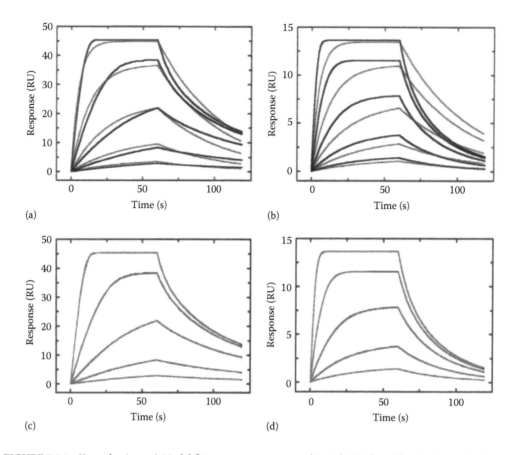

FIGURE 7.24 **(See color insert.)** Model fitting to mass-transport-limited SPR data. The data for probe density R_{T1} in (a) and (c) and density R_{T2} in (b) and (d) are shown in black—the model fits are shown in red. Langmuir fits to the data are shown in (a) and (b), and two-compartment model fits to the same data are shown in (c) and (d). Because reactions were mass-transport-limited, the curves having a one-to-one correspondence (same target concentration) between sets have different shapes, unlike in Figure 7.22. As seen in (a) and (b), the Langmuir model fits mass-transport-limited data poorly. Since, at equal target concentration, equilibrium is reached faster for a lower probe density, it follows that $R_{T1} > R_{T2}$. (From Myszka, D.G. et al., *Biophys. J.*, 75(2), 583, 1998.)

In microfluidics, flow is generally *laminar* ($Re \ll 100$ typically, with $Re < 1$ in many cases). In the context of a surface-based sensing in a microfluidic channel, the Reynolds number is very useful in understanding the mechanisms of target transport to the probes on the sensing surface.

   In turbulent flow, target supply to the surface is replenished by *convection* (transport of particles by the fluid); self-mixing is sufficient to maintain a constant target concentration, C_0, throughout the fluid volume.

   In laminar flow, fluid moves straight through the microfluidic channel with little or no lateral movement. The innermost parts of the fluid flow the fastest, and the fluid touching the channel walls is static, resulting in a *parabolic* velocity profile, or *Poiseuille* flow, as shown in Figure 7.25.

Since flow is generally laminar in microfluidics, there is little or no transport of target molecules by self-mixing in the fluid—target molecules rely solely on diffusion to migrate perpendicularly to the direction of fluid flow toward the sensing surface. Consequently, as targets are consumed by the probes on the

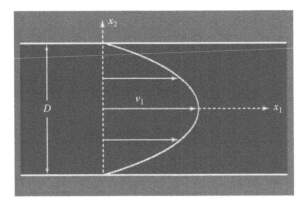

FIGURE 7.25 Parabolic flow profile. (From Squires, T.M. et al., *Nat. Biotechnol.*, 26(4), 417, 2008.)

sensing surface, the target supply in the immediate neighborhood of the surface may not be efficiently replenished, thus resulting in mass-transport-limited kinetics (see following section).

7.2.3.2.2 Péclet Number (Pe_H): Convection versus Diffusion in Mass Transport

The Péclet number is a second useful dimensionless parameter expressing the relative importance of mass transport by diffusion versus convection in a fluid. The Péclet number can be expressed as the ratio between the time, Δt_{conv}, taken by a target to move a given distance by convection and the time, Δt_{diff}, taken by the target to diffuse that same distance. The Péclet number, Pe_H, is defined as

$$Pe_H = \frac{\Delta t_{diff}}{\Delta t_{conv}} = \frac{Q}{DW} \tag{7.21}$$

where
   Q is the volumetric flow rate
   D is the diffusivity (diffusion coefficient) of the target molecules in the fluid
   W is the channel width (see Figure 7.26)

When convection is much faster than diffusion ($Pe_H \gg 1$), flow is considered *fast*, which is generally the case in microfluidics.

In the context of targets in solution and surface-immobilized probes in a microfluidic channel, the combination of a low Reynolds number (laminar flow) and a high Péclet number (fast flow) leads to the following: (1) because flow is laminar, targets are carried by the fluid along mainly linear trajectories down the length of the channel, with any lateral movement toward the sensing surface due to diffusion only, and (2) transport by the fluid is so fast relative to diffusion that most targets are transported down the channel without having sufficient time to diffuse down to the sensing surface.

In this case, a *depletion zone* forms above the sensing surface where targets are consumed by the probes faster than they can be replenished (Figure 7.26). The depletion zone *thickness* is defined as the height above the sensing surface where target replenishment by convection exactly balances consumption by diffusion to the sensing surface. The depletion zone thickness is typically less than 1 µm in microfluidic biosensing systems.

For a sensor in a microchannel with dimension defined as in Figure 7.26, the target diffusive flux, F, through the depletion zone and the depletion zone thickness, δ, are [106]

$$F \approx O\left\{\left(\frac{L_s}{H}\right)^{2/3}\left(\frac{Q}{DW}\right)^{1/3}\right\} \approx O\left\{\left(\frac{L_s}{H}\right)^{2/3}(Pe_H)^{1/3}\right\} \tag{7.22}$$

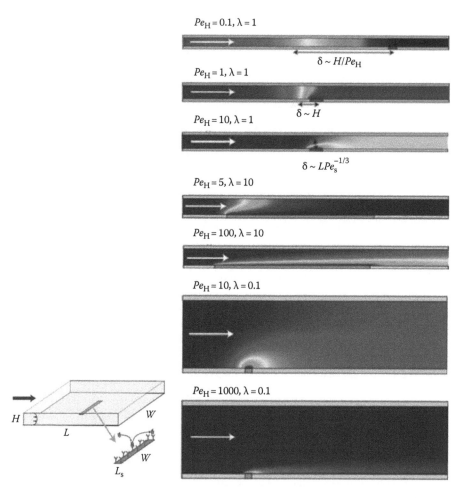

FIGURE 7.26 **(See color insert.)** (a) Strip biosensor (dimensions, $L_s \times W$) in a microfluidic channel; (b) depletion zone profile as a function of Pe_H (blue, low target concentration; red, high concentration). Sensor length, L_s, is shown in green; λ is the ratio of sensor length to channel height (L/H). (From Squires, T.M. et al., *Nat. Biotechnol.*, 26(4), 417, 2008.)

$$\delta \approx O\left\{\left(\frac{L_s W H^2 D}{Q}\right)^{1/3}\right\} \approx O\left\{\left(\frac{L_s H^2}{Pe_H}\right)^{1/3}\right\} \tag{7.23}$$

where the fluid of viscosity, μ, in *thin* ($H \ll W$) rectangular cross-sectional channel under a pressure differential, ΔP, will have a volumetric flow rate, Q, defined as

$$Q = \frac{WH^3}{12\mu}\left(\frac{\Delta P}{L}\right) \tag{7.24}$$

Under these circumstances (thin rectangular cross-sectional channel), (7.23) shows that an increase in volumetric flow rate, Q, reduces the thickness, δ, of the depletion zone via an accentuation of the parabolic profile (Figure 7.26), thereby decreasing the distance over which freshly supplied targets in the fluid must diffuse to the sensing surface. However, (7.22) indicates that the mass transport diffusive flux, F, to the surface varies only weakly with flow rate. Indeed, the volumetric flow rate must be increased by 10^3 to enhance the diffusive flux by 10×, resulting in greatly reduced target capture efficacy. Simply increasing flow rate, therefore, is a very inefficient method of increasing target diffusive flux to the sensor.

A final important situation to consider is the complete absence of flow, for example, in a microwell. Diffusive flux is proportional to the concentration gradient, that is, the target concentration difference divided by distance ($\sim C_0/\delta$, assuming zero concentration at the sensor surface). As the depletion zone thickness, δ, increases, the diffusive flux gets ever smaller, and collection ever slower. Hence, in the absence of flow, *steady state is never reached in 2D systems*. Note, however, that this result is specific to 1D and 2D systems. Sensors whose size is limited in all three dimensions do reach steady state—for example, spherical beads or microarray spots.

7.2.3.2.3 Damkohler Number (D_a): Mass-Transport-Limited versus Reaction-Limited Kinetics

The Damkohler number, D_a, is the third very useful dimensionless parameter that expresses the relative importance of the *reactive* flux (rate of targets consumed by the probes on the sensor surface per unit area) to the *diffusive* flux (rate of targets supplied by diffusion to the sensor per unit area). The Damkohler number is defined as

$$D_a = \frac{\text{Reactive flux}}{\text{Diffusive flux}} = \frac{k_a R_T \delta}{D} \tag{7.25}$$

If $D_a \ll 1$, the chemical reaction is *slow* and the system is reaction-limited. Diffusive flux maintains a constant concentration of free targets, C_0, in solution close to the surface. The Langmuir model is applicable.

If $D_a \gg 1$, the chemical reaction is *fast* and the system is mass-transport-limited. The Langmuir model is *not* applicable.

Note, however, that D_a is a function of the probe surface concentration, R_T, which is not always known with precision a priori.

7.2.3.3 Other Implications on Experiments

7.2.3.3.1 Time to Equilibrium

We now consider the time taken for the chemical reaction to reach equilibrium. Equation 7.13 can be rewritten slightly by replacing the term $1/(k_a C_0 + k_d)$ in the exponential by a characteristic time constant, τ_R:

$$\frac{B(t)}{R_T} = \frac{k_a C_0}{k_a C_0 + k_d}[1 - e^{-(k_a C_0 + k_d)t}] = \frac{k_a C_0}{k_a C_0 + k_d}[1 - e^{-t/\tau_R}] \tag{7.26}$$

In the *reaction-limited* case ($D_a \ll 1$), $\tau_R = (k_d + k_a C_0)^{-1} = k_d^{-1}(1 + C_0/K_D)^{-1}$, two cases arise:

In *dilute conditions* ($C_0 \ll K_D$), the characteristic time constant is a function of the *dissociation* rate constant:

$$\tau_R = k_d^{-1} \tag{7.27}$$

In *concentrated conditions* ($C_0 \gg K_D$), the characteristic time constant is a function of the *association* rate constant:

$$\tau_R = (k_a C_0)^{-1} \tag{7.28}$$

In the *mass-transport-limited* case ($D_a \gg 1$), which is most often encountered in the context of surface-based biosensing in a microfluidic channel, the characteristic time constant, τ_{CRD}, is equal to the reaction-limited time constant *scaled by the Damkohler number* [106]:

$$\tau_{CRD} \approx \tau_R D_a \tag{7.29}$$

7.2.3.3.2 How Much Material Is Needed to Bind at Least One Target to the Surface?

This question is especially important nowadays with so many results targeting ever more sensitive assays. If a target concentration, K_D, yields 50% probe occupancy, what must be the target concentration, C^*, to ensure that at least one target molecule is bound on average at all times to a sensor of surface of area, A, and probe density, R_T? The answer, derived in [106], is

$$C^* = \frac{K_D}{R_T A} \tag{7.30}$$

As an example, assuming an (optimal) antibody binding affinity of $K_D = 1$ nM and a (relatively high) surface binding site density of $R_T = 2 \times 10^{12}$ cm^{-2},

For a 50 μm × 50 μm microsensor, $C^* = 20 \times 10^{-18}$ M
For a 2 μm × 10 nm nanowire, $C^* = 10^{-12}$ M

Therefore, larger surface-area sensors have potentially lower detection limits, and decisions to miniaturize a device must be made carefully.

7.2.3.4 Target Homogenization

7.2.3.4.1 Microfluidic Mixing

A low Reynolds number means that flow is laminar with no turbulence to intermix the fluid strata in the microfluidic channel. Flow is fastest down the center of the channel and very slow close the surface (parabolic profile). A high Péclet number means that increasing flow rate has little effect on target diffusive flux (mass transport) to the sensing surface and increasing flow rate causes an even greater proportion of targets to be flushed down the channel without ever having a chance to come into contact with the sensing surface. Though recirculation eliminates target waste, capture efficacy and time to equilibrium are unchanged. In the low Reynolds and high Péclet number regime, the time scales for diffusive mixing of biomolecules can be extremely slow—for example, the time to equilibrium for a typical DNA hybridization assay can be in the order of 10^5 s [110].

In addition to speed, the sensitivity of a biosensor is also affected by the lack of adequate mixing. Indeed, the two-compartment model will fit the data poorly when there is too high a difference (over 10× according to [111]) between the rate at which targets diffuse to the sensing surface and the rate at which they are consumed by the assay (large Damkohler numbers). If diffusion is too slow, a *fast* reaction will appear to be instantaneous, and poor estimates of the $k_a R_T$ product will result. Mass-transport flux therefore effectively sets an upper limit on the reaction speeds and/or surface density of probes that can be estimated. Consequently, the range of measurable rate constants under mass-transport-limiting conditions could be extended in direct proportion to increasing the rate of mass transport to the surface [111].

As a result, extensive research has been devoted to microfluidic mixing in order to both increase the speed and improve the sensitivity of biosensors in microfluidic devices [112].

Figure 7.27 presents an interesting graph of publications as a function of Péclet number versus Reynolds number.

7.2.3.4.2 Coupled SPR Biosensing and SAW-Induced Mixing

Surface acoustic waves (SAWs) are mechanical oscillations that propagate on the surface of a material. They can be generated with interdigited transducers (IDTs) fabricated using thin-film metal deposition

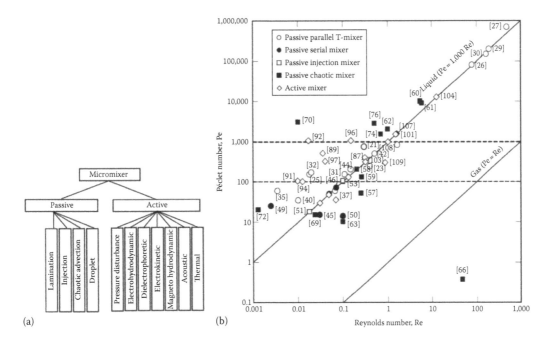

FIGURE 7.27 Micromixing technologies. (a) Mixing types; (b) graph of micromixing publications as a function of Péclet number versus Reynolds number. (From Nguyen, N.T. and Wu, Z.G., *J. Micromech. Microeng.*, 15(2), R1, 2005.)

on a piezoelectric substrate. Shear-vertical (Rayleigh) SAWs deform the substrate in the direction normal to the surface and transmit mechanical energy onto the fluid both by deformation of the surface and via the electric field, inducing turbulent flow within the fluid with *acoustic streaming* [113]. SAWs have proven very effective for microfluidic mixing in the context of biosensing [114].

We have developed a device combining biosensing via SPR and micromixing via SAW on a single platform [115]. Since both the SPR sensor and SAW transducer can be fabricated using low-cost microfabrication methods simultaneously on a single substrate, the design is well suited to chip-based biosensing applications. As an added bonus, high-intensity SAW has been shown to reduce and/or remove molecules nonspecifically bound to the surface, thereby increasing the measurement signal-to-noise ratio [116,117]. Figure 7.28 shows a schematic diagram of the device with the SPR sensing surface and IDT electrodes on the common $LiNbO_3$ piezoelectric substrate. The IDT electrodes and SPR sensing surface were fabricated from 48 nm thick Au thin films with a 3 nm thick Cr adhesion layer.

Figure 7.29 illustrates the performance of the SPR/SAW chip for measuring assay binding kinetics. SPR reflectance variations are shown as a function of time at a fixed angle of interrogation for a standard assay: biotin–avidin in PBS. Starting at the time of avidin introduction (time = 0 in the graphs), SAW excitation was applied in 5 s duration pulses followed by 120 s relaxation intervals, for a range of SAW power levels (27, 30, and 36 dBm). These experiments show that SAW action results in accelerated kinetics due to microfluidic mixing (~5× compared to the negative control for these particular experiments). Experiments performed with higher SAW power levels resulted in curves with an envelope that was identical to that of the 36 dBm curve, indicating that the chip had achieved a maximum mixing efficiency for that particular SAW/SPR design. Power levels of 30 and 27 dBm also resulted in accelerated kinetics but with intermediate levels of mixing efficiency.

The downward spikes in the SPR signal visible in the 36 dBm data are due to parasitic heat injection into the fluid by the SAW pulses, since the refractive index of the fluid changes with temperature (in the case of water, there is a 10^{-5} refractive index unit (RIU) refractive index change for every 0.1°C of temperature

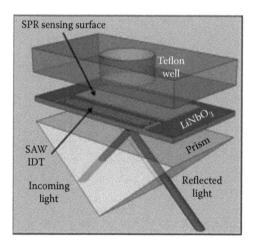

FIGURE 7.28 Schematic diagram showing the SPR sensing surface and IDT SAW electrodes on a common LiNbO₃ piezoelectric substrate. Also shown are the SPR excitation and reflected light paths that are coupled to the sensing surface via the prism, as well as the microfluidic well atop the SPR sensing surface.

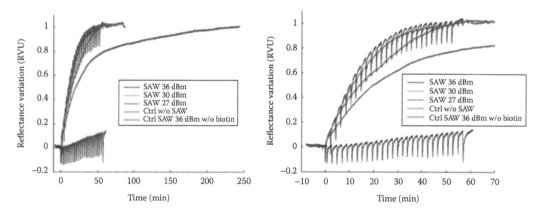

FIGURE 7.29 SPR reflectance variations at a fixed angle of interrogation as a function of time for a biotin–avidin assay in PBS (zoomed view on the right). Periodic SAW excitation was applied in 5 s duration pulses followed by 120 s relaxation intervals, for a range of SAW power levels (27, 30, and 36 dBm). A negative control without the application of SAW in the avidin–biotin assay is shown (*Ctrl w/o SAW*). A second negative control where unbiotinylated BSA was adsorbed onto the surface followed by injection of avidin under 36 dBm SAW is also shown (*Ctrl SAW 36 dBm w/o biotin*). The downward spikes visible in the 36 dBm data are due to parasitic heat injection into the fluid by the SAW pulses. Results are given in reflectance variation units (RVUs), where 1 RVU equals 100% reflectance change. (From Charette, P.G. et al., *Lab Chip*, 10(1), 111, 2010.)

change, an easy measurement signal for SPR). The results also demonstrate that the chip nevertheless recovers well from the heat injection pulses with the binding curve maintaining an exponential envelope, as expected for this type of assay.

7.2.4 Modeling and Data Processing

7.2.4.1 Thin-Film Modeling for Sensitivity Calculations

Reflectance, R, from a layered structure can be calculated with the Fresnel equations either using the transfer matrix method [118] or the Rouard method modified for complex refractive indices [119,120]. Note that the Rouard method yields faster computations because of the recursive nature of the algorithm.

However, since there is no analytical solution for multilayered structures such as SPR chip, the equation must be evaluated numerically either using the full rigorous expression based on the Fresnel equations or using the often-quoted Lorentzian approximation about resonance [17]. Alternatively, approximations with simpler models such as [20], yield good results within a scale factor for most metals.

7.2.4.2 Signal Processing of SPR Measurement Results

Most existing SPR systems are based either on varying the angle of incidence at a fixed excitation wavelength or on varying the excitation wavelength at a fixed angle of incidence. As such, the great majority of SPR signal processing algorithms that have been published are designed to identify the minimum in the reflectance curve corresponding to the angle/wavelength of resonance [121–124].

Angulo-spectral SPR systems produce 2D data maps of incidence angle versus wavelength, requiring more sophisticated algorithms for the analysis of multidimensional SPR data. In the work by [125], a linear algebra-based data analysis method is used to achieve a measurement resolution of 5×10^{-9} RIU from angulo-spectral SPR data. This result, which is superior or equal to phase-based SPR methods, is achieved while retaining the large measurement dynamic range typical of reflectance-based SPR methods.

In this work, a basis function set is determined by performing an eigenvector analysis on a training set of reflectance/dispersion (angulo-spectral) images corresponding to known refractive indices distributed across the solution space. The *inverse problem*, by which the refractive index of a candidate reflectance/dispersion image is calculated, proceeds by projecting the candidate image against the basis to obtain a vector of weights associated with the reflectance/dispersion images in the training set. The weights thus correspond to the relative degree of similarity between the candidate reflectance/dispersion image and each of the images in the original training set. The elements of the weights vector can be considered as sampled values of a continuous objective function to be maximized over the solution space. If desired, the dimensionality of the problem can be reduced by retaining only a subset of most significant vectors in the basis, as in the method of principal component analysis (PCA).

The authors evaluated the robustness of the method with respect to variations in experimental parameters such as random intensity additive noise, CCD camera spatial resolution, and intensity-level resolution (A/D quantization noise). Figure 7.30 shows results with respect to both the CCD spatial resolution and intensity-level quantization. The upper set of curves is for an 8-bit CCD, while the lower set is for a 16-bit CCD. Each set consists of three separate curves for pixel resolutions of 256 × 256, 512 × 512, and 1024 × 1024. While it is clear that high-resolution CCDs outperform low-resolution CCDs, the gain in performance is modest. A more significant difference is the A/D quantization, where 16-bit CCDs outperform 8-bit devices by more than an order of magnitude.

7.2.5 Performance Summary

In *classical* SPRI systems, the changes in the spatial reflectivity, $R(x, y, T)$, are generally monitored at fixed wavelength and coupling angle, θ_0, λ_0. This is illustrated in Figure 7.31 showing a *plasmonic movie* of the biochip surface evolution, as governed by the microfluidic and biochemical interactions. The imaging information is processed to extract kinetics interactions information from each individual probe/target interaction.

Step index sensitivities, Δn, in the range of 10^{-5} to 10^{-6} can be obtained, and 10^{-7} or slightly better has been achieved in the some cases. Refractive index changes, however, are not of direct interest for biosensing. Rather, it is the sensitivity to biological film thickness changes ($\delta R/\delta e$) that is generally of interest. As pointed out previously, these quantities are linked in a spectrally dependent way in the case of propagating plasmons. Also of particular interest is the evolution of the measured output, ΔR (or $\Delta \lambda$ or $\Delta \theta$), as a function of target concentration C, $\Delta R = f(C)$ for each given probe–target interaction.

It is generally agreed upon that even with the best instrumentation, the main cause of noise in the experimental data originates from issues related to the surface functionalization such as the inhomogeneity of the biofunctionalization, biomolecular cross-reactivity, and overly complex binding

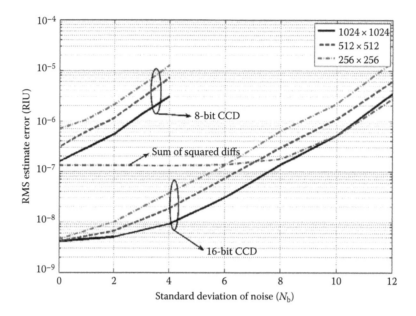

FIGURE 7.30 Performance of the algorithm as a function of the number of bits of additive Gaussian noise in the reflectance/dispersion images, calculated for a series of candidate test images over index values ranging from 1.305 to 1.375. Results are shown for both 8-bit and 16-bit cameras, at three different resolutions (256×256, 512×512, and 1024×1024). Note the graph labeled "Sum of squared diffs" that indicates the best-case performance (1024×1024 16-bit camera) of a variation of the algorithm that uses a simple sum of squared differences as the error measure between training set and candidate test images for building the weights vector, rather than the full method involving the projection against the basis. (Taken from Leavitt, D.A. et al., *Urology*, 80(4), 914, 2012.)

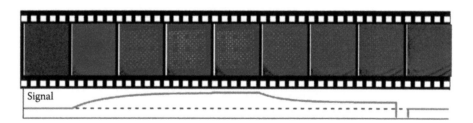

FIGURE 7.31 **(See color insert.)** SPRI movie—surface reflectivity changes with time as ssDNA target sequences bind to complementary surface ssDNA—functionalized probe spots. From each spot area, an interaction signal curve is extracted.

kinetics. As pointed out in the biochip functionalization section and further developed with an example in the medical application and model case of CF genotyping section, a self-calibration methodology is generally required to quantify and correct for such sources of noise.

As discussed previously, more sophisticated plasmonic imaging systems can be designed using a greater number of parameters to characterize the plasmonic resonance, in order to improve sensitivity and yield a richer set of data. For example, a single value in the spatiotemporal dimension such as $R(x, y, T)$ can be replaced by a more complete set of data by simultaneously varying the incident wavelength and coupling angle, as well as the propagation direction, P: $R(x, y, T, \theta, \lambda, P)$. For example, in an a spectro-angular imaging configuration [126] where the reflectivity spectrum of a 1D array of spots is acquired in parallel, spectral resolution on the resonance shift is of the order of a few picometers. This allows the clear discrimination of point mutation on 20 base oligonucleotides at a concentration as low as 100 pmol.

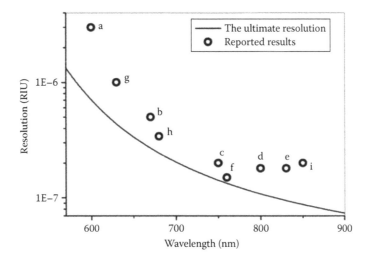

FIGURE 7.32 The ultimate resolution of an SPR sensor calculated and compared with the best experimental results reported by (a) Stemmler et al. [133], (b) Thirstrup et al. [123], (c) Piliarik et al. [134], (d) Nenninger et al. [122], (e) Chinowsky et al. [135], (f) Biacore 3000 (GE Healthcare, United States), (g) Wu and Pao [136], (h) Bardin et al. [126], and (i) Piliarik et al. [137]. (From Piliarik, M. and J. Homola, *Opt. Express*, 17(19), 16505, 2009.)

In addition, SPR systems based on interferometry have also been demonstrated [127,128], gaining another order of amplitude in sensitivity but at the cost of reduced dynamic range. Other investigators have also pointed out that the use of markers can significantly enhance the plasmonic sensor system response [129]. A totally different but important field, outside the scope of this chapter, involves SPR fluorescence-enhanced sensing [130,131]. The reader is referred to the paper from Piliarik and Homola, entitled *Surface plasmon resonance sensor—reaching their limits?* [132], which reviews the state of the art of such plasmonic sensors based on propagating plasmon along continuous interface obtained from homogeneous thick metal films (Figure 7.32).

The plasmonic optical reader system has been optimized in many ways; a great deal of research effort is now devoted to the biochip itself where surface nanostructuring is expected to further enhance the response of biochip systems. Such work is outside the scope of this chapter, but we may however point out that work on the spatial structuration of the evanescent wave with the localization of hot spots and colocalization of probes in locations where the binding of target will most affect the plasmon mode is very promising.

7.3 Application of SPRI to Genotyping

7.3.1 Challenges of DNA Characterization

Of all the biomedical/biomolecular possible fields, that of DNA–DNA interactions is certainly the one that has been the most investigated and used with the biochip SPRI reader systems [5–9,28,29, 51,91,97,138,139]. This is due to the tremendous importance of the potential applications of genotyping in both the medical domain (it has to be kept in mind that the human genome is diploid), for the search of either hereditary or acquired disease signatures, and the health and food industry, especially quality assessments, including traceability, of raw material, in particular with the growing importance of genetically modified organisms (GMOs). It is also helped by the fact that DNA materials are now readily available products, are fairly stable, and, as such, can be routinely used in the physics and engineering laboratory where the biochip reader systems are being developed. In this context, such DNA hybridization/dehybridization reactions are also used as model systems for all types of biomolecular specific interactions as far as the plasmonic biochip reader system development is concerned.

In this DNA–DNA interaction field, depicted Figure 7.33, the relatively easiest task consists in ascertaining the presence or absence of a given sequence in the DNA target material.

The next level of difficulty is to actually determine the three possible genotypes, even at the level of one nucleotide (point mutation or single-nucleotide polymorphisms [SNPs]), in discriminating unambiguously the homozygote from the heterozygote genotypes, where both types of sequences, wild type and mutant, are present in equal 1:1 proportion.

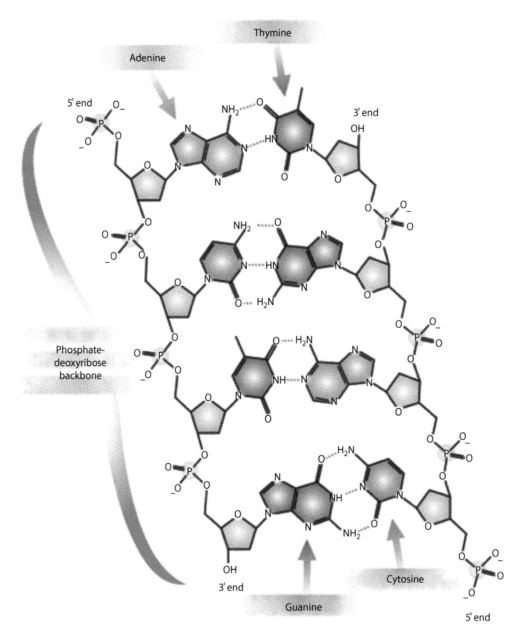

FIGURE 7.33 Illustration of DNA–DNA interaction—the stabilized genetic material being the well-known double helix structure of complementary matched nucleotide sequences, based on the four blocks two by two complementaries: adenine (A) and cytosine (C), thymine (T), and guanine (G). (Courtesy of Price Ball, M., DNA chemical structure. Wikimedia Commons, 2010.)

TABLE 7.9 Increasing Difficulty Levels in Instrumental Tasks, from 1A to 5abC, in Discriminating Known DNA Sequences in a Target Solution to Analyze

Difficulty Level Increases as One Goes Down and Left in This Table	A in Clean Target-Containing Solution	B in Mixed Target-Containing Solution	C in as Prepared PCR Bioanalytical Solution
1	Ascertaining the presence of a given sequence compared to nonrelevant ones		
2	Discriminating the homozygous wild type from the homozygous mutant sequence		
3	Discriminating the heterozygous from the homozygous genotypes		
4	Quantifying the relative concentration of the various target sequences		
5a	Diminishing the required concentration/quantity of target material		
5b	Increasing the number of SNPs that are addressed on the chip		

The relatively hardest task consists in recognizing and quantifying the normal and mutant DNA sequences in as large as possible concentration ratio (away from the 1/0, 0/1, and 1/1 diploid genotype cases), with as close as possible resemblance, up to the nucleotide or base pair level. This is of primary importance, for example, if one attempts to detect specific cancer-type signatures in a sample in which the mutation is more or less diluted, depending on the nature of the biological sample. This will also be the case for ascertaining the quality of *GMO-free* or in the other case *GMO-only* material (although this type of testing will address relatively large change in DNA sequences, one should note that the European limit for GMO-free is currently set at *less than 0.01 fraction*).

Table 7.9 summarizes the difficulty levels in discriminating a given DNA sequence in a given target solution, from 1, present alone or not, to 5, present in a DNA mixture at relatively low concentration, from A, clean ideal solution, to C, as prepared analytical solution; note that clinical genotyping demonstration starts at case 4C not 1A as sometime claimed in nonmedical application-oriented publication!

As explained in the precedent section, the entire system consists in a biochip containing an array of ssDNA probes complementary to specific target DNA sequences, the ssDNA solution to be analyzed, a microfluidic system allowing these complementary sequences to come into contact, a SPRI system that will convert the surface interaction binding events into grayscale levels of the biochip image, and a computer and software that will process the data. To actually make it to the market application, the systems have to possess many qualities including being user-friendly, fast, reliable, and low cost to run.

Progresses in the knowledge of the human genome and, as a result, in the understanding of the molecular bases of an increasing number of hereditary diseases have unraveled the underlying complexity of many of these monogenic or oligogenic conditions. Indeed, the picture that is emerging is that several layers of complexity determine the phenotypic diversity observed for some of these disorders, with a wide variety of primary mutations at the main gene(s) and some at other characterized modifying loci. This picture complicates the clinician's task, both to make the precise diagnosis and to give a prognosis. To face these difficulties, novel diagnostic strategies are needed, and higher-throughput mutation detection methods, suited to simultaneously analyze various sets of mutations in different genes, must be developed and implemented.

With a few exceptions, most of the existing molecular diagnostics tests remain cumbersome, relatively low throughput, and expensive; they are sequential in nature, requiring significant amounts of time and labor to evaluate just a single gene. In addition, they often rely upon skills mainly found in specialized research or diagnostic laboratories. Semiautomated DNA sequencing is still labor intensive, and interpretation of the results can be demanding. Although Next Generation Sequencing (NGS) methods are becoming more and more used in clinical molecular diagnostics, patient-focused diagnosis, as well as population screening, still needs the availability of high-throughput systems allowing simultaneous analysis of sets of mutations with 100% accuracy and reliability. To increase the speed and throughput of the diagnostic assays, DNA chips or microarrays are being progressively implemented in the diagnostics setting. To evaluate the interest of these novel approaches, we have focused our effort on a genetic disease, CF, used as a model system.

7.3.2 Cystic Fibrosis Mutation Screening: A Model Case

Over the past 15 years, there has been a dramatic increase in the number of disorders for which gene identification has been successful, based in part upon tools provided by the Human Genome Project. This has resulted in the proliferation and rapid integration of molecular genetic tests into clinical practice. Molecular diagnostic services are now in operation in many medical centers and are increasingly used to detect gene mutations, to monitor treatment of infectious diseases and cancers, and to determine disease susceptibility. In this context, a major focus is the development of appropriate, cost-effective, and high-throughput systems for the detection of gene mutations that are sensitive, rapid, and robust.

To this aim, in the last few years, a number of microarray-based sequencing and genotyping techniques have been developed. Currently, in most of these systems, observation of DNA hybridization relies on radiolabeled or fluorescent probes. Such *active* labeling, due to low background noise, has a high sensitivity but requires the use of costly reagents and time-consuming labeling procedures. Also, currently available instruments are based on end-point reaction detection. In this work, we have used SPRI as a DNA sensor for the detection of gene mutations. SPRI system allows simultaneous real-time monitoring of hybridization dynamics on an array of immobilized oligonucleotides probes. In an SPRI experiment, local changes in the reflectivity from a thin metal film are exploited to monitor the hybridization kinetics.

To evaluate the interest of these novel approaches, we have focused our effort on a genetic disease, CF, used as a model system.

7.3.2.1 Cystic Fibrosis and CFTR Gene Mutations

CF (MIM 219700) is one of the most common autosomal recessive diseases in Caucasians. It affects about 1 in 2500 births and approximately 1 in 25 individuals are heterozygotes, with marked regional variations (as indicated on the "Cystic Fibrosis Mutation Database", www.genet.sickkids.on.ca/cftr). It is caused by mutations of the CF transmembrane conductance regulator (CFTR or ABCC7) gene (MIM 602421), which is also involved in a broad spectrum of phenotypes, including male infertility by congenital bilateral absence of the vas deferens (CBAVD), disseminated bronchiectasis (DB), and chronic pancreatitis. So far, over 1000 CFTR gene mutations have been described throughout the gene, along with geographic and ethnic variations in their distribution and frequency (www.genet.sickkids.on.ca/cftr; Figure 7.34).

The most common causal mutation is F508del, which accounts for approximately two thirds of all CFTR alleles in patients with CF, with a decreasing prevalence from Northwest to Southeast Europe. The remaining third of alleles are substantially heterogeneous, with fewer than 20 mutations occurring at a worldwide frequency of more than 0.1%. Some mutations can reach a higher frequency in certain populations, due to a founder effect.

The majority of CFTR mutations have been associated with European-derived populations. There are also CFTR mutations in non-European populations, such as African and East Asian populations, but no alleles have reached the high frequency of F508del.

To date, more than 1500 sequence alterations have been identified in the CFTR gene and their listing is continuously updated within the Cystic Fibrosis Genetic Analysis Consortium (CFGAC) database. In the database, missense mutations account for 42%, frameshift for 15%, splicing for 12%, nonsense for around 10%, inframe insertions/deletions for 2%, large insertions/deletions for 3%, promoter mutations for 0.5%, and sequence variations that are not predicted to be disease causing for 15% of all alleles.

7.3.2.2 CF Molecular Diagnosis

CFTR molecular testing mainly relies on direct gene analysis procedures, which are based on our knowledge of CFTR molecular pathology and on the availability of a wide range of techniques, but there is no gold standard for routine testing.

Methods used in CFTR testing can be divided into two groups: those targeted at known mutations (i.e., testing DNA samples for the presence or absence of specific mutation(s)) and scanning methods

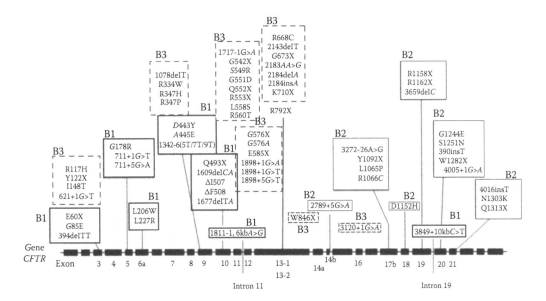

FIGURE 7.34 Location of the 68 most common CF point mutations tested by the Henri Mondor CF diagnosis center. The gene fragments containing these mutations are amplified by multiplex PCR in three different batches (respectively framed in bold, thin, and dash) and subsequently analyzed by SPRI.

(i.e., screening samples for any deviation from the standard sequence). These now include searching for large unknown CFTR rearrangements, including large deletions, insertions, and duplications, using assays based on semiquantitative polymerase chain reaction (PCR), including multiplex ligation-dependant probe amplification (MLPA) or quantitative fluorescent multiplex PCR.

The CF molecular tests currently performed in clinical laboratory hospitals are able to identify 30–35 mutations, including the most frequently found in the Caucasian population. These diagnostic kits allow detection of about 85% of the defects in this population. Such coverage level is insufficient in some situations, in particular when non-Caucasian or mixed populations are studied, as their spectrum of mutations is different. To reach 85%–90% coverage independently of the population, a genetic test able to screen for at least 100 mutations is necessary.

To develop a better tool for CF mutation screening, we devised a novel detection system based on SPRI. In preliminary studies, the target DNAs consisted in short oligonucleotides complementary to the normal (wild type) or mutant probes bound to the sensor surface in an array format. We then carried out similar experiments using PCR products obtained from DNAs of patients with CF mutations. We also evaluated the quality of the response obtained when the probes are immobilized on the sensor surface using two different chemistries, that is, 11-mercaptoundecanoic acid-poly(ethylenimine) (MUA-PEI) and dextran. Altogether, the results demonstrate that our SPRI sensor system allows, without the need for labeling, unambiguous detection of gene mutations in an array format, taking advantages of kinetic monitoring of the molecular interactions (Figure 7.35).

At the time the first experiments were started, the three kits that were available were addressing 30–35 point mutations. This resulted in 15% false-negative answers due to the huge number of rarely occurring, and therefore untested, point mutations related to CF. Such overall performance was mostly the consequence of a trade-off between quality and cost. In this context, the potential of dedicated bio-chip systems is great.

The generalization to other genetic illnesses would be quasi-immediate, and CF serves here as model case; lots of other works have been devoted to other diseases such as in particular the thalassemia, as well as different types of cancer signatures, and also mediated applications such as Asian flu signature recognition.

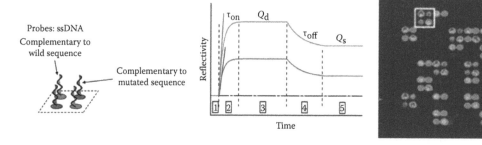

FIGURE 7.35 **(See color insert.)** Schematic representation of the four spots' diagnosis scheme—one diagonal (in green) is spotted using the ssDNA wild-type sequence, while the other one (in red) uses the ssDNA mutated sequence. If wild-type target sequences are interacting with the probes, one expects the perfectly complementary interaction signal (with the wild-type probe spot) to be stronger than the partial match interaction signal (with the mutant probe spot)—this is further illustrated by the biochip SPRI measurement on the right.

7.3.3 Interaction Monitoring Using Oligonucleotide DNA

Initial experiments targeted known mutations of particular clinical importance, in particular the most frequent molecular defect identified, F508del, and other surrounding mutations and polymorphisms. F508del is a deletion of 3 bases occurring in position 1519–1524* of exon 10 of gene CFTR (www.genet. sickkids.on.ca/cftr).

This first set of mutation/polymorphism on which were carried most of our experiments is given in Table 7.10.

In all the following data of this section, the probe and target sequences used were between 8 bases and 39 bases and centered on the mutations to characterize. In particular, the oligonucleotide set to study the impact of sequence length set was performed using, respectively, 8, 9, 10, 11, 12, 13, 15, 17, 19, 29, and 39 bases, and the diagnostic arrays set (as detailed further) were performed choosing length that set the melting temperatures of the perfectly complementary interactions to around 40°C, as calculated using SantaLucia nearest method online calculations.

In order to perform the genotyping, we use ssDNA probes, both the normal wild-type sequences and the mutant ones. We chose to arrange them, as illustrated in Figure 7.35, in a square pattern, with the two diagonals corresponding, one to the wild-type sequence and the other one to the variant sequence. Once the biochip surface is put in contact with the solution containing the ssDNA targets, the goal is to quantify if the target products have more affinity with

- The wild-type sequences (i.e., corresponding to the normal homozygote genotype)
- The mutated sequences (i.e., corresponding to a mutated homozygote genotype)
- Both in a more or less equilibrated manner (i.e., corresponding to a heterozygote genotype)

In Figures 7.35, 7.36a through d, 7.37a, and 7.40 (bottom), the interactions monitoring with the wild-type probe sequences will be presented in light gray, the ones with the mutated probe sequences in dark gray.

As one varies the length of the corresponding sequences (PhD Nathalie Bassil 2005), one expects to see different behaviors: first, the longer the complementary sequences, the larger the interaction binding energy and the more stable the corresponding dsDNA duplex; second, for the same molar

---

* The nucleotide change of p.F508del—"deletion of 3 bp between nucleotides 1519 and 1524" means any three consecutive nucleotides in this range of four nucleotides: either T(1520)C(1521)T(1522) or C(1521)T(1522)T(1523). Both 3 bp deletions lead to the same DNA sequence: A(1519)TTT(1524)G(1525).

TABLE 7.10 List of Initial Set of Sequences Containing Point Mutations Tested on the Exon 10 of Gene CFTR

Mutation Acronym (Type)	Position on Gene CFTR Exon/Location	Wild-Type and Mutated Sequences: Probes Then Targets
ΔF508(p.Phe508del, F508del) (3 bases deletion: CTT)	10/c.1521_1523del	5'-ATATCAT**CTT**TGGTG-3' 5'-AATATCATTGGTGTT-3'
		5'-CACCA**AAG**ATGATAT-3' 5'-AACACCAATGATATT-3' (shifted from DF508)
ΔF507(p.Ile507del, I507del)	10/c.1519_1521del	
Q493X(p.Gln493X, Q493X)	10/c.1477C > T	5'-TGTTCT**C**AGTTTT-3' 5'-TGTTCT**T**AGTTTT-3'
		5'-AAAACT**G**AGAACA-3' 5'-AAAACT**A**AGAACA-3'
MV470(p.Met470Val, M470V)	10/c.1408A > G	5'-CTT CTA ATG **A**TG ATT ATG G-3' 5'-CTT CTA ATG **G**TG ATT ATG G-3'
		5'-C CAT AAT CA**T** CAT TAG AAG-3' 5'-C CAT AAT CA**C** CAT TAG AAG-3'
V520F	10/	5'-GAAGC**G**TCATC-3' 5'-GAAGC**T**TCATC-3'
		5'-GATGA**C**GCTTC-3' 5'-GATGA**A**GCTTC 3'
1716	10/	5'-GAAGC**G**TCATC-3' 5'-GAAGC**T**TCATC-3'
		5'-TCTTAC**C**TCTTCT-3' 5'-TCTTAC**T**TCTTCT-3'

Note: Point mutations are bolded and underlined.

quantity of target, the longer the sequence, the stronger the signal, which, for a given optical index contrast, is going to be proportional to the actual mass of DNA binding to the surface. Also, it can be anticipated that, the longer the interacting sequences, the greater its stability and the relatively smaller impact a given SNP will induce. Basically, one would expect a strong difference signal on very weak detected signals for very short sequences and a very small difference signal on very strong signal for long sequences. One must therefore expect an optimum sequence length to exist to allow efficient discrimination of genotypes, and one goal is therefore to pinpoint such optimal case. Figure 7.36 presents a set of data corresponding to probe and target pairs of, respectively, 8, 11, 17, and 29 oligonucleotides, using the sequences centered on the ΔF508 site and a relatively high target concentration of 15 μmol, allowing to reach equilibrium fairly rapidly. One can indeed observe the anticipated effects. Firstly, the signal amplitude increases with sequence length. Secondly, the discrimination between the perfect match case and the partially complementary case is very different on the four cases. As the sequence length is increased, such discrimination is first more and more efficient during the target flow (cases a and b); then the amplitude of both types of signals saturates at even values (case c), but then strong discrimination can be made after rinsing—if the sequences are too long, strong signals are effectively obtained during target flow and after rinsing, but discrimination of both types of signals, perfect match and partial match, is indeed difficult (case d). Clearly interacting sequence length is, all things given, a way to optimize individually many different point mutations to address on a single biochip. Furthermore, the discrimination can be optimized for different parts of the dynamical signal: hybridization, quasi-equilibrium with targets in solution, rinsing, or quasi-equilibrium without targets in solution.

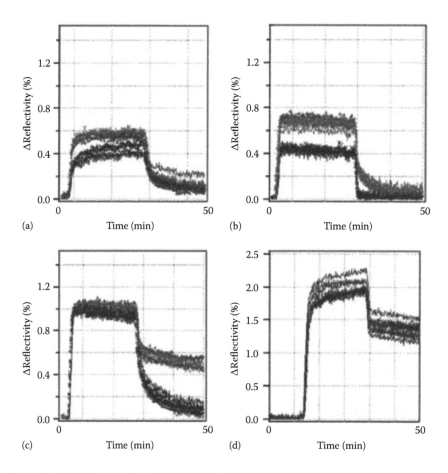

FIGURE 7.36 Example of DNA–DNA interaction data—perfect match and partial matches—for different sequence lengths, respectively, (a) 8-, (b) 11-, (c) 17-, and (d) 29-oligonucleotide long section. Sequences are those centered on the DF508 site—probes are mutated, targets are either mutated (gray) or wild type (black), the buffer is PBS 1×, and the target concentration was 15 µmol.

Although this behavior is general, it is of course dependent on the actual buffer solution that is used as interacting medium. A better parameter taking such effect into account is described in the next section that aims in quantifying the interaction energy and the associated duplex temperature stability.

7.3.3.1 Importance of Melting Temperature T_m

An important parameter when studying DNA–DNA hybridization is the melting temperature, T_m, of the given duplex. At low temperature, the duplex is stable and the DNA is in its double-stranded form. As the temperature is increased, the thermal activation is sufficient to break enough of the physical bonds that link the bases and dissociate the dsDNA duplex. At high temperature, the DNA is only present in its single-stranded ssDNA form. This is illustrated in Figure 7.37. The T_m is defined, in solution, as the temperature at which at thermodynamical equilibrium half of the dsDNA has been denatured into ssDNA. Note that this value is of course dependent on the initial DNA concentration and the stringency of the buffer solution (its salt contents)—see, for example, [140–143].

Basically, if the measurement is performed at a temperature well above the T_m, only a small hybridization signal will be detectable, and if the measurement is performed under the melting temperature, a strong saturated signal will be obtained. This saturated signal is reached when maximum coverage of the surface is achieved.

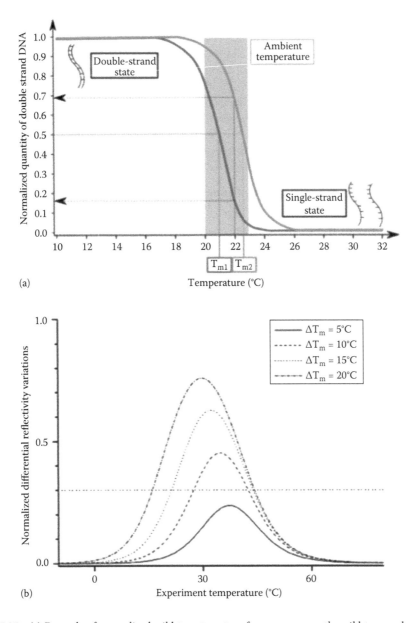

(a)

(b)

FIGURE 7.37 (a) Example of normalized wild-type target surface coverage on the wild-type and mutated spot as a function temperature T for, respectively, T_{m1} (partial match case) and T_{m2} (perfect match case); (b) example of normalized discrimination signal as a function of T, T_m, and ΔT_m ($= T_{m2} - T_{m1}$).

For the short sequences (up to about 30 oligonucleotides), where both the effects of secondary structures and steric hindrance are minimal, the equilibrium that is reached during target flow is consistent with duplex hybridization melting temperature, as calculated using the nearest neighbor method, as explained by SantaLucia et al. [141–143]. These experiments and calculations concerned four different probe sequences annealed with either their perfectly or their partially complementary targets. For the estimation of T_ms, we used the calculator web pages accessible on John SantaLucia websites, as well as Michael Zucker's site, and wrote our own software codes based on SantaLucia published values (such calculations are now more common and can now be found on many laboratory and company web pages). For the 40-oligonucleotide long sequences, secondary structures and/or steric hindrance led to slightly smaller normalized to size (i.e., length) plasmonic signals.

One should note that this T_m parameter is clearly defined as an equilibrium temperature $(PT \leftrightarrow P + T)$ between a duplex (PT) and its single-stranded components (probe + target) and as such concerns a volumic solution environment. For a biochip, one of the species, the probe, P, is bound to the surface. At some time, a surface effect correction was offered on some of the online calculator; it then disappeared. However, such T_m proves to be a useful parameter for the surface interactions also, and what is important is that the real effective T_m and the calculated T_m, whatever methods are used, are closely related by a continuous bijective function. Systems and protocols have to be benchmarked versus any calculations, leading to the necessity of using a temperature offset correction function.

7.3.3.2 Optimization of Specific Probe Sequences

As a consequence of Figure 7.37, it is clear that in order to maximize the genotyping discrimination potential of any given couple of wild-type and mutated probes sequences, one has to choose perfect matches with T_ms above the temperature at which the experiment is run T_{exp} (so that the concentration of perfect match duplexes is relatively high, >0.5) and T_ms of the mismatch below T_{exp} (so that the concentration of partial match duplexes is relatively low, <0.5) with as large as possible differences ΔT_ms (so that the difference in concentration of perfect match and partial match duplexes is relatively as high as possible). This is illustrated in Figure 7.37b. Quite naturally, the higher the ΔT_m, typically between 2°C and 20°C for an SNP, the greater the discrimination signal of the properly temperature-tuned experiment. The optimized experimental temperature corresponds to the average of the two T_ms: $(T_{m1} + T_{m2})/2$.

Practically, for any given point mutation one wishes to diagnose, we calculate the perfect match T_m of both the *wild-type probe/wild-type target* (T_mWW) and the *mutated probe/mutated target* (T_mMM) duplexes as a function of sequence length, keeping the point mutation to analyze centered. We stopped when the calculated T_ms were above 40°C. We then calculated the partial match TMs, corresponding to the *wild-type probe/mutated target* (T_mWM) and *mutated probe/wild-type target* (T_mMW), to check that the corresponding values were both below 35°C. This insured that all point mutations would be analyzed in such a way that one would have to differentiate hybridization reactions of ΔT_m of at least 5°C. In practice for the 70 point mutations tentatively addressed, these ΔT_ms were typically in the 5°C–15°C range.

One can graphically visualize the discrimination potential of the plasmonic biochip system using an abacus, as presented Figure 7.38. This represents as a function of both the T_m of the perfect match and the partial match the discrimination signal that can be expected for a given experimental temperature. Note that as the partial match T_m being always smaller than the perfect match T_m and in order to extend the graph visibility, the representation uses as x-axis the perfect match T_m and as y-axis the ΔT_m, difference between the perfect match and partial match T_ms. For very low T_m, no hybridization is expected in either perfect or partial match, or therefore there are no discrimination signals; for high T_m, a strong hybridization is expected on the corresponding perfect match spot and dependently on the ΔT_m strong to null on the partial match spot.

Lines of isodiscrimination signals are plotted on the abacus, no discrimination is expected on the left-down corner and on the respective edges, and the top-right corner and the associated triangular plateau are where the maximum discrimination can be expected.

For a given point mutation, if one starts considering a long sequence (usually the mutation is centered although it is not of paramount importance), both perfect match and partial match T_ms will be highly relative to the experimental conditions, around 30°C, for example, and in the representation, the associated data location will correspond to high T_m and small ΔT_m (right-down area). As the sequence length is progressively shortened, the estimated T_ms are going to decrease, the partial match in a quicker way than the perfect match—therefore, the trajectory of the data point in this representation is going to move from right to left and from bottom to top—clearly, it is going to go first up and then down the levels across the isodiscrimination lines. Following this method, an optimal sequence length and associated discriminating

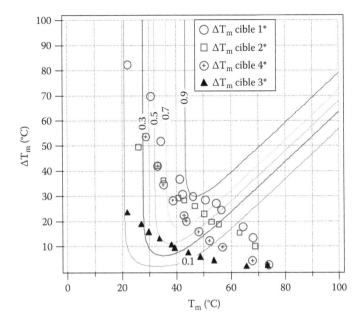

FIGURE 7.38 Calculated abacus of discrimination signal as a function of T_m and relative ΔT_m—lines are isosignal ones, 0 no discrimination, 1 maximum discrimination—data points correspond to the sequences of 2 different point mutations, respectively, DF508 (1 wild, 2 mutated) and M470V (3 wild, 4 mutated) analyzing both the wild-type and mutated probes cases versus both the wild-type and mutated targets, that is, with given T_m and ΔT_m. The wild M470V case (filled triangle) will clearly be the most difficult to discriminate.

signal can be calculated for each individual probe and point mutation considered. Figure 7.38 gives an example for two different point mutations, DF508 and M470V, corresponding to four probes. One can clearly see that the wild-type and mutated probes do not have symmetrical behaviors and that the best expected discriminating signals can sometime be relatively small, less than 0.5 (blue filled triangle corresponding to the M470V wild-type probe sequence), yet still clearly noticeable, more than 0.3. We performed such calculations for all 68 mutations, 136 probes, under consideration in our study. All could be discriminated above the 0.3 level.

7.3.4 Demonstration Using PCR Products Issued from Patient Sequences

7.3.4.1 PCR-Prepared Materials for Targets

In order to secure optimal hybridization conditions between target and probe DNA sequences, the target DNA sequences are prepared as ssDNA molecules using enzymatic digestion by λ-exonuclease. Indeed, the hybridization characteristics of DNA targets to solid-phase-bound probes depend on the probe–target position and on target renaturation if a dsDNA target is used. To prepare the ssDNA, the target is first amplified by PCR making use of specific primers and Taq polymerase, and the PCR product is subsequently incubated with λ-exonuclease, an enzyme that digests one of the two DNA strands.

Such long sequence, of several hundred bases, may of course interact with itself (its parts are of course always in close vicinity!) and partially hybridize some parts of the sequence leading to so-called secondary structures—an example is given in Figure 7.39. As for the hybridization/denaturation, this strongly depends on temperature and buffer solution stringency, and at any moment, many of these secondary structures may coexist; although the warmer, the less of them are probable to occur.

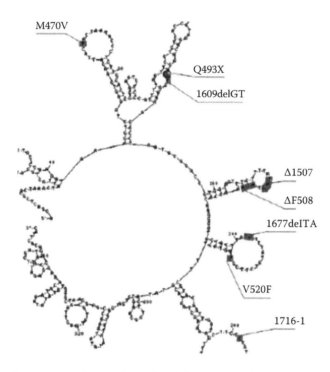

FIGURE 7.39   Secondary structure of a 377-oligonucleotide long section of exon 10 of gene CFTR. Depending on temperature and solution, many different secondary structures can coexist. Accessibility and effective concentration of the target sequence site are therefore strongly affected.

During experiments, some precautions can be taken. Preheating the solution and cooling it just before injecting it onto the biochip surface is one often recommended; operating in condition of high stringency is an advantage. Other solutions sometimes suggested include chopping the single strand PCR (ssPCR)-prepared strand into multiple fragments. This may be done either methodologically using specific enzymes or randomly using technique such as sonication. In the following section giving experimental demonstration of hybridization of such ssPCR strands, no such protocols were used and the 377-base long product was used as is.

7.3.4.2 Mutation Diagnostic on Patient DNA Amplified by PCR

Figure 7.40 (left) is a plasmonic reflectivity difference image of biochip allowing quantifying the hybridization reaction of such PCR from patient-prepared target material. The subsquares with diagonal only signals are related to the three-base deletion mutation with therefore strong discrimination potential. The more or less equilibrated diagonals are due to SNPs. Figure 7.40 (right) is a representation of such wild-type and mutated probe spot signals for 6 polymorphism of this exon 20 of gene CFTR around the most frequent ΔF507 mutation. The patient was effectively of MV470 mutated type [29].

7.3.4.3 Instrumental Mutation Diagnostic Potential

As would have now been understood, the instrumental goal is to monitor and quantify the interaction signals of a target DNA material with both wild-type (S_W) and mutated (S_M) sequences and compare ($S_D = S_W - S_M$) with reliability these data, in order to allow unambiguous genotyping. This is illustrated in Figure 7.41. Firstly, the biomolecular chemistry laws and application to each specific case will impose its reality and effective difference and asymmetry of the interactions, that is, the three main directions corresponding to the three genotypes will not necessarily be symmetrically distributed and far apart. Secondly, the instrumental transducer will inherently be limited by noise and drifts, leading to a widening of the area. Quality, especially including homogeneity, of the biochip and target material will also lead to such widening effect.

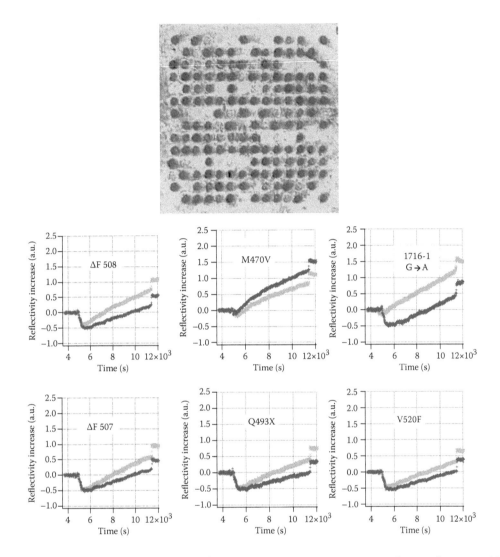

FIGURE 7.40 **(See color insert.)** Example of DNA–DNA interactions using PCR products as characterized by the SPRI biochip. (Left) Image of the plasmonic reflectivity difference of the diagnostic biochip after submitting the surface to a solution containing the target PCR materials and rinsing. (Right) Kinetics of the PCR material solution-induced binding events (for each point mutation characterized: in green the wild sequence spots and in red the mutated sequence spots). In the case presented here, the patient was indeed diagnosed with the MV470 CF point mutation—for which the red (MT) experimental curve is above the green one (WT) (middle-top graph).

From a system point of view, it is of primary importance that there exist a time after which all three areas are clearly separated. If this minimum time of interaction is too long, it can severally reduce the throughput of the system. Note that such abacus has to be quantified for all the mutations, which are addressed by the biochips, whose goals would be several tens to hundreds, depending on the specific applications.

7.3.5 Diagnostic Reliability Using Self-Calibration Procedure

As explained previously in the instrumental section 7.2, the transducer spatial response can be quantified and normalized using a step index procedure, and the biochip spot reactivities (which depends a lot on probe concentration homogeneity) can be quantified and normalized using a common calibration binding reaction based on a given probe structure, as sketched in Figure 7.42.

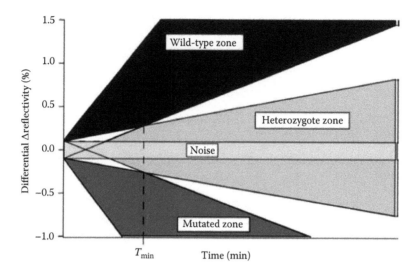

FIGURE 7.41   Instrumental diagnostic abacus principle—three possible genotypes, each with its own biomolecular type of response, whose quantification is limited by reader and biochip instrumental imperfections, drift, and noise.

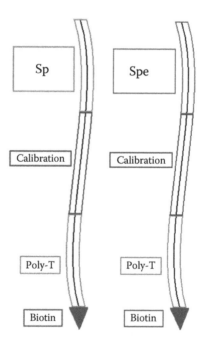

FIGURE 7.42   Sketch of probe structure; in addition from the linker group (here a biotin), the spacer (here a ssDNA sequence) and probe-specific group (here a ssDNA), which is different for the different spots of the biochip, a common calibration group, in our case, another ssDNA sequence, is used for all the probes used on the different spots—it allows quantification of biochip spot spatial inhomogeneities.

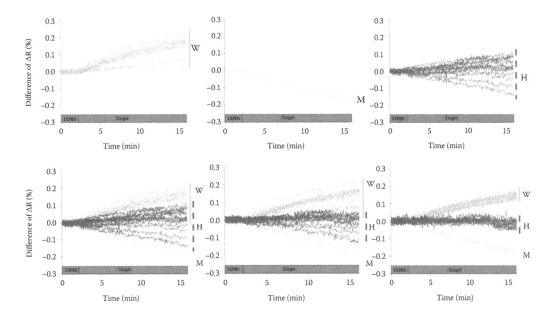

FIGURE 7.43 Data from self-calibration genotyping. Top line (left to right): homozygote wild ("W", gray), homozygote mutated ("M", light gray) and heterozygote ("H", black) target mimicking ssDNA solutions. Bottom line all three cases together (left) initial data, (middle) optical transducer step index corrected and (right) biochip inhomogeneity corrected.

The following example illustrates the potential of the self-calibration methodology [20]. Wild-type and mutated sequences of M470V were used for the biochip, and many replicates of the four spots' spatial organization were realized. To mimic patient genotype, complementary sequences, wild type only (homozygous wild-type case), mutated only (homozygous mutated case), and wild type and mutated at equal concentration (heterozygote case) were sequentially used (regeneration of the biochip was performed in between each target injection). Figure 7.43 top shows a typical example of the distribution of uncorrected response $S_D = S_W - S_M$ given by the system, from left to right, homozygote wild type indeed positive, homozygote mutated indeed negative, and heterozygote indeed in between.

Figure 7.43 bottom left shows the superposition of such sets of data and demonstrates that even if clearly on average, there is no way of mistaking one case for the other and if one was not using so many replicates and just selecting at random one of each set of data, no such unambiguous discrimination of the three possible genotypes would be possible. This would be a severe limitation in information spatial density and would limit total signature analysis throughput. As previously pointed out, the self-calibration method allows to go beyond the frontiers (CNRS) as demonstrated by the next two subfigures. Figure 7.43 bottom center and bottom right, respectively, shows the same set of experimental data after processing using firstly the step index data and secondly the calibration target data. As can be seen in the last representation, no ambiguity would arise even if one only had one of the experimental curves to assign a genotype to [46].

Normalized data and genotyping can be realized using either the discriminating level reached after a given time or the dynamics, that is, the slope, of such signal (Figure 7.44).

7.3.6 Envisioned Systems and Bottlenecks

The future dedicated biochip analytical systems will be capable of having an attractive trade-off in terms of throughput and cost. They will have to be further integrated to make little use of consumable and of exterior manipulation entering the field of so-called LOC. In the particular

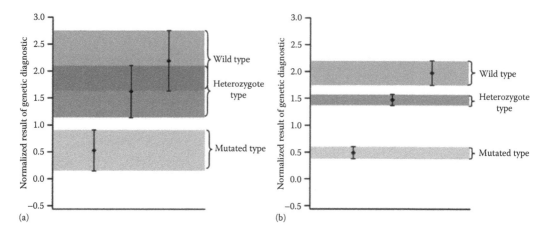

FIGURE 7.44 Graphical representation of the genetic diagnostic capability of the plasmonic CF biochip sensor, respectively, without (a) and with (b) the self-calibration protocol used; y-axis quantifies the spatial (spot-to-spot) variation in reflectivity temporal variations ($\Delta R_W / \Delta R_M$). Demonstration was done using the M470V point mutation. Note that as anticipated the two homozygote genotypes are clearly distinguished and that it is the overlap of the heterozygote genotype with one of the homozygotes, the wild one in the case of M470V, which is difficult to diagnose and for which the self-calibration methodology is especially effective.

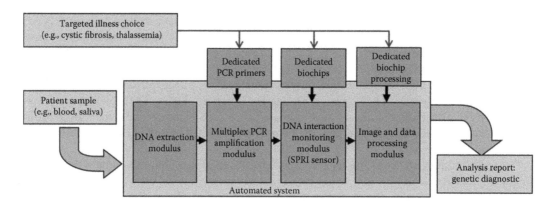

FIGURE 7.45 Schematic of the main module of envisioned dedicated systems.

case of genotyping, either hereditary or acquired, this will imply that the DNA amplification and all associated microfluidics will have to be performed on the chip as already demonstrated with success in many cases such as Christopoulos (2003). The overall system would work as depicted in Figure 7.45.

An example of expected responses is given in Figure 7.46.

The most critical point to address lies in the specific development of the multiple-interactions protocol that has to deal with the question of intra- and inter-ssDNA target interactions, in particular taking into account the PCR secondary structures—this difficulty increases, nonlinearly, faster than the number of genetic signatures to be identified and can lead to work with shorter sequences.

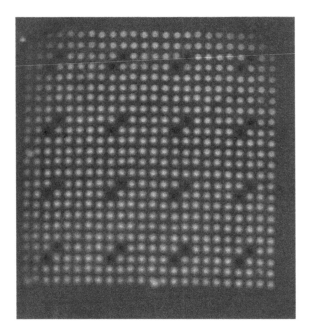

FIGURE 7.46 Theoretical responses of the envisioned CF 65 mutations.

7.4 Conclusions

Propagating SPR is an optical phenomenon that is localized around a metal–dielectric interface and that is very sensitive to minute changes in the optical indices of the surrounding materials that support its propagation. It is therefore particularly well suited to be taken advantage of as the basis of sensing devices. Using an optical imaging setup, it is possible to monitor surface evolution with subnanometric resolution in average thickness, typically corresponding to few atograms (ag—10^{-18} g) of material deposited per square micron area—corresponding to a small population of (bio)molecules (the larger the target molecules, the lesser the captured number needed for detection). Such label-free sensitivity is very well suited to the characterization of biomolecular surface interactions—yet adding labels allows extra sensitivity keeping all the other advantage if proven necessary. Furthermore, the ease of the data collection allows monitoring the temporal evolution of the surface, therefore the kinetics of the interactions and not only their end-point states. Providing proper microfluidic conditions and data processing, this will provide either precise new thermodynamical data, in particular affinity constant about the interactions under study, or signature recognition of specific targets in an unknown solution to characterize.

Such setups are the basis of label-free dynamical biochip SPRI systems that can be applied to many fields, especially including genotyping, as discussed herein, but have also been demonstrated to be useful for a wide variety of other biomedical applications.

Genetic characterization of the three possible genotypes of polymorphism and in particular SNP can be performed and was demonstrated on many clinical cases, in particular CF, using PCR prepared from patient DNA material.

For such systems to be fully developed, it is mandatory to master many fields, including plasmonics, surface functionalization, biomolecular interactions, fluidics, imaging, engineering, and data processing, but must be routinely used without specialized knowledge as for any classical laboratory equipment. It seems therefore promised to a bright future!

Acknowledgments

The authors would like to acknowledge the work from current and previous colleagues of their respective institutions. The basis of this work was also partially funded by the support from different funding agencies and organizations, including CNRS, INSERM, association VLM (Vaincre la Mucoviscidose—Defeat Cystic Fibrosis), Ecole Centrale de Lyon, CNANO–Région Ile de France, Région Rhône–Alpes, Agence Nationale de la Recherche, and the spin-off start-up GenOptics, recently acquired by Horiba Scientific. The IOGS–CNRS partner is also core member of the European Network of Excellence in BioPhotonics, Photonics for Life, P4L, http://www.photonics4life.eu. Authors are also involved in the newly created international CNRS laboratory UMI LN2 on nanotechnologies and nanosystems.

References

1. Waggoner, P.S. and H.G. Craighead, Micro- and nanomechanical sensors for environmental, chemical, and biological detection. *Lab on a Chip*, 2007. **7**(10): 1238–1255.
2. Chao, C.Y. and L.J. Guo, Biochemical sensors based on polymer microrings with sharp asymmetrical resonance. *Applied Physics Letters*, 2003. **83**(8): 1527–1529.
3. Patolsky, F., G.F. Zheng, and C.M. Lieber, Fabrication of silicon nanowire devices for ultrasensitive, label-free, real-time detection of biological and chemical species. *Nature Protocols*, 2006. **1**(4): 1711–1724.
4. Bakker, E. and Y. Qin, Electrochemical sensors. *Analytical Chemistry*, 2006. **78**(12): 3965–3983.
5. Nelson, B.P. et al., Surface plasmon resonance imaging measurements of DNA and RNA hybridization adsorption onto DNA microarrays. *Analytical Chemistry*, 2001. **73**(1): 1–7.
6. Bassil, N. et al., One hundred spots parallel monitoring of DNA interactions by SPR imaging of polymer-functionalized surfaces applied to the detection of cystic fibrosis mutations. *Sensors and Actuators B: Chemical*, 2003. **94**(3): 313.
7. Manera, M.G. et al., Real-time monitoring of carbonarius DNA structured biochip by surface plasmon resonance imaging. *Journal of Optics A: Pure and Applied Optics*, 2008. **10**(6): 064018.
8. Manera, M.G. et al., Surface plasmon resonance imaging technique for nucleic acid detection. *Sensors and Actuators B: Chemical*, 2008. **130**(1): 82–87.
9. Mariotti, E., M. Minunni, and M. Mascini, Surface plasmon resonance biosensor for genetically modified organisms detection. *Analytica Chimica Acta*, 2002. **453**(2): 165–172.
10. Wegner, G.J., H.J. Lee, and R.M. Corn, Characterization and optimization of peptide arrays for the study of epitope–antibody interactions using surface plasmon resonance imaging. *Analytical Chemistry*, 2002. **74**(20): 5161–5168.
11. Giakoumaki, E. et al., Combination of amplification and post-amplification strategies to improve optical DNA sensing. *Biosensors & Bioelectronics*, 2003. **19**(4): 337–344.
12. Kanda, V. et al., Label-free reading of microarray-based immunoassays with surface plasmon resonance imaging. *Analytical Chemistry*, 2004. **76**(24): 7257–7262.
13. Smith, E.A. et al., Surface plasmon resonance imaging studies of protein–carbohydrate interactions. *Journal of the American Chemical Society*, 2003. **125**(20): 6140–6148.
14. Wegner, G.J. et al., Real-time surface plasmon resonance imaging measurements for the multiplexed determination of protein adsorption/desorption kinetics and surface enzymatic reactions on peptide microarrays. *Analytical Chemistry*, 2004. **76**(19): 5677–5684.
15. Maillart, E. et al., Versatile analysis of multiple macromolecular interactions by SPR imaging: Application to p53 and DNA interaction. *Oncogene*, 2004. **23**(32): 5543.
16. Chabot, V. et al., Biosensing based on surface plasmon resonance and living cells. *Biosensors & Bioelectronics*, 2009. **24**(6): 1667.
17. Valicenti-McDermott, M. et al., Age at diagnosis of autism spectrum disorders. *Journal of Pediatrics*, 2012. **161**(3): 554–556.

18. Homola, J., *Surface Plasmon Resonance Based Sensors*. Springer Series on Chemical Sensors and Biosensors, ed. O.S. Wolfbeis, Springer, Berlin, Germany, 2006, p. 247.

19. Liedberg, B., C. Nylander, and I. Lundstrom, Surface-plasmon resonance for gas-detection and biosensing. *Sensors and Actuators*, 1983. **4**(2): 299–304.

20. Hottin, J. et al., Biochip data normalization using multifunctional probes. *Analyst*, 2012. **137**(13): 3119–3125.

21. Giebel, K.F. et al., Imaging of cell/substrate contacts of living cells with surface plasmon resonance microscopy. *Biophysical Journal*, 1999. **76**(1): 509–516.

22. Huang, B., F. Yu, and R.N. Zare, Surface plasmon resonance imaging using a high numerical aperture microscope objective. *Analytical Chemistry*, 2007. **79**(7): 2979–2983.

23. Berger, C.E.H., R.P.H. Kooyman, and J. Greve, Resolution in surface-plasmon microscopy. *Review of Scientific Instruments*, 1994. **65**(9): 2829–2836.

24. Mitsushio, M., K. Miyashita, and M. Higo, Sensor properties and surface characterization of the metal-deposited SPR optical fiber sensors with Au, Ag, Cu, and Al. *Sensors and Actuators A: Physical*, 2006. **125**(2): 296–303.

25. Palik, E.D., Handbook of optical-constants. *Journal of the Optical Society of America A, Optics Image Science, and Vision*, 1984. **1**(12): 1297–1297.

26. Kano, H., S. Mizuguchi, and S. Kawata, Excitation of surface-plasmon polaritons by a focused laser beam. *Journal of the Optical Society of America B, Optical Physics*, 1998. **15**(4): 1381–1386.

27. Watanabe, K., N. Horiguchi, and H. Kano, Optimized measurement probe of the localized surface plasmon microscope by using radially polarized illumination. *Applied Optics*, 2007. **46**(22): 4985–4990.

28. Hottin, J. et al., Plasmonic DNA: Towards genetic diagnosis chips. *Plasmonics*, 2007. **2**(4): 201–215.

29. Mannelli, I. et al., Surface plasmon resonance imaging (SPRI) system and real-time monitoring of DNA biochip for human genetic mutation diagnosis of DNA amplified samples. *Sensors and Actuators B: Chemical*, 2006. **119**(2): 583–591.

30. Thariani, R. and P. Yager, Novel, high-quality surface plasmon resonance microscopy. *Sensors and Actuators B: Chemical*, 2008. **130**(2): 765–770.

31. Piliarik, M., H. Vaisocherova, and J. Homola, A new surface plasmon resonance sensor for high-throughput screening applications. *Biosensors & Bioelectronics*, 2005. **20**(10): 2104–2110.

32. De Feijter, J.A., J. Benjamins, and F.A. Veer, Ellipsometry as a tool to study the adsorption behavior of synthetic and biopolymers at the air–water interface. *Biopolymers*, 1978. **17**(7): 1759–1772.

33. Gordus, A. and G. MacBeath, Circumventing the problems caused by protein diversity in microarrays: Implications for protein interaction networks. *Journal of the American Chemical Society*, 2006. **128**(42): 13668.

34. Rusk, N., Overcoming protein diversity on arrays. *Nature Methods*, 2006. **3**(12): 966.

35. Jones, R.B. et al., A quantitative protein interaction network for the ErbB receptors using protein microarrays. *Nature*, 2006. **439**(7073): 168–174.

36. Calevro, F. et al., Assessment of 35mer amino-modified oligonucleotide based microarray with bacterial samples. *Journal of Microbiological Methods*, 2004. **57**(2): 207.

37. Everett, D.H., Manual of symbols and terminology for physicochemical quantities and units, Appendix II: Definitions, terminology and symbols in colloid and surface chemistry. *Pure and Applied Chemistry*, 1972. **31**(4): 577–638.

38. Burwell Jr., R.L., Manual of symbols and terminology for physicochemical quantities and units—Appendix II. Definitions, terminology and symbols in colloid and surface chemistry. Part II: Heterogeneous catalysis. *Pure and Applied Chemistry*, 1976. **46**(4): 71–90.

39. Atkins, P. and J.D. De Paula, eds. *Physical Chemistry*. W.H. Freeman and Co., New York, 2009.

40. Goldfarb, D., *Biophysics DeMYSTiFieD*. McGraw-Hill, New York, 2011.

41. Gabler, R. and T. Shiro, Electrical interactions in molecular biophysics: An introduction. *Physics Today*, 1978. **31**(12): 52.

42. Folkers, J.P., P.E. Laibinis, and G.M. Whitesides, Self-assembled monolayers of alkanethiols on gold: Comparisons of monolayers containing mixtures of short- and long-chain constituents with methyl and hydroxymethyl terminal groups. *Langmuir*, 1992. **8**(5): 1330.

43. Kakiuchi, T. et al., Miscibility of adsorbed 1-undecanethiol and 11-mercaptoundecanoic acid species in binary self-assembled monolayers on Au(111). *Langmuir*, 2001. **17**(5): 1599.

44. Li, L., S. Chen, and S. Jiang, Protein adsorption on alkanethiolate self-assembled monolayers: Nanoscale surface structural and chemical effects. *Langmuir*, 2003. **19**(7): 2974.

45. Briand, E. et al., Functionalisation of gold surfaces with thiolate SAMs: Topography/bioactivity relationship—A combined FT-RAIRS, AFM and QCM investigation. *Surface Science*, 2007. **601**(18): 3850–3855.

46. Hottin, J. et al., Biochip data normalization using multifunctional probes, *Analyst*, 2012, 137: 3119–3125.

47. Fiche, J.B. et al., Point mutation detection by surface plasmon resonance imaging coupled with a temperature scan method in a model system. *Analytical Chemistry*, 2008. **80**(4): 1049.

48. Descamps, E. et al., Fabrication of oligonucleotide chips by using parallel cantilever-based electrochemical deposition in picoliter volumes. *Advanced Materials*, 2007. **19**(14): 1816–1821.

49. Grosjean, L. et al., A polypyrrole protein microarray for antibody–antigen interaction studies using a label-free detection process. *Analytical Biochemistry*, 2005. **347**(2): 193.

50. Maillart, E. et al., Surface plasmon resonance imaging and versatile surface functionalization for real time comparisons of biochemical interactions, Biophotonics New Frontier: From Genome to Proteome. *Proceedings of SPIE*, 2004. 5461: 69–77.

51. Livache, T. et al., Polypyrrole based DNA hybridization assays: Study of label free detection processes versus fluorescence on microchips. *Journal of Pharmaceutical and Biomedical Analysis*, 2003. **32**(4–5): 687.

52. Livache, T. et al., Polypyrrole electrospotting for the construction of oligonucleotide arrays compatible with a surface plasmon resonance hybridization detection. *Synthetic Metals*, 2001. **121**(1–3): 1443.

53. Lassalle, N. et al., Electronically conductive polymer grafted with oligonucleotides as electrosensors of DNA: Preliminary study of real time monitoring by in situ techniques. *Journal of Electroanalytical Chemistry*, 2001. **509**(1): 48.

54. Livache, T. et al., Electroconducting polymers for the construction of DNA or peptide arrays on silicon chips. *Biosensors and Bioelectronics*, 1998. **13**(6): 629.

55. Livache, T., H. Bazin, and G. Mathis, Conducting polymers on microelectronic devices as tools for biological analyses. *Clinica Chimica Acta*, 1998. **278**(2): 171.

56. Livache, T. et al., Preparation of a DNA matrix via an electrochemically directed copolymerization of pyrrole and oligonucleotides bearing a pyrrole group. *Nucleic Acids Research*, 1994. **22**(15): 2915–2921.

57. Love, J.C. et al., Self-assembled monolayers of thiolates on metals as a form of nanotechnology. *Chemical Reviews*, 2005. **105**(4): 1103.

58. Laibinis, P.E. et al., Comparison of the structures and wetting properties of self-assembled monolayers of normal-alkanethiols on the coinage metal-surfaces, Cu, Ag, Au. *Journal of the American Chemical Society*, 1991. **113**(19): 7152–7167.

59. Ulman, A., *An Introduction to Ultrathin Organic Films: From Langmuir–Blodgett to Self-Assembly*, Academic Press, London, U.K., 1991, 442pp.

60. Ulman, A., Formation and structure of self-assembled monolayers. *Chemical Reviews*, 1996. **96**(4): 1533.

61. Boujday, S. et al., Detection of pathogenic *Staphylococcus aureus* bacteria by gold based immunosensors. *Microchimica Acta*, 2008. **163**(3–4): 203–209.

62. Boujday, S. et al., Innovative surface characterization techniques applied to immunosensor elaboration and test: Comparing the efficiency of Fourier transform-surface plasmon resonance, quartz crystal microbalance with dissipation measurements, and polarization modulation-reflection absorption infrared spectroscopy. *Analytical Biochemistry*, 2009. **387**(2): 194–201.

63. Boujday, S. et al., In-depth investigation of protein adsorption on gold surfaces: Correlating the structure and density to the efficiency of the sensing layer. *Journal of Physical Chemistry B*, 2008. **112**(21): 6708–6715.

64. Tielens, F. et al., Stability of binary SAMs formed by omega-acid and alcohol functionalized thiol mixtures. *Langmuir*, 2009. **25**(17): 9980–9985.

65. Ben Ali, M. et al., Use of ultra-thin organic silane films for the improvement of gold adhesion to the silicon dioxide wafers for (bio)sensor applications. *Materials Science and Engineering C: Biomimetic and Supramolecular Systems*, 2008. **28**(5–6): 628–632.

66. Skaife, J.J. and N.L. Abbott, Quantitative interpretation of the optical textures of liquid crystals caused by specific binding of immunoglobulins to surface-bound antigens. *Langmuir*, 2000. **16**(7): 3529.

67. Skaife, J.J. and N.L. Abbott, Influence of molecular-level interactions on the orientations of liquid crystals supported on nanostructured surfaces presenting specifically bound proteins. *Langmuir*, 2001. **17**(18): 5595.

68. Skaife, J.J., J.M. Brake, and N.L. Abbott, Influence of nanometer-scale topography of surfaces on the orientational response of liquid crystals to proteins specifically bound to surface-immobilized receptors. *Langmuir*, 2001. **17**(18): 5448.

69. Ahn, W. et al., Electroless gold island thin films: Photoluminescence and thermal transformation to nanoparticle ensembles. *Langmuir*, 2008. **24**(8): 4174.

70. Boussert, S. et al., An intramolecular O–N migration reaction on gold surfaces: Toward the preparation of well-defined amyloid surfaces. *ACS Nano*, 2009. **3**(10): 3091.

71. Hostetler, M.J., A.C. Templeton, and R.W. Murray, Dynamics of place-exchange reactions on monolayer-protected gold cluster molecules. *Langmuir*, 1999. **15**(11): 3782.

72. Poirier, G.E. et al., Molecular-scale characterization of the reaction of ozone with decanethiol monolayers on Au(111). *Journal of the American Chemical Society*, 1999. **121**(41): 9703.

73. Poirier, G.E. and M.J. Tarlov, Molecular ordering and gold migration observed in butanethiol self-assembled monolayers using scanning tunneling microscopy. *The Journal of Physical Chemistry*, 1995. **99**(27): 10966.

74. Lauer, M.E. et al., Formation and healing of micrometer-sized channel networks on highly mobile Au(111) surfaces. *Langmuir*, 2007. **23**(10): 5459–5465.

75. Poirier, G.E. and M.J. Tarlov, The c(4X2) superlattice of n-alkanethiol monolayers self-assembled on Au(111). *Langmuir*, 1994. **10**(9): 2853.

76. Maalouf, R. et al., Label-free detection of bacteria by electrochemical impedance spectroscopy: Comparison to surface plasmon resonance. *Analytical Chemistry*, 2007. **79**(13): 4879–4886.

77. Cloarec, J.P. et al., A multidisciplinary approach for molecular diagnostics based on biosensors and microarrays. *IRBM*, 2008. **29**(2–3): 105–127.

78. Löfås, S. and A. Mcwhirter, The art of immobilization for SPR biosensors, *Surface Plasmon Resonance Based Biosensors*, Springer Series on Chemical Sensors and Biosensors 2006, vol. 4, Springer, Berlin, Germany, 2006, pp. 117–151.

79. Hermanson, G.T., *Bioconjugate Techniques*, 2nd edn., Elsevier, Burlington, MA, 2008, 1323pp.

80. Löfås, S. and B. Johnsson, A novel hydrogel matrix on gold surfaces in surface plasmon resonance sensors for fast and efficient covalent immobilization of ligands. *Chemical Communications*, 1990. 21: 1526–1528.

81. Soultani-Vigneron, S. et al., Immobilisation of oligo-peptidic probes for microarray implementation: Characterisation by FTIR, atomic force microscopy and 2D fluorescence. *Journal of Chromatography B: Analytical Technologies in the Biomedical and Life Sciences*, 2005. **822**(1–2): 304–310.

82. Dugas, V. et al., Immobilization of single-stranded DNA fragments to solid surfaces and their repeatable specific hybridization: Covalent binding or adsorption? *Sensors and Actuators B: Chemical*, 2004. **101**(1–2): 112–121.

83. Blanchard, A.P., R.J. Kaiser, and L.E. Hood, High-density oligonucleotide arrays. *Biosensors & Bioelectronics*, 1996. **11**(6–7): 687.

84. Brès, J.C. et al., New method for DNA microarrays development: Applied to human platelet antigens polymorphisms. *Biomedical Microdevices*, 2005. **7**(2): 137.

85. El Khoury, G. et al., Acid deprotection of covalently immobilized peptide probes on glass slides for peptide microarrays, in *2007 Annual International Conference of the IEEE Engineering in Medicine and Biology Society*, vols. 1–16, Lyon, France, 2007, pp. 2242–2246.

86. El Khoury, G. et al., A generic surface chemistry for peptide microarrays implementation: Application to the detection of anti-H3 antibody. *Biosensors & Bioelectronics*, 2010. **26**(4): 1320–1325.

87. Wieczerzak, E. et al., Monitoring of native chemical ligation on solid substrate by surface plasmon resonance. *Peptide Science*, 2008. **90**(3): 415–420.

88. Maskos, U. and E.M. Southern, Parallel analysis of oligodeoxyribonucleotide (oligonucleotide) interactions. 1. Analysis of factors influencing oligonucleotide duplex formation. *Nucleic Acids Research*, 1992. **20**(7): 1675–1678.

89. Maskos, U. and E.M. Southern, Oligonucleotide hybridizations on glass supports—A novel linker for oligonucleotide synthesis and hybridization properties of oligonucleotides synthesized in situ. *Nucleic Acids Research*, 1992. **20**(7): 1679–1684.

90. Southern, E.M. et al., Arrays of complementary oligonucleotides for analyzing the hybridization behavior of nucleic-acids. *Nucleic Acids Research*, 1994. **22**(8): 1368–1373.

91. Spadavecchia, J. et al., New cysteamine based functionalization for biochip applications. *Sensors and Actuators B: Chemical*, 2009. **143**(1): 139.

92. Gray, D.E. et al., Ellipsometric and interferometric characterization of DNA probes immobilized on a combinatorial array. *Langmuir*, 1997. **13**(10): 2833–2842.

93. Bras, M. et al., Optimisation of a silicon/silicon dioxide substrate for a fluorescence DNA microarray. *Biosensors & Bioelectronics*, 2004. **20**(4): 797–806.

94. Bessueille, F. et al., Assessment of porous silicon substrate for well-characterised sensitive DNA chip implement. *Biosensors & Bioelectronics*, 2005. **21**(6): 908–916.

95. Mazurczyk, R. et al., Low-cost, fast prototyping method of fabrication of the microreactor devices in soda-lime glass. *Sensors and Actuators B: Chemical*, 2008. **128**(2): 552.

96. Babacan, S. et al., Evaluation of antibody immobilization methods for piezoelectric biosensor application. *Biosensors & Bioelectronics*, 2000. **15**(11–12): 615–621.

97. Mannelli, I. et al., DNA immobilisation procedures for surface plasmon resonance imaging (SPRI) based microarray systems. *Biosensors & Bioelectronics*, 2007. **22**(6): 803–809.

98. Storri, S. et al., Surface modifications for the development of piezoimmunosensors. *Biosensors & Bioelectronics*, 1998. **13**(3–4): 347–357.

99. Tombelli, S., M. Mascini, and A.P.F. Turner, Improved procedures for immobilisation of oligonucleotides on gold-coated piezoelectric quartz crystals. *Biosensors & Bioelectronics*, 2002. **17**(11–12): 929–936.

100. Cui, X. et al., Layer-by-layer assembly of multilayer films composed of avidin and biotin-labeled antibody for immunosensing. *Biosensors & Bioelectronics*, 2003. **18**(1): 59.

101. Hou, Y. et al., Immobilization of rhodopsin on a self-assembled multilayer and its specific detection by electrochemical impedance spectroscopy. *Biosensors & Bioelectronics*, 2006. **21**(7): 1393.

102. Trevisan, M. et al., Evanescent wave fluorescence biosensor combined with DNA bio-barcode assay for platelet genotyping. *Biosensors & Bioelectronics*, 2010. **26**(4): 1631–1637.

103. Grubor, N.M. et al., Novel biosensor chip for simultaneous detection of DNA-carcinogen adducts with low-temperature fluorescence. *Biosensors & Bioelectronics*, 2004. **19**(6): 547–556.

104. Cloarec, J.P. et al., Immobilization of homooligonucleotide probe layers onto Si/SiO_2 substrates: Characterization by electrochemical impedance measurements and radiolabelling. *Biosensors & Bioelectronics*, 2002. **17**(5): 405–412.

105. Storri, S., T. Santoni, and M. Mascini, A piezoelectric biosensor for DNA hybridisation detection. *Analytical Letters*, 1998. **31**(11): 1795–1808.

106. Squires, T.M., R.J. Messinger, and S.R. Manalis, Making it stick: Convection, reaction and diffusion in surface-based biosensors. *Nature Biotechnology*, 2008. **26**(4): 417–426.

107. Rich, R.L. and D.G. Myszka, Grading the commercial optical biosensor literature-class of 2008: 'The Mighty Binders'. *Journal of Molecular Recognition*, 2010. **23**(1): 1–64.

108. Myszka, D.G. et al., Extending the range of rate constants available from BIACORE: Interpreting mass transport-influenced binding data. *Biophysical Journal*, 1998. **75**(2): 583–594.

109. Karlsson, R. et al., Kinetic and concentration analysis using BIA technology. *Methods*, 1994. **6**(2): 99–110.

110. Frommelt, T. et al., Microfluidic mixing via acoustically driven chaotic advection. *Physical Review Letters*, 2008. **100**(3): 034502.

111. Roper, D.K., Enhancing lateral mass transport to improve the dynamic range of adsorption rates measured by surface plasmon resonance. *Chemical Engineering Science*, 2006. **61**(8): 2557–2564.

112. Nguyen, N.T. and Z.G. Wu, Micromixers—A review. *Journal of Micromechanics and Microengineering*, 2005. **15**(2): R1–R16.

113. Sritharan, K. et al., Acoustic mixing at low Reynold's numbers. *Applied Physics Letters*, 2006. **88**(5): 054102.

114. Coakley, W.T. and L.A. Kuznetsova, Applications of ultrasound streaming and radiation force in biosensors. *Biosensors & Bioelectronics*, 2007. **22**(8): 1567–1577.

115. Charette, P.G. et al., Integrated active mixing and biosensing using surface acoustic waves (SAW) and surface plasmon resonance (SPR) on a common substrate. *Lab on a Chip*, 2010. **10**(1): 111–115.

116. Cular, S. et al., Removal of nonspecifically bound proteins on microarrays using surface acoustic waves. *IEEE Sensors Journal*, 2008. **8**(3–4): 314–320.

117. Meyer, G.D. et al., Nonspecific binding removal from protein microarrays using thickness shear mode resonators. *IEEE Sensors Journal*, 2006. **6**(2): 254–261.

118. Hottin, A. et al., Iminosugar-ferrocene conjugates as potential anticancer agents. *Organic and Biomolecular Chemistry*, 2012. **10**(29): 5592–5597.

119. Lecaruyer, P., M. Canva, and J. Rolland, Metallic film optimization in a surface plasmon resonance biosensor by the extended Rouard method. *Applied Optics*, 2007. **46**(12): 2361–2369.

120. Lecaruyer, P. et al., Generalization of the Rouard method to an absorbing thin-film stack and application to surface plasmon resonance. *Applied Optics*, 2006. **45**(33): 8419–8423.

121. Omuro, A. et al., Phase II trial of continuous low-dose temozolomide for patients with recurrent malignant glioma. *Neuro Oncology*, 2013. **15**(2): 242–250.

122. Nenninger, G.G., M. Piliarik, and J. Homola, Data analysis for optical sensors based on spectroscopy of surface plasmons, *Measurement Science and Technology*, 2002. 13(12): 2038–2046.

123. Thirstrup, C. and W. Zong, Data analysis for surface plasmon resonance sensors using dynamic baseline algorithm, *Sensors & Actuators B: Chemical*, 2005. 106(2): 796–802.

124. Hottinger, A.F. et al., Decision making and management of gliomas: Practical considerations. *Annals of Oncology*, 2012. **23**(Suppl. 10): x33–x40.

125. Leavitt, D.A. et al., A case series of genital vascular anomalies in children and their management: Lessons learned. *Urology*, 2012. **80**(4): 914–918.

126. Bardin, F., A. Bellemain, G. Roger, and M. Canva, Surface plasmon resonance spectro-imaging sensor for biomolecular surface interaction characterization, *Biosensors & Bioelectronics*, 2009. 24(7): 2100–2105.

127. Grigorenko, A.N., P.I. Nikitin, and A.V. Kabashin, Phase jumps and interferometric surface plasmon resonance imaging. *Applied Physics Letters*, 1999. **75**(25): 3917–3919.

128. Nikitin, P.I. et al., Surface plasmon resonance interferometry for micro-array biosensing. *Sensors and Actuators A: Physical*, 2000. **85**(1–3): 189–193.

129. Lee, G.B. et al., Microfluidic systems integrated with two-dimensional surface plasmon resonance phase imaging systems for microarray immunoassay. *Biosensors & Bioelectronics*, 2007. **23**(4): 466–472.
130. Lakowicz, J.R., Radiative decay engineering 5: Metal-enhanced fluorescence and plasmon emission. *Analytical Biochemistry*, 2005. **337**(2): 171–194.
131. Liebermann, T. and W. Knoll, Surface-plasmon field-enhanced fluorescence spectroscopy. *Colloids and Surfaces A: Physicochemical and Engineering Aspects*, 2000. **171**(1–3): 115–130.
132. Piliarik, M. and J. Homola, Surface plasmon resonance (SPR) sensors: Approaching their limits? *Optics Express*, 2009. **17**(19): 16505–16517.
133. Stemmler, I., A. Brecht, and G. Gauglitz, Compact surface plasmon resonance-transducers with spectral readout for biosensing applications. *Sensors and Actuators B: Chemical*, 1999. **54**(1–2): 98–105.
134. Piliarik, M., L. Parova, and J. Homola, High-throughput SPR sensor for food safety. *Biosensors & Bioelectronics*, 2009. **24**(5): 1399–1404.
135. Chinowsky, T.M. et al., Performance of the Spreeta 2000 integrated surface plasmon resonance affinity sensor. *Sensors and Actuators B: Chemical*, 2003. **91**(1–3): 266–274.
136. Wu, C.M. and M.C. Pao, Sensitivity-tunable optical sensors based on surface plasmon resonance and phase detection. *Optics Express*, 2004. **12**(15): 3509–3514.
137. Piliarik, M. et al., Compact and low-cost biosensor based on novel approach to spectroscopy of surface plasmons. *Biosensors & Bioelectronics*, 2009. **24**(12): 3430–3435.
138. Guedon, P. et al., Characterization and optimization of a real-time, parallel, label-free, polypyrrole-based DNA sensor by surface plasmon resonance imaging. *Analytical Chemistry*, 2000. **72**(24): 6003.
139. Rothenhausler, B. and W. Knoll, Surface-plasmon microscopy. *Nature*, 1988. **332**(6165): 615–617.
140. Fotin, A.V. et al., Parallel thermodynamic analysis of duplexes on oligodeoxyribonucleotide microchips. *Nucleic Acids Research*, 1998. **26**(6): 1515–1521.
141. Bommarito, S., N. Peyret, and J. SantaLucia, Jr., Thermodynamic parameters for DNA sequences with dangling ends. *Nucleic Acids Research*, 2000. **28**(9): 1929–1934.
142. Allawi, H.T. and J. SantaLucia, Jr., Nearest neighbor thermodynamic parameters for internal G.A mismatches in DNA. *Biochemistry*, 1998. **37**(8): 2170–2179.
143. Allawi, H.T. and J. SantaLucia, Jr., Thermodynamics of internal C.T mismatches in DNA. *Nucleic Acids Research*, 1998. **26**(11): 2694–2701.
144. Haddour, N., Y. Chevolot, M. Trévisan, E. Souteyrand, and J.P. Cloarec, Use of magnetic field for addressing, grafting onto support and actuating permanent magnetic filaments applied to enhanced biodetection. *Journal of Materials Chemistry*, 2010. **20**(38): 8266–8271.
145. Balladur, V., A. Theretz, and B. Mandrand, Determination of the main forces driving DNA oligonucleotide adsorption onto aminated silica wafers. *Journal of Colloid and Interface Science*, 1997. **194**(2): 408–418.
146. Bras, M., V. Dugas, F. Bessueille, J.P. Cloarec, J.R. Martin, M. Cabrera, and M. Garrigues, Optimisation of a silicon/silicon dioxide substrate for a fluorescence DNA microarray. *Biosensors and Bioelectronics*, 2004. **20**(4): 797–806.
147. Brès, J.C., Y. Merieux, V. Dugas, J. Broutin, E. Vnuk, M. Jaber, and J.P. Cloarec, New method for DNA microarrays development applied to human platelet antigens polymorphisms. *Biomedical microdevices*, 2005. **7**(2): 137–141.
148. Calevro, F., H. Charles, N. Reymond, V. Dugas, J.P. Cloarec, J. Bernillon, and J.M. Fayard, Assessment of 35mer amino-modified oligonucleotide based microarray with bacterial samples. *Journal of Microbiological Methods*, 2004. **57**(2): 207–218.
149. Li, L., S. Chen, S. Oh, and S. Jiang, In situ single-molecule detection of antibody-antigen binding by tapping-mode atomic force microscopy. *Analytical Chemistry*, 2002. **74**(23): 6017–6022.
150. Wang, H., S. Chen, L. Li, and S. Jiang, Improved method for the preparation of carboxylic acid and amine terminated self-assembled monolayers of alkanethiolates. *Langmuir*, 2005. **21**(7): 2633–2636.

151. Mosquet, M., Y. Chevalier, P. Le Perchec, and J.P. Guicquero, Synthesis of poly (ethylene oxide) with a terminal amino group by anionic polymerization of ethylene oxide initiated by aminoalcoholates. *Macromolecular Chemistry and Physics*, 1997. **198**(8): 2457–2474.

152. Cosnier, S. Biomolecule immobilization on electrode surfaces by entrapment or attachment to electrochemically polymerized films. A review. *Biosensors and Bioelectronics*, 1999. **14**(5): 443–456.

153. Haddour, N., J. Chauvin, C. Gondran, and S. Cosnier, Photoelectrochemical immunosensor for label-free detection and quantification of anti-cholera toxin antibody. *Journal of the American Chemical Society*, 2006. **128**(30): 9693–9698.

154. Vidic, J., M. Pla-Roca, J. Grosclaude, M.A. Persuy, R. Monnerie, D. Caballero, and J. Samitier, Gold surface functionalization and patterning for specific immobilization of olfactory receptors carried by nanosomes. *Analytical Chemistry*, 2007. **79**(9): 3280–3290.

155. Briand, E., M. Salmain, J.M. Herry, H. Perrot, C. Compère, and C.M. Pradier, Building of an immunosensor: How can the composition and structure of the thiol attachment layer affect the immunosensor efficiency? *Biosensors and Bioelectronics*, 2006. **22**(3): 440–448.

156. Lu, B., M.R. Smyth, and R. O'Kennedy, Oriented immobilization of antibodies and its applications in immunoassays and immunosensors. *Analyst*, 1996. **121**(3): 29R–32R.

8

Surface-Enhanced Raman Scattering for Biomedical Diagnostics

Tuan Vo-Dinh
Duke University

David L. Stokes
EOIR Technologies

8.1 Introduction

Raman spectroscopy is based on vibrational transitions that yield very narrow spectral features that are characteristic of the investigated sample. Thus, it has long been regarded as a valuable tool for the identification of chemical and biological samples as well as the elucidation of molecular structure, surface processes, and interface reactions. Despite such advantages, Raman scattering suffers the disadvantage of extremely poor efficiency. Compared to luminescence-based processes, Raman spectroscopy has an inherently small cross section (e.g., 10^{-30} cm^2 per molecule), thus precluding the possibility of analyte detection at low concentration levels without special enhancement processes. Some modes of signal enhancement have included resonance Raman scattering and nonlinear processes such as coherent anti-Stokes Raman scattering. However, the need for high-power, multiple-wavelength excitation sources has limited the widespread use of these techniques.

Nevertheless, there has been a renewed interest in Raman techniques in the past three decades due the discovery of the surface-enhanced Raman scattering (SERS) effect, which results from the adsorption of molecules on specially textured metallic surfaces. The giant enhancement was first reported in 1974 by Fleischmann et al., who observed the effect for pyridine molecules adsorbed on electrochemically roughened silver electrodes.[1] It was initially believed that the enhancement resulted from the increased surface area produced by the electrochemical roughening, giving rise to increased probed sample density.

The teams of Jeanmaire and Van Duyne[2] and Albrecht and Creighton[3] later confirmed the enhancement (up to 10^8) but attributed the effect to more complex surface enhancement processes, which continue to be the subject of intense theoretical studies. More recent reports have cited SERS enhancements from 10^{13} to 10^{15}, thus demonstrating the potential for single-molecule detection with SERS.[4–14] In fact, studies have demonstrated single-molecule detection of compounds of biomedical interest.[10–14]

In the early years following the discovery of SERS (mid-1970s), the focus of SERS studies was on the development of theoretical models to account for the SERS effect.[15–21] However, these studies were limited to a small number of highly polarizable molecules in the 1–100 mM concentration range. As a result, despite the great theoretical progress achieved in early SERS studies, interest in SERS as a practical analytical tool was delayed largely because of the common belief that the SERS effect occurred only for a few compounds under specific experimental conditions. Nevertheless, the 1980s marked the beginning of a new phase of SERS evolution, which was characterized by the development of a wide variety of SERS-inducing media and applications to a wide range of chemicals. For example, the use of planar solid-surface-based substrates for SERS-based measurements of a variety of chemicals, including several homocyclic and heterocyclic polyaromatic compounds, was first reported in 1984.[22] These substrates were composed of a planar support material that was covered with dielectric nanoparticles to impart the roughness required for the SERS effect and then overcoated with a layer of silver. In a similar approach, silver-coated frosted glass was demonstrated to be SERS active.[23] Silver colloids were investigated for analytical applications.[24–27] Indeed, silver colloids were a popular media for early SERS-based applications due to the fact that, with some skill and patience, they could be prepared with chemical reagents available in most common analytical laboratories. In addition, research demonstrated that silver colloids could be used in solid[28,29] as well as free-solution matrices. Researchers also found that through a variety of innovative techniques, the reduction process for producing elemental silver colloids could be made to match the chemical and environmental conditions of specific applications. For example, SERS-active *photocolloids* were produced through in situ laser-induced photoreduction of silver nitrate solutions.[30] The development of a wide variety of additional SERS-inducing media had been described in the early 1980s; these included electrolyte interfaces, mechanically ground silver, matrix-isolated metal clusters, holographic gratings, silver island films, gold colloids, and tunnel junctions with a silver electrode on a rough surface.[14] Because of the aggressive development of SERS substrates and application to a wide range of chemicals, the potential of SERS as a routine analytical technique was recognized by the mid-1980s.

The SERS technique has since continued to receive increased interest, as is evidenced by the large number of papers and review articles.[15–19,31–37] Furthermore, the scope of SERS has been extended to include other surface-enhanced spectroscopies such as surface-enhanced second-harmonic generation[38] and surface-enhanced hyper-Raman scattering.[39]

This chapter provides a brief theoretical background on the SERS effect, followed by a synopsis of the development of SERS-inducing media that have demonstrated repeated success and show great potential for use in biomedical analysis. The chapter also summarizes some of the most significant applications of SERS to date, with a focus on both chemical and biomedical areas. Some highlights of this chapter include reports of various fiber-optic SERS monitors, SERS nanoprobes, near-field SERS probes, SERS-based bioassays, and single-molecule detection.

8.2 Theoretical Background

Since the discovery of the SERS effect in the 1970s, extensive fundamental studies have been undertaken to gain a better understanding of the enhancement mechanisms. Nevertheless, it is believed that our current understanding of SERS is still incomplete. For instance, the most established theoretical models predict maximum Raman enhancements on the order of 10^6–10^8 for the SERS effect. However, recent near-field SERS measurements have shown evidence of SERS enhancement factors as high as 10^{13}.[8,9] Single-molecule studies have further indicated that enhancement factors on the order of 10^{14}–10^{15} may be possible at specific sites referred to as *hot spots*.[4–7,40] Although new experimental observations in SERS studies are expected to spur the development of new or refined theoretical models, several current theoretical models could explain some of the more general observations associated with the SERS effect.

A qualitative understanding of the SERS process can be gained through the classical theory of light scattering. Consider an incident light beam inducing an oscillating dipole, Φ, in a particle that scatters light at the frequency of the dipole oscillation.[41] The dipole moment consists generally of many different harmonic frequency components; each component may be represented by the following equation:

$$\Phi(t) = \Phi° \cos(2\pi v t) \tag{8.1}$$

where

v is the dipole oscillation (i.e., scattering) frequency

$\Phi°$ is the maximum induced dipole moment for a given frequency component of Φ

For the case where the magnitude of the incident electric field E_{inc} is not too large, the induced dipole moment can be approximated as

$$\Phi(t) = P \cdot E_{inc}(t) \tag{8.2}$$

where P is the polarizability of the molecule. The polarizability, which is a tensor quantity, can be qualitatively described as the ease with which molecular orbitals are distorted in the presence of an external field.

Because Raman intensity is proportional to the square of the induced dipole, Φ, it can be inferred from Equation 8.2 that enhancements of either the incident field or the molecular polarizability or both can contribute to Raman enhancements observed via SERS. As a result, theoretical models generally involve two major types of enhancement mechanisms: (1) an *electromagnetic effect* (sometimes referred to as the field effect) in which the molecule experiences large local fields caused by electromagnetic resonances occurring near metal surface structures and (2) a *chemical effect* (also referred to as the molecular effect) in which the molecular polarizability is affected by interactions between the molecule and the metal surface.

The relative contributions of the two mechanisms can vary widely for different molecules, largely because of the specificity of the *chemical effect*. Electromagnetic interactions, which are more general and relatively long range (i.e., inversely dependent on the distance cubed between the adsorbed molecule and the metal surface), have been extensively investigated and are reasonably well understood. On the other hand, short-range *chemical effects*, which may be dependent on atomic-scale features of both the metal surface and the adsorbed molecule, are less well known and are currently topics of extensive research. A detailed summary of these studies is far beyond the scope of this chapter but can be found in a number of excellent reviews.[15–20,32,35,42]

8.3 Development of SERS Substrates

The first SERS-active surfaces to be discovered—roughened metal electrodes—served as the basis for extensive theoretical studies. Subsequently, metal colloids gained widespread use in SERS studies because they could easily be prepared chemically with commonly used reagents. While the popularity of metal colloids has persisted since the early 1980s, alternative media—metal nanoparticle films and nanostructured probes—have since been developed for a wide variety of applications with improved reproducibility. Etched quartz posts coated with silver have also exhibited a great deal of reproducibility. In an effort to simplify fabrication of solid SERS probes, materials have been mechanically roughened to induce the SERS effect. Inherently, rough silver membranes requiring little additional preparation, have also been investigated. Many of these technologies have been the basis of recently developed innovative probes, such as silver nanoparticle-embedded solgels and polymers, in situ photoreduced sols, and a variety of fiber-optic-based SERS probes.

Some particularly exciting movements in SERS probe development have focused on SERS nanoprobes and near-field probes, which have introduced the possibility of extremely spatially specific SERS analysis as well as single-molecule detection. Another area of intense research has been the development of highly specific solid SERS probes that incorporate coatings of polymers, self-assembled monolayers (SAMs), and bioreceptors. As a result of the extensive development of SERS-based probes, the scope of applications of SERS has been dramatically expanded to include solid, liquid, and airborne samples in many major areas (e.g., environmental, biotechnical, biomedical, remote-sensing analyses).

8.3.1 Metal Electrodes

Electrochemically roughened electrodes were the first media with which the SERS effect was observed.[1] The observation of this effect resulted in further inaugural studies to confirm it and to establish enhancement factors.[2,3,19] While several metals have been investigated for SERS activity in electrochemical cells,[21,43–46] silver has been most commonly used. During electrochemical preparation, silver at the electrode surface is first oxidized by the reaction $Ag \rightarrow Ag^+ + e^-$; then, elemental silver is redeposited in the ensuing reduction process, $Ag^+ + e^- \rightarrow Ag$. This oxidation–reduction procedure generally produces protrusions on the electrode surface in the size range of 25–500 nm. Strong SERS signals appear only after several electrochemical oxidation–reduction cycles, often referred to as *activation cycles*.

Other metal electrodes roughened by oxidation–reduction cycles have been investigated for use as SERS substrates; these include platinum[44] and copper.[47,48] A distinct advantage of roughened metal electrodes is that they allow selective detection in situ by promoting adsorption of particular compounds at specific applied voltages. For example, both SERS and surface-enhanced hyper-Raman spectroscopy (SEHRS) have been reported for pyrazine and pyridine adsorbed on silver electrodes at varying potentials.[49] Oxidized forms of metal electrodes have also been demonstrated to promote enhanced adsorption of compounds otherwise exhibiting low SERS intensity. For example, oxidized silver electrodes have made possible enhanced detection of nerve agent simulants.[50] In addition, aluminum oxide surfaces have been used for the detection of phthalic acid isomers and phenylphosphate in the near-infrared (NIR) region.[51,52]

8.3.2 Metal Colloids

SERS-active suspensions of elemental metal colloids or nanoparticles of various sizes can be chemically formed in solution. Hence, they can be readily used in suspension for in situ solution SERS measurements. Alternatively, they can be immobilized on various solid media for use as surface-based SERS substrates. As with roughened metal electrodes, silver is the most commonly used material. Silver colloids can easily be prepared by reducing a solution of $AgNO_3$ with ice-cold $NaBH_4$,[24–30,53–55] trisodium citrate,[56,57] or hydrogen peroxide under basic conditions.[58] Other more innovative techniques that reduce the need for wet chemistry have been demonstrated. For example, Ahern and Garrell described a unique in situ photoreduction method to produce photocolloids in solutions,[30] while another innovative method involved laser ablation of colloids from silver foils into aqueous solutions.[59]

Gold colloids have also been investigated as SERS-active media. Because gold is virtually bioinert, it may prove to be a valuable material for biomedical applications of SERS. Furthermore, gold produces large SERS enhancement factors when NIR excitation sources are used. NIR excitation radiation is particularly useful in biomedical studies because it allows greater penetration depths in tissues while causing less fluorescence background relative to visible radiation. Gold sols have been used for the SERS detection of various dyes.[11,60,61] In particular, Kneipp et al. have observed extremely large enhancement factors (up to 10^{14}) for dyes adsorbed on gold colloids when using NIR excitation.[7] Silver-encapsulated gold nanoparticles[62] and silver oxide sols[63] have also been reported to induce SERS activity. Silver-encapsulated gold nanoparticles in particular have shown great potential for biomedical applications.[64–66]

A primary advantage of colloid hydrosols is that they make SERS an accessible technology. For example, they are easily produced with common chemical reagents. Furthermore, they can be readily characterized by simple UV absorption spectroscopy. The production of hydrosols does not require the use of expensive, bulky vacuum evaporation chambers, which are common to the production of solid silver-coated nanoparticle-based substrates (see Sections 8.3.3.2 and 8.3.3.3). On the other hand, this wet chemistry-based procedure is vulnerable to environmental factors as well as experimental error. As a result, the reproducibility in hydrosol sizes can be problematic. Furthermore, the size range can be quite large for particles produced in a single batch. The selection of colloidal particles with optimal sizes requires a tedious procedure.[67] Although some reports have indicated that carefully prepared colloid solutions can last for more than 3 weeks,[25–27,68] they more often tend to be unstable. More specifically, the colloids have a propensity to aggregate into particles that are too large to induce the SERS effect. In order to offset this disadvantage, stabilizers such as poly(vinylalcohol), poly(vinylpyrrolidone) (PVPL), and sodium dodecyl sulfate have been used to hinder this coagulation process.[69–71]

As mentioned earlier, bimetallic nanoparticles have been developed to improve compatibility with biological systems while preserving giant SERS enhancements. Other examples of multiple-layer and heterogeneous composite nanoparticles have recently been reported. For example, silica-coated metallic nanoparticles have been developed for stability and a basis for imparting functionality for biomedical diagnosis.[72–74] Furthermore, dye-embedded nanoparticles such as SERS dots and composite organic–inorganic nanoparticles (COINS) have proven to yield exceptional sensitivity and selectivity in bioassays.[75–79] Functionalized gold nanoshells have been demonstrated to serve as both a vehicle of therapeutic drug delivery and a medium to potentially monitor such delivery through SERS.[80] The combined attributes of high sensitivity, selectivity, and stability afforded by recent developments in various SERS-active nanoparticles have made them amenable to multiplex bioassay formats[75,79,81,82] including conventional lateral flow platforms and microfluidic lab-on-a-chip formats.[83–86] They have also been applied to SERS-based imaging of cells[64,87] and analysis of tissues.[79,88]

Metal colloids have also been adapted for use in solid-surface-based substrates. For example, silver colloids have been immobilized on filter paper supports (cellulose, glass, and quartz fibers) for the SERS detection of various dyes.[28,29] However, the SERS effect was found to depend highly on the specific type of filter paper that was used. In a similar approach, filter paper treated with silver colloids has been used for the collection and detection of trace amounts of atmospheric contaminants in aerosols.[89] Extensive studies have been devoted to the immobilization of colloids on various substrates pretreated with organic coatings having affinities for both silver and gold. For example, Freeman et al. have demonstrated self-assembly of monodisperse silver and gold colloid polymers on substrates coated with polymers having cyanide, amine, and thiol functional groups.[90] SAMs of *p*-aminothiophenol[91,92] and *p*-mercaptopyridine[93] have also been used to adsorb gold colloids onto solid gold surfaces. A disadvantage to using SAMs to immobilize colloids is an inherent background SERS signal yielded by the underlying SAM. Nevertheless, such signals have been the basis for fundamental studies regarding the self-assembly of the colloid overlayer. For example, kinetic studies of the assembly of silver and gold colloids on organosilane-polymer-treated surfaces have been pursued.[94,95] Results of these studies have permitted the control and optimization of intercolloid spacing in the production of SAM-based SERS probes. In an innovative method for producing patterns of gold nanoparticles, microcontact printing has been used to deposit corresponding patterns of the underlying poly(dimethyl)siloxane SAMs with amine and thiol functionalities.[96] Finally, SAMs of 3-aminopropyl trimethoxysilane have even been used to immobilize silver colloids on optical fibers for the production of SERS-active fiber-optic sensors.[97]

8.3.3 Solid SERS Substrates Based on Metallic Nanostructures

In addition to immobilized colloids, researchers have developed a variety of solid-surface-based SERS substrates that are produced entirely from solid materials, as depicted schematically in Figure 8.1. In contrast to immobilized colloids, the solid SERS-based probes described in this section exhibit a high degree of reproducibility. Figures 8.2 and 8.3 are SEM photographs that illustrate the highly uniform surface features achievable with various solid-surface-based substrate technologies, several of which are described in the following section.

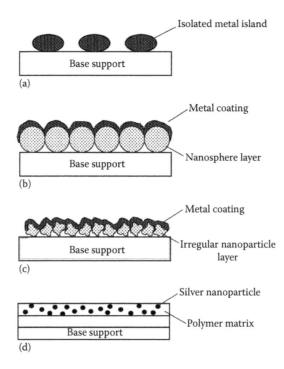

FIGURE 8.1 Schematic representation of various types of solid-surface-based SERS substrates. (a) Metal island films, (b) metal-coated nanospheres, (c) metal-coated random nanostructures, and (d) polymer coatings embedded with metal nanoparticles. (From Vo-Dinh, T. et al., *J. Raman Spectrosc.*, 30(9), 785, 1999.)

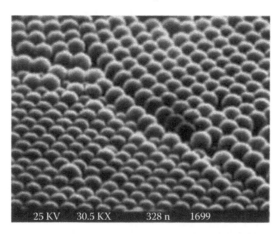

FIGURE 8.2 SEM photograph of a silver-coated substrate having 261 nm radius nanospheres.

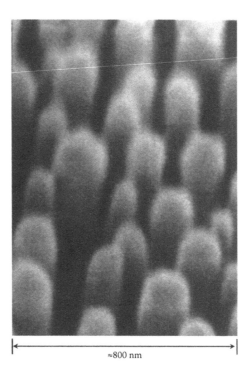

≈800 nm

FIGURE 8.3 SEM photograph of acid-etched quartz posts.

8.3.3.1 Metal Nanoparticle Island Films

Metallic nanostructured SERS substrates based on metal island films (Figure 8.1a) are among the most easily prepared surface-based media, granted the availability of a vacuum evaporation system. Such systems are commonly equipped with crystal microbalances for monitoring metal film thickness. Metal island films can be produced by depositing a thin (<10 nm) layer of a metal directly onto a smooth solid base support via sputter deposition[54] or vacuum evaporation. At such a small thickness, the metal layer forms as aggregated, isolated metal islands, the size and shape of which can be influenced largely by the metal thickness, deposition rate, geometry, and temperature, as well as postdeposition annealing. In order to optimize the production of SERS-active metal island films, various diagnostic techniques have been used, including optical absorption, atomic force microscopy (AFM), SERS, or combinations thereof.[98,99] Silver island films have been characterized by combining scanning near-field optical microscopy (SNOM) with Raman spectroscopy, thereby achieving <70 nm resolution.[100] A disadvantage of metal island films is that they are easily disturbed by solvents encountered in typical biomedical analyses.[101,102] To minimize this disadvantage, buffer metal layers, (3-mercaptopropyl)-trimethoxysilane (MCTMS) layers, and organometallic paint layers have been applied to glass supports to stabilize gold island films.[103] Likewise, support media investigated for SERS-active silver islands have included sapphire, carbon, stochastically distributed posts, optical gratings, mica, glass, derivatized glass, and formvar-coated glass.[101,104]

In addition to gold and silver, indium[105,106] and copper[107] have been used in SERS-active metal island films. Among these metals, silver is the most commonly used. Extensive evaluations of silver island films have included comparisons to a variety of other silver nanostructured SERS substrates.[108,109] Nevertheless, the less commonly used gold and copper island films have been developed for use with NIR (1064.1 nm) excitation.[107] This report is especially promising for biomedical applications because of minimal incidence of fluorescent background in the NIR region. Furthermore, NIR radiation can be propagated through greater distances in tissues than UV or visible light.

8.3.3.2 Metal-Coated Nanosphere Substrates

In our laboratory, we have developed a very dependable solid-surface-based SERS substrate technology that can be generally described as metal-coated dielectric nanospheres (Figure 8.1b) supported by various planar support media. Nanospheres within a specific size range (e.g., 50–500 nm) are spin coated on a solid support in order to produce the roughness required to induce the SERS effect. The resulting nanostructured plate is then coated with a layer of silver (50–150 nm), which provides the conduction electrons required for the surface plasmon mechanisms. All factors of surface morphology are easily controlled, enabling high batch-to-batch reproducibility. An additional advantage is that the relatively thick layer of silver is less vulnerable to air oxidation than silver islands. Furthermore, the surface is highly resistant to disturbance by sample solvents, making this type of SERS substrate very practical for biomedical applications. Teflon and latex are particularly well suited for SERS substrates because they are commercially available in a wide variety of sizes, which can be selected for optimal enhancement.

The preparation of a nanosphere substrate is relatively easy. A 50 μL aliquot of a suspension of nanospheres is deposited evenly over the surface of a dielectric planar support medium, such as filter paper, cellulosic membrane, glass, or quartz.[22,36,110–113] Using a photoresist spinner to produce uniform monolayer coverage, the substrate is then spun at 800–2000 rpm for about 20 s. The spheres adhere to the glass surface, providing uniform coverage. The nanosphere-coated support is then placed in a vacuum evaporator, where silver is deposited on the roughened surface at a rate of 0.15–0.2 nm/s. Figure 8.2 shows a scanning electron micrograph (SEM) of a silver-coated substrate having 261 nm radius nanospheres (deposited from a 10% suspension). As demonstrated by the figure, the sphere surfaces exhibit excellent uniformity with respect to nanosphere size, shape, and surface coverage.

Nanosphere-based substrates were among the first to be applied to the detection of a wide variety of compounds of health and environmental interest, including organophosphorus agents, chlorinated pesticides, polynuclear aromatic hydrocarbons (PNAs), and DNA adducts.[114–118]

8.3.3.3 Metal-Coated Nanoparticle Substrates

Nanoparticles with irregular shapes (Figure 8.1c) can also be used in place of regularly shaped nanospheres in the production of dependable, cost-effective SERS substrates. Dielectric nanoparticle materials investigated in our laboratory have included alumina,[119] titanium dioxide,[120] and fumed silica.[111] The production of irregular nanoparticle-based substrates is achieved with an ease equivalent to that for nanosphere-based substrates described earlier. Generally, 5%–10% (wt/vol) aqueous suspensions of the nanoparticles are spin coated onto solid support media, then coated by 75–150 nm of silver via vacuum evaporation. As an alternative to the vacuum evaporation process, other groups have investigated silver coating via chemical processes.[121,122] Nevertheless, substrates prepared via vacuum evaporation yield exceptional reproducibility.

Alumina-based substrates produced by vacuum evaporation have proven to be among the most dependable, with a batch-to-batch variability of typically <10% for induced signals of selected model compounds. The surface of an alumina-based substrate consists of randomly distributed surface agglomerates and protrusions in the 10–100 nm range. These structures produce large electromagnetic fields on the surface when the incident photon energy is in resonance with the localized surface plasmons. Alumina-based substrates have numerous applications.[117,118,121,123–128] In studies performed in our laboratory, these substrates have been incorporated in a passive vapor dosimeter for the detection of airborne chemicals[123,129] and used for the detection of SERS-active gene probes.[128] Gold coating has also been applied to alumina-coated plates for use in the visible to NIR region,[130] hence demonstrating greater utility in biomedical applications.

Silver-coated titanium dioxide[120] and fumed silica[111] surfaces also provide efficient SERS-active substrates. Titanium dioxide provides the necessary nanosized surface roughness for the SERS effect; the nominal particle diameter of TiO_2 used in our probes is 0.2 μm. When coated with 50–100 nm of silver, this type of probe can yield exceptional SERS enhancement with limits of detection of various compounds in the parts-per-billion (ppb) range.[120] Fumed silica substrates have allowed trace detection of PNAs and pesticides.[114,120]

8.3.4 SERS Substrates Based on Lithographically Prepared Nanoarrays

Lithographic techniques have been used to control the surface roughness to a degree suitable for testing the electromagnetic model of SERS.[131–134] For example, silver-coated, regularly spaced submicron posts formed in quartz substrates have proven to be a dependable, yet labor-intensive SERS substrate. While these surfaces produce a Raman enhancement on the order of 10^7, they are difficult to produce with a large surface area. However, an alternative etching procedure for producing quartz posts overcomes this limitation by using an island film as an etching mask on a SiO_2.[22,108,109,132,135] The preparation of SiO_2 prolate posts is a multistep operation, as depicted in Figure 8.4. A 500 nm layer of SiO_2 is first thermally evaporated onto a fused quartz base support at a rate of 0.1–0.2 nm/s. The resulting thermally deposited crystalline quartz is annealed at 950°C to the fused quartz for 45 min. A 5 nm silver layer is then evaporated onto the thermal SiO_2 layer, and the substrate is flash-heated (500°C) for 20 s, causing the thin silver layer to bead up in small globules. These isolated silver globules act as etch masks when the substrate is subsequently etched for 30–60 min in a CHF_3 plasma. This etching produces submicron prolate SiO_2 posts under the silver globules. Since fused quartz is etched much more slowly than is thermally deposited quartz, the fused quartz base survives the etching process. The posts are then cleaned to remove the silver etch mask and coated with either a continuous 80 nm silver layer[135] or a discontinuous layer with

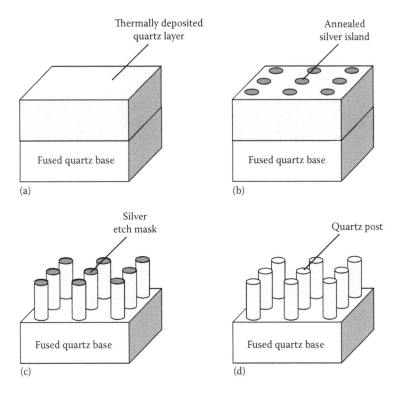

FIGURE 8.4 Schematic diagram of the production of quartz post-based SERS-active substrates. (a) After thermal deposition of quartz on fused quartz base, (b) after deposition and annealing of silver island film, (c) after plasma etching, and (d) after removal of silver etch mask.

the silver deposition restricted to the tips of the quartz posts.[108,109] Figure 8.3 shows the SEM photograph of the resulting uniformly shaped and distributed quartz posts.

A disadvantage of quartz post-based substrates is the difficult, time-consuming etching procedure required for post fabrication. Nevertheless, optimized quartz posts can serve as the base for a reusable SERS substrate, provided the silver coating is replaced between uses. It is worthwhile to note, however, that the posts are fragile, and hence, not amenable to field studies. In contrast, the nanosphere- and nanoparticle-based substrates described earlier are generally simpler to prepare and very simple to handle. Furthermore, comparative studies indicate that the simple fumed silica-, alumina-, or nanosphere-based probes provide SERS enhancements similar or superior to quartz post-based probes. Consequently, practical applications involving quartz post-based SERS probes have been extremely limited.

Another technique to produce highly ordered nanoarrays involves electron beam lithographic (EBL) fabrication.[134,136] For example, EBL fabrication of polymer structures designed and manifested through AutoCAD software has been reported.[134] With this graphical approach, a great deal of control is offered with respect to structure size, shape, geometric arrangement, and packing density. Patterns produced in AutoCAD have been directly etched in methacrylate-based e-beam resist films (ma-N 2403) via EBL. Using this technique, arrays of square, hexagonal, and elliptical pillars have been prepared, then coated with silver or gold films via thermal evaporation. The attributes of reproducibility and control of morphology achievable through this technique make it a powerful tool for theoretical and optimization studies.

8.3.5 SERS Substrates Based on Chemically and Abrasively Roughened Solid Surfaces

Smooth surfaces can be roughened by chemical and abrasive techniques to impart the required roughness for the SERS effect. In several cases, SERS substrates have been produced through a one-step procedure of roughening metal foils, analogous to redox-roughened metal electrodes. Because the foils act as a source of surface plasmons, no metallic overlayer is required. Copper[137,138] and silver[139–143] foils have been acid etched to impart roughness. These SERS substrates exhibit exceptional thermal stability, are cost effective, and can be reused. As a result, the SERS activity of acid-etched silver foils compare favorably with a variety of other types of SERS substrates.[139–143]

Another procedure involves a combination of sandblasting and acid-etching steps to produce 10–100 nm scale surface features. In a more innovative technique, silver foils have been selectively etched with ferrocyanide(III) and potassium thiocyanate using SAMs as etch masks,[144] producing 100 nm surface features with excellent uniform coverage. Dielectric materials have also been chemically and mechanically roughened to induce SERS, but with the requirement of subsequent metal-coating steps. For example, silver-coated, chemically etched polymer supports have been developed and compared to SERS-active crossed gratings and posted quartz wafers.[145] In an exciting development toward biomedical applications, Mullen and Carron have described abrasively roughened optical fibers coated with silver.[146] This integration of a SERS-active surface fiber-optic tip could be useful in a single-fiber SERS probe for low-volume measurements.

8.3.6 SERS Substrates Based on Inherently Rough Materials

Certain planar support materials have inherent roughness suitable for inducing the SERS effect. For example, direct metal coating of special cellulosic filter papers produces useful substrates.[32,116,147] SEMs of these cellulosic materials have shown that these surfaces consist of fibrous 10 μm strands with numerous tendrils that provide the necessary protrusions required for the SERS enhancement. For example, silver-coated paper substrates have been used to detect approximately 3 ng/mL methyl red.[148] Solid-phase extraction membranes and thin-layer chromatographic (TLC) plates have also been SERS activated through silver coating via chemical reduction.[149,150] Furthermore, such SERS probes have been used for combined TLC separation and detection of sulfonamides,[149,150] illicit drugs,[151] and nucleic purine derivatives.[55]

Inherently rough materials can sometimes induce the SERS effect with little or no additional preparation. One such example investigated in our laboratory is a silver membrane used for air particulate sampling.[32] The membrane already has micropores and interstices that provide the roughness features required to induce SERS. Furthermore, because it is solid silver, it can be used directly as an SERS-active substrate without applying any additional silver. Another example is black-and-white photographic paper, for which SERS activation is achieved simply through low-level light illumination and development steps.[152] It is important to note, however, that inherently rough materials suitable for SERS are a very rare find.

8.3.7 SERS Substrates Based on Metal Nanoparticle-Embedded Media

Silver nanoparticles embedded in various solid porous media (Figure 8.1d) have recently been investigated as stable SERS substrates with the potential for selective detection. The in situ production of these nanoparticles in solid matrices provides several advantages. For example, a solid matrix not only spatially stabilizes but also physically protects the colloids. In addition, the porosity of such materials as solgels, cellulose acetate gels, and polycarbonate films permits interaction of analyte compounds with the embedded metal nanoparticles. Furthermore, control of pore size and matrix polarity through simple chemical means (particularly when using the solgel technique) can impart selectivity. Finally, the chemical processes generally used to prepare such substrates make the SERS technique accessible for general analytical laboratories.

A silver nanoparticle-embedded solgel substrate produced through the chemical reduction of silver halide particles distributed in the solgel matrix has been reported for the detection of neurotransmitters and dopamine.[153,154] In situ precipitation of silver chloride nanoparticles via reaction of silver nitrate with trichloroacetic acid throughout the solgel matrix was performed before curing. Immediately prior to use, the silver chloride particles were reduced to elemental silver nanoparticles with $FeSO_4 \cdot 7H_2O$. An advantage of this technique is that the solgel can be stored for long periods in the nonreduced form, precluding vulnerability to air oxidation. In a similar approach, chemically reduced silver and gold colloids have been produced in solgel-derived xerogel,[155] and silver-doped solgel films have been formed through in situ chemical reduction of $[Ag(NH_3)_2^+]$.[156] Polycarbonate films doped with silver via chemical reduction have been reported as well.[157] As an alternative to chemical reduction, photodeposited gold particles have been produced through UV irradiation of organometallic gold precursors dispersed in solgels.[158] In a quite different approach, a counterdiffusion technique has been used to embed cellulose acetate films through impregnation with preformed fine silver particles.[159,160]

8.3.8 Overcoatings on SERS Substrates

The application of a wide variety of coatings to many of the SERS substrates described in the previous sections has been the focus of extensive research in recent years, with the goals of imparting selectivity and/or robustness to the SERS technology. These coatings have generally been in the form of organic coatings distributed as relatively thick polymer layers or SAMs, ultrathin metal films, dielectric films, and monolayers of bioreceptors. These coatings have improved detection selectivity through enhanced adsorption or selective permeability mechanisms. In some cases, coatings have stabilized SERS-active surface features, hence extending their shelf lives.

8.3.8.1 General Organic, Metallic, and Dielectric Overcoatings

Polymer coatings have been applied to a variety of solid-surface-based SERS substrates. In one study, a relatively thick layer (~10 μm) of PVPL was applied to alumina-based silver SERS substrates.[161] In addition to prolonging shelf life, this procedure was demonstrated to preserve surface features vital to the SERS effect by offering resistance to physical disturbance. Furthermore, chemical selectivity was imparted via selective permeability, particularly for compounds having hydrogen-bonding properties. The procedure involved simply dipping the bare silver SERS probes into a 5% (wt/vol) methanolic solution of the polymer, followed by room-temperature curing on a level surface for ~30 min. PVPL coatings have also been applied to silver-island-based SERS probes for selective detection of airborne chemicals.[129,162] In this study, the coating was observed to preserve the delicate silver island films over a 20-day period.

A combination of polybenzimidazole and mercaptobenzimidazole has been applied to SERS-active, nitric-acid-etched copper foils.[163] This coating was determined to inhibit corrosion and thus prolong the shelf life of the SERS-active substrate. In addition, treatment of silver SERS substrates with various thiols can provide long-term stability, even for substrates stored in water for a month.[164] Propanethiol-coated silver SERS substrates, investigated as potential SERS-based detectors in gas chromatography, have also exhibited enhanced adsorption and detection of hydrophilic compounds.[165] In order to promote enhanced adsorption of metal ions (Cu^{2+}, Pb^{2+}, Cd^{2+}), 4-(2-pyridylazo) resorcinol coatings have been applied to SERS-active silver.[166] As an example of the enhanced selectivity offered by reactive coatings in the analysis of complex biological matrices, bilirubin and salicylate has been detected at below normal therapeutic levels via direct SERS analysis of whole blood.[167] In this study, application of the coating, diazonium, precluded the need for a time-consuming and possibly risky preparation of a less complex serum sample. A reactive coating has also been proposed for the one-step detection of the illicit drugs amphetamine and methamphetamine.[168]

Extensive efforts have also been devoted toward the development of coatings based on inorganic materials. For example, transition metals (Pd, Rh, Pt, Ir, Ru) have been applied to gold substrates as pinhole-free, ultrathin (2–3 monolayers) films to enhance adsorption of CO and NO while preserving the SERS-inducing properties of the underlying gold substrates.[169,170] The ultrathin coatings were achieved through a special electrodeposition process. SiO_2-coated silver-island-based substrates have also been reported as viable SERS substrates.[171–173] These dielectric-coated substrates have made possible the quantitative detection of dyes adsorbed from solutions. Furthermore, they have been used in fundamental analyte adsorption kinetics studies. SiO_2-coated substrates could prove especially useful in SERS-based biosensors because of the well-defined hydrophilic and stabilizing properties of the coating. For example, silica-coated metallic nanoparticles have been reported as a basis for imparting functionality for biomedical diagnosis.[72–74] Such substrates could also be resistant to oxidation and physical damage, hence both prolonging shelf life and offering the potential for reuse.

8.3.8.2 Self-Assembled Monolayer Overcoatings

SAMs have proven to be a valuable factor in SERS substrate development and theoretical applications of SERS. For example, they have been used to immobilize SERS-active metal colloids on planar supports in a highly ordered fashion.[92,93,96,157] In fact, specific colloidal patterns have been prepared by microcontact printing of SAMs on planar surfaces before exposure to SERS-active colloids.[96] SAMs have also been used for the production of UV-induced SERS-active photopatterns on silver films coated with *p*-nitrophenol.[174] In more fundamental studies, the inherent SERS signals of SAMs have been used to evaluate the surface uniformity of SERS probe surfaces, including electrochemically roughened gold electrodes and immobilized gold colloids.[175] Adlayers of mercaptoalkalinic acids formed on silver surfaces have been studied as well.[176,177] The application of SAMs to SERS substrate surfaces also allows selective detection. For example, SAMs of mercaptoalkalinic acids on colloidal silver substrates have been used for the SERS detection of selectively adsorbed cytochrome c[178] and have formed the basis for anchoring capture DNA probes for SERS-active hybridization platforms.[179,180] SAMs of *N*-acetylalanine have also been proposed as a biocompatible functional interface for biosensors.[181] Monolayers of cysteamine on silver SERS substrates have also been reported.[182,183] Such monolayers could promote the selective adsorption of proteins. The effects of electrolytes and pH on the molecular structure and distribution of *N*-acetylalanine,[181] cysteamine,[182,183] and mercaptopurine[184] layers have been investigated. The application of various SAMs as partition layers in reusable glucose sensors has been reported.[185–190] These glucose sensors have exhibited great selectivity[186] and have been demonstrated in vivo.[189]

8.3.8.3 Bioreceptor Monolayer Overcoating

The potential use of SERS in biodiagnostic tests has been demonstrated through the use of immobilized monolayers of bioreceptors, including oligonucleotides and antibodies. The use of surface-enhanced Raman gene (SERG) probes for medical diagnostics[128,179,191–194] is covered in greater detail in following sections. In the production of SERG probes, SERS-active dye labels can be attached to oligonucleotide primers used in polymerase chain reaction (PCR) amplification of specific target DNA sequences. Following PCR, the resulting labeled target DNA can be denatured, allowing hybridization of specific, single-stranded, labeled DNA to oligonucleotide capture probes, which can be immobilized on solid supports. Contact with SERS-active media permits subsequent detection of the SERG probe. This method combines the high sensitivity of the SERS technique with the inherent molecular specificity offered by DNA sequence hybridization.

Antibody monolayers have also been the basis of SERS detection with molecular selectivity[64–66,72,76–78,195–203] thus demonstrating the potential for SERS in immunoassays. In one study, Ni et al. demonstrated the simultaneous detection of two antigens in a single-sandwich immunoassay using two reporter molecules.[196] Capture antibodies selective for the target antigens were bound to gold colloids. The capture antibody-coated colloids were then exposed to a mixture of target antigens. Finally, reporter antibodies specific to the immobilized target antigens were immobilized on the colloid via interaction with the target antigens. SERS-active markers on the reporter antibodies permitted extrinsic detection of the immobilized antigens. Each antigen was assigned a different marker, yet both reporters could be detected in a single measurement because of minimal overlap of the respective Raman spectra. In another study, Dou et al. demonstrated the potential for an SERS-based immunoassay with no need for reporter molecules.[195] Instead, they monitored the native SERS signatures of antimouse immunoglobulin-G (IgG) antibodies adsorbed on gold nanoparticles. Because of the structure-specific nature of Raman scattering, they were able to directly confirm conjugation with antigens through the observation of changes in relative intensities of spectral features of the IgG spectrum. Neither reporter probes nor rinsing steps to remove unbound antigens were required in this assay. In another label-free approach, SERS detection of multiple proteins on a single platform was based on Western blot assay.[204]

The expanding interest in implementation of SERS in immunoassays has spurred fundamental studies for optimization of immunoassay substrates as well as conjugation conditions. For example, an in-depth study of sandwich assay architecture as well as nanoparticle shapes has been performed for SAMs.[205] An innovative approach to increasing conjugation efficiency using a rotating capture substrate has been investigated.[206] Control of mass transfer using a rotating capture substrate has been demonstrated.[207] Finally, a comparison between surface-enhanced resonance Raman scattering (SERRS) and more commonly used fluorescence for detection of a labeled antibody has been reported.[208]

8.4 Biomedical Applications of SERS Probes

8.4.1 SERS Bioanalysis

The extensive progress in the development of dependable SERS substrates over the past few decades has promoted the application of SERS in the rapidly expanding field of biotechnology, as is demonstrated in several excellent reviews.[209–216] The variety of substrates has made these applications far reaching indeed, spanning liquid and gas phase samples from the meso- to nanovolume scale. For example, various SERS-active fiber-optic probes have been developed for analyzing biological samples, as is discussed in the succeeding text. Furthermore, the development of nanoscale fiber-optic probe tips offers the potential for intracellular measurements as well as the integration of SERS with SNOM via an effect now termed as tip-enhanced Raman scattering (TERS).[8,9,191,209–212,217–221] Reliable substrates have been the basis for SERS-based screening for illicit drugs,[151,168,222–226] as well as bioassays based on DNA[84,128,180,191,192,227–236] and antibody[64–66,72,76–78,195,196,237–239] probes. SERS has been applied to the low-level detection of therapeutic drugs[25,240–259] and has even been used to evaluate the interaction between drugs and target species as well as complex matrices,[260–274] sometimes within cells.[275–278] A host of biological compounds (e.g., proteins, amino acids, lipids, fats, fatty acids, DNA, RNA, antibodies, enzymes) and systems (e.g., lipid bilayers and intracellular environments) have been studied via SERS. Such studies could provide valuable insights into cellular processes (some of which promote diseases), thereby aiding in establishing the mechanisms of therapeutic drugs and in the development and evaluation of new therapeutic species.

8.4.1.1 SERS-Based Bioassays

Among the most innovative biomedical applications of SERS have been bioassays. DNA-based bioassays are discussed in great detail in Section 8.4.2. Immunoassays have also received considerable interest for the past two decades.[64–66,72,76–78,195–203] For example, an early example of an SERS-based immunoassay was reported by Rohr et al.[239] The same year, Grabbe and Buck reported on SERS studies of native human IgG.[279] More recently, SERS signatures of native antibodies have been the basis for a simplified immunoassay[195] in which conjugation of the antibody with a target antigen was confirmed through observance of alterations of the SERS spectrum for the native antibody. In another label-free approach, SERS detection of multiple proteins on a single platform was based on Western blot assay.[204]

As an alternative, extremely sensitive detection can be achieved with reporter antibody probes tagged with intensely SERS-active compounds or with enzymes that react with substrates to yield SERS-active products. These methods often involve sandwich immunoassay techniques, which increase the number of required steps but offer the advantages of excellent sensitivity and the potential for *label multiplexing*. For example, Ni et al. recently reported the simultaneous detection of two types of antigens in a single assay by using two reporter antibodies.[196] The labels of the reporter probes yielded SERS spectral features with minimal overlap, permitting exploitation of a label multiplex advantage. In a sandwich assay format, one set of antibodies immobilized the target antigens on gold colloids, while the reporter antibody probes were subsequently immobilized at allosteric sites of the target antigens.

In other studies, reporter antibodies have been tagged with the enzyme peroxidase.[237,238] Once the peroxidase-labeled antigen was immobilized on the target, it could be exposed to the substrates, *o*-phenylenediamine and hydrogen peroxide. A sustained reaction of the enzyme with a multitude of substrate molecules yielded an extremely high yield of the SERS-active product, azoaniline. This method has thus far been limited to sandwich immunoassay formats. For example, in a study to detect membrane-bound enzymes in cells, cells were first exposed to primary antibodies specific to the membrane-bound enzymes, then exposed to a peroxidase-tagged reporter antibody specific to the primary antibody.[237] A format that uses a capture antibody to immobilize a target antigen, and a reporter antibody to bind to an allosteric site of the immobilized target antigen, has also been reported.[238]

As a result of the development of a variety of SERS-based immunoassays, SERS has been successfully applied to cellular and tissue diagnosis, often with the selective detection of disease markers. For example, prostate-specific antigen detection has been achieved with SERS,[197] including within tissue samples using COINs conjugated with antibodies.[78] SERS dots have been used for an immunoassay for bronchoaveolar stem cells in murine lung.[77] Immunogold nanoparticles have been used for the detection of hepatitis B.[202,280] Several examples of SERS-based immunoassays for tracking cancer markers have been reported.[72,76] In fact, SERS nanoparticle tags have been used for in vivo tumor targeting and detection.[88] Furthermore, recent developments in various SERS-active nanoparticles have been highlighted by application to multiplex immunoassay formats.[75,79] They have also been applied to SERS-based imaging of cells[64,87] and analysis of tissues.[79,88]

8.4.1.2 SERS Detection of Illicit Drugs

Another potential biomedical application of SERS-based analysis is drug screening. Several studies have demonstrated SERS detection of illicit drugs on a variety of substrates.[151,168,222–225] These works have collectively yielded SERS spectra for cocaine·HCl, crack cocaine, amphetamine, methamphetamine, mefenorex, pentylenetetrazole, pemoline, heroin, codeine, and other drugs banned in sports. In one study, stimulant drugs were detected in human urine spiked at μg/mL levels.[226] In other works, SERS was used to distinguish between cocaine and common cutting agents and impurities, including benzocaine and lidocaine.[222]

While these studies have demonstrated the potential for direct analysis of complex media with SERS, other efforts have been directed toward the development of reactive coatings to enhance selectivity. For example, Sulk et al. have proposed a reactive coating for the selective detection of amphetamine and methamphetamine.[168] Silver colloids have been most commonly used for this application, but some solid-surface-based media have also been reported, including colloidal silver supported by cellulose paper and ion-exchange paper, as well as acid-etched silver foils.[224] TLC plates coated with silver through vacuum evaporation have also been used for the detection of illicit drugs. TLC plates have a unique advantage in that they not only provide the roughness needed to induce SERS but also serve as a separation medium. In the TLC study, a mixture of heroin, codeine, and cocaine was separated on bare TLC plates, which were subsequently coated with silver to allow detection at approximately 0.2 μg/mm².[151] Separation-based SERS detection of drugs banned in sports has also been achieved through the coupling of SERS with liquid chromatography (LC) via a postcolumn windowless detection flow cell that was supplied with a stream of silver colloids.[225]

8.4.1.3 SERS Studies of Therapeutic Drugs

SERS has been used to detect a large number of therapeutic drugs, as indicated in Table 8.1. A key advantage of SERS spectroscopy is the structural information it provides. In several studies, this advantage has been exploited to confirm interactions between therapeutic drugs and targets. In many cases, such studies have even yielded the establishment of interaction mechanisms, including the identification of specific active sites, complex molecules, and modes of bonding. Observable changes in SERS spectra for drugs and/ or targets before and after interactions have served as the basis for such determinations. Fortunately, interaction between the complexes and the SERS-inducing medium (e.g., silver colloids) often has negligible effects on the drug/target interactions. There have been extensive studies of interactions between a variety of antitumor drugs and DNA, including doxorubicin,[271,278] fagaronine,[268] ethoxidine,[268] mitoxantrone,[252] intoplicine,[272,277] aclacinomycin,[273] saintopin,[273] acridines,[281] danthron,[258] quinizarin,[258] and various ellipticines.[254,274,282,283] Several studies of interactions between topoisomerases and topoisomerase-inhibiting antitumor drugs, including amsacrine[276] and intoplicine,[272,277] have been reported as well. For both drugs, interactions have been confirmed in K562 cancer cells.[276,277] Furthermore, interactions within ternary complexes of topoisomerase-inhibiting drugs, DNA, and topoisomerases have been reported for intoplicine.[272,277] In other in vivo studies, the interaction between the antitumor drug doxorubicin and targets has been studied in K562 cancer cells.[278] Interaction between another antitumor drug, dimethylcrocetin, and the retinoic acid receptor, RAR-gamma, has been confirmed in HL60 cancer cells.[275] Both ionic bonds and ring stacking have been determined via SERS as modes of interaction between 9-amino acridine and the metastasis-related protease guanidobenzoatase.[260,261] SERS has been used to identify active sites for the interaction between the antiviral/antiparkinsonian drug amantadine and histidine.[263] The antiviral drugs hypocrellin A[267] and hypericin[269] have been evaluated for interaction with human serum albumin. Another interesting study has demonstrated that SERS spectral changes resulting from the interaction between the antimalarial drug quinacrine and oligonucleotides are dependent on the nucleotide sequence.[264] Finally, the influence of pH and anion concentrations on SERS spectra of the antimicrobial drug rifampicin, adsorbed on silver colloids, has been reported.[257]

TABLE 8.1 SERS Studies of Therapeutic Drugs

Drug	Study
Antitumoral drugs	
9-Aminoacridine	[241,247,260,261]
Quinacrine	[241,264]
6-Mercaptopurine	[243]
Hypocrellin A	[267]
Fagaronine	[268]
Ethoxidine	[268]
Dimethylcrocetin	[275]
Camptothecins	[248]
Amsacrine	[276]
Ellipticines	[254,274,282,283]
Doxorubicin or adriamycin	[271,278]
Mitoxantrone	[252]
Aclacinomycin	[273]
Saintopin	[273]
Intoplicine	[272,277]
4'-o-Tetrahydropyranyl-adriamycin	[278]
Danthron	[258]
Quinizarin	[258]
Antiviral drugs	
Amantadine	[240,263]
Hypocrellin A	[267]
Antiretroviral drugs	
Hypericin	[249,269]
Emodin	[249]
Antiparkinsonian drugs (e.g., amantadine)	[240,263]
Antimalarial drugs (e.g., quinacrine)	[241,264]
Antitubercle bacillus drugs (e.g., pyrazinamide, isoniazid, and isonicotinamide)	[242]
Beta blockers (e.g., propranolol, alprenolol, acebutolol, and atenolol)	[250]
Diuretic drugs	
Triamterene	[141]
Amiloride	[225,253]
Sulfa drugs	[255,256]
Antimicrobial drugs (e.g., pefloxacin)	[251,270]
Nitrogen-containing drugs	[25]
Others	
Diazepam	[244]
Nitrazepam	[244]
Amphotericin B	[245]
2-Mercaptopyridine	[225]
Pemoline	[225]
Triamterene	[225]
Rifampicin	[257]

8.4.2 SERS Genomics

Over the last few years, there has been a great deal of interest in the development of optical techniques for genomics analysis such as nonradioactive DNA probes for use in biomedical diagnostics, pathogen detection, gene identification, gene mapping, and DNA sequencing. This section presents an overview of SERS methods and instruments, such as DNA mapping and sequencing applications that can be used in genomics analysis. The hybridization of a nucleic acid probe to DNA biotargets (e.g., gene sequences, bacteria, viral DNA) permits a very high degree of accuracy in identifying DNA sequences complementary to that probe. The possibility of using SERS for low-level detection of the DNA base and oligonucleotides was demonstrated in several studies in the 1980s.[55,284–289] More recently, the possibility of using Raman and/or SERS labels for extremely sensitive detection of DNA has been demonstrated.[84,128,179,180,191,192,194,227–231,233–236] For example, Graham et al. have claimed adequate sensitivity for single-molecule DNA detection via SERRS.[194] With the use of labeled DNA as gene probes, the SERS technique has been applied to the detection of DNA fragments of the human immunodeficiency virus (HIV)[73,192,228] as well as oncogenes.[179,180,229,230]

A critical aspect of sequencing the entire human genome involves defining and identifying large insert clones of DNA corresponding to specific regions of the human genome. These maps will be composed of overlapping fragments of human DNA and will allow the direct acquisition of DNA fragments that correspond to specific genes.[290–293] An approach that facilitates large-scale genomic sequencing involves developing maps of human chromosomes into maps based on large insert bacterial clones, such as bacterial artificial chromosomes (BACs).[291–293] A time-saving method for detecting multiple BAC-clone-labeled probes simultaneously would be especially appealing for the BAC approach to genome sequencing and mapping. The SERS technique can provide this label multiplex capability. The SERG probes described in this section preclude the need for radioactive labels and have great potential to provide sensitivity, selectivity, and label multiplexing for DNA sequencing as well as clinical assays. For example, multiplex DNA-based assays have been reported over the past decade.[82,229,233,294–297] A variety of sampling platforms have been developed to support such multiplex assays, including conventional lateral flow platforms or biochips[229] and microfluidic lab-on-a-chip systems.[84,85,233]

8.4.2.1 Instrumental Systems for SERS Genomics

In this section, two detection systems are described, which allow two different recording modes: (1) spectral recording of individual spots and (2) imaging of an entire 2D hybridization array plate. An example of a 2D hybridization platform that has been developed in our laboratory consists of a microspot array of capture probes for the breast cancer susceptibility gene BRCA1.[179,229]

A detection system used for recording the SERS spectrum of individual spots is illustrated in Figure 8.5. An individual spot could correspond to an individual microdot on a hybridization platform. This system can readily be assembled using commercially available or off-the-shelf components. A focused, low-power laser beam is used to excite an individual spot on the hybridization platform. In our studies, a helium–neon laser is used to provide 632.8 nm excitation with approximately 5 mW power. A band-pass filter is used to isolate the 632.8 nm line prior to sample excitation. A signal collection optical module is used to collect the SERS signal at 180° with respect to propagation of the incident laser beam. The collection module includes a Raman holographic filter, which rejects the Rayleigh-scattered radiation before it enters the collection fiber. Finally, the collection fiber is coupled to a spectrograph (ISA, HR-320), which is equipped with a Princeton Instruments RE-ICCD-576S detection system. The signal collection module can be coupled directly to the spectrograph, bypassing the optical fiber. However, the optical fiber greatly simplifies measurements and improves reproducibility by minimizing critical optical alignment steps.

Since the SERG probe hybridization platform consists of a 2D array of DNA hybridization spots,[179,229] a method for recording signals from all spots simultaneously would be highly advantageous, reducing analysis time as well as precluding the need for platform scanning. For analysis of SERG probe-based assays,

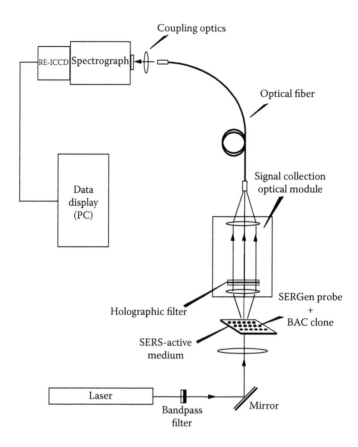

FIGURE 8.5 Schematic diagram of the instrumental setup for spectral acquisition from individual spots on a bioassay platform. (From Vo-Dinh, T. et al., *J. Raman Spectrosc.*, 30(9), 785, 1999.)

this feat can be accomplished through multispectral imaging (MSI). The concept of MSI is illustrated in Figure 8.6. With conventional imaging, the optical emission from every pixel of an image is without tunable wavelength selection capability (Figure 8.6a). With conventional spectroscopy, the signal at every wavelength within a spectral range can be recorded, but for only a single analyte spot. This condition is the basis for the single-point analysis system described earlier. The MSI concept (Figure 8.6c) combines these two recording modalities, thereby allowing the acquisition of a Raman spectrum for every hybridization spot on the assay platform, provided that the entire platform can be included in the instrument field of view. Critical to the success of this concept is an imaging spectrometer. In our studies, a rapid-scanning solid-state device, an acousto-optic tunable filter (AOTF), is used for tunable wavelength selection with image-preserving capability. This compact solid-state device has an effective wavelength range from 450 to 700 nm with a spectral resolution of 2 Å and a diffraction efficiency of 70%. Wavelength tuning is achieved simply by supplying the AOTF with a tunable RF signal.

A system developed to implement the MSI concept is illustrated in Figure 8.7. In this system, an expanded, collimated laser beam is used to stimulate a 0.5 cm diameter region of the assay array platform. In these studies, a krypton ion laser (Coherent, I-70) is used as the excitation source (at 25–50 mW). A band-pass filter is used to isolate the 647.1 nm line of the laser. After passing through a band-pass filter (Corion), the laser beam is expanded and collimated using a spatial filter/beam expansion module. An imaging optical module collects and projects the image of the back-illuminated SERG probe hybridization platform through an AOTF (Brimrose, Model TEAF 10-45-70-S) and onto a charge-coupled device (CCD) camera (Photometrics, Model CH210). A holographic notch filter (Kaiser, HNPF-647-1.0) is

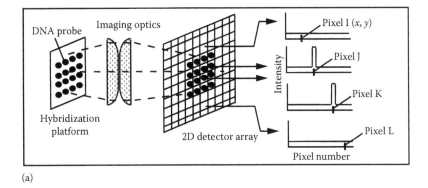

(a)

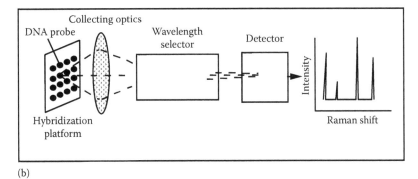

(b)

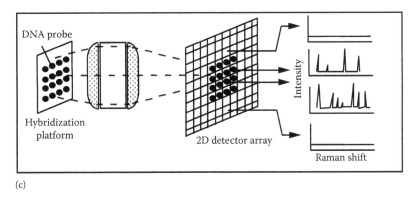

(c)

FIGURE 8.6   Various modes of data acquisition from bioassay platforms. (a) Imaging in which intensity is recorded for every pixel at one single wavelength, (b) spectroscopy in which intensity is recorded for a single spot at multiple wavelengths, and (c) multispectral imaging in which intensity is recorded at multiple wavelengths for every pixel. (From Vo-Dinh, T. et al., *J. Raman Spectrosc.*, 30(9), 785, 1999.)

placed in front of the CCD detector for rejection of laser Rayleigh scatter. For these studies, the imaging optical module is a microscope (Nikon, Microphot, SA) that is equipped with an image port to which the AOTF/CCD detection complex is attached. The image is collected with a 10× objective lens.

Figure 8.8 shows the 2D SERS image of an array pattern of *p*-aminobenzoic acid (PABA), acquired with the MSI system.[191] The diameter of each spot observed in this image is approximately 500 μm. This result demonstrates the capability of the MSI system to detect a SERS label spot array deposited on the 5 × 5 mm substrate. The MSI technique has also been used for imaging cresyl fast violet (CFV)-based SERS patterns at a much smaller scale.[191] For example, pattern features with <20 μm diameters and 75 μm spacing were fully resolved when using a 50× objective lens. CFV has been successfully used as a SERS label for the

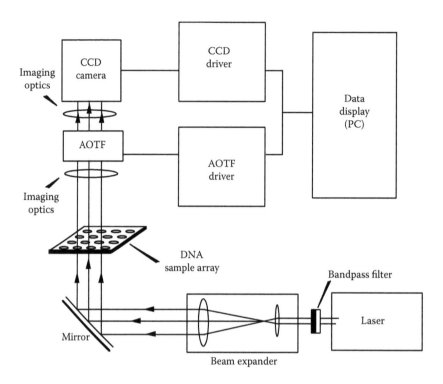

FIGURE 8.7 Schematic diagram of an instrument for MSI of bioassay platforms. (From Vo-Dinh, T. et al., *J. Raman Spectrosc.*, 30(9), 785, 1999.)

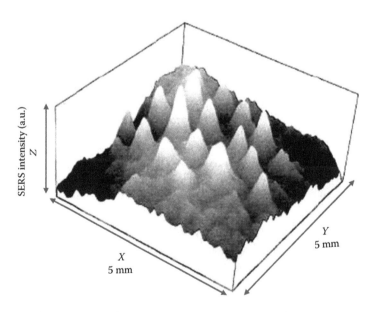

FIGURE 8.8 Image of a 2D SERS signal pattern for PABA spots acquired with a MSI system. (From Vo-Dinh, T. et al., *J. Raman Spectrosc.*, 30(9), 785, 1999.)

detection of the HIV gene system.[192] These examples, though not based on true hybridizations, illustrate the possibility of performing MSI on DNA hybridization array platforms with high resolution.

8.4.2.2 SERS Advantage in Label Multiplexing

In order to fully exploit the label multiplex advantage for DNA hybridization and SERG detection, several factors must be considered. First, a label must be selected that is SERS active and compatible with the hybridization platform. The ideal label would exhibit a strong SERS signal when used with the SERS-active substrate of interest (Figure 8.9a). Second, the strong SERS signal should not be affected by being attached to the oligonucleotide selected for the gene probe (Figure 8.9b). Third, the unlabeled oligonucleotide should not exhibit a significant SERS signal relative to the label's signal (Figure 8.9c). Finally, the SERS signal from the labeled probe should not be affected by the hybridization process (Figure 8.9d).

Luminescence labels have been shown to have adequate sensitivity for gene detection.[298] Nevertheless, a more desirable technique would both offer better spectral selectivity than is yielded by broadband luminescence and overcome the need for radioactive labels. The SERG probe is an excellent alternative to the other spectroscopy-based probes. For example, Figure 8.10 compares the fluorescence and SERS spectra of CFV, a SERG probe label. As shown in the figure, the spectral bandwidth of the CFV label in the fluorescence spectrum is relatively broad (approximately 50–60 nm halfwidth), whereas the bandwidth of a characteristic

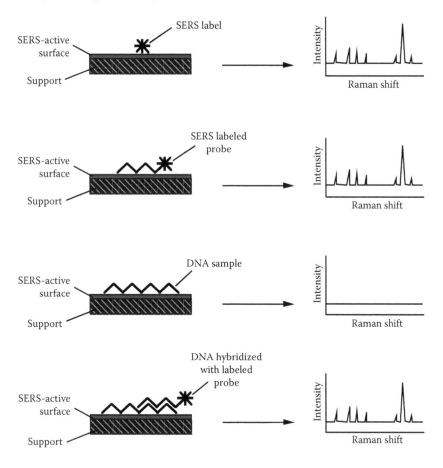

FIGURE 8.9 Factors considered for development of the SERG probe technology. (From Vo-Dinh, T. et al., *J. Raman Spectrosc.*, 30(9), 785, 1999.)

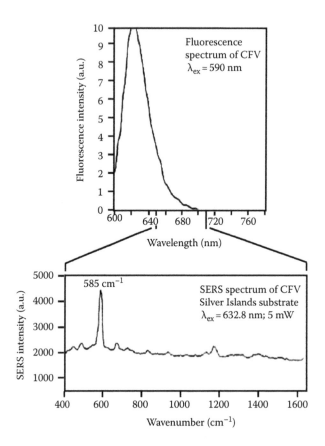

FIGURE 8.10 Comparison of fluorescence and SERS spectra for the SERG probe label. (From Vo-Dinh, T. et al., *J. Raman Spectrosc.*, 30(9), 785, 1999.)

feature (e.g., 585 cm^{-1} band) of the corresponding SERS spectrum of the same CFV label is orders of magnitude narrower (<0.5 nm halfwidth). This observation clearly illustrates the advantage of using SERS for label multiplexing. More specifically, this example demonstrates a 100-factor increase in label multiplexing capacity relative to fluorescence. In a typical Raman spectrum, a 2000 cm^{-1} spectral range can provide approximately 1000 resolvable spectral *intervals* at any given time. Assuming a deduction factor of 10 due to possible spectral overlap, it should be possible to find 100 labels that can be used for the detection of multiple SERG probes simultaneously. This multiplex advantage is particularly useful in high-throughput analyses where multiple gene targets can be screened in a highly parallel multiplex modality.

Exploitation of the multiplex advantage offered by SERS-based gene probes has been demonstrated in several works over the past decade.[82,229,233,294–297] For example, the first use of SERRS probes for highly sensitive multiplex genotyping was reported by Graham et al.[296] The multiplex detection of three different dye-labeled oligonucleotides in a microfluidic lab-on-a-chip format was first demonstrated by Docherty et al. in 2004.[233] The potential for multiplex genotyping on a 2D biochip sampling platform was demonstrated in our laboratory using microdot arrays of capture probes for the breast cancer oncogene BRCA1.[179,229]

8.4.2.3 SERS Detection of SERS-Labeled DNA on Solid SERS Substrates

The importance of BAC clone DNA in genome sequencing and mapping has been discussed in previous sections. We recently demonstrated the potential of using SERG probes for BAC clone DNA detection.[191] In this study, CFV was covalently attached to a 20mer oligonucleotide (5′-TAA-TAC-GAC-TCA-CTA-TAG-GG-3′) of a BAC clone model system. The labeled probe was then spotted on a SERS-active substrate

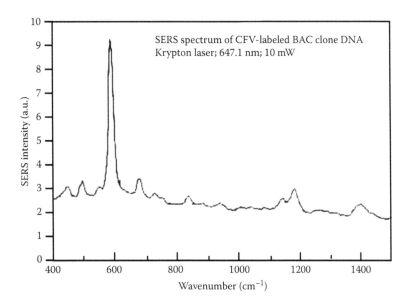

FIGURE 8.11 SERS spectrum of CFV-labeled BAC clone DNA. (From Vo-Dinh, T. et al., *J. Raman Spectrosc.*, 30(9), 785, 1999.)

for analysis. Figure 8.11 illustrates the SERS spectrum of this CFV-labeled BAC clone DNA fragment. This spectrum exhibits a series of narrow lines characteristic of CFV, with the strongest at 590 cm^{-1}. This intense, sharp line can be attributed to the benzene ring deformation mode. Another less intense but also sharp line at 1195 cm^{-1} could be related to benzene ring breathing vibrations. Another group of small peaks between 1000 and 1400 cm^{-1} could be associated with aromatic ring substitution-sensitive modes. Finally, several peaks that could correspond to benzene stretch vibrations occur between 1500 and 1650 cm^{-1}.

To further demonstrate the applicability of the SERS method in DNA gene probe technology, we have performed hybridization and SERS detection experiments with BAC clone probes. Hybridization, which involves the joining of a strand of nucleic acid with its corresponding complementary-sequence strand, is a powerful technique for identifying DNA sequences of interest. BAC clone capture probes were immobilized in the wells of an Immuno Maxisorp 96-well plate using Reacti-Bind DNA coating solution (Pierce, Rockford, IL). The capture probes were then incubated with the CFV-labeled BAC clone SERG probes. After stringency washes, silver colloids were added to the wells for SERS detection of the hybridized probes. Hybridization of the labeled probe to BAC DNA could be readily detected via the CFV spectral signature. Selective detection of HIV via hybridization of SERG probes has also been demonstrated.[192]

8.4.2.4 Selective Amplification and Detection of SERS Gene Probes via PCR with Labeled Primers

Isola et al. have demonstrated that primers labeled with SERS-active compounds can be implemented in the PCR process.[192] Furthermore, these researchers hybridized PCR-amplified products to DNA capture probes immobilized on *N*-oxysuccinimide (NOS)-derivatized polystyrene plates (DNA-BIND, Corning-Costar). Following hybridization, the plates were SERS activated through the deposition of a silver island coating. This method has the potential for combining the spectral selectivity and high sensitivity of SERS with the inherent molecular specificity of PCR and the ensuing DNA sequence hybridization. The effectiveness of this technique has been demonstrated using the *gag* gene sequence of HIV. This is an especially encouraging result because there is a need for a direct nucleic-acid-based test for the detection of HIV. For example, standard HIV serologic tests, including the enzyme-linked immunoassay and the Western blot assay, do not provide a useful diagnosis of HIV in early infancy because of the overwhelming presence of transplacentally derived maternal antibody in the infant's blood.

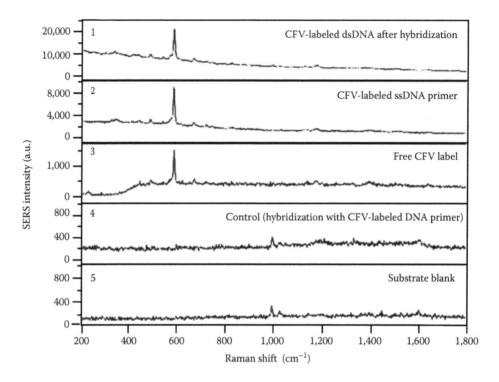

FIGURE 8.12 Demonstration of the SERG probe technology for the selective detection of the HIV1 *gag* gene using via hybridization after PCR amplification. (From Isola, N.R. et al., *Anal. Chem.*, 70(7), 1352, 1998.)

Figure 8.12 illustrates the results of the HIV *gag* gene hybridization following PCR amplification with a primer labeled with CFV. Curve 1 shows the SERS spectrum of the hybridized CFV-labeled probe. For comparison, the detection of a nonhybridized CFV-labeled probe (ssDNA) is also shown in curve 2. Curve 3 illustrates a SERS spectrum of free CFV. This study showed that no major alteration in the CFV spectrum occurs as a result of being bound to single- or double-stranded DNA. Furthermore, the researchers observed no CFV spectrum for hybridization evaluation for nonspecific binding between noncomplementary DNA strands. This is demonstrated by the hybridization control spectrum illustrated in curve 4. In this case, the CFV-labeled DNA was a single-stranded primer (designed for PCR). Without the PCR step, there was no complementarity between the CFV-labeled primer and the immobilized capture probe. Curve 5, a blank spectrum for a SERS-activated NOS plate with immobilized DNA capture probes, exhibits no major spectral background in the region of interest.

In a more recent study, the feasibility of coupling SERS with PCR was investigated as a means of selective amplification of a diagnostic DNA probe for Chlamydia.[84] As an alternative to using a solid hybridization platform, however, a microfluidic lab-on-a-chip format was used with SERS-inducing nanoparticles.

8.4.2.5 Selective Detection of Labeled DNA Probes via Hybridization on SERS-Active Bioassay Platforms

We have recently developed in our laboratory SERS-active DNA hybridization platforms that greatly enhance the utility of the SERS gene probe technology.[179,180,229] In previous work, hybridization of labeled DNA probes was performed on conventional commercially available platforms (e.g., DNA-bind plates), followed by SERS activation of the platforms.[191,192] To make the SERS gene probe technology more practical, we developed inherently SERS-active hybridization platforms. No SERS activation of the assay was required following the hybridization step. The new DNA assay platform was an array of oligonucleotide capture probes immobilized directly on a silver-island-based substrate prepared on glass. The capture

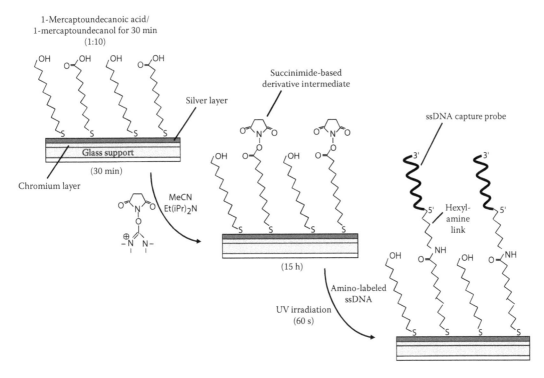

FIGURE 8.13 Schematic diagram of the production of a SERS-active hybridization platform using a SAM of mercaptoundecanoic acid.

probes were anchored directly to the silver surface via reaction with a SAM of alkyl mercaptans, as illustrated in Figure 8.13. The coupling approach involved the esterification under mild conditions of a carboxylic acid (immobilized mercaptoundecanoic acid) with a labile group, an *N*-hydroxysuccinimide (NHS) derivative, and further reaction with a 5′-amine-labeled DNA capture probe, producing a stable amide.[299] Our studies have demonstrated the potential of this technology in cancer gene detection (BRCA1 and BAX genes).[179,180,229]

The breast cancer susceptibility genes BRCA1 and BRCA2 are associated with genetically predisposed breast cancer development. Breast cancer is diagnosed annually in about 180,000 women in the United States.[300] Of these cases, only 5%–10% are estimated to arise from genetic predisposition. Nevertheless, within the population with a family history of breast cancer, germ line mutations in BRCA1 account for a predisposing genetic factor >80% for breast and/or ovarian cancers.[301] Therefore, intense research has been conducted on the principle of action of BRCA1 and BRCA2 genes, as well as their detection.[302,303]

In our laboratory, we have demonstrated the potential for detecting the BRCA1 gene through hybridization of a rhodamine-B-labeled SERG probe on the new SERS-active hybridization platform. Figure 8.14 illustrates the results of this study. Curve (a) is the SERS spectrum of the rhodamine-B-labeled gene probe after hybridization with the BAC clone capture probe, which was previously immobilized on the SERS-active platform. This spectrum is a clear signature of the rhodamine-B label. For example, the majority of the peaks in 1200–1500 cm^{-1} region can be attributed to Raman-active aromatic vibrations. Furthermore, no new spectral features are observed in the hybridized probe spectrum, indicating that neither the ssDNA capture probe nor the reagents used in the capture probe anchoring steps contribute significant background signals. In contrast, the spectrum for the hybridization control, illustrated in curve (b), shows no spectral features characteristic of rhodamine-B. The hybridization control was a silver surface modified with alkylthiol SAMS but lacking the BRCA1 DNA

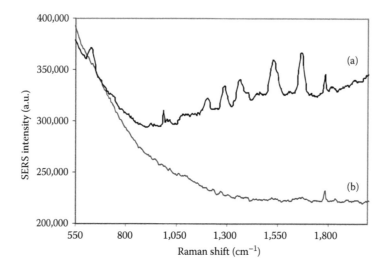

FIGURE 8.14 Demonstration of the SERG probe technology for the detection of the oncogene, BRCA-1, via hybridization on a prefabricated SERS-active hybridization platform. (From Vo-Dinh, T. et al., *J. Raman Spectrosc.*, 33, 511, 2002.)

capture probes, and hence ideally offering no means for attracting the BRCA1 gene probe during the hybridization step. Indeed, the lack of the spectral features characteristic of rhodamine-B indicates that nonspecific binding is insignificant. Similar results have been reported for BAX gene detection using a rhodamine-110-labeled SERG probe.[179]

8.4.3 Fiber-Optic SERS Monitors for Bioanalysis

SERS-based fiber-optic probes have been developed for remote and in situ monitoring for a wide variety of applications.[124,217,304–306] The general interest in fiber-optic sensors has arisen from the development of SERS substrates that allow direct measurements in liquid samples. The direct measurement of potentially complex samples is afforded by the spectral selectivity of SERS, which can allow discrimination of multiple components detected simultaneously. Such SERS substrates have been incorporated in remote fiber-optic monitors.

The first SERS-based fiber-optic probes developed in our laboratory had a dual-fiber design in which the SERS-inducing substrate was a separate entity to which the fibers were optically coupled.[124,304–306] One optical fiber was used to transmit the laser excitation to the SERS substrate, and a second fiber was used to collect the scattered radiation from the sample.[124] The SERS substrate was a glass-backed, translucent medium based on silver-coated nanoparticles. With this substrate, the excitation and collection fibers could be configured with one of two geometries: either head on (with the fibers positioned on opposite sides of the SERS substrate) or side by side (with the two fibers on the glass-backed side of the substrate). The collection fiber was coupled to a spectrograph. Using a red-enhanced intensified CCD (RE-ICCD), we were able to detect trace levels of various analytes in milliseconds, even using excitation and collection fibers as long as 20 m. Dual-fiber systems have also been the basis for several remote sensors based on normal Raman detection, but these systems typically have much lower sensitivity.[307,308]

More recently, several studies have reported use of SERS-based fiber-optic sensors with single-fiber designs in which the SERS-inducing medium is integrated on the tip of the optical fiber.[97,146,217,306,309,310] In an early report of integrated single-fiber SERS sensors, Mullen and Carron abrasively roughened the optical fiber before applying a metal layer directly to the tip.[146] More recently, we have applied a nanoparticle layer directly to an optical fiber to impart a uniform and reproducible roughness, which is critical to the SERS effect. The fiber was simply dipped in an aqueous suspension of 0.1 μm alumina nanoparticles and then coated with a 100 nm layer of silver via vacuum evaporation.[309] Integrated single-fiber SERS sensors have also been fabricated through immobilization of silver colloid particles on the tips of optical fibers pretreated with (3-aminopropyl)-trimethoxysilane.[97] The simplicity of these integrated single-fiber SERS sensors may enable nanoscale fabrication for more practical biomedical applications (e.g., probing single cells). While nanoscale fibers are not commercially available, it is possible to use a special, commercially available fiber tapering device (Sutter Instrument Co., Model P-2000) to routinely taper fibers with core diameters as large as 600 μm down to tips of approximately 25 nm diameter. In our laboratory, we used this laser-based fiber tapering technology as a basis for producing a SERS nanoprobe.[217] The tapered fiber-optic tip was coated with a SERS-active silver layer via thermal evaporation. The resulting nanoprobe was used to induce SERS through contact with dry surfaces. Alternatively, a tapered tip can be formed more passively through etching with HF. The tapered end can then be SERS activated with a dependable SERS-inducing medium (e.g., silver islands or immobilized colloids).

8.4.4 SERS-Scanning Near-Field Optical Microscopy

SNOM has received considerable attention in recent years, largely because of the exceptional resolution offered by this new technology. Indeed, SNOM routinely provides optical imaging with resolutions exceeding the diffraction limit.[311,312] Furthermore, SNOM has been coupled with molecular spectroscopy, most commonly through the use of luminescence. Recently, the combination of SNOM and SERS was reported.[8,9,311,312] In this study, researchers used a planar silver-island-based SERS substrate to generate SERS signals and a chemically etched, 200 nm optical fiber tip to deliver the excitation radiation from an argon ion laser (488 nm). The tapered sides of the fiber tip were coated with a thick, opaque layer of metal to limit escape of the excitation radiation to the 200 nm tip, hence permitting extremely localized sample excitation. This factor, combined with a substrate-to-fiber tip spacing of approximately 0.1 nm, enabled the acquisition of spectral and spatial information, with subwavelength lateral resolution, for CFV and rhodamine-6G molecules distributed on the silver island substrate. Furthermore, the SERS/SNOM technique demonstrated exceptional sensitivity. Spectra from as few as 300 molecules have been recorded.

A variation of SERS/SNOM has been enabled by the recent emergence of TERS. With TERS, a SERS-active nanoprobe is used to induce the SERS effect on molecules located within the near field. The tip is SERS activated with a silver or gold layer and typically has a diameter of 20–30 nm. There is no need for adsorption of the sample to a planar SERS substrate as is required with SERS/SNOM. As a result, TERS is more practical for nondestructive analysis of unaltered samples. As an early demonstration in our laboratory of the possibility of TERS, a silver-coated tapered nanoprobe was used to induce SERS on a dry sample of a DNA marker molecule distributed on a planar surface.[217] More recently, TERS has been applied for the detection of DNA components.[218] Furthermore, the potential for probing bacterial surfaces at the nanometer scale has been reported.[220,221]

8.4.5 SERS Single-Molecule Detection

There have been several reports of single-molecule detection using SERS in recent years.[4–14,194] A critical factor in these milestone studies has been the development of exceptional SERS substrates. Most of the reports of single-molecule SERS detection have involved the use of metal colloids in suspensions. For example, Kneipp et al. demonstrated single-molecule detection of dyes in both silver[5,6] and gold colloid suspensions.[7] In these studies, an effective cross section of approximately 10^{-16} cm^2 per molecule was observed, corresponding to a 10^{14} enhancement factor. The gold nanoparticles were commercially available but required proper agglomeration through the addition of NaCl. These results are promising because these dyes could be used as bioassay markers.

In some cases, bioassay markers can be resonance enhanced in addition to benefiting from SERS. For example, a DNA marker, 2,5,1′,3′,7′,9′-hexachloro-6-carboxyfluorescein (HEX) has been used to achieve single-molecule detection via SERRS in a silver colloid suspension.[194] The HEX signature was observed for 8×10^{-13} M DNA, which corresponded to less than 1 molecule per probed volume at any time required for measurement. Single-molecule detection has also been demonstrated on planar surface-based substrates. For example, enhancements factors of $10^{14}–10^{15}$ have been observed for rhodamine-6G molecules adsorbed on silver colloids that had been immobilized on a polylysine-coated substrate.[4] Similarly, $10^{14}–10^{15}$ factor enhancements have been reported for hemoglobin molecules adsorbed on silver nanoparticles immobilized on a polymer-coated silicon wafer.[13] Researchers in this study reported, however, that single-molecule detection was observed only for hemoglobin molecules situated between and adsorbed to two silver nanoparticles.

In our group, we have progressed toward the goal of single-molecule detection using silver-island-based SERS substrates.[40] We have demonstrated extremely low-level detection of CFV, which is a label we normally use for SERS gene probes. In addition to the giant SERS enhancement produced by the silver islands, a He–Ne laser enabled an additional resonance enhancement factor at 632.8 nm. Furthermore, the detection system utilized a spectrograph equipped with a RE-ICCD. A confocal excitation/collection geometry was implemented with a 100× objective lens. The 0.9 numerical aperture of this lens helped ensure a tight focus and efficient signal collection. Sample preparation for the low-level CFV detection simply involved spotting a 1 μL aliquot of 5×10^{-11} M CFV solution (i.e., 3×10^7 molecules) on the silver island SERS substrate and allowing it to spread to a 6.5 mm diameter spot. Assuming a laser spot diameter of 10 μm and even distribution of CFV molecules within the 6.5 mm diameter spot, we estimated the number of probed molecules to be approximately 70. Nevertheless, signal-to-noise levels on this measurement indicated that this number could be reduced by at least a factor of 3. Furthermore, we observed *hot spots* in the area of sample deposition, or micron-scale points of enhanced SERS signal. This phenomenon along with an improved collection optics and longer signal integration times may allow detection of single CFV molecules on silver-island-based solid substrates.

8.5 Conclusions

The development of dependable SERS substrates has spurred renewed interest in Raman scattering as a practical analytical tool in biomedical applications. Until such developments were achieved, there was little interest in Raman scattering-based analysis because the cross section of normal Raman scattering is miniscule (10^{-30} cm² per molecule) relative to the cross sections available through other molecular spectroscopies, particularly luminescence. In the past, high laser powers were used to compensate for this shortcoming. However, this procedure had limited effectiveness, largely because it induced photodecomposition on probed molecules, particularly at trace-level concentrations. By contrast, SERS-inducing media enable trace-level detection with relatively low laser powers.

Both liquid- and solid-based SERS-inducing media are now being used for the detection of biomedically significant compounds; moreover, innovative SERS-based biomedical applications are being developed. The development of such substrates and their use in practical analytical applications has required a triumph over the daunting challenge of producing nanoscale structures in reproducible and cost-effective ways. A significant portion of recent efforts has been devoted toward investigating SERS coatings to improve selectivity, longevity, and ruggedness. As a result of this work, the scope of applications of SERS has been greatly expanded in the past two decades, evolving from environmental to biomedical applications. Some highlights of SERS-based applications have included single-molecule detection, SERS-based fiber-optic probes and nanoprobes, SERS-based bioassays, and hyphenated techniques such as SNOM/SERS and LC/SERS. As we go forward into this new century, researchers continue to explore the potential of SERS, opening new horizons in the development of biophotonic probes.

Acknowledgments

This work was jointly sponsored by the Federal Bureau of Investigation (Project No. 2051-II18-Y1) and the Office of Biological and Environmental Research, US Department of Energy, under Contract DE-AC05-00OR22725 with UT-Battelle, LLC, and by the Laboratory Directed Research and Development Program (Advanced Nanosystems Project) at Oak Ridge National Laboratory. David L. Stokes was also supported by an appointment to the Oak Ridge National Laboratory administered by the Oak Ridge Institute for Science and Education.

References

1. Fleischmann, M., Hendra, P. J., and McQuillan, A. J., Raman-spectra of pyridine adsorbed at a silver electrode, *Chemical Physics Letters* 26(2), 163–166, 1974.
2. Jeanmaire, D. L. and Van Duyne, R. P., Surface Raman spectroelectrochemistry. 1. Heterocyclic, aromatic, and aliphatic-amines adsorbed on anodized silver electrode, *Journal of Electroanalytical Chemistry* 84(1), 1–20, 1977.
3. Albrecht, M. G. and Creighton, J. A., Anomalously intense Raman-spectra of pyridine at a silver electrode, *Journal of the American Chemical Society* 99(15), 5215–5217, 1977.
4. Nie, S. M. and Emery, S. R., Probing single molecules and single nanoparticles by surface-enhanced Raman scattering, *Science* 275(5303), 1102–1106, 1997.
5. Kneipp, K., Wang, Y., Kneipp, H., Perelman, L. T., Itzkan, I., Dasari, R., and Feld, M. S., Single molecule detection using surface-enhanced Raman scattering (SERS), *Physical Review Letters* 78(9), 1667–1670, 1997.
6. Kneipp, K., Kneipp, H., Deinum, G., Itzkan, I., Dasari, R. R., and Feld, M. S., Single-molecule detection of a cyanine dye in silver colloidal solution using near-infrared surface-enhanced Raman scattering, *Applied Spectroscopy* 52(2), 175–178, 1998.
7. Kneipp, K., Kneipp, H., Manoharan, R., Hanlon, E. B., Itzkan, I., Dasari, R. R., and Feld, M. S., Extremely large enhancement factors in surface-enhanced Raman scattering for molecules on colloidal gold clusters, *Applied Spectroscopy* 52(12), 1493–1497, 1998.
8. Deckert, V., Zeisel, D., Zenobi, R., and Vo-Dinh, T., Near-field surface enhanced Raman imaging of dye-labeled DNA with 100-nm resolution, *Analytical Chemistry* 70(13), 2646–2650, 1998.
9. Zeisel, D., Deckert, V., Zenobi, R., and Vo-Dinh, T., Near-field surface-enhanced Raman spectroscopy of dye molecules adsorbed on silver island films, *Chemical Physics Letters* 283(5–6), 381–385, 1998.
10. Kneipp, K., Kneipp, H., Kartha, V. B., Manoharan, R., Deinum, G., Itzkan, I., Dasari, R. R., and Feld, M. S., Detection and identification of a single DNA base molecule using surface-enhanced Raman scattering (SERS), *Physical Review E* 57, R6281–R6284, 1998.
11. Bjerneld, E. J., Johansson, P., and Kaell, M., Single molecule vibrational fine-structure of tyrosine adsorbed on Ag nano-crystals, *Single Molecule* 1, 239–248, 2000.
12. Bjerneld, E. J., Foldes-Papp, Z., Kaell, M., and Rigler, R., Single-molecule surface-enhanced Raman and fluorescence correlation spectroscopy of horseradish peroxidase, *Journal of Physical Chemistry B* 106, 1213–1218, 2002.
13. Xu, H., Bjerneld, E. J., Kaell, M., and Boerjesson, L., Spectroscopy of single hemoglobin molecules by surface enhanced Raman scattering, *Physical Review Letters* 83(21), 4357–4360, 1999.
14. Kneipp, J., Kneipp, H., and Kneipp, K., SERS—A single-molecule and nanoscale tool for bioanalytics, *Chemical Society Reviews* 37, 1052–1060, 2008.
15. Moskovits, M., Surface-enhanced spectroscopy, *Reviews of Modern Physics* 57(3), 783–826, 1985.
16. Wokaun, A., Surface-enhanced electromagnetic processes, *Solid State Physics—Advances in Research and Applications* 38, 223–294, 1984.
17. Schatz, G. C., Theoretical-studies of surface enhanced Raman-scattering, *Accounts of Chemical Research* 17(10), 370–376, 1984.

18. Kerker, M., Electromagnetic model for surface-enhanced Raman-scattering (SERS) on metal colloids, *Accounts of Chemical Research* 17(8), 271–277, 1984.

19. Chang, R. K. and Furtak, T. E., *Surface Enhanced Raman Scattering*, Plenum Press, New York, 1982.

20. Pockrand, I., *Surface-Enhanced Raman Vibrational Studies at Solid/Gas Interfaces*, Springer, Berlin, Germany, 1984.

21. Pemberton, J. E. and Buck, R. P., Detection of low concentrations of a colored adsorbate at silver by surface-enhanced and resonance-enhanced Raman spectrometry, *Analytical Chemistry* 53(14), 2263–2267, 1981.

22. Vodinh, T., Hiromoto, M. Y. K., Begun, G. M., and Moody, R. L., Surface-enhanced Raman spectrometry for trace organic-analysis, *Analytical Chemistry* 56(9), 1667–1670, 1984.

23. Ni, F. and Cotton, T. M., Chemical procedure for preparing surface-enhanced Raman-scattering active silver films, *Analytical Chemistry* 58(14), 3159–3163, 1986.

24. Sheng, R. S., Zhu, L., and Morris, M. D., Sedimentation classification of silver colloids for surface-enhanced Raman-scattering, *Analytical Chemistry* 58(6), 1116–1119, 1986.

25. Torres, E. L. and Winefordner, J. D., Trace determination of nitrogen-containing drugs by surface enhanced Raman-scattering spectrometry on silver colloids, *Analytical Chemistry* 59(13), 1626–1632, 1987.

26. Laserna, J. J., Torres, E. L., and Winefordner, J. D., Studies of sample preparation for surface-enhanced Raman spectrometry on silver hydrosols, *Analytica Chimica Acta* 200(1), 469–480, 1987.

27. Berthod, A., Laserna, J. J., and Winefordner, J. D., Surface enhanced Raman-spectrometry on silver hydrosols studied by flow-injection analysis, *Applied Spectroscopy* 41(7), 1137–1141, 1987.

28. Tran, C. D., Subnanogram detection of dyes on filter-paper by surface-enhanced Raman-scattering spectrometry, *Analytical Chemistry* 56(4), 824–826, 1984.

29. Tran, C. D., In situ identification of paper chromatogram spots by surface enhanced Raman-scattering, *Journal of Chromatography* 292(2), 432–438, 1984.

30. Ahern, A. M. and Garrell, R. L., In situ photoreduced silver-nitrate as a substrate for surface-enhanced Raman-spectroscopy, *Analytical Chemistry* 59(23), 2813–2816, 1987.

31. Garrell, R. L., Surface-enhanced Raman-spectroscopy, *Analytical Chemistry* 61(6), 401A–411A, 1989.

32. Vo-Dinh, T., Surface-enhanced Raman spectrometry, in *Chemical Analysis of Polycyclic Aromatic Compounds*, Vo-Dinh, T. (ed.), Wiley, New York, 1989, pp. 451–486.

33. Pemberton, J. E., in *Electrochemical Interfaces: Modern Techniques for In-Situ Characterization*, Abruna, H. D. (ed.), VCH Verlag Chemie, Berlin, Germany, 1991, pp. 193–263.

34. Cotton, T. M. and Brandt, E. S., *Physical Methods of Chemistry*, Wiley, New York, 1992.

35. Otto, A., Mrozek, I., Grabhorn, H., and Akemann, W., Surface-enhanced Raman-scattering, *Journal of Physics—Condensed Matter* 4(5), 1143–1212, 1992.

36. Vo-Dinh, T., Surface-enhanced Raman spectroscopy, in *Photonic Probes of Surfaces*, Halevi, P. (ed.), Elsevier, New York, 1995, pp. 65–95.

37. Ruperez, A. and Laserna, J. J., Surface-enhanced Raman spectroscopy, in *Modern Techniques in Raman Spectroscopy*, Laserna, J. J. (ed.), Wiley, New York, 1996, pp. 227–264.

38. Haller, K. L., Bumm, L. A., Altkorn, R. I., Zeman, E. J., Schatz, G. C., and Van Duyne, R. P., Spatially resolved surface enhanced 2nd harmonic-generation—Theoretical and experimental-evidence for electromagnetic enhancement in the near-infrared on a laser microfabricated Pt surface, *Journal of Chemical Physics* 90(2), 1237–1252, 1989.

39. Golab, J. T., Sprague, J. R., Carron, K. T., Schatz, G. C., and Van Duyne, R. P., A surface enhanced hyper-Raman scattering study of pyridine adsorbed onto silver—Experiment and theory, *Journal of Chemical Physics* 88(12), 7942–7951, 1988.

40. Stokes, D. L., Hueber, D., and Vo-Dinh, T., Towards single-molecule detection with SERS using solid substrates, *1998 Pittsburgh Conference*, New Orleans, LA, March 1–5, 1998, Abstract 683.

41. Stevenson, C. L. and Vo-Dinh, T., Signal expressions in Raman spectroscopy, in *Modern Techniques in Raman Spectroscopy*, Laserna, J. J. (ed.), Wiley, New York, 1996, pp. 1–39.

42. Kambhampati, P., Child, C. M., Foster, M. C., and Campion, A., On the chemical mechanism of surface enhanced Raman scattering: Experiment and theory, *Journal of Chemical Physics* 108(12), 5013–5026, 1998.

43. Pettinger, B., Wenning, U., and Wetzel, H., Surface-plasmon enhanced Raman-scattering frequency and angular resonance of Raman scattered-light from pyridine on Au, Ag and Cu electrodes, *Surface Science* 101(1–3), 409–416, 1980.

44. Loo, B. H., Surface-enhanced Raman-spectroscopy of platinum. 2. Enhanced light-scattering of chlorine adsorbed on platinum, *Journal of Physical Chemistry* 87(16), 3003–3007, 1983.

45. Fleischmann, M., Graves, P. R., and Robinson, J., The Raman-spectroscopy of the ferricyanide ferrocyanide system at gold, beta-palladium hydride and platinum-electrodes, *Journal of Electroanalytical Chemistry* 182(1), 87–98, 1985.

46. Carrabba, M. M., Edmonds, R. B., and Rauh, R. D., Feasibility studies for the detection of organic-surface and subsurface water contaminants by surface-enhanced Raman-spectroscopy on silver electrodes, *Analytical Chemistry* 59(21), 2559–2563, 1987.

47. Kudelski, A., Bukowska, J., Janik-Czachor, M., Grochala, W., Szummer, A., and Dolata, M., Characterization of the copper surface optimized for use as a substrate for surface-enhanced Raman scattering, *Vibrational Spectroscopy* 16(1), 21–29, 1998.

48. Barber, T. E., List, M. S., Haas, J. W., and Wachter, E. A., Determination of nicotine by surface-enhanced Raman-scattering (SERS), *Applied Spectroscopy* 48(11), 1423–1427, 1994.

49. Li, W. H., Li, X. Y., and Yu, N. T., Surface-enhanced hyper-Raman spectroscopy (SEHRS) and surface-enhanced Raman spectroscopy (SERS) studies of pyrazine and pyridine adsorbed on silver electrodes, *Chemical Physics Letters* 305(3–4), 303–310, 1999.

50. Taranenko, N., Alarie, J. P., Stokes, D. L., and VoDinh, T., Surface-enhanced Raman detection of nerve agent simulant (DMMP and DIMP) vapor on electrochemically prepared silver oxide substrates, *Journal of Raman Spectroscopy* 27(5), 379–384, 1996.

51. Haigh, J. A., Hendra, P. J., and Forsling, W., Extension of a novel method for the examination of oxidized aluminum surfaces using near-infrared (NIR) Fourier-transform surface-enhanced Raman-Spectroscopy (FT-SERS), *Spectrochimica Acta. Part A, Molecular and Biomolecular Spectroscopy* 50(11), 2027–2034, 1994.

52. Klug, O., Szaraz, I., Forsling, W., and Ranheimer, M., A novel method for investigation of dibasic aromatic acids on oxidized aluminium surfaces by NIR-FT-SERS, *Mikrochimica Acta* 14, 649–651, 1997.

53. Freeman, R. D., Hammaker, R. M., Meloan, C. E., and Fateley, W. G., A detector for liquid-chromatography and flow-injection analysis using surface-enhanced Raman-spectroscopy, *Applied Spectroscopy* 42(3), 456–460, 1988.

54. Ni, F., Sheng, R. S., and Cotton, T. M., Flow-injection analysis and real-time detection of RNA bases by surface-enhanced Raman-spectroscopy, *Analytical Chemistry* 62(18), 1958–1963, 1990.

55. Sequaris, J. M. L. and Koglin, E., Direct analysis of high-performance thin-layer chromatography spots of nucleic purine derivatives by surface-enhanced Raman-scattering spectrometry, *Analytical Chemistry* 59(3), 525–527, 1987.

56. Munro, C. H., Smith, W. E., Garner, M., Clarkson, J., and White, P. C., Characterization of the surface of a citrate-reduced colloid optimized for use as a substrate for surface-enhanced resonance Raman-scattering, *Langmuir* 11(10), 3712–3720, 1995.

57. Tarabara, V. V., Nabiev, I. R., and Feofanov, A. V., Surface-enhanced Raman scattering (SERS) study of mercaptoethanol monolayer assemblies on silver citrate hydrosol. Preparation and characterization of modified hydrosol as a SERS-active substrate, *Langmuir* 14(5), 1092–1098, 1998.

58. Li, Y. S., Cheng, J. C., and Coons, L. B., A silver solution for surface-enhanced Raman scattering, *Spectrochimica Acta. Part A, Molecular and Biomolecular Spectroscopy* 55(6), 1197–1207, 1999.

59. Prochazka, M., Mojzes, P., Stepanek, J., Vlckova, B., and Turpin, P. Y., Probing applications of laser ablated Ag colloids in SERS spectroscopy: Improvement of ablation procedure and SERS spectral testing, *Analytical Chemistry* 69(24), 5103–5108, 1997.
60. Lee, P. C. and Meisel, D., Adsorption and surface-enhanced Raman of dyes on silver and gold sols, *Journal of Physical Chemistry* 86(17), 3391–3395, 1982.
61. Hildebrandt, P. and Stockburger, M., Surface-enhanced resonance Raman-spectroscopy of Rhodamine-6g adsorbed on colloidal silver, *Journal of Physical Chemistry* 88(24), 5935–5944, 1984.
62. Bright, R. M., Walter, D. G., Musick, M. D., Jackson, M. A., Allison, K. J., and Natan, M. J., Chemical and electrochemical Ag deposition onto preformed Au colloid monolayers: Approaches to uniformly-sized surface features with Ag-like optical properties, *Langmuir* 12(3), 810–817, 1996.
63. Li, Y. S., Surface-enhanced Raman-scattering at colloidal silver-oxide surfaces, *Journal of Raman Spectroscopy* 25(10), 795–797, 1994.
64. Lee, S. Y., Kim, S. Y., Choo, J. B., Shin, S. Y., Lee, Y. H., Choi, H. Y., Ha, S. H., Kang, K. H., and Oh, C. H., Biological imaging of HEK293 cells expressing PLCγ1 using surface-enhanced Raman microscopy, *Analytical Chemistry* 79, 916–922, 2007.
65. Cui, Y., Ren, B., Yao, J. L., Gu, R. A., and Tian, Z. Q., Synthesis of AgcoreAushell bimetallic nanoparticles for immunoassay based on surface-enhanced Raman spectroscopy, *Journal of Physical Chemistry B* 110, 4002–4006, 2006.
66. Ji, X. H., Xu, S. P., Wang, L. Y., Liu, M., Pan, K., Yuan, H., Ma, L. et al., Immunoassay using the probe-labeled Au/Ag core-shell nanoparticles based on surface-enhanced Raman scattering, *Colloids and Surfaces A* 257–258, 171–175, 2005.
67. Emory, S. R. and Nie, S., Screening and enrichment of metal nanoparticles with novel optical properties, *Journal of Physical Chemistry B* 102(3), 493–497, 1998.
68. Vodinh, T., Alak, A., and Moody, R. L., Recent advances in surface-enhanced Raman spectrometry for chemical-analysis, *Spectrochimica Acta. Part B, Atomic Spectroscopy* 43(4–5), 605–615, 1988.
69. Siiman, O., Bumm, L. A., Callaghan, R., Blatchford, C. G., and Kerker, M., Surface-enhanced Raman-scattering by citrate on colloidal silver, *Journal of Physical Chemistry* 87(6), 1014–1023, 1983.
70. Heard, S. M., Grieser, F., and Barraclough, C. G., Surface-enhanced Raman-scattering from amphiphilic and polymer-molecules on silver and gold sols, *Chemical Physics Letters* 95(2), 154–158, 1983.
71. Lee, P. C. and Meisel, D., Surface-enhanced Raman-scattering of colloid stabilizer systems, *Chemical Physics Letters* 99(3), 262–265, 1983.
72. Gong, J. L., Liang, Y., Huang, Y., Chen, J. W., Jiang, J. H., Shen, G. L., and Yu, R. Q., Ag/SiO$_2$ core-shell nanoparticle-based surface-enhanced Raman probes for immunoassay of cancer markers using silica-coated magnetic nanoparticles as separation tools, *Biosensors and Bioelectronics* 22, 1501–1507, 2007.
73. Liang, Y., Huang, Y., Zheng, Y., Jiang, J. H., Shen, G. L., and Yu, R. Q., Biocompatible core-shell nanoparticle-based surface-enhanced Raman scattering probes for detection of DNA related to HIV gene using silica-coated magnetic nanoparticles as separation tools, *Talanta* 72, 443–449, 2007.
74. Gong, J. L., Jiang, J. H., Yang, H. F., Shen, G. L., Yu, R. Q., and Ozaki, Y., Novel dye-embedded core-shell nanoparticles as surface-enhanced Raman scattering tags for immunoassay, *Analytica Chimica Acta* 564, 151–157, 2006.
75. Yu, K. N., Lee, S.-M., Han, J. Y., Park, H. M., Woo, M.-A., Noh, M. S., Hwang, S.-K. et al., Multiplex targeting, tracking and imaging of apoptosis by fluorescent surface enhanced Raman spectroscopic dots, *Bioconjugate Chemistry* 18, 1155–1162, 2007.
76. Kim, J.-H., Kim, J.-S., Choi, H. J., Lee, S.-M., Jun, B.-H., Yu, K.-N., Kuk, E. Y. et al., Nanoparticle probes with surface enhanced Raman spectroscopic tags for cellular cancer targeting, *Analytical Chemistry* 78, 6967–6973, 2006.
77. Woo, M.-A., Lee, S.-M., Kim, G., Baek, J., Noh, M. S., Kim, J. E., Park, S. J. et al., Multiplex immunoassay using fluorescent-surface enhanced Raman spectroscopic dots for the detection of bronchioaveolar stem cells in murine lung, *Analytical Chemistry* 81, 1008–1015, 2009.

78. Lutz, B., Dentinger, C., Sun, L., Nguyen, L. C., Zhang, J. W., Chmura, A. J., Allen, A., Chan, S., and Knudsen, B. J., Raman nanoparticle probes for antibody-based protein detection in tissues, *Histochemistry and Cytochemistry* 56, 371–379, 2008.

79. Su, X., Zhang, J. W., Sun, L., Koo, T. W., Chan, S., Sundararajan, N., Yamakawa, M., and Berlin, A. A., Composite organic–inorganic nanoparticles (COINs) with chemically encoded optical signatures, *Nano Letters* 5, 49–54, 2005.

80. Levin, C. S., Bishnoi, S. W., Grady, N. K., and Halas, N. J., Determining the conformation of thiolated poly(ethylene glycol) on Au nanoshells by surface-enhanced Raman scattering spectroscopic assay, *Analytical Chemistry* 78, 3277–3281, 2006.

81. Brown, L. O. and Doorn, S. K., A controlled and reproducible pathway to dye-tagged, encapsulated silver nanoparticles as substrates for SERS multiplexing, *Langmuir* 24, 2277–2280, 2008.

82. Docherty, F. T., Clark, M., McNay, G., Graham, D., and Smith, W. E., Multiple labelled nanoparticles for bio detection, *Faraday Discussions* 126, 281–288, 2004.

83. Doering, W. E., Piotti, M. E., Natan, M. J., and Freeman, R. G., SERS as a foundation for nanoscale, optically detected biological labels, *Advanced Materials* 19, 3100–3108, 2007.

84. Monaghan, P. B., McCarney, K. M., Ricketts, A., Littleford, R. E., Docherty, F., Smith, W. E., Graham, D., and Cooper, J. M., Bead-based DNA diagnostic assay for chlamydia using nanoparticle-mediated surface-enhanced resonance Raman scattering detection within a lab-on-a-chip format, *Analytical Chemistry* 79, 2844–2849, 2007.

85. Park, T., Lee, S., Seong, G. H., Choo, J., Lee, E. K., Kim, Y. S., Ji, W. H., Hwang, S. Y., Gweon, D. G., and Lee, S., Highly sensitive signal detection of duplex dye-labelled DNA oligonucleotides in a PDMS microfluidic chip: Confocal surface-enhanced Raman spectroscopic study, *Lab Chip* 5, 437–442, 2005.

86. Cao, Y. C., Jin, R., and Mirkin, C. A., Nanoparticles with Raman spectroscopic fingerprints for DNA and RNA detection, *Science* 297, 1536–1540, 2002.

87. Hu, Q., Tay, L. L., Noestheden, M., and Pezacki, J. P., Mammalian cell surface imaging with nitrile-functionalized nanoprobes: Biophysical characterization of aggregation and polarization anisotropy in SERS imaging, *Journal of the American Chemical Society* 129, 14–15, 2007.

88. Qian X., Peng, X. H., Anasari, D. O., Yin-Goen, Q., Chen, G. Z., Shin, D. M., Yang, L., Young, A. N., Wang, M. D., and Nie, S., In vivo tumor targeting and spectroscopic detection with surface-enhanced Raman nanoparticle tags, *Nature Biotechnology* 26, 83–90, 2008.

89. Ayora, M. J., Ballesteros, L., Perez, R., Ruperez, A., and Laserna, J. J., Detection of atmospheric contaminants in aerosols by surface-enhanced Raman spectrometry, *Analytica Chimica Acta* 355(1), 15–21, 1997.

90. Freeman, R. G., Grabar, K. C., Allison, K. J., Bright, R. M., Davis, J. A., Guthrie, A. P., Hommer, M. B. et al., Self-assembled metal colloid monolayers—An approach to SERS substrates, *Science* 267(5204), 1629–1632, 1995.

91. Wang, J., Zhu, T., Fu, X. Y., and Liu, Z. F., Study of chemical enhancement in SERS from Au nanoparticles assembly, *Acta Physico-Chimica Sinica* 14(6), 485–489, 1998.

92. Fu, X. Y., Mu, T., Wang, J., Zhu, T., and Liu, Z. F., pH-dependent assembling of gold nanoparticles on p-aminothiophenol modified gold substrate, *Acta Physico-Chimica Sinica* 14(11), 968–974, 1998.

93. Zhu, T., Zhang, X., Wang, J., Fu, X. Y., and Liu, Z. F., Assembling colloidal Au nanoparticles with functionalized self-assembled monolayers, *Thin Solid Films* 329, 595–598, 1998.

94. Grabar, K. C., Smith, P. C., Musick, M. D., Davis, J. A., Walter, D. G., Jackson, M. A., Guthrie, A. P., and Natan, M. J., Kinetic control of interparticle spacing in Au colloid-based surfaces: Rational nanometer-scale architecture, *Journal of the American Chemical Society* 118(5), 1148–1153, 1996.

95. Park, S. H., Im, J. H., Im, J. W., Chun, B. H., and Kim, J. H., Adsorption kinetics of Au and Ag nanoparticles on functionalized glass surfaces, *Microchemical Journal* 63(1), 71–91, 1999.

96. He, H. X., Zhang, H., Li, Q. G., Zhu, T., Li, S. F. Y., and Liu, Z. F., Fabrication of designed architectures of Au nanoparticles on solid substrate with printed self-assembled monolayers as templates, *Langmuir* 16(8), 3846–3851, 2000.

97. Polwart, E., Keir, R. L., Davidson, C. M., Smith, W. E., and Sadler, D. A., Novel SERS-active optical fibers prepared by the immobilization of silver colloidal particles, *Applied Spectroscopy* 54(4), 522–527, 2000.

98. Van Duyne, R. P., Hulteen, J. C., and Treichel, D. A., Atomic-force microscopy and surface-enhanced Raman-spectroscopy. 1. Ag island films and Ag film over polymer nanosphere surfaces supported on glass, *Journal of Chemical Physics* 99(3), 2101–2115, 1993.

99. Semin, D. J. and Rowlen, K. L., Influence of vapor-deposition parameters on SERS active Ag film morphology and optical-properties, *Analytical Chemistry* 66(23), 4324–4331, 1994.

100. Stockle, R. M., Deckert, V., Fokas, C., Zeisel, D., and Zenobi, R., Sub-wavelength Raman spectroscopy on isolated silver islands, *Vibrational Spectroscopy* 22(1–2), 39–48, 2000.

101. Roark, S. E. and Rowlen, K. L., Thin Ag films—Influence of substrate and postdeposition treatment on morphology and optical-properties, *Analytical Chemistry* 66(2), 261–270, 1994.

102. Roark, S. E., Semin, D. J., Lo, A., Skodje, R. T., and Rowlen, K. L., Solvent-induced morphology changes in thin silver films, *Analytica Chimica Acta* 307(2–3), 341–353, 1995.

103. Mosier-Boss, P. A. and Lieberman, S. H., Comparison of three methods to improve adherence of thin gold films to glass substrates and their effect on the SERS response, *Applied Spectroscopy* 53(7), 862–873, 1999.

104. Mrozek, I. and Otto, A., Quantitative separation of the classical electromagnetic and the chemical contribution to surface enhanced Raman-scattering, *Journal of Electron Spectroscopy and Related Phenomena* 54, 895–911, 1990.

105. Jennings, C., Aroca, R., Hor, A. M., and Loutfy, R. O., Surface-enhanced Raman-scattering from copper and zinc phthalocyanine complexes by silver and indium island films, *Analytical Chemistry* 56(12), 2033–2035, 1984.

106. Aroca, R. and Martin, F., Trace analysis of tetrasulfonated copper phthalocyanine by surface enhanced Raman-spectroscopy, *Journal of Raman Spectroscopy* 17(3), 243–247, 1986.

107. Jennings, C. A., Kovacs, G. J., and Aroca, R., Fourier-transform surface-enhanced Raman-scattering of Langmuir–Blodgett monolayers on copper and gold island substrates, *Langmuir* 9(8), 2151–2155, 1993.

108. Meier, M., Wokaun, A., and Vodinh, T., Silver particles on stochastic quartz substrates providing tenfold increase in Raman enhancement, *Journal of Physical Chemistry* 89(10), 1843–1846, 1985.

109. Vodinh, T., Meier, M., and Wokaun, A., Surface-enhanced Raman-spectrometry with silver particles on stochastic-post substrates, *Analytica Chimica Acta* 181, 139–148, 1986.

110. Goudonnet, J. P., Begun, G. M., and Arakawa, E. T., Surface-enhanced Raman-scattering on silver-coated Teflon sphere substrates, *Chemical Physics Letters* 92(2), 197–201, 1982.

111. Alak, A. M. and Vodinh, T., Silver-coated fumed silica as a substrate material for surface-enhanced Raman-scattering, *Analytical Chemistry* 61(7), 656–660, 1989.

112. Moody, R. L., Vodinh, T., and Fletcher, W. H., Investigation of experimental parameters for surface-enhanced Raman-scattering (SERS) using silver-coated microsphere substrates, *Applied Spectroscopy* 41(6), 966–970, 1987.

113. Alak, A. M. and Vodinh, T., Surface-enhanced Raman spectrometry of chlorinated pesticides, *Analytica Chimica Acta* 206(1–2), 333–337, 1988.

114. Vodinh, T., Miller, G. H., Bello, J., Johnson, R., Moody, R. L., Alak, A., and Fletcher, W. R., Surface-active substrates for Raman and luminescence analysis, *Talanta* 36(1–2), 227–234, 1989.

115. Alak, A. M. and Vodinh, T., Surface-enhanced Raman-spectrometry of organophosphorus chemical-agents, *Analytical Chemistry* 59(17), 2149–2153, 1987.

116. Vodinh, T., Uziel, M., and Morrison, A. L., Surface-enhanced Raman analysis of benzo [a] pyrene-DNA adducts on silver-coated cellulose substrates, *Applied Spectroscopy* 41(4), 605–610, 1987.

117. Helmenstine, A. M., Li, Y. S., and Vodinh, T., Surface-enhanced Raman-scattering analysis of etheno adducts of adenine, *Vibrational Spectroscopy* 4(3), 359–364, 1993.

118. Helmenstine, A., Uziel, M., and Vodinh, T., Measurement of DNA-adducts using surface-enhanced Raman-spectroscopy, *Journal of Toxicology and Environmental Health* 40(2–3), 195–202, 1993.

119. Bello, J. M., Stokes, D. L., and Vodinh, T., Silver-coated alumina as a new medium for surfaced-enhanced Raman-scattering analysis, *Applied Spectroscopy* 43(8), 1325–1330, 1989.

120. Bello, J. M., Stokes, D. L., and Vodinh, T., Titanium-dioxide based substrate for optical monitors in surface-enhanced Raman-scattering analysis, *Analytical Chemistry* 61(15), 1779–1783, 1989.

121. Li, Y. S., Vodinh, T., Stokes, D. L., and Yu, W., Surface-enhanced Raman analysis of P-nitroaniline on vacuum evaporation and chemically deposited silver-coated alumina substrates, *Applied Spectroscopy* 46(9), 1354–1357, 1992.

122. Li, Y. S. and Wang, Y., Chemically prepared silver alumina substrate for surface-enhanced Raman-scattering, *Applied Spectroscopy* 46(1), 142–146, 1992.

123. Vodinh, T. and Stokes, D. L., Surface-enhanced Raman vapor dosimeter, *Applied Spectroscopy* 47(10), 1728–1732, 1993.

124. Alarie, J. P., Stokes, D. L., Sutherland, W. S., Edwards, A. C., and Vodinh, T., Intensified charge coupled device-based fiberoptic monitor for rapid remote surface-enhanced Raman-scattering sensing, *Applied Spectroscopy* 46(11), 1608–1612, 1992.

125. Narayanan, V. A., Begun, G. M., Bello, J. M., Stokes, D. L., and Vodinh, T., Analysis of the plant-growth regulator Alar (Daminozide) and its hydrolysis products using Raman-spectroscopy, *Analysis* 21(2), 107–112, 1993.

126. Narayanan, V. A., Begun, G. M., Stump, N. A., Stokes, D. L., and Dinh, T. V., Vibrational-spectra of fluvalinate, *Journal of Raman Spectroscopy* 24(3), 123–128, 1993.

127. Narayanan, V. A., Stokes, D. L., and Tuan, V. D., Vibrational spectral-analysis of eosin-Y and erythrosin-B—Intensity studies for quantitative detection of the dyes, *Journal of Raman Spectroscopy* 25(6), 415–422, 1994.

128. Vodinh, T., Houck, K., and Stokes, D. L., Surface-enhanced Raman gene probes, *Analytical Chemistry* 66(20), 3379–3383, 1994.

129. Vo-Dinh, T. and Stokes, D. L., Surface-enhanced Raman detection of chemical vapors with the use of personal dosimeters, *Field Analytical Chemistry and Technology* 3(6), 346–356, 1999.

130. Ibrahim, A., Oldham, P. B., Stokes, D. L., and VoDinh, T., Determination of enhancement factors for surface-enhanced FT-Raman spectroscopy on gold and silver surfaces, *Journal of Raman Spectroscopy* 27(12), 887–891, 1996.

131. Wachter, E. A., Storey, J. M. E., Sharp, S. L., Carron, K. T., and Jiang, Y., Hybrid substrates for real-time SERS-based chemical sensors, *Applied Spectroscopy* 49(2), 193–199, 1995.

132. Liao, P. F., Silver structures produced by microlithography, in *Surface Enhanced Raman Scattering*, Chang, R. K. and Furtak, T. E. (eds.), Plenum Press, New York, 1982, pp. 379–390.

133. Haynes, C. L. and Van Duyne, R. P., Nanosphere lithography: A versatile nanofabrication tool for studies of size-dependent nanoparticle optics, *Journal of Physical Chemistry B* 5599–5611, 2001.

134. De Jesus, M. A., Giesfeldt, K. S., Oran, J. M., Abu-Hatab, N. A., Lavrik, N. V., and Sepaniak, M. J., Nanofabrication of densely packed metal–polymer arrays for surface-enhanced Raman spectrometry, *Applied Spectroscopy* 59, 1501–1508, 2005.

135. Enlow, P. D., Buncick, M., Warmack, R. J., and Vodinh, T., Detection of nitro polynuclear aromatic-compounds by surface-enhanced Raman-spectrometry, *Analytical Chemistry* 58(6), 1119–1123, 1986.

136. Felidj, N., Aubard, J., Levi, G., Krenn, J. R., Hohenau, A., Schider, G., Leitner, A., and Aussenegg, F. R., Optimized surface-enhanced Raman scattering on gold nanoparticle arrays, *Applied Physics Letters* 82, 3095–3097, 2003.

137. Xue, G., Dong, J., and Zhang, M. S., Surface-enhanced Raman-scattering (SERS) and surface-enhanced resonance Raman-scattering (SERRS) on HNO_3-roughened copper foil, *Applied Spectroscopy* 45(5), 756–759, 1991.

138. Miller, S. K., Baiker, A., Meier, M., and Wokaun, A., Surface-enhanced Raman-scattering and the preparation of copper substrates for catalytic studies, *Journal of the Chemical Society, Faraday Transactions I* 80, 1305–1312, 1984.

139. Ruperez, A. and Laserna, J. J., Surface-enhanced Raman-spectrometry on a silver substrate prepared by the nitric-acid etching method, *Analytica Chimica Acta* 291(1–2), 147–153, 1994.

140. Ruperez, A. and Laserna, J. J., Surface-enhanced Raman sensor, *Analysis* 23(2), 91–93, 1995.

141. Ruperez, A. and Laserna, J. J., Surface-enhanced Raman spectrometry of triamterene on a silver substrate prepared by the nitric acid etching method, *Talanta* 44(2), 213–220, 1997.

142. Lu, Y., Xue, G., and Dong, J., HNO_3 etched silver foil as an effective substrate for surface-enhanced Raman-scattering (SERS) analysis, *Applied Surface Science* 68(4), 485–489, 1993.

143. Norrod, K. L., Sudnik, L. M., Rousell, D., and Rowlen, K. L., Quantitative comparison of five SERS substrates: Sensitivity and limit of detection, *Applied Spectroscopy* 51(7), 994–1001, 1997.

144. Cao, Y. H. and Li, Y. S., Constructing surface roughness of silver for surface-enhanced Raman scattering by self-assembled monolayers and selective etching process, *Applied Spectroscopy* 53(5), 540–546, 1999.

145. Szabo, N. J. and Winefordner, J. D., Surface enhanced Raman scattering from an etched polymer substrate, *Analytical Chemistry* 69(13), 2418–2425, 1997.

146. Mullen, K. I. and Carron, K. T., Surface-enhanced Raman-spectroscopy with abrasively modified fiber optic probes, *Analytical Chemistry* 63(19), 2196–2199, 1991.

147. Sutherland, W. S. and Winefordner, J. D., Preparation of substrates for surface-enhanced Raman microprobe spectroscopy, *Journal of Raman Spectroscopy* 22(10), 541–549, 1991.

148. Xue, G., Lu, Y., and Zhang, J. F., Stable SERS substrates used for in-situ studies of the polymer–metal interface at elevated-temperature, *Macromolecules* 27(3), 809–813, 1994.

149. Szabo, N. J. and Winefordner, J. D., Evaluation of two commercially available TLC materials as SER substrates, *Applied Spectroscopy* 51(7), 965–975, 1997.

150. Szabo, N. J. and Winefordner, J. D., Evaluation of a solid-phase extraction membrane as a surface-enhanced Raman substrate, *Applied Spectroscopy* 52(4), 500–512, 1998.

151. Horvath, E., Mink, J., and Kristof, J., Surface-enhanced Raman spectroscopy as a technique for drug analysis, *Mikrochimica Acta* 14, 745–746, 1997.

152. Gliemann, H., Nickel, U., and Schneider, S., Application of photographic paper as a substrate for surface-enhanced Raman spectroscopy, *Journal of Raman Spectroscopy* 29(12), 1041–1046, 1998.

153. Volkan, M., Stokes, D. L., and Vo-Dinh, T., A new surface-enhanced Raman scattering substrate based on silver nanoparticles in sol-gel, *Journal of Raman Spectroscopy* 30(12), 1057–1065, 1999.

154. Volkan, M., Stokes, D. L., and Tuan, V. D., Surface-enhanced Raman of dopamine and neurotransmitters using sol-gel substrates and polymer-coated fiber-optic probes, *Applied Spectroscopy* 54(12), 1842–1848, 2000.

155. Murphy, T., Schmidt, H., and Kronfeldt, H. D., Use of sol-gel techniques in the development of surface-enhanced Raman scattering (SERS) substrates suitable for in situ detection of chemicals in sea-water, *Applied Physics B: Lasers and Optics* 69(2), 147–150, 1999.

156. Lee, Y. H., Dai, S., and Young, J. P., Silver-doped sol-gel films as the substrate for surface-enhanced Raman scattering, *Journal of Raman Spectroscopy* 28(8), 635–639, 1997.

157. Wang, K. and Li, Y. S., Silver doping of polycarbonate films for surface-enhanced Raman scattering, *Vibrational Spectroscopy* 14(2), 183–188, 1997.

158. Akbarian, F., Dunn, B. S., and Zink, J. I., Surface-enhanced Raman-spectroscopy using photodeposited gold particles in porous sol-gel silicates, *Journal of Physical Chemistry* 99(12), 3892–3894, 1995.

159. Imai, Y., Tamai, Y., and Kurokawa, Y., Surface-enhanced Raman scattering of benzoic and thiosalicylic acids adsorbed on fine Ag particle-impregnated cellulose gel films, *Journal of Sol-Gel Science and Technology* 11(3), 273–278, 1998.

160. Imai, Y., Kurokawa, Y., Hara, M., and Fukushima, M., Observation of SERS of picolinic acid and nicotinic acid using cellulose acetate films doped with Ag fine particles, *Spectrochimica Acta. Part A, Molecular and Biomolecular Spectroscopy* 53(11), 1697–1700, 1997.

161. Pal, A., Stokes, D. L., Alarie, J. P., and Vodinh, T., Selective surface-enhanced Raman-spectroscopy using a polymer-coated substrate, *Analytical Chemistry* 67(18), 3154–3159, 1995.

162. Stokes, D. L., Pal, A., Narayanan, V. A., and Vo-Dinh, T., Evaluation of a chemical vapor dosimeter using polymer-coated SERS substrates, *Analytica Chimica Acta* 399(3), 265–274, 1999.

163. Carron, K. T., Lewis, M. L., Dong, J. A., Ding, J. F., Xue, G., and Chen, Y., Surface-enhanced Raman-scattering and cyclic voltammetry studies of synergetic effects in the corrosion inhibition of copper by polybenzimidazole and mercaptobenzimidazole at high-temperature, *Journal of Materials Science* 28(15), 4099–4103, 1993.

164. Deschaines, T. O. and Carron, K. T., Stability and surface uniformity of selected thiol-coated SERS surfaces, *Applied Spectroscopy* 51(9), 1355–1359, 1997.

165. Carron, K. T. and Kennedy, B. J., Molecular-specific chromatographic detector using modified SERS substrates, *Analytical Chemistry* 67(18), 3353–3356, 1995.

166. Crane, L. G., Wang, D. X., Sears, L. M., Heyns, B., and Carron, K., SERS surfaces modified with a 4-(2-pyridylazo)resorcinol disulfide derivative—Detection of copper, lead, and cadmium, *Analytical Chemistry* 67(2), 360–364, 1995.

167. Sulk, R., Chan, C., Guicheteau, J., Gomez, C., Heyns, J. B. B., Corcoran, R., and Carron, K., Surface-enhanced Raman assays (SERA): Measurement of bilirubin and salicylate, *Journal of Raman Spectroscopy* 30(9), 853–859, 1999.

168. Sulk, R. A., Corcoran, R. C., and Carron, K. T., Surface enhanced Raman scattering detection of amphetamine and methamphetamine by modification with 2-mercaptonicotinic acid, *Applied Spectroscopy* 53(8), 954–959, 1999.

169. Zou, S. Z. and Weaver, M. J., Surface-enhanced Raman scattering an uniform transition metal films: Toward a versatile adsorbate vibrational strategy for solid-nonvacuum interfaces? *Analytical Chemistry* 70(11), 2387–2395, 1998.

170. Wilke, T., Gao, X. P., Takoudis, C. G., and Weaver, M. J., Surface-enhanced Raman-spectroscopy as a probe of adsorption at transition metal-high-pressure gas interfaces—NO, CO, and oxygen on platinum-coated gold, rhodium-coated gold, and ruthenium-coated gold, *Langmuir* 7(4), 714–721, 1991.

171. Tarcha, P. J., DeSaja-Gonzalez, J., Rodriguez-Llorente, S., and Aroca, R., Surface-enhanced fluorescence on SiO$_2$-coated silver island films, *Applied Spectroscopy* 53(1), 43–48, 1999.

172. Lacy, W. B., Olson, L. G., and Harris, J. M., Quantitative SERS measurements on dielectric-overcoated silver-island films by solution deposition control of surface concentrations, *Analytical Chemistry* 71(13), 2564–2570, 1999.

173. Lacy, W. B., Williams, J. M., Wenzler, L. A., Beebe, T. P., and Harris, J. M., Characterization of SiO$_2$-overcoated silver-island films as substrates for surface-enhanced Raman scattering, *Analytical Chemistry* 68(6), 1003–1011, 1996.

174. Yang, X. M., Tryk, D. A., Ajito, K., Hashimoto, K., and Fujishima, A., Surface-enhanced Raman scattering imaging of photopatterned self-assembled monolayers, *Langmuir* 12(23), 5525–5527, 1996.

175. Zhu, T., Yu, H. Z., Wang, J., Wang, Y. Q., Cai, S. M., and Liu, Z. F., Two-dimensional surface enhanced Raman mapping of differently prepared gold substrates with an azobenzene self-assembled monolayer, *Chemical Physics Letters* 265(3–5), 334–340, 1997.

176. Castro, J. L., Lopez-Ramirez, M. R., Arenas, J. F., and Otero, J. C., Surface-enhanced Raman scattering of 3-mercaptopropionic acid adsorbed on a colloidal silver surface, *Journal of Raman Spectroscopy* 35, 997–1000, 2004.

177. Wrzosek, B., Bukowska, J., and Kudelski, A., Raman study on the structure of adlayers formed on silver from mixtures of 2-aminoethanethioland 3-mercaptopropionic acid, *Journal of Raman Spectroscopy* 36, 1040, 2005.

178. Maeda, Y., Yamamoto, H., and Kitano, H., Self-assembled monolayers as novel biomembrane mimetics. 1. Characterization of cytochrome-c bound to self-assembled monolayers on silver by surface-enhanced resonance Raman-spectroscopy, *Journal of Physical Chemistry* 99(13), 4837–4841, 1995.

179. Vo-Dinh, T., Allain, L. R., and Stokes, D. L., Cancer gene detection using surface-enhanced Raman scattering (SERS), *Journal of Raman Spectroscopy* 33, 511–516, 2002.

180. Culha, M., Stokes, D., Allain, L. R., and Vo-Dinh, T., Surface-enhanced Raman scattering substrate based on a self-assembled monolayer for use in gene diagnostics, *Analytical Chemistry* 75, 6196–6201, 2003.

181. Yang, H. F., Zhu, J., Sheng, C., Sun, X. J., Ji, J. H., and Ma, X. L., pH-dependent surface-enhanced Raman scattering studies of *N*-acetylalanine monolayers self-assembled on a silver surface, *Journal of Raman Spectroscopy* 38, 890–895, 2007.

182. Michota, A., Kudelski, A., and Bukowska, J., Chemisorption of cysteamine on silver studied by surface-enhanced Raman scattering, *Langmuir* 16(26), 10236–10242, 2000.

183. Michota, A., Kudelski, A., and Bukowska, J., Influence of electrolytes on the structure of cysteamine monolayer on silver studied by surface-enhanced Raman scattering, *Journal of Raman Spectroscopy* 32(5), 345–350, 2001.

184. Szeghalmi, A. V., Leopold, L., Pinzaru, S., Chis, V., Silaghi-Dumitrescu, I., Schmitt, M., Popp, J., and Kiefer, W., Adsorption of 6-mercaptopurine and 6-mercaptopurine riboside on silver colloid: A pH dependent surface enhanced Raman spectroscopy and density functional theory study. Part I. 6-Mercaptopurine, *Journal of Molecular Structure* 735–736, 103–113, 2005.

185. Shafer-Peltier, K. E., Haynes, C. L., Glucksberg, M. R., and Van Duyne, R. P., Toward a glucose biosensor based on surface-enhanced Raman scattering, *Journal of the American Chemical Society* 125, 588–593, 2003.

186. Yonzon, C. R., Haynes, C. L., Zhang, X., Walsh, J. T., and Van Duyne, R. P., A glucose biosensor based on surface-enhanced Raman scattering: Improved partition layer, temporal stability, reversibility, and resistance to serum protein interference, *Analytical Chemistry* 76, 78–85, 2004.

187. Stuart, D. A., Yonzon, C. R., Zhang, X., Lyandres, O., Shah, N. C., Glucksberg, M. R., Walsh, J. T., and Van Duyne, R. P., Glucose sensing using near infrared surface-enhanced Raman spectroscopy: Gold surfaces, 10-day stability, and improved accuracy, *Analytical Chemistry* 77, 4013–4019, 2005.

188. Lyandres, O., Shah, N. C., Yonzon, C. R., Walsh, J. T. Jr., Glucksberg, M. R., and VanDuyne, R. P., Real-time glucose sensing by surface-enhanced Raman spectroscopy in bovine plasma facilitated by a mixed decanethiol/mercaptohexanol partition layer, *Analytical Chemistry* 77, 6134–6139, 2005.

189. Stuart, D. A., Yuen, J. M., Shah, N., Lyandres, O., Yonzon, C. R., Glucksberg, M. R., Walsh, J. T., and VanDuyne, R. P., In vivo glucose measurement by surface-enhanced Raman spectroscopy, *Analytical Chemistry* 78, 7211–7215, 2006.

190. Shah, N. C., Lyanders, O., Walsh, J. T., Jr., Glucksberg, M. R., and Van Duyne, R. P., Lactate and sequential lactate-glucose sensing using surface-enhanced Raman spectroscopy, *Analytical Chemistry* 79, 6927–6932, 2007.

191. Vo-Dinh, T., Stokes, D. L., Griffin, G. D., Volkan, M., Kim, U. J., and Simon, M. I., Surface-enhanced Raman scattering (SERS) method and instrumentation for genomics and biomedical analysis, *Journal of Raman Spectroscopy* 30(9), 785–793, 1999.

192. Isola, N. R., Stokes, D. L., and Vo-Dinh, T., Surface enhanced Raman gene probe for HIV detection, *Analytical Chemistry* 70(7), 1352–1356, 1998.

193. Brown, R., Smith, W. E., and Graham, D., Synthesis of a benzotriazole phosphoramidite for attachment of oligonucleotides to metal surfaces, *Tetrahedron Letters* 42(11), 2197–2200, 2001.

194. Graham, D., Smith, W. E., Linacre, A. M. T., Munro, C. H., Watson, N. D., and White, P. C., Selective detection of deoxyribonucleic acid at ultralow concentrations by SERRS, *Analytical Chemistry* 69(22), 4703–4707, 1997.

195. Dou, X., Yamaguchi, Y., Yamamoto, H., Doi, S., and Ozaki, Y., NIR SERS detection of immune reaction on gold colloid particles without bound/free antigen separation, *Journal of Raman Spectroscopy* 29(8), 739–742, 1998.

196. Ni, J., Lipert, R. J., Dawson, G. B., and Porter, M. D., Immunoassay readout method using extrinsic Raman labels adsorbed on immunogold colloids, *Analytical Chemistry* 71(21), 4903–4908, 1999.

197. Grubisha, D. S., Lipert, R. J., Park, H.-Y., Driskell, J., and Porter, M. D., Femtomolar detection of prostate-specific antigen: An immunoassay based on surface-enhanced Raman scattering and immunogold labels, *Analytical Chemistry* 75, 5936–5943, 2003.

198. Grow, A. E., Wood, L. L., Claycomb, J. L., and Thompson, P. A., New biochip technology for label-free detection of pathogens and their toxins, *Microbiological Methods* 53, 221–233, 2003.

199. Narayanan, R., Lipert, R. J., and Porter, M. D., Cetyltrimethylammonium bromide-modified spherical and cube-like gold nanoparticles as extrinsic Raman labels in surface-enhanced Raman spectroscopy based heterogeneous immunoassays, *Analytical Chemistry* 80, 2265–2272, 2008.

200. Xu, S. P., Ji, X. H., Xu, W. Q., Li, X. L., Wang, L. Y., Bai, Y. B., Zhao, B., and Ozaki, Y., Immunoassay using probe-labelling immunogold nanoparticles with silver staining enhancement via surface-enhanced Raman scattering, *Analyst* 129, 63–68, 2004.

201. Manimaran, M. and Jana, N. R., Detection of protein molecules by surface-enhanced Raman spectroscopy-based immunoassay using 2–5 nm gold nanoparticle labels, *Journal of Raman Spectroscopy* 38, 1326–1331, 2007.

202. Xu, S., Ji, X., Xu, W., Zhao, B., Dou, X., Bai, Y., and Ozaki, Y., Surface-enhanced Raman scattering studies on immunoassay, *Journal of Biomedical Optics* 10, 031112/1, 2005.

203. Park, H. Y., Driskell, J. D., Kwarta, K. M., Lipert, R. J., Porter, M. D., Schoen, C., Neill, J. D., and Ridpath, J. F., Ultrasensitive immunoassays based on surface-enhanced Raman scattering by immunogold labels, *Topics in Applied Physics* 103, 427–446, 2006.

204. Han, X. X., Jia, H. Y., Wang, Y. F., Lu, Z. C., Wang, C. X., Xu, W. Q., Zhao, B., and Ozaki, Y., Analytical technique for label-free multi-protein detection based on western blot and surface-enhanced Raman scattering, *Analytical Chemistry* 80, 2799–2801, 2008.

205. Orendorff, C. J., Gole, A., Sau, T. K., and Murphy, C. J., Surface enhanced Raman spectroscopy of self-assembled monolayers: Sandwich architecture and nanoparticle shape dependence, *Analytical Chemistry* 77, 3261–3266, 2005.

206. Driskell, J. D., Uhlenkamp, J. M., Lipert, R. J., and Porter, M. D., Surface-enhanced Raman scattering immunoassays using a rotated capture substrate, *Analytical Chemistry* 79, 4141–4148, 2007.

207. Driskell, J. D., Kwarta, K. M., Lipert, R. J., Vorwald, A., Neill, J. D., Ridpath, J. F., and Porter, M. D., Control of antigen mass transfer via capture substrate rotation: An absolute method for the determination of viral pathogen concentration and reduction of heterogeneous immunoassay incubation times, *Journal of Virological Methods* 138, 160–169, 2006.

208. Sabatte, G., Keir, R., Lawlor, M., Black, M., Graham, D., and Smith, W. E., Comparison of surface-enhanced resonance Raman scattering and fluorescence for detection of a labeled antibody, *Analytical Chemistry* 80, 2351–2356, 2008.

209. Nabiev, I. and Manfait, M., Industrial applications of the surface-enhanced Raman-spectroscopy, *Revue De L Institut Francais Du Petrole* 48(3), 261–285, 1993.

210. Nabiev, I., Chourpa, I., and Manfait, M., Applications of Raman and surface-enhanced Raman-scattering spectroscopy in medicine, *Journal of Raman Spectroscopy* 25(1), 13–23, 1994.

211. Kneipp, K., Kneipp, H., Itzkan, I., Dasari, R. R., and Feld, M. S., Surface-enhanced Raman scattering: A new tool for biomedical spectroscopy, *Current Science* 77(7), 915–924, 1999.

212. Koglin, E. and Sequaris, J. M., Surface enhanced Raman-scattering of biomolecules, *Topics in Current Chemistry* 134, 1–57, 1986.

213. Haynes, C. L., McFarland, A. D., and Van-Duyne, R. P., Surface-enhanced Raman spectroscopy, *Analytical Chemistry* 77, 338A–346A, 2005.

214. Vo-Dinh, T., Surface-enhanced Raman spectrometry using metallic nanostructures, *Trends in Analytical Chemistry* 17, 557–582, 1998.

215. Vo-Dinh, T., Yan, F., Stokes, D. L., Plasmonics-based nanostructures for surface-enhanced Raman scattering bioanalysis, *Methods in Molecular Biology* 300, 255–283, 2005.

216. El-Kouedi, M., and Keating, C. D., Biofunctionalized nanoparticles for SERS and SPR, in *Nanobiotechnology: Concepts, Applications, and Perspectives*, Niemeyer, C. and Mirkin, C. A. (eds.), Wiley-VCH Verlag GmbH & Co., Weinheim, Germany, 2004, pp. 429–443.

217. Stokes, D. L., Chi, Z., and Vo-Dinh, T., Surface-enhanced-Raman-scattering-inducing nanoprobe for spectrochemical analysis, *Applied Spectroscopy* 58, 292–298, 2004.

218. Ichimura, T., Hayazawa, N., Hashimoto, M., Inouye, Y., and Kawata, S., Tip-enhanced coherent anti-stokes Raman scattering for vibrational nanoimaging, *Physical Review Letters* 92, 220801, 2004.

219. Rasmussen, A. and Deckert, V., Surface and tip-enhanced Raman scattering of DNA components, *Journal of Raman Spectroscopy* 37, 311–317, 2006.

220. Neugebauer, U., Rosch, P., Schmitt, M., Popp, J., Julien, C., Rasmussen, A., Budich, C., and Deckert, V., On the way to nanometer-sized information of the bacterial surface by tip-enhanced Raman spectroscopy, *ChemPhysChem* 7, 1428–1430, 2006.

221. Neugebauer, U., Schmid, U., Baumann, K., Ziebuhr, W., Kozitskaya, S., Deckert, V., Schmitt, M., and Popp, J., Towards a detailed understanding of bacterial metabolism—Spectroscopic characterization of *Staphylococcus epidermidis*, *ChemPhysChem* 8, 124–137, 2007.

222. Carter, J. C., Brewer, W. E., and Angel, S. M., Raman spectroscopy for the in situ identification of cocaine and selected adulterants, *Applied Spectroscopy* 54(12), 1876–1881, 2000.

223. Angel, S. M., Carter, J. C., Stratis, D. N., Marquardt, B. J., and Brewer, W. E., Some new uses for filtered fiber-optic Raman probes: In situ drug identification and in situ and remote Raman imaging, *Journal of Raman Spectroscopy* 30(9), 795–805, 1999.

224. Perez, R., Ruperez, A., and Laserna, J. J., Evaluation of silver substrates for surface-enhanced Raman detection of drugs banned in sport practices, *Analytica Chimica Acta* 376(2), 255–263, 1998.

225. Cabalin, L. M., Ruperez, A., and Laserna, J. J., Surface-enhanced Raman-spectrometry for detection in liquid-chromatography using a windowless flow cell, *Talanta* 40(11), 1741–1747, 1993.

226. Ruperez, A., Montes, R., and Laserna, J. J., Identification of stimulant-drugs by surface-enhanced Raman-spectrometry on colloidal silver, *Vibrational Spectroscopy* 2(2–3), 145–154, 1991.

227. Vo-Dinh, T., Yan, F., and Wabuyele, M. B., Surface-enhanced Raman scattering for medical diagnostics and biological imaging, *Journal of Raman Spectroscopy* 36, 640–647, 2005.

228. Wabuyele, M. B. and Vo-Dinh, T., Detection of human immunodeficiency virus type 1 DNA sequence using plasmonics nanoprobes, *Analytical Chemistry* 77, 7810–7815, 2005.

229. Allain, L. R. and Vo-Dinh, T., Surface-enhanced Raman scattering detection of the breast cancer susceptibility gene BRCA1 using a silver-coated microarray platform, *Analytica Chimica Acta* 469, 149–154, 2002.

230. Pal, A., Isola, N. R., Alarie, J. P., Stokes, D. L., and Vo-Dinh, T., Synthesis and characterization of SERS gene probe for BRCA-1 (breast cancer), *Faraday Discussions* 132, 293–301, 2006.

231. Faulds, K., Smith, W. E., and Graham, D., DNA detection by surface enhanced resonance Raman scattering (SERRS), *Analyst* 130, 1125–1131, 2005.

232. Faulds, K., Smith, W. E., Robson, D. C., Thompson, D. G., Enright, A., Smith, E. W., and Graham, D., A new approach for DNA detection by SERRS, *Faraday Discussions* 132, 261–268, 2006.

233. Docherty, F. T., Monaghan, P. B., Keir, R., Graham, D., Smith, W. E., and Cooper, J. M., The first SERRS multiplexing from labelled oligonucleotides in a microfluidic lab-on-a-chip, *Journal of Chemical Communications,* 1, 118–119, 2004.

234. Faulds K., Smith, W. E., and Graham, D., Evaluation of surface-enhanced resonance Raman scattering for quantitative DNA analysis, *Analytical Chemistry* 76, 412–417, 2004.

235. Fabris, L., Dante, M., Braun, G., Lee, S. J., Reich, N. O., Moskovits, M., Nguyen, T. Q., and Bazan, G. C., A heterogeneous PNA-based SERS method for DNA detection, *Journal of the American Chemical Society* 129, 6086–6087, 2007.

236. Thompson, D. G., Enright, A., Faulds, K., Smith, W. E., and Graham, D., Ultrasensitive DNA detection using oligonucleotide-silver nanoparticle conjugates, *Analytical Chemistry* 80, 2805–2810, 2008.

237. Hawi, S. R., Rochanakij, S., Adar, F., Campbell, W. B., and Nithipatikom, K., Detection of membrane-bound enzymes in cells using immunoassay and Raman microspectroscopy, *Analytical Biochemistry* 259(2), 212–217, 1998.

238. Dou, X., Takama, T., Yamaguchi, Y., Yamamoto, H., and Ozaki, Y., Enzyme immunoassay utilizing surface-enhanced Raman scattering of the enzyme reaction product, *Analytical Chemistry* 69(8), 1492–1495, 1997.

239. Rohr, T. E., Cotton, T., Fan, N., and Tarcha, P. J., Immunoassay employing surface-enhanced Raman-spectroscopy, *Analytical Biochemistry* 182(2), 388–398, 1989.

240. Rivas, L., Sanchez-Cortes, S., Stanicova, J., Garcia-Ramos, J. V., and Miskovsky, P., FT-Raman, FTIR and surface-enhanced Raman spectroscopy of the antiviral and antiparkinsonian drug amantadine, *Vibrational Spectroscopy* 20(2), 179–188, 1999.

241. Rivas, L., Murza, A., Sanchez-Cortes, S., and Garcia-Ramos, J. V., Adsorption of acridine drugs on silver: Surface-enhanced resonance Raman evidence of the existence of different adsorption sites, *Vibrational Spectroscopy* 25(1), 19–28, 2001.

242. Wang, Y., Li, Y. S., Wu, J., Zhang, Z. X., and An, D. Q., Surface-enhanced Raman spectra of some anti-tubercle bacillus drugs, *Spectrochimica Acta. Part A, Molecular and Biomolecular Spectroscopy* 56(14), 2637–2644, 2000.

243. Vivoni, A., Chen, S. P., Ejeh, D., and Hosten, C. M., Determination of the orientation of 6-mercaptopurine adsorbed on a silver electrode by surface-enhanced Raman spectroscopy and normal mode calculations, *Langmuir* 16(7), 3310–3316, 2000.

244. Cinta, S., Iliescu, T., Astilean, S., David, L., Cozar, O., and Kiefer, W., 1,4-benzodiazepine drugs adsorption on the Ag colloidal surface, *Journal of Molecular Structure* 483, 685–688, 1999.

245. Ridente, Y., Aubard, J., and Bolard, J., Absence in amphotericin B-spiked human plasma of the free monomeric drug, as detected by SERS, *FEBS Letters* 446(2–3), 283–286, 1999.

246. Sockalingum, G. D., Beljebbar, A., Morjani, H., Angiboust, J. F., and Manfait, M., Characterization of island films as surface-enhanced Raman spectroscopy substrates for detecting low antitumor drug concentrations at single cell level, *Biospectroscopy* 4(5), S71–S78, 1998.

247. Murza, A., Sanchez-Cortes, S., and Garcia-Ramos, J. V., Fluorescence and surface-enhanced Raman study of 9-aminoacridine in relation to its aggregation and excimer emission in aqueous solution and on silver surface, *Biospectroscopy* 4(5), 327–339, 1998.

248. Chourpa, I., Beljebbar, A., Sockalingum, G. D., Riou, J. F., and Manfait, M., Structure-activity relation in camptothecin antitumor drugs: Why a detailed molecular characterisation of their lactone and carboxylate forms by Raman and SERS spectroscopies? *Biochimica et Biophysica Acta: General Subjects* 1334(2–3), 349–360, 1997.

249. Sanchez-Cortes, S., Jancura, D., Miskovsky, P., and Bertoluzza, A., Near infrared surface-enhanced Raman spectroscopic study of antiretroviraly drugs hypericin and emodin in aqueous silver colloids, *Spectrochimica Acta. Part A, Molecular and Biomolecular Spectroscopy* 53(5), 769–779, 1997.

250. Ruperez, A. and Laserna, J. J., Surface-enhanced Raman spectrometry of chiral beta-blocker drugs on colloidal silver, *Analytica Chimica Acta* 335(1–2), 87–94, 1996.

251. Lecomte, S., Moreau, N. J., Manfait, M., Aubard, J., and Baron, M. H., Surface-enhanced Raman spectroscopy investigation of fluoroquinolone DNA/DNA gyrase Mg^{2+} interactions. 1. Adsorption of pefloxacin on colloidal silver—Effect of drug concentration, electrolytes, and pH, *Biospectroscopy* 1(6), 423–436, 1995.

252. Nabiev, I., Baranov, A., Chourpa, I., Beljebbar, A., Sockalingum, G. D., and Manfait, M., Does adsorption on the surface of a silver colloid perturb drug–DNA interactions—Comparative SERS, FT-SERS, and resonance Raman-study of mitoxantrone and its derivatives, *Journal of Physical Chemistry* 99(5), 1608–1613, 1995.

253. Calvo, N., Montes, R., and Laserna, J. J., Surface-enhanced Raman-spectrometry of amiloride on colloidal silver, *Analytica Chimica Acta* 280(2), 263–268, 1993.

254. Levi, G., Pantigny, J., Marsault, J. P., Christensen, D. H., Nielsen, O. F., and Aubard, J., Surface-enhanced Raman-spectroscopy of ellipticines adsorbed onto silver colloids, *Journal of Physical Chemistry* 96(2), 926–931, 1992.

255. Montes, R. and Laserna, J. J., Fingerprinting and activity of sulpha drugs in surface-enhanced Raman-spectrometry on silver hydrosols, *Analyst* 115(12), 1601–1605, 1990.

256. Sutherland, W. S., Laserna, J. J., Angebranndt, M. J., and Winefordner, J. D., Surface-enhanced Raman analysis of sulfa drugs on colloidal silver dispersion, *Analytical Chemistry* 62(7), 689–693, 1990.

257. Howes, B. D., Guerrini, L., Sanchez-Cortes, S., Marzocchi, M. P., Garcia-Ramos, J. V., and Smulevich, G., The influence of pH and anions on the adsorption mechanism of rifampicin on silver colloids, *Journal of Raman Spectroscopy* 38, 859–864, 2007.

258. Fabriciova, G., Garcia-Ramos, J. V., Miskovsky, P., and Sanchez-Cortes, S., Adsorption and acidic behavior of anthraquinone drugs quinizarin and danthron on Ag nanoparticles studied by Raman spectroscopy, *Vibrational Spectroscopy* 34, 273–281, 2004.

259. McLaughlin, C., MacMillan, D., McCardle, C., and Smith, W. E., Quantitative analysis of mitoxantrone by surface-enhanced resonance Raman scattering, *Analytical Chemistry* 74, 3160–3167, 2002.

260. Murza, A., Sanchez-Cortes, S., Garcia-Ramos, J. V., Guisan, J. M., Alfonso, C., and Rivas, G., Interaction of the antitumor drug 9-aminoacridine with guanidinobenzoatase studied by spectroscopic methods: A possible tumor marker probe based on the fluorescence exciplex emission, *Biochemistry* 39(34), 10557–10565, 2000.

261. Murza, A., Sanchez-Cortes, S., and Garcia-Ramos, J. V., Surface-enhanced Raman and steady fluorescence study of interaction between antitumoral drug 9-aminoacridine and trypsin-like protease related to metastasis processes, guanidinobenzoatase, *Biopolymers* 62(2), 85–94, 2001.

262. Shen, J. K., Ye, Y., Hu, J. M., Shen, H. Y., and Le, Z. F., Surface-enhanced Raman spectra study of metal complexes of *N*-D-glucosamine beta-naphthaldehyde and glycine and their interaction with DNA, *Spectrochimica Acta. Part A, Molecular and Biomolecular Spectroscopy* 57(3), 551–559, 2001.

263. Stanicova, J., Kovalcik, P., Chinsky, L., and Miskovsky, P., Pre-resonance Raman and surface-enhanced Raman spectroscopy study of the complex of the antiviral and antiparkinsonian drug amantadine with histidine, *Vibrational Spectroscopy* 25(1), 41–51, 2001.

264. Rivas, L., Murza, A., Sanchez-Cortes, S., and Garcia-Ramos, J. V., Interaction of antimalarial drug quinacrine with nucleic acids of variable sequence studied by spectroscopic methods, *Journal of Biomolecular Structure & Dynamics* 18(3), 371–383, 2000.

265. Ye, Y., Hu, J. M., and Zeng, Y. N., Comparison of different spectroscopic methods for the interaction of antitumour compounds with deoxyribonucleic acid, *Chinese Journal of Analytical Chemistry* 28(7), 798–804, 2000.

266. Ermishov, M., Sukhanova, A., Kryukov, E., Grokhovsky, S., Zhuze, A., Oleinikov, V., Jardillier, J. C., and Nabiev, I., Raman and surface-enhanced Raman scattering spectroscopy of bis-netropsins and their DNA complexes, *Biopolymers* 57(5), 272–281, 2000.

267. Kocisova, E., Jancura, D., Sanchez-Cortes, S., Miskovsky, P., Chinsky, L., and Garcia-Ramos, J. V., Interaction of antiviral and antitumor photoactive drug hypocrellin A with human serum albumin, *Journal of Biomolecular Structure & Dynamics* 17(1), 111–120, 1999.

268. Ianoul, A., Fleury, F., Duval, O., Waigh, R., Jardillier, J. C., Alix, A. J. P., and Nabiev, I., DNA binding by fagaronine and ethoxidine, inhibitors of human DNA topoisomerases I and II, probed by SERS and flow linear dichroism spectroscopy, *Journal of Physical Chemistry B* 103(11), 2008–2013, 1999.

269. Miskovsky, P., Jancura, D., Sanchez-Cortes, S., Kocisova, E., and Chinsky, L., Antiretrovirally active drug hypericin binds the IIA subdomain of human serum albumin: Resonance Raman and surface-enhanced Raman spectroscopy study, *Journal of the American Chemical Society* 120(25), 6374–6379, 1998.

270. Lecomte, S. and Baron, M. H., Surface-enhanced Raman spectroscopy investigation of fluoroquinolones–DNA–DNA gyrase-Mg^{2+} interactions. 2. Interaction of pefloxacin with Mg^{2+} and DNA, *Biospectroscopy* 3(1), 31–45, 1997.
271. Beljebbar, A., Sockalingum, G. D., Angiboust, J. F., and Manfait, M., Comparative FT SERS, resonance Raman and SERRS studies of doxorubicin and its complex with DNA, *Spectrochimica Acta. Part A, Molecular and Biomolecular Spectroscopy* 51(12), 2083–2090, 1995.
272. Nabiev, I., Chourpa, I., Riou, J. F., Nguyen, C. H., Lavelle, F., and Manfait, M., Molecular-interactions of DNA topoisomerase-I and topoisomerase-II inhibitor with DNA and topoisomerases and in ternary complexes—Binding modes and biological effects for intoplicine derivatives, *Biochemistry* 33(30), 9013–9023, 1994.
273. Nabiev, I., Chourpa, I., and Manfait, M., Comparative-studies of antitumor DNA intercalating agents, aclacinomycin and saintopin, by means of surface-enhanced Raman-scattering spectroscopy, *Journal of Physical Chemistry* 98(4), 1344–1350, 1994.
274. Aubard, J., Schwaller, M. A., Pantigny, J., Marsault, J. P., and Levi, G., Surface-enhanced Raman-spectroscopy of ellipticine, 2-*N*-methylellipticinium and their complexes with DNA, *Journal of Raman Spectroscopy* 23(7), 373–377, 1992.
275. Beljebbar, A., Morjani, H., Angiboust, J. F., Sockalingum, G. D., Polissiou, M., and Manfait, M., Molecular and cellular interaction of the differentiating antitumour agent dimethylcrocetin with nuclear retinoic acid receptor as studied by near-infrared and visible SERS spectroscopy, *Journal of Raman Spectroscopy* 28(2–3), 159–163, 1997.
276. Chourpa, I., Morjani, H., Riou, J. F., and Manfait, M., Intracellular molecular interactions of antitumor drug amsacrine (m-AMSA) as revealed by surface-enhanced Raman spectroscopy, *FEBS Letters* 397(1), 61–64, 1996.
277. Morjani, H., Riou, J. F., Nabiev, I., Lavelle, F., and Manfait, M., Molecular and cellular interactions between intoplicine, DNA, and topoisomerase-II studied by surface-enhanced Raman-scattering spectroscopy, *Cancer Research* 53(20), 4784–4790, 1993.
278. Nabiev, I. R., Morjani, H., and Manfait, M., Selective analysis of antitumor drug-interaction with living cancer-cells as probed by surface-enhanced Raman-spectroscopy, *European Biophysics Journal* 19(6), 311–316, 1991.
279. Grabbe, E. S. and Buck, R. P., Surface-enhanced Raman-spectroscopic investigation of human immunoglobulin-G adsorbed on a silver electrode, *Journal of the American Chemical Society* 111(22), 8362–8366, 1989.
280. Xu, W., Xu, S., Ji, X., Strong, B., Yuan, H., Ma, L., and Bai, Y., Preparation of gold colloid monolayer by immunological identification, *Colloids and Surfaces B* 40, 169–172, 2005.
281. Chourpa, I. and Manfait, M., Specific molecular-interactions of acridine drugs in complexes with topoisomerase-II and DNA—SERS and resonance Raman-study of M-AMSA in comparison with O-AMSA, *Journal of Raman Spectroscopy* 26(8–9), 813–819, 1995.
282. Bernard, S., Schwaller, M. A., Moiroux, J., Bazzaoui, E. A., Levi, G., and Aubard, J., SERS identification of quinone-imine species as oxidation products of antitumor ellipticines, *Journal of Raman Spectroscopy* 27(7), 539–547, 1996.
283. Bernard, S., Schwaller, M. A., Levi, G., and Aubard, J., Metabolism of the antitumor drug *N*(2)-methyl-9-hydroxy ellipticinium: Identification by surface-enhanced Raman spectroscopy of adducts formed with amino acids and nucleic acids, *Biospectroscopy* 2(6), 377–389, 1996.
284. Koglin, E. and Sequaris, J. M., Interaction of proflavine with DNA studied by colloid surface enhanced resonance Raman-spectroscopy, *Journal of Molecular Structure* 141, 405–409, 1986.
285. Koglin, E., Sequaris, J. M., Fritz, J. C., and Valenta, P., Surface enhanced Raman-scattering (SERS) of nucleic-acid bases adsorbed on silver colloids, *Journal of Molecular Structure* 114(March), 219–223, 1984.
286. Koglin, E., Sequaris, J. M., and Valenta, P., Surface Raman-spectra of nucleic-acid components adsorbed at a silver electrode, *Journal of Molecular Structure* 60, 421–425, 1980.

287. Koglin, E., Sequaris, J. M., and Valenta, P., Surface enhanced Raman-spectroscopy of nucleic-acid bases on Ag electrodes, *Journal of Molecular Structure* 79(1–4), 185–189, 1982.

288. Ervin, K. M., Koglin, E., Sequaris, J. M., Valenta, P., and Nurnberg, H. W., Surface enhanced Raman-spectra of nucleic-acid components adsorbed at a silver electrode, *Journal of Electroanalytical Chemistry* 114(2), 179–194, 1980.

289. Sequaris, J. M., Fritz, J., Lewinsky, H., and Koglin, E., Surface enhanced Raman-scattering spectroscopy of methylated guanine and DNA, *Journal of Colloid and Interface Science* 105(2), 417–425, 1985.

290. Foote, S., Vollrath, D., Hilton, A., and Page, D. C., The human Y-chromosome—Overlapping DNA clones spanning the euchromatic region, *Science* 258(5079), 60–66, 1992.

291. Kim, U. J., Shizuya, H., Deaven, L., Chen, X. N., Korenberg, J. R., and Simon, M. I., Selection of a sublibrary enriched for a chromosome from total human bacterial artificial chromosome library using DNA from flow-sorted chromosomes as hybridization probes, *Nucleic Acids Research* 23(10), 1838–1839, 1995.

292. Kim, U. J., Birren, B. W., Slepak, T., Mancino, V., Boysen, C., Kang, H. L., Simon, M. I., and Shizuya, H., Construction and characterization of a human bacterial artificial chromosome library, *Genomics* 34(2), 213–218, 1996.

293. Kim, U. J., Shizuya, H., Kang, H. L., Choi, S. S., Garrett, C. L., Smink, L. J., Birren, B. W., Korenberg, J. R., Dunham, I., and Simon, M. I., A bacterial artificial chromosome-based framework contig map of human chromosome 22q, *Proceedings of the National Academy of Sciences of the United States of America* 93(13), 6297–6301, 1996.

294. Sun, L., Yu, C., and Irudayaraj, J., Surface-enhanced Raman scattering based nonfluorescent probe for multiplex DNA detection, *Analytical Chemistry* 79, 3981–3988, 2007.

295. Graham, D., Mallinder, B. J., Whitcombe, D., Watson, N. D., and Smith, W. E., Simple multiplex genotyping by surface-enhanced resonance Raman scattering, *Analytical Chemistry* 74, 1069–1074, 2002.

296. Graham, D., Mallinder, B. J., Whitcombe, D., and Smith, W. E., Surface enhanced resonance Raman scattering (SERRS)—A first example of its use in multiplex genotyping, *ChemPhysChem* 12, 746–748, 2001.

297. Faulds, K., McKenzie, F., Smith, W. E., and Graham, D., Quantitative simultaneous multianalyte detection of DNA by dual-wavelength surface-enhanced resonance Raman scattering, *Angewandte Chemie International Edition* 46, 1829–1831, 2007.

298. Richterich, P. and Church, G. M., DNA-sequencing with direct transfer electrophoresis and nonradioactive detection, *Methods in Enzymology* 218, 187–222, 1993.

299. Boncheva, M., Scheibler, L., Lincoln, P., Vogel, H., and Akerman, B., Design of oligonucleotide arrays at interfaces, *Langmuir* 15(13), 4317–4320, 1999.

300. Kelsey, J. L. and Hornross, P. L., Breast-cancer—Magnitude of the problem and descriptive epidemiology—Introduction, *Epidemiologic Reviews* 15(1), 7–16, 1993.

301. Martin, A. M. and Weber, B. L., Genetic and hormonal risk factors in breast cancer, *Journal of the National Cancer Institute* 92(14), 1126–1135, 2000.

302. Staff, S., Nupponen, N. N., Borg, A., Isola, J. J., and Tanner, M. M., Multiple copies of mutant BRCA1 and BRCA2 alleles in breast tumors from germ-line mutation carriers, *Genes Chromosomes & Cancer* 28(4), 432–442, 2000.

303. Boyd, J., Sonoda, Y., Federici, M. G., Bogomolniy, F., Rhei, E., Maresco, D. L., Saigo, P. E. et al., Clinicopathologic features of BRCA-linked and sporadic ovarian cancer, *Journal of the American Medical Association* 283(17), 2260–2265, 2000.

304. Bello, J. M., Narayanan, V. A., Stokes, D. L., and Vodinh, T., Fiberoptic remote sensor for in situ surface-enhanced Raman-scattering analysis, *Analytical Chemistry* 62(22), 2437–2441, 1990.

305. Bello, J. M. and Vodinh, T., Surface-enhanced Raman fiberoptic sensor, *Applied Spectroscopy* 44(1), 63–69, 1990.

306. Stokes, D. L., Alarie, J. P., Ananthanarayanan, V., and Vo-Dinh, T., Fiber optics SERS sensors for environmental monitoring, in *Proc. SPIE* 3534, Environmental Monitoring and Remediation Technologies, Boston, MA, 1998, pp. 647–654.

307. McCreery, R. L., Instrumentation for dispersive Raman spectroscopy, in *Modern Techniques in Raman Spectroscopy*, Laserna, J. J. (ed.), Wiley, New York, 1996, pp. 41–72.

308. Myrick, M. L., Angel, S. M., and Desiderio, R., Comparison of some fiber optic configurations for measurement of luminescence and Raman-scattering, *Applied Optics* 29(9), 1333–1344, 1990.

309. Stokes, D. L. and Vo-Dinh, T., Development of an integrated single-fiber SERS sensor, *Sensors and Actuators B: Chemical* 69(1–2), 28–36, 2000.

310. Stokes, D. L., Alarie, J. P., and Vo-Dinh, T., Surface-enhanced Raman fiberoptic sensors for remote monitoring, *Proceedings of SPIE* 2504, 552–558, 1995.

311. Pohl, D. W., Denk, W., and Lanz, M., Optical stethoscopy—Image recording with resolution lambda/20, *Applied Physics Letters* 44(7), 651–653, 1984.

312. Betzig, E., Trautman, J. K., Harris, T. D., Weiner, J. S., and Kostelak, R. L., Breaking the diffraction barrier—Optical microscopy on a nanometric scale, *Science* 251(5000), 1468–1470, 1991.

9

Functional Imaging with Diffusing Light

Arjun G. Yodh
University of Pennsylvania

David A. Boas
Harvard Medical School and Massachusetts General Hospital and Athinoula A. Martinos Center for Biomedical Imaging

9.1 Introduction

Many materials are visually opaque because photons traveling within them are predominantly scattered rather than absorbed. Some common examples of these highly scattering media include white paint, foam, mayonnaise, and human tissue. Indeed, anyone who has held a flashlight up to his or her hand will notice some of this light is transmitted, albeit after experiencing many scattering events. Light travels through these materials in a process similar to heat diffusion.

What does it mean to say light transport is diffusive? Consider a simple experiment in which an optical fiber is used to inject light into a highly scattering material such as paint or tissue. Microscopically, the injected photons experience thousands of elastic scattering events in the media. A few of the photons will be absorbed by chromophores and will be lost. The remaining photons travel along pathways that resemble a random walk. These individual trajectories are composed of straight-line segments with sudden interruptions where the photon propagation direction is randomly changed. The average length of the straight-line segments is called the random walk steplength of the traveling photon. By summing all trajectories one can compute the photon concentration or photon fluence rate as a function of time and position within the media.

It is then straightforward to show that the collective migration of photon concentration is described by a diffusion equation. In practice one can carry out a variety of measurements to confirm the diffusive nature of light transport. For example, if a short pulse of light is injected into the medium and a second optical fiber is used to detect transmitted photons, then, when the transport is diffusive, the most probable arrival times for the detected photons will scale with the square of the source–detector separation divided by the random walk steplength.

Diffuse light imaging and spectroscopy aims to investigate tissue physiology millimeters to centimeters below the tissue surface.[1-5] The cost of this goal is that we must abandon traditional optical spectroscopies and traditional microscopy because traditional methodologies require optically thin samples. In addition, light penetration must be large in order to reach tissue located centimeters below the surface. Fortunately, a spectral window exists within tissues in the near-infrared from 700 to 900 nm, wherein photon transport is dominated by scattering rather than absorption. The absorption of hemoglobin and water is small in the near-infrared, but elastic scattering from organelles and other microscopic interfaces is large. These are precisely the conditions required for application of the diffusion model. The recognition and widespread acceptance that light transport over long distances in tissues is well approximated as a diffusive process has propelled the field. Using this physical model it is possible to separate tissue scattering from tissue absorption quantitatively, and to incorporate the influence of boundaries, such as the air–tissue interface, into the transport theory accurately. The diffusion approximation also provides a tractable basis for tomographic approaches to image reconstruction using highly scattered light. Tomographic methods were not employed in early transillumination patient studies, and are crucial for recovery of information about tissue optical property heterogeneity.

Even though absorption in the near-infrared is relatively small, the spectra of major tissue chromophores, particularly oxy- and deoxyhemoglobin and water, differ significantly in the near-infrared. As a result, the diffuse optical methods are sensitive to blood dynamics, blood volume, blood oxygen saturation, and water and lipid content of interrogated tissues. In addition, one can induce optical contrast in tissues with exogenous contrast agents, for example, chemical species that occupy vascular and extravascular space and preferentially accumulate in diseased tissue. Together these sensitivities provide experimenters with access to a wide spectrum of biophysical problems. The greater blood supply and metabolism of tumors compared to surrounding tissues provides target heterogeneity for tissue maps based on absorption.[6-25] Similar maps can be applied for studies of brain bleeding[26-28] and cerebral oxygen dynamics associated with activation by mental and physical stimulation.[29-41] Other applications of the deep tissue methods include the study of mitochondrial diseases,[42-44] of muscle function and physiology,[45,46] and of photodynamic therapy.[47-51]

Biomedical applications for diffusing near-infrared light probes parallel the application of nuclear magnetic resonance to tissue study. Generally, the categories of measurement can be termed spectroscopy and imaging. Spectroscopy is useful for measurement of time-dependent variations in the absorption and scattering of large tissue volumes. For example, brain oximetry (hemoglobin spectroscopy) of the frontal, parietal, or occipital regions can reveal reduced brain perfusion caused by head injury. Imaging is important when a localized heterogeneity of tissue is involved, for example, an early breast or brain tumor, a small amount of bleeding in the brain, or an early aneurysm. Images enable one to identify the site of the trauma and differentiate it from background tissue. Imaging is also important because it improves the accuracy of a spectroscopic measurement. Typically, spectroscopic methods employ oversimplified assumptions about the scattering media. Imaging relaxes some of these assumptions, usually at the cost of a more complex experimental instrument and computation, and ultimately improves the fidelity of the gathered optical property information.

The purpose of this chapter is to discuss functional imaging with diffusing photons. Our emphasis will be on imaging rather than spectroscopy, but it will be necessary to briefly review the basics of diffuse optical spectroscopy. This chapter is intended as a tutorial about what can be done with diffuse optical imaging, how to do it, and how to understand it. We intend to give a tutorial snapshot of the field with selected examples, but not a comprehensive review of research in the field. The remainder of this tutorial consists of sections on theory, instrumentation, and imaging examples, and a discussion about limitations and compromises associated with the technique.

9.2 Theory

9.2.1 Diffusion Approximation

Many researchers (e.g., Refs. [52–56] and others) have shown that the photon fluence rate, $\Phi(\mathbf{r},t)$ (photons/[cm² · s]), obeys the following diffusion equation in highly scattering media:

$$\nabla \cdot D(r)\nabla\Phi(r,t) - v\mu_a(r)\Phi(r,t) + vS(r,t) = \frac{\partial\Phi(r,t)}{\partial t} \tag{9.1}$$

$\Phi(\mathbf{r},t)$ is proportional to the photon number density $U(\mathbf{r},t)$ (photons/cm³), that is, $\Phi(\mathbf{r},t) = vU(\mathbf{r},t)$. The turbid medium is characterized by a speed of light, v, an absorption coefficient μ_a (i.e., the multiplicative inverse of the photon absorption length), and a photon diffusion coefficient, $D = v/3(\mu_s' + \mu_a) \cong v/3(\mu_s')$; the dependence of D on μ_a is a subject of recent debate,[53,57–68] but the latter relation follows in most tissues wherein $\mu_s' \gg \mu_a$. The medium's reduced scattering coefficient is defined as $\mu_s' = (1 - g)\mu_s$ and represents the multiplicative inverse of the photon random walk steplength, l^*. Here μ_s is the reciprocal of the photon scattering length, l, and $g = \langle\cos\theta\rangle$ is the ensemble-averaged cosine of the scattering angle θ associated with a typical single scattering event in the sample; g accounts for the fact that light is more typically scattered in the forward direction, so that many scattering events are required before the initial photon propagation direction is truly randomized. $S(r,t)$ is an isotropic source term that gives the number of photons emitted at position r and time t per unit volume per unit time.

The right-hand side of Equation 9.1 represents the rate of increase of photons within a sample volume element. This rate equals the number of photons scattered into the volume element per unit time from its surroundings, *minus* the number of photons absorbed per unit time within the volume element, *plus* the number of photons emitted per unit time from any sources in the volume element.

The diffusion equation is based upon the *P*1 approximation of the linear transport equation.[69,70] It is valid when the reduced albedo $\alpha' = \mu_s'/(\mu_a + \mu_s')$ is close to unity, that is, the reduced scattering coefficient is much greater than the absorption coefficient ($\mu_s' \gg \mu_a$). The near-infrared (NIR) spectral window (commonly called the "therapeutic" window) of biological tissue lies between the intense visible absorption bands of hemoglobin and the NIR absorption band of water. In this window the reduced scattering coefficient is often 10–1000 times greater than the absorption coefficient,[71] for example, $\mu_s' \approx 10$ cm⁻¹ and $\mu_a \approx 0.03$ cm⁻¹ at 800 nm in human breast tissues. Of course tissues are not homogeneous, but they can be accurately divided into domains of piecewise homogeneous turbid media, each obeying Equation 9.1. Measurements are accomplished using sources and detectors arranged on the surfaces of or embedded within the tissue. Strictly speaking, it is also important for the source-detector separation to be of order three photon random walk steps (i.e., $3l^*$) or larger; otherwise the photon scattering angles will not be sufficiently randomized at the point of detection for rigorous application of the diffusion approximation.[72,73]

9.2.2 Sources of Diffusing Photons

Three types of sources are commonly employed in diffusive light measurements (see Figure 9.1). The simplest and easiest method to use is the continuous-wave (CW) device. In this case the source amplitude is constant, and the transmitted amplitude is measured as a function of source-detector separation or wavelength. The second method is the pulsed-time or time-resolved technique. In this scheme a short, usually subnanosecond light pulse is launched into the medium, and the temporal point spread function of the transmitted pulse is measured. The third method is the intensity modulated or frequency-domain technique. In this case the amplitude of the input source is sinusoidally modulated, producing a diffusive wave within the medium. The amplitude and phase of the transmitted diffuse light wave are then measured. These methods are related; the time-resolved and frequency-domain approaches are Fourier

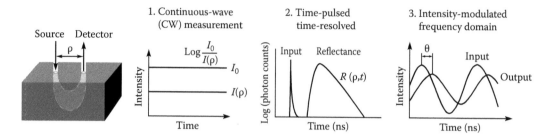

FIGURE 9.1 Three source-detector schemes are generally employed in the photon migration field. On the far left we illustrate a typical remission geometry: (1) continuous wave, called CW spectroscopy; (2) time-pulsed or time-resolved technique (often called TRS); (3) intensity amplitude modulation, that is, often referred to as the frequency-domain method.

transformations of one another, and the CW approach is a special case of the frequency-domain approach wherein the modulation frequency is zero. Each of these approaches has strengths and weaknesses.

Briefly, the CW scheme is inexpensive and provides for rapid data collection. However, because it measures amplitude only, it lacks the capability for characterizing simultaneously the absorption and scattering of even a homogeneous medium from a measurement using only a single source-detector pair. The more expensive time-resolved scheme collects the full temporal point spread function, which is equivalent to a frequency domain measurement over a wide range of modulation frequencies. In this case, when the medium is homogeneous, μ_a and μ'_s can be obtained simultaneously from a single source-detector separation. The photon counting, however, can be slow and the technique is often limited by shot noise. The frequency domain technique is a compromise between CW and time-resolved techniques, with respect to cost and speed. It concentrates all the light energy into a single modulation frequency. It measures amplitude and phase, which ideally enable us to obtain μ_a and μ'_s for a homogeneous medium using a single source-detector separation. In practice all of these methods benefit significantly from use of many source-detector pairs and many optical wavelengths. In this chapter we focus on frequency domain sources, but the results can be applied to time-resolved and CW methods.

9.2.3 Diffuse Photon Density Waves in Homogeneous Turbid Media

Consider a light source at the origin with its intensity sinusoidally modulated at a modulation frequency f, for example, the source term in Equation 9.1 is $S(\mathbf{r},t) = (M_{\mathrm{DC}} + M_{\mathrm{AC}}e^{-i\omega t})\,\delta(\mathbf{r})$, where $\omega = 2\pi f$ is the angular source modulation frequency, M_{DC} and M_{AC} are the source strengths of the DC and AC source components. The diffusion equation continues to be valid for light derived from these highly modulated sources as long as the modulation frequency ω is significantly smaller than the scattering frequency $v_{\mu's}$; that is, photons must experience many scattering events during a single modulation period. Photons leaving the source and traveling along different random walk trajectories within the turbid medium will add incoherently to form a macroscopic scalar wave of photon concentration or fluence rate.

The total fluence rate consists of a DC and an AC component, that is, $\Phi_{total}(\mathbf{r},t) = \Phi_{\mathrm{DC}}(\mathbf{r}) + \Phi_{\mathrm{AC}}(\mathbf{r},t)$. We focus on the AC component $\Phi_{\mathrm{AC}}(\mathbf{r},t) = \Phi(\mathbf{r})e^{-i\omega t}$. The photon fluence will oscillate at the source of modulation frequency ω. Plugging the AC source term into Equation 9.1 we obtain the following Helmholtz equation for the oscillating part of the photon fluence:

$$(\nabla^2 + k^2)\Phi(r) = -\left(\frac{vM_{\mathrm{AC}}}{D}\right)\delta(r) \qquad (9.2)$$

We refer to this disturbance as a diffuse photon density wave (DPDW).[74,75] The DPDW has wavelike properties; for example, refractive,[76] diffractive,[77] and dispersive[78] behaviors of the DPDW have been demonstrated.

The photon density wave has a simple spherical wave solution for an infinite homogeneous highly scattering medium of the form:

$$\Phi_{AC}(r,t) = \left(\frac{vM_{AC}}{4\pi Dr}\right) \exp(ikr)\exp(-i\omega t) \tag{9.3}$$

The diffuse photon density wave wavenumber is complex, $k = k_r + ik_i$, and $k^2 = (-v_{\mu a} + i\omega)/D$. The real and imaginary parts of the wavenumber are

$$k_r = \left(\frac{v\mu_a}{2D}\right)^{1/2}\left(\left(1+\left(\frac{\omega^2}{v\mu_a}\right)\right)^{1/2} - 1\right)^{1/2}$$
$$k_i = \left(\frac{v\mu_a}{2D}\right)^{1/2}\left(\left(1+\left(\frac{\omega^2}{v\mu_a}\right)\right)^{1/2} + 1\right)^{1/2} \tag{9.4}$$

In Figure 9.2, the measured wave is demonstrated within a tank of homogeneous highly scattering Intralipid. Constant-phase contours are shown in 20° intervals about the source at the origin. We see that the wave contours are circular and that their radii can be extrapolated back to the source. In the inset we exhibit the phase shift and a simple function of the wave amplitude plotted versus the source-detector separation. From the slopes of these linear position-dependent measurements, one can deduce the wavelength of the disturbance, as well as the absorption and scattering factors of the homogeneous turbid medium via Equations 9.3 and 9.4.

For homogeneous media in more complex geometries, one can still derive a set of phase and amplitude curves as a function of source-detector separation. The functional relationships may not be linear,

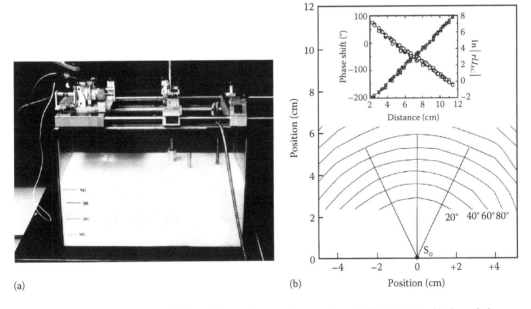

(a) (b)

FIGURE 9.2 (a) An aquarium used for model experiments. The aquarium is filled with Intralipid, a polydisperse emulsion whose absorption and scattering coefficients in the NIR region can be adjusted to approximate those of tissue. (b) Constant-phase contours of diffuse photon-density waves in the homogeneous sample of Intralipid. The source for this measurement is a 1 mW laser diode operating at 780 nm and modulated at 200 MHz. Inset: measured phase-shift and a dimensionless (logarithmic) function of the amplitude as a function of source-detector separation.

but it is still readily possible to derive the average absorption and scattering factors of the underlying media by fitting to this data.

9.2.4 Spectroscopy of Homogeneous Turbid Media

The absorption factor, μ_a, depends on the chromophore concentrations, and their extinction coefficients. The predominant endogenous absorbers in tissues are oxy- and deoxyhemoglobin, and water. The scattering factor, μ_s', depends on other tissue properties such as organelle (e.g., mitochondria) concentration and the index of refraction of the background fluids. If the medium is sufficiently homogenous, then by measuring the absorption and scattering coefficients as a function of light wavelength, one generates a set of simultaneous equations that can be solved to yield the concentrations of the tissue chromophores.

The simplest and most commonly used physical model for tissue spectroscopy treats the sample as a semi-infinite medium. In this case the sources and detectors are placed on the "air side" of the tissue surface (see, e.g., Figure 9.3). Emission and detection take place through optical fibers placed flush with the surface. The quantity measured in practice at position $\mathbf{r}$, time t, and along the direction n is the radiance integrated over the collection solid angle. Within the diffusion approximation, the radiance consists of an isotropic fluence rate ($\Phi(\mathbf{r},t)$) and a directional photon flux ($J(\mathbf{r},t)$) that is proportional to the gradient of Φ.

Diffusion theory for semi-infinite media predicts the reflectivity $R(\rho; \mu_a, \mu_s')$ as a function of ρ, where ρ is the source-detector separation along the sample surface. $R(\rho; \mu_a, \mu_s')$ is derived from photon flux and fluence rate at the boundary[79,80]

$$R(\rho;\mu_a,\mu_s') = C_1\Phi(\rho) + C_2 J_z(\rho) \tag{9.5}$$

where

$$\Phi(\rho) = \frac{1}{4\pi D}\left(\frac{\exp(-\mu_{eff}r_1(\rho))}{r_1(\rho)} - \frac{\exp(-\mu_{eff}r_2(\rho))}{r_2(\rho)}\right) \tag{9.6a}$$

and

$$J_z(\rho) = \frac{1}{4\pi\mu_t}\left[\left(\mu_{eff} + \frac{1}{r_1(\rho)}\right)\frac{\exp(-\mu_{eff}r_1(\rho))}{r_1^2(\rho)} + \left(\frac{1}{\mu_t} + 2z_b\right)\left(\mu_{eff} + \frac{1}{r_2(\rho)}\right)\frac{\exp(-\mu_{eff}r_2(\rho))}{r_2^2(\rho)}\right] \tag{9.6b}$$

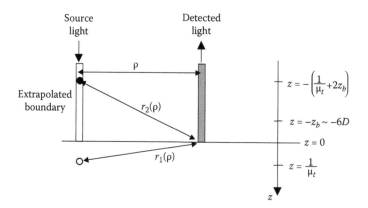

FIGURE 9.3 Schematic of the experimental fiber configuration showing the relative positions of surface boundary ($z = 0$), extrapolated boundaries, $r_1(\rho)$ and $r_2(\rho)$ as defined in Equations 9.5 and 9.6a and b.

Here, $\mu_t = \mu_a + \mu_s'$, and $\mu_{eff} = [3\mu_a(\mu_a + \mu_s')]^{1/2}$. C_1 and C_2 are constants that depend on the relative refractive index mismatch between the tissue and the detector fiber, and the numerical aperture of the detection fibers. The parameters $r_i(\rho)$ are defined in Figure 9.2. Briefly, $r_1(\rho)$ is the distance from the point of contact of the detector fiber on the tissue surface to the effective source position in the tissue located $1/\mu_t'$ directly beneath the source fiber; $r_2(\rho)$ is the distance between the point of contact of the detector fiber and a point located $1/\mu_t + 2z_b$ directly above the source; z_b is the extrapolated boundary length above the surface of the medium. Here the z-direction has been taken normal to the tissue surface (located at $z = 0$), so that J_z is the directional flux normal to the surface.

The tissue optical properties at a fixed wavelength are derived from the measured reflectance by fitting with Equation 9.5. Many schemes have been developed to search for the optimal parameters[80–82]; their relative success depends on the measurement signal-to-noise ratio and the accuracy of the physical model. When everything works, one obtains a best estimate of the absorption factor and scattering factor at one or more optical wavelengths. We then decompose the absorption coefficient into contributions from different tissue chromophores, that is,

$$\mu_a(\lambda) = \sum_i \varepsilon_i(\lambda)c_i \tag{9.7}$$

Here the sum is over the different tissue chromophores; $\varepsilon_i(\lambda)$ is the extinction coefficient as a function of wavelength for the ith chromophore and c_i is the concentration of the ith chromophore. The c_i are unknowns to be reconstructed from the wavelength-dependent absorption factors. Three unknowns require measurements at a minimum of three optical wavelengths (generally more, because tissue scattering is also an unknown).

Oxy- and deoxyhemoglobin concentrations (e.g., c_{HbO_2}, c_{Hb}, respectively) along with water concentration are the most significant tissue absorbers in the NIR. They can be combined to obtain blood volume (which is proportional to total hemoglobin concentration ($[c_{Hb} + c_{HbO_2}]$) and blood oxygen saturation (i.e., $[c_{HbO_2}/(c_{Hb} + c_{HbO_2})] \times 100$), which in turn provide useful physiological information. The same schemes are often extended to derive information about exogenous agents such as photodynamic therapy (PDT) drugs, indocyanine green (ICG), etc.; in such cases the effect of these other chromophores is accounted for by adding their contribution to the sum in Equation 9.7.

9.2.5 Imaging in Heterogeneous Media

9.2.5.1 Brief History

Tissue is often quite heterogeneous, so it is natural to contemplate making images with the diffusive waves. While high spatial resolution is desirable (e.g., a few millimeters), resolutions of about 1 cm are useful for many problems. A simple example of the utility of imaging is the early localization of a head injury that causes brain bleeding or hematomas. Tumors are another type of structural anomaly that one wants to detect, localize, and classify. The diffuse optical methods probe a variety of properties associated with tumor growth: larger blood volume resulting from a larger number density and volume fraction of blood vessels residing within the tumor; blood deoxygenation arising from relatively high metabolic activity within the tumor; increased concentration of the intracellular organelles necessary for the energy production associated with rapid growth; and the accumulation of highly scattering calcium precipitates.

Some of these properties may prove helpful in classifying tumors as benign or malignant. In the long term it should be possible to design contrast agents that respond to specific tumor properties. Other types of tissue of interest for functional imaging include the neonatal brain and a variety of animal models. For example, physiological studies of hemodynamics in relation to the oxygen demand probe important changes in the functional brain, especially during mental activity. In Section 9.4, we describe current research that investigates many of the clinical issues just outlined.

Optical characterization of the heterogeneous tissues has been attempted since 1929[83] when the term *diaphanography* was applied to shadowgraphs of breast tissue. This class of transillumination measurement was renewed in the early 1980s.[84-95] Even in the region of low tissue absorption, however, the high degree of tissue scattering distorted spectroscopic information and blurred optical images as a result of the large distribution of photon pathways through the tissue. Widebeam transillumination proved largely inadequate for clinical use because the two-dimensional "photographic" data were poorly suited for image reconstruction. The mathematical modeling of light transport in tissues was not developed sufficiently for optical tomography to be readily employed.

The diffusion approximation now provides a tractable basis for tomographic approaches to image reconstruction using highly scattered light. Tomographic methods crucial for recovery of information about breast heterogeneities were not employed in the early transillumination patient studies. Several approaches have been developed for diffuse optical tomography; these include backprojection methods,[96,97] diffraction tomography in *k*-space,[98-101] perturbation approaches,[102-107] the Taylor series expansion approach,[108-113] gradient-based iterative techniques,[114] elliptic systems method (ESM),[115,116] and Bayesian conditioning.[117] Backprojection methods, borrowed from CT, produce images quickly and use few computational resources. However, they lack quantitative information and rely on simple geometries. Perturbation approaches based on Born or Rytov approximations can use analytic forms or iterative techniques based on numerical solutions. The analytic forms are relatively fast, but require the use of simple boundary conditions and geometries, and generally underestimate the properties of the perturbations. The numerical solutions are relatively slow and computationally intensive; however, in principle, realistic boundaries present no significant limitations for these methods.

9.2.5.2 Formulation of the Imaging Problem

In this section we formulate the imaging problem in the frequency domain. The starting point of this analysis is the time-independent form of the diffusion equation (Equation 9.1), where we have divided out all of the $e^{i\omega t}$ dependencies:

$$\nabla \cdot D(r)\nabla\Phi(r) - (v\mu_a(r) - i\omega)\Phi(r) = -vS(r,\omega) \tag{9.8}$$

The problem is difficult because the diffusion coefficient and the absorption coefficient vary with spatial position. We write $D(\mathbf{r}) = D_o + \delta D(\mathbf{r})$, and $\mu_a(\mathbf{r}) = \mu_{ao} + \delta\mu_a(\mathbf{r})$; here D_o and μ_{ao} are constant, "background" optical properties. The source can have any form, but typically we assume point sources of the form $A\delta(\mathbf{r} - \mathbf{r}_s)$.

The goal of diffuse optical imaging is to derive $D(\mathbf{r})$ and $\mu_a(\mathbf{r})$ from measurements of $\Phi(\mathbf{r})$ on the sample surface. Two common forms are used for $\Phi(\mathbf{r})$ in the formulation of the inversion problem. The Born-type approach writes $\Phi(\mathbf{r}) = \Phi_o(\mathbf{r}) + \Phi_{sc}(\mathbf{r})$; traditionally one can view $\Phi_o(\mathbf{r})$ as the incident wave and $\Phi_{sc}(\mathbf{r})$ as the wave produced by the scattering of this incident wave off the absorptive and diffusive heterogeneities. The Rytov approach writes $\Phi(\mathbf{r}) = \Phi_o(\mathbf{r})\exp[\Phi_{sc}(\mathbf{r})]$. We will focus on the Born approximation for our analysis, and indicate when possible the corresponding Rytov results.

We next substitute $D(\mathbf{r})$, $\mu_a(\mathbf{r})$, and $\Phi(\mathbf{r}) = \Phi_o(\mathbf{r}) + \Phi_{sc}(\mathbf{r})$ into Equation 9.8 to obtain a differential equation for $\Phi_{sc}(\mathbf{r})$ with general solution:

$$\Phi_{sc}(\mathbf{r}_d,\mathbf{r}_s) = \int\left(\frac{-v\delta\mu_a(\mathbf{r})}{D_o}\right)G(\mathbf{r}_d,\mathbf{r})\Phi(\mathbf{r},\mathbf{r}_s)d\mathbf{r} + \int\left(\frac{\delta D(\mathbf{r})}{D_o}\right)\nabla G(\mathbf{r}_d,\mathbf{r})\cdot\nabla\Phi(\mathbf{r},\mathbf{r}_s)d\mathbf{r} \tag{9.9}$$

where
  $\mathbf{r}_s$ is the source position
  $\mathbf{r}_d$ is the detector position
  $\mathbf{r}$ is a position within the sample

The integration is over the entire sample volume. $G(\mathbf{r},\mathbf{r}')$ is the Green's function associated with Equation 9.8. Examination of Equation 9.9 reveals some of the intrinsic challenges of the inverse problem. In a typical experiment, one measures Φ on the sample surface and then extracts Φ_{sc} on the surface by subtracting Φ_o from Φ. The problem of deriving $\delta\mu_a(\mathbf{r})$ and $\delta D(\mathbf{r})$ from Φ is intrinsically nonlinear because Φ and G are nonlinear functions of $\delta\mu_a(\mathbf{r})$ and $\delta D(\mathbf{r})$.

9.2.5.2.1 The Linearized Problem

The simplest and most direct route to inverting Equation 9.9 starts by replacing Φ by Φ_o and G by G_o. Here Φ_o and G_o are solutions of the homogeneous version of Equation 9.8 with $D(\mathbf{r}) = D_o$, and $\mu_a(\mathbf{r}) = \mu_{ao}$. This approximation is good when $\Phi_o \ll \Phi$, and when the perturbations are very small compared to the background. It is also important that we have accurate estimates of D_o and μ_{ao}. In this case, Equation 9.9 is readily discretized in Cartesian coordinates and written in the following form:

$$\Phi_{sc}(\mathbf{r}_d,\mathbf{r}_s) = \sum_{j=1}^{NV}(W_{a,j}\delta\mu_a(\mathbf{r}_j) + W_{s,j}\delta D(\mathbf{r}_j)) \qquad (9.10)$$

The sum is taken over NV volume elements (i.e., voxels) within the sample; the absorption and scattering weights are, respectively, $W_{a,j} = G_o(\mathbf{r}_d,\mathbf{r}_j)\Phi_o(\mathbf{r}_j,\mathbf{r}_s)(-v\Delta x\Delta y\Delta z/D_o)$, and $W_{s,j} = \nabla G_o(\mathbf{r}_d,\mathbf{r}_j) \cdot \nabla\Phi_o(\mathbf{r}_j,\mathbf{r}_s)$ $(\Delta x\Delta y\Delta z/D_o)$. In any practical situation there will be NS sources and ND detectors, and so there will be up to $NM = NS \times ND$ measurements of Φ on the sample surface. For the multisource-detector problem one naturally transforms Equation 9.10 into a matrix equation, that is,

$$[W_{a,jt},W_{s,ij}]\{\delta\mu_a(\mathbf{r}_j),\delta D(\mathbf{r}_j)\}^T = \{\Phi_{sc}(\mathbf{r}_d,\mathbf{r}_s)_i\} \qquad (9.11)$$

Here, the index i refers to source-detector pair, and the index j refers to position within the sample. The perturbation vector $\{\delta\mu_a(\mathbf{r}_j), \delta D(\mathbf{r}_j)\}^T$ is $2NV$ in length, the measurement vector $\{\Phi_{sc}(\mathbf{r}_d,\mathbf{r}_s)_i\}$ is NM in length, and the matrix $[W]$ has dimensions $NM \times (2NV)$. In the Rytov scheme, the formulation in the weak perturbation limit is almost exactly the same, except that $W_{a,j} = G_o(\mathbf{r}_d,\mathbf{r}_j)\Phi_o(\mathbf{r}_j,\mathbf{r}_s)$ $(-v\Delta x\Delta y\Delta z/\Phi_o(\mathbf{r}_d,\mathbf{r}_s)D_o)$, $W_{s,j} = \nabla G_o(\mathbf{r}_d,\mathbf{r}_j)...\nabla\Phi_o(\mathbf{r}_j,\mathbf{r}_s)(\Delta x\Delta y\Delta z/\Phi_o(\mathbf{r}_d,\mathbf{r}_s)D_o)$, and the vector $\{\Phi_{sc}(\mathbf{r}_d,\mathbf{r}_s)_i\}$ is set equal to $\{\ln[\Phi(\mathbf{r}_d,\mathbf{r}_s)/\surd_o(\mathbf{r}_d,\mathbf{r}_s)]_i\}$ rather than $\{[\Phi(\mathbf{r}_d,\mathbf{r}_s) - \Phi_o(\mathbf{r}_d,\mathbf{r}_s)]_i\}$. The Rytov scheme has some experimental advantages because it is intrinsically normalized (the Born scheme, however, can be modified so that it is normalized in essentially the same way); the major approximations of the Rytov scheme are associated with the gradients of Φ, in particular that $(\nabla\Phi_{sc})^2$ is small relative to the perturbation terms in Equation 9.9. Thus both Born and Rytov approaches give rise to an inverse problem of the form $[W]\{x\} = \{b\}$; the unknown vector $\{x\}$ can be determined from this set of linear equations by a number of standard mathematical techniques. The numerical elements in $[W]$ are often assigned in simple geometries using analytic forms of G_o and Φ_o (e.g., Equation 9.3 and variants), or more generally by numerically solving Equation 9.8 and its Green's function analog for Φ_o and G_o.

9.2.5.2.2 The Nonlinear Problem

The linear formulation described above works well when perturbations are small and isolated, and when the background media are relatively uniform. However, Equation 9.9 is intrinsically nonlinear because Φ and G are also functions of the variables we are trying to determine by inversion. The most broadly useful image reconstruction schemes are iterative. These approaches follow similar algorithms: (1) the optical properties (μ_a and D) are initialized; (2) the forward problem is solved; (3) a chi-squared is calculated and convergence is checked; (4) the inverse problem is set up; (5) the inverse problem is solved; (6) the optical properties are updated and a return to step 1 occurs.

The forward problem is defined as calculating the diffuse photon density, $\Phi_C(\mathbf{r},\mathbf{r}_s)$, for each source position $\mathbf{r}_s$ and is typically found using finite elements or finite difference methods using Equation 9.8. The boundary conditions are defined as

$$\frac{\partial \Phi_C}{\partial \hat{n}} = -\alpha \Phi_C, \alpha = \frac{(1-R_{eff})}{(1+R_{eff})} \frac{3\mu_s'}{2} \tag{9.12}$$

R_{eff} is the effective reflection coefficient and can be approximated by $R_{eff} = -1.440n^{-2} + 0.710n^{-1} + 0.668 + 0.0636n$, $n = n_{in}/n_{out}$ the relative index of refraction.[55] The chi-squared (χ^2) is generally defined as:

$$\chi^2 = \sum_{NM} \left(\frac{\Phi_M(\mathbf{r}_d^i) - \Phi_C(\mathbf{r}_d^i)}{\sigma^i} \right)^2 \tag{9.13}$$

Here

NM = number of measurements
M = measured photon density wave
C = calculated photon density wave
$\mathbf{r}_d^i$ is the *i*th detector position
σ^i is the *i*th measurement error

By comparing χ^2 to some defined ε, a convergence criterion is defined and checked.

We then need a way of updating the optical properties from their previous values. A standard Taylor method expands Φ_C about its assumed optical property distribution, which is a perturbation away from another distribution presumed closer to the true value. In particular we set the measured photon density wave for each source-detector pair equal to the calculated photon density wave at the corresponding source-detector pair plus the first-order Taylor series perturbation expansion terms in μ_a and D, that is, $\Phi_M = \Phi_C + (\partial \Phi_C/\partial \mu_a)\Delta\mu_a + (\partial \Phi_C/\partial D)\Delta D$.

The inverse problem is defined from this relationship:

$$[J]\{\Delta\mu_a, \Delta D\}^T = -\{\Phi_M(\mathbf{r}_d) - \Phi_C(\mathbf{r}_d)\} \tag{9.14}$$

Here, $[J] = [\partial \Phi_C/\partial \mu_a, \partial \Phi_C/\partial D]$ is called the Jacobian. The Jacobian matrix will have the following entries:

$$\left[\frac{\partial \Phi_C}{\partial \mu_a} \right]_{ij} = \frac{-v\Delta x\Delta y\Delta z}{D_o} G(\mathbf{r}_{di}, \mathbf{r}_j) \Phi_C(\mathbf{r}_j, \mathbf{r}_{si}) \tag{9.15a}$$

$$\left[\frac{\partial \Phi_C}{\partial D} \right]_{ij} = \frac{\Delta x\Delta y\Delta z}{D_o} \nabla G(\mathbf{r}_{di}, \mathbf{r}_j) \cdot \nabla \Phi_C(\mathbf{r}_j, \mathbf{r}_{si}) \tag{9.15b}$$

It is illuminating at this point to compare Equation 9.14 with Equation 9.11. The two expressions are essentially the same if we associate Φ_M with Φ, Φ_C with Φ_o, $\Delta\mu_a$ with $\delta\mu_a$, ΔD with δD, and if we use the true Green's function G rather than G_o. The same set of substitutions in the Rytov formulation gives a Rytov version of the nonlinear inversion scheme. Thus the iterative formulation of the inverse problem is based on the same underlying integral relationship (Equation 9.9), and one readily sees that each step of the "nonlinear" iteration process is a linear inverse problem of the form $[J]\{x\} = \{b\}$.

9.2.5.3 Methods for Solving the Inverse Problem

The inverse problem may be solved using a wide range of methods (an excellent review of these methods was given by Arridge[118]). The solution method chosen depends in part on the determination of the *implicit* or *explicit* Jacobian. For the explicit Jacobian two methods are commonly employed: the Newton–Raphson and the conjugate gradient techniques. It is also possible to combine these methods with Bayesian conditioning or regularization to improve reconstruction. For the implicit Jacobian, the methods of choice are the gradient-based iterative technique and ART (algebraic reconstruction technique).

There are essentially two ways to construct the Jacobian, $[J]$ *explicitly*: direct and adjoint. The *direct* approach explicitly takes the derivative of the forward problem (Equation 9.8) with respect to the optical properties to determine the Jacobian. For example, suppose $[A]\{\sqrt{C}\} = \{S\}$ is the forward problem; here $[A]$ is the operator on the left side of Equation 9.8 and $\{S\}$ is the source on the right side of Equation 9.8. Then the equation $[A]\{\partial \sqrt{C}/\partial \mu_a\} = \{\partial S/\partial \mu_a\}[\partial A/\partial \mu_a]\{\sqrt{C}\}$ enables one to compute $\partial \Phi_C/\partial \mu_a$ (and a similar forward problem enables the computation of $\partial \Phi_C/\partial D$).[108] This approach is optimal with finite elements; because the numerical formulation lends itself easily to taking the derivative of $[A]$. Φ_C, $[A]$ and $[A]^{-1}$ are updated on each iteration. The *adjoint* approach solves the forward problem $[A]\{\sqrt{C}\} = \{S\}$ to determine Φ_C, and an adjoint problem $[A^*]\{G\} = \{S'\}$ to determine Green's function $G(\mathbf{r}_d,\mathbf{r})$ due to a unit source at the detector position.[1,102–105,107,119,120] G and Φ_C then fix the elements of $[J]$ according to Equation 9.15. Both Φ_C and G are updated at each iteration. The impact of the two different approaches on convergence and accuracy is not well understood. However, from the computational perspective, for each iteration the direct approach requires 3*NS* solves per iteration, while the adjoint Born or Rytov approach requires *NS* plus *ND* solves per iteration.

The inverse problem, $[J] \{\Delta\mu_a, \Delta D\}^T = \{\Phi_M - \Phi_C\}$, which is also a matrix equation, is significantly more costly than these other subproblems because the Jacobian is a full nonsquare matrix $\{NM \times 2NV\}$. However, the inverse problem only needs to be solved once per iteration cycle. The Jacobian is ill-conditioned and is thus singular or close to singular, which makes it difficult to invert directly. Generally, the approach to address these issues is twofold. First, the matrix is made square by multiplying the inverse problem by the transpose of the Jacobian, that is,

$$[J]^T[J]\{\Delta\mu_a, \Delta D\}^T = [J]^T\{\Phi_M - \Phi_C\} \tag{9.16}$$

Unfortunately, by squaring the Jacobian the equation becomes even more ill conditioned. This problem is solved by regularization[121,122] so that the equation becomes

$$([J]^T[J] + \lambda[C]^T[C])\{\Delta\mu_a, \Delta D\}^T = [J]^T\{\Phi_M - \Phi_C\} \tag{9.17}$$

where
  λ is the regularization parameter
  $[C]$ is the regularizing operator, which is sometimes taken to be the identity matrix

The regularization parameter generally is related to the measurement signal-to-noise. It is a theoretical "knob" that can be adjusted and it will affect image quality by introducing a trade-off between spatial resolution and contrast.[122,123] Nevertheless, its use converts the inverse problem into a readily solvable problem. $\{\Delta\mu_a, \Delta D\}^T$ can now be determined using Equation 9.17 and any number of mathematical techniques that solve systems of linear equations. A particularly useful and common solution scheme is the conjugate gradient method.

A qualitatively different scheme due to Arridge involves the implicit determination of the Jacobian. Briefly, this technique utilizes the Born or Rytov approximation for the inverse problem, and has at least two known solution methods: gradient-based iterative technique and ART (algebraic reconstruction technique). The Jacobian is not calculated; instead an objective function (e.g., a chi-square function) is defined whose gradient, for example, can be used to derive subsequent search directions (see the original papers, Refs. [114] and [118], for details.) Note that the implicit formulation is particularly attractive for experimental systems that rely on many detectors rather than many sources.

9.2.5.4 Challenges for Implementation

The main barrier for full three-dimensional reconstruction is the significant memory and processing time it requires. There are three costly steps of the algorithms: (1) solving the forward problem for each source position, (2) determining the Jacobian, and (3) solving the inverse problem. The forward problem requires the solution of a matrix equation banded in finite difference or sparse in finite elements. The solvers in three-dimensional reconstruction are necessarily iterative because direct solvers require very large storage space for full matrices. Subsequently, multiple source positions demand multiple forward solves. Determination of the Jacobian requires additional matrix equation solutions. For explicit determination, the Green's function for each detector position is needed or the vectors $\partial\Phi_C/\partial\mu_a$ and $\partial\Phi_C/\partial D$ are needed.

Consider a system with one frequency—NS sources and ND detectors; assume further that all the detectors are used for each source. The number of measurements is $NM = NS \times ND$. For each iteration we require NS forward solves and, depending on the Jacobian determination, either ND Green's function or $2NS$ solves for the vectors $\partial\Phi_C/\partial\mu_a$ and $\partial\Phi_C/\partial D$ (implicit would require NS solves). The final costly step of the algorithm is the solution of the inverse problem. However, the inverse problem only needs to be solved once per iteration cycle. For many practical problems the calculations take a long time, and limited memory is available to store the Jacobian explicitly. An important solution to this large-scale computational problem is parallel computing—the execution of many computations at one time using many processors. It has been used successfully in areas of medical imaging, such as positron emission tomography (PET),[124-128] single photon emission computed tomography (SPECT),[129,130] computed tomography (CT),[131-133] electrical impedance tomography (EIT),[134] and optical sectioning microscopy (OSM).[135] It is just beginning to catch on in the diffuse optical tomography (DOT) community.[136,137] In Figure 9.4, we illustrate how the problem is parallelized at the University of Pennsylvania.

9.2.6 Diffusion of Light Correlations: Blood Flow

Thus far our discussion has centered around the determination of tissue absorption and scattering properties. Among other things, these measurements provide access to concentrations of oxygenated and deoxygenated hemoglobin. Even more information, however, is impressed upon these diffusing light fields. Speckle fluctuations of the scattered light are sensitive to the motions of scatterers such as red blood cells.

The means for using light fluctuations and light frequency shifts to study motions have appeared with numerous names over the years.[138-158] In most of these experiments the quantity of interest is the electric field temporal autocorrelation function $G_1(\mathbf{r},\tau) = \langle E(\mathbf{r},t)E^*(\mathbf{r},t+\tau)\rangle$ or its Fourier transform. Here the angle brackets $\langle\;\rangle$ denote ensemble averages or averages over time for most systems of practical interest. τ is called the correlation time. The field correlation function is explicitly related to the motions of scatterers within the samples that we study.

The study of these motions in deep tissues is possible because the electric field temporal autocorrelation function for light traveling in highly scattering media also obeys a diffusion equation.[152] In steady-state (i.e., $\omega = 0$) and in homogeneous media, this correlation diffusion equation is quite simple:

$$(D\nabla^2 - v\mu_a - \alpha k_o^2 \mu_s' \langle\Delta\mathbf{r}^2(\tau)\rangle/3)G_1(\mathbf{r},\tau) = -vS(\mathbf{r}) \qquad (9.18)$$

Here k_o is the wavevector of the photons in the medium and $\langle\Delta\mathbf{r}^2(\tau)\rangle$ is the mean-square displacement in time τ of the scattering particles (e.g., blood cells); it can have different forms depending on

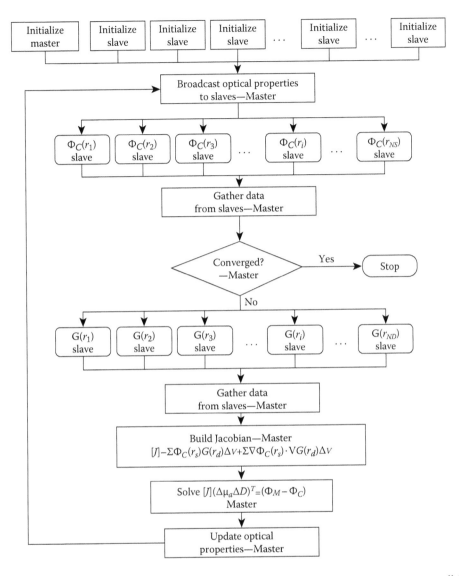

FIGURE 9.4 Schematic of the University of Pennsylvania algorithm for image reconstruction using parallel computing. In the first step each node has its own set of arrays and variables that are initialized. The master must initialize the Jacobian array, the forward solution vector array, and the Green's function vector array. In the second step the master sends out the optical properties, which (in the first iteration) are just the background values. In the third step, the slaves calculate the solutions to the forward problem; *NS* slaves are used in this step. The solution vectors are then returned to the master and at this point the master checks for convergence. If convergence has not been achieved then the slaves calculate the solutions to the Green's function; *ND* slaves are used in this step. The solution vectors are returned to the master and the Jacobian is determined. Next the master solves the inverse problem, in this case by using a spatially variant regularized conjugate gradient optimization method. Finally, the optical properties are updated on the master and the algorithm repeats until convergence has been achieved.

the nature of the particle motion and can also vary with position. $S(\mathbf{r})$ is the source light distribution, and α represents the fraction of photon scattering events in the tissue that occur from moving cells or particles.

Notice that, for $\tau \to 0$, $\langle \Delta \mathbf{r}^2(\tau) \rangle \to 0$, and Equation 9.18 reduces to the steady-state diffusion equation for diffuse photon fluence rate (i.e., Equation 9.8 with $\omega = 0$). Notice also that the homogenous version of

Equation 9.18 can be recast as a Helmholtz-like equation for the temporal field autocorrelation function, $G_1(\mathbf{r}, \tau)$, that is,

$$(\nabla^2 + K^2(\tau))G_1(\mathbf{r}, \tau) = \frac{-S(\mathbf{r})}{D} \tag{9.19a}$$

$$K^2(\tau) = \left(\frac{-\nu}{D}\right)(\mu_a + \alpha k_o^2 \mu_s' \langle \Delta \mathbf{r}^2(\tau) \rangle / 3) \tag{9.19b}$$

For an infinite homogenous medium with a point source at the origin, this equation will also have the well known spherical-wave solution, that is, $\sim [\exp\{-K(\tau)\mathbf{r}\}/D4\pi \mathbf{r}]$.

The mean-square displacement $\langle \Delta \mathbf{r}^2(\tau) \rangle = 6D_B \tau$ for organelles or cells undergoing Brownian motion with "particle" diffusion coefficient D_B. For the important case of random flow that can arise in the tissue vasculature, $\langle \Delta \mathbf{r}^2(\tau) \rangle = \langle V^2 \rangle \tau^2$, where $\langle V^2 \rangle$ is the second moment of the cell speed distribution. In the latter case the correlation function will decay exponentially as τ.

Multidistance measurements of $G_1(\mathbf{r}, \tau)$ provide dynamical information about the motions within the sample in exactly the same way that diffusive waves provide information about scattering and absorption properties. The layout of the sources and detectors is similar to the diffusive wave schemes, but the correlation measurements are a little more complex. For the measurements, one needs a special piece of equipment called an autocorrelator, which takes the detector output and uses the photon arrival times to compute $G_1(\mathbf{r}, \tau)$ or (more precisely) its light *intensity* analog.

The entire set of formalisms for imaging outlined in Sections 9.2.5.2 and 9.2.5.3 is applicable to diffuse light temporal correlations. The technique is attractive because it enables us to measure the blood flow (i.e., $\langle \Delta \mathbf{r}^2(\tau) \rangle$ within deep tissues. The ability to measure relative changes concurrently in blood flow, hemoglobin concentration, and hemoglobin oxygenation within a single instrument makes possible a range of cerebral studies in animal models and in infants and neonates (see Refs. [159–161]).

9.2.7 Contrast Agents

The use of contrast agents in DOT and spectroscopy for disease diagnostics and for probing tissue functionality follows established clinical imaging modalities such as magnetic resonance imaging (MRI),[162–164] ultrasound,[164–166] and x-ray computed tomography (CT).[164,167,168] Contrast agent administration provides for accurate difference images of the same heterogenous tissue volume under nearly identical experimental conditions; this approach often yields superior diagnostic information. Although contrast agents most commonly induce changes in absorption, recently fluorescent/phosphorescent agents have also been considered as means to increase specificity and sensitivity for tumor detection and imaging.[77,169–184] In addition to concentration changes, fluorophore lifetime is sensitive to physiological environment, for example, through oxygen quenching or pH. Most contrast agent schemes rely on the fact that the exogenous macromolecular structures accumulate preferentially in abnormal tissues.

9.2.7.1 Fluorescent Contrast Agents

A chapter in this handbook already reviews contrast agents in photon migration, so we will be very brief. (Our discussion follows from Refs. [185–187].) Suppose a heterogeneous turbid medium with fluorophore distribution $N(\mathbf{r})$ is excited by an excitation diffusive wave, $\Phi(\mathbf{r}, \mathbf{r}_s)$, emitted from $\mathbf{r}_s$ and whose optical wavelength is in the absorption band of the fluorophore. A fluorescent diffuse photon density wave, $\Phi_{fl}(\mathbf{r}, \mathbf{r}_s)$, is produced in the medium, and

$$\Phi_{fl}(\mathbf{r}, \mathbf{r}_s) = \int G_{fl}(\mathbf{r}, \mathbf{r}')T(\mathbf{r}')\Phi(\mathbf{r}', \mathbf{r}_s)d\mathbf{r} \tag{9.20a}$$

where

$$T(\mathbf{r}') = \varepsilon \frac{\tau}{\tau_o} \frac{\eta N(\mathbf{r})}{1-\omega\tau} \qquad (9.20b)$$

The integration is over the sample volume. Here $T(\mathbf{r})$ is a fluorescence transfer function, which depends on the fluorophore radiative and total lifetimes, τ_o and τ respectively, the source modulation frequency ω, the fluorophore extinction coefficient ε, the fluorescence quantum yield η, and the fluorophore distribution $N(\mathbf{r})$. In principle, τ_o and τ (and even ε and η) can also depend on position. The Green's function $G_{fl}(\mathbf{r}, \mathbf{r}')$ is derived with a diffusion equation (Equation 9.8) for the fluorescent diffuse photon density wave at the emission wavelength, that is, the absorption and scattering coefficients in this diffusion equation are defined at the fluorescent emission wavelength. Equation 9.20 is very similar to the equations we inverted in Sections 9.2.5.2 and 9.2.5.3. However, it is deceptively simple because heterogeneity information is embedded in $\mathbf{\Phi}$ and G_{fl}, in addition to N and τ. Nevertheless, it can be inverted numerically using similar techniques.

9.2.7.2 Differential Absorption

In these measurements, optical data are typically obtained before and after administration of the absorbing optical contrast agent (e.g., the intravenous administration of ICG). In principle, DOT images taken before and after administration may be reconstructed and subtracted; however, in practice a more robust approach derives images of the differential changes due to the extrinsic perturbtion. In the latter case experimental measurements use the exact same geometry within a short time of one another, thereby minimizing positional and movement errors and instrumental drift. Furthermore, the use of differential measurements eliminates systematic errors associated with the different medium often required to calibrate operational parameters of the instrument or to provide a baseline measurement for independent reconstructions. Finally, the effect of surface absorbers such as hair- or skin-color variation is also minimized.

The main analytical difficulties of the differential approach arise because the media are inhomogeneous. Thus the total diffuse light field in the contrast agent perturbation problem does not separate into a homogeneous background field and a scattered field in a straightforward way. Furthermore, the average background optical properties, particularly the absorption, can change as a result of contrast agent administration.

In the typical experiment, relative absorption changes are much larger than scattering changes and one can ignore the relative changes in scattering. Under these circumstances the differential signal $\Delta\Phi$, can be related to the differential absorption $\Delta\mu_a$ via the integral relation[188]:

$$\Delta\Phi(\mathbf{r},\mathbf{r}_s) = \int W_a'(\mathbf{r},\mathbf{r}',\mathbf{r}_s)\Delta\mu_a(\mathbf{r}')d\mathbf{r} + C \qquad (9.21)$$

Here W_a' is a weight function very similar to the functions discussed in Section 9.2.5.2. C is a correction; it is an integral that depends on source-detector geometry and on the weight function before and after administration of the contrast agent. For many geometries (e.g., the transmission geometry) C is small and can be ignored. In those cases we can directly invert Equation 9.21 according to the ideas described in Sections 9.2.5.2 and 9.2.5.3, and thus obtain the differential absorption changes directly from difference measurements.

9.3 Instrumentation

The basic imaging geometry for diffuse optical tomography consists of a set of distinguishable point-like sources and a set of photodetectors, each covering a small area of <10 mm² on the surface of the medium. In general some type of source encoding strategy must be used so that the origin of the detected signals can be traced to specific sources. In this way, measurements with differing spatial sensitivities are obtained, and an image can be reconstructed.

There are three common measurement geometries: (1) planar transillumination measurements, (2) cylindrical measurements, and (3) reflectance measurements. All three are used for breast imaging (transillumination,[10–13,189] cylindrical,[15,190–192] and reflectance[119,137,193]). The cylindrical and reflectance geometries are used for imaging animals, human baby heads,[28,194–197] and limbs on the human body (e.g., arm or leg). The reflectance geometry is used for imaging human adult heads.[159,198–200]

In Section 9.2.2 we identified three diffuse light excitation schemes: (1) illumination by subnanosecond pulses of light, (2) CW illumination, and (3) radio-frequency (RF) amplitude-modulated illumination. Short-pulse systems[201–205] detect the temporal distribution of photons as they leave the tissue. The shape of the distribution provides information about tissue optical parameters. Although these systems provide the most information per source-detector pair for characterizing optical properties, their relatively poor signal-to-noise ratio (SNR) leads to longer image acquisition times (typically a few minutes in systems used today).

CW systems[195,206–208] emit light of constant intensity or amplitude. (Sometimes the emitted intensity is amplitude modulated at frequencies less than a few tens of kilohertz.) Detectors measure the amplitude of the light transmitted through the tissue. These systems are simple to build and provide fast image rates (presently up to 100 Hz), but their lack of temporal information makes quantitation of tissue absorption and scattering more difficult. In RF systems[209–211] the light source intensity is amplitude modulated at frequencies of tens to hundreds of megahertz. Information about the absorption and scattering properties of tissue is obtained by recording amplitude decay and phase shift (delay) of the detected signal with respect to the incident wave.[211,212] These systems offer the fast image acquisition rate of CW systems and contain information sufficient for quantitative characterization of absorption and scattering optical properties. The advantages and disadvantages of the three systems are outlined in Table 9.1.

In DOT it is desirable to make a large number of measurements for image reconstruction in a short period of time so that the data are not confounded by physiological or movement artifacts. The balance between number of measurements and image acquisition time is dictated by application. CW systems are popular for imaging spatial variations of absorption changes on timescales of seconds to minutes, for example, imaging muscle[213,214] and brain activation.[195,196,198] CW systems usually have the best SNR and lend themselves well to several encoding strategies enabling massively parallel measurements. Furthermore, although CW systems are poor at quantifying static absorption and scattering properties uniquely, they excel at quantifying spectroscopic changes in absorption and scattering, particularly when a priori knowledge of the spectroscopic features is available. On the other hand, RF and time-domain systems are popular for imaging static optical properties when quantitative accuracy is required and when data acquisition times of one to several minutes are acceptable.

TABLE 9.1 Comparison of Relative Advantages and Disadvantages of Time-Domain, Frequency-Domain, and Continuous-Wave Instrumentation

Instrumentation	Advantages	Disadvantages
Time domain	Full temporal impulse response Quantitative	Difficult to maintain Expensive optoelectronics
Frequency domain	Diffusive wave phase and amplitude Faster than time domain Lower cost than time domain	Difficult RF electronics

Continuous wave	Lowest cost
	Easy electronics
	Fastest
	Accurate for differential
	    measurements of optical properties
		Diffuse light amplitude only
		Less accurate for extimates of absolute
		    optical properties

9.3.1 Source Encoding Strategies

If cost is not an issue, then increasing the number of parallel detectors or detection systems is a straightforward approach to increasing the number of measurements per unit time. Often, however, measurements with multiple source wavelengths and source positions are desired. In this case an encoding strategy enabling the separation of source wavelengths and positions must be employed. The encoding strategies currently used in CW systems and applicable to RF systems are switched-source time-division multiplexing (SS-TDM), phase-division multiplexing (PDM), pulse-modulated time-division multiplexing (PM-TDM), frequency-division multiplexing (FDM), and wavelength-division multiplexing (WDM). SS-TDM and WDM are applicable to time-domain imaging systems as well.

For SS-TDM, sources are modulated at the same frequency and cycled through consecutively; the detectors synchronously obtain the source signal through their own demodulators. This is the easiest system to design and build. Because at any given time only a single source illuminates the sample, interchannel crosstalk is low, and simple circuit construction techniques (point-to-point wiring, Protoboards, etc.) can be used successfully.

For PDM, two sources are modulated with a square-wave at the same frequency, but in phase quadrature (i.e., at a 90° phase difference). Each of the detectors synchronously detects each source through two separate demodulators and low-pass filters, each of which is "tuned" to the in-phase source. Source pairs can then be cycled through consecutively. This is an easy system to design and build, but component layout affects performance, particularly interchannel crosstalk.

For PM-TDM, M sources are cycled on and off in sequence, but at a rapid (~kHz) rate. For N detectors, each source is synchronously detected through individual demodulators, each of which is time-gated to one source. This approach has all the benefits of SS-TDM, but with no temporal skew. The system can be difficult to design and construct due to the complex interdigitation and fast switching speeds. Because only one source operates at any one time, the background level is very low.

For FDM, each of the sources is modulated at one of a number of anharmonically related frequencies (to minimize the effects of intermodulation distortion). For each of the detectors, the sources are demodulated coherently (synchronous detection) or incoherently (envelope detection). This is the most complex system to design and build due to the high potential for interchannel crosstalk. The high background flux arising because all sources are on simultaneously raises the shot noise floor and can saturate photo-detectors. However, because each source is "on" all the time, the scheme is more parallel than the sequential approaches described previously.

WDM simply uses bandpass optical filters in front of the photodetectors to distinguish different wavelength sources. This method can be used in combination with any of the encoding strategies described earlier to distinguish light from different spatial locations.

9.3.1.1 Continuous-Wave Imaging System

As an example of the CW imaging system, we consider one used at the Massachusetts General Hospital-Nuclear Magnetic Resonance (MGH-NMR) Center. This system employs the FDM scheme to detect 32 lasers with 32 detectors (see Figure 9.5). At present, the 32 lasers are divided into 16 lasers at 690 nm and 16 at 830 nm. These 16 laser pairs are fiber coupled and deliver light to 16 positions on the medium to be imaged. The detectors are avalanche photodiodes (APDs, Hamamatsu C5460-01). A master clock generates the 32 distinct frequencies between 6.4 and 12.6 kHz in approximately 200 Hz steps. These frequencies are then used to drive the individual lasers with current stabilized square-wave modulation. Following each APD module is a bandpass filter, cut-on frequency of ~500 Hz to reduce 1/f noise and the 60 Hz room light signal, and a cut-off frequency of ~16 kHz to reduce the third harmonics of the square-wave signals. After the bandpass filter is a programmable gain stage to match the signal levels with the acquisition level on the analog-to-digital converter within the computer. Each detector is digitized at ~45 kHz and the individual source signals are then obtained by use of a digital bandpass filter—for example, a discrete Fourier transform or an infinite-impulse-response filter.

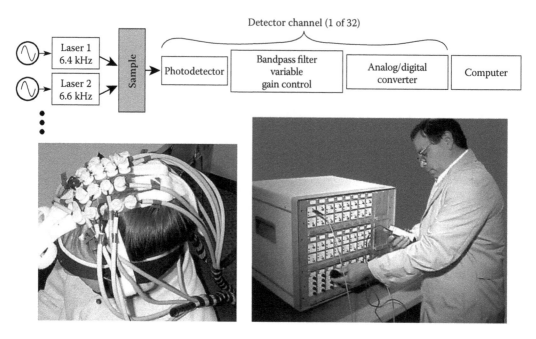

FIGURE 9.5 The MGH-NMR Center CW imaging system with 32 lasers and 32 detectors along with a block diagram indicating the frequency encoded sources and electronic processing steps from the photodetector to the computer memory.

9.3.1.2 Frequency-Domain Imaging System

A typical frequency-domain imaging system is illustrated in Figure 9.6. Developed at Dartmouth College,[215] this system modulates the intensity of a laser diode at 100,000 MHz and couples the light sequentially into different fiber optics (the SS-TDM encoding scheme). Diffusely remitted light is captured by detector fibers that are coupled into a single photomultiplier tube (PMT). The PMT is time-shared between the individual detector fibers, so the instrument employs a TDM encoding scheme. A filter wheel is positioned before the PMT to prevent saturation of the detector by stronger optical signals coming from closer to the source. The photo-electric signal within the PMT is modulated at 100,001 MHz to heterodyne the signal down to 1 kHz. The 1 kHz signal is acquired by an analog-to-digital converter, from which a computer calculates the relative amplitude and phase of the detected 100 MHz diffuse photon density wave.

9.3.1.3 Time-Domain Imaging System

Figure 9.7 shows a diagram of the time-domain image system developed at University College London.[216] The light source is a subpicosecond pulsed Ti:Sapphire laser with wavelength tunable from approximately 750 to 850 nm. Laser pulses are fiber coupled and fiber-optically multiplexed between 32 fibers that deliver source light to 32 independent positions. Photons exiting the sample are received by 32 large diameter detector fibers that relay the light to 32 individual time-correlated single photon counting channels. Computer controlled variable optical attenuators ensure that the detected light intensity does not saturate the photodetectors. The arrival time of detected photons is histogrammed by a picosecond time analyzer, which simultaneously produces histograms of the measured TPSF for all 32 detector channels. The full set of TPSFs for all source-detector pairs represents the raw data used for reconstructing images.

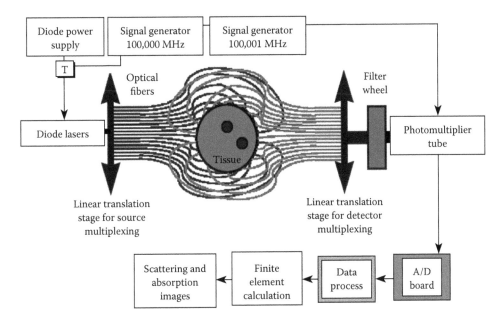

FIGURE 9.6 Schematic of the frequency-domain imaging system developed at Dartmouth College. (From Pogue, B.W. et al., *Opt. Express*, 1, 391, 1997. With permission.)

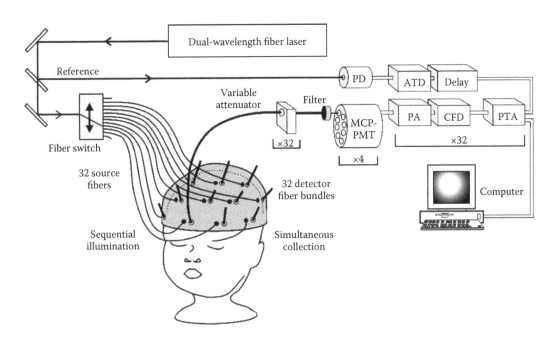

FIGURE 9.7 Schematic diagram of the time-domain imaging system. For clarity, only one detector fiber bundle is shown. PD, photo diode; PA, pre-amplifier; ATD, amplitude timing discriminator; CFD, constant fraction discriminator; PTA, picosecond time analyzer.

9.4 Experimental Diffuse Optical Tomography: Functional Breast and Brain Imaging

The imaging systems described previously and others like them have been used in phantom, animal, and human subject studies. In this section we provide a coherent snapshot of these activities. We begin with a tissue phantom experiment in order to illustrate image reconstruction on a controlled sample; the DOT reconstructions produce acceptable images by striking a balance between image noise, contrast, and resolution. Next we review the application to breast imaging, with recent clinical results. We describe measurements of normal breast optical properties, of tumors based on endogenous contrast, and of tumors using exogenous contrast agents to enhance tumor absorption characteristics preferentially.

Finally, we review the application to functional brain imaging. In this case we show images of blood flow, blood volume, and oxygen saturation changes in a rat stroke model. Then we show images that reveal localized variations in cerebral hemodynamics due to a sensory stimulation of a rat. Finally, we provide an example of functional brain imaging in adult humans with motor-sensory stimuli. The experiments presented are not exhaustive and do not represent the full range of results from the community. Nevertheless, the selected experiments indicate the promise of DOT for in vivo functional imaging.

9.4.1 Multiple Absorbers in a Slab Phantom

In this section we show how DOT is able to resolve multiple perturbations in the optical properties of a highly scattering medium. We also illustrate the trade-off between image resolution and the contrast-to-noise ratio. This type of experiment is important because it validates DOT techniques in well controlled samples.

The experimental data were collected using a hybrid CW and RF system developed at the University of Pennsylvania[217,218] (see Figure 9.8). Laser light is multiplexed to 45 positions (a 9×5 array) on one

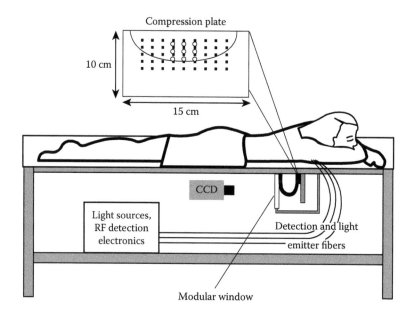

FIGURE 9.8 Phantom geometry for the transillumination measurements. The array of 9×5 light sources is indicated in the compression plate by the black squares. The 3×3 array of frequency-domain photodetectors intermingled with the source fibers is indicated by the open circles. A CCD camera images the transmission of the CW light from each source position individually. A slightly modified version of this experimental system was used for the clinical measurements described in Section 9.4.1, with the CCD camera replaced by a scanning frequency-domain photodetector.

side of the slab phantom (i.e., parallel planes, see Figure 9.8). Nine detector fibers are interspersed within the 9 × 5 array to receive a 70 MHz frequency-domain signal, simultaneously, from which the amplitude and phase is determined by an IQ-homodyne demodulation.[219] This frequency-domain information was used to determine the background optical properties of the medium. A 16-bit CCD camera (Roper Scientific, NTE1340) was positioned to image the CW light transmitted through the phantom. The CCD camera had 800 × 1120 pixels, which were binned 24 × 24. The measurements were cropped to within a radius of 6 cm of the maximum transmitted signal producing approximately 250 independent measurements (i.e., a 21 × 13 detector array) per source position.

For the phantom experiment, the breast tank was filled with an Intralipid/ink solution (see Figure 9.8)[220,221] with $\mu_s' = 8$ cm^{-1} and $\mu_a = 0.05$ cm^{-1}. In one experiment, two highly absorbing spheres ($\mu_a = 2$ cm^{-1} and $\mu_s' = 8$ cm^{-1}) were suspended in the Intralipid solution with a 5 cm separation; in another experiment many more spheres were suspended in the Intralipid solution. The image reconstruction algorithm was formulated using the Rytov approximation to the integral solution of the diffusion equation (see Section 9.2.5.2). A finite difference scheme was used to solve the forward problem in the rectangular geometry, and a conjugate gradient method was used to solve the inverse problem. Regularization was used for the inverse problem (see Section 9.2.5.3), and the entire scheme was iterative. Convergence was consistently obtained after 15 iterations.

An image of the two spheres was reconstructed with optimal regularization (see Figure 9.9). The three-dimensional image shows that two absorbers are easily resolved. The optimal regularization parameter was determined by examining the dependence of the regularization parameter on image norm, image variance, full-width at half-maximum (FWHM) of the imaged absorber, and measurement residual (see Figure 9.10). When the numerical value of the regularization parameter was increased, the image norm and image variance decreased, but at the expense of decreased image resolution (i.e., an increase in FWHM of the spheres) and increased measurement residual. A plot of the image contrast-to-noise ratio

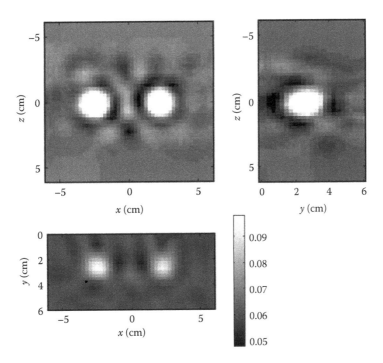

FIGURE 9.9 Three slices of the three-dimensional absorption image reconstructed from the phantom data are shown. The x–z plane is parallel to the measurement planes of the phantom. The scale bar indicates the range of values for the absorption coefficient.

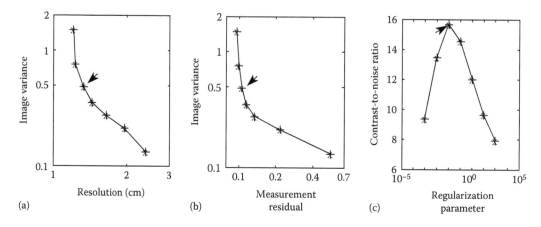

FIGURE 9.10 The dependence of objective measures of image quality on the regularization parameter is shown. (a) Increasing the regularization parameter controls the trade-off between image noise and resolution. (b) Increasing the regularization parameter also increases the residual of the fit to the experimental data. (c) The optimal regularization parameter as determined by the maximum image contrast to noise ratio corresponds to the points in (a) and (b) that balance image noise and resolution/measurement residual (indicated by the arrows in each figure).

versus the regularization parameter indicates that contrast-to-noise ratio is optimized with a regularization parameter that balances image noise and resolution (see arrows in Figure 9.10).[217] Similar trade-offs between image noise and resolution can be expected when imaging animals and human subjects. Culver et al.[217] also demonstrated images of many (i.e., >10) spheres in the same sample volume, thus indicating the potential of DOT for reconstructing multiple heterogeneities (as opposed to isolated heterogeneities in a homogenous background).

9.4.2 Breast Imaging

The use of light to detect tumors in the breast was first proposed by Cutler,[83] who hoped to be able to distinguish between solid tumors and cysts in the breast by illuminating the breast and shadowing the tumors. However, he found it difficult to produce the necessary light intensity without exposing the patient's skin to extreme heat, while the low resolution of the technique severely limited its clinical applications. With the advent of more modern optical sources and detectors, optical transillumination breast imaging was tried again in the 1970s and 1980s, but was abandoned because of lack of sensitivity and specificity.[93,222,223] The burst of activity in the 1990s can be traced to widespread acceptance of the diffusion approximation, which provides a tractable basis for tomographic approaches to image reconstruction using highly scattered light. Tomographic methods are crucial for recovery of information about heterogeneous breast tissues.

Functional, tomography-based diffuse optical breast imaging has been demonstrated, but further understanding and improvements are needed in order for it to become clinically useful. Current research is focusing on the construction of imaging systems with higher resolution and increased quantitative accuracy, as well as on the improvement of the algorithms used in image reconstruction. Thus far three general patient positions have been used: (1) the patient lies prone on a cot with a breast (or breasts) in a pendant position for imaging[15,190–192]; (2) the patient sits or stands with a breast held in compression similar to x-ray mammography[10–13]; and (3) the patient lies supine and is imaged with a hand-held probe that is moved to different positions on the breast.[119,193] The advantages of one approach over another for extraction of optical properties have not been fully explored.

Current research is also focusing more closely on the physiological information available to the technique. For example, quantitative hemoglobin images of the female breast showed localized increases in hemoglobin concentration that corresponded with biopsy-confirmed pathological abnormalities, suggesting that NIRS is capable of characterizing tumors as small as 0.8 ± 0.1 cm.[15] Other investigators have focused on the intrinsic sensitivity of the optical method to blood, water, and adipose—the principal components of the breast. Many of these researchers are studying the changes in breast optical properties associated with age, exogenous hormone levels, and menopausal status as well as, to a lesser extent, fluctuations in menstrual cycles.[14,224] Still other researchers are exploring the use of contrast agents[13,225,226] and the combination of DOT with other imaging techniques such as MRI and ultrasound.

In this section we briefly review some recent advances in the application of DOT to breast imaging. Our first example establishes the baseline optical properties of the normal breast; such information provides a useful benchmark about the requirements for detection of tumors based on endogenous (and exogenous) contrast. Then we describe experiments that image the endogeneous properties of the breast, revealing tumor signals, and we describe experiments that utilize contrast agents to create images with improved tumor sensitivity.

9.4.2.1 Endogenous Properties of Normal Breast

Our group at the University of Pennsylvania has collected optical breast data with the subject in a prone position, using essentially the same system discussed in Ref. [218] (see Figure 9.8). The goal of these measurements was to establish in-vivo the baseline optical and physiological properties of the normal breast. The experimental system employed diode lasers at three wavelengths (750, 786, and 830 nm), each modulated at 140 MHz. The source light was delivered to the moveable breast-stabilization plate through an optical fiber. For detection, the CCD camera in Figure 9.8 was not used; instead a fiber-coupled PMT was scanned to multiple positions on the breast with the source fiber fixed at the center of the tissue and scan region. Prior to collecting data, the tank surrounding the breast is filled with a scattering liquid whose optical properties closely approximated the breast tissue. The amplitude and phase of the transmitted DPDW was measured using a homodyne IQ demodulation scheme.[219] In 15 min, 153 measurements (17 × 9) are obtained over an area of 10 cm × 7 cm (x,y).

Measurements were collected on 52 healthy volunteers. The analysis had one new innovative feature: the data were fit simultaneously at all three wavelengths and "reconstructed" using spectral responses of oxy- and deoxyhemoglobin, and a Mie-based model for the wavelength dependence of the scattering coefficient. This spectroscopically self-consistent approach reduced crosstalk between scattering and absorption, overcoming some of the limitations of the homogeneous tissue model often used for characterization. The average absorption and scattering coefficients of the normal breast tissue were found to be 0.041 ± 0.025 cm^{-1} and 8.5 ± 2.1 cm^{-1}, respectively, at 786 nm. The mean blood volume and blood oxygen saturation were found to be 34 ± 9 μM and $68\% \pm 8\%$, respectively.

A scatter plot of the blood volume and blood saturation results is shown in Figure 9.11. We see from this plot that the optical method will be sensitive to tumors with large blood volume and low blood saturation (outside the dashed lines); this condition might prevail in many tumors. A weak correlation of total hemoglobin concentration and scattering with body mass index (BMI) was found (i.e., decreasing with increasing BMI), but no statistically significant correlation with age was observed (20–65 years). This information provides insight into the types of intrinsic contrast available to optical breast imaging and, importantly, indicates the range of values that malignant tumors must have to be clearly distinguishable from the typical variation of normal breast tissue.

9.4.2.2 Clinical Optical Images of Breast Lesions

The optical breast imaging system developed by the group at Dartmouth is shown in Figure 9.12.[15,191] It is a pendant system, similar in many respects to the one at the University of Pennsylvania, but it obtains a coronal image of one breast at a time with a ring of interspersed 16 source and 16 detector fibers. The fiber ring is vertically positioned by a translation stage to image different planes of interest. The laser diodes emit light at 761, 785, 808, and 826 nm, are modulated at 100 MHz, and are optically combined before being serially multiplexed to each of the 16 source fibers. The lasers are driven sequentially so that the signal at each of the 16 photodetectors distinguishes different wavelengths and positions by time-division multiplexing. At each of the four wavelengths, 256 independent measurements are

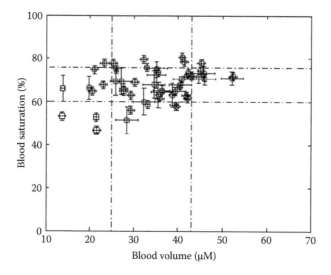

FIGURE 9.11   Hemoglobin saturation versus total hemoglobin concentration; the dashed lines indicate the ranges for normal tissue from the mean and standard deviation of the healthy breast tissue.

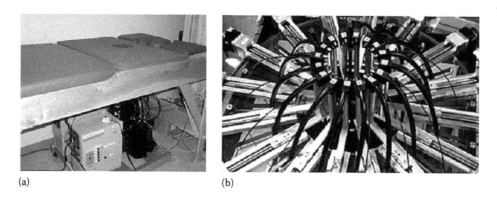

(a)   (b)

FIGURE 9.12   (a) Patient bed for the optical breast imaging system developed at Dartmouth. (b) The fiber optic array for coupling light to and from the patient. The larger black cables are the detector fibers. The fibers are mounted on posts that translate radially for making contact with the tissue.

obtained and then processed by a finite element program to reconstruct absorption and scattering images (as described in Pogue et al.[15] and McBride et al.[191]).

Figure 9.13 shows optical images for a 73-year-old female volunteer who had undergone routine mammography that demonstrated a 2.5 cm focal density with a larger ~6 cm diameter area of associated architectural distortion. The imaged lesion corresponded to a palpable mass; needle biopsy subsequently diagnosed the mass as an invasive ductal carcinoma. The optical image was acquired 2 weeks after the biopsy and was aligned such that the coronal imaging plane was centered on the palpable lump. From the scattering and absorption information, images were derived of the scatter power,[191,227] water concentration, lipid concentration, total hemoglobin concentration, and oxygen saturation. A lesion is clearly visible in the total hemoglobin image, which shows a threefold contrast-to-background ratio. In comparison to the variation of total hemoglobin concentration observed in normal tissue (Figure 9.11), the tumor has significantly greater total hemoglobin concentration. Structures in the other physiological images do not correspond well to the hemoglobin image; however, sensitivity to water and lipid percentages is expected

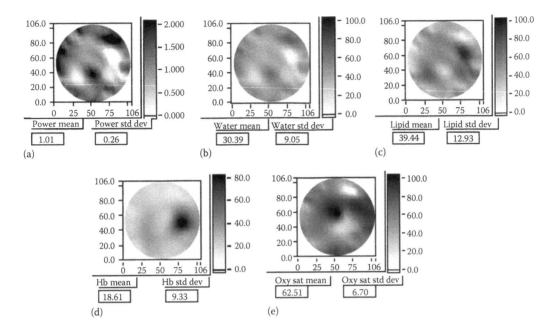

FIGURE 9.13 Clinical breast images are shown of (a) scattering power, (b) water (%), (c) lipids (%), (d) total hemoglobin concentration (μM), and (e) hemoglobin oxygen saturation (%). (From McBride, T.O. et al., *J. Biomed. Opt.*, 7, 72, 2002. With permission.)

to be weak because of the chosen wavelengths. The similarity between the scattering power, water, and lipid images suggests that water and lipid images are susceptible to crosstalk from the scattering power image.

9.4.2.3 Contrast Agents to Enhance Breast Lesion Detection

Another experiment at the University of Pennsylvania employed a time-domain imaging system in transmission mode to acquire *contrast enhanced* breast images while simultaneously obtaining magnetic resonance images. The time-domain optical imager has been described in detail in Refs. [13] and [228]. The instrument uses time-correlated single photon counting to measure the TPSF of photons diffusing through the breast tissue. The TPSF is then Fourier transformed to produce data at multiple modulation frequencies, which are then used to reconstruct differential absorption images[188] of the contrast agent ICG. The 830 nm pulsed laser source is coupled to 24 source fibers through a fiber optic switch. The detection collects light from eight positions simultaneously. Thus images are obtained using 24 × 8 measurements times the number of modulation frequencies. All source fibers are mounted on one plate forming a 3 × 8 array of fibers spaced by intervals of 1.25 cm. The detector fibers are mounted on the other plate to form a 2 × 4 array with a 2.5 cm separation. These two plates stabilize the breast and also contain the RF coils for the MRI. The MR studies were performed with a 1.5 T Signa, GE Medical Systems imager.

Figure 9.14 shows the results from a 70-year-old patient with an infiltrating ductal carcinoma about 1 cm in diameter. The pre-gadolinium (Gd) enhanced sagittal MR image slice passing through the carcinoma is shown in Figure 9.14a in gray scale, while the relative signal increase due to the Gd is shown in color. A rectangle surrounding the carcinoma indicates the sagittal cut of the region of interest that was reconstructed in the optical image (shown in Figure 9.14b) in the coronal plane, and the corresponding MR coronal slice shown in Figure 9.14c. A strong optical contrast-induced absorption increase is seen in the upper right of the optical image, congruent with the position of the carcinoma revealed in the coronal MR image. Another lesion is revealed in the left of the optical image, congruent with the Gd enhancement observed in the MR image, but with a different size and shape. The differences

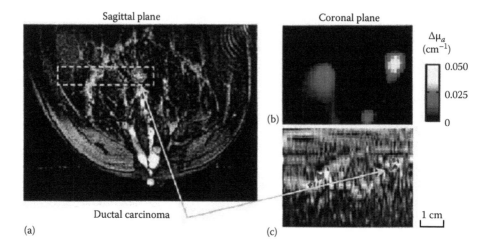

FIGURE 9.14 **(See color insert.)** A dynamic MRI and contrast-enhanced DOT image of a ductal carcinoma. (a) A dynamic sagittal MR image after Gd contrast enhancement passing through the center of the malignant lesion. (b) The coronal DOT image, perpendicular to the plane of the MRI image in (a), but in the volume of interest indicated in (a) by the dashed-line box. (c) The dynamic MR coronal image resliced from the same volume of interest and same dimensions as (b).

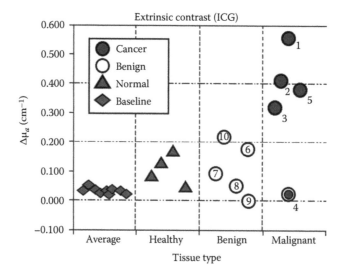

FIGURE 9.15 The ICG-induced absorption enhancement in healthy tissue and benign and malignant lesions compared with the nonenhanced absorption coefficient of normal healthy tissue.

in size and shape can be explained by the low spatial resolution of this implementation of DOT and the chosen threshold level for displaying the images. Similar results were seen in other patients with malignant and benign lesions. A summary of tissue ICG absorption enhancement seen in a group of patients is shown in Figure 9.15. This summary suggests that malignant lesions enhance absorption more than benign lesions by a factor of 2, and more than normal tissue by a factor of 3–4.

9.4.3 Diffuse Optical Imaging of Brain Function

DOT of the brain affords continuous, in vivo deep tissue[159,161] measurements of cerebral oxyhemoglobin (HbO), deoxyhemoglobin (Hb), total hemoglobin (HbT = HbO + Hb), and even blood flow.[197,229–231] It is therefore a potentially new and important noninvasive technique for bedside monitoring. For example, optical spectroscopy can provide crucial information about cerebral hemodynamics and oxygenation during acute and chronic brain conditions, and optical imaging enables the detection of brain ischemia, necrosis, and hemorrhage.[232,233] Knowledge of the most appropriate optical parameters to use clinically, and how they reflect the pathophysiology of such conditions, is still evolving. It is unlikely that DOT will achieve the anatomical resolution of CT or MRI, but its noninvasive nature, low cost, and capability to obtain continuous, real-time information on cerebral hemodynamics and oxygenation under various physiological and pathophysiological conditions constitute a major advantage over other techniques.

Knowledge about how optical parameters reflect tissue pathophysiology is still evolving, but it is clear that application areas for DOT are associated with stroke, brain trauma, and the basic science of brain activation. We elaborate briefly on each of these target areas next.

Diffuse optical tomography offers an attractive alternative for diagnosing and monitoring internal bleeding and ischemic stroke when CT and MRI are not available. There are several possible optical signal indications of stroke. Using a bolus of intravascular contrast agent, it is possible to monitor mean cortical transit times; transit time changes there can reveal flow variations associated with ischemic stroke. Quantitative differential spectroscopy can indicate alterations in hemoglobin saturation in affected tissue due to reduced perfusion or modulated metabolic demand. Bleeding stroke can also be detected spectroscopically, in this case via a large blood volume increase. Scattering contrasts are also possible. Edema and swelling may provide heterogeneities in images of tissue scattering.

The feasibility of near-infrared spectroscopy (NIRS) to detect brain hemorrhage in patients with head trauma has been demonstrated.[27] Studies that compare primitive diffuse optical measurements of brain hematomas with CT images clearly demonstrate a correlation between the optical signal and hematoma location.[26,27,234] These correlation studies have shown that subcortical hemorrhages as deep as 3 cm beneath the cortical surface and as small as 5 mm in diameter can be detected. Furthermore, the different classes of hemorrhages give characteristically different signals. These pilot NIRS results are promising, but they are based on simple relative NIRS measures. Quantitative images of hemoglobin saturation and fast hemodynamics will provide great improvement in available diagnostic information over the data involved in these pilot studies. A means to detect early hemorrhage in at-risk patients—i.e., those treated with thrombolysis or anticoagulants—would have tremendous value. In addition, swelling and edema may be detectable through alterations in the scattering coefficient of the tissue.

Beyond the clinical uses described previously, DOT is experiencing widespread application in functional brain imaging. Since the first demonstrations of noninvasive optical measures of brain function,[29-31] studies have been performed on adult humans using visual,[32] auditory,[33] and somatosensory stimuli.[34] In addition, a number of studies have investigated the motor system.[35-37] Other areas of scientific investigation have included language,[38] higher cognitive function, and functional studies of patient populations.[39-41] Following in the footsteps of functional MRI,[235,236] DOT is likely to play an important role in increasing our knowledge of brain activity associated with various stimulation paradigms, as well as our understanding of cerebral physiology, particularly the coupling between neuronal activity and the associated metabolic and vascular response. Interestingly, optical imaging is potentially the only neuroimaging modality that can measure the hemodynamic (see references above) and metabolic response[237-243] associated with neuronal activity, and measure neuronal activity directly.[209,244,245]

In the remainder of this section we describe three recent experiments. The first experiments measure flow, hemoglobin saturation, and hemoglobin concentration in a rat during stroke; this combination of parameters ultimately makes possible the assignment of oxygen metabolism changes to specific tissue volumes. The second and third sets of experiments image functional activation in the rat and in humans, with high spatial and temporal resolution.

9.4.3.1 Flow and Blood Oxygen Saturation Images of Rat Stroke

Experimenters at the University of Pennsylvania have used DOT to examine the spatial–temporal evolution of focal ischemia in a rat model.[197] Their measurements probe through the *intact* rat skull and combine "static" diffuse photon density wave measurements of Hb and HbO concentrations with "dynamic" diffuse correlation flowmetry (see Section 9.2.6). Their results are the first application of DOT correlation flowmetry to experimental stroke models.

Figure 9.16a shows the TTC stain of the infarct region of a focal ischemia induced in the rats by intra-luminal suture occlusion of the middle cerebral artery. After 60 min of occlusion the suture was retracted for reperfusion. The animals recovered and, at 24 h after occlusion, were sacrificed for TTC staining.

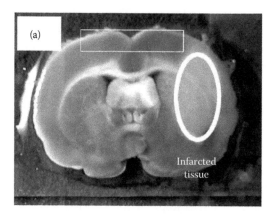

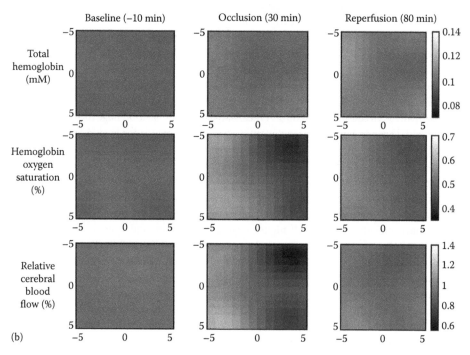

FIGURE 9.16 (a) TTC staining of infarct area; rectangle indicates slice position of DOT image reconstruction. (b, c) Diffuse optical tomography images of total hemoglobin concentrations, tissue averaged hemoglobin satura-tion, and relative cerebral blood flow (rCBF). A middle cerebral artery occlusion was performed during the time from $t = -5$ min to $t = 0$. The suture was retracted at $t = 60$ min resulting in reperfusion. (b) Images at baseline, during occlusion (+30 min) and +80 min. The spatial dimensions are given in millimeters. The scale bars indicate the concentration of hemoglobin, the percent oxygen saturation, and the relative blood flow change where 1 is no change and 1.4 is a 40% change.

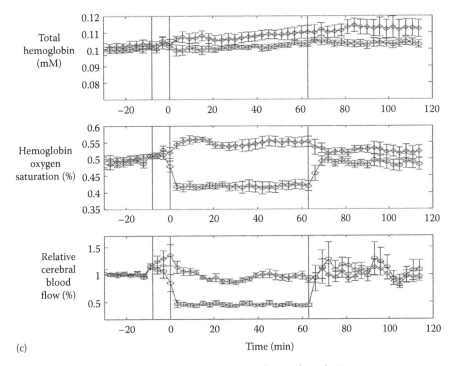

(c)

Time (min)

FIGURE 9.16 (continued) (c) The time traces for ipsilateral and contralateral ROIs.

Differential images of the concentrations were reconstructed in a slice at a depth of 2 mm below the skull surface, extending 5 mm either side of midline and from 2 mm anterior of bregma to 8 mm posterior of bregma. The hemoglobin and flow images were obtained using the linear Rytov approach described in Sections 9.2.5.2 and 9.2.5.3.

Figure 9.16b shows image slices of total hemoglobin concentration (HbT), blood oxygen saturation StO_2, and relative changes in cerebral blood flow (rCBF) reconstructed with DOT. Note that the measurements cover the predominantly penumbral tissue and an equivalent tissue volume on the contralateral side. Image stacks were reconstructed from measurements averaged over five animals. Images are shown for time points representing baseline (−8 min), occlusion (+30 min), and reperfusion (+80 min). Regions of interest (ROIs) were defined for the contralateral and ipsilateral sides, consisting of 4 mm × 8 mm areas centered in the respective half of each image; the time traces for [Hb], StO_2, and (rCBF) in these regions are plotted in Figure 9.16c. Occlusion and saturation decreased by about 40% from baseline in the affected hemisphere. The numbers for flow are in reasonable agreement with near-surface laser Doppler measurements of penumbral tissues. The cerebral blood volume, on the other hand, showed much smaller percentage changes during occlusion.

These images demonstrate the feasibility of continuously imaging an integrated set of hemodynamic parameters through the time course of ischemia and reperfusion in experimental focal ischemia models. The combined measurements also offer the possibility to make quantitative maps of differential oxygen metabolism. A simplified model for oxygen metabolism relates two of the measurements made. If we assume that the product of the blood perfusion rate with the difference in oxyhemoglobin concentration between the artery perfusing the tissue and the vein draining the tissue equals the oxygen consumption rate, then the measured changes enable us to construct a map of local variations in cerebral oxygen metabolism in deep tissues.[197] This exciting prospect further enhances the attractiveness of the diffuse optical method.

9.4.3.2 Activation Imaging of Brain Function in a Rat Model

In this section we describe applications to functional activation of the rat brain. By using classical functional stimulation paradigms, these studies provide an opportunity to evaluate the imaging capabilities of diffuse optical tomography through comparisons with exposed cortex and fMRI studies.

These studies employed the CW system developed at the MGH-NMR center (see Section 9.3.1.1). The dual wavelength sources were positioned on a 3 × 3 grid interspersed within the 4 × 4 grid of detectors. In accordance with standard procedures used in exposed cortex studies of functional activation, the baseline hemoglobin concentrations were assumed—i.e., [Hb] = [HbO] = 50 µM.[246] Absorption coefficients were calculated using published spectra. The scattering coefficient was assumed to be equal to 10.0 cm^{-1}.

The experiments were performed on adult male Sprague-Dawley rats weighing 300–325 g. The rats were fasted overnight before measurements. The animals were anesthetized (Halothane 1%–1.5%, N_2O 70%, O_2 30%) and catheters were placed into a femoral artery to monitor the arterial blood pressure and into a femoral vein for drug delivery. The animals were tracheotomized, mechanically ventilated, and fixed on a stereotaxic frame. The probe was then placed symmetrically about midline. It covered a region from 2 mm anterior to 6 mm posterior of the rhinal fissure. After the surgical procedures, Halothane was discontinued, and anesthesia was maintained with a 50 mg/kg intravenous bolus of αchloralose followed by continuous intravenous infusion at 40 mg/kg/h.

Electrical forepaw stimulation was performed using two subdermal needle electrodes inserted into the dorsal forepaw. The stimulus pattern was relayed to an isolated, pulsed current supply to provide 300 µ$_s$ constant current pulses at programmed times. The current was maintained at 1.0 mA. A 3 Hz, 6 s stimulus was provided with 54 s interstimulus interval. The measurements were then averaged over 42 stimulus intervals. The final averaged temporal data stack was reconstructed frame by frame using the methods described in Sections 9.2.5.2 and 9.2.5.3. Each slice was reconstructed at a depth of 2 mm from the skull surface extending 5 mm either side of midline, and from 2 mm anterior of bregma to 8 mm posterior of bregma. The absorption image stacks were then converted to oxy- and deoxyhemoglobin image stacks.

The series of DOT [Hb] and [HbO] images show focal activation contralateral to the stimulated forepaw. The images are frames taken every 5 s. The time traces were extracted for a 3 mm × 3 mm area centered at maximal activation (see Figure 9.17). The oscillations seen after stimulus are similar to vasomotion signals seen by optical studies in exposed cortex.[247]

9.4.3.3 Images of Brain Function in Humans

The same MGH CW imaging system described in Section 9.3.2.1 was used to study 15 subjects during finger tapping, finger tactile stimulation, and median nerve electrical stimulation. The finger tapping and finger tactile protocols consisted of series of 10 stimulation/rest sequences for each hand (i.e., 20 s stimulation and 20 s rest), wherein the stimulation occurs at a frequency of ~4–5 Hz (the stimulus frequency of each subject was adjusted so as to be anharmonic with the heart rate). The median nerve electrical stimulation protocol consisted of a series of 18 stimulation/rest sequences (i.e., 10 s stimulation and 20 s rest) with stimulus intensity slightly above the motor threshold (i.e., using rectangular electrical pulses, current peak: <10 mA, duration: 0.2 ms, repetition rate: 4–5 Hz). Motion sensors were used on the fingers of the subjects to synchronize the stimuli with the optical signals recorded on the head.

The optical data were band-pass filtered between 0.02 and 0.50 Hz to correct for slow drifts and to reduce the ~1 Hz arterial pulsation amplitude. Finally, the multiple stimulation sequences were block averaged to achieve better statistics. This resulted in a time series of the measured signal intensity for each source-detector pair. Source-detector pairs near a region of brain activation showed changes similar to those seen in a rat as shown in Figure 9.18, while the other source-detector pairs showed little signal variation. Absorption images at the different wavelengths were converted into images of changes in oxy- and deoxyhemoglobin concentrations.

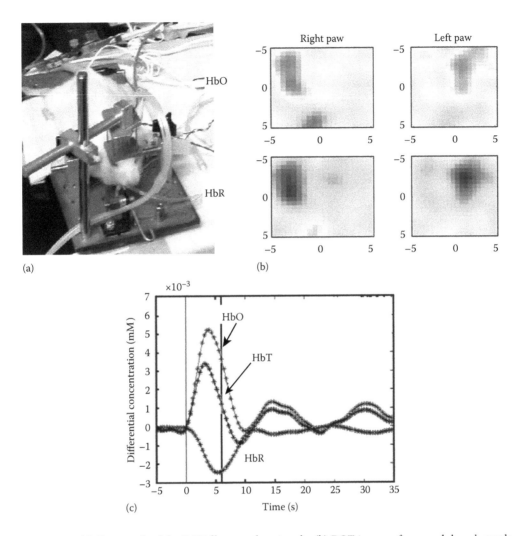

FIGURE 9.17 (a) Photograph of the DOT fibers on the rat scalp. (b) DOT images of oxy- and deoxyhemoglobin concentrations during functional activation of the somatosensory cortex. The oxyhemoglobin (HbO) images exhibit a concentration increase. The deoxyhemoglobin (HbR) images exhibit a concentration decrease. Images are shown for left- and right-forepaw stimulation, the activation showing up on the contralateral side. (c) Time-course of the hemoglobin concentration changes in the region of interest defined by the significant focal concentration change seen in (b).

The hemodynamic response to stimulation was always visible in the optical data. During the finger tapping experiment, the oxy- and deoxyhemoglobin concentration variations were not sharply localized. This is probably because of a systemic elevation in blood volume, presumably resulting from a corresponding heart rate increase. During finger tactile stimulation, oxyhemoglobin increases were two to three times smaller than during finger tapping; also, oxy- and deoxyhemoglobin were sharply localized. During electrical stimulation, the hemoglobin changes were sharply localized and had a magnitude comparable with finger tactile stimulation. In the latter experiments a peculiar feature of ipsilateral decrease in blood volume was observed during the stimulation period (see Figure 9.19). By contrast, magnetoencephaolography (MEG) and functional magnetic resonance imaging (fMRI) studies during median nerve stimulation have shown an activation of only the contralateral primary sensory-motor cortex.[248,249] A deactivation of the ipsilateral primary sensory-motor cortex has been observed in

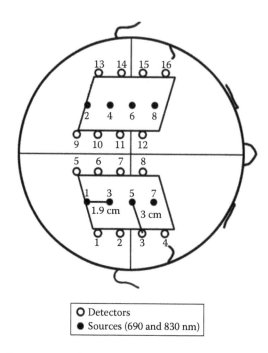

FIGURE 9.18   Geometrical arrangement of source and detector fibers on the head.

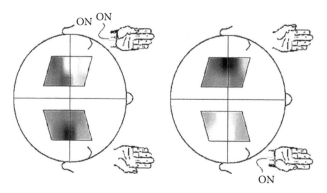

FIGURE 9.19   Block average hemoglobin maps at the end of the electrical stimulation period. Top panels: deoxy-hemoglobin changes; bottom panels: oxyhemoglobin changes. Left panels: left wrist median nerve stimulation; right panels: right wrist median nerve stimulation.

previous fMRI experiments during finger tapping[250]; these optical results suggest that a similar decrease in blood flow occurs in the ipsilateral cortex during electrical somatosensory stimulation.

In summary, DOT offers an exciting new method for studying human brain function, and should play an important role in the brain sciences when other imaging modalities (e.g., fMRI, EEG, MEG) are not attractive because of cost, sensitivity to motion artifacts, or confinement of the research subject.

9.5   Fundamental and Practical Issues: Problems and Solutions

In this final section we touch on some of the fundamental and practical difficulties associated with DOT. In particular, we discuss the fundamental limits of detection, characterization, and resolution, we discuss practical problems of source-detector calibration, and we briefly outline some of the ways researchers are overcoming these barriers.

9.5.1 Detection, Localization, Characterization, and Resolution Limits

The detection limits of DOT are set by the smallest signal perturbation that can be detected above the noise level. The spatial localization limit is generally the same as the detection limit because the maximum signal perturbation often occurs when an object is located directly between a source and detector. Full characterization of object optical properties, shape, size, and position is more difficult than detection and localization. For example, a fixed signal perturbation can be caused by a small, strongly absorbing object or a large, weakly absorbing object. The distinction between the large and small object must be derived from relative spatial differences in the perturbation of the measured fluence.

These limits have been extensively explored[251] for a transmission geometry applicable to breast imaging. In this work, a best-case scenario noise model assumed shot noise and small positional uncertainties gave rise to a random noise on the order of 0.1% of the signal intensity. Measurements were simulated in the transmission geometry with a single modulation frequency. With these assumptions about the noise, it was possible to detect 3 mm diameter-absorbing objects that possessed a threefold greater absorption than the background. A similar analysis of the characterization limits indicated that simultaneous determination of object diameter and absorption coefficient required that object diameters were a minimum of 8–10 mm (for a 100% contrast); see Ref. [251] for details. Another investigation,[252] focusing on resolution (defined as the FWHM of the fluence point-spread function caused by a localized perturbation,[252-254]) found that, if proper deconvolution of the measured data is performed, then resolutions of order 5–7 mm are possible with DOT.

There are potentially many ways to overcome some of these barriers, and many researchers are exploring the following possibilities, as well as other ideas. The brute force approach is to increase the number of measurements or decrease the measurement noise. This can be done, by increasing numbers of source-detector pairs, modulation frequencies, or optical wavelengths. The use of many optical wavelengths is beneficial because relatively few significant chromophores are in tissue and their spectra are well known. The use of prior spatial information, for example, the assignment of particular tissue types to specific volume elements of the image,[106,137,194] enables one to reduce the number of unknowns in the inverse problem and thus can effectively improve images. Optical techniques can also be combined with other imaging modalities (e.g., ultrasound[119,137,255] or MRI[13,106,256]) to constrain the DOT problem. Singular-value analysis of the tomographic weight matrix associated with specific data types, geometries, and optode arrangements has been developed recently[123] and should provide experimenters with quantitative tools to optimize for the spatial sampling interval, field-of-view parameters, resolution trade-offs, and, ultimately, physiology. Finally, it is now possible to reduce the systematic errors associated with source-detector amplitudes by directly incorporating these unknowns into the image reconstruction problem. This is the subject of the last section of this chapter.

9.5.2 Calibration of Source and Detector Amplitudes

The modeling of the DOT forward problem requires accurate knowledge of source and detector amplitudes and their positions. Systematic errors in the calibration of these parameters will result in absorption and scattering image artifacts, for example, image spikes near the positions of the sources and detectors. This type of artifact has been observed by a number of groups.[257] Some schemes to minimize these artifacts include median filtering[258] and spatial regularization; the latter approach penalizes the reconstruction near sources and detectors with a weight that varies exponentially from the sample surfaces.[113,257,259] The result is an image with suppressed variations near the sources and detectors, but with improved image quality further from the boundaries. However, the scheme has the undesirable effect of biasing the reconstruction away from the boundaries of the medium.

A recent and relatively simple solution to this problem models the uncertainties of source and detector amplitude and includes them in the inverse problem.[260] Within the linear Rytov approximation, the unknown source and detector amplitudes can be solved simultaneously with the unknown optical

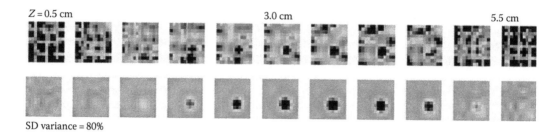

FIGURE 9.20 A three-dimensional absorption image without (top row) and with (bottom row) modeling the unknown source and detector amplitudes. The images span X and Y from −3 to 3 cm; Z-slices are indicated from 0.5 to 5.5 cm. The absorbing object is observable in the image with modeling of the 80% source and detector variance; however, its contrast is obscured by the large amplitude variation near the boundaries. Modeling for the unknown variance provides an image with significantly improved image quality.

properties of the medium. We briefly outline this procedure next, assuming for simplicity a sample with absorption heterogeneities, but without scattering heterogeneities.

Recall the linear approximation for calculating fluence perturbations from spatial variation in the absorption and scattering coefficients, discussed in Section 9.2.5.2. The problem was written in the form $[W]\{x\} = \{b\}$ where $[W]$ represented the weight matrix, $\{x\}$ represented the unknown optical properties, and $\{b\}$ represented the difference between experiment and calculation (or the scattered wave). If we include the unknown source and detector amplitudes into the model, then the matrix equation can be reformulated as $[B]\{\xi\} = \{b\}$ where $[B] = [W'SD]$ and

$$\{\xi\} = \left\{ \frac{\delta\mu_{a,1}}{\mu_{ao}} \cdots \frac{\delta\mu_{a,NV}}{\mu_{ao}} \ln s_1 \cdots \ln s_{NS} \ln d_1 \cdots \ln d_{ND} \right\} \tag{21.22}$$

Here, s_i and d_i represent the amplitude of the ith source and detector, respectively, NV is the number of voxels, NS is the number of sources, and ND is the number of detectors. Scaling $\delta\mu_{a,j}$ by μ_{ao} makes the elements dimensionless and of the same order as $\ln s$ and $\ln d$. $\mathbf{W'} = \mu_{ao}\mathbf{W}$ is the rescaling of the standard weight matrix. $\mathbf{S}$ and $\mathbf{D}$ are simple, well-defined matrices with block diagonal form that have 1 or 0 in the elements corresponding to particular sources and detectors.

Simulation results have demonstrated that incorporation of the unknown source and detector amplitudes into the inverse problem maintains image quality despite amplitude uncertainties greater than 50%. This is illustrated in Figure 9.20; a simulation of transmission through a 6 cm slab was considered with background optical properties of $\mu'_{so} = 10$ cm^{-1} and $\mu_{ao} = 0.05$ cm^{-1} and a 1.6 cm diameter absorbing sphere with $\mu_a = 0.15$ cm^{-1}, centered at $(x,y,z) = (1,1,3)$ cm. Measurements were made with 16 sources and 16 detectors equally spaced from −3 to 3 cm, and CW measurements were simulated. There was no additive measurement noise (i.e., shot or detector electronic noise) in the simulated data, only the multiplicative model error associated with the source and detector amplitudes.

Acknowledgments

We have benefited from discussions with many colleagues and collaborators and many of their observations are found in this chapter. In particular, we thank Joe Culver, Maria Angela Franceschini, and Gary Boas for significant assistance in the preparation of this chapter. We also thank Turgut Durduran, Jeremy Hebden, Vasilis Ntziachristos, and Brian Pogue for discussion and for providing figures for the chapter. For other useful discussions over many years we thank Simon Arridge, Britton Chance, Regine Choe, Alper Corlu, Anders Dale, Joel Greenberg, Monica Holboke, Xingde Li, Eric Miller, Bruce Tromberg, Guoqiang Yu, and Tim Zhu.

D.A.B. acknowledges funding from Advanced Research Technologies, from National Institutes of Health grants R29-NS38842 and P41-RR14075, from the Center for Innovative Minimally Invasive Therapies, and from the US Army under Cooperative Agreement DAMD17-99-2-9001. The material presented does not necessarily reflect the position or the policy of the government, and no official endorsement should be inferred. A.G.Y. acknowledges partial support from NIH grants 2-R01-CA-75124-04 and 2-RO1-HL-57835-04.

References

1. Yodh, A. and Chance, B. Spectroscopy and imaging with diffusing light. *Phys. Today* 48: 34, 1995.
2. Tromberg, B., Yodh, A., Sevick, E., and Pine, D. Diffusing photons in turbid media: Introduction to the feature. *Appl. Opt.* 36: 9, 1997.
3. Yodh, A., Tromberg, B., Sevick-Muraca, E., and Pine, D. Diffusing photons in turbid media. *J. Opt. Soc. Am. A* 14: 136, 1997.
4. Boas, D.A., Brooks, D.H., Miller, E.L., DiMarzio, C.A., Kilmer, M., Gaudette, R.J., and Zhang, Q. Imaging the body with diffuse optical tomography. *IEEE Signal Process. Mag.* 18: 57, 2001.
5. Miller, E. Focus issue: Diffuse optical tomography—Introduction. *Opt. Express* 7: 461, 2000.
6. Chance, B. Near-infrared images using continuous, phase-modulated, and pulsed light with quantitation of blood and blood oxygenation. *Ann. N.Y. Acad. Sci.* 838: 19, 1998.
7. Kang, K.A., Chance, B., Zhao, S., Srinivasan, S., Patterson, E., and Trouping, R. Breast tumor characterization using near-infrared spectroscopy. *Proc. SPIE* 1888, 1993.
8. Suzuki, K., Yamashita, Y., Ohta, K., and Chance, B. Quantitative measurement of optical-parameters in the breast using time-resolved spectroscopy—Phantom and preliminary in-vivo results. *Invest. Radiol.* 29: 410, 1994.
9. Fishkin, J.B., Coquoz, O., Anderson, E.R., Brenner, M., and Tromberg, B. Frequency-domain photon migration measurements of normal and malignant tissue optical properties in a human subject. *Appl. Opt.* 36: 10, 1997.
10. Grosenick, D., Wabnitz, H., Rinneberg, H.H., Moesta, K.T., and Schlag, P.M. Development of a time-domain optical mammograph and first in vivo applications. *Appl. Opt.* 38: 2927, 1999.
11. Franceschini, M.A., Moesta, K.T., Fantini, S., Gaida, G., Gratton, E., Jess, H., Mantulin, W.W., Seeber, M., Schlag, P.M., and Kaschke, M. Frequency-domain techniques enhance optical mammography: Initial clinical results. *Proc. Natl. Acad. Sci. USA* 94: 6468, 1997.
12. Nioka, S., Miwa, M., Orel, S., Shnall, M., Haida, M., Zhao, S., and Chance, B. Optical imaging of human breast cancer. *Adv. Exp. Med. Biol.* 361: 171, 1994.
13. Ntziachristos, V., Yodh, A.G., Schnall, M., and Chance, B. Concurrent MRI and diffuse optical tomography of breast after indocyanine green enhancement. *Proc. Natl. Acad. Sci. USA* 97: 2767, 2000.
14. Cerussi, A.E., Berger, A.J., Bevilacqua, F., Shah, N., Jakubowski, D., Butler, J., Holcombe, R.F., and Tromberg, B.J. Sources of absorption and scattering contrast for near-infrared optical mammography. *Acad. Radiol.* 8: 211, 2001.
15. Pogue, B.W., Poplack, S.P., McBride, T.O., Wells, W.A., Osterman, K.S., Osterberg, U.L., and Paulsen, K.D. Quantitative hemoglobin tomography with diffuse near-infrared spectroscopy: Pilot results in the breast. *Radiology* 218: 261, 2001.
16. McBride, T.O., Pogue, B.W., Gerety, E.D., Poplack, S.B., Osterberg, U.L., and Paulsen, K.D. Spectroscopic diffuse optical tomography for the quantitative assessment of hemoglobin concentration and oxygen saturation in breast tissue. *Appl. Opt.* 38: 5480, 1999.
17. Delpy, D.T. and Cope, M. Quantification in tissue near-infrared spectroscopy. *Philos. Trans. R. Soc. London B* 352: 649, 1997.
18. Painchaud, Y., Mailloux, A., Harvey, E., Verreault, S., Frechette, J., Gilbert, C., Vernon, M.L., and Beaudry, P. Multi-port time-domain laser mammography: Results on solid phantom and volunteers. *Int. Symp. Biomed. Opt.* 3597: 548, 1999.

19. Tromberg, B., Coquoz, O., Fishkin, J., Pham, T., Anderson, E.R., Butler, J., Cahn, M., Gross, J.D., Venugopalan, V., and Pham, D. Non-invasive measurements of breast tissue optical properties using frequency-domain photon migration. *Philos. Trans. R. Soc. London B* 352: 661, 1997.

20. Sickles, E.A. Breast cancer detection with transillumination and mammography. *Am. J. Roentgenol.* 142: 841, 1984.

21. Hoogenraad, J.H., van der Mark, M.B., Colak, S.B., Hooft, G.W., and van der Linden, E.S. First results from the Phillips Optical Mammoscope, in *Photon Propagation of Tissues III*, 31294, Benaron, D.A., Chance, B., and Ferrari, M., eds. New York: Plenum Press, 1997, p. 184.

22. Ntziachristos, V., Ma, X.H., and Chance, B. Time-correlated single photon counting imager for simultaneous magnetic resonance and near-infrared mammography. *Rev. Sci. Instrum.* 69: 4221, 1998.

23. Ntziachristos, V., Yodh, A.G., Schnall, M., and Chance, B. Comparison between intrinsic and extrinsic contrast for malignancy detection using NIR mammography. *Proc. SPIE* 3597: 565, 1999.

24. Pogue, B.W., Poplack, S.D., McBride, T.O., Jiang, S., Osterberg, U.L., and Paulsen, K.D. Breast tissue and tumor hemoglobin and oxygen saturation imaging with multi-spectral near infrared computed tomography, in *Advances in Experimental Medicine and Biology Series*. New York: Plenum Press, 2001.

25. Pogue, B.W., Poplack, S.D., McBride, T.O., Jiang, S., Osterberg, U.L., and Paulsen, K.D. Near-infrared tomography: Status of Dartmouth imaging studies and future directions, in progress.

26. Gopinath, S.P., Robertson, C.S., Grossman, R.G., and Chance, B. Near-infrared spectroscopic localization of intracranial hematomas. *J. Neurosurg.* 79: 43, 1993.

27. Robertson, C.S., Gopinath, S.P., and Chance, B. A new application for near-infrared spectroscopy: Detection of delayed intracranial hematomas after head injury. *J. Neurotrauma* 12: 591, 1995.

28. Hintz, S.R., Cheong, W.F., Van Houten, J.P., Stevenson, D.K., and Benaron, D.A. Bedside imaging of intracranial hemorrhage in the neonate using light: Comparison with ultrasound, computed tomography, and magnetic resonance imaging. *Pediatr. Res.* 45: 54, 1999.

29. Hoshi, Y. and Tamura, M. Detection of dynamic changes in cerebral oxygenation coupled to neuronal function during mental work in man. *Neurosci. Lett.* 150: 5, 1993.

30. Villringer, A., Planck, J., Hock, C., Schleinkofer, L., and Dirnagl, U. Near infrared spectroscopy (NIRS): A new tool to study hemodynamic changes during activation of brain function in human adults. *Neurosci. Lett.* 154: 101, 1993.

31. Okada, F., Tokumitsu, Y., Hoshi, Y., and Tamura, M. Gender- and handedness-related differences of forebrain oxygenation and hemodynamics. *Brain Res.* 601: 337, 1993.

32. Ruben, J., Wenzel, R., Obrig, H., Villringer, K., Bernarding, J., Hirth, C., Heekeren, H., Dirnagl, U., and Villringer, A. Haemoglobin oxygenation changes during visual stimulation in the occipital cortex. *Adv. Exp. Med. Biol.* 428: 181, 1997.

33. Sakatani, K., Chen, S., Lichty, W., Zuo, H., and Wang, Y.P. Cerebral blood oxygenation changes induced by auditory stimulation in newborn infants measured by near infrared spectroscopy. *Early Hum. Dev.* 55: 229, 1999.

34. Obrig, H., Wolf, T., Doge, C., Hulsing, J.J., Dirnagl, U., and Villringer, A. Cerebral oxygenation changes during motor and somatosensory stimulation in humans, as measured by near-infrared spectroscopy. *Adv. Exp. Med. Biol.* 388: 219, 1996.

35. Colier, W.N., Quaresima, V., Oeseburg, B., and Ferrari, M. Human motor-cortex oxygenation changes induced by cyclic coupled movements of hand and foot. *Exp. Brain Res.* 129: 457, 1999.

36. Kleinschmidt, A., Obrig, H., Requardt, M., Merboldt, K.D., Dirnagl, U., Villringer, A., and Frahm, J. Simultaneous recording of cerebral blood oxygenation changes during human brain activation by magnetic resonance imaging and near-infrared spectroscopy. *J. Cereb. Blood Flow Metab.* 16: 817, 1996.

37. Hirth, C., Obrig, H., Villringer, K., Thiel, A., Bernarding, J., Muhlnickel, W., Flor, H., Dirnagl, U., and Villringer, A. Non-invasive functional mapping of the human motor cortex using near-infrared spectroscopy. *Neuroreport* 7: 1977, 1996.

38. Sato, H., Takeuchi, T., and Sakai, K.L. Temporal cortex activation during speech recognition: An optical topography study. *Cognition* 73: B55, 1999.

39. Hock, C., Villringer, K., Muller-Spahn, F., Wenzel, R., Heekeren, H., Schuh-Hofer, S., Hofmann, M. et al. Decrease in parietal cerebral hemoglobin oxygenation during performance of a verbal fluency task in patients with Alzheimer's disease monitored by means of near-infrared spectroscopy (NIRS)—Correlation with simultaneous rCBF-PET measurements. *Brain Res.* 755: 293, 1997.

40. Hock, C., Villringer, K., Heekeren, H., Hofmann, M., Wenzel, R., Villringer, A., and Muller-Spahn, F. A role for near infrared spectroscopy in psychiatry? *Adv. Exp. Med. Biol.* 413: 105, 1997.

41. Fallgatter, A.J. and Strik, W.K. Reduced frontal functional asymmetry in schizophrenia during a cued continuous performance test assessed with near-infrared spectroscopy. *Schizophr. Bull.* 26: 913, 2000.

42. Bank, W. and Chance, B. Diagnosis of mitochondrial disease by NIRS. *Proc. SPIE* 2383, 1995.

43. Bank, W. and Chance, B. An oxidative defect in metabolic myopathies: Diagnosed by non-invasive tissue oximetry. *Ann. Neurol.* 36: 830, 1994.

44. Chance, B. and Bank, W. Genetic disease of mitochondrial function evaluated by NMR and NIR spectroscopy of skeletal tissue. *Biochim. Biophys. Acta* 1271: 7, 1995.

45. Nioka, S., Moser, D., Lech, G., Evengelisti, M., Verde, T., Chance, B., and Kuno, S. Muscle deoxygenation in aerobic and anaerobic exercise. *Adv. Exp. Med. Biol.* 454: 63, 1998.

46. Nioka, S., Chance, B., and Nakayama, K. Possibility of monitoring mitochondrial activity in isometric exercise using NIRS, in *Oxygen Transport to Tissue*, Chance, B., ed. New York: Plenum Press, 1998, p. 454.

47. Dougherty, T.J., Gomer, C.J., Henderson, B.W., Jori, G., Kessel, D., Korbelik, M., Moan, J., and Peng, Q. Photodynamic therapy. *J. Nat. Cancer Inst.* 90: 889, 1998.

48. Patterson, M.S., Wilson, B.C., and Graff, R. In vivo tests of the concept of photodynamic threshold dose in normal rat liver photosensitized by aluminum chlorosulphonated phthalocyanine. *Photochem. Photobiol.* 51: 343, 1990.

49. van Gemert, J.C., Berenbaum, M.C., and Gijsberg, G.H.M. Wavelength and light dose dependence in tumor phototherapy with haematoporphyrin derivative. *Br. J. Cancer* 52: 43, 1985.

50. Farrell, T.J., Wilson, B.C., Patterson, M.S., and Olivio, M.C. Comparison of the in vivo photodynamic threshold dose for photofrin, mono- and tetrasulfonated aluminum phthalocyanine using a rat liver model. *Photochem. Photobiol.* 68: 394, 1998.

51. Lilge, L., Olivo, M.C., Shatz, S.W., MaGuire, J.A., Patterson, M.S., and Wilson, B.C. The sensitivity of the normal brain and intracranially implanted VX2 tumour to intestinal photodynamic therapy. *Br. J. Cancer* 73: 332, 1996.

52. Johnson, C.C. Optical diffusion in blood. *IEEE Trans. Biomed. Eng.* 17: 129, 1970.

53. Ishimaru, A. *Wave Propagation and Scattering in Random Media*. San Diego, CA: Academic Press, 1978.

54. Furutsu, K. On the diffusion equation derived from the space-time transport equation. *J. Opt. Soc. Am. A* 70: 360, 1980.

55. Groenhuis, R.A.J., Ferwerda, H.A., and Ten Bosch, J.J. Scattering and absorption of turbid materials determined from reflection measurements. I. Theory. *Appl. Opt.* 22: 2456, 1983.

56. Patterson, M.S., Chance, B., and Wilson, B.C. Time resolved reflectance and transmittance for the noninvasive measurement of tissue optical properties. *Appl. Opt.* 28: 2331, 1989.

57. Durduran, T., Chance, B., Yodh, A.G., and Boas, D.A. Does the photon diffusion coefficient depend on absorption? *J. Opt. Soc. Am. A* 14: 3358, 1997.

58. Case, K.M. and Zweifel, P.F. *Linear Transport Theory*. Boston, MA: Addison-Wesley, 1967.

59. Furutsu, K. and Yamada, Y., Diffusion approximation for a dissipative random medium and the applications. *Phys. Rev. E* 50: 3634, 1994.

60. Furutsu, K. Pulse wave scattering by an absorber and integrated attenuation in the diffusion approximation. *J. Opt. Soc. Am.* 14: 267, 1997.

61. Aronson, R. and Corngold, N. Photon diffusion coefficient in an absorbing medium. *J. Opt. Soc. Am. A* 16: 1066, 1999.
62. Durian, D.J. The diffusion coefficient depends on absorption. *Opt. Lett.* 23: 1502, 1998.
63. Glasstone, S. and Edlund, M.C. *The Elements of Nuclear Reactor Theory.* New York: Van Nostrand, 1952.
64. Star, W.M., Marijnissen, J.P.A., and van Gemert, M.J.C. Light dosimetry in optical phantoms and in tissues: I. Multiple flux and transport theory. *Phys. Med. Biol.* 33: 437, 1988.
65. Davidson, B. *Neutron Transport Theory.* Oxford, U.K.: Clarendon, 1957.
66. Duderstadt, J.J. and Martin, W.R. *Transport Theory.* New York: Wiley, 1979.
67. Graaff, R. and Ten Bosch, J.J. Diffusion coefficient in photon density theory. *Opt. Lett.* 25: 43, 2000.
68. Martelli, F., Bassani, M., Alianelli, L., Zangheri, L., and Zaccanti, G. Accuracy of the diffusion equation to describe photon migration through an infinite medium: Numerical and experimental investigation. *Phys. Med. Biol.* 45: 2235, 2000.
69. Boas, D. Diffuse photon probes of structural and dynamical properties of turbid media: Theory and biomedical applications. PhD dissertation, University of Pennsylvania, Philadelphia, PA, 1996.
70. Li, X. Fluorescence and diffusive wave diffraction tomographic probes in turbid media. PhD dissertation, University of Pennsylvania, Philadelphia, PA, 1998.
71. Wilson, B.C. and Patterson, M.S. The physics of photodynamic therapy. *Phys. Med. Biol.* 31: 327, 1986.
72. Kaplan, P.D., Kao, M.H., Yodh, A.G., and Pine, D.J. Geometric constraints for the design of diffusing-wave spectroscopy experiments. *Appl. Opt.* 32: 3828, 1993.
73. Kaplan, P.D. Optical studies of the structure and dynamics of opaque colloids. PhD dissertation, University of Pennsylvania, Philadelphia, PA, 1992.
74. Barbieri, B., Piccoli, F.D., van de Ven, M., and Gratton, E. What determines the uncertainty of phase and modulation measurements in frequency domain fluorometry? *SPIE Time Resolved Laser Spectrosc. Biochem. II* 1204: 158, 1990.
75. Fishkin, J.B. and Gratton, E. Propagation of photon density waves in strongly scattering media containing an absorbing "semi-infinite" plane bounded by a straight edge. *J. Opt. Soc. Am. A* 10: 127, 1993.
76. O'Leary, M.A., Boas, D.A., Chance, B., and Yodh, A.G. Refraction of diffuse photon density waves. *Phys. Rev. Lett.* 69: 2658, 1992.
77. Boas, D.A., Oleary, M.A., Chance, B., and Yodh, A.G. Scattering and wavelength transduction of diffuse photon density waves. *Phys. Rev. E* 47: R2999, 1993.
78. Tromberg, B.J., Svaasand, L.O., Tsay, T., and Haskell, R.C. Properties of photon density waves in multiple-scattering media. *Appl. Opt.* 32: 607, 1993.
79. Farrell, T.J., Patterson, M.S., and Wilson, B. A diffusion theory model of spatially resolved, steady state diffuse reflectance for the noninvasive determination of tissue optical properties in vivo. *Med. Phys.* 19: 879, 1992.
80. Hull, E.L., Nichols, M.G., and Foster, T.H. Quantitative broadband near-infrared spectroscopy of tissue-simulating phantoms containing erthrocytes. *Phys. Med. Biol.* 43: 2281, 1998.
81. Solonenko, M., Cheung, R., Busch, T.M., Kachur, A., Griffin, G.M., Vulcan, T., Zhu, T.C., Wang, H.-W., Hahn, S.M., and Yodh, A.G. In vivo reflectance measurement of optical properties, blood oxygenation and motexafin lutetium uptake in canine large bowel, kidneys and prostates. *Phys. Med. Biol.* 47: 1, 2002.
82. Fantini, S., Franceschini, M.A., Maier, J.S., Walker, S., and Gratton, E. Frequency domain multi-source optical spectrometer and oximeter, *Proc. SPIE* 2326: 108, 1994.
83. Cutler, M. Transillumination of the breast. *Surg. Gynecol. Obstet.* 48: 721, 1929.
84. Watmough, D.J. Transillumination of breast tissues: Factors governing optimal imaging of lesions. *Radiology* 147: 89, 1983.
85. Sickles, E.A. Periodic mammographic follow-up of probably benign lesions: Results in 3184 consecutive cases. *Radiology* 179: 463, 1991.

86. Wallberg, H., Alveryd, A., Bergvall, U., Nasiell, K., Sundelin, P., and Troel, S. Diaphanography in breast carcinoma. *Acta Radiol. Diagn.* 26: 33, 1985.

87. Profio, A.E. and Navarro, G.A. Scientific basis of breast diaphanography. *Med. Phys.* 16: 60, 1989.

88. Pera, A. and Freimanis, A.K. The choice of radiologic procedures in the diagnosis of breast disease. *Obstet. Gynecol. Clin. North Am.* 14: 635, 1987.

89. Homer, M.J. Breast imaging: Pitfalls, controversies, and some practical thoughts. *Radiol. Clin. North Am.* 14: 635, 1985.

90. Gisvold, J.J., Brown, L.R., Swee, R.G., Raygor, D.J., Dickerson, N., and Ranfranz, M.K. Comparison of mammography and transillumination light scanning in the detection of breast lesions. *Am. J. Roentgenol.* 147: 191, 1986.

91. Bartrum, R.J.J. and Crow, H.C. Transillumination lightscanning to diagnose breast cancer: A feasibility study. *Am. J. Roentgenol.* 142: 409, 1984.

92. Merrit, C.R.B., Sullivan, M.A., and Segaloff, A. Real time transillumination lightscanning of the breast. *Radiographics* 4: 989, 1984.

93. Carlsen, E.N. Transillumination light scanning. *Diagn. Imaging* 4: 28, 1982.

94. Marshall, V., Williams, D.C., and Smith, K.D. Diaphanography as a means of detecting breast cancer. *Radiology* 150: 339, 1984.

95. Monsees, B., Destouet, J.M., and Totty, W.G. Light scanning versus mammography in breast cancer detection. *Radiology* 163: 463, 1987.

96. Walker, S.A., Fantini, S., and Gratton, E. Image reconstruction by back-projection from frequency-domain optical measurements in highly scattering media. *Appl. Opt.* 36: 170, 1997.

97. Colak, S.B., Papaioannou, D.G., 't Hooft, G.W., van der Mark, M.B., Schomberg, H., Paasschens, J.C.J., Melissen, J.B.M., and Van Asten, N.A.A.J. Tomographic image reconstruction from optical projections in light-diffusing media. *Appl. Opt.* 36: 180, 1997.

98. Schotland, J.C. Continuous-wave diffusion imaging. *J. Opt. Soc. Am.* 14: 275, 1997.

99. Li, X.D., Durduran, T., Yodh, A.G., Chance, B., and Pattanayak, D.N. Diffraction tomography for biochemical imaging with diffuse-photon density waves. *Opt. Lett.* 22: 573, 1997.

100. Cheng, X. and Boas, D.A. Diffuse optical reflectance tomography with continuous-wave illumination. *Opt. Express* 3: 118, 1998.

101. Matson, C.L. and Liu, H.L. Analysis of the forward problem with diffuse photon density waves in turbid media by use of a diffraction tomography model. *J. Opt. Soc. Am. A* 16: 455, 1999.

102. Schotland, J.C., Haselgrove, J.C., and Leigh, J.S. Photon hitting density. *Appl. Opt.* 32: 448, 1993.

103. O'Leary, M.A., Boas, D.A., Chance, B., and Yodh, A.G. Experimental images of heterogeneous turbid media by frequency-domain diffusing-photon tomography. *Opt. Lett.* 20: 426, 1995.

104. Arridge, S.R. Photo-measurement density functions. Part 1: Analytical forms. *Appl. Opt.* 34: 7395, 1995.

105. Arridge, S.R. and Schweiger, M. Photon-measurement density-functions. 2. Finite-element-method calculations. *Appl. Opt.* 34: 8026, 1995.

106. Barbour, R.L., Graber, H.L., Chang, J., Barbour, S.S., Koo, P.C., and Aronson, R. MRI-guided optical tomography: Prospects and computation for a new imaging method. *IEEE Comput. Sci. Eng.* 2: 63, 1995.

107. Yao, Y., Wang, Y., Pei, Y., Zhu, W., and Barbour, R.L. Frequency-domain optical imaging of absorption and scattering distributions using a Born iterative method. *J. Opt. Soc. Am. A* 14: 325, 1997.

108. Paulsen, K.D. and Jiang, H. Spatially varying optical property reconstruction using a finite element diffusion equation approximation. *Med. Phys.* 22: 691, 1995.

109. Jiang, H., Paulsen, K.D., Osterberg, U.L., Pogue, B.W., and Patterson, M.S. Optical image reconstruction using frequency-domain data: Simulations and experiments. *J. Opt. Soc. Am. A* 13: 253, 1996.

110. Paulsen, K.D. and Jiang, H. Enhanced frequency-domain optical image reconstruction in tissues through total variation minimization. *Appl. Opt.* 35: 3447, 1996.

111. Jiang, H.B., Paulsen, K.D., Osterberg, U.L., and Patterson, M.S. Frequency-domain optical image reconstruction in turbid media: An experimental study of single-target detectability. *Appl. Opt.* 36: 52, 1997.

112. Jiang, H., Paulsen, K.D., Osterberg, U.L., and Patterson, M.S. Improved continuous light diffusion imaging in single- and multi-target tissue-like phantoms. *Phys. Med. Biol.* 43: 675, 1998.

113. Pogue, B.W., McBride, T.O., Prewitt, J., Osterberg, U.L., and Paulsen, K.D. Spatially variant regularization improves diffuse optical tomography. *Appl. Opt.* 38: 2950, 1999.

114. Arridge, S.R. and Schweiger, M. A gradient-based optimisation scheme for optical tomography. *Opt. Express* 2: 213, 1998.

115. Klibanov, M.V., Lucas, T.R., and Frank, R.M. A fast and accurate imaging algorithm in optical/diffusion tomography. *Inverse Probl.* 13: 1341, 1997.

116. Gryazin, Y.A., Klibanov, M.V., and Lucas, T.R. Imaging the diffusion coefficient in a parabolic inverse problem in optical tomography. *Inverse Probl.* 1: 373, 1999.

117. Eppstein, M.J., Dougherty, D.E., Troy, T.L., and Sevick-Muraca, E.M. Biomedical optical tomography using dynamic parameterization and Bayesian conditioning on photon migration measurements. *Appl. Opt.* 38: 2138, 1999.

118. Arridge, S.R. Optical tomography in medical imaging. *Inverse Probl.* 15: R41, 1999.

119. Zhu, Q., Durduran, T., Ntziachristos, V., Holboke, M., and Yodh, A.G. Imager that combines near-infrared diffusive light and ultrasound. *Opt. Lett.* 24: 1050, 1999.

120. Yao, Y., Pei, Y., Wang, Y., and Barbour, R.L. A Born type iterative method for imaging of heterogeneous scattering media and its application to simulated breast tissue. *Proc. SPIE* 2979: 232, 1997.

121. Lagendijk, A. and Biemond, J. *Iterative Identification and Restoration of Images.* Dordrecht, the Netherlands: Kluwer Academic, 1991.

122. Hansen, P.C. *Rank-Deficient and Discrete Ill-Posed Problems.* Philadelphia, PA: SIAM, 1998.

123. Culver, J.P., Ntziachristos, V., Holboke, M.J., and Yodh, A.G. Optimization of optodearrangements for diffuse optical tomography: A singular-value analysis. *Opt. Lett.* 26: 701, 2001.

124. Atkins, M.S., Murray, D., and Harrop, R. Use of transputers in a three-dimensional positron emission tomograph. *IEEE Trans. Med. Imaging* 10: 276, 1991.

125. Rajan, K., Patnaik, L.M., and Ramakrishna, J. High-speed computation of the EM algorithm for PET image reconstruction. *IEEE Trans. Nucl. Sci.* 41: 1721, 1994.

126. Chen, C.-M. An efficient four-connected parallel system for PET image reconstruction. *Parallel Comput.* 24: 1499, 1998.

127. Gregor, J. and Huff, D.A. A computational study of the focus-of-attention EM-ML algorithm for PET reconstruction. *Parallel Comput.* 24: 1481, 1998.

128. Zaidi, H., Labbe, C., and Morel, C. Implementation of an environment for Monte Carlo simulation of fully three-dimensional positron tomography on a high-performance parallel platform. *Parallel Comput.* 24: 1523, 1998.

129. Miller, M.I. and Butler, C.S. Three-dimensional maximum a posteriori estimation for single photon emission computed tomography on massively-parallel computers. *IEEE Trans. Med. Imaging* 12: 560, 1993.

130. Butler, C.S., Miller, M.I., Miller, T.R., and Wallis, J.W. Massively parallel computers for three-dimensional single-photon-emission computed tomography. *Phys. Med. Biol.* 39: 575, 1994.

131. Chen, C.M., Lee, S.-Y., and Cho, Z.H. A parallel implementation of three-dimensional image reconstruction on hypercube multiprocessor. *IEEE Trans. Nucl. Sci.* 37: 1333, 1990.

132. Rajan, K., Patnaik, L.M., and Ramakrishna, J. High-speed implementation of a modified PBR algorithm on DSP-based EH topology. *IEEE Trans. Nucl. Sci.* 44: 1658, 1997.

133. Laurent, C., Peyrin, F., Chassery, J.-M., and Amiel, M. Parallel image reconstruction on MIMD computers for three-dimensional cone-beam tomography. *Parallel Comput.* 24: 1461, 1998.

134. Woo, E.J., Hua, P., Webster, J.G., and Tompkins, W.J. A robust image reconstruction algorithm and its parallel implementation in electrical impedance tomography. *IEEE Trans. Med. Imaging* 12: 137, 1993.

135. Joshi, S. and Miller, M. Maximum a posteriori estimation with Good's roughness for three-dimensional optical-sectioning microscopy. *J. Opt. Soc. Am.* 10: 1078, 1993.

136. Schweiger, M., Zhukov, L., Arridge, S.R., and Johnson, C.R. Optical tomography using the SCIRun problem solving environment: Preliminary results for three-dimensional geometries and parallel processing. *Opt. Express* 4: 263, 1999.

137. Holboke, M.J., Tromberg, B.J., Li, X., Shah, N., Fishkin, J., Kidney, D., Butler, J., Chance, B., and Yodh, A.G. Three-dimensional diffuse optical mammography with ultrasound localization in a human subject. *J. Biomed. Opt.* 5: 237, 2000.

138. Boas, D.A. and Yodh, A.G. Spatially varying dynamical properties of turbid media probed with diffusing temporal light correlation. *J. Opt. Soc. Am. A* 14: 192, 1997.

139. Clark, N.A., Lunacek, J.H., and Benedek, G.B. A study of Brownian motion using light scattering. *Am. J. Phys.* 38: 575, 1970.

140. Berne, P.J. and Pecora, R. *Dynamic Light Scattering.* New York: Wiley, 1976.

141. Fuller, G.G., Rallison, J.M., Schmidt, R.L., and Leal, L.G. The measurement of velocity gradients in laminar flow by homodyne light-scattering spectroscopy. *J. Fluid Mech.* 100: 555, 1980.

142. Tong, P., Goldburg, W.I., Chan, C.K., and Sirivat, A. Turbulent transition by photon-correlation spectroscopy. *Phys. Rev. A* 37: 2125, 1988.

143. Bertolotti, M., Crosignani, B., Di Porto, P., and Sette, D. Light scattering by particles suspended in a turbulent fluid. *J. Phys. A* 2: 126, 1969.

144. Bourke, P.J., Butterworth, J., Drain, L.E., Egelstaff, P.A., Jakeman, E., and Pike, E.R. A study of the spatial structure of turbulent flow by intensity-fluctuation spectroscopy. *J. Phys. A* 3: 216, 1970.

145. Tanaka, T., Riva, C., and Ben-Sira, I. Blood velocity measurements in human retinal vessels. *Science* 186: 830, 1974.

146. Stern, M.D. In vivo evaluation of microcirculation by coherent light scattering. *Nature* 254: 56, 1975.

147. Bonner, R. and Nossal, R. Model for laser Doppler measurements of blood flow in tissue. *Appl. Opt.* 20: 2097, 1981.

148. Pine, D.J., Weitz, D.A., Chaikin, P.M., and Herbolzheimer, E. Diffusing-wave spectroscopy. *Phys. Rev. Lett.* 60: 1134, 1988.

149. MacKintosh, F.C. and John, S. Diffusing-wave spectroscopy and multiple scattering of light in correlated random media. *Phys. Rev. B* 40: 2382, 1989.

150. Maret, G. and Wolf, P.E. Multiple light scattering from disordered media. The effect of Brownian motion of scatterers. *Z. Phys. B* 65: 409, 1987.

151. Pusey, P.N. and Vaughan, J.M. *Dielectric and Related Molecular Processes X XKW*, Vol. 2. Specialist Periodical Report, Davies, M., ed. London, U.K.: Chemical Society, 1975.

152. Boas, D.A., Campbell, L.E., and Yodh, A.G. Scattering and imaging with diffusing temporal field correlations. *Phys. Rev. Lett.* 75: 1855, 1995.

153. Berne, B.J. and Pecora, R. *Dynamic Light Scattering with Applications to Chemistry, Biology, and Physics.* Malabar, FL: Krieger, 1990.

154. Brown, W. *Dynamic Light Scattering: The Method and Some Applications.* New York: Clarendon, 1993.

155. Cummings, H.Z. and Pike, E.R. *Photon Correlation and Light-Bearing Spectroscopy.* New York: Plenum, 1974.

156. Val'kov, A.Y. and Romanov, V.P. Characteristics of propagation and scattering of light in nematic liquid crystals. *Sov. Phys. JETP* 63: 737, 1986.

157. Rice, S.O. Mathematical analysis of random noise, in *Noise and Stochastic Processes*, Wax, N., ed. New York: Dover, 1954, p. 133.

158. Hackmeier, M., Skipetrov, S.E., Maret, G., and Maynard, R. Imaging of dynamic heterogeneities in mulitiple-scattering media. *J. Opt. Soc. Am. A* 14: 185, 1997.

159. Benaron, D.A., Hintz, S.R., Villringer, A., Boas, D., Kleinschmidt, A., Frahm, J., Hirth, C. et al. Noninvasive functional imaging of human brain using light. *J. Cereb. Blood Flow Metab.* 20: 469, 2000.

160. Danen, R.M., Wang, Y., Li, X.D., Thayer, W.S., and Yodh, A.G. Regional imager for low-resolution functional imaging of the brain with diffusing near-infrared light. *Photochem. Photobiol.* 67: 33, 1998.

161. Villringer, A. and Chance, B. Non-invasive optical spectroscopy and imaging of human brain function. *Trends Neurosci.* 20: 435, 1997.

162. Kelcz, F. and Santyr, G. Gadolinium-enhanced breast MRI. *Crit. Rev. Diagn. Imaging* 36: 287, 1995.

163. Barkhof, F., Valk, J., Hommes, O.R., and Scheltens, P. Meningeal Gd-DTPA enhancement in multiple-sclerosis. *Am. J. Neuroradiol.* 13: 397, 1992.

164. Tilcock, C. Delivery of contrast agents for magnetic resonance imaging, computed tomography, nuclear medicine and ultrasound. *Adv. Drug Deliv. Rev.* 37: 33, 1999.

165. Kedar, R.P., Cosgrove, D., McCready, V.R., Bamber, J.C., and Carter, E.R. Microbubble contrast agent for color Doppler US: Effect on breast masses. *Radiology* 198: 679, 1996.

166. Melany, M.L., Grant, E.G., Farooki, S., McElroy, D., and Kimme-Smith, C. Effect of US contrast agents on spectral velocities: In vitro evaluation. *Radiology* 211: 427, 1999.

167. Thompson, S.E., Raptopoulos, V., Sheiman, R.L., McNicholas, M.M.J., and Prassopoulos, P. Abdominal helical CT: Milk as a low-attenuation oral contrast agent. *Radiology* 211: 870, 1999.

168. Jain, R., Sawhney, S., Sahni, P., Taneja, K., and Berry, M. CT portography by direct intrasplenic contrast injection: A new technique. *Abdom. Imaging* 24: 272, 1999.

169. Knuttel, A., Schmitt, J.M., Barnes, R., and Knutson, J.R. Acousto-optic scanning and interfering photon density waves for precise localization of an absorbing (or fluorescent) body in a turbid medium. *Rev. Sci. Instrum.* 64: 638, 1993.

170. O'Leary, M.A., Boas, D.A., Chance, B., and Yodh, A.G. Reradiation and imaging of diffuse photon density waves using fluorescent inhomogeneities. *J. Luminesc.* 60: 789, 1994.

171. Li, X.D., Beauvoit, B., White, R., Nioka, S., Chance, B., and Yodh, A.G. Tumor localization using fluorescence of indocyanine green (ICG) in rat model. *SPIE Proc.* 2389: 789, 1995.

172. Wu, J., Wang, Y., Perelman, L., Itzkan, I., Dasari, R.R., and Feld, M.S. Time-resolved multichannel imaging of fluorescent objects embedded in turbid media. *Opt. Lett.* 20: 489, 1995.

173. Bambot, S.B., Lakowicz, J.R., Sipior, J., Carter, G., and Rao, G. Bioprocess and clinical monitoring using lifetime-based phase-modulation fluorometry. *Abst. Papers Am. Chem. Soc.* 209: 11-BTEC Part 2, 1995.

174. Rumsey, W.L., Vanderkooi, J.M., and Wilson, D.F. Imaging of phosphorescence: A novel method for measuring oxygen distribution in perfused tissue. *Science* 241: 1649, 1988.

175. Vinogradov, S.A., Lo, L.W., Jenkins, W.T., Evans, S.M., Koch, C., and Wilson, D.F. Noninvasive imaging of the distribution of oxygen in tissue in vivo using infrared phosphors. *Biophys. J.* 70: 1609, 1996.

176. Lakowicz, J.R. *Principles of Fluorescence Spectroscopy.* New York: Plenum Press, 1983.

177. Mordon, S., Devoisselle, J.M., and Maunoury, V. In-vivo pH measurement and imaging of tumor-issue using a pH-sensitive fluorescent-probe (56-carboxyfluorescein)—Instrumental and experimental studies. *Photochem. Photobiol.* 60: 274, 1994.

178. Russell, D.A., Pottier, R.H., and Valenzeno, D.P. Continuous noninvasive measurement of in-vivo pH in conscious mice. *Photochem. Photobiol.* 59: 309, 1994.

179. Sevick-Muraca, E.M. and Burch, C.L. The origin of phosphorescent and fluorescent signals in tissues. *Opt. Lett.* 19: 1928, 1994.

180. Hutchinson, C.L., Lakowicz, J.R., and Sevick-Muraca, E.M. Fluorescence lifetime-based sensing in tissues—A computational study. *Biophys. J.* 68: 1574, 1995.

181. Patterson, M.S. and Pogue, B.W. Mathematical-model for time-resolved and frequency-domain fluorescence spectroscopy in biological tissue. *Appl. Opt.* 33: 1963, 1994.

182. Wu, J., Feld, M.S., and Rava, R.P. Analytical model for extracting intrinsic fluorescence in turbid media. *Appl. Opt.* 32: 3585, 1993.

183. Hull, E.L., Nichols, M.G., and Foster, T.H. Localization of luminescent inhomogeneities in turbid media with spatially resolved measurements of CW diffuse luminescence emittance. *Appl. Opt.* 37: 2755, 1998.

184. Feldmann, H.J., Molls, M., and Vaupel, P.W. Blood flow and oxygenation status of human tumors—Clinical investigations. *Strahlenther. Onkol.* 175: 1, 1999.

185. O'Leary, M.A., Boas, D.A., Li, X.D., Chance, B., and Yodh, A.G. Fluorescent lifetime imaging in turbid media. *Opt. Lett.* 21: 158, 1996.

186. Li, X.D., O'Leary, M.A., Boas, D.A., Chance, B., and Yodh, A.G. Fluorescent diffuse photon density waves in homogenous and heterogeneous turbid media: Analytic solutions and applications. *Appl. Opt.* 35: 3746, 1996.

187. Li, X.D., Chance, B., and Yodh, A.G. Fluorescent heterogeneities in turbid media: Limits for detection, characterization, and comparison with absorption. *Appl. Opt.* 37: 6833, 1998.

188. Ntziachristos, V., Chance, B., and Yodh, A.G. Differential diffuse optical tomography. *Opt. Express* 5: 230, 1999.

189. Chernomordik, V., Hattery, D.W., Grosenick, D., Wabnitz, H., Rinneberg, H., Moesta, K.T., Schlag, P.M., and Gandjbakhche, A. Quantification of optical properties of a breast tumor using random walk theory. *J. Biomed. Opt.* 7: 80, 2002.

190. Colak, S.B., van der Mark, M.B., Hooft, G.W., Hoogenraad, J.H., van der Linden, E.S., and Kuijpers, F.A. Clinical optical tomography and NIR spectroscopy for breast cancer detection. *IEEE J. Sel. Top. Quant. Electron.* 5: 1143, 1999.

191. McBride, T.O., Pogue, B.W., Poplack, S., Soho, S., Wells, W.A., Jiang, S., Osterberg, U.L., and Paulsen, K.D. Multispectral near-infrared tomography: A case study in compensating for water and lipid content in hemoglobin imaging of the breast. *J. Biomed. Opt.* 7: 72, 2002.

192. Jiang, H., Iftimia, N.V., Xu, Y., Eggert, J.A., Fajardo, L.L., and Klove, K.L. Near-infrared optical imaging of the breast with model-based reconstruction. *Acad. Radiol.* 9: 186, 2002.

193. Nioka, S., Yung, Y., Shnall, M., Zhao, S., Orel, S., Xie, C., Chance, B., and Solin, L. Optical imaging of breast tumor by means of continuous waves. *Adv. Exp. Med. Biol.* 411: 227, 1997.

194. Pogue, B.W. and Paulsen, K.D. High-resolution near-infrared tomographic imaging simulations of the rat cranium by use of a priori magnetic resonance imaging structural information. *Opt. Lett.* 23: 1716, 1998.

195. Siegel, A.M., Marota, J.J.A., and Boas, D.A. Design and evaluation of a continuous-wave diffuse optical tomography system. *Opt. Express* 4: 287, 1999.

196. Hintz, S.R., Benaron, D.A., Siegel, A.M., Zourabian, A., Stevenson, D.K., and Boas, D.A. Bedside functional imaging of the premature infant brain during passive motor activation. *J. Perinat. Med.* 29: 335, 2001.

197. Cheung, C., Culver, J.P., Takahashi, K., Greenberg, J.H., and Yodh, A.G. In vivo cerebrovascular measurement combining diffuse near-infrared absorption and correlation spectroscopies. *Phys. Med. Biol.* 46: 2053, 2001.

198. Maki, A., Yamashita, Y., Ito, Y., Watanabe, E., Mayanagi, Y., and Koizumi, H. Spatial and temporal analysis of human motor activity using noninvasive NIR topography. *Med. Phys.* 22: 1997, 1995.

199. Takahashi, K., Ogata, S., Atsumi, Y., Yamamoto, R., Shiotsuka, S., Maki, A., Yamashita, Y., Yamamoto, T., Koizumi, H., Hirasawa, H., and Igawa, M. Activation of the visual cortex imaged by 24-channel near-infrared spectroscopy. *J. Biomed. Opt.* 5: 93, 2000.

200. Franceschini, M.A., Toronov, V., Filiaci, M., Gratton, E., and Fanini, S. On-line optical imaging of the human brain with 160-ms temporal resolution. *Opt. Express* 6: 49, 2000.

201. Benaron, D.A. and Stevenson, D.K. Optical time-of-flight and absorbance imaging of biologic media. *Science* 259: 1463, 1993.

202. Chance, B., Leigh, J. S., Miyake, H., Smith, D.S., Nioka, S., Greenfeld, R., Finander, M. et al. Comparison of time-resolved and unresolved measurements of deoxyhemoglobin in brain. *Proc. Natl. Acad. Sci. USA* 85: 4971, 1988.

203. Cubeddu, R., Pifferi, A., Taroni, P., Torricelli, A., and Valentini, G. Time-resolved imaging on a realistic tissue phantom: μ'_s and μ_a images versus time-integrated images. *Appl. Opt.* 35: 4533, 1996.

204. Hebden, J. C., Arridge, S.R., and Delpy, D.T. Optical imaging in medicine: I. Experimental techniques. *Phys. Med. Biol.* 42: 825, 1997.

205. Grosenick, D., Wabnitz, H., and Rinneberg, H. Time-resolved imaging of solid phantoms for optical mammography. *Appl. Opt.* 36: 221, 1997.

206. Nioka, S., Luo, Q., and Chance, B. Human brain functional imaging with reflectance CWS. *Adv. Exp. Med. Biol.* 428: 237, 1997.

207. Maki, A., Yamashita, Y., Watanabe, E., and Koizumi, H. Visualizing human motor activity by using non-invasive optical topography. *Front. Med. Biol. Eng.* 7: 285, 1996.

208. Colier, W., van der Sluijs, M.C., Menssen, J., and Oeseburg, B. A new and highly sensitive optical brain imager with 50 Hz sample rate. *NeuroImage* 11: 542, 2000.

209. Gratton, E., Fantini, S., Franceschini, M.A., Gratton, G., and Fabiani, M. Measurements of scattering and absorption changes in muscle and brain. *Philos. Trans. R. Soc. London B: Biol. Sci.* 352: 727, 1997.

210. Pogue, B.W., Patterson, M.S., Jiang, H., and Paulsen, K.D. Initial assessment of a simple system for frequency domain diffuse optical tomography. *Phys. Med. Biol.* 40: 1709, 1995.

211. Chance, B., Cope, M., Gratton, E., Ramanujam, N., and Tromberg, B. Phase measurement of light absorption and scattering in human tissues. *Rev. Sci. Instrum.* 689: 3457, 1998.

212. Fishkin, J.B., So, P.T.C., Cerussi, A.E., Fantini, S., Franceschini, M.A., and Gratton, E. A frequency-domain method for measuring spectral properties in multiply scattering media: Methemoglobin absorption spectrum in a tissue-like phantom. *Appl. Opt.* 34: 1143, 1995.

213. Quaresima, V., Colier, W.N., van der Sluijs, M., and Ferrari, M. Non-uniform quadriceps O_2 consumption revealed by near infrared multipoint measurements. *Biochem. Biophys. Res. Commun.* 285: 1034, 2001.

214. Miura, H., McCully, K., Hong, L., Nioka, S., and Chance, B. Exercise-induced changes in oxygen status in calf muscle of elderly subjects with peripheral vascular disease using functional near infrared imaging machine. *Ther. Res.* 2: 1585, 2000.

215. Pogue, B.W., Testorf, M., McBride, T., Osterberg, U., and Paulsen, K. Instrumentation and design of a frequency-domain diffuse optical tomography imager for breast cancer detection. *Opt. Express* 1: 391, 1997.

216. Schmidt, F.E., Fry, M.E., Hillman, E.M.C., Hebden, J.C., and Delpy, D.T. A 32-channel time-resolved instrument for medical optical tomography. *Rev. Sci. Instrum.* 71: 256, 2000.

217. Culver, J.P., Choe, R., Holboke, M.J., Zubkov, L., Durduran, T., Slemp, A., Ntziachristos, V., Chance, B., and Yodh, A.G. 3D diffuse optical tomography in the plane parallel transmission geometry: Evaluation of a hybrid frequency domain/continuous wave clinical system for breast imaging. *Med. Phys.,* accepted.

218. Durduran, T., Choe, R., Culver, J. P., Zubkov, L., Holboke, M.J., Giammarco, J., Chance, B., and Yodh, A.G. Bulk optical properties of healthy female breast tissue. *Phys. Med. Biol.* 47: 2847, 2002.

219. Yang, Y., Liu, H., Li, X., and Chance, B. Low-cost frequency-domain photon migration instrument for tissue spectroscopy, oximetry and imaging. *Opt. Eng.* 36: 1562, 1997.

220. Flock, S.T., Jacques, S.L., Wilson, B.C., Star, W.M., and van Gemert, M.J.C. Optical properties of Intralipid: A phantom medium for light propagation studies. *Lasers Surg. Med.* 12: 510, 1992.

221. van Staveren, H.J., Moes, C.J.M., van Marle, J., Prahl, S.A., and van Gemert, M.J.C. Light scattering in Intralipid—10% in the wavelength range of 400 to 1100 nm. *Appl. Opt.* 30: 4507, 1991.

222. Gros, C., Quenneville, Y., and Hummel, Y. Breast diaphanology. *J. Radiol. Electrol. Med. Nucl.* 53: 297, 1972.

223. Alveryd, A., Andersson, I., Aspegren, K., Balldin, G., Bjurstam, N., Edstrom, G., Fagerberg, G. et al. Lightscanning versus mammography for the detection of breast cancer in screening and clinical practice. A Swedish multicenter study. *Cancer* 65: 1671, 1990.

224. Shah, N., Cerussi, A., Eker, C., Espinoza, J., Butler, J., Fishkin, J., Hornung, R., and Tromberg, B. Noninvasive functional optical spectroscopy of human breast tissue. *Proc. Natl. Acad. Sci. USA* 98: 4420, 2001.

225. Sevick-Muraca, E.M., Reynolds, J. S., Troy, T.L., Lopez, G., and Paithankar, D.Y. Fluorescence lifetime spectroscopic imaging with measurements of photon migration. *Ann. N.Y. Acad. Sci.* 838: 46, 1998.

226. Hawrysz, D.J. and Sevick-Muraca, E.M. Developments toward diagnostic breast cancer imaging using near-infrared optical measurements and fluorescent contrast agents. *Neoplasia* 2: 388, 2000.

227. Tromberg, B.J., Shah, N., Lanning, R., Cerussi, A., Espinoza, J., Pham, T., Svaasand, L., and Butler, J. Non-invasive in vivo characterization of breast tumors using photon migration spectroscopy. *Neoplasia* 2: 26, 2000.

228. Ntziachristos, V., Ma, X.H., Yodh, A.G., and Chance, B. Multichannel photon counting instrument for spatially resolved near infrared spectroscopy. *Rev. Sci. Instrum.* 70: 193, 1999.

229. Boas, D.A., Meglinsky, I.V., Zemany, L., Campbell, L.E., Chance, B., and Yodh, A.G. Diffusion of temporal field correlation with selected applications. *Proc. SPIE* 2732: 34, 1996.

230. Briers, J.D. Laser Doppler and time-varying speckle: A reconciliation. *J. Opt. Soc. Am. A* 13: 345, 1996.

231. Dunn, A.K., Bolay, H., Moskowitz, M.A., and Boas, D.A. Dynamic imaging of cerebral blood flow using laser speckle. *J. Cereb. Blood Flow Metab.* 21: 195, 2001.

232. Kuebler, W.M., Sckell, A., Habler, O., Kleen, M., Kuhnle, G.E.H., Welte, M., Messmer, K., and Goetz, A.E. Noninvasive measurement of regional cerebral blood flow by near-infrared spectroscopy and indocyanine green. *J. Cereb. Blood Flow Metab.* 18: 445, 1998.

233. Patel, J., Marks, K., Roberts, I., Azzopardi, D., and Edwards, A.D. Measurement of cerebral blood flow in newborn infants using near infrared spectroscopy with indocyanine green. *Pediatr. Res.* 43: 34, 1998.

234. Gopinath, S.P., Robertson, C.S., Contant, C.F., Narayan, R.K., Grossman, R.G., and Chance, B. Early detection of delayed traumatic intracranial hematomas using near-infrared spectroscopy. *J. Neurosurg.* 83: 438, 1995.

235. Ogawa, S., Tank, D., Menon, R., Ellermann, J., Kim, S.-G., Merkel, H., and Ugurbil, K. Intrinsic signal changes accompanying sensory stimulation: Functional brain mapping with magnetic resonance imaging. *Proc. Natl. Acad. Sci. USA* 89: 5951, 1992.

236. Kwong, K.K., Belliveau, J.W., Chesler, D.A., Goldberg, I.E., Weisskoff, R.M., Poncelet, B.P., Kennedy, D.N. et al. Dynamic magnetic resonance imaging of human brain activity during primary sensory stimulation. *Proc. Natl. Acad. Sci. USA* 89: 5675, 1992.

237. Jobsis, F.F. Nonivasive, infrared monitoring of cerebral and myocardial oxygen sufficiency and circulatory parameters. *Science* 198: 1264, 1977.

238. Wyatt, J.S., Cope, M., Delpy, D.T., Wray, S., and Reynolds, E.O.R. Quantification of cerebral oxygenation and haemodynamics in sick newborn infants by near infrared spectrophotometry. *Lancet* ii: 1063, 1986.

239. Chance, B. and Williams, G.R. The respiratory chain and oxidative phosphorylation. *Adv. Enzymol.* 17: 65, 1956.

240. Lockwood, A.H., LaManna, J.C., Snyder, S., and Rosenthal, M. Effects of acetazolamide and electrical stimulation on cerebral oxidative metabolism as indicated by cytochrome oxidase redox state. *Brain Res.* 308: 9, 1984.

241. Wong Riley, M.T. Cytochrome oxidase: An endogenous metabolic marker for neuronal activity. *Trends Neurosci.* 12: 94, 1989.

242. Kohl, M., Nolte, C., Heekeren, H.R., Horst, S., Scholz, U., Obrig, H., and Villringer, A. Changes in cytochrome-oxidase oxidation in the occipital cortex during visual stimulation: Improvement in sensitivity by the determination of the wavelength dependence of the differential pathlength factor. *Proc. SPIE* 3194: 18, 1998.

243. Wobst, P., Wenzel, R., Kohl, M., Obrig, H., and Villringer, A. Linear aspects of changes in deoxygenated hemoglobin concentration and cytochrome oxidase oxidation during brain activation. *Neuroimage* 13: 520, 2001.

244. Steinbrink, J., Kohl, M., Obrig, H., Curio, G., Syre, F., Thomas, F., Wabnitz, H., Rinneberg, H., and Villringer, A. Somatosensory evoked fast optical intensity changes detected non-invasively in the adult human head. *Neurosci. Lett.* 291: 105, 2000.

245. Stepnoski, R.A., LaPorta, A., Raccuia-Behling, F., Blonder, G.E., Slusher, R.E., and Kleinfeld, D. Noninvasive detection of changes in membrane potential in cultured neurons by light scattering. *Proc. Natl. Acad. Sci. USA* 88: 9382, 1991.

246. Mayhew, J., Johnston, D., Martindale, J., Jones, M., Berwick, J., and Zheng, Y. Increased oxygen consumption following activation of brain: Theoretical footnotes using spectroscopic data from barrel cortex. *Neuroimage* 13: 975, 2001.

247. Mayhew, J., Zheng, Y., Hou, Y., Vuksanovic, B., Berwick, J., Askew, S., and Coffey, P. Spectroscopic analysis of changes in remitted illumination: The response to increased neural activity in brain. *Neuroimage* 10: 304, 1999.

248. Simoes, C.H.R. Relationship between responses to contra- and ipsilateral stimuli in the human second somatosensory cortex SII. *Neuroimage* 10: 408, 1999.

249. Spiegel, J.T.J., Gawehn, J., Stoeter, P., and Treede, R.D. Functional MRI of human primary somatosensory and motor cortex during median nerve stimulation. *Clin. Neurophysiol.* 110: 47, 1999.

250. Allison, J.D.M.K., Loring, D.W., Figueroa, R.E., and Wright, J.C. Functional MRI cerebral activation and deactivation during finger movement. *Neurology* 54: 135, 2000.

251. Boas, D.A., O'Leary, M.A., Chance, B., and Yodh, A.G. Detection and characterization of optical inhomogeneities with diffuse photon density waves: A signal-to-noise analysis. *Appl. Opt.* 36: 75, 1997.

252. Matson, C.L. Deconvolution-based spatial resolution in optical diffusion tomography. *Appl. Opt.* 40: 5791, 2001.

253. Moon, J.A. and Reintjes, J. Image resolution by use of multiply scattered light. *Opt. Lett.* 19: 521, 1994.

254. Moon, J.A., Mahon, R., Duncan, M.D., and Reintjes, J. Resolution limits for imaging through turbid media with diffuse light. *Opt. Lett.* 18, 1591: 1993.

255. Zhu, Q., Conant, E., and Chance, B. Optical imaging as an adjunct to sonograph in differentiating benign from malignant breast lesions. *J. Biomed. Opt.* 5: 229, 2000.

256. Ntziachristos, V., Yodh, A.G., Schnall, M., and Chance, B. MRI-guided diffuse optical spectroscopy of malignant and benign breast lesions. *Neoplasia* 4: 347, 2002.

257. Arridge, S.R., Schweiger, M., Hiraoka, M., and Delpy, D.T. Performance of an iterative reconstruction algorithm for near infrared absorption and scatter imaging. *Proc. SPIE* 1888: 360, 1993.

258. Schweiger, M., Arridge, S.R., and Delpy, D.T. Application of the finite-element method for the forward and inverse models in optical tomography. *J. Math. Imaging Vision* 3: 263, 1993.

259. Arridge, S.R. and Schweiger, M. Inverse methods for optical tomography, in *Information Processing in Medical Imaging (IPMI'93 Proceedings)*, Lecture Notes in Computer Science, 687, Springer-Verlag, Berlin, Germany, 1993, p. 259.

260. Boas, D.A., Gaudette, T.J., and Arridge, S.R. Simultaneous imaging and optode calibration with diffuse optical tomography. *Opt. Express* 8: 263, 2001.

Molecular Contrast Optical Coherence Tomography

Oscar
Carrasco-Zevallos
Duke University

Joseph A. Izatt
Duke University

10.1 Introduction

Optical coherence tomography (OCT) is a well-developed imaging modality that achieves structural imaging of tissue via interferometric detection of backscattered light [1]. Because of its high-resolution tomographic imaging, OCT was quickly adopted by ophthalmologists after its inception in 1991. Ever since, OCT has revolutionized the field of ophthalmology and is now the gold standard retinal imaging modality. OCT structural imaging enables the visualization of tissue with micron-scale resolution by probing refractive index discontinuities. However, because the real part of the refractive index does not vary significantly among molecular species, OCT has inherently poor molecular contrast. Akin to CT/PET imaging, simultaneous structural and molecular OCT imaging may allow for more complete diagnostic analysis, since many pathological processes stem in biochemical abnormalities before progressing to structural deformations.

To this date, a clinically accepted functional OCT extension has yet to be developed. The primary reason hindering molecular contrast OCT is the interferometric detection scheme vital in coherence imaging. Popular optical techniques, including fluorescence contrast microscopy [2], Forster resonance energy transfer (FRET) [3], and evanescent wave fluorescence [4], typically utilize fluorescence for molecular specificity. However, because fluorescence is not a coherent phenomenon, it is inherently incompatible with OCT. Furthermore, there are a limited number of FDA-approved optical contrast agents, the most popular of which is indocyanine green (ICG) [5].

Yet the benefits of merging molecular imaging with OCT are substantial. Conventional molecular imaging techniques suffer from shallow penetration depth (300–400 µm) [6]. Because the axial and lateral resolutions are decoupled, OCT employs low NA objectives to provide a long depth of focus for increased penetration depth while preserving fine axial resolution via coherence gating. Therefore, molecular specificity in OCT would enable molecular imaging depths of several millimeters with micron-level axial and lateral resolution. A well-developed molecular contrast OCT system would thus be attractive to biologists and clinicians as an alternative to fluorescence-based imaging. To this end, a variety of different molecular contrast OCT schemes have been pursued and will be discussed in this chapter.

10.2 Engineered Contrast Agents for OCT

Recently, there has been considerable interest in developing contrast agents to alter the scattering properties of the sample and provide localized signal enhancement in OCT. Furthermore, these contrast agents can be readily targeted to molecules, cells, and different tissue types of interest to provide molecular specificity in OCT. Such targeted imaging can improve diagnostic capabilities in a wide range of applications.

One of the most prevalent OCT scattering contrast agents, microspheres can be manufactured from a variety of different materials, including gold and carbon. In particular, gold-shelled microspheres filled with oil and coated with scattering silica nanoparticles were utilized for enhanced contrast in liver tissue [7]. The vegetable oil embedded in the microsphere's core increased stability and lifetime (from several days to several months) of the nanoparticle compared to air-filled microspheres. The gold-embedded microspheres were injected intravenously into anesthetized mice and liver tissue was imaged with conventional OCT.

In this particular case, the contrast agents were localized to liver tissue without the need for functionalization or targeting since the liver is the physiological collection site after the microspheres are cleared from the circulatory system. Mice livers with and without the contrast agents were imaged to illustrate the enhanced contrast provided by the microspheres, as depicted in Figure 10.1.

Silica-gold nanoshells are also an attractive choice for an OCT contrast agent because of their increased diffusion rates compared to microspheres. In essence, because gold nanoshells are smaller than microspheres, the particles can reach the desired target faster. Specifically, silica-gold nanoshells (gold shell with a silica core) have been fabricated for optimum backscatter in the NIR region—the typical OCT

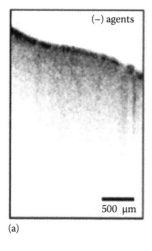
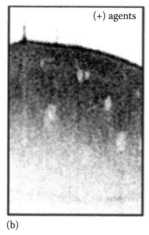

(–) agents   (+) agents

500 µm

(a)   (b)

FIGURE 10.1   Gold-shelled oil-filled microspheres were delivered into a mouse via the tail vein utilizing passive targeting. Contrast agents accumulated in liver tissue after clearance from the bloodstream. The figure depicts the OCT image enhancement with the contrast agents. (a) OCT image of liver tissue without nanoparticles. (b) OCT image of liver tissue after nanoparticle delivery. (From Lee, T.M. et al., *Opt. Lett.*, 28(17), 1546, September 2003. With permission.)

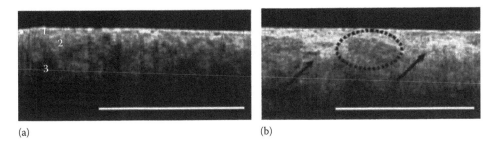

(a)   (b)

FIGURE 10.2 OCT images of rabbit skin before (a) and after (b) application of silica-gold nanoshells. 1, 2, and 3 depict the epidermis, the superficial part of the dermis, and deep layers of the dermis, respectively. Arrows indicate the border between the deeper layers and the superficial parts of the dermis, while a hair follicle is encircled. Because the silica-gold nanoshells do not diffuse past the superficial part of the dermis, OCT contrast of 2 is enhanced after application of contrast agent. Differentiation of 2 and 3 is easier using contrast agent. (From Zagaynova, E.V. et al., *Phys. Med. Biol.*, 53(18), 4995, September 2008. With permission.)

wavelength range [8]. The shell thickness of the nanoshells can also be tuned for greater scattering than absorption in the NIR range to increase OCT contrast [9]. Fabrication details of these nanoshells and other OCT contrast agents can be found in [10]. These gold nanoshells were utilized to enhance contrast in rabbit thigh tissue to help differentiate tissue layers. OCT images appear brighter in the superficial part of the dermis where the nanoparticles are situated after introduction into the tissue, allowing for easier differentiation between the top layers of the dermis and deeper layers, as depicted in Figure 10.2 [8].

In regard to contrast agent delivery, there are two broadly defined approaches: active and passive targeting. In passive targeting, the nanoparticles are delivered into the body, usually intravenously, and diffuse until they reach an end-organ site. Passively targeted nanoparticles injected into the bloodstream readily end up in the liver. Therefore, in order to ensure that a sufficient amount of contrast agent reaches the desired destination, the particles must be introduced at a nearby location. However, localizing passively targeted nanoparticles is difficult if the desired location is not close to the surface of the skin. Typically, passive targeting results in a low concentration of contrast agent at the target site. The OCT contrast agents discussed earlier all utilize passive targeting.

Active targeting contrast agent delivery refers to functionalizing the nanoparticles, typically via surface conjugation with target-specific ligands. Compared to passive targeting, active targeting typically results in a much larger nanoparticle concentration at the target site [11]. Specifically, there is considerable interest in functionalizing nanoparticles to target tumors to allow for added imaging contrast and thereby improved diagnostic potential. Gold nanoshells, via active targeting, have been utilized to image cancerous tumors. Epidermal growth factor receptors (EGFR) were conjugated to the surface of the nanoshells to decrease delivery time and increase particle concentration at the target site [12–14]. The benefits of active targeting versus passive targeting are depicted in Figure 10.3. Furthermore, the dependence of OCT contrast enhancement on nanoparticle concentration has also been investigated [15].

There are a variety of other nanostructures, each with their own advantages and disadvantages, that can be utilized as OCT contrast agents, including gold nanorods (GNRs) and gold nanocages. GNRs can be synthesized at dimensions below 100 nm, enhancing their diffusion properties relative to nanoshells or nanospheres. Furthermore, the longitudinal plasmon resonance can be tailored to the NIR frequencies by adjusting the ratio of length to width of the nanorods [16]. Gold nanocages can also be engineered to have surface plasmon resonance at NIR frequencies for enhanced OCT contrast. However, in contrast to the previously discussed nanostructures, nanocages are hollow with porous walls that allow for faster diffusion. Moreover, nanocages can be engineered at dimensions as small as 40 nm while still maintaining optical resonances at the frequencies of interest [17,18]. These structures,

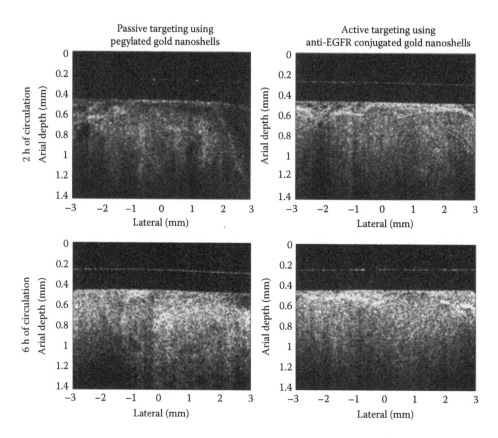

FIGURE 10.3   Comparison of OCT images of tumor tissue with nontargeted gold nanoshells (left column) and anti-EGFR conjugated gold nanoshells (right column). Images were taken after 2 h (top row) and 6 h (bottom row) of circulation. As evident, OCT contrast when using active targeting is much higher than when using passive targeting after 2 h of circulation. After 6 h of circulation, OCT images are comparable. Therefore, functionalizing gold nanoshells results in faster delivery to target site. (From Kah, J.C.Y. et al., *J. Biomed. Opt.*, 14(5), 1, 2009. With permission.)

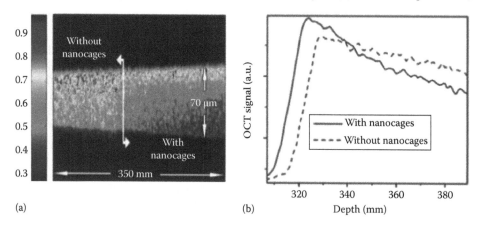

FIGURE 10.4   (See color insert.) Comparison of OCT images of gelatin phantom before and after application of gold nanocages (a). Plots of the averaged of OCT signal as a function of depth with and without gold nanocages (b). Application of nanocages results in enhanced OCT signal only at shallow depths. OCT signal from the phantom with the nanocages decays faster than the phantom without the nanocages. (From Chen, J. et al., *Nano Lett.*, 5(3), 473, March 2005. With permission.)

along with GNRs, can also be surface functionalized for target-specific delivery for tumor imaging. Increased OCT contrast utilizing gold nanocages is illustrated in Figure 10.4.

Lastly, the use of polypyrrole nanoparticles as OCT contrast agents has also been explored. Polypyrrole is an organic compound that can be tailored to have strong absorption in the NIR. As opposed to the aforementioned nanostructures, polypyrrole nanoparticles act as negative contrast agents since they reduce OCT backscattered contrast [19].

Contrast agents have proven vital for diagnostic imaging in a variety of different imaging modalities. While OCT structural imaging has been proven clinically useful, OCT contrast agents can help improve diagnostic capabilities. Gold nanostructures have the potential for in vivo imaging of a variety of different structures either through active or passive targeting.

10.3 Magnetomotive OCT

While the contrast agents discussed in the previous section can be considered passive scattering agents, magnetomotive OCT (MMOCT) utilizes active scattering contrast agents since their scattering properties can be externally modulated. This external modulation can help differentiate contrast agent scattering from background scattering. In MMOCT, superparamagnetic iron oxide (SPIO) particles, which have large magnetic susceptibility, can be manipulated with an external magnetic field. These magnetic nanoparticles are widely used as negative contrast agents in MRI [20]. Recently, a new imaging modality termed magnetic particle imaging (MPI) was specifically developed for the detection of magnetic nanoparticles [21]. Furthermore, FDA approval makes SPIO particles an attractive choice for image enhancement.

The premise of MMOCT is the following: a small electromagnetic added to the sample arm of a conventional OCT system is used to magnetostimulate SPIO particles introduced into the sample. The magnetic nanoparticles undergo both translational and rotational movement controlled by the external magnetic field [22,23]. The system schematic is illustrated in Figure 10.5.

The magnetomotion of the SPIO particles induces the movement of the neighboring tissue, thereby resulting in local scattering changes. In an elastic medium, the magnetic nanoparticle will undergo translation when the magnetic field is applied and return to its original location when the magnetic field is turned off. Therefore, modulating the magnetic field at a certain frequency results in an oscillatory

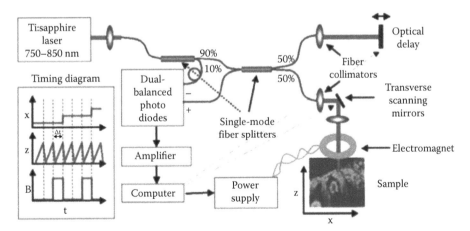

FIGURE 10.5 MMOCT system schematic. A typical time-domain OCT system is depicted utilizing a balanced-detection configuration. The electromagnet required for magnetostimulation of SPIO particles is placed in the sample arm, with the imaging beam directed through the center of the solenoid. The timing diagram depicts the image acquisition strategy. Three axial scans are obtained at the same lateral location of the sample; the electromagnet is turned on only during the third axial scan. (From Oldenburg, A. et al., *Opt. Express*, 13(17), 6597, August 2005. With permission.)

movement of the magnetic nanoparticles that induces modulation of the local scattering at the same frequency. Furthermore, because the magnetic susceptibility of tissue is small compared to magnetic nanoparticles, the effects of the external magnetic field on tissue are negligible. Any large locoregional scattering changes in the presence of the magnetic field can be attributed to SPIO particles.

The first implementation of MMOCT utilized difference imaging, in which an image without the enhancement of the contrast agents, termed a background image, is obtained and subtracted from the contrast-enhanced image to improve SNR. Specifically, difference imaging in MMOCT is achieved by obtaining three axial scans at the same lateral location on the sample. With the external magnetic field off, the first scan and the second scan are taken with a time Δt between scans. Between these two measurements, the so-called structure function, which is a measure of the intrinsic background fluctuations in the image due to speckle, can be measured. A third axial scan is taken at time Δt after the second scan with the external magnetic field turned on. The third axial scan is then normalized by the structure function to obtain the magnetomotive signal. Furthermore, the difference imaging scheme allows for simultaneously obtaining structural data from the OCT background images and molecular contrast from the magnetomotive signal [23].

External modulation of the scattering agents in MMOCT introduces new system design considerations. First, the axial scanning rate in MMOCT is limited by the completion time of magnetomotion. That is, after the magnetic particles are stimulated and undergo magnetomotion, enough time must be allotted for them to return to their original location after the magnetic field has been turned off before another axial scan can be taken. This relaxation time primarily depends on the intrinsic material properties of the surround medium. For example, the elastic modulus, or stiffness of the sample, will determine the oscillation speed of the magnetic nanoparticles after magnetostimulation. For tissue phantoms, the relaxation time was measured to be less than 1 ms; therefore, MMOCT line rate is inherently limited to 1 kHz. However, the magnetomotion dependence on tissue stiffness enables characterization of material properties via analysis of the oscillatory motion of the nanoparticles [24]. Additionally, hyperthermia induced by high-frequency modulated magnetic fields must also be considered in MMOCT. While magnetically induced hyperthermia therapy is beneficial in other scenarios, MMOCT is a diagnostic tool; therefore, the modulation of magnetic fields must be kept below 100 kHz to prevent thermal tissue damage. Furthermore, since the magnetic field induced by the electromagnet is a function of axial position, the solenoid must be placed as close as possible to the sample. Because positioning of sample relative to the electromagnet can affect signal, MMOCT is currently limited to small samples applications. To further optimize accuracy of magnetomotive signal, calibration of the magnetic field axial position dependence is typically necessary. A more recent application of MMOCT utilized a pulsed magnetic field to reduce hyperthermia risk and enable imaging of samples as far as 30 mm away from the electromagnet [25].

In the first application of MMOCT, SPIO particles were injected into *Xenopus laevis* tadpoles via passive targeting. The magnetic particles were introduced into the bloodstream and quickly uptaken by the reticuloendothelium system and finally deposited in the liver and intestines. Several sample locations were imaged with MMOCT. The majority of contrast enhancement was located in the intestines and tail, as evident in Figure 10.6 [23].

SPIO particles can also be functionalized for tissue-specific delivery. Although challenging, magnetic particles have been conjugated with proteins, enzymes, antibodies, nucleotides, and peptide ligands. One of the most popular MMOCT applications, tumor imaging with active targeted magnetic nanoparticles has been demonstrated [26]. The magnetic nanoparticles were antibody functionalized to target EFGR proteins, which are overexpressed in the presence of a tumor. The rats utilized as the animal models were injected with targeted nanoprobes, nontargeted nanoprobes, and saline solution through the tail vein. In vivo MMOCT imaging utilizing targeted nanoprobes indicated much greater concentration of contrast agent at the delivery site. The location of the magnetic particles was confirmed using histology. Clearly, using targeted nanoprobes can help reduce the amount of contrast agent needed to successfully image the site of interest, as seen in Figure 10.7.

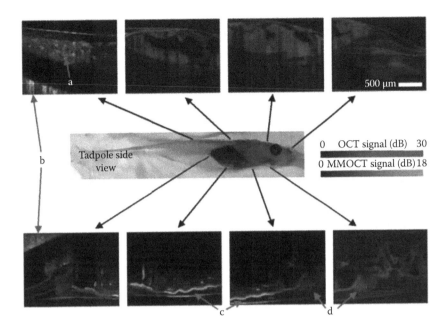

FIGURE 10.6 **(See color insert.)** MMOCT imaging of *X. laevis* tadpole at different locations. MMOCT B-scans are referenced to a microscopy image of the tadpole. (b) Magnetic particles accumulated in molding clay situated underneath tadpole. (c) MMOCT signal in the intestines of the tadpole. Accumulation of magnetic particles in the intestines is probably a result of clearance from the bloodstream. (a) MMOCT signal from the tail of the tadpole. (d) The lack of MMOCT signal from the beating heart. In MMOCT, it is important to consider that movement within the sample can result in locoregional scattering modulation and therefore might contribute to image artifacts. The lack of MMOCT signal demonstrates the effectiveness of background subtraction in difference imaging. (From Oldenburg, A. et al., *Opt. Express*, 13(17), 6597, August 2005. With permission.)

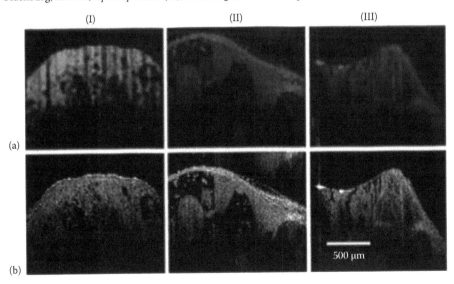

FIGURE 10.7 MMOCT imaging of breast tumors in animal model. (a) MMOCT B-scans and (b) conventional, coregistered OCT B-scans. (I) Imaging with targeted nanoprobes, (II) imaging with nontargeted nanoprobes, and (III) imaging without nanoprobes. As evident, using active targeting results in much greater nanoprobe concentration at the location of interest. Passive targeting results in almost no MMOCT signal, indicating that nanoprobes may have been cleared to another location of the body. (From John, R. et al., *Proc. Natl. Acad. Sci. U.S.A.*, 107(18), 8085, May 2010. With permission.)

Magnetic particles have been used to image a variety of different tissue types and cells. Interestingly, tissue-based macrophages can readily uptake SPIO particles, making them attractive targets for MMOCT imaging [27]. Furthermore, imaging endothelial damage is also facilitated using magnetic particles. Specifically, SPIO particles can be inserted into platelets, which are then introduced into the circulatory system. Platelets release growth factors to stimulate growth of extracellular matrix for tissue repair and are functionalized to target locations of endothelial damage. Therefore, once inserted into platelets, the SPIO particles are automatically targeted to sites of vascular tissue damage allowing identification of such sites via MMOCT [28,29], as seen in Figure 10.8. Lastly, Doppler analysis in MMOCT can help improve Doppler OCT imaging of blood flow. Because hemoglobin contains iron, a modulating magnetic field will induce magnetomotion of RBCs, which can be utilized to help differentiate the Doppler signal from background noise. Furthermore, the Doppler shift can be altered using the externally modulated magnetic field to help increase Doppler OCT SNR [30]. A similar approach can also be utilized to analyze and quantify flow of magnetic nanoparticles [31].

Since its inception in 2005, MMOCT has quickly developed into a modality with potential for *in vivo* diagnostic imaging. Imaging of a variety of tissue with targeted nanoprobes illustrates the capabilities of MMOCT. Furthermore, FDA approval of SPIO particles may expedite the transition from bench side to bedside of MMOCT in the near future.

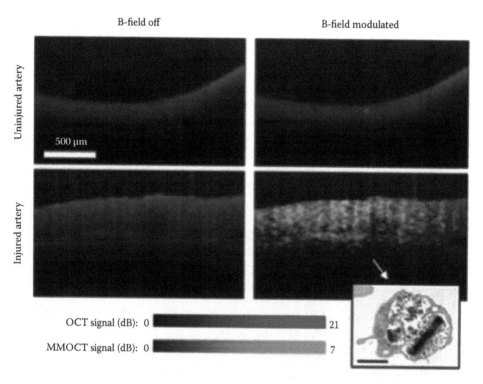

FIGURE 10.8   (See color insert.) MMOCT imaging of injured and uninjured arteries with and without the magnetic field. Top row are MMOCT B-scans of uninjured artery. Bottom row are MMOCT B-scans of injured artery. Left column shows images with magnetic field off. Right column shows images with magnetic field on. Ex vivo porcine arteries were exposed to platelets laden with SPIO particles. MMOCT signal is restricted to injured artery site, while no MMOCT signal is present from the uninjured artery. (From Oldenburg, A.L. et al., *IEEE J. Select. Top. Quantum Electron.*, 18(3), 1100, May 2012. With permission.)

10.4 Photothermal OCT

Photothermal OCT (PTOCT), similar to MMOCT, employs nanoparticles for additional molecular contrast. However, unlike the aforementioned techniques in which scattering contrast were utilized, photothermal relies on absorption of light to induce regional thermal expansion. Furthermore, PTOCT signal is independent of the inherent mechanical tissue properties and allows for lock-in detection; molecular contrast is achieved either through active or passive targeting of nanoparticles. PTOCT imaging necessitates a *heating beam* added to a conventional SD-OCT system. The heating beam is aligned using a dichroic mirror (DM) such that it copropagates with the OCT beam to ensure overlap at the sample, as depicted in Figure 10.9. PTOCT signal arises from the detection of photothermal heating.

Thermal heating of a nanoparticle induces local temperature changes that lead to thermal expansion of the surrounding tissue. Consequently, the local index of refraction of the tissue is altered, leading to changes in optical path length that are measured in the phase of the OCT interferogram. The heating beam amplitude is modulated, causing subsequent modulation of optical path length for detection of the PTOCT signal [33]. Contrast agents are chosen or engineered to have their plasmon resonance peak to coincide with the heating beam frequency. Furthermore, because PTOCT utilizes absorption rather than scattering as its contrast mechanism, photothermal detection is largely insensitive to intrinsic background fluctuations in the image [34].

The processing required to extract the PTOCT signal is as follows: the amplitude of the heating beam is modulated at a certain frequency, thereby modulating the optical path length at the same frequency. A conventional OCT M-scan is obtained and the phase data as a function of time is analyzed. A Fourier transform across the time axis is filtered about the modulation frequency of the heating beam (the phase modulation peak), giving rise to a PTOCT A-line.

Furthermore, similar to the previous molecular contrast OCT techniques discussed, the nanoparticles can be surface functionalized for active delivery to ensure a sufficient concentration is present at the target site. In a particular application of PTOCT, gold nanospheres with absorption at 532 nm were conjugated with anti-EGFR to target tumor tissue [33]. Another implementation utilized gold nanoshells—tailored for a surface plasmon resonance peak at 808 nm—and a laser diode modulated up to 60 kHz as the heating beam [35]. Similarly, gold nanoshells were employed for PTOCT imaging of ex vivo breast tissue using 830 nm excitation [36]. The relationship between photothermal particle concentration and photothermal signal can also be determined, enabling depth profiling of the photothermal compound concentration [37].

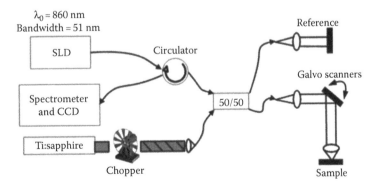

FIGURE 10.9 Schematic of PTOCT system. A Ti:sapphire laser, amplitude modulated using an optical chopper, is utilized as the heating beam. Coupling the OCT heating beam into a 50/50 fiber coupler ensures overlap of both beams at the sample. (From Tucker-Schwartz, J.M. et al., *Biomed. Opt. Express*, 3(11), 2881, November 2012. With permission.)

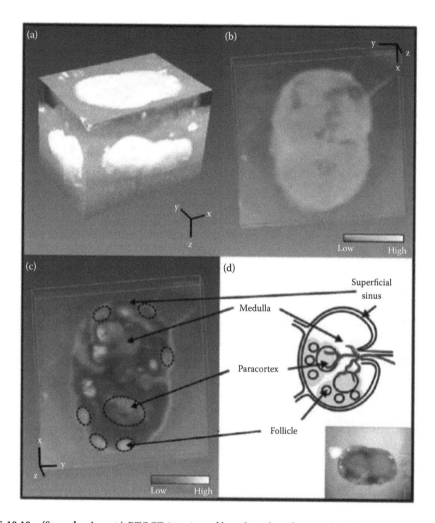

FIGURE 10.10 **(See color insert.)** PTOCT imaging of lymph nodes after uptake of passively targeted GNRs. (a) The OCT volumetric image, (b) a cross-sectional cut at around 240 μm below the surface, (c) PTOCT image at the same location, and (d) a diagram of different depicting structures of the lymph node. After uptake of GNRs, a variety of features are delineated using PTOCT. The GNRs accumulate in the cortex surrounding the follicles. (From Jung, Y. et al., *Nano Lett.*, 11, 2938, 2011. With permission.)

In a recent study, the photothermal signal in relation to GNR (using passive targeting) uptake rates at different locations in sentinel lymph nodes have been evaluated *in situ*. Such analysis can elucidate the different structures of the lymph node and how their diffusion properties vary, as seen in Figure 10.10 [38]. Other exogenous contrast agents utilized with PTOCT include nanorose for detection of macrophages [39], ICG-encapsulated PLGA nanoparticles [40], and carbon nanotubes [41].

Furthermore, the first *in vivo* implementation of PTOCT using exogenous contrast agents was recently published [32]. Nude mice were anesthetized and GNRs mixed in a Matrigel solution were injected into the ear. For a control, the Matrigel solution only was also injected into a mouse ear and imaged with PTOCT. A heating beam tuned to 795 nm was utilized. Moreover, because hemoglobin absorbs at 795 nm and might give rise to photothermal signal, Doppler OCT imaging was performed concurrently to ensure that PTOCT contrast stemmed from the GNRs and not hemoglobin absorption. Results show that PTOCT signal is not dependent on the presence of vasculature, as evident in Figure 10.11. Also, there is almost negligible PTOCT signal when GNRs are not present.

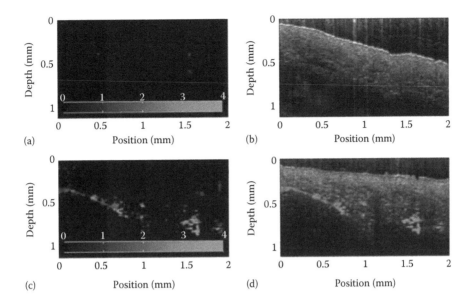

FIGURE 10.11 (See color insert.) PTOCT in vivo imaging of GNRs injected into mouse ears. (a) PTOCT and (b) OCT images without GNRs and (c, d) with GNRs. Right column depicts the OCT B-scans. Doppler OCT, depicted by the red and blue channels, is overlaid on the OCT B-scans. PTOCT B-scans are also overlaid on the OCT images. As depicted, there is PTOCT signal at locations where there are no blood vessels present as indicated by Doppler OCT. Furthermore, there is very little PTOCT signal when the GNRs are not present, indicating that PTOCT signal arises primarily from GNR absorption of the heating beam. (From Tucker-Schwartz, J.M. et al., *Biomed. Opt. Express*, 3(11), 2881, November 2012. With permission.)

Another implementation of PTOCT exploits the different absorption properties of oxyhemoglobin and deoxyhemoglobin. As opposed to other OCT techniques that capture the intensity of the backscattered spectra to analyze the absorption properties of hemoglobin (such as spectroscopic OCT [SOCT]; see Section 10.5), PTOCT is encoded through the modulation of optical path length that is detected from the phase of the interferometric OCT signal. Therefore, PTOCT detection of hemoglobin absorption is largely insensitive to speckle or other intensity variations that may otherwise contribute to noise. Furthermore, because of its dependence solely of light absorption of the targeted chromophores, PTOCT can resolve small changes in hemoglobin absorption of the heating beam. By employing dual-wavelength excitation, where wavelengths are chosen to coincide with the absorption spectra of oxyhemoglobin and deoxyhemoglobin, blood oxygen saturation levels can be measured based on PTOCT signal fluctuations. Depth-resolved blood oxygen saturation levels of microvasculature in a murine brain were measured noninvasively and compared to the current gold standard, pulse oximetry [42,43].

PTOCT is a promising imaging technology that images both endogenous and exogenous contrast agents. Because it relies on light absorption rather than scattering, PTOCT has greater sensitivity than scattering-based molecular imaging OCT techniques. A variety of different applications, including tumor imaging using functionalized contrast agents and blood oxygen saturation measurements, make PTOCT an attractive imaging modality.

10.5 Spectroscopic OCT

In addition to structural imaging provided by conventional OCT, SOCT enables spectroscopic analysis and imaging of the sample. Spectroscopy entails characterizing the absorption spectra of the different constituents of the sample of interest. Depending on the implementation, little to no hardware in addition to the traditional OCT setup is required; spectral analysis of OCT images is embedded in the software processing. Utilizing a traditional SD-OCT system, the spectral content of the sample is captured via the backscattered spectrum in a single shot. The broadband light source—required for adequate axial resolution in OCT—enables acquisition over a large bandwidth for spectroscopic analysis.

When discussing SOCT, it is important to note the inherent trade-off between coherence length and spectral resolution. Conventional OCT systems employ a broad bandwidth source to minimize the coherence length, thereby improving axial resolution of the system and worsening spectral resolution. However, in spectroscopic analysis, high spectral resolution is sometimes required to differentiate between samples that might have almost overlapping absorption spectra.

This trade-off is prominent in SOCT, where spectra of the backscattered light along the axial scanning direction vary both in time (depth) and frequency (wavelength) [44]. Therefore, if a conventional Fourier transform of the backscattered signal is used for spectroscopic analysis, the time varying information will be lost. To circumvent this problem, methods such as short-time Fourier transforms and wavelet transforms have been utilized. However, implementation of these transforms introduces the trade-off between spectral and time (depth) resolution as dictated by the time–frequency uncertainty principle or Gabor limit. In essence, a signal cannot be bounded both in the time and frequency domain. Consequently, there are a variety of time–frequency distributions arising from different processing techniques that are acceptable for different situations.

Several approaches, both processing techniques and hardware alterations, to avoid or improve the trade-off between spatial resolution and spectral resolution in SOCT have been implemented. Spectral domain spectroscopic optical coherence microscopy (SOCM) aims to decouple the spectral resolution from the spatial resolution by utilizing a high NA objective. Because a long depth of focus is desired in conventional OCT to maximize axial imaging range, the coherence length of the source limits the axial resolution. Employing high NA optics in an OCT setup, termed optical coherence microscopy (OCM), limits the depth imaging range but may improve axial resolution, which is now limited by the optics. Spectral detection in OCM allows spectroscopic analysis without the hindrance by the Gabor limit since the spectral window is physically bounded to a small focal volume. However, imaging depth range is sacrificed [45]. A more recent approach focused on processing rather than hardware to improve performance of SOCT. The so-called dual-window method refers to using two orthogonal analysis windows, one determining the temporal (spatial) resolution and the second determining the spectral resolution. The two windows are utilized to reconstruct time–frequency distributions that yield high resolution in both domains. The theoretical treatment justifying the dual-window method is found here [46,47].

The first implementation of SOCT utilized a time-domain system to allow analysis of the entire backscattered spectra at each pixel [48]. Rather than collecting solely the envelope of the interferogram, corresponding to the coherence length of the source and OCT axial resolution, the entire interferometric signal is obtained and processed for spectroscopic analysis. Reduction of backscattered signal at certain wavelength range yields information about the absorption spectra of the sample contents. SOCT B-scans of *X. laevis* in which mesenchymal cells of different sizes are present were obtained. In the SOCT image, melanocytes tend to appear red due to enhanced absorption at shorter wavelengths as shown in Figure 10.12.

Furthermore, a second early implementation of SOCT utilized a spectrometer detector to capture the backscattered spectra directly instead of capturing light intensities. Similar to backscatter spectral interferometry, capturing the spectra directly allowed access to the Fourier components of weakly scattered objects to yield information about particle sizes in the sample [49].

SOCT also enables access functional information such as absorption coefficients of hemoglobin, hemoglobin concentrations, and blood oxygen saturation measurements [50–54]. A recent SOCT implementation, utilizing a visible broad bandwidth source and the dual-window processing method previously discussed enabled en face OCT vasculature maps in addition to blood oxygen saturation measurements from specific vessels [55]. While the source spectrum in the visible range enabled higher

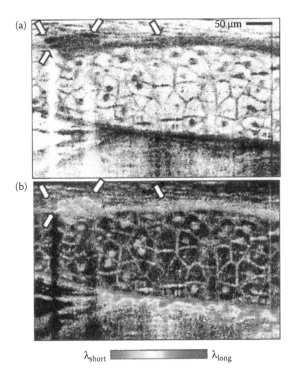

λ_{short} ▬▬▬ λ_{long}

FIGURE 10.12 (See color insert.) In vivo OCT and SOCT imaging of *X. laevis*. OCT B-scan is shown in (a), while SOCT B-scan is shown in (b). The green hue in the SOCT image indicates a short-wavelength shift of the center of the spectrum, while a red hue indicates a long-wavelength shift. Melanocytes, indicated by arrows, appear red in the SOCT due to their absorbance of short wavelengths. As evident, the melanocytes are difficult to visualize in the OCT B-scan, but are readily visible in the SOCT B-scan. (From Morgner, U. et al., *Opt. Lett.*, 25(2), 111, January 2000. With permission.)

spectral sensitivity to fluctuations in blood oxygen saturation, penetration depth of the imaging beam was sacrificed. En face SOCT images of vasculature were obtained from an in vivo mouse model, as shown in Figure 10.13. The image depicts two major blood vessels along with a network of capillaries. Four points in the image corresponding to vasculature were chosen for spectroscopic analysis. At these points, a spectral window from 520 to 585 nm was used to obtain the extinction coefficients for oxy- and deoxyhemoglobin. The measured absorption spectra for hemoglobin measured were found to match the theoretical spectra.

Furthermore, exogenous contrast agents, such as near-infrared dyes [56], gold nanocages [18], and GNRs [57], have also been utilized for enhanced contrast in SOCT. Since these contrast agents absorb, their presence can be measured through spectral analysis in SOCT. In particular, a suspension containing GNRs was injected into human breast tumor tissue. Volumetric SOCT images were taken before and after the injection of the GNRs. Utilizing spectral analysis, the location and relative density of the GNRs were measured and superimposed onto the coregistered OCT B-scans as shown in Figure 10.14. Moreover, the GNR density required for sufficient SOCT molecular contrast was calculated.

Lastly, SOCT also allows access to wavelength-dependent scattering information, similar to light scattering spectroscopy (LSS). Because the majority of cellular organelles can be interpreted as spherical models, Mie theory, in conjunction with LSS, can elucidate sample properties such as particle size and particle spatial distribution [58]. The same principle is applied in SOCT, where the modulation

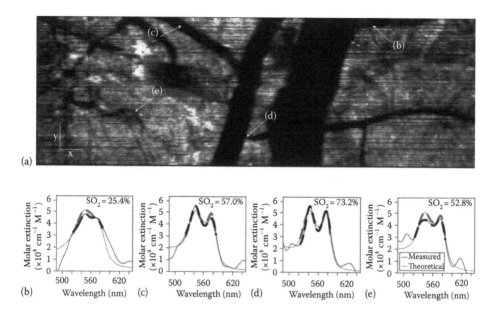

FIGURE 10.13 In vivo SOCT image of a mouse model in which vasculature is depicted. (a) Several spots in the image, denoted by arrows, are chosen for spectroscopic analysis to calculate blood oxygen saturations. The theoretical and measured molar extinction spectra are plotted for each of the four points. (b) Corresponds to a vein, while (c) and (d) correspond to arteries, and (e) corresponds to a capillary plexus. Blood oxygen saturation measurements indicate lower blood oxygenation in the veins than the arteries and capillary network. (From Robles, F.E. et al., *Nat. Photonics*, 5(12), 744, December 2011. With permission.)

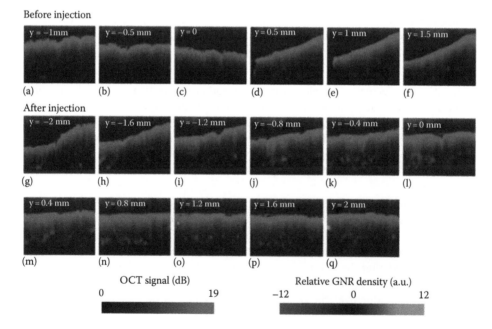

FIGURE 10.14 (**See color insert.**) GNRs were injected into excised breast carcinoma tumor tissue and OCT and SOCT volumetric were obtained before and after injection. Relative GNR density determined from SOCT signal. (a–f) depict B-scans of the same volumetric image with SOCT contrast overlaid. (g–q) show OCT B-scans of volumetric image after injection of GNRs. As evident, SOCT contrast is more apparent after injection of GNRs. (From Oldenburg, A.L. et al., *J. Mater. Chem.*, 19, 6407, January 2009. With permission.)

properties of the backscattered spectrum are dependent on size and density of the scattering particles [59]. Wavelength scattering dependence can enable contrast enhancement in SOCT [60,61] and also provide quantitative information such as scattering particle sizes [62,63].

SOCT is a fast method to evaluate the spectroscopic properties of the sample. Although there is an evident trade-off between spectral and spatial resolution, different processing techniques and hardware modifications can optimized spectroscopic analysis. Endogenous chromophores, such as oxygenated and deoxygenated hemoglobin, as well as exogenous contrast agents, can be utilized in SOCT contrast. Finally, in addition to access to absorption properties, SOCT's access to wavelength-dependent scattering information enables particle sizing.

10.6 Pump–Probe OCT

Pump–probe OCT (PPOCT) is a technique that utilizes the premise of pump–probe spectroscopy for additional molecular contrast in OCT. Pump–probe spectroscopy is used to probe different molecular energy level transition states and can provide information about the lifetime dynamics of the different excited states by varying the pump–probe delay. In essence, pump excitation causes population changes of different energy levels. A second illumination source can probe these electron population changes to provide molecular specificity. Pump–probe spectroscopy has been utilized to characterize the vibrational and orientational dynamics of hydrogen-bonded molecules [64] and to study different electron spin characteristics of heme proteins [65]. In PPOCT, the pump–probe physical process allows transient absorption of the OCT beam to enable additional molecular contrast.

In addition to the conventional OCT hardware, an additional light source to serve as the pump is necessary while the OCT beam serves as the probe in the pump–probe spectroscopy scheme. Figure 10.15 depicts the PPOCT system. A pulsed source is used for both the pump and probe to allow for pump–probe pulse delay control. Copropagation of the probe and OCT beam is ensured using a DM.

In the first implementation of PPOCT, methylene blue was the molecule of interest [66]. Methylene blue has a triplet–triplet energy level transition that can be exploited with a pump–probe scheme.

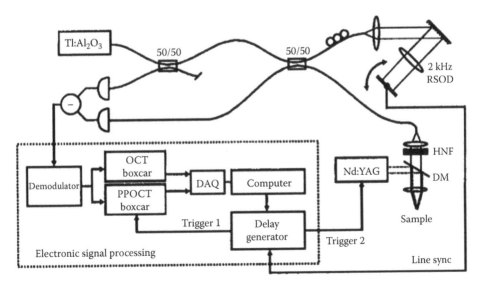

FIGURE 10.15 PPOCT system schematic. A pulsed Nd:YAG laser at 532 nm is used as the pump source and coupled onto OCT beam using a DM. A delay generator is utilized to control the interpulse pump–probe delay. A pulsed Ti:sapphire laser is used as the OCT/probe source. (From Rao, K.D. et al., *Opt. Lett.*, 28(5), 340, March 2003. With permission.)

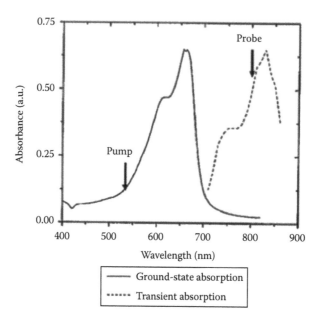

FIGURE 10.16 Ground-state absorption and transient absorption spectra of methylene blue, a commonly used biological dye. Pump and probe wavelengths are denoted. Note that the pump wavelength coincides with the ground-state absorption spectra, while the probe wavelength coincides with the transient absorption spectra. Via the pump–probe mechanism, absorption of the probe is only possible after pump excitation. (From Rao, K.D. et al., *Opt. Lett.*, 28(5), 340, March 2003. With permission.)

A 532 nm probe illuminates the chromophore exciting electrons into a triplet–triplet state. The populated lower triplet state then allows absorption of the 830 nm OCT beam/probe. Therefore, transient absorption of the probe/OCT beam is only possible after the pump has excited the chromophores. Figure 10.16 depicts the ground-state and transient absorption spectra resulting from the pump–probe interaction. Therefore, when the two beams are scanned over the chromophores of interest, transient absorption of the OCT/probe beam results in a loss of the backscattered signal measured in OCT. Amplitude modulation of the pump at a specific frequency results in modulation of the OCT signal only in the presence of chromophores, thereby allowing molecular specific contrast.

A delay generator can be utilized to control the pump–probe interpulse delay to measure lifetime dynamics of the different excited states. The process to extract the PPOCT signal from the OCT data is as follows: as mentioned before, amplitude modulation of the pump results in modulation of the OCT signal at the same frequency in the presence of the chromophore. Using a conventional OCT M-scan, the OCT amplitude modulation can be recovered. Fourier transforms along the time axis of the M-scan at every pixel depth reveal the modulation frequency, which can be extracted by filtering, ultimately yielding a PPOCT A-scan. The PPOCT signal depends on several design parameters, including pump power, concentration of the targeted chromophores, and pump–probe overlap, in addition to the traditional contributors to OCT signal degradation. Moreover, because the state populated by the pump allowing absorption of the probe has a finite lifetime, the pump–probe delay must be set accordingly to optimize PPOCT signal.

PPOCT was first used to image methylene blue in several phantoms, including a two-level well phantom containing water and the chromophore. Furthermore, a capillary tube containing methylene blue dye and submerged in a scattering medium was imaged. Figure 10.17 illustrates the experiment results. PPOCT A-lines are evident only once the pump beam has traversed the methylene blue, as shown in (a) and (b). Furthermore, PPOCT signal of the dye is present only when the pump is on. Finally, a PPOCT

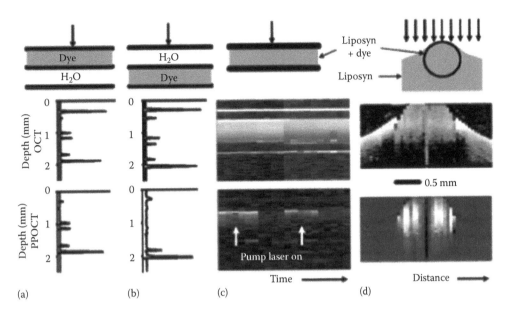

FIGURE 10.17 PPOCT imaging of different methylene blue samples. (a) and (b) Show the two-well phantom containing pure water and methylene blue in alternate locations, along with the respective OCT and PPOCT A-lines. (c) Shows OCT and PPOCT M-scans with pump laser amplitude modulated. (d) Shows OCT and PPOCT B-scans of a capillary tube filled with methylene blue and submerged in a Liposyn solution. As evident in (a) and (b), PPOCT signal is obtained only once the beams traverse the methylene blue solution. The dependence of PPOCT signal on the pump laser is demonstrated in (c). A PPOCT B-scan shown in (d) shows only contrast from the methylene blue in the capillary tube, while the OCT B-scan shows additional scattering signal from the surrounding scattering solution. (From Rao, K.D. et al., *Opt. Lett.*, 28(5), 340, March 2003. With permission.)

image depicts contrast solely from the dye in the capillary tube and not from the surrounding scattering medium, unlike in the conventional OCT B-scan.

A variety of different chromophores and pump–probe physical mechanisms have been explored in PPOCT. Using a degenerate pump–probe scheme—in which both sources have the same optical frequency—and a ground-state recovery pump–probe mechanism, dsRed, rhodamine 6G, hemoglobin, and whole blood have been imaged [67]. In ground-state recovery PPOCT (gsrPPOCT), a triplet–triplet transition is not excited, unlike PPOCT imaging of methylene blue. Instead, gsrPPOCT probes electron population differences in the original ground state after absorption of the pump using 530 nm light. gsrPPOCT was utilized to image a variety of endogenous and exogenous chromophores. Specifically, hemoglobin was imaged in wild-type zebra fish, as seen in Figure 10.18. A 3D image set of the gills after surgical removal of the operculum was obtained. Using a total power of 4 mW on the sample, no photodamage was detected. Some volume projections were also obtained from the 3D volume sets. In the OCT images, the arteries are visualized as dark lines, corresponding to low OCT signal due to hemoglobin absorption of the 530 nm illumination. However, in the gsrPPOCT images, the arteries appear bright due to the added molecular contrast. A thresholded gsrPPOCT image superimposed on the OCT images demonstrates the corregistration of the two.

Other implementations of PPOCT investigated the use of ICG, one of the few FDA-approved exogenous optical contrast agents. ICG was imaged using PPOCT in *X. laevis* [68]. Furthermore, while previous implementations of PPOCT utilized a time-domain OCT setup, the first Fourier-domain PPOCT system was recently demonstrated for imaging of melanin ex vivo in a porcine iris [69]. This system offered several advantages over previous implementations, including faster line rates and access to the interferometric phase information enabled by the phase stability of an FD-OCT system. Furthermore,

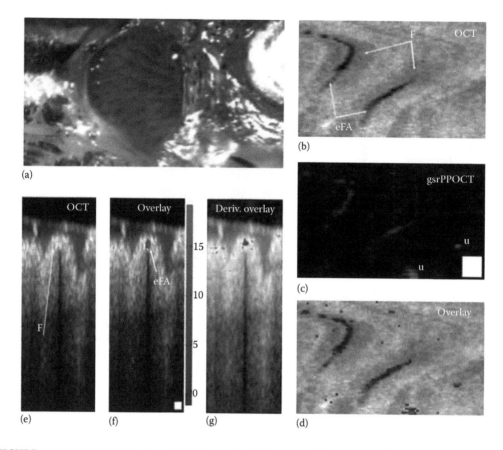

FIGURE 10.18 gsrPPOCT imaging of wild-type zebra fish arteries. (a) Depicts a photo of the gills. (b–d) are volume projections to provide an *en face* view of the gills. (c) is the corresponding gsrPPOCT image, while (d) is the superimposed OCT and PPOCT image. (e) and (f) are the OCT and PPOCT B-scans depicting an artery, respectively. (g) is the derivative image from (f). Notice how, in the convectional B-scans, arteries are depicted with negative contrast due to absorption of the 532 nm OCT beam. However, with the additional gsrOCT contrast, the arteries are clearly defined with positive contrast and can be overlaid on the OCT B-scans to give both structural and molecular information. (From Applegate, B.E. and Izatt, J.A., *Opt. Express*, 14(20), 9142, October 2006. With permission.)

while some of the previous PPOCT implementations utilized a 530 nm probe source, this system utilized a 532 nm pump and an 830 nm probe/OCT beam, exploiting the longer penetration depth afforded by IR illumination. The large concentration of melanin in a porcine iris was imaged with both OCT and PPOCT. Moreover, since PPOCT signal is a function of chromophore concentration, melanin concentration maps were readily derived from the PPOCT data, as depicted in Figure 10.19. Additional work in Fourier Domain PPOCT included *in vivo* imaging of *Xenopus* vasculature using hemoglobin as the contrast agent [70].

PPOCT enables molecular specificity by exploiting pump–probe physical mechanisms inherent to the target chromophore. Furthermore, varying the pump–probe delay and recording the change in PPOCT signal can measure the relaxation dynamics of the different excited electronic states. PPOCT ex vivo imaging of a variety of different exogenous and endogenous chromophores, including methylene blue, dsRed, rhodamine 6G, melanin, hemoglobin, and whole blood, has been demonstrated.

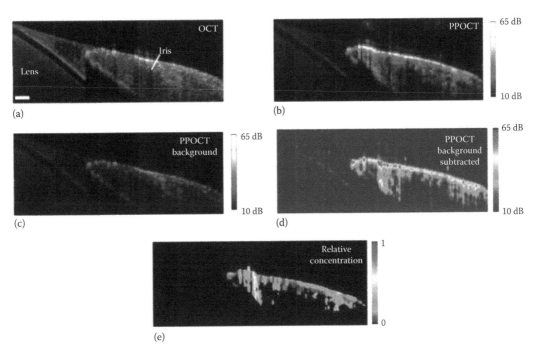

FIGURE 10.19 **(See color insert.)** Fourier-domain PPOCT ex vivo imaging of melanin in a porcine iris. (a) Shows the conventional OCT image, (b) shows the PPOCT image, (c) shows the PPOCT background image, (d) shows the PPOCT image after background subtraction, and (e) shows a melanin relative concentration map. The PPOCT signal clearly shows additional molecular contrast from melanin. The ratio of the PPOCT image after background subtraction and the OCT image yields a reflectivity-independent relative concentration map of melanin. 1 indicates maximum concentration. (From Jacob, D. et al., *Opt. Express*, 18(12), 12399, July 2010. With permission.)

10.7 Second Harmonic Generation OCT

Second harmonic generation (SHG) of tissue is a well-studied phenomenon. The tissue sample emits light at twice the frequency of the excitation source due to nonlinear optical susceptibility in the sample. This nonlinear process is determined by the molecule's specific structure and orientation, thereby enabling the potential for molecular specific contrast. Using a ruby 694 nm laser, SHG was first demonstrated in corneas, scleras, skin, whole blood, and tumor melanosomes in different animal models [71]. Furthermore, collagen, skeletal muscle, and microtubules were shown to exhibit SHG, where the SHG efficiency is dependent of the structure orientation relative to the illumination. In particular, SHG microscopy was utilized to image collagen in tendons and cartilage [72,73]. Since SHG is a coherent process, interferometric detection of the phenomena is possible and can provide added sensitivity. SHG generation from the sample can be interfered with SHG of a nonlinear crystal in the sample arm of an interferometer [74].

Because it is a coherence process, SHG is an attractive method for additional molecular contrast in OCT (SHOCT). In SHOCT, a conventional OCT system is utilized and a sample that exhibits SHG is placed at the sample arm, while a nonlinear crystal is placed at the reference arm to produce SHG at the same frequency. It is interesting to note that the axial resolution of the SHOCT image now depends on the properties of the frequency-doubled light and not the fundamental frequency. The topology of a conventional OCT system can be modified slightly to enable concurrent acquisition of the interferometric fringes from both light frequencies to enable simultaneous OCT and SHOCT imaging [75,76]. Because SHG is only possible in noncentrosymmetric highly ordered structures, such as collagen, the polarization state of the frequency-doubled emitted light can elucidate the orientation of the sample.

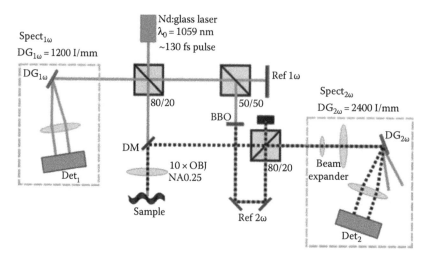

FIGURE 10.20 The schematic of a spectral domain SHOCT setup. The solid line delineates the fundamental beam's path, while the dashed line indicates the SH light. Two different spectrometers are used to detect the fundamental and the SH beam simultaneously (Det₁, Det₂). A nonlinear crystal (BBO) was used to generate the second harmonic reference light. A DM separated the two beams. (From Sarunic, M.V. et al., *Opt. Lett.*, 30(18), 2391, September 2005. With permission.)

While the original SHOCT implementation utilized a time-domain scheme, spectral domain SHOCT for greater sensitivity has also been demonstrated [77]. The schematic of the system is depicted in Figure 10.20. Second harmonic light generated from the sample is interfered with second harmonic light generated from a nonlinear crystal and directed to a spectrometer detector. The fundamental light is decoupled from the second harmonic generated light using a DM, and the interference of the fundamental light is detected using a separate spectrometer, thus allowing simultaneous acquisition of both frequency signals.

To demonstrate the molecular imaging capabilities of the SHG system, fish skin and a chicken wing containing collagen were imaged. SHOCT imaging of the fish skin clearly delineates the location of scales, which are composed of collagen. Furthermore, the molecular contrast enabled by SHOCT enabled differentiation of cartilage, periosteum, and bone from the chicken wing. SHG signal is evident from the cartilage and periosteum containing collagen, while bone is only visible via conventional OCT signal, as illustrated in Figure 10.21. Other implementations of SHOCT include imaging collagen in a rat tail [78] and pig leg tendon [79].

As previously mentioned, SHG signal depends on the orientation and anisotropy of the tissue. Therefore, the polarization of the incident beam relative to the orientation of the collagen fibrils affects SHG efficiency. Specifically, polarized incident light parallel to the collagen fibrils yields maximum SHG signal. Conversely, collagen fibrils oriented perpendicularly to the incident light polarization yield the minimum SHG signal. Therefore, by varying the polarization of the incident light, the fibrillar alignment of the collagen can be deduced. The SH polarization in both arms of the OCT system can be controlled with half-wave plates. The polarization anisotropy of fish scales and rabbit-eye sclera was imaged with SHOCT by varying the polarization of the fundamental beam incident on the sample, as shown in Figure 10.22 [79]. The signal intensities of the SHG light using orthogonal polarization states of the fundamental beam can be utilized to calculate the anisotropy of the sample.

SH-OCT utilizes endogenous contrast agents—primarily collagen—for molecular specificity. Utilizing a nonlinear crystal in the sample arm enables the interferometric detection of SHG. Furthermore, simultaneous collection of the fundamental and SGH light enables structural and molecular imaging concurrently. The polarization dependences of the SGH signal can elucidate fibril orientation as well.

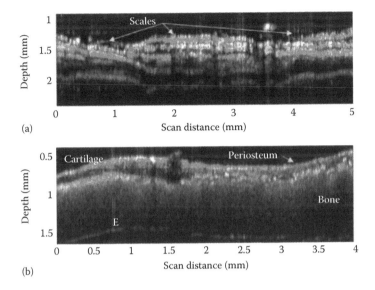

(a)

(b)

FIGURE 10.21 Second harmonic images of fish skin (a) and chicken wing bone (b). SHG from collagen is visualized. Using the added molecular contrast from SHG OCT, the scales containing collagen can be differentiated from the rest of the fish skin. Furthermore, the cartilage and periosteum containing collagen can be differentiated from the chicken wing bone. (From Sarunic, M.V. et al., *Opt. Lett.*, 30(18), 2391, September 2005. With permission.)

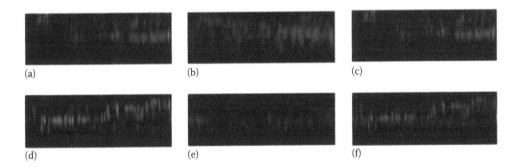

FIGURE 10.22 SH-OCT images of fish scales and rabbit-eye sclera illustrating polarization anisotropy. (a–c) SH-OCT images of fish scales with the fundamental at different polarizations. (d–f) SH-OCT images of rabbit-eye sclera. Left column are images when polarization of fundamental and second harmonic radiation are perpendicular. Middle column are images when polarization of fundamental and second harmonic radiation are parallel. Left column shows overlay of the two polarization-resolved SH-OCT images. The orientation of the collagen fibrils can be deduced from the polarization-resolved images. (From Su, J. et al., *Appl. Opt.*, 46(10), 1770, 2007. With permission.)

10.8 Conclusion

Although not yet clinically accepted, molecular imaging OCT presents substantial benefits over conventional fluorescence-based imaging, including a longer depth of focus and enhanced penetration depth. To this end, a variety of schemes to merge molecular specificity with OCT have been developed and discussed here. By exploiting the different absorption and scattering properties of a variety of exogenous contrast agents, techniques such as MMOCT, PPOCT, and SOCT provide molecular specificity in conjunction with structural imaging. Furthermore, endogenous molecules and structures, such as hemoglobin, collagen, and melanin, can be probed for functional imaging. In addition, quantitative diagnostic parameters, including blood oxygen saturation, can be obtained from the OCT molecular specificity. While conventional OCT is a well-accepted imaging modality, additional molecular contrast may help enhance its diagnostic capabilities and provide a more complete analysis of pathology.

References

1. D. Huang, E. A. Swanson, C. P. Lin, J. S. Schuman, W. G. Stinson, W. Chang, M. R. Hee et al., Optical coherence tomography, *Science*, 254, 1178–1181, 1991.
2. P. T. C. So, C. Y. Dong, B. R. Masters, and K. M. Berland, Two-photon excitation fluorescence microscopy, *Annual Review of Biomedical Engineering*, 2, 399–429, 2000.
3. P. R. Selvin, The renaissance of fluorescence resonance energy transfer, *Nature Structural Biology*, 7(9), 730–734, September 2000.
4. D. Loerke, B. Preitz, W. Stühmer, and M. Oheim, Super-resolution measurements with evanescent-wave fluorescence excitation using variable beam incidence, *Journal of Biomedical Optics*, 5(1), 23–30, January 2000.
5. E. M. Sevick-Muraca, W. J. Akers, B. P. Joshi, G. D. Luker, C. S. Cutler, L. J. Marnett, C. H. Contag, T. D. Wang, and A. Azhdarinia, Advancing the translation of optical imaging agents for clinical imaging, *Biomedical Optics Express*, 4(1), 160–170, January 2013.
6. C. Yang, Molecular contrast optical coherence tomography: A review, *Photochemistry and Photobiology*, 81, 215–237, 2005.
7. T. M. Lee, A. L. Oldenburg, S. Sitafalwalla, D. L. Marks, W. Luo, F. J.-J. Toublan, K. S. Suslick, and S. A. Boppart, Engineered microsphere contrast agents for optical coherence tomography, *Optics Letters*, 28(17), 1546–1548, September 2003.
8. E. V. Zagaynova, M. V. Shirmanova, M. Y. Kirillin, B. N. Khlebtsov, A. G. Orlova, I. V. Balalaeva, M. A. Sirotkina, M. L. Bugrova, P. D. Agrba, and V. A. Kamensky, Contrasting properties of gold nanoparticles for optical coherence tomography: Phantom, *in vivo* studies and Monte Carlo simulation, *Physics in Medicine and Biology*, 53(18), 4995–5009, September 2008.
9. Y. Xia, N. J. Halas, and G. Editors, Shape-controlled surface plasmonic nanostructures, *Chemical Physics Letters*, 2–4(May), 243–247, 1988.
10. S. Oldenburg, R. Averitt, S. Westcott, and N. Halas, Nanoengineering of optical resonances, *Chemical Physics Letters*, 288(2–4), 243–247, May 1998.
11. R. John and S. A. Boppart, Magnetomotive molecular nanoprobes, *Current Medicinal Chemistry*, 18(14), 2103–2114, January 2011.
12. J. C. Y. Kah, M. Olivo, T. H. Chow, K. S. Song, K. Z. Y. Koh, S. Mhaisalkar, and C. J. R. Sheppard, Control of optical contrast using gold nanoshells for optical coherence tomography imaging of mouse xenograft tumor model in vivo, *Journal of Biomedical Optics*, 14(5), 1–13, 2009.
13. K. Sokolov, M. Follen, J. Aaron, I. Pavlova, A. Malpica, R. Lotan, and R. Richards-Kortum, Real-time vital optical imaging of precancer using anti-epidermal growth factor receptor antibodies conjugated to gold nanoparticles, *Cancer Research*, 63, 1999–2004, 2003.
14. A. M. Gobin, M. H. Lee, N. J. Halas, W. D. James, R. A. Drezek, and J. L. West, Near-infrared resonant nanoshells for combined optical imaging and photothermal cancer therapy, *Nano Letters*, 7(7), 1929–1934, July 2007.
15. J. C. Y. Kah, T. H. Chow, B. K. Ng, S. G. Razul, M. Olivo, and C. J. R. Sheppard, Concentration dependence of gold nanoshells on the enhancement of optical coherence tomography images: A quantitative study, *Applied Optics*, 48(10), D96–D108, April 2009.
16. A. L. Oldenburg, M. N. Hansen, D. A. Zweifel, A. Wei, and S. A. Boppart, Plasmon-resonant gold nanorods as low backscattering albedo contrast agents for optical coherence tomography, *Optics Express*, 14(15), 6724–6738, July 2006.

17. J. Chen, F. Saeki, B. J. Wiley, H. Cang, M. J. Cobb, Z.-Y. Li, L. Au, H. Zhang, M. B. Kimmey, X. Li, and Y. Xia, Gold nanocages: Bioconjugation and their potential use as optical imaging contrast agents, *Nano Letters*, 5(3), 473–477, March 2005.

18. H. Cang, T. Sun, Z.-Y. Li, J. Chen, B. J. Wiley, Y. Xia, and X. Li, Gold nanocages as contrast agents for spectroscopic optical coherence tomography, *Optics Letters*, 30(22), 3048–3050, November 2005.

19. K. M. Au, Z. Lu, S. J. Matcher, and S. P. Armes, Polypyrrole nanoparticles: A potential optical coherence tomography contrast agent for cancer imaging, *Advanced Materials* (Deerfield Beach, FL), 23(48), 5792–5795, December 2011.

20. E. M. Shapiro, S. Skrtic, K. Sharer, J. M. Hill, C. E. Dunbar, and A. P. Koretsky, MRI detection of single particles for cellular imaging, *Proceedings of the National Academy of Sciences of the United States of America*, 101(30), 10901–10906, July 2004.

21. P. W. Goodwill and S. M. Conolly, The X-space formulation of the magnetic particle imaging process: 1-D signal, resolution, bandwidth, SNR, SAR, and magnetostimulation, *IEEE Transactions on Medical Imaging*, 29(11), 1851–1859, 2010.

22. A. L. Oldenburg, J. R. Gunther, and S. A. Boppart, Imaging magnetically labeled cells with magnetomotive optical coherence tomography, *Optics Letters*, 30(7), 747–749, April 2005.

23. A. Oldenburg, F. Toublan, K. Suslick, A. Wei, and S. Boppart, Magnetomotive contrast for in vivo optical coherence tomography, *Optics Express*, 13(17), 6597–6614, August 2005.

24. A. L. Oldenburg and S. A. Boppart, Resonant acoustic spectroscopy of soft tissues using embedded magnetomotive nanotransducers and optical coherence tomography, *Physics in Medicine and Biology*, 55(4), 1189–1201, February 2010.

25. J. Koo, C. Lee, H. W. Kang, Y. W. Lee, J. Kim, and J. Oh, Pulsed magneto-motive optical coherence tomography for remote cellular imaging, *Optics Letters*, 37(17), 3714–3716, September 2012.

26. R. John, R. Rezaeipoor, S. G. Adie, E. J. Chaney, A. L. Oldenburg, M. Marjanovic, J. P. Haldar, B. P. Sutton, and S. A. Boppart, In vivo magnetomotive optical molecular imaging using targeted magnetic nanoprobes, *Proceedings of the National Academy of Sciences of the United States of America*, 107(18), 8085–8090, May 2010.

27. J. Oh, M. D. Feldman, J. Kim, H. W. Kang, P. Sanghi, and T. E. Milner, Magneto-motive detection of tissue-based macrophages by differential phase optical coherence tomography, *Lasers in Surgery and Medicine*, 39(3), 266–272, March 2007.

28. A. L. Oldenburg, C. M. Gallippi, F. Tsui, T. C. Nichols, K. N. Beicker, R. K. Chhetri, D. Spivak, A. Richardson, and T. H. Fischer, Magnetic and contrast properties of labeled platelets for magnetomotive optical coherence tomography, *Biophysical Journal*, 99(7), 2374–2383, October 2010.

29. A. L. Oldenburg, G. Wu, D. Spivak, F. Tsui, A. S. Wolberg, and T. H. Fischer, Imaging and elastometry of blood clots using magnetomotive optical coherence tomography and labeled platelets, *IEEE Journal of Selected Topics in Quantum Electronics*, 18(3), 1100–1109, May 2012.

30. J. Kim, J. Oh, T. E. Milner, and J. S. Nelson, Hemoglobin contrast in magnetomotive optical Doppler tomography, *Optics Letters*, 31(6), 778, 2006.

31. J. Kim, J. Oh, T. E. Milner, and J. S. Nelson, Imaging nanoparticle flow using magneto-motive optical Doppler tomography, *Nanotechnology*, 18(3), 035504, January 2007.

32. J. M. Tucker-Schwartz, T. A. Meyer, C. A. Patil, C. L. Duvall, and M. C. Skala, In vivo photothermal optical coherence tomography of gold nanorod contrast agents, *Biomedical Optics Express*, 3(11), 2881–2895, November 2012.

33. M. C. Skala, M. J. Crow, A. Wax, and J. A. Izatt, Photothermal optical coherence tomography of epidermal growth factor receptor in live cells using immunotargeted gold nanospheres, *Nano Letters*, 8(10), 3461–3467, October 2008.

34. D. Boyer, P. Tamarat, A. Maali, B. Lounis, and M. Orrit, Photothermal imaging of nanometer-sized metal particles among scatterers, *Science*, 297(5584), 1160–1163, 2002.

35. D. C. Adler, S.-W. Huang, R. Huber, and J. G. Fujimoto, Photothermal detection of gold nanoparticles using phase-sensitive optical coherence tomography, *Optics Express*, 16(7), 4376–4393, March 2008.

36. C. Zhou, T.-H. Tsai, D. C. Adler, H.-C. Lee, D. W. Cohen, A. Mondelblatt, Y. Wang, J. L. Connolly, and J. G. Fujimoto, Photothermal optical coherence tomography in ex vivo human breast tissues using gold nanoshells, *Optics Letters*, 35(5), 700–702, March 2010.

37. G. Guan, R. Reif, Z. Huang, and R. K. Wang, Depth profiling of photothermal compound concentrations using phase sensitive optical coherence tomography, *Journal of Biomedical Optics*, 16(12), 126003, 2011.

38. Y. Jung, R. Reif, Y. Zeng, and R. K. Wang, Three-dimensional high-resolution imaging of gold nanorods uptake in sentinel lymph nodes, *Nano Letters*, 11, 2938–2943, 2011.

39. A. S. Paranjape, R. Kuranov, S. Baranov, L. L. Ma, J. W. Villard, T. Wang, K. V. Sokolov, M. D. Feldman, K. P. Johnston, and T. E. Milner, Depth resolved photothermal OCT detection of macrophages in tissue using nanorose, *Biomedical Optics Express*, 1(1), 2, June 2010.

40. H. M. Subhash, H. Xie, J. W. Smith, and O. J. T. Mccarty, Optical detection of indocyanine green encapsulated acid nanoparticles with photothermal optical coherence tomography, *Optics Letters*, 37(5), 981–983, 2012.

41. J. M. Tucker-Schwartz, T. Hong, D. C. Colvin, Y. Xu, and M. C. Skala, Dual-modality photothermal optical coherence tomography and magnetic-resonance imaging of carbon nanotubes, *Optics Letters*, 37(5), 872, February 2012.

42. R. V. Kuranov, J. Qiu, A. B. Mcelroy, A. Estrada, J. Kiel, A. K. Dunn, T. Q. Duong, and T. E. Milner, Depth-resolved blood oxygen saturation measurement by dual-wavelength photothermal (DWP) optical coherence tomography, *Biomedical Optics Express*, 2(12), 491–504, 2011.

43. R. V. Kuranov, S. Kazmi, A. B. McElroy, J. W. Kiel, A. K. Dunn, T. E. Milner, and T. Q. Duong, In vivo depth-resolved oxygen saturation by dual-wavelength photothermal (DWP) OCT, *Optics Express*, 19(24), 23831–23844, November 2011.

44. C. Xu, F. Kamalabadi, and S. A. Boppart, Comparative performance analysis of time-frequency distributions for spectroscopic optical coherence tomography, *Applied Optics*, 44(10), 1813–1822, May 2005.

45. C. Xu, C. Vinegoni, T. S. Ralston, W. Luo, W. Tan, and S. A. Boppart, Spectroscopic spectral-domain optical coherence microscopy, *Optics Letters*, 31(8), 1079–1081, May 2006.

46. F. Robles, R. N. Graf, and A. Wax, Dual window method for processing spectroscopic optical coherence tomography signals with simultaneously high spectral and temporal resolution, *Optics Express*, 17(8), 6799–6812, May 2009.

47. R. N. Graf and A. Wax, Temporal coherence and time-frequency distributions in spectroscopic optical coherence tomography, *Journal of the Optical Society of America A*, 24(8), 2186–2195, 2007.

48. U. Morgner, W. Drexler, F. X. Kärtner, X. D. Li, C. Pitris, E. P. Ippen, and J. G. Fujimoto, Spectroscopic optical coherence tomography, *Optics Letters*, 25(2), 111–113, January 2000.

49. R. Leitgeb, M. Wojtkowski, A. Kowalczyk, C. K. Hitzenberger, M. Sticker, and A. F. Fercher, Spectral measurement of absorption by spectroscopic frequency-domain optical coherence tomography, *Optics Letters*, 25(11), 820–822, July 2000.

50. D. J. Faber and T. G. van Leeuwen, Are quantitative attenuation measurements of blood by optical coherence tomography feasible? *Optics Letters*, 34(9), 1435–1437, May 2009.

51. D. J. Faber, E. G. Mik, M. C. G. Aalders, and T. G. van Leeuwen, Light absorption of (oxy-)hemoglobin assessed by spectroscopic optical coherence tomography, *Optics Letters*, 28(16), 1436–1438, August 2003.

52. F. E. Robles, S. Chowdhury, and A. Wax, Assessing hemoglobin concentration using spectroscopic optical coherence tomography for feasibility of tissue diagnostics, *Biomedical Optics Express*, 1(1), 310–317, January 2010.

53. D. J. Faber, E. G. Mik, M. C. G. Aalders, and T. G. van Leeuwen, Toward assessment of blood oxygen saturation by spectroscopic optical coherence tomography, *Optics Letters*, 30(9), 1015–1017, May 2005.

54. J. Yi and X. Li, Estimation of oxygen saturation from erythrocytes by high-resolution spectroscopic optical coherence tomography, *Optics Letters*, 35(12), 2094–2096, July 2010.

55. F. E. Robles, C. Wilson, G. Grant, and A. Wax, Molecular imaging true-colour spectroscopic optical coherence tomography, *Nature Photonics*, 5(12), 744–747, December 2011.

56. C. Xu, J. Ye, D. L. Marks, and S. A. Boppart, Near-infrared dyes as contrast-enhancing agents for spectroscopic optical coherence tomography, *Optics Letters*, 29(14), 1647–1649, July 2004.

57. A. L. Oldenburg, M. N. Hansen, T. S. Ralston, A. Wei, and S. A. Boppart, Imaging gold nanorods in excised human breast carcinoma by spectroscopic optical coherence tomography, *Journal of Materials Chemistry*, 19, 6407–6411, January 2009.

58. P. M. A. Sloot, A. G. Hoekstra, and C. G. Figdor, Osmotic response of lymphocytes measured by means of forward light scattering: Theoretical considerations, *Cytometry*, 9, 636–641, 1988.

59. A. Wax, C. Yang, and J. A. Izatt, Fourier-domain low-coherence interferometry for light-scattering spectroscopy, *Optics Letters*, 28(14), 1230–1232, 2003.

60. C. Xu, D. Marks, M. Do, and S. Boppart, Separation of absorption and scattering profiles in spectroscopic optical coherence tomography using a least-squares algorithm, *Optics Express*, 12(20), 4790–4803, October 2004.

61. D. Adler, T. Ko, P. Herz, and J. Fujimoto, Optical coherence tomography contrast enhancement using spectroscopic analysis with spectral autocorrelation, *Optics Express*, 12(22), 5487–5501, December 2004.

62. C. Xu, P. Carney, and S. Boppart, Wavelength-dependent scattering in spectroscopic optical coherence tomography, *Optics Express*, 13(14), 5450–5462, July 2005.

63. J. Yi, J. Gong, and X. Li, Analyzing absorption and scattering spectra of micro-scale structures with spectroscopic optical coherence tomography, *Optics Express*, 17(15), 13157–13167, July 2009.

64. S. Woutersen, U. Emmerichs, and H. J. Bakker, Femtosecond Mid-IR pump-probe spectroscopy of liquid water: Evidence for a two-component structure, *Science*, 278(5338), 658–660, October 1997.

65. F. Rosca, A. T. N. Kumar, D. Ionascu, T. Sjodin, A. A. Demidov, and P. M. Champion, Wavelength selective modulation in femtosecond pump–probe spectroscopy and its application to heme proteins, *The Journal of Chemical Physics*, 114(24), 10884–10898, 2001.

66. K. D. Rao, M. A. Choma, S. Yazdanfar, A. M. Rollins, and J. A. Izatt, Molecular contrast in optical coherence tomography by use of a pump–probe technique, *Optics Letters*, 28(5), 340–342, March 2003.

67. B. E. Applegate and J. A. Izatt, Molecular imaging of endogenous and exogenous chromophores using ground state recovery pump–probe optical coherence tomography, *Optics Express*, 14(20), 9142–9155, October 2006.

68. Z. Yaqoob, E. McDowell, J. Wu, X. Heng, J. Fingler, and C. Yang, Molecular contrast optical coherence tomography: A pump–probe scheme using indocyanine green as a contrast agent, *Journal of Biomedical Optics*, 11(5), 054017, 2006.

69. D. Jacob, R. L. Shelton, and B. E. Applegate, Fourier domain pump–probe optical coherence tomography imaging of melanin, *Optics Express*, 18(12), 12399–12410, July 2010.

70. O. Carrasco-Zevallos, R. L. Shelton, W. Kim, J. Pearson, and B. E. Applegate, In vivo pump–probe optical coherence tomography imaging in *Xenopus laevis*, *Journal of Biophotonics*, 2013, doi: 10.1002/jbio.201300119. [Epub ahead of print].

71. S. Fine and W. P. Hansen, Optical second harmonic generation in biological systems, *Applied Optics*, 10(10), 2350–2353, October 1971.

72. I. Freund and M. Deutsch, Second-harmonic microscopy of biological tissue, *Optics Letters*, 11(2), 94–96, February 1986.

73. W. R. Zipfel, R. M. Williams, R. Christie, A. Y. Nikitin, B. T. Hyman, and W. W. Webb, Live tissue intrinsic emission microscopy using multiphoton-excited native fluorescence and second harmonic generation, *Proceedings of the National Academy of Sciences of the United States of America*, 100(12), 7075–7080, June 2003.

74. S. Yazdanfar, L. Laiho, and P. So, Interferometric second harmonic generation microscopy, *Optics Express*, 12(12), 2739–2745, June 2004.

75. Y. Jiang, I. Tomov, Y. Wang, and Z. Chen, Second harmonic optical coherence tomography, *Optics Letters*, 29(10), 1090–1092, January 2004.

76. B. E. Applegate, C. Yang, A. M. Rollins, and J. A. Izatt, Polarization-resolved second-harmonic-generation optical coherence tomography in collagen, *Optics Letters*, 29(19), 2252–2254, October 2004.

77. M. V. Sarunic, B. E. Applegate, and J. A. Izatt, Spectral domain second-harmonic optical coherence tomography, *Optics Letters*, 30(18), 2391–2393, September 2005.

78. Y. Jiang, I. V. Tomov, Y. Wang, and Z. Chen, High-resolution second-harmonic optical coherence tomography of collagen in rat-tail tendon, *Applied Physics Letters*, 86(13), 133901, 2005.

79. J. Su, I. V. Tomov, Y. Jiang, and Z. Chen, High-resolution frequency-domain second-harmonic optical coherence tomography, *Applied Optics*, 46(10), 1770–1775, 2007.

11

Multiscale Photoacoustic Microscopy and Macroscopy

Song Hu
Washington University in St. Louis

Lihong V. Wang
Washington University in St. Louis

11.1 Introduction

Optical imaging, providing physiologically specific optical absorption, scattering, polarization, and molecular contrasts with nonionizing radiation, is a promising tool for medical diagnosis. Moreover, it complements the established nonoptical clinical modalities (e.g., magnetic resonance imaging, x-ray computed tomography, positron emission tomography, and ultrasound imaging) by providing insights at the cell and organelle levels (Figure 11.1). However, in vivo optical imaging is challenging due to strong tissue scattering and absorption. There are two fundamental depth limits for pure optical imaging. The first is near one transport mean free path (TMFP), the depth dimension of the quasiballistic regime in biological tissues (~1 mm; yellow dashed line in Figure 11.1).[1] To reach the depth of one TMFP, incident photons may undergo as many as tens of scattering events, which disable effective optical focusing. Thus, TMFP presents as the *soft* depth limit (also called the diffusion limit) for all ballistic optical microscopy (e.g., confocal microscopy, two-photon microscopy [TPM], and optical coherence tomography [OCT]). The second depth limit is around 5–7 cm (red dashed line in Figure 11.1), which corresponds to a 43 dB one-way decay in light intensity.[1] Beyond this limit, referred to as the *hard* depth limit for all optical imaging modalities, there are simply not enough photons to provide sufficient signal-to-noise ratio.

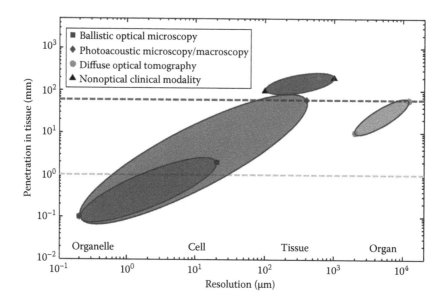

FIGURE 11.1 (**See color insert.**) Spatial resolution and tissue penetration depth of modern biomedical imaging technologies.

Mainstream optical imaging modalities operate at two distinct spatial scales: ballistic optical microscopy provides cell-level resolution within the soft limit and diffuse optical tomography (DOT) provides organ-level resolution toward the hard limit (Figure 11.1). The spatial resolution and penetration differences between optical microscopy and DOT are 2–3 orders of magnitude, leaving high-resolution (tissue level) imaging at the quasidiffusive and diffusive regimes inaccessible. Photoacoustic tomography (PAT) ultrasonically breaks through the soft depth limit and bridges the spatial gap.

PAT optically excites biological tissues with short-pulsed or intensity-modulated light and then acoustically detects pressure waves generated from an optical-absorption-induced transient temperature rise. The conversion of optical absorption into ultrasonic waves enables PAT to achieve high acoustic resolution beyond the soft limit. Moreover, with the one-way optical path rather than the round trip in pure optical modalities, PAT experiences less optical attenuation and thus holds the potential to operate beyond the hard depth limit. Besides the excellent spatial scalability of PAT, its exclusive sensitivity to optical absorption (i.e., 100%) makes it a unique complement to other optical imaging modalities, which are primarily sensitive to optical scattering, polarization, and fluorescence.

In this chapter, we focus on multiscale and multicontrast photoacoustic microscopy and macroscopy (PAM and PAMac), an emerging PAT implementation with spatial resolution spanning from submicrons in the ballistic regime to submillimeters in the diffusive regime (Figure 11.1). Photoacoustic computed tomography (PACT), another major PAT implementation, will not be discussed here in detail. First, the principle and the instrumentation of multiscale PAM and PAMac are illustrated, and then major photoacoustic contrast sources are discussed. After that, a wide spectrum of biomedical applications in neurology, ophthalmology, dermatology, oncology, cardiology, and gastroenterology are introduced, and a few future directions are proposed in the conclusion of the chapter.

11.2 Spatial Scalability of PAM and PAMac

PAM and PAMac, similar to OCT, are based on 2D raster scanning for 3D imaging. To maximize detection sensitivity, optical irradiation and ultrasonic detection are configured confocally in PAM and PAMac. Depending on the depth, one of the dual foci primarily determines the lateral resolution.[2]

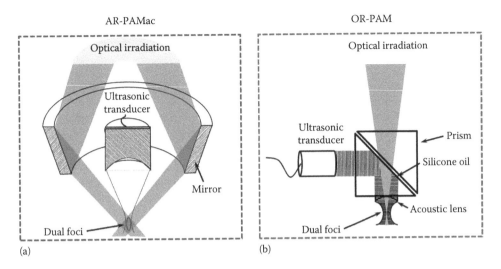

FIGURE 11.2 Multiscale PAM and PAMac. Acousto-optical confocal configurations of (a) AR-PAM and AR-PAMac and (b) OR-PAM.

Carefully choosing the two focal diameters offers PAM and PAMac the freedom to seamlessly scale between optical resolution and ultrasonic resolution for the desired tissue penetration.

Acoustic-resolution PAM and PAMac (AR-PAM and AR-PAMac) operate in the quasidiffusive and diffusive regime, respectively, where optical focusing is too blurred to provide high spatial resolution. In AR-PAM and AR-PAMac, a conical lens and an optical condenser are usually utilized to weakly focus light into tissues, producing a dark-field irradiation (Figure 11.2a).[3] In an optically clear medium, the dark-field irradiation has a solid focal spot (2 mm in diameter) but is donut-shaped elsewhere, thereby providing an optically dark zone on the tissue surface for ultrasonic detection and also mitigating surface interference. The ultrasonic transducer positioned in the dark zone is tightly focused in the optical focal volume and preferentially picks up the photoacoustic signal generated within its focus at each scanning position. Thus, the lateral resolution of AR-PAM and AR-PAMac is determined ultrasonically. With a 50 MHz ultrasonic center frequency and a 0.44 acoustic numerical aperture (NA), a 45 μm lateral resolution was achieved in the quasidiffusive regime (~3 mm penetration).[3] With a 5 MHz ultrasonic center frequency and a 0.38 acoustic NA, a 560 μm lateral resolution was achieved deep in the diffusive regime (~4 cm penetration).[4] Tissue penetration approaching the hard limit has been achieved by further compromising the acoustic resolution.[5]

AR-PAM and AR-PAMac have broad biomedical applications in the mesoscopic and macroscopic domains.[6-9] However, to resolve cellular or subcellular structures, higher spatial resolution is desired. Improving the lateral resolution acoustically to such resolution is impractical because at the required high frequencies (>300 MHz), the ultrasonic attenuation within tissue (~80 dB/mm) limits acoustic penetration to ~100 μm. Alternatively, achieving fine later resolution by diffraction-limited optical focusing is more feasible within the soft limit of penetration, which led to the invention of optical-resolution PAM (OR-PAM).[10] In OR-PAM (Figure 11.2b), the optical irradiation and ultrasonic detection are aligned coaxially and confocally via an acousto-optical beam splitter containing two right-angle glass prisms and a thin layer of silicone oil in between. The similar optical refractive indices but distinct acoustic impedances between glass and silicone oil make the beam splitter optically transmissive but acoustically reflective. Thus, at each scanning position, the photoacoustic signal is exclusively generated within the diffraction-limited optical focal zone, which determines the lateral resolution of OR-PAM. With a 1.23 NA objective, a 200 nm resolution was recently achieved in the ballistic regime (~100 μm penetration).[11] With a 0.1 NA microscope objective, a 5 μm lateral resolution was achieved in the quasiballistic regime (~1 mm penetration).[10] Note that the penetration of OR-PAM is not strictly limited to one TMFP. Although having undergone multiple scattering events and having been defocused, photons beyond the soft limit can still be absorbed by biological tissues to generate photoacoustic signals.

11.3 Major Optical Contrasts

Intrinsic optical absorbers, such as hemoglobin, melanin, and water, carry important physiological/pathological information and are ideal contrasts for label-free PAM and PAMac. Hemoglobin is the primary oxygen carrier in the circulation system and plays an integral role in tissue metabolism. Taking advantage of the strong yet spectrally distinct absorption of oxyhemoglobin (HbO_2) and deoxyhemoglobin (HbR) in the visible spectral range, PAM and PAMac are able to image the concentration of total hemoglobin (HbT),[12,13] hemoglobin oxygen saturation (sO_2),[9,14] and blood flow velocity.[15]

Figure 11.3 illustrates three contrast mechanisms. Figure 11.3a shows a representative OR-PAM image of the vascular anatomy in a living mouse ear. Acquired at an isosbestic optical wavelength (570 nm) where the absorption coefficients of HbO_2 and HbR are identical, Figure 11.3a also reflects the relative distribution of HbT. Melanin, the primary pigment in human skin, has a high concentration in skin melanoma. Taking advantage of the distinct absorption spectra of melanin and hemoglobin, multiwavelength PAM and PAMac can simultaneously image the skin melanoma and the surrounding tumor vasculature (Figure 11.3b),[3] thereby holding great clinical potential for noninvasive melanoma detection and staging. Water, the primary body content, is an important disease indicator. Changes in body water under pathological states give clues to the nature of the problem. Taking advantage of the significant water absorption in the near-infrared (NIR) range, ex vivo photoacoustic imaging of a water phantom embedded in fat tissues was recently demonstrated (Figure 11.3c).[16] In vivo mapping of water distribution in pathological tissues has also been demonstrated using PACT in our lab (data unpublished). Note that there are more intrinsic optical absorbers that can potentially serve as photoacoustic contrasts. For example, deoxyribonucleic acid and nicotinamide adenine dinucleotide have strong ultraviolet absorption, while lipid has considerable NIR absorption.

Exogenous biomarkers are highly desired to extend the scope of PAM and PAMac and have been intensively explored in recent years. Till now, nanoparticles, organic dyes, and reporter genes have been successfully applied as photoacoustic contrast agents.[17] Nanoparticles are ideal photoacoustic

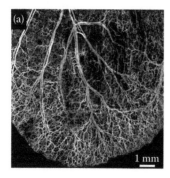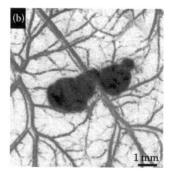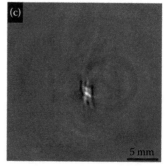

FIGURE 11.3 Endogenous photoacoustic contrasts. (a) OR-PAM of hemoglobin in a living mouse ear. (b) Simultaneous AR-PAM of hemoglobin and melanin (dark lump at the center) in a living mouse skin melanoma. (From Zhang, H.F. et al., *Nat. Biotechnol.*, 24(7), 848, 2006.) (c) PACT of a water–agar mixture (bright spot) embedded in fat tissue. (From Xu, Z. et al., *J. Biomed. Opt.*, 15(3), 036019, 2010.)

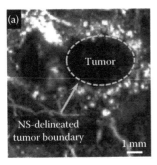 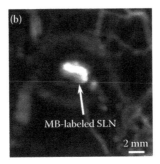 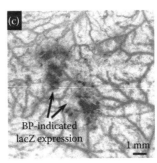

FIGURE 11.4 Exogenous photoacoustic contrasts. (a) AR-PAM of NS extravasation from the vasculature of a murine colon tumor xenograft under a living mouse scalp. (From Li, M.L. et al., *J. Biomed. Opt.*, 14(1), 010507, 2009.) (b) AR-PAMac of MB-labeled SLN in a living rat. (From Song, K.H. et al., *J. Biomed. Opt.*, 13(5), 054033, 2008.) (c) AR-PAM of BP-indicated lacZ reporter gene expression in a gliosarcoma tumor xenograft under a living rat scalp. (From Li, L. et al., *J. Innov. Opt. Health Sci.*, 1(2), 207, 2008.)

contrast agents because their absorption peaks can be tuned to the NIR optical window (700–800 nm) to minimize the endogenous-absorption-induced background and to maximize tissue penetration. Moreover, its effective bioconjugation capability is ideal for delivering,[18] targeting,[19] and therapy.[20] Figure 11.4a shows an in vivo PAM image of nanoshell (NS) extravasation from the vasculature of a murine colon tumor xenograft.[21] Taking advantage of the leaky nature of tumor vasculature (enhanced permeability and retention), PAM can clearly identify the NS-rich tumor boundary by injecting NSs via the tail vein of a mouse. Organic dyes with a vast range of colors (i.e., different optical absorption spectra) have also been widely used as photoacoustic contrast agents. The small molecule size of organic dye leads to an efficient clearance from the body. Figure 11.4b shows an in vivo noninvasive PAMac image of a rat sentinel lymph node (SLN) labeled by methylene blue (MB), a clinically used organic dye for breast cancer staging.[22] PAM and PAMac can also be applied to image gene expression with the aid of exogenous reporter genes. Figure 11.4c shows an in vivo PAM image of lacZ reporter gene expression in a gliosarcoma tumor xenograft under a rat scalp.[23] The lacZ reporter gene encodes β-galactosidase, which produces a blue product (BP) by cleaving the glycosidic linkage of 5-bromo-4-chloro-3-indolyl-β-D-galactoside (X-gal) and thereby provides optical absorption contrast for photoacoustic imaging. Fluorescent dyes and proteins, which have been widely used in molecular imaging, can also serve as photoacoustic contrast agents.[24] The non-unity fluorescence quantum yield (usually less than 50%) suggests that a remarkable portion of the absorbed photon energy undergoes nonradiative relaxation and is dissipated as heat, which can be utilized for photoacoustic imaging. This can be a promising direction for molecular imaging because the high volumetric resolution and deep penetration offered by PAM and PAMac provide valuable extensions to existing fluorescence imaging technologies.

11.4 Photoacoustic Microscopy of Neuronal Disorder

Amyloid-β, the primary constituent of senile plaques, is hypothesized to play an essential role in the pathogenesis of Alzheimer's disease.[25] Neuropathologic changes of amyloid plaques are microscopic, and TPM is currently the mainstay of imaging tools to study such changes in murine models.[26] However, effective two-photon excitation requires the skull to be thinned or even removed, which limits the imaging region and may alter the behavior of the underlying brain.[27]

OR-PAM, capable of utilizing multiple-scattered photons, shows greater tolerance for optical scattering of the skull. Recently, OR-PAM has demonstrated in vivo transcranial imaging of single capillaries,[14] which are similar to or smaller than the average plaque size. With the aid of amyloid-specific photoacoustic biomarkers, transcranial OR-PAM of amyloid plaques is highly likely. As an initial step, we compared and validated OR-PAM with TPM for intravital imaging of amyloid plaques labeled with Congo red, a widely used amyloid-specific dye for fluorescence imaging.[28] A 10-month-old APPswe/PS1dE9 mouse was injected with Congo red through the cisterna magna. Twenty-four hours after injection, an open-skull cranial window was created over the parietal cortex, and dye labeling was confirmed by fluorescence microscopy (Figure 11.5a). A region of interest (ROI) containing a variety of amyloid plaques and blood vessels (enclosed by a red dashed box in Figure 11.5a) was selected for both TPM (Figure 11.5b) and dual-wavelength (570 and 523 nm) OR-PAM imaging (Figure 11.5c and d). Taking advantage of the distinct optical absorption spectra of Congo red and hemoglobin (the absorption of Congo red at 523 nm is 6 times higher than that at 570 nm; however, hemoglobin absorption at these two wavelengths differs by only 40%), we can clearly separate them, as shown in Figure 11.5e (plaques were labeled in green, and blood vessels were in red). OR-PAM and TPM images were directly compared, revealing excellent correlation in plaque distribution (arrows in Figure 11.5b–e). Note that the current system sensitivity is not yet adequate for transcranial imaging of amyloid plaques labeled by Congo red. Further optimization of system parameters (e.g., irradiation wavelength and detection mechanism) and development of photoacoustic-specific amyloid contrast agents are highly desired.

Besides molecular imaging of neuronal disorders, PAM and PAMac are also an ideal research tool for neurovascular coupling—the interaction between neuronal activities and cerebral hemodynamics.[29] The attractive features—including label-free detection, noninvasiveness/minimal invasiveness, functional imaging capability (HbT, sO_2, and flow), and scalable tissue penetration—make PAM and PAMac well suited for neurovascular imaging.

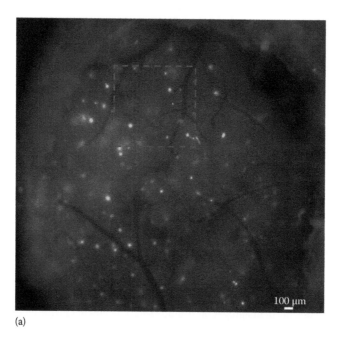

(a)

FIGURE 11.5 **(See color insert.)** Intravital imaging of a Congo-red-injected APPswe/PS1dE9 mouse through an open-skull cranial window. (a) Conventional fluorescence microscopic image of an exposed cortical brain region.

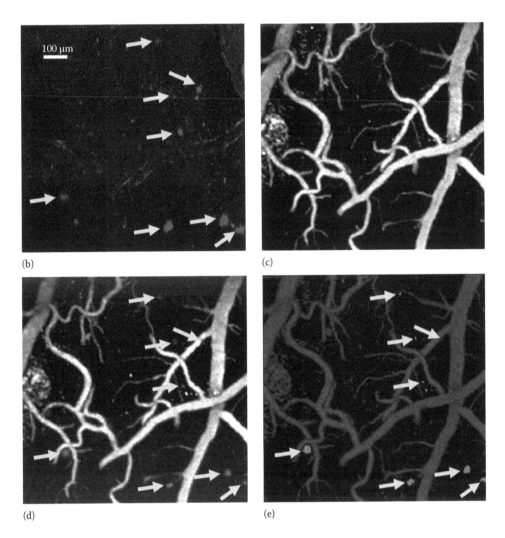

FIGURE 11.5 (continued) **(See color insert.)** Intravital imaging of a Congo-red-injected APPswe/PS1dE9 mouse through an open-skull cranial window. The ROI marked by a red dashed box was imaged by (b) multiphoton microscopy and dual-wavelength OR-PAM at (c) 570 nm and (d) 523 nm. (e) Composite dual-contrast OR-PAM image, where amyloid plaques are colored green and blood vessels are colored red. Arrows indicate amyloid plaques. Scale bar in (b) applies to panels (b–e). (From Hu, S. et al., *Opt. Lett.*, 34(24), 3899, 2009.)

11.5 Photoacoustic Ocular Angiography

Visual impairment is highly prevalent worldwide, and a majority of vision problems are manifested in the ocular vasculature.[30] Fluorescence angiography is the current gold standard in ophthalmology; however, the required injection of contrast agents can cause pain and a variety of complications.[31] Moreover, the agents may fail to perfuse in the presence of conspicuous vascular leakage. Thus, the development of label-free ocular angiography is warranted.

Recently, OR-PAM has successfully demonstrated label-free imaging of both the anterior segment (Figure 11.6a, iris vasculature)[32] and the posterior segment (Figure 11.6b, retina vasculature)[33] of living mouse eyes. Compared with conventional fluorescence angiography, OR-PAM has multiple advantages.[32] First, the diffraction-limited optical focusing and the high nonradiative quantum yield

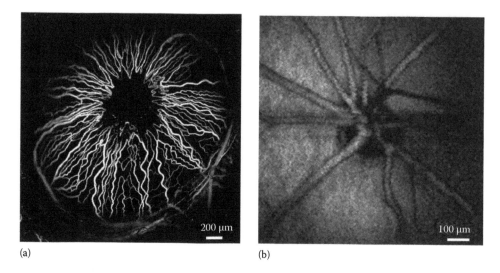

(a)   (b)

FIGURE 11.6 In vivo label-free OR-PAM of (a) mouse iris vasculature (From Hu, S. et al., *Opt. Lett.*, 35(1), 1, 2010.); and (b) rat retina vasculature. (From Jiao, S. et al., *Opt. Express*, 18(4), 3967, 2010.)

of hemoglobin enable single red blood cell resolution and sensitivity with a laser exposure level well within the American National Standards Institute (ANSI) safety limits. Second, the label-free feature enables repetitive imaging, which is highly desirable for disease monitoring and drug evaluation. Third, spectroscopic measurement of blood oxygenation is essential for the early diagnosis of ocular vessel malfunctions.

Although promising, OR-PAM for ophthalmic imaging is still at an initial stage. Substantial efforts should be devoted to high-resolution real-time imaging of ocular vascular anatomy, sO_2, and flow.

11.6 Photoacoustic Dermoscopy

11.6.1 Skin Melanoma

The 10-year survival rate of patients with early-stage skin melanoma is very high (99%), but it rapidly drops to 40% after nodal metastases.[19] Thus, early and accurate diagnosis of skin melanoma is of crucial clinical importance. Although PAM and PAMac can visualize melanoma via the intrinsic melanin contrast,[3,34] it remains challenging to assess melanoma at its early stage.

Recently, a melanoma-specific, optical-absorbing gold nanocage (AuNC) has been developed as an effective biomarker for PAM and PAMac of early-stage melanomas with high sensitivity and specificity.[19] Figure 11.7 compares two molecular photoacoustic studies of B-16 melanomas. The top row (Figure 11.7a–c) shows in vivo PAM and PAMac of melanomas labeled with the newly developed melanoma-specific AuNCs (bioconjugated with [Nle4,d-Phe7]-α-melanocyte-stimulating hormone), and the bottom row (Figure 11.7d–f) shows PAM and PAMac of melanomas labeled with the conventional PEGylated AuNCs. Prior to the AuNC injection, two control melanoma images were acquired (Figure 11.7a and d) by using a combination of 10 MHz PAMac (operating at 778 nm, where melanin has strong absorption while hemoglobin has low absorption) and 50 MHz PAM (operating at 570 nm, where hemoglobin has strong absorption). Deep-penetrating PAMac was used to see through the entire thickness of the melanoma, and high-resolution PAM was used to resolve tumor vasculature. Then, 100 μL of either bioconjugated or PEGylated AuNCs (particle concentration, 10 nM) was injected into two experimental mice via the tail veins, and the accumulation of AuNCs was quantified by pixel-wise subtracting the baseline melanoma images from the postinjection images acquired 3 and 6 h later. The differential melanoma images were overlaid on the images of blood vessels (Figure 11.7b, c, e, and f). Although both

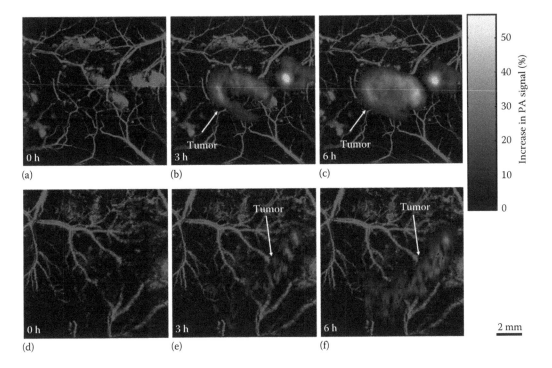

FIGURE 11.7 In vivo noninvasive PAM and PAMac of AuNC-labeled B16 melanomas. (a–c) Sequential images of melanoma and surrounding vasculature before, 3 h after, and 6 h after [Nle4,d-Phe7]-α-MSH-AuNC injection. (d–f) Sequential images of melanoma and surrounding vasculature before, 3 h after, and 6 h after PEGylated AuNC injection. Melanomas are indicated by white arrows. (From Kim, C. et al., *ACS Nano*, 4(8), 4559, 2010.)

types of AuNCs proved themselves capable of enhancing melanoma signals, the bioconjugated AuNCs show a threefold greater enhancement. The much improved specificity of the bioconjugated AuNC is expected to promote the accurate diagnosis of skin melanomas.

11.6.2 Skin Burns

The clinical significance of skin burns depends on the percentage of total body involved and the depth of the burn, both of which are crucial for planning proper treatments. Taking advantage of the distinct optical absorption properties between normal tissues and burned tissues (blood tends to accumulate along the burn boundaries), AR-PAM can accurately determine the 3D profile of an acute thermal burn.[35]

Figure 11.8a shows the photograph of an acute burn of pig skin induced in vivo with cautery. A 10×10 mm^2 ROI was excised and imaged by AR-PAM. The hyperemic ring on the skin surface is clearly shown in the maximum-amplitude-projection photoacoustic image (Figure 11.8b). The depth profile of the burn can be further extracted from a cross-sectional (B-scan) AR-PAM image (Figure 11.8d), which shows a good agreement with the cross-sectional histological photograph (Figure 11.8c). The ratios of the photoacoustic amplitude of the hyperemic bowl to that of the inner coagulated tissue and to that of the outer normal tissue are ~20 and ~10, respectively, providing excellent contrasts to accurately identify the boundary of the burn. The burn depth can be further quantified based on the distance between the skin surface and the inner boundary of the hyperemic bowl. Figure 11.8e shows a representative depth profile (A-line) within the B-scan image. The two peaks in the A-line profile correspond to the skin surface and to the inner boundary of the hyperemic bowl, respectively. Thus, the distance between these two peaks reflects the burn depth, which is ~1.73 mm.

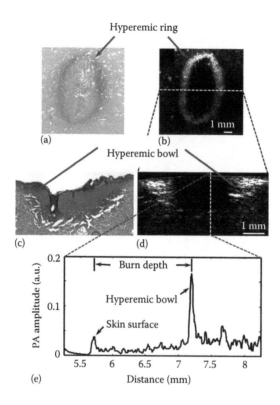

FIGURE 11.8 AR-PAM image of an acute skin burn heated at 175°C for 20 s. (a) Photograph of the burn from the epidermal side. (b) Maximum-amplitude-projection image showing the morphology of the hyperemic ring. (c) Hematoxylin- and eosin-stained histological section showing the depth profile of the burn. (d) B-scan image of the hyperemic bowl at the location marked by the white dashed line in panel (b). (e) A-line profile at the location marked by the white dashed line in panel (d). (From Zhang, H.F. et al., *J. Biomed. Opt.*, 11(5), 054033, 2006.)

11.7 Photoacoustic Mapping of Sentinel Lymph Nodes

SLN is the first lymph node receiving drainage from tumors, serving as a crucial indicator for cancer metastases. SLN biopsy (SLNB), possessing high identification rates (90%–97%) and low false-negative rates (5%–10%), is the preferred method for axillary lymph node staging of breast cancer patients. However, SLNB remains an invasive surgical procedure with potential postoperative complications, including lymphedema, seroma formation, sensory nerve injury, and range-of-motion limitations.[36] Moreover, SLNB requires ionizing radiation for SLN identification.

PAT is ideal for in vivo noninvasive and nonionizing SLN mapping because clinically used SLN markers (e.g., isosulfan blue and MB dyes) are strong optical absorbers. Recently, PAMac has been applied for rat SLN mapping[22]; however, the slow imaging speed limits its clinical applicability. To improve the imaging speed, an ultrasonic-array-based PAMac system (UA-PAMac) was built by adapting a clinical ultrasound imaging system.[36] The dynamic focusing capability of ultrasonic array avoids time-consuming mechanical scanning and thereby improves the off-line imaging speed to 10 B-scan fp/s (the online B-scan rate, limited by the data transfer, is only 1 fps), which can be further increased with faster laser repetition. The online imaging speed can also be improved through faster data transfer. Because photoacoustic reconstruction is used, this modality, strictly speaking, belongs to PACT in limited view of detection. Photoacoustic and ultrasonic imaging were performed before and after MB injection in a Sprague-Dawley rat. The preinjection B-mode UA-PAMac image

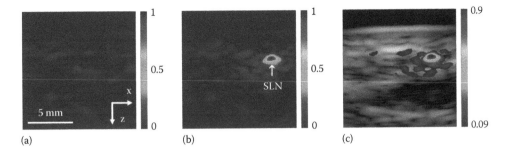

FIGURE 11.9 **(See color insert.)** Noninvasive photoacoustic and ultrasonic B-mode imaging of a living rat SLN. (a) Control photoacoustic image acquired before MB injection. (b) Photoacoustic image acquired 20 min following MB injection. (c) Coregistered photoacoustic and ultrasonic images acquired 20 min following MB injection. (From Erpelding, T.N. et al., *Radiology*, 256(1), 102, 2010.)

(Figure 11.9a) showed superficial blood vessels, which provide fairly weak photoacoustic signals at 658 nm. Twenty minutes after injection, UA-PAMac clearly imaged the SLN through the accumulation of MB (Figure 11.9b). Coregistered photoacoustic and ultrasonic images (Figure 11.9c) demonstrate the capability to combine functional (photoacoustic) and structural (ultrasonic) mapping of SLNs. The combination of photoacoustic SLN mapping and fine-needle biopsy could be a viable, minimally invasive alternative to SLNB.

11.8 Real-Time Photoacoustic Monitoring of Cardiac Dynamics

The vascular system, serving as a distributing conduit for the heart to supply oxygen and nutrients to the vital parts of the body, carries important cardiac information. For instance, the pulsatile nature of blood flow, remaining throughout the microcirculation, is essential for the synchronicity and efficiency of the cardiac system.[37] Ultrasonic-array-based PAM (UA-PAM) is able to perform real-time (50 Hz B-scan rate) vascular imaging, thereby enabling noninvasive monitoring of human pulsatile dynamics.[38]

As shown in Figure 11.10a, a 9×7 mm² ROI near the wrist of a volunteer was imaged by UA-PAM. A representative B-scan across an apparent artery (Figure 11.10b) was selected for real-time pulsatile monitoring. The artery pulsatility was clearly captured in the recorded B-mode movie.[38] To show the pulsatile motion in a static image, the time course (Figure 11.10c) of a representative A-line across the center of the artery (yellow dashed line "A" in Figure 11.10b) was extracted from the B-mode movie. The pulsatile rate recorded by UA-PAM was estimated to be 66 min⁻¹, consistent with the pulse oximeter readout (65 ± 2 min⁻¹). In contrast, the time course of an A-line (yellow dashed line "B" in Figure 11.10b) of a nearby vein shows much weaker pulsatility (Figure 11.10d).

11.9 Photoacoustic Endoscopy of Internal Organs

Although PAM and PAMac have approached the hard depth limit in biological tissues, there are still a variety of vital organs that remain inaccessible. With the recently developed photoacoustic endoscopy (PAE), a miniaturized implementation of PAM, efficient optical illumination, and ultrasonic detection of interior organs can be achieved at distances from the body surface far beyond the hard limit.[39]

In the endoscopic probe shown in Figure 11.11a, the pulsed laser beam from a high-repetition-rate short-pulsed laser is delivered by a multimode optical fiber and emitted through the central hole in an ultrasonic transducer. A mirror, driven by a micromotor through two magnets, rotates both the optical illumination and the ultrasonic detection modules at 2.6 Hz to accomplish circular B-scans. As shown in Figure 11.11b, part of the circular field of view (~110°) is blocked by the stainless-steel housing bridge.

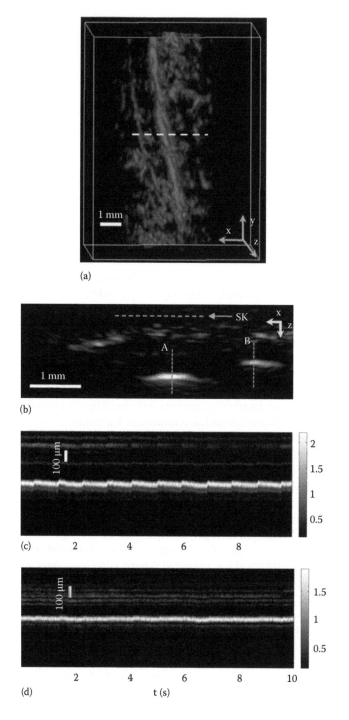

FIGURE 11.10 In vivo noninvasive UA-PAM monitoring of vascular pulsatility. (a) 3D UA-PAM of a human hand. (b) The selected B-scan labeled by the dashed line in panel (a) for pulsatile monitoring. (c) The time course of a representative A-line across the center of the artery marked by the dashed line "A" in panel (b). (d) The time course of a representative A-line across the center of the vein marked by the dashed line "B" in panel (b). (From Song, L. et al., *J. Biomed. Opt.*, 15(2), 021303, 2010.)

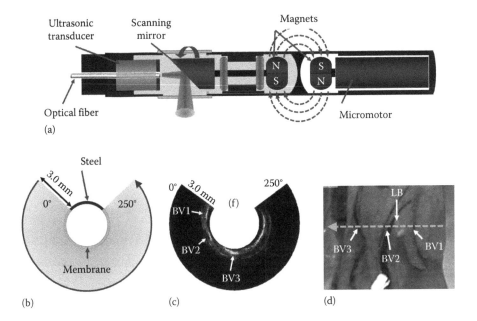

FIGURE 11.11 (a) Schematic of the PAE system. (b) The circular field of view of PAE. (c) Ex vivo PAE image and (d) in situ photograph of a rat intestinal tract. BV, blood vessel; LB, laser beam for photoacoustic irradiation. Dashed arrow, scanning direction and range. (From Yang, J.M. et al., *Opt. Lett.*, 34(10), 1591, 2009.)

To demonstrate the endoscopic potential, a large intestinal tract of a rat was imaged ex vivo (Figure 11.11c). The three major vessels imaged by PAE are validated by a corresponding in situ photograph (Figure 11.11d).

Note that the current PAE implementation has an outer diameter of 4.2 mm, which needs to be reduced to be compatible with generic endoscopes. Moreover, its spatial resolutions need further improvements to visualize microvessels.

11.10 Perspectives

Possessing highly scalable spatial resolution and tissue penetration as well as fruitful contrast sources, PAM and PAMac have poised themselves as enabling technologies in medical diagnosis, especially in the cardiovascular field. Two future directions are envisaged as follows.

11.10.1 Portable Multiscale Photoacoustic Dermoscopy

Strictly confined within the ANSI safety standards, PAT has been demonstrated to be safe for human applications.[3,38,40] AR-PAM has imaged the subcutaneous microvasculature in a human palm with a high contrast-to-noise ratio of 51 dB (Figure 11.12),[3] and several pilot clinical studies of port-wine stains have been reported.[41-43] However, technical improvement is required to facilitate an effective clinical translation. For dermatological applications (e.g., skin cancer and cutaneous vascular lesions), multiscale photoacoustic dermoscopy spanning both the optical and ultrasonic scales is highly desired. It would allow physicians to select an optimal trade-off between spatial resolution and tissue penetration for specific diseases. Moreover, a portable handheld probe rather than a bulky microscopy station is essential for effective translation from benchtop to bedside, where UA-PAM may serve as an enabling technology.

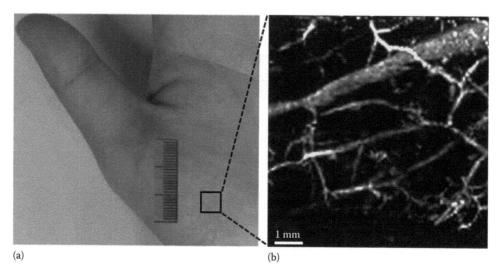

(a)   (b)

FIGURE 11.12 (a) Photograph and (b) in vivo label-free AR-PAM image of the subcutaneous vasculature of a human palm. (From Zhang, H.F. et al., *Nat. Biotechnol.*, 24(7), 848, 2006.)

11.10.2 In Vivo Label-Free Lipid Imaging

Lipid, a vital constituent for all biomembranes, is essential for energy storage and cell signaling. However, progress in understanding lipid function is hampered by methodological limitations because only a few antilipid antibodies and specific lipid-binding protein domains are available for fluorescence microscopy.[44] Taking advantage of the distinct optical absorption spectrum of lipid from other intrinsic tissue absorbers (e.g., hemoglobin, melanin, and water), multiwavelength PAM and PAMac, in principle, are able to perform label-free lipid imaging. Recently, ex vivo photoacoustic imaging of lipid has been demonstrated in rabbit atherosclerotic vessels.[45] In vivo label-free lipid imaging is highly possible given further improvements in photoacoustic detection sensitivity and spectroscopic analysis.

Although holding great potential in medical diagnosis, PAM and PAMac have not yet matured into a mainstream imaging technology. Much effort still needs to be invested for technological innovation and standardization.

Acknowledgments

The authors appreciate Dr. Lynnea Brumbaugh's close reading of the manuscript. This work was sponsored by the National Institutes of Health Grants R01 EB000712, R01 EB008085, R01 CA134539, U54 CA136398, and 5P60 DK02057933. Prof. Lihong V. Wang has a financial interest in Microphotoacoustics, Inc., and Endra, Inc., which, however, did not support this work.

References

1. L. V. Wang and H. Wu, *Biomedical Optics: Principles and Imaging*, Wiley, Hoboken, NJ (2007).
2. S. Hu and L. V. Wang, Photoacoustic imaging and characterization of the microvasculature, *J. Biomed. Opt.* 15(1), 011101 (2010).
3. H. F. Zhang, K. Maslov, G. Stoica, and L. V. Wang, Functional photoacoustic microscopy for high-resolution and noninvasive in vivo imaging, *Nat. Biotechnol.* 24(7), 848–851 (2006).
4. K. H. Song and L. V. Wang, Deep reflection-mode photoacoustic imaging of biological tissue, *J. Biomed. Opt.* 12(6), 060503 (2007).

5. C. Kim, T. N. Erpelding, L. Jankovic, M. D. Pashley, and L. V. Wang, Deeply penetrating in vivo photoacoustic imaging using a clinical ultrasound array system, *Biomed. Opt. Express* 1(1), 278–284 (2010).

6. E. W. Stein, K. Maslov, and L. V. Wang, Noninvasive mapping of the electrically stimulated mouse brain using photoacoustic microscopy, *Proc. SPIE* 6856, 68561J (2008).

7. E. W. Stein, K. Maslov, and L. V. Wang, Noninvasive, in vivo imaging of blood-oxygenation dynamics within the mouse brain using photoacoustic microscopy, *J. Biomed. Opt.* 14(2), 020502 (2009).

8. H. F. Zhang, K. Maslov, M. L. Li, G. Stoica, and L. H. V. Wang, In vivo volumetric imaging of subcutaneous microvasculature by photoacoustic microscopy, *Opt. Express* 14(20), 9317–9323 (2006).

9. H. F. Zhang, K. Maslov, M. Sivaramakrishnan, G. Stoica, and L. H. V. Wang, Imaging of hemoglobin oxygen saturation variations in single vessels in vivo using photoacoustic microscopy, *Appl. Phys. Lett.* 90(5), 3 (2007).

10. K. Maslov, H. F. Zhang, S. Hu, and L. V. Wang, Optical-resolution photoacoustic microscopy for in vivo imaging of single capillaries, *Opt. Lett.* 33(9), 929–931 (2008).

11. C. Zhang, K. Maslov, and L. V. Wang, Subwavelength-resolution label-free photoacoustic microscopy of optical absorption in vivo, *Opt. Lett.* 35(19), 3195–3197 (2010).

12. S. Hu, K. Maslov, and L. V. Wang, Noninvasive label-free imaging of microhemodynamics by optical-resolution photoacoustic microscopy, *Opt. Express* 17(9), 7688–7693 (2009).

13. Z. Guo, S. Hu, and L. V. Wang, Calibration-free absolute quantification of optical absorption coefficients using acoustic spectra in 3D photoacoustic microscopy of biological tissue, *Opt. Lett.* 35(12), 2067–2069 (2010).

14. S. Hu, K. Maslov, V. Tsytsarev, and L. V. Wang, Functional transcranial brain imaging by optical-resolution photoacoustic microscopy, *J. Biomed. Opt.* 14(4), 040503 (2009).

15. J. J. Yao, K. I. Maslov, Y. F. Shi, L. A. Taber, and L. H. V. Wang, In vivo photoacoustic imaging of transverse blood flow by using Doppler broadening of bandwidth, *Opt. Lett.* 35(9), 1419–1421 (2010).

16. Z. Xu, C. Li, and L. V. Wang, Photoacoustic tomography of water in phantoms and tissue, *J. Biomed. Opt.* 15(3), 036019 (2010).

17. C. Kim, C. Favazza, and L. V. Wang, In vivo photoacoustic tomography of chemicals: High-resolution functional and molecular optical imaging at new depths, *Chem. Rev.* 110(5), 2756–2782 (2010).

18. M. S. Yavuz, Y. Cheng, J. Chen, C. M. Cobley, Q. Zhang, M. Rycenga, J. Xie et al., Gold nanocages covered by smart polymers for controlled release with near-infrared light, *Nat. Mater.* 8(12), 935–939 (2009).

19. C. Kim, E. C. Cho, J. Chen, K. H. Song, L. Au, C. Favazza, Q. Zhang et al., In vivo molecular photoacoustic tomography of melanomas targeted by bioconjugated gold nanocages, *ACS Nano* 4(8), 4559–4564 (2010).

20. K. Homan, J. Shah, S. Gomez, H. Gensler, A. Karpiouk, L. Brannon-Peppas, and S. Emelianov, Silver nanosystems for photoacoustic imaging and image-guided therapy, *J. Biomed. Opt.* 15(2), 021316 (2010), Article No. 10, 10.3389/fnene.2010.00010.

21. M. L. Li, J. C. Wang, J. A. Schwartz, K. L. Gill-Sharp, G. Stoica, and L. V. Wang, In-vivo photoacoustic microscopy of nanoshell extravasation from solid tumor vasculature, *J. Biomed. Opt.* 14(1), 010507 (2009).

22. K. H. Song, E. W. Stein, J. A. Margenthaler, and L. V. Wang, Noninvasive photoacoustic identification of sentinel lymph nodes containing methylene blue in vivo in a rat model, *J. Biomed. Opt.* 13(5), 054033 (2008).

23. L. Li, H. F. Zhang, R. J. Zemp, K. Maslov, and L. Wang, Simultaneous imaging of a lacZ-marked tumor and microvasculature morphology in vivo by dual-wavelength photoacoustic microscopy, *J. Innov. Opt. Health Sci.* 1(2), 207–215 (2008).

24. D. Razansky, C. Vinegoni, and V. Ntziachristos, Multispectral photoacoustic imaging of fluorochromes in small animals, *Opt. Lett.* 32(19), 2891–2893 (2007).

25. M. E. McLellan, S. T. Kajdasz, B. T. Hyman, and B. J. Bacskai, In vivo imaging of reactive oxygen species specifically associated with thioflavine S-positive amyloid plaques by multiphoton microscopy, *J. Neurosci.* 23(6), 2212–2217 (2003).

26. B. J. Bacskai, W. E. Klunk, C. A. Mathis, and B. T. Hyman, Imaging amyloid-beta deposits in vivo, *J. Cereb. Blood Flow Metab.* 22(9), 1035–1041 (2002).

27. H. T. Xu, F. Pan, G. Yang, and W. B. Gan, Choice of cranial window type for in vivo imaging affects dendritic spine turnover in the cortex, *Nat. Neurosci.* 10(5), 549–551 (2007).

28. S. Hu, P. Yan, K. Maslov, J.-M. Lee, and L. V. Wang, Intravital imaging of amyloid plaques in a transgenic mouse model using optical-resolution photoacoustic microscopy, *Opt. Lett.* 34(24), 3899–3901 (2009).

29. S. Hu and L. V. Wang, Neurovascular photoacoustic tomography, *Front. Neuroenerg.* 2(10), doi:10.3389/fnene.2010.00010 (2010).

30. L. P. Aiello, R. L. Avery, P. G. Arrigg, B. A. Keyt, H. D. Jampel, S. T. Shah, L. R. Pasquale et al., Vascular endothelial growth factor in ocular fluid of patients with diabetic retinopathy and other retinal disorders, *N. Engl. J. Med.* 331(22), 1480–1487 (1994).

31. B. R. Hurley and C. D. Regillo, Fluorescein angiography: General principles and interpretation, in: J. F. Arevalo (ed.), *Retinal Angiography and Optical Coherence Tomography*, Springer, New York (2009).

32. S. Hu, B. Rao, K. Maslov, and L. V. Wang, Label-free photoacoustic ophthalmic angiography, *Opt. Lett.* 35(1), 1–3 (2010).

33. S. L. Jiao, M. S. Jiang, J. M. Hu, A. Fawzi, Q. F. Zhou, K. K. Shung, C. A. Puliafito, and H. F. Zhang, Photoacoustic ophthalmoscopy for in vivo retinal imaging, *Opt. Express* 18(4), 3967–3972 (2010).

34. J. T. Oh, M. L. Li, H. F. Zhang, K. Maslov, G. Stoica, and L. V. Wang, Three-dimensional imaging of skin melanoma in vivo by dual-wavelength photoacoustic microscopy, *J. Biomed. Opt.* 11(3), 34032 (2006).

35. H. F. Zhang, K. Maslov, G. Stoica, and L. V. Wang, Imaging acute thermal burns by photoacoustic microscopy, *J. Biomed. Opt.* 11(5), 054033 (2006).

36. T. N. Erpelding, C. Kim, M. Pramanik, L. Jankovic, K. Maslov, Z. Guo, J. A. Margenthaler, M. D. Pashley, and L. V. Wang, Sentinel lymph nodes in the rat: Noninvasive photoacoustic and US imaging with a clinical US system, *Radiology* 256(1), 102–110 (2010).

37. J. K.-J. Li, *Dynamics of the Vascular System*, World Scientific, Singapore (2004).

38. L. Song, K. Maslov, K. K. Shung, and L. V. Wang, Ultrasound-array-based real-time photoacoustic microscopy of human pulsatile dynamics in vivo, *J. Biomed. Opt.* 15(2), 021303 (2010).

39. J.-M. Yang, K. Maslov, H.-C. Yang, Q. F. Zhou, K. K. Shung, and L. V. Wang, Photoacoustic endoscopy, *Opt. Lett.* 34(10), 1591–1593 (2009).

40. E. Z. Zhang, J. G. Laufer, R. B. Pedley, and P. C. Beard, In vivo high-resolution 3D photoacoustic imaging of superficial vascular anatomy, *Phys. Med. Biol.* 54(4), 1035–1046 (2009).

41. J. A. Viator, G. Au, G. Paltauf, S. L. Jacques, S. A. Prahl, H. Ren, Z. Chen, and J. S. Nelson, Clinical testing of a photoacoustic probe for port wine stain depth determination, *Lasers Surg. Med.* 30(2), 141–148 (2002).

42. J. A. Viator, B. Choi, M. Ambrose, J. Spanier, and J. S. Nelson, In vivo port-wine stain depth determination with a photoacoustic probe, *Appl. Opt.* 42(16), 3215–3224 (2003).

43. R. G. Kolkman, M. J. Mulder, C. P. Glade, W. Steenbergen, and T. G. van Leeuwen, Photoacoustic imaging of port-wine stains, *Lasers Surg. Med.* 40(3), 178–182 (2008).

44. L. Kuerschner, C. S. Ejsing, K. Ekroos, A. Shevchenko, K. I. Anderson, and C. Thiele, Polyene-lipids: A new tool to image lipids, *Nat. Methods* 2(1), 39–45 (2005).

45. B. Wang, J. L. Su, J. Amirian, S. H. Litovsky, R. Smalling, and S. Emelianov, Detection of lipid in atherosclerotic vessels using ultrasound-guided spectroscopic intravascular photoacoustic imaging, *Opt. Express* 18(5), 4889–4897 (2010).

12

Polarized Light for Medical Diagnostics

Steven L. Jacques
Oregon Health &
Science University

12.1 Introduction

Optical imaging can be conducted on both the microscopic scale and the macroscopic scale. Microscopic examination can observe cellular structure and biomarkers, using absorptive and fluorescent dyes and phase-sensitive techniques, and observe tissue architecture using optical coherence tomography. Practical clinical optical imaging, however, must still survey large tracts on tissue, on the scale of many millimeters or centimeters. Yet such macroscopic surveillance must remain sensitive to the microscale structure of the tissue in order to achieve meaningful contrast. Toward this surveillance task, several investigative groups are developing label-free imaging based on light scattering. While a pixel in a macroscopic image does not *image* the microscale, it can *characterize* the microscale of tissue within that pixel by the absorption, fluorescence, and scattering behavior. In order to use label-free scattering as a contrast mechanism, an understanding of the relation between light scattering and tissue microscale structure, from the sub-nm to several μm scale, is being developed.

Polarized light adds another dimension to optical imaging. Rather than simply measuring the intensity of light escaping a tissue, polarized light imaging also measures the polarization state of the escaping light. The sensitivity of polarized light to birefringence is well known and has been long exploited in polarization microscopes. Light scattering also affects the polarization state of light in a manner that characterizes the scatterers within a tissue. This chapter discusses the use of polarized light for biomedical imaging.

Polarized light offers two opportunities in biomedical imaging: gating and characterization.

1. *Gating*: Polarized light can select only superficially scattered photons and reject multiply scattered photons and hence provide an image of superficial tissues that is independent of underlying tissue structure.
2. *Characterization*: The change in polarized light caused by transport through a tissue can characterize the tissue. Hence, a fingerprint for the tissue structure can be acquired, which can serve as a mechanism of contrast.

These two aspects of polarized light imaging combine to enable the development of medical diagnostics. As an example application, we have developed a handheld polarized light camera to image skin cancer margins prior to excision in the Mohs surgery suite at Oregon Health & Science University (Ramella-Roman et al. 2004, Jacques et al. 2008). The normal-light image of the skin looks featureless, while the polarized light image gates the photons to create an image that displays the *fabric pattern* of the superficial skin layers. Skin cancer disrupts the fabric pattern such that the margin between normal and cancerous skin becomes visible. Our clinical trial is testing the sensitivity and specificity of this polarized-light camera prediction of basal cell and squamous cell skin cancer margins. The concept can be extended to cancer margins during the surveillance of any large tract of tissue that presents a superficial surface, such as esophagus, bronchus, colon, and the oral cavity.

12.2 Basics of Polarized Light

This chapter does not provide a full introduction to polarized light. There are text books (Tuchin et al. 2006, Goldstein 2010) and book chapters (Jacques 2011, Ghosh et al. 2010) for that purpose. Rather, this chapter discusses the gating and characterization modes of optical measurement. But a brief mention of the basics of polarized light is appropriate. The electric field (E field) of a photon oscillates with some orientation relative to the reference plane of an observer as the photon propagates. Assume one places a light source, a light-scattering sample, and a detector on an optical bench, such that the source delivers light to the sample and the detector observes light scattered by the sample. In this case, it is convenient to choose the frame of reference to be the scattering plane specified by the source–sample–detector triangle. In other words, the optical bench is the frame of reference. If the E field oscillates parallel to the scattering plane, the light is called horizontal linearly polarized light (I_H, the intensity of such light). If the E field oscillates perpendicular to the scattering plane, the light is called vertical linearly polarized light (I_V). If the E field oscillation is oriented at either +45° (a counterclockwise rotation as viewed by an observer watching the light approach the observer) or −45° relative to the bench, the light is called I_{+45} or I_{-45}, respectively. If the E field orientation rotates as it propagates, the light is called either right circularly polarized (I_R) (E field moves as right-handed corkscrew) or left circularly polarized (I_L) (E field moves as left-handed corkscrew). To describe a population of photons, the balance between the different types of polarization is specified: $Q = I_H - I_V$, $U = I_{+45} - I_{-45}$, $R = I_R - I_L$. A four-element vector called a *Stokes vector* summarizes the polarization state of a population of photons:

$$S = \begin{vmatrix} I \\ Q \\ U \\ V \end{vmatrix} = \begin{vmatrix} I_H + I_V \\ I_H - I_V \\ I_{+45} + I_{-45} \\ I_R + I_L \end{vmatrix} \tag{12.1}$$

As incident light transmits through an optical element, such as a thin slab of tissue, the incident Stokes vector (S_{in}) is transformed into the output Stokes vector (S_{out}). A Mueller matrix (M) relates S_{in} to S_{out}, $S_{out} = MS_{in}$:

$$S_{out} = \begin{vmatrix} I \\ Q \\ U \\ V \end{vmatrix}_{out} = \begin{vmatrix} M_{11} & M_{12} & M_{13} & M_{14} \\ M_{21} & M_{22} & M_{23} & M_{24} \\ M_{31} & M_{32} & M_{33} & M_{34} \\ M_{41} & M_{42} & M_{43} & M_{44} \end{vmatrix} \times \begin{vmatrix} I \\ Q \\ U \\ V \end{vmatrix}_{in} = MS_{in} \tag{12.2}$$

Hence, the Mueller matrix is analogous to a transmittance T, $T = \exp(-\mu L)$, where μ (cm^{-1}) is an attenuation coefficient and L (cm) is the thickness of the tissue slab. (*Note:* The path length of a photon [L_{photon}]

in the tissue is approximately equal to the slab thickness L for a thin tissue slab. For thicker tissues, L_{photon} will exceed L_{slab} due to multiple scattering that creates a tortuous photon path, which is illustrated later.) The T does not characterize the tissue, since changing L will change T. Rather, the μ characterizes the tissue. So the task of tissue characterization requires identifying μ. Each element of the Mueller matrix is like a particular type of transmittance measurement and can be used for imaging (Jiao and Wang 2002b). This chapter does not discuss the possibilities for imaging using the Mueller matrix. Instead, as an entré to this task, this chapter discusses the delivery of I_H light to a tissue:

$$S_{in \cdot H} = \begin{vmatrix} 1 \\ 1 \\ 0 \\ 0 \end{vmatrix} \tag{12.3}$$

and the collection of transmitted I_H and I_V light:

$$I_H = \begin{vmatrix} 0.5 & 0.5 & 0 & 0 \\ 0.5 & 0.5 & 0 & 0 \\ 0 & 0 & 0 & 0 \\ 0 & 0 & 0 & 0 \end{vmatrix} \times \begin{vmatrix} M_{11} & M_{12} & M_{13} & M_{14} \\ M_{21} & M_{22} & M_{23} & M_{24} \\ M_{31} & M_{32} & M_{33} & M_{34} \\ M_{41} & M_{42} & M_{43} & M_{44} \end{vmatrix} \times \begin{vmatrix} 1 \\ 1 \\ 0 \\ 0 \end{vmatrix} \tag{12.4a}$$

$$I_V = \begin{vmatrix} 0.5 & -0.5 & 0 & 0 \\ -0.5 & 0.5 & 0 & 0 \\ 0 & 0 & 0 & 0 \\ 0 & 0 & 0 & 0 \end{vmatrix} \times \begin{vmatrix} M_{11} & M_{12} & M_{13} & M_{14} \\ M_{21} & M_{22} & M_{23} & M_{24} \\ M_{31} & M_{32} & M_{33} & M_{34} \\ M_{41} & M_{42} & M_{43} & M_{44} \end{vmatrix} \times \begin{vmatrix} 1 \\ 1 \\ 0 \\ 0 \end{vmatrix} \tag{12.4b}$$

In Equation 12.4a, a horizontal linear polarizer is represented by the left-most matrix that multiplies $MS_{in \cdot H}$. In Equation 12.4b, a vertical linear polarizer is represented by the left-most matrix. In practice, these are the simplest of measurements. If one shines light onto an object through the lens of a common pair of Polaroid™ glasses held sideways, one has created I_H illumination. The lens acts as a linear polarizing filter. Observing the object through the lens of a second pair of Polaroid glasses held either sideways or normal yields the observed I_H or I_V light, respectively.

The *degree of linear polarization* (DOLP) is defined as

$$DOLP = \frac{Q}{I} = e^{-\mu_{LP}L} \tag{12.5}$$

12.2.1 Gating

Gating allows imaging of superficial tissue structure. The method selects or *gates* the subset of all reflected photons escaping a tissue, which have only interacted with the superficial tissue layer. Photons that have penetrated more deeply into the tissue are rejected. The image formed enhances the contrast found in the superficial tissue layer and avoids image information from underlying tissue layers. This section discusses the gating method.

When photons propagate through tissue, they usually encounter microdomains of homogenous tissue. For example, these microdomains may be local regions within which birefringent collagen fibers are oriented in one direction and fibers in neighboring microdomains are oriented differently. A photon can propagate through a variety of local microdomains, each microdomain affecting the E field of the photon. Additionally, the photon is multiply scattered by the tissue, with each scattering event redirecting the photon from its current trajectory into a new trajectory. A reflected photon has undergone anywhere from one to many scattering events in order to be redirected toward the tissue surface where it can escape and be observed. Optical measurements detect populations of photons. In general, the different photons within a detected population will have experienced a different path through the tissue, encountering a unique sequence of microdomain scattering events and escaping with its own unique polarization state. A measurement, however, will characterize the population of photons.

Figure 12.1a schematically illustrates a polarized light imaging system. White light is passed through a linear polarizer to illuminate the tissue (delivery of *horizontal* linearly polarized light, with E field parallel to the source–tissue–camera scattering plane). This illumination is delivered obliquely to the tissue, at about 30° off the normal, so that specular reflectance or *glare* from the tissue surface reflects off-axis and does not enter the camera. A glass plate is optically coupled to the tissue by saline or gel to enforce a flat surface and reduce surface glare. The camera views the tissue from above, along the axis normal to this tissue. Hence, the RGB color camera only collects light scattered from within the tissue.

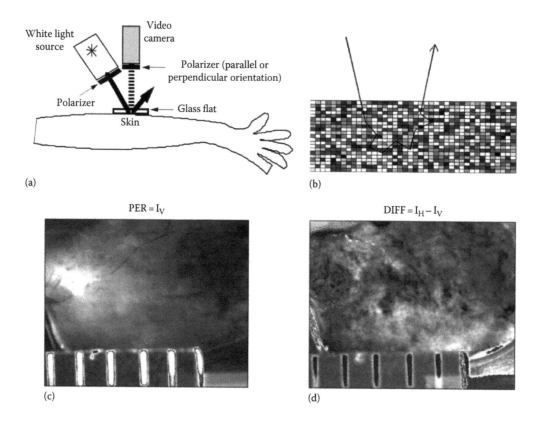

(a)   (b)   (c)   (d)

PER = I_V

DIFF = $I_H - I_V$

FIGURE 12.1   (a) Schematic of polarized light imaging system. White light is delivered through a linear polarizer oriented parallel to the scattering plane (source/tissue/camera plane) to illuminate the tissue. A glass flat is coupled by water or gel to the tissue, which causes surface glare to reflect away from the camera. The camera views the tissue orthogonally through a second polarizer that is oriented either parallel or perpendicular to the scattering plane. (b) Schematic of light propagating through many microdomains within the tissue, each microdomain having different optical properties. (c) PER image of mouse muscle using I_V light. (d) DIFF image based on $Q = I_H - I_V$, which reveals the heterogeneity of the tissue. (The original image is an RGB color image. The grayscale image adequately depicts the microdomains where the density and orientation of muscle fibers vary. The ruler shows 1 mm spacings. The field of view is 5 mm × 6.5 mm.)

The backscattered light is passed through a second linear polarizer before collection by the camera. Two images are taken, one image (PAR = I_H) with the second polarizer parallel with the orientation of the illumination's polarization and one image (PER = I_V) with the second polarizer perpendicular to the illumination. The difference image, DIFF, is calculated:

$$DIFF = PAR - PER = I_H - H_V = Q \tag{12.6}$$

The significance of the DIFF or Q image is better appreciated by the expressions:

$$PAR = \frac{1}{2}R_{deep} + R_{superficial} \tag{12.7a}$$

$$PAR = \frac{1}{2}R_{deep} \tag{12.7b}$$

$$DIFF = PAR - PER = R_{superficial} \tag{12.7c}$$

where
   R_{deep} is the reflectance signal from photons that propagate into the tissue and are multiply scattered and/or pass through a variety of microdomains
   $R_{superficial}$ is the reflectance signal from photons that scatter from the superficial tissue layer

The polarization of the population of photons comprising R_{deep} has been randomized and on average there is no net polarization, that is, the population has been *depolarized*. The population of photons comprising $R_{superficial}$ have only scattered once or a few times and still retain some orientation of polarization. Both the PAR and PER images collect 1/2 of the R_{deep} photons since the analyzing polarizer in front of the camera passes half the unpolarized light regardless of the polarizer's orientation. The DIFF image subtracts this common signal and thereby rejects the depolarized light associated with R_{deep}. Therefore, the DIFF image retains the $R_{superficial}$ signal, which yields an image of the superficial tissue layer. This process of generating a DIFF or Q image is here called *gating*.

Figure 12.1 shows experimental PER and DIFF images of mouse liver coupled by saline to a glass plate. The PAR and DIFF images were calculated separately for each of the red, blue, and green channels. Images were normalized by the average image of a white reflectance standard, then recombined to yield a color image. Figure 12.1c and d are shown in black-and-white, but the original images are in color and properly color-balanced so that the colors perceived are true colors. Such color images show wavelength-dependent differences in the DIFF image, indicating a wavelength-dependent interaction of polarized light with the tissue. The black-and-white DIFF image reveals the microdomains of the tissue, seen as local regions on the order of 10–100 μm. The magnitude of the pixels in the DIFF image is typically about 5%–20% of the pixel values in the normal-light image, PAR + PER. Consequently, one's eye normally does not clearly see the colors and structure in the DIFF image since one is blinded by the strong R_{deep} signal. The rejection of the 80%–95% of R_{deep} light allows the superficial detail to be seen.

Following Equation 12.5, the DOLP is defined: DOLP = (PAR − PER)/(PAR + PER). Using DOLP for imaging has some advantages: (1) DOLP decreases from 1 to 0 (dimensionless) and hence is well defined regardless of the imaging system. (2) Calculating DOLP cancels any spatial variation in the illumination intensity over the field of view, which improves the image. The disadvantage is that the denominator, I = PAR + PER, contains information from the R_{deep} photons and hence complicates the image. For example, a large underlying blood vessel may decrease R_{deep} while not influencing $R_{superficial}$, and the calculation of DOLP will be sensitive to the presence or absence of the blood vessel.

This disadvantage, in our opinion, outweighs the advantages. In our work imaging the superficial skin layer to identify cancer margins, we use Q = PAR − PER. The advantage is its exclusive superficial imaging. The disadvantage is that it is in the arbitrary units of the camera. It is possible to normalize by the total reflectance of a reflectance standard, R_{std}, averaged over the field of view, $\langle PAR_{std} + PER_{std} \rangle$, so that the DOPL image is DOLP = (PAR − PER)R_{std}/$\langle PAR_{std} + PER_{std} \rangle$ = QR_{std}/$\langle I_{std} \rangle$. This normalization yields an image that has dimensionless units, thereby correcting for the uniqueness of a particular camera. In general, we routinely use the DIFF image to view $R_{superficial}$ and use the PER image to view R_{deep}.

12.3 Characterization

The characterization of a tissue by the attenuation coefficient for DOLP, μ_{LP} (cm^{-1}), is discussed in this section. The depolarization of DOLP occurs due to two dominant mechanisms: scattering and birefringence.

12.3.1 Mechanism 1: Scattering

The process of attenuation of DOLP by scattering is discussed by (1) a simple model, (2) a simulated experiment that mimics experimental data for chicken or pig muscle, and (3) Monte Carlo simulations.

12.3.1.1 Simple Model

When a photon is scattered, the orientation of its E field is modified as its trajectory is deflected by the scattering event within the tissue. Let θ indicate the orientation of the photon's E field relative to the orientation of the linear polarization of the incident light. Let $\theta = 0$ radians indicate a horizontal orientation that is parallel to the scattering plane, and light is delivered as horizontal linearly polarized light, I_H. As each photon is multiply scattered by the tissue, its orientation θ randomly walks away from its original orientation in θ-space. In other words, with each additional scatter event, the orientation of the photon's E field incrementally changes. The population of transmitted photons is observed to have a distribution of E field orientations, which is described by a probability density function for the angle of orientation, p(θ) (radian^{-1}). The random walk in θ-space by each photon causes the DOLP of the population of photons to decrease from an initial value of unity at launch toward a final value of zero at large tissue thickness L. This random walk has been described (Jacques et al. 2000):

$$p(\theta) = \frac{e^{-(\theta^2/2\sigma^2)}}{2\sigma\sqrt{\pi/2}} \tag{12.8}$$

where
  θ (radians) is the angle of orientation relative to the orientation of the incident population
  $\sigma^2 = \chi\tau$ is the variance

The factor χ is a diffusivity in θ-space (radian^2/mfp), where mfp = 1/μ_s is the mean free path between scattering events, and μ_s is the scattering coefficient (cm^{-1}). The factor τ is the optical depth of the tissue, $\tau = \mu_s L$, and L is the tissue slab thickness (cm).

The light transmitted through the slab is detected through a second analyzing linear polarizer oriented either parallel to the incidence, yielding PAR or I_H, or perpendicular to the incidence, yielding PER or I_V. The collected PAR and PER can be calculated by integrating the expectation values for

$(\cos \theta)^2$ and $(\sin \theta)^2$, respectively, since intensity equals the square of E field amplitude, over the entire range of angles in the random walk:

$$PAR = I_H = \int_{\theta=-\infty}^{+\infty} p(\theta)(\cos\theta)^2 d\theta \qquad (12.9a)$$

$$PER = I_V = \int_{\theta=-\infty}^{+\infty} p(\theta)(\sin\theta)^2 d\theta \qquad (12.9b)$$

Then DOLP is calculated as in Equation 12.5. The DOLP decays exponentially as L increases, which specifies the coefficient μ_{LP}.

The relationship between μ_{LP} and χ can be determined by inserting a variety of values of χ versus a range of slab thicknesses L into Equations 12.8, 12.9a, 12.9b, and 12.5 to yield a value of μ_{LP}. The μ_s (cm^{-1}) values were set to [1 10 50 100 200 300 500 1000]. The χ (radians^2/mfp) values were set to [0.010 0.050 0.080 0.100 0.500 1]. For each choice of μ_s and χ, the DOLP was calculated for a series of L values from 30 μm to 1.5 mm. Fitting the 48 DOLP versus L curves to yield 48 values of μ_{LP}, the results indicated that

$$\mu_{LP} = 2\mu_s\chi \qquad (12.10)$$

The units of the product $\mu_s\chi$ are (cm^{-1})(radian^2/mfp), where mfp is dimensionless. The units of μ_{LP} are cm^{-1}. Hence, the factor 2 has units of (radians^{-2}).

12.3.1.2 Simulation of Experimental Data

Figure 12.2 illustrates a simulated example of DOLP for polarized light at 633 nm wavelength in muscle tissue (as reported for chicken and pig [Jacques et al. 2000]), where the diffusivity χ is ~0.060 radians^2/mfp and the scattering coefficient μ_s is ~250 cm^{-1}. Figure 12.2a shows the broadening of p(θ) as L increases. Figure 12.2b shows the behavior of PAR and PER, in which PAR decreases toward a value of 1/2 and PER increases from zero to a value of 1/2. One-half of unpolarized light will pass through a linear polarizer regardless of its orientation; hence, PAR and PER approach the same value of 1/2. Figure 12.2c shows the behavior of DOLP as a function of L. The DOLP decreases exponentially, with μ_{LP} = 30.0 cm^{-1}. An *efficiency of depolarization* k_{LP} can be defined:

$$k_{LP} = \frac{\mu_{LP}}{\mu_s} \qquad (12.11)$$

For this example of muscle at 633 nm wavelength, k_{LP} = (30 cm^{-1})/(250 cm^{-1}) = 0.120. In other words, it is expected that 1/0.12 = 8.3 scattering events, on average, are required to cause DOLP to drop to e^{-1} or 0.37.

12.3.1.3 Monte Carlo Simulations

Simulated experiments were used to test the earlier approximate model for how DOPL attenuates versus tissue slab thickness (L). A polarized Monte Carlo model (Ramella-Roman et al. 2005) simulated the transmission and reflectance of light from a slab of tissue composed of 300 nm diameter microspheres of lipid in cytoplasm at a concentration (volume fraction v_f = 0.130) that yielded μ_s = 250 cm^{-1} at 633 nm wavelength. The simulation ignored any packing factor effect due to the high v_f. Horizontally polarized light was delivered to a slab of simulated tissue of varying thickness (L)

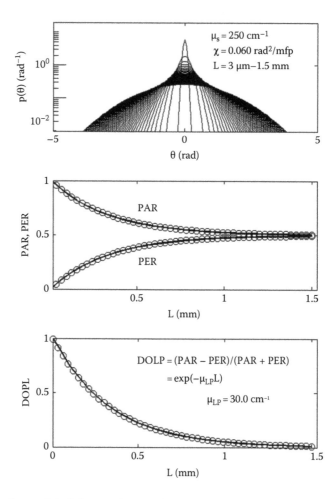

FIGURE 12.2 Simulation of the behavior of DOLP for a population of 633 nm wavelength photons transmitting through a tissue slab of chicken muscle of thickness L. (a) The probability density function for the angle θ of orientation of the E field of photons, where incident light has $\theta = 0$ (horizontal orientation, I_H). As L increases from 10 µm to 1 cm, the $p(\theta)$ broadens. (b) The intensity of transmitted light selected by a linear polarizer oriented either horizontal (PAR = I_H) or vertical (PER = I_V), as a function of L. (c) The DOPL as a function of L, and an exponential fit to the behavior, specifying that the attenuation coefficient for DOPL is $\mu_{LP} = 30$ cm^{-1}.

between 10 and 700 µm. Figure 12.3 shows the spatial distribution of reflectance R(x, y) from the slab and transmittance T(x, y) through the slab, for the case of a 100 µm thick slab. The spatial patterns of the intensities I, Q, U, and V are shown. The DOPL equals Q/I, and the integrated value of Q/I for all pixels was 0.225 for reflected light (R) and 0.669 for transmitted light (T). Figure 12.4 shows the behavior of total DOPL versus slab thickness L. The initial attenuation of DOPL indicates $\mu_{LP} = 30.2$ cm^{-1}, which matches the value 30.0 specified by the simple model for the same tissue conditions. However, for L > 100 µm, the DOPL decays faster, as if $\mu_{LP} = 80.9$ cm^{-1}. The likely explanation is that larger tissue thicknesses, L $\gg$ mfp, cause the photon path length within the tissue, L_{photon}, to become greater than the tissue slab thickness, L, due to multiple scattering, which yields a tortuous photon path. Therefore, when measuring light transport in thicker tissues, one should analyze using the following expression: DOPL = $\exp(-\mu_{LP}L_{photon})$. Proper interpretation of DOPL in a reflectance image should also utilize L_{photon}.

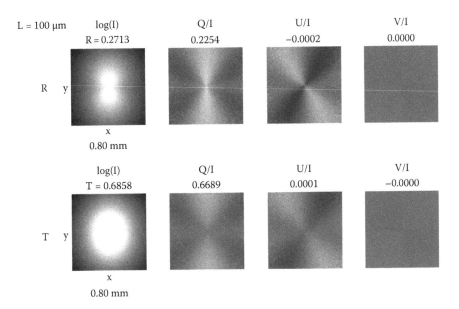

FIGURE 12.3 Monte Carlo simulation of reflectance (R) and transmittance (T) through a 100 μm thick slab of scattering medium with 300 nm diameter microspheres mimicking lipid droplets in cytoplasm ($n_{particle}$ = 1.46, n_{medium} = 1.35, v_f = 0.1302 such that g = 0.6364, μ_s = 250 cm^{-1}, and $\mu_s(1 - g)$ = 10 cm^{-1} at 633 nm wavelength). The images show the x, y spatial distribution of the Stokes vector elements I, Q, U, and V, for both R and T (field of view is 0.800 mm × 0.800 mm). The first column shows log(I) (same color bar for R and T), and other columns show Q/I, U/I, and V/I on −1 to +1 scale (black = −1, white = +1, gray = 0). The total R and T values (0.0214 and 0.9684) are the integral of all pixel values divided by the number of photons launched.

It should also be noted that the simulation used the total reflectance and transmission, but experiments usually involve a smaller solid angle of collection, which can influence the result. More work on the effect of solid angle of collection on such polarized light measurements is needed.

In summary, the simple model still needs some refinement to account for the transition from a few scattering events to many scattering events. Analysis should use DOPL(L_{photon}) rather than DOPL(L) to specify μ_{LP}. A well-trained student of biomedical optics knows how to measure the optical properties of a tissue with respect to unpolarized light in order to document the absorption coefficient (μ_a), the scattering coefficient (μ_s), and the anisotropy of scattering (g). The student can then deduce the photon path L_{photon} for light escaping the tissue at some position. Then, the interpretation of DOLP(L_{photon}) for light escaping at that position would yield a value for μ_{LP} despite multiple scattering. Then, the ratio $k_{LP} = \mu_{LP}/\mu_s$ would characterize the depolarization efficiency of scatterers in that tissue.

12.3.2 Mechanism 2: Birefringence

The second mechanism of depolarization is due to the birefringence of the microdomains in a tissue. When the x and y components of the E field of a photon encounter different refractive indices in a microdomain, for example, due to the orientation of collagen fibers, the x and y components transit the local microdomain at different speeds. The speed of light with its E field oriented parallel to the axis of the fibers is slower than the speed of light oriented perpendicular to the fibers. Therefore, the x and y components become differentially delayed in phase after passing through the microdomain, which causes linearly polarized light to transition toward circularly polarized light. When the photon encounters the next microdomain with a different orientation of collagen fibers, the x and y components of the E field will again alter their respective phases but in a manner unique to that microdomain. Hence, as the photon passes through multiple microdomains, the phases of the x and y components

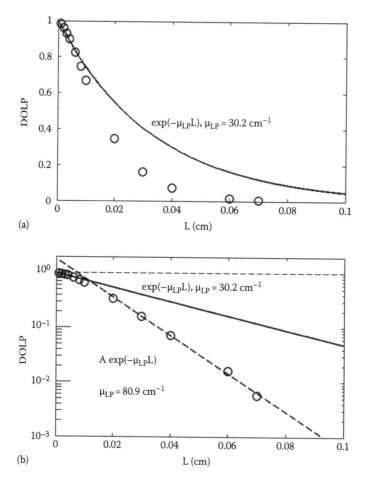

FIGURE 12.4 DOLP for total transmitted light versus thickness of tissue slab. The tissue is the simulated medium cited in Figure 12.3. The initial slope within the first 60 μm specifies $\mu_{LP} = 30.2$ cm^{-1}, in agreement with the prediction of Equations 12.5, 12.8, 12.9a, and 12.9b for $\mu_s = 250$ cm^{-1}, $\chi = 0.060$ rad^2/mfp. Beyond 100 μm where multiple scattering dominates, the DOLP drops faster with $\mu_{LP} = 80.9$ cm^{-1}.

will become unpredictably randomized. A population of photons will sample a variety of sequences of microdomains, and the polarization of the population of photons as observed by a detector will grow increasingly randomized. The apparent DOLP of the transmitted population will have decayed toward zero. Hence, the birefringence of randomly oriented microdomains causes depolarization of a population of initially linearly polarized photons, and the rate of depolarization specifies a value of μ_{LP}.

To illustrate the process, consider incident linearly polarized light (I_H) propagating through a series of very thin incremental slabs of nonscattering but birefringent material (Figure 12.5). Each incremental slab is 10 μm thick and corresponds to a microdomain with a local birefringence Δn. For example, let each microdomain be a region of oriented collagen fibers. This local birefringence is defined as $\Delta n = n_e - n_o$, where n_e (subscript e indicates *extraordinary*) is the refractive index of the microdomain tissue for photons with their E field oriented parallel to the collagen fibers and n_o (subscript o indicates *ordinary*) is the refractive index of the microdomain for photons with their E field oriented perpendicular to the collagen fibers. A typical value of Δn for skin at 630 nm wavelength light is ~3 × 10^{-3} (Jiao and Wang 2002a). Let the fibers in each microdomain be randomly oriented for each photon that is launched, which simulates a population of photons propagating

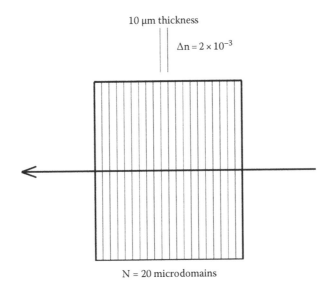

10 μm thickness

$\Delta n = 2 \times 10^{-3}$

N = 20 microdomains

FIGURE 12.5 Passing 633 nm wavelength photons through 20 incremental slabs of nonscattering medium with birefringence comparable to collagen. Each slab is a microdomain with a random orientation of its fast axis. The photons are launched as linearly polarized light, I_H. Each photon that is launched experiences a unique sequence of randomly oriented microdomains. The population of transmitted photons is consequently depolarized to some degree (see Figure 12.6).

through different paths in a tissue, thereby intersecting different microdomains. The transmitted photons can be detected in terms of the Stokes vector $[I\ Q\ U\ V]^T$.

To briefly describe the simulation method, a Stokes vector of incident light I_H, $S_{in} = [1\ 1\ 0\ 0]^T$, was multiplied by a Mueller matrix, M, corresponding to a 10 μm thick retarder with a phase delay of $2\pi(3 \times 10^{-3})(10\ \mu m)/(0.633\ \mu m)$ for 633 nm light, for which the fast axis of the retarder was randomly oriented, which mimicked a microdomain of collagen fibers. The output Stokes vector, $S_{out} = MS_{in}$, then became the new S_{in} and was passed through a second Mueller matrix defined by a similar retarder that was reoriented randomly. The process was iterated until the light had been multiplied by N unique Mueller matrices, that is, N randomly oriented microdomains of collagen fibers. This method has been discussed elsewhere (Jacques 2002).

Figure 12.6 uses the Poincaré sphere to indicate the polarization state of the Stokes vector $[I\ Q\ U\ V]^T$ after transmission through an increasing number of birefringent microdomains. The values of Q, U, and V in the Stokes vector of each transmitted photon are indicated by a point on the Poincaré sphere surface. The axes of the sphere (x, y, z) indicate the values of the Stokes vector elements Q, U, and V, which lay between −1 and +1. The north pole indicates the detected intensity of purely right circular polarization (I_R), the south pole indicates purely left circular polarization (I_L), and the z-axis is labeled $V = I_R - I_L$, which is the balance between right and left circularly polarized detected intensity. The x-axis dimension indicates $Q = I_H - I_V$, which is the balance between horizontal (I_H) and vertical (I_V) linearly polarized detected intensity. The y-axis dimension indicates $U = I_{P_+} - I_{P_-}$, which is the balance between +45° (I_{P_+}) and −45° (I_{P_-}) linearly polarized detected intensity. Hence, the polarization of any photon can be described as a point on the Poincaré sphere. The incident light is I_H light, so the photons are initiated at one end of the sphere ([Q, U, V] = [1, 0, 0]). In Figure 12.6a, the photons have passed through just one microdomain, causing the photons to move along a longitudinal meridian toward either right circular polarization (toward north pole) or left circular polarization (toward south pole), and the average $\langle Q \rangle$ for the population is 0.97. In Figure 12.6b, they have propagated through N = 3 incremental slabs, and the photons have begun to also spread longitudinally, yielding $\langle Q \rangle = 0.91$. In Figure 12.6c, they have propagated through N = 10 incremental slabs, and the photons have

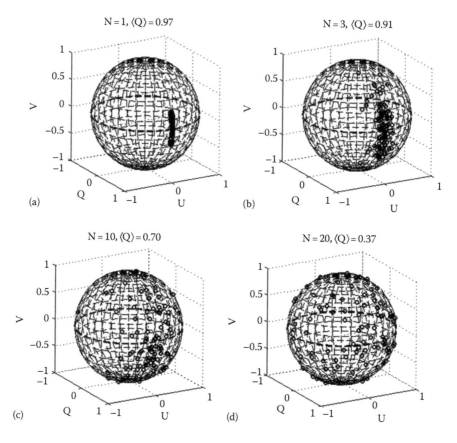

FIGURE 12.6   The depolarization of photons by the series of incremental birefringent slabs of Figure 12.5 is depicted as a spreading on the Poincaré sphere, which describes the polarization state as $Q = H - V$, $U = P^+ - P^-$, and $V = R - L$, where $S = [I\ Q\ U\ V]^T$ is the Stokes vector describing the photons' polarization state. Incident light is horizontal linear polarization, I_H, or $[Q, U, V] = [+1, 0, 0]$. The population of transmitted photons becomes increasingly spread out on the sphere as the number of incremental slabs increases, $N = 0, 3, 10, 20$. The average value $\langle Q \rangle$ falls exponentially from an initial value of 1.0 toward a final value of zero as N increases. (a) After transmission through 1 microdomain, (b) after 3 microdomains, (c) after 10 microdomains, and (d) after 20 microdomains.

begun to spread over the surface of the sphere, $\langle Q \rangle = 0.70$. In Figure 12.6d, they have propagated through $N = 20$ incremental slabs, and they have become even more randomized, $\langle Q \rangle = 0.37$. The polarization state of each photon is unique because each photon has passed through a different sequence of microdomains; hence, each photon appears on the sphere as a point. The average $\langle Q \rangle$ for the population of photons, however, has decayed exponentially toward zero as N increased and the photons' final states become more uniformly distributed on the Poincaré sphere. Recalling that the ΔL for each microdomain is 10 μm, and since $\langle Q \rangle = 0.37$ for $N = 20$, the value of μ_{LP} is $-\ln(0.37)/(20 \times 10\ \mu m) = 50\ cm^{-1}$.

12.4 Experimental Studies

12.4.1 Tissue Properties

The value of μ_{LP} due to birefringence (50 cm^{-1} for skin, 633 nm) in Section 12.3.2 is comparable in magnitude to the μ_{LP} due to scattering (30 cm^{-1} for muscle, 633 nm) in Section 12.3.1.2. Fibrous tissues that present both birefringent fibers and scattering will have a net μ_{LP} with contributions from both mechanisms of depolarization. Tissues that lack birefringence will have a μ_{LP} due only to scattering.

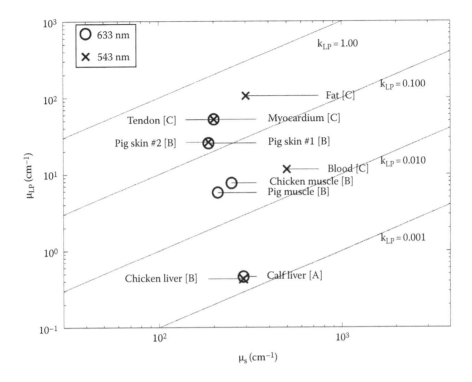

FIGURE 12.7 The efficiency (k_{LP}) of depolarization of linearly polarized light by various tissues differs by two orders of magnitude. The coefficient of depolarization (μ_{LP} [cm⁻¹]) is plotted versus the scattering coefficient (μ_s [cm⁻¹]). (The μ_s data for tendon, myocardium, blood, and fat were estimated, since data were not available from the reference.) (Circles indicate 633 nm wavelength; crosses indicate 543 nm wavelength. Data [A] is from Jarry et al 1998, [B] from Jacques et al 2000, [C] from Sankaran et al 2002.)

Figure 12.7 summarizes a recent review (Jacques 2002) of experimental values (Jarry et al. 1998, Jacques et al. 2000, Sankaran et al. 2002) for the μ_{LP} of biological tissues, which illustrates that the efficiency of depolarization differs for various tissue types by two orders of magnitude. The figure plots μ_{LP} versus μ_s, and constant k_{LP} lines (Equation 12.11) are also plotted. Liver has the lowest μ_{LP} and fat has the highest μ_{LP}. Tissues that are birefringent, like skin and tendon containing a high density of collagen fibers, have a high efficiency of depolarization. The μ_s values for tendon and myocardium were estimated to be $\mu_s \approx 200$ cm⁻¹. The μ_s value for blood was estimated to be $\mu_s \approx 500$ cm⁻¹ with a very high anisotropy of scattering, $g \approx 0.98$, such that $\mu_s(1 - g) \approx 10$ cm⁻¹, which is the approximate observed value for whole blood (Kienle et al. 1996, Steinke and Shepherd 1988). The μ_s and g values for fat were estimated to be 300 cm⁻¹ and 0.975, respectively (Peters et al. 1990). These estimates were made because μ_s data for these tissues were not available from the reference and should be regarded as tentative.

For any particular tissue, it is not clear whether scattering or the birefringence is the dominant mechanism of depolarization. The previous section suggested that both mechanisms equally contribute to the DOPL in strongly birefringent tissues like skin, muscle, myocardium, and tendon. For nonbirefringent tissues like blood, fat, and liver, the scattering is the major mechanism of depolarization.

12.4.2 Polystyrene Microspheres

To illustrate the relationship between scatterer size and depolarization by scattering, experiments were conducted with aqueous suspensions of polystyrene microspheres (Jacques et al. 2000). Measurements of collimated PAR and PER transmission through a cuvette holding the microspheres were made, with a

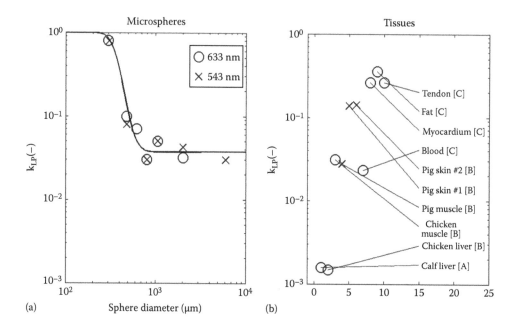

FIGURE 12.8 The efficiency, k_{LP} (dimensionless), of depolarization of linearly polarized light. (a) k_{LP} versus sphere diameter for polystyrene microspheres. (b) k_{LP} for various tissue types. The y-axis is the same for both figures, allowing comparison of the efficiencies for tissues versus spheres of varying size. (Circles indicate 633 nm wavelength; crosses indicate 543 nm wavelength. Data [A] is from Jarry et al 1998, [B] from Jacques et al 2000, [C] from Sankaran et al 2002.)

limited numerical aperture of collection. The DOLP was calculated as the concentration of microspheres was varied. The results yielded values for μ_{LP} and μ_s, allowing the efficiency k_{LP} to be specified. Figure 12.8a shows the values of k_{LP} experimentally determined for suspensions of polystyrene microsphere of varying diameters. The smallest spheres (diameter $\ll$ wavelength λ) are the most efficient in achieving depolarization. Once the spheres become large (diameter $\approx >\lambda$), the efficiency k_{LP} drops over an order of magnitude.

Figure 12.8b shows the values of k_{LP} for the tissues in Figure 12.7, using the same y-axis as Figure 12.8a. Hence, the k_{LP} in Figure 12.8a and b can be easily compared. The high k_{LP} for tendon, skin, and fat suggests that very small particles (diam. $\leq$ 400 nm) dominate the scattering and achieve the depolarization. Yet fat droplets in adipose tissue are typically rather large (diam. $> \lambda$). So the high k_{LP} for fat is surprising. Also, the high k_{LP} for myocardium relative to the moderate k_{LP} for skeletal muscle is noted. There is definitely need for more experimental work on the DOPL of biological tissues.

12.5 Summary

In summary, there is a great need for more work on the depolarization properties of biological tissues. The experimental data available for the analysis of this chapter were limited. Such work should take care to document both the scattering coefficient μ_s (cm^{-1}) and the depolarization coefficient μ_{LP} (cm^{-1}), allowing the ratio $k_{LP} = \mu_{LP}/\mu_s$ to be calculated as a characteristic of each tissue.

The strategy of measuring the μ_{LP} and k_{LP} for DOPL can also be applied to circular polarization. The behavior of circular polarization is considered elsewhere (Jacques 2002). Similarly, the elements of the Mueller matrix are analogous to transmittance between the elements of the input Stokes vector S_{in} and the elements of the output Stokes vector S_{out}. Hence, the incremental decrease in the elements of the Mueller matrix per incremental increase in the path length of photons through a tissue can be described by a depolarization coefficient. In short, the simple and familiar concept of optical attenuation offers a simple approach toward characterizing the polarization properties of biological tissues.

Acknowledgment

This work was supported by the National Institutes of Health (R01-CA80985).

References

Goldstein D. H. 2010. *Polarized Light*, 3rd edn., CRC Press, Boca Raton, FL.

Ghosh, N., M. Wood, and A. Vitkin. 2010. Polarized light assessment of complex turbid media such as biological tissues using Mueller matrix decomposition, in *Handbook of Photonics for Biomedical Science,* Series in Medical Physics and Biomedical Engineering, ed. V. V. Tuchin, CRC Press, Boca Raton, FL.

Jacques S. L. 2011. Polarized light imaging of biological tissues, in *Handbook of Biomedical Optics*, eds. D. A. Boas, C. Pitris, N. Ramanujam, CRC Press, Boca Raton, FL, Vol. 27(2), pp. 101–103.

Jacques S. L., J. R. Roman, and K. Lee. 2000. Imaging superficial tissues with polarized light. *Lasers Surg. Med.* 26: 119–129.

Jacques S. L., R. Samatham, S. Isenhath, and K. Lee. 2008. Polarized light camera to guide surgical excision of skin cancers. *Proc. SPIE* 6842: 68420I.

Jarry G., E. Steimer, V. Damaschini et al. 1998. Coherence and polarization of light propagating through scattering media and biological tissues. *Appl. Opt.* 37: 7357–7367.

Jiao S. and L. V. Wang. 2002a. Jones-matrix imaging of biological tissues with quadruple-channel optical coherence tomography. *J. Biomed. Opt.* 7(3): 350–358.

Jiao S. and L. V. Wang. 2002b. Two-dimensional depth-resolved Mueller matrix of biological tissue measured with double-beam polarization-sensitive optical coherence tomography. *Opt. Lett.* 27(2): 101–103.

Kienle A., L. Lilge, M. S. Patterson, R. Hibst, R. Steiner, and B. C. Wilson. 1996. Spatially resolved absolute diffuse reflectance measurements for noninvasive determination of the optical scattering and absorption coefficients of biological tissue. *Appl. Opt.* 35(13): 2304–2314.

Peters V. G., D. R. Wymant, M. S. Patterson, and G. L. Frank. 1990. Optical properties of normal and diseased human breast tissues in the visible and near infrared. *Phys. Med. Biol.* 35(9): 1317–1334.

Ramella-Roman J. C., K. Lee, S. A. Prahl, and S. L. Jacques. 2004. Design, testing, and clinical studies of a handheld polarized light camera. *J. Biomed. Opt.* 9(6): 1305–1310.

Ramella-Roman J. C., S. A. Prahl, and S. L. Jacques. 2005. Three Monte Carlo programs of polarized light transport into scattering media: Part I. *Opt. Express* 13(12): 4420–4438.

Sankaran V., J. T. Walsh Jr., and D. J. Maitland. 2002. Comparative study of polarized light propagation in biologic tissues. *J Biomed. Opt.* 7(3): 300–306.

Steinke J. M. and A. P. Shepherd. 1988. Comparison of Mie theory and the light scattering of red blood cells. *Appl. Opt.* 27(19): 4027–4033.

Tuchin V. V., L. Wang, and D. A. Zimnyakov. 2006. *Optical Polarization in Biomedical Applications*, Springer, Berlin, Germany.

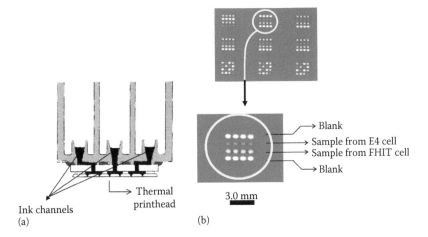

Ink channels
(a)

Thermal printhead

Blank
Sample from E4 cell
Sample from FHIT cell
Blank

3.0 mm
(b)

FIGURE 3.5 (a) Schematic diagram of a generic bubble-jet cartridge illustrating the connection of ink channels to the printhead. (b) Membrane printed with biological materials using the bubble-jet technology. For purposes of better visualization of the spotting, different fluorescent dyes were added for the preparation of this sample. (From Allain, L.R. et al., *Fresenius J. Anal. Chem.*, 371(2), 146, 2001.)

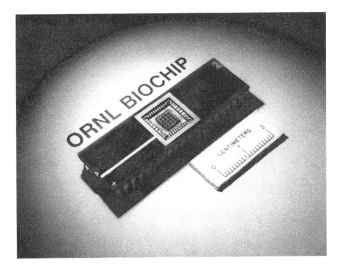

FIGURE 3.6 Photograph of an IC microchip for a biochip with 4 × 4 sensor array. (From Vo-Dinh, T., *Sens. Actuat. B*, 51, 52, 1998.)

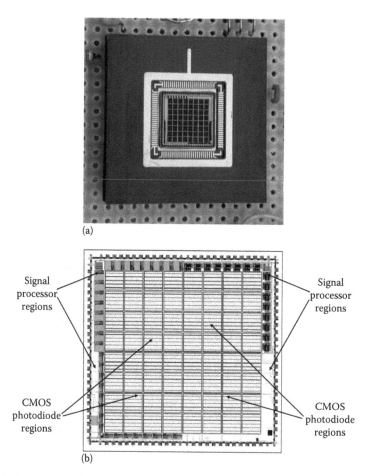

(a)

(b)

FIGURE 3.7 (a) Photograph of the 8 × 8 IC microchip. (b) Schematic of the electronic design of the 8 × 8 microchip with CMOS photodiode regions and signal processor regions.

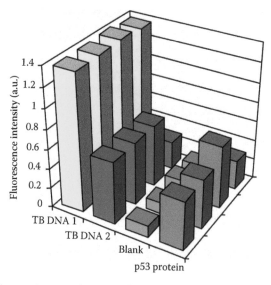

FIGURE 3.8 MFB used for simultaneous detection of the p53 protein (antibody probe) and the *M. tuberculosis* gene (DNA probe).

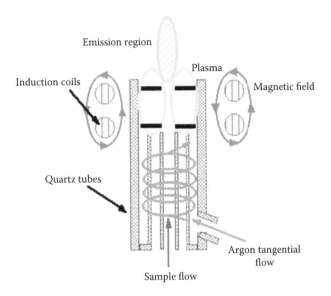

FIGURE 4.5 ICP torch.

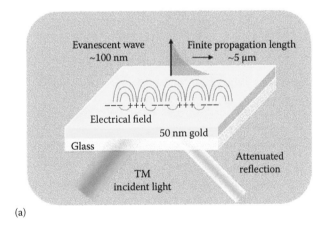

(a)

FIGURE 7.3 (a) Diagram of the SPR effect where TM monochromatic light is reflected from a 50 nm gold layer through a glass substrate. At the resonance angle, an evanescent surface wave is created and a drop in reflectivity is observed.

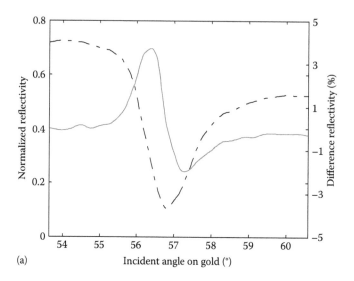

(a)

FIGURE 7.4 (a) Solid line, angular reflectivity curve for an incident wavelength of 633 nm extracted from Figure 7.1; dashed line, variation of reflectivity due to the binding of BSA on the gold surface.

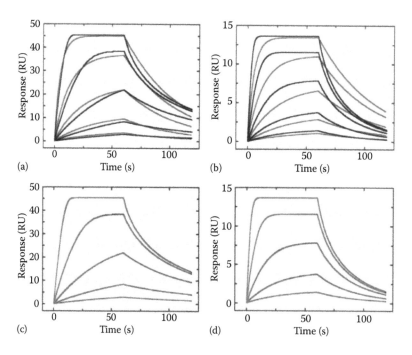

FIGURE 7.24 Model fitting to mass-transport-limited SPR data. The data for probe density R_{T1} in (a) and (c) and density R_{T2} in (b) and (d) are shown in black—the model fits are shown in red. Langmuir fits to the data are shown in (a) and (b), and two-compartment model fits to the same data are shown in (c) and (d). Because reactions were mass-transport-limited, the curves having a one-to-one correspondence (same target concentration) between sets have different shapes, unlike in Figure 7.22. As seen in (a) and (b), the Langmuir model fits mass-transport-limited data poorly. Since, at equal target concentration, equilibrium is reached faster for a lower probe density, it follows that $R_{T1} > R_{T2}$. (From Myszka, D.G. et al., *Biophys. J.*, 75(2), 583, 1998.)

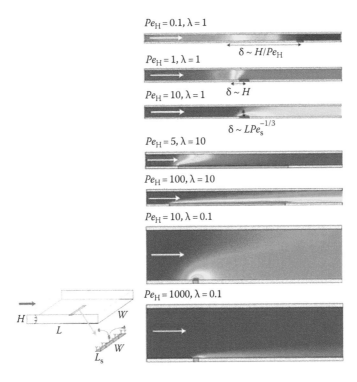

$Pe_H = 0.1, \lambda = 1$

$\delta \sim H/Pe_H$

$Pe_H = 1, \lambda = 1$

$\delta \sim H$

$Pe_H = 10, \lambda = 1$

$\delta \sim LPe_s^{-1/3}$

$Pe_H = 5, \lambda = 10$

$Pe_H = 100, \lambda = 10$

$Pe_H = 10, \lambda = 0.1$

$Pe_H = 1000, \lambda = 0.1$

FIGURE 7.26 (a) Strip biosensor (dimensions, $L_s \times W$) in a microfluidic channel; (b) depletion zone profile as a function of Pe_H (blue, low target concentration; red, high concentration). Sensor length, L_s, is shown in green; λ is the ratio of sensor length to channel height (L/H). (From Squires, T.M. et al., *Nat. Biotechnol.*, 26(4), 417, 2008.)

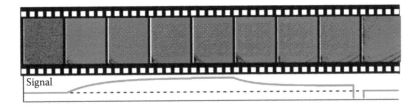

FIGURE 7.31 SPRI movie—surface reflectivity changes with time as ssDNA target sequences bind to complementary surface ssDNA—functionalized probe spots. From each spot area, an interaction signal curve is extracted.

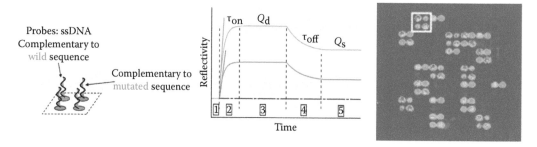

FIGURE 7.35 Schematic representation of the four spots' diagnosis scheme—one diagonal (in green) is spotted using the ssDNA wild-type sequence, while the other one (in red) uses the ssDNA mutated sequence. If wild-type target sequences are interacting with the probes, one expects the perfectly complementary interaction signal (with the wild-type probe spot) to be stronger than the partial match interaction signal (with the mutant probe spot)—this is further illustrated by the biochip SPRI measurement on the right.

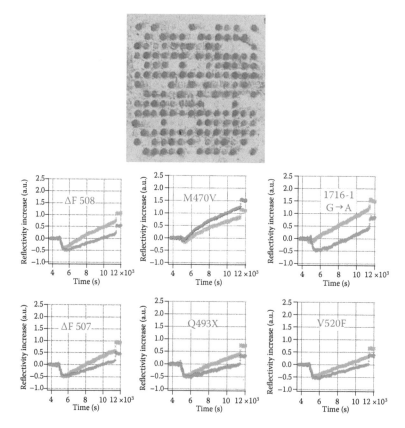

FIGURE 7.40 Example of DNA–DNA interactions using PCR products as characterized by the SPRI biochip. (Left) Image of the plasmonic reflectivity difference of the diagnostic biochip after submitting the surface to a solution containing the target PCR materials and rinsing. (Right) Kinetics of the PCR material solution-induced binding events (for each point mutation characterized: in green the wild sequence spots and in red the mutated sequence spots). In the case presented here, the patient was indeed diagnosed with the MV470 CF point mutation—for which the red (MT) experimental curve is above the green one (WT) (middle-top graph).

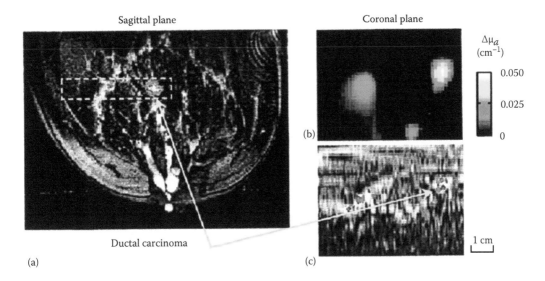

FIGURE 9.14 A dynamic MRI and contrast-enhanced DOT image of a ductal carcinoma. (a) A dynamic sagittal MR image after Gd contrast enhancement passing through the center of the malignant lesion. (b) The coronal DOT image, perpendicular to the plane of the MRI image in (a), but in the volume of interest indicated in (a) by the dashed-line box. (c) The dynamic MR coronal image resliced from the same volume of interest and same dimensions as (b).

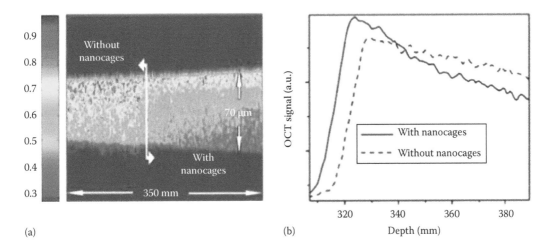

FIGURE 10.4 Comparison of OCT images of gelatin phantom before and after application of gold nanocages (a). Plots of the averaged of OCT signal as a function of depth with and without gold nanocages (b). Application of nanocages results in enhanced OCT signal only at shallow depths. OCT signal from the phantom with the nanocages decays faster than the phantom without the nanocages. (From Chen, J. et al., *Nano Lett.*, 5(3), 473, March 2005. With permission.)

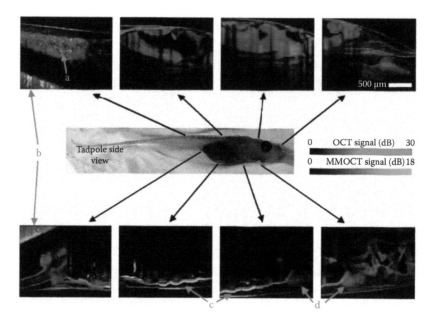

FIGURE 10.6 MMOCT imaging of *X. laevis* tadpole at different locations. MMOCT B-scans are referenced to a microscopy image of the tadpole. (b) Magnetic particles accumulated in molding clay situated underneath tadpole. (c) MMOCT signal in the intestines of the tadpole. Accumulation of magnetic particles in the intestines is probably a result of clearance from the bloodstream. (a) MMOCT signal from the tail of the tadpole. (d) The lack of MMOCT signal from the beating heart. In MMOCT, it is important to consider that movement within the sample can result in locoregional scattering modulation and therefore might contribute to image artifacts. The lack of MMOCT signal demonstrates the effectiveness of background subtraction in difference imaging. (From Oldenburg, A. et al., *Opt. Express*, 13(17), 6597, August 2005. With permission.)

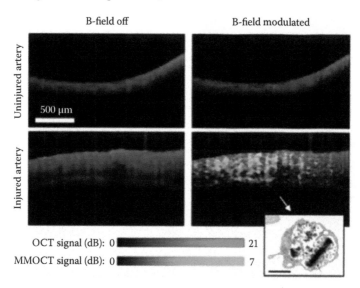

FIGURE 10.8 MMOCT imaging of injured and uninjured arteries with and without the magnetic field. Top row are MMOCT B-scans of uninjured artery. Bottom row are MMOCT B-scans of injured artery. Left column shows images with magnetic field off. Right column shows images with magnetic field on. Ex vivo porcine arteries were exposed to platelets laden with SPIO particles. MMOCT signal is restricted to injured artery site, while no MMOCT signal is present from the uninjured artery. (From Oldenburg, A.L. et al., *IEEE J. Select. Top. Quantum Electron.*, 18(3), 1100, May 2012. With permission.)

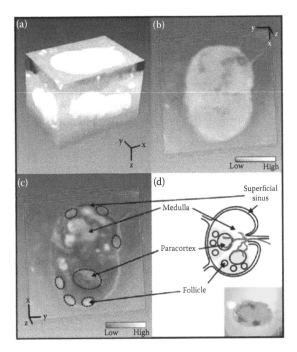

FIGURE 10.10 PTOCT imaging of lymph nodes after uptake of passively targeted GNRs. (a) The OCT volumetric image, (b) a cross-sectional cut at around 240 μm below the surface, (c) PTOCT image at the same location, and (d) a diagram of different depicting structures of the lymph node. After uptake of GNRs, a variety of features are delineated using PTOCT. The GNRs accumulate in the cortex surrounding the follicles. (From Jung, Y. et al., *Nano Lett.*, 11, 2938, 2011. With permission.)

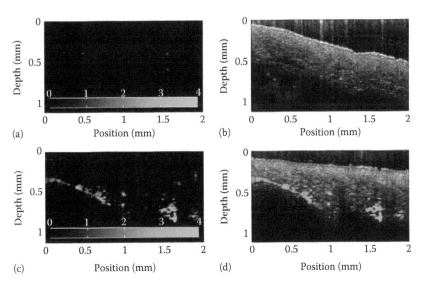

FIGURE 10.11 PTOCT in vivo imaging of GNRs injected into mouse ears. (a) PTOCT and (b) OCT images without GNRs and (c, d) with GNRs. Right column depicts the OCT B-scans. Doppler OCT, depicted by the red and blue channels, is overlaid on the OCT B-scans. PTOCT B-scans are also overlaid on the OCT images. As depicted, there is PTOCT signal at locations where there are no blood vessels present as indicated by Doppler OCT. Furthermore, there is very little PTOCT signal when the GNRs are not present, indicating that PTOCT signal arises primarily from GNR absorption of the heating beam. (From Tucker-Schwartz, J.M. et al., *Biomed. Opt. Express*, 3(11), 2881, November 2012. With permission.)

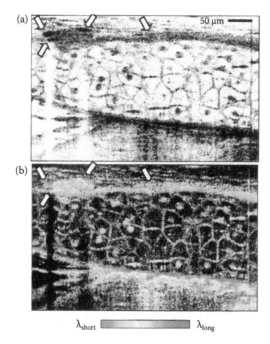

FIGURE 10.12 In vivo OCT and SOCT imaging of *X. laevis*. OCT B-scan is shown in (a), while SOCT B-scan is shown in (b). The green hue in the SOCT image indicates a short-wavelength shift of the center of the spectrum, while a red hue indicates a long-wavelength shift. Melanocytes, indicated by arrows, appear red in the SOCT due to their absorbance of short wavelengths. As evident, the melanocytes are difficult to visualize in the OCT B-scan, but are readily visible in the SOCT B-scan. (From Morgner, U. et al., *Opt. Lett.*, 25(2), 111, January 2000. With permission.)

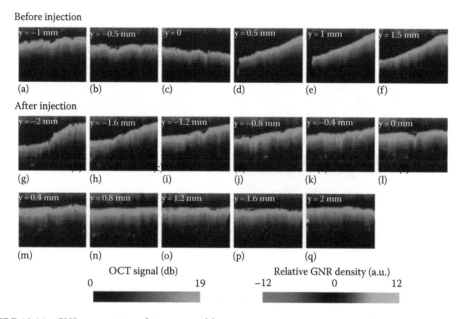

FIGURE 10.14 GNRs were injected into excised breast carcinoma tumor tissue and OCT and SOCT volumetric were obtained before and after injection. Relative GNR density determined from SOCT signal. (a–f) depict B-scans of the same volumetric image with SOCT contrast overlaid. (g–q) show OCT B-scans of volumetric image after injection of GNRs. As evident, SOCT contrast is more apparent after injection of GNRs. (From Oldenburg, A.L. et al., *J. Mater. Chem.*, 19, 6407, January 2009. With permission.)

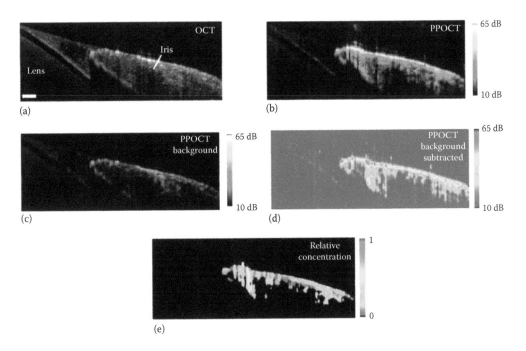

FIGURE 10.19 Fourier-domain PPOCT ex vivo imaging of melanin in a porcine iris. (a) Shows the conventional OCT image, (b) shows the PPOCT image, (c) shows the PPOCT background image, (d) shows the PPOCT image after background subtraction, and (e) shows a melanin relative concentration map. The PPOCT signal clearly shows additional molecular contrast from melanin. The ratio of the PPOCT image after background subtraction and the OCT image yields a reflectivity-independent relative concentration map of melanin. 1 indicates maximum concentration. (From Jacob, D. et al., *Opt. Express*, 18(12), 12399, July 2010. With permission.)

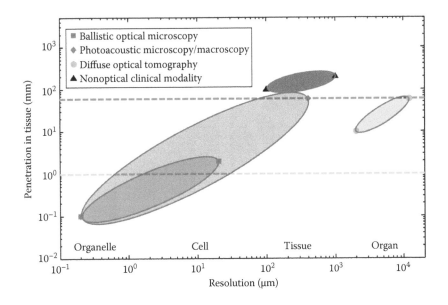

FIGURE 11.1 Spatial resolution and tissue penetration depth of modern biomedical imaging technologies.

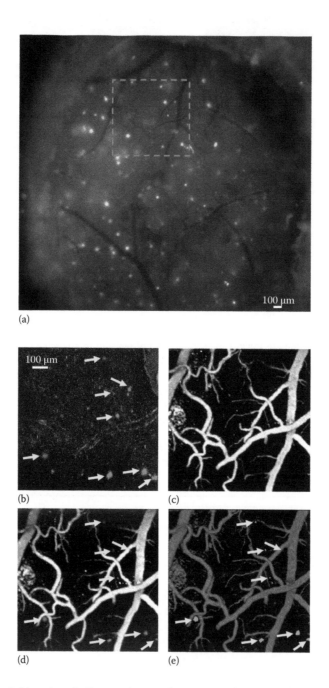

(a)

(b)

(c)

(d)

(e)

FIGURE 11.5 Intravital imaging of a Congo-red-injected APPswe/PS1dE9 mouse through an open-skull cranial window. (a) Conventional fluorescence microscopic image of an exposed cortical brain region. The ROI marked by a red dashed box was imaged by (b) multiphoton microscopy and dual-wavelength OR-PAM at (c) 570 nm and (d) 523 nm. (e) Composite dual-contrast OR-PAM image, where amyloid plaques are colored green and blood vessels are colored red. Arrows indicate amyloid plaques. Scale bar in (b) applies to panels (b–e). (From Hu, S. et al., *Opt. Lett.*, 34(24), 3899, 2009.)

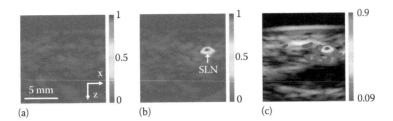

FIGURE 11.9 Noninvasive photoacoustic and ultrasonic B-mode imaging of a living rat SLN. (a) Control photoacoustic image acquired before MB injection. (b) Photoacoustic image acquired 20 min following MB injection. (c) Coregistered photoacoustic and ultrasonic images acquired 20 min following MB injection. (From Erpelding, T.N. et al., *Radiology*, 256(1), 102, 2010.)

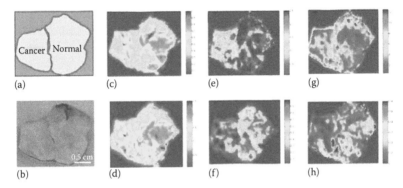

FIGURE 17.5 Breast tissue images obtained with the MIT margin scanner. (a) Diagram of normal and breast cancer tissues placed on glass plate during scanning; (b) gross photograph of breast tissues; (c) DRS spectral intensity map of normal and cancer tissues at 545 nm; (d–f) scattering parameters a (related to the amount of Mie scatterers), b (related to the size of the scatterers), and c (related to the amount of Rayleigh scatterers); (g) Hb concentration (mg/mL) map; and (h) β-carotene concentration (mg/mL) map. (From Lue, N. et al., *PLoS One*, 7, e30887, 2012.)

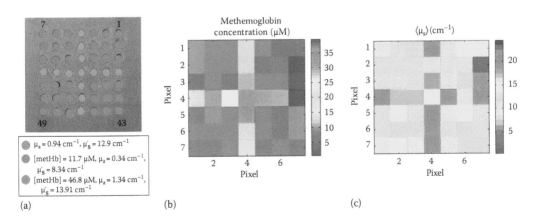

FIGURE 17.13 Quantitative image of a heterogeneous phantom target. (a) Forty-nine holes matching the probe geometry were drilled in a homogeneous solid phantom. The holes were filled with liquid phantoms. The red holes have higher concentrations of metHb and microspheres than the blue ones. (b) Extracted metHb concentration. (c) Extracted scattering coefficient.

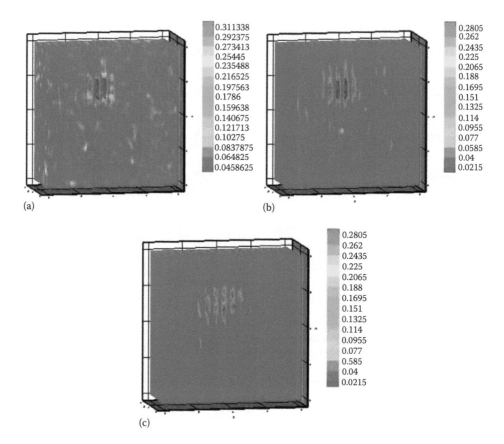

FIGURE 18.21 A 3D reconstruction from simply bound truncated Newton's method. (a) Actual distribution of fluorophore absorption coefficient of background tissue variability of endogenous (50%) and exogenous (500%) properties; (b) reconstructed fluorophore absorption coefficient of background tissue variability of endogenous (50%) and exogenous (500%) properties using relative measurement of the emission fluence with respect to the excitation fluence at the same detector point, $\varepsilon = 0.0001$; (c) reconstructed fluorophore absorption coefficient of background tissue variability of endogenous (50%) and exogenous (500%) properties using relative measurement of the emission fluence with respect to the excitation fluence at the same detector point. (Reproduced from Roy, R. et al., *IEEE Trans. Med. Imaging*, 22, 824, 2003. With permission.)

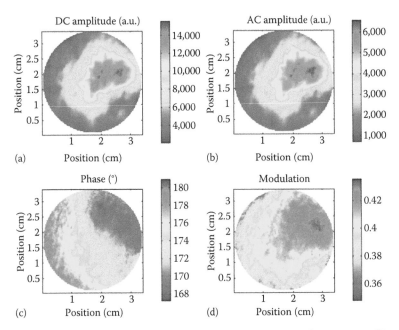

FIGURE 18.23 The 128 × 128 pixel-based imaging of 830 nm fluorescence of (a) CW DC, (b) amplitude I_{AC}, (c) phase delay, and (d) modulation ratio of the detected fluorescence generated from the area cranial of the left fourth mammary gland of a canine. Illumination was accomplished with an expanded 780 nm laser diode. Modulation frequency was 100 MHz. (Reproduced from Reynolds, J.S. et al., *Photochem. Photobiol.*, 70, 87, 1999. With permission.)

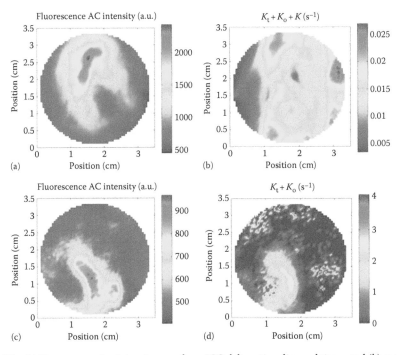

FIGURE 18.25 (a) Fluorescence I_{AC} intensity map from ICG delineating diseased tissue and (b) map of pharmacokinetic uptake parameters obtained from fitting the time sequences of fluorescence intensity images showing no specific uptake of ICG in diseased tissue. (c) Fluorescence AC intensity map from HPPH-car delineating diseased tissue and (d) map of pharmacokinetic uptake parameters obtained from fitting the time sequences of fluorescence intensity images showing specific uptake of HPPH-car in diseased tissue. (Reproduced from Gurfinkel, M. et al., *Photochem. Photobiol.*, 72, 94, 2000. With permission.)

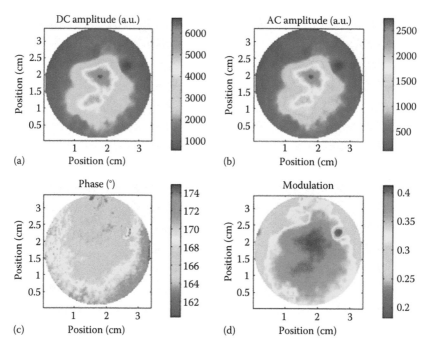

FIGURE 18.26 The 128 × 128 pixel-based imaging of 830 nm fluorescence of (a) CW I_{DC}, (b) amplitude I_{AC}, (c) phase delay, and (d) modulation ratio of the detected fluorescence generated from the area cranial of the left fifth mammary gland of a canine. Illumination was accomplished with an expanded 780 nm laser diode. Modulation frequency was 100 MHz. (Reproduced from Reynolds, J.S. et al., *Photochem. Photobiol.*, 70, 87, 1999. With permission.)

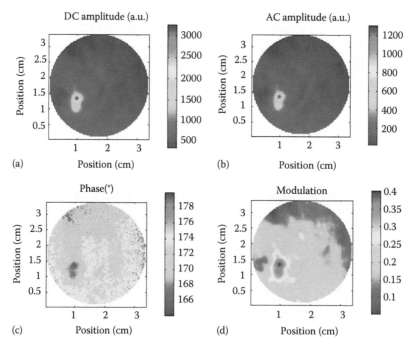

FIGURE 18.27 The 128 × 128 pixel-based imaging of 830 nm fluorescence of (a) CW DC, (b) amplitude I_{AC}, (c) phase delay, and (d) modulation ratio of the detected fluorescence generated from a lymph node in the area of the right fifth mammary gland. Illumination was accomplished with an expanded 780 nm laser diode. Modulation frequency was 100 MHz. (Reproduced from Reynolds, J.S. et al., *Photochem. Photobiol.*, 70, 87, 1999. With permission.)

13

X-Ray Diagnostic Techniques

Xizeng Wu
University of Alabama at Birmingham

Molly Donovan Wong
University of Oklahoma

Abby E. Deans
University of California, San Francisco

Hong Liu
University of Oklahoma

13.1 Introduction

X-ray diagnostic imaging is one of the most important tools in modern medicine. Approximately 120,000 x-ray systems are in operation in the United States, performing an estimated 240 million x-ray procedures each year. X-ray diagnostic imaging is based on the tissue-differential contrast generated by x-ray and tissue interaction. In Section 13.2, x-ray–tissue interaction and tissue contrast are presented. In addition to the traditional coverage of x-ray attenuation-based tissue contrast, the section also details x-ray phase-based tissue contrast arising from the nature of x-ray as a wave, which is especially appropriate due to the recent research focus on x-ray phase imaging. Next, Section 13.3 examines x-ray generation, spectra, and exposure control, followed by projection x-ray imaging, both radiography and fluoroscopy (R&F); digital imaging detectors; examines x-ray generation, spectra and exposure control. Section 13.4 details projection x-ray imaging, both radiography and fluoroscopy, as well as digital imaging detectors, x-ray image intensifiers (IIs) and signal-to-noise ratio (SNR) analysis of projection imaging. Finally, Section 13.5 presents in-line phase-contrast imaging, which is an emerging x-ray imaging modality with great potential for biomedical applications.

13.2 Biological Tissue–X-Ray Interaction and Tissue Contrast

13.2.1 Attenuation-Based Tissue Contrast

X-rays are ionizing and invisible electromagnetic radiation with much shorter wavelengths than light. A simple relationship exists between the energy E and the wavelength λ of an x-ray photon:

$$\lambda = \frac{12.4}{E\,(\text{keV})}\,(\text{Å}).\tag{13.1}$$

For example, in medical diagnostic imaging, the energy of an x-ray photon ranges from approximately 10 to 150 keV, which corresponds to wavelengths ranging from 1.2 to 0.083 Å. The amount of x-ray radiation exposure is often quantified by the amount of ionization generated by the x-ray exposure or, more specifically, by the electric charge generated per unit mass of air. The unit of x-ray exposure is defined as the Roentgen (R), where $1\ R = 2.58 \times 10^{-4}$ coulomb/kg.

Through interactions with atomic electrons of biological tissue, x-ray photons can be absorbed, scattered (i.e., deflected), or transmitted by the tissue. Absorption and scattering result in attenuation of the incident x-ray intensity I_0, and the remaining x-ray is transmitted with an intensity I, which is defined as follows:

$$I = I_0 \exp\left(-\frac{\mu}{\rho}\rho t\right) = I_0 \exp(-\mu t), \tag{13.2}$$

where
　μ/ρ is the mass attenuation coefficient
　ρ is the mass density
　μ is the linear attenuation coefficient of the tissue
　t is the thickness of the tissue

Thus, x-ray attenuation is dependent on the tissue's elemental composition (μ/ρ), mass density (ρ), and thickness (t). It follows that x-ray attenuation increases with increasing μ/ρ, ρ, and t. A biological tissue's mass attenuation coefficient can be calculated as the weighted sum of the coefficients for its constituent elements:

$$\left(\frac{\mu}{\rho}\right)_{Tissue} = \sum_i w_i \left(\frac{\mu}{\rho}\right)_i, \tag{13.3}$$

where
　$(\mu/\rho)_i$ is the mass attenuation coefficient for the ith element
　w_i is the corresponding weight fraction

This mixture rule ignores any effects of changes in the atomic wave functions as a result of the molecular, chemical, and crystalline environment; however, the resulting errors are less than a few percent. Biological tissues with different elemental compositions and mass densities have different linear attenuation coefficients. Coupled with differences in tissue thickness, the differences in tissue linear attenuation coefficients result in attenuation-based tissue contrast according to Equation 13.2. For example, the values of μ/ρ and ρ are larger for bone than soft tissue. Thus, bone attenuates many more x-ray photons than soft tissue of comparable thickness, providing high contrast between bone and tissue in x-ray images. However, the μ/ρ and ρ values for infiltrating invasive breast carcinoma are only slightly higher than the values for glandular breast tissue; the small attenuation difference presents mammography with the greatest technical challenge among the radiological imaging modalities. A comprehensive compilation of attenuation may be found in the literature.[1] Table 13.1 provides the mass attenuation coefficients of water from 10 to 150 keV. The data have been interpolated from the data of the referenced compilation.

The primary goal of x-ray diagnostic imaging is to provide adequate tissue contrast while maintaining the lowest possible radiation dose. In order to achieve this, it is important to understand that tissue attenuation-based contrast is dependent on the x-ray photon energy, because the mass attenuation coefficient μ/ρ of a given tissue depends on the x-ray photon energy. In fact, three effects contribute to the attenuation for photon energies up to 1 MeV (i.e., below the threshold for pair production): coherent scattering, incoherent scattering, and the photoelectric effect. Consequently, the mass attenuation coefficient μ/ρ has three factors:

$$\left(\frac{\mu}{\rho}\right)_{Total} = \left(\frac{\mu}{\rho}\right)_{Coh} + \left(\frac{\mu}{\rho}\right)_{Incoh} + \left(\frac{\mu}{\rho}\right)_{Photoel}. \tag{13.4}$$

TABLE 13.1 Mass Attenuation Coefficients of Water

X-Ray Photon, E (keV)	μ/ρ (m²/kg)
10	0.5232
20	0.0795
30	0.0376
40	0.0268
50	0.0228
60	0.0207
70	0.0193
80	0.0183
90	0.0175
100	0.0169
110	0.0164
120	0.0159
130	0.0155
140	0.0152
150	0.0149

Coherent scattering is considered elastic because the x-ray photon does not lose energy when it is deflected from its original path. On the other hand, incoherent scattering is referred to as inelastic, due to the fact that the x-ray photon transfers energy to the tissue while it is being deflected. With the photoelectric effect, the x-ray photon is absorbed by an atom within the tissue, which releases a bound electron from the atom. Table 13.2 demonstrates the different dependence of the three contributions on the x-ray photon energy E and on the atomic number Z and the atomic weight A.[2] Radiological techniques utilize these relationships to determine optimal x-ray techniques. More specifically, tissue attenuation contrast in x-ray imaging is determined by the subject contrast (SC):

$$SC = \ln \frac{E_2}{E_1},\qquad(13.5)$$

where E_1 and E_2 are the absorbed x-ray energy fluences in the detector corresponding to the two tissue projection areas. If μ_1 and μ_2 are the linear attenuation coefficients for the two tissues, each of thickness t, then the SC between these two tissues for a monoenergetic incident x-ray can be calculated with Equation 13.2 as follows:

$$SC = \ln \frac{\exp(-\mu_2 t)}{\exp(-\mu_1 t)} = (\mu_1 - \mu_2)t.\qquad(13.6)$$

For polychromatic x-rays, the difference $(\mu_1 - \mu_2)$ in this formula should be weighted by the x-ray spectrum. Figure 13.1 illustrates the SC between a 0.5 mm thick microcalcification and breast glandular tissue as a function of x-ray photon energy. The figure demonstrates that the tissue SC decreases rapidly with increasing x-ray photon energy, which is because tissue μ/ρ decreases with increasing x-ray photon energy. Therefore, tissue contrast decreases with increasing x-ray photon energy. In addition,

TABLE 13.2 Dependence of Mass Attenuation Coefficients on X-Ray Photon Energy E and on Atomic Number Z and Atomic Weight A

Mass Attenuation Coefficients	Dependence on E	Dependence on Z and A
$(\mu/\rho)_{coherent}$	$E^{-1.8}$	$Z^{2.8}/A$
$(\mu/\rho)_{incoherent}$	$E^{-0.2}$	Z/A
$(\mu/\rho)_{photoelectric}$	$E^{-3.5}$	$Z^{4.5}/A$

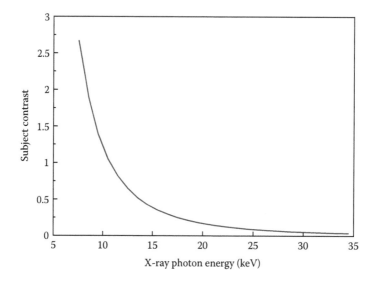

FIGURE 13.1 The SC between a 0.5 mm microcalcification and breast glandular tissue as a function of x-ray photon energy.

the contrast between two tissues increases as the differences between their relative atomic numbers increase. Therefore, different x-ray energy values are typically employed to provide optimal imaging for different body parts. As detailed previously, tissue contrast is low in breast imaging; thus, photons of low energies from 15 to 25 keV are optimal for maintaining adequate tissue contrast and a relatively low radiation dose.[3] Alternatively, high tissue contrast exists among bone, soft tissue, and air. Thus, photons of much higher energies (up to 150 keV) are used in modalities such as chest imaging, in order to maintain a low radiation dose and provide a reasonable dynamic range.

In general, increasing the photon energy reduces the μ/ρ value. However, the photon absorption amount experiences a dramatic increase when the photon energy equals the binding energy of the atomic electrons of the tissue. This is due to the increasing atom ionization, which results in a corresponding increase in the mass attenuation μ/ρ. The photon energies causing this increase in μ/ρ are called the absorption edges. The existence of absorption edges is of great significance for designing x-ray imaging detectors and spectrum-shaping filters, which will be detailed in the following sections.

13.2.2 Phase-Based Tissue Contrast

In addition to attenuation, tissue contrast can be produced by the x-ray phase change generated within tissues. Attenuation-based tissue contrast has been utilized in medical imaging for more than 100 years, but the concept of phase-based tissue contrast was not recognized until recently.[4] X-ray phase change does not arise from new x-ray–tissue interaction but instead is a result of coherent x-ray scattering. As detailed previously, x-ray is an electromagnetic wavelike light and thus can be described as a coherent x-ray wave field propagating along the *z*-axis:

$$\psi(x,z) = \sqrt{I(x)}\,\exp(ikz), \tag{13.7}$$

where
    x is the coordinate for the transverse direction
    λ is the x-ray wavelength
    $k = 2\pi/\lambda$
    $I(x)$ is the x-ray intensity

In this case, the phase of the x-ray wave is equal to kz. When x-ray scatters from tissue, the phase of the x-ray wave field has been changed. This phase change results from coherent scattering through small angles and contains both diffraction and refraction effects. The amount of the phase change is determined by the biological tissue dielectric susceptibility or, equivalently, by the refractive index of the tissue. The refractive index n for x-ray is a complex quantity:

$$n = 1 - \delta - i\beta, \tag{13.8}$$

where
  δ is the refractive index decrement, which is responsible for the x-ray phase shift
  β is responsible for the x-ray absorption

The following formula for calculating δ is given by Wilkins et al.[4]:

$$\delta = \left(\frac{r_e \lambda^2}{2\pi}\right) \sum_k N_k (Z_k + f_k^r), \tag{13.9}$$

where
  r_e is the classical electron radius
  N_k is the atomic density for the element k
  Z_k is the atomic number for the element k
  f_k is the real part of the anomalous atomic scattering factor for the element k

If the x-ray energy value is far from the absorption edge of tissue, the aforementioned formula can be simplified as follows:

$$\delta = \left(\frac{r_e \lambda^2}{2\pi}\right) \sum_k N_k (Z_k + f_k^r) \cong (4.49 \times 10^{-16}) \lambda^2 N_e, \tag{13.10}$$

where N_e is the electron density. While x-ray absorption by the body is frequently acknowledged, the fact that human tissue actually refracts x-ray is not as widely recognized. This is not because the value of δ for tissue is much smaller as compared to β; on the contrary, the value of δ for tissue (10^{-6}–10^{-8}) is approximately 1000 times greater than the value of β (10^{-9}–10^{-11}) for x-ray in the energy range from 10 to 100 keV. It is therefore ironic that the existing x-ray clinical imaging techniques were designed to image tissue β only. Using the formula for the refractive index decrement δ, the amount of the x-ray phase change in biological tissue can then be calculated:

$$\phi = \frac{2\pi}{\lambda} \int \delta(s) ds, \tag{13.11}$$

where s is the distance traveled by the x-ray beam along the vacuum propagation direction.

At this stage of development, there are three primary methods of phase imaging: x-ray interferometry, diffraction-enhanced imaging, and in-line phase-contrast imaging. X-ray interferometry[5] directly images the phase ϕ, through the use of monochromatic x-rays from synchrotron radiation and a monochromator crystal. Diffraction-enhanced imaging[6] measures the phase gradient $\nabla\phi$ directly, also with monochromatic x-rays from synchrotron radiation. In-line phase-contrast imaging[4] directly measures the Laplacian of the phase $\nabla^2\phi$ and can be implemented with polychromatic x-rays from an x-ray tube, which are compact and readily available. Thus, in-line phase-contrast imaging has great potential for clinical applications and will be discussed in detail in Section 13.5.

13.3 X-Ray Spectra and Exposure Control

13.3.1 Bremsstrahlung and Characteristic Radiation

X-ray attenuation and tissue contrast are dependent on the x-ray photon energy; thus, it is very important to utilize x-ray photons of appropriate energies to image specific parts of the body. This is achieved by controlling the x-ray spectrum used for imaging. X-rays are typically generated through the interaction of electromagnetic fields with charged particles such as electrons. A charged particle in uniform motion of any velocity cannot produce an electromagnetic wave, even if the particle is surrounded by an electromagnetic field. Only charged particles undergoing acceleration or deceleration can emit x-ray radiation. In medical imaging, x-rays are generally produced by bombarding a metal target with energetic electrons. Upon impact with the metal target, the incident electrons collide with the electrons and nuclei of the metal atoms, and the collisions slow down and deflect the incident electrons. The electrostatic attractive force between the nuclei of the metal atoms and the incident electrons primarily results in swift deflections, which rapidly increase the momentum of the incident electrons, producing large acceleration values. As a result, the deflected incident electrons emit x-rays. Repeated collisions with the metal atoms eventually slow down the incident electrons to a resting state in the metal, which ends their ability to emit x-rays. X-ray radiation generated by the deceleration of energetic electrons in metal is referred to as Bremsstrahlung, which typically contains x-ray photons of different wavelengths; thus, it is polychromatic. According to Kramers' law,[2] the Bremsstrahlung intensity $I_{br}(E)$ at photon energy E is defined as follows:

$$I_{br}(E) = CZI_{tube}(E_o - E), \quad \text{for } E < E_o,$$

$$I_{br}(E) = 0, \quad \text{for } E > E_o,$$

(13.12)

where

Z is the atomic number of the metal target
I_{tube} is the current of the incident electrons
E_o is the kinetic energy of the incident electrons

In medical x-ray imaging equipment, incident electrons are accelerated by an applied voltage before striking the metal target. In Equation 13.12, a Bremsstrahlung energy E_o is therefore equal to eV_o, where V_o is the applied acceleration voltage and e is the electron charge. For energy values less than E_o, Kramers' law predicts that the spectral intensity increases with decreasing E. However, due to x-ray attenuation by the metal target, the output Bremsstrahlung energy typically peaks near $E_o/2$, as illustrated in Figure 13.2. The actual value is dependent on the target material and the use of filtration, which will be further detailed in the following sections. The total Bremsstrahlung intensity I_{br-t} can be approximated by integrating Equation 13.12 over E, which results in the following:

$$I_{br-t} = CZI_{tube}V_o^2 = CZI_{tube}PV_o,$$

(13.13)

where P is the power loading of the tube. Equation 13.13 demonstrates that the total Bremsstrahlung intensity is approximately proportional to the square of the applied acceleration voltage V_o, the tube current I_{tube}, and the atomic number Z of the metal target material. Therefore, increasing the Bremsstrahlung intensity is accomplished by applying a high acceleration voltage, increasing the current, and adopting a high-Z target material. In fact, these three factors are among the most important considerations in the design of x-ray-generating devices.

In addition to Bremsstrahlung radiation, another important mechanism of x-ray generation is referred to as characteristic radiation. The atomic electrons of the target are removed from their atomic shells by the collisions from the incident electrons, which cause the inner-shell ionization of the metal atoms. X-ray photons can then be emitted when the ionized atoms return to their ground states. This mechanism of x-ray radiation is known as characteristic radiation, because the energies of the emitted x-ray

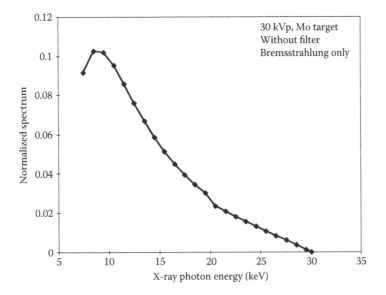

FIGURE 13.2 X-ray Bremsstrahlung spectrum for an Mo target at 30 kVp.

photons are discrete values that are equal to the binding energy differences of the atomic shells. The type of characteristic radiation indicates the relevant inner atomic shells, such as K-shell and L-shell. For example, K-characteristic radiation results from the removal of a K-shell electron by an incident electron. If eV_b represents the binding energy of an atomic shell, characteristic radiation from this shell can only be generated if the applied voltage V is greater than V_b. A larger difference $(V - V_b)$ produces more characteristic radiation. The total output x-ray consists of both Bremsstrahlung and characteristic radiation, which produces a combined spectrum as shown in Figure 13.3. The spikes in the figure are produced by the superposition of the two types of x-ray radiation.

For tubes utilized in general R&F, the metal target layer is generally made up of tungsten (W) alloyed with 5%–10% of rhenium (Re). However, the target material used in mammography is conventionally

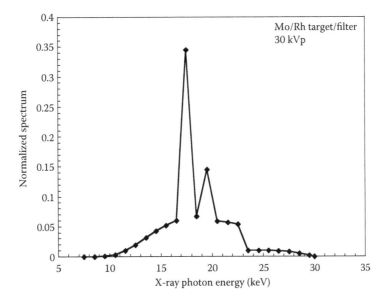

FIGURE 13.3 X-ray spectrum for an Mo target with an Rh filter at 30 kVp.

molybdenum (Mo) or rhodium (Rh). The atomic numbers for W, Mo, and Rh are 74, 42, and 45, respectively; thus, Equation 13.13 indicates that a W target would generate much more Bremsstrahlung radiation than an Mo target or an Rh target. However, Mo and Rh targets are utilized in mammography applications because they generate K-characteristic radiation photons in the range of 17–23 keV, which is optimal for breast imaging.

In addition to the metal target material, another method utilized to shape the output x-ray spectrum is referred to as a filter, which is a metal sheet placed directly in the path of the x-ray beam. During an x-ray exposure, many low-energy photons are produced in the Bremsstrahlung spectrum, as shown in Figure 13.2. These photons will be absorbed by the patient's body before reaching the imaging detector; thus, they do not contribute useful information in producing the image. An aluminum filter can reduce the number of low-energy photons, which increases the penetrating ability of the x-ray beam and therefore reduces the radiation dose to the patient. This method of shaping the x-ray spectra is referred to as beam hardening by filtration. An aluminum filter with a thickness of 1 mm or more is typically used for this purpose, although a copper filter with a thickness of 0.1 mm or more can be used in fluoroscopy to significantly reduce the patient dose. In mammography, absorption-edge filters are also used to shape the beam spectrum. As detailed previously, the mass attenuation coefficient μ/ρ increases dramatically at the absorption edge. The use of an absorption-edge filter provides the ability to selectively attenuate photons with energies above the absorption edge, thereby shaping the output x-ray spectrum. For example, Mo and Rh have absorption edges at 19.97 and 23.19 keV, respectively. Therefore, a larger portion of x-ray photons within the optimal energy range from 18 to 23 keV can be generated by using either an Mo or an Rh filter with an Mo target, which produces improved tissue contrast along with a reduced radiation dose to the breast glandular tissue.[7-9]

13.3.2 X-Ray Tubes

An x-ray tube is a device designed to generate x-rays through the principles discussed previously. As illustrated in Figure 13.4, an x-ray tube consists of a cathode emitting the electrons, a rotating anode disc acting as the metal target, and a glass or metal envelope providing structural support, which maintains a vacuum of approximately 5×10^{-7} torr inside the tube. The cathode is composed of a focusing cup and a filament, which consists of a tungsten wire helix with a diameter of 0.2–0.3 mm. When heated to approximately 2400°C by the filament current, the filament emits electrons. With the exception of low tube potentials, the tube current I_A resulting from the emitted electrons is almost independent of the tube potential and can be determined as a function of the filament temperature:

$$I_A = CT^2 \exp\left(\frac{-W}{kT}\right) A_f,$$
(13.14)

where
    C is a material-dependent constant
    T is the temperature in K
    W is the work function of the filament, which is 4.5 eV for tungsten
    A_f is the area of the filament
    k is the Boltzmann constant

The equation indicates that the tube current I_A increases with increasing filament temperature. For radiography, the filament current is approximately 5 A, and the tube current ranges from 20 to 1000 mA. Equation 13.14 is invalid for tube potentials less than 50 kV, due to the fact that all of the electrons emitted by the filament are not drawn to the anode for low tube potentials. In these cases, the tube current

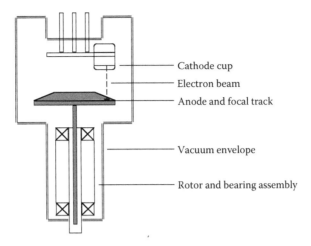

FIGURE 13.4 Schematic of an x-ray tube with a rotating anode.

I_A is lower than the value predicted by Equation 13.14, and it becomes dependent on the tube potential. This behavior of I_A is referred to as the space-charge effect. In breast imaging, the tube potentials vary from 25 to 35 kVp; thus, the achievable I_A is limited by the space-charge effect, especially for x-ray tubes with small focal spots. This low I_A value imposes a technical challenge on mammography applications.

The focusing cup maintains a small focal spot on the anode surface, which is necessary to achieve good spatial resolution. In projection x-ray imaging, the size of the x-ray focal spot determines the amount of blurring in the image as follows:

$$B = (M - 1)f, \tag{13.15}$$

where
  M is the geometric magnification factor, which is the ratio of the source-to-detector distance (SDD) to the source-to-object distance (SOD)
  f is the focal spot size

For example, in magnification mammography where M has a value of 2, B is therefore equal to f, and features smaller than f at the image plane cannot be recognized in the image. In general, a diagnostic x-ray tube provides the ability to select one of two or three available focal spot sizes. In general radiography, the typical sizes are 1–1.2 mm for the large focal spot and 0.5–0.6 mm for the small focal spot. However, in mammography, the typical sizes are 0.3 mm for the large focal spot and 0.1 mm for the small focal spot.

The tube anode is a rotating metal alloy disc. In addition to the metal target layer discussed in the previous subsection, the remainder of the anode disc is made up of a graphite or molybdenum (Mo) material. Since approximately 99% of the energy from incident electrons is transformed into heat in the anode, the anode disc materials must have high melting points and good thermal conductivity. During an x-ray exposure, the temperature of the focal spot is higher than that of the focal track, which in turn is higher than that of the anode body, due to the fact that the anode is rotating during an exposure. The anode operates as a rotor, which is driven by the stator through magnetic induction and runs as an asynchronous motor. The stator driving current is provided by the high-speed starter of the x-ray generator, which will be discussed in detail in the next subsection. The anode rotation speed generally ranges from 1,200 to 3,600 rpm, although speeds up to 10,800 rpm can be used for the high-speed mode. For *dry*

operation in a vacuum at such high temperatures, the ball bearing must satisfy exceptional specifications. To extend its life, the anode starts to rotate immediately before each exposure and is brought to
rest quickly after the exposure by a braking circuit of the generator. The electron impact time decreases
with the velocity ωr, where ω is the anode angular velocity and r is the anode radius. Therefore, the focal
spot temperature increases with the input power and x-ray exposure time and decreases with increasing
focal spot size, rotation speed, and anode diameter. The practical limit of the focal spot temperature is
2500°C, although the melting point of tungsten is 3370°C, which is the highest of all metals. Therefore,
an x-ray tube is assigned a specific maximum power loading based on the aforementioned parameters,
which is known as the tube power rating. During an exposure, the average power loading P_{Load} to an
x-ray tube is determined by

$$P_{\text{Load}} = wVI, \tag{13.16}$$

where
  w is the kV-wave-shape factor
  V is the tube kVp, which is the peak voltage in kV
  I is the tube current in mA

The kV-wave-shape factor w depends on the kV-wave form, because the tube kVp is not equal to the average tube potential. For 3-phase 12-pulse, or high-frequency (HF) generators, the value of w is 0.99, while
it is only 0.95 for 3-phase 6-pulse generators, and 0.74 for single-phase generators. For tube operation,
the power loading of an exposure should always be lower than the tube power rating, which increases
with increasing focal spot size, rotation speed, and anode diameter but decreases with exposure time.
The power ratings for a specific exposure time can be determined from the manufacturer-supplied tube
rating chart or the single-exposure rating chart. For R&F applications, the tube power rating is 100 kW
for a 0.1 s exposure with an anode rotation of 10,800 rpm and a focal spot of 1.2 mm. However, decreasing the focal spot size to 0.6 mm reduces the tube power rating to 30 kW.

In addition to the power rating, x-ray tube specifications also include the anode heat capacity, which
is the maximum anode heat loading amount. The heat loading H_L generated during an exposure, which
is expressed in heat units (HU), where 1 J = 1.35 HU, is given as follows:

$$H_L = 1.35 P_{\text{Load}} T_{\text{exp}}, \tag{13.17}$$

where
  P_{Load} is the power loading of the exposure
  T_{exp} is the exposure time in s

Increasing the mass of the anode provides a higher anode heat capacity. For R&F applications, the
tube anode heat capacity is typically greater than 400 kHU. Although the power loading is not
high for x-ray tubes in computed tomography (CT) applications, the heat loading can be as high
as 6.5 MHU or more, due to long continuous scan times. The amount of tube heating during multiple exposures depends also on heat dissipation; in fact, the anode cools by releasing heat. In order
to increase the amount of heat dissipation, the anode surface area can be increased to utilize the
additional emissive coating. In addition, the tube housing is limited by a separate maximum heat
loading specification. Exceeding this value can result in housing or tube failure, due to the thermal
expansion of the insulation oil surrounding the tube. For applications such as digital subtraction
angiography (DSA), a tube assembly may be equipped with an external oil-to-air or oil-to-water heat
exchanger to allow faster cooling.

13.3.3 X-Ray Generators

The main function of an x-ray generator is to provide high and controllable tube voltages and tube currents to facilitate x-ray generation and exposure control. A generator is specified by the kVp rating, the power rating, and the kV-ripple. The kVp rating indicates the maximum kVp allowed, which refers to the peak tube voltage in kV. The power rating specifies the maximum power loading for a 0.1 s exposure. During an exposure, the actual tube voltage value is not a strict constant but instead oscillates around a mean value. The amount of this oscillation is referred to as the kV-ripple, which is usually specified as a percentage of the peak voltage. As mentioned previously, the tube voltage determines the highest energy of the output x-ray photons. Therefore, in addition to tube voltage and tube current, the amount of kV-ripple also affects x-ray radiation output and x-ray spectra shape. A small amount of kV-ripple is desirable in order to provide x-ray exposure reproducibility, consistency of image quality, and radiation dose reduction.

In general, higher kVp values produce a more penetrating x-ray beam, but they also result in lower image contrast; thus, the optimal tube kVp value varies depending on the part of the body being imaged. Typically, clinical systems utilize 125–150 kVp for chest x-rays, 110–130 kVp for CT, 75–85 kVp for abdomen exams, 65–75 kVp for skull exams, and 24–35 kVp for mammography. X-ray generator kVp ratings are generally specified accordingly as 150 kVp for R&F generators and 45 kVp for mammography generators. Typical power ratings are 60–100 kW for DSA generators, 50–60 kW for R&F generators, and approximately 5 kW for mammography generators.

The core of an x-ray generator is a high-power, high-voltage circuit. A basic single-phase generator is shown in Figure 13.5. The autotransformer TF1, which is powered by the line ac, functions as the kVp controller. The low input ac voltage is transformed into high ac voltage by the high-voltage transformer HTF. The diode bridge provides full-wave rectification of the high-voltage ac. The step-down transformer TF2 provides filament current control. The kV-ripple value could be as high as 100% with a single-phase generator. However, if the line supply is replaced by a three-phase line supply, then the rectified sine waves from different phases can be interleaved, and the kV-ripple can be reduced to 13%–25% for 6-pulse interleaving and 5%–10% for 12-pulse interleaving. The tube kVp generated by single- or three-phase generators also depends on the input line regulation, and the kVp reproducibility is easily compromised by unstable line supply conditions. Another drawback of single- or three-phase generators is the slow response time in controlling the tube kVp.

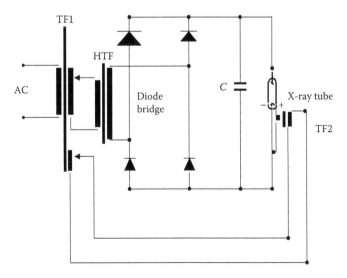

FIGURE 13.5 Circuit schematic of a single-phase x-ray generator.

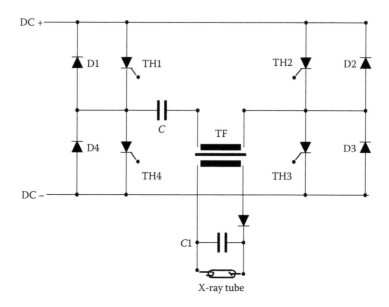

FIGURE 13.6 Circuit schematic of an HF inverter.

Another important specification for medical imaging equipment is compactness. The high-voltage transformers of single- and three-phase generators are especially bulky in size and weight. However, the voltage U induced by a transformer is proportional to the product of the operating frequency f, the core cross-sectional area A, and the number of turns n. Thus, increasing f reduces the values of A and n, and a generator operating at a higher frequency can be much smaller in size and lighter in weight. For this reason, HF generators operating at a frequency of a few to tens or even 100 kHz have proliferated in recent years. As compared to single- and three-phase generators, these generators are 50%–80% smaller in size and weight, which also reduces the manufacturing cost. Moreover, HF generators provide a faster response and a greatly reduced kV-ripple amount.

HF generators are based on converter technology, in which the key is to convert the conventional ac power of 60 Hz and a few hundred volts to an HF power supply providing tens of kHz. This task is accomplished by the HF inverter. Conventional ac power is first rectified and filtered into dc power, which is then inverted to HF pulses. A basic dc to HF inverter is shown in Figure 13.6. Four thyristors, which are denoted TH1 to TH4, operate as controlled switches. A thyristor functions as a diode with a control gate, and the trigger pulses applied to the gate control whether the current flows through the thyristor. The high-voltage transformer TF couples the x-ray tube as a load to the inverter and provides high voltage to the tube. The HF pulses are generated by a series RLC resonant circuit, which denotes a circuit having a resistor (R), and inductor (L), and a capacitor (C).

In this case, the coupling capacitor C, the inductance L of transformer TF, and the tube load form a series RLC resonant circuit, which is controlled by thyristors TH1 to TH4. When the gates of TH1 and TH3 are enabled, they operate as two closed switches. DC voltage is then applied to the RLC circuit. It is a well-known fact that a capacitor tends to oppose voltage changes and an inductor tends to resist current changes. This is because the capacitor stores electric energy and the inductor stores magnetic energy, and energy transfer is not instantaneous. The interchange of stored electric and magnetic energy results in an oscillation of the current in the thyristors and the RLC circuit. Due to the energy dissipation to the load R, the oscillating current functions as a damped sinusoidal current. The frequency of the oscillating current is referred to as the resonant frequency f_{res}, which is given by

$$f_{res} = \frac{1}{2\pi\sqrt{LC}}.$$

(13.18)

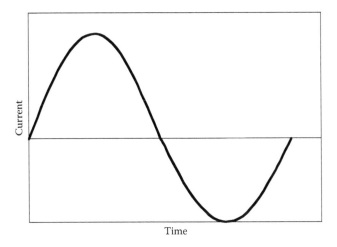

FIGURE 13.7 Current pulse waveform in an HF inverter.

During the negative half of the sinusoidal cycle, current flows through the antiparallel diodes D1 and D3 instead of through thyristors TH1 and TH3, due to the fact that thyristors do not allow a reverse current. Damping the load results in a second peak value that is smaller than that of the first peak in the cycle. However, when the full sinusoidal cycle is completed, the RLC resonator cannot start its second cycle, because thyristors TH1 and TH3 have already been disabled through self-communication during the reversing half cycle. Therefore, as illustrated in Figure 13.7, a single current pulse is generated for each pair of trigger pulses to the gates of TH1 and TH3. To degauss the transformer core, TH2 and TH4 alternate to produce the next current pulse in a similar way. The difference lies in the fact that the polarity of the applied dc power is now reversed; hence, the RLC resonance process leads to a *reversed* current pulse. The frequency at which the two trigger pulse pairs are applied is denoted the driving frequency f_d. A higher driving frequency value produces a more dense current pulse train.

The secondary coil of the transformer TF couples a rectifying circuit with the RLC circuit. The rectifying circuit consists of a diode bridge and a capacitor C_l for filtering. The tube voltage is equal to the voltage across C_l, which is therefore referred to as the load capacitor. The rectifying circuit converts the HF current pulses into charge pockets, which are stored in the load capacitor. At the beginning of an exposure, the driving frequency is very high in order to charge the load capacitor rapidly to build up the desired tube voltage. The voltage of the load capacitor can be measured by a precision resistor voltage divider. When the desired tube voltage is established, a feedback signal will be sent to the voltage–frequency converter *V/F*, the output of which controls the driving frequency of the gate trigger pulse circuit. The driving frequency will then be reduced to deliver the exact amount of charge pockets to the load capacitor to compensate for the discharge consumed by the tube current. Therefore, although the value of the resonant frequency f_{res} is fixed by the coupling capacitance C and the inductance L through Equation 13.18, the driving frequency varies during exposures. However, the maximum driving frequency value is equal to the resonant frequency. Using the closed-loop feedback control described previously, the tube voltage control mechanism is very fast and accurate, and the kV-ripple ranges from 2% to 15%, depending on the power rating. For a given resonant frequency, the amount of ripple decreases with increasing power. Therefore, in order to maintain a constant kV-ripple value, an x-ray generator may need to employ different coupling capacitors depending on the focal spot size, due to the fact that the tube power rating with the small focal spot size is much lower than the rating with the large focal spot size. Another advantage of HF generators involves the flexibility to use either a single-phase or a three-phase line supply, due to the fact that the inverter circuits of the generators are powered by dc power. The inverter circuit described earlier can also provide power to the filament. In a filament inverter, the filament transformer provides a step-down in voltage or a step-up in current, and the secondary coil of the transformer is coupled directly with the tube filament without the need for rectifying circuitry. A precision resistor in series with the x-ray tube detects the tube current in real time, and the sensed signal is used as the feedback for controlling the driving frequency of the filament inverter. In this way, the tube current control is much faster and more accurate than with single- or three-phase generators.

In addition to providing high voltage and power to the tube, an x-ray generator should also provide a reliable method for x-ray exposure control. As indicated by Equation 13.13, the exposure rate is proportional to the tube current, and the total exposure is proportional to the integral of I_{tube} over the exposure time, which is denoted the total mAs, or mA × seconds, of the exposure. X-ray generators must include an mAs switch to control the total mAs delivered during an exposure. The mAs switch circuitry might consist of a simple electronic timer that ensures a constant mA during exposure or a current integrator that facilitates a decreasing I_{tube} during exposure. However, typical x-ray generators use automatic exposure control (AEC) circuitry as the mAs switch. With AEC, exposures are terminated when a preset amount of exposure incident on the image receptor is reached. Thus, AEC ensures that the imaging detector always receives a similar amount of radiation exposure, regardless of the amount of object attenuation. A typical AEC circuit consists of an x-ray sensor, a current integrator, and a comparator. The x-ray sensor generates a sensing current, which is proportional to the exposure rate incident on the image receptor. The current integrator measures the total exposure to the image receptor, and the comparator transmits the exposure termination signal when the output of the current integrator reaches the preset exposure value. The radiation sensor might be an ionization chamber that transforms x-ray to electric current, or it could also be a fluorescent screen coupled with a photodiode. In this case, the fluorescent screen transforms x-ray to light, and the photodiode functions as a light sensor.

13.4 Projection X-Ray Imaging

13.4.1 Conventional Radiography

Projection radiography is the conventional technique performed in radiological imaging. It uses an x-ray beam to generate a 2D transmission image of the patient anatomy. As shown in Figure 13.8, the x-ray beam passes through the body of the patient during x-ray exposure and is recorded by a 2D detector. Within the body, the x-ray radiation experiences attenuation, through absorption and scattering, as well as diffraction. The x-ray beam is attenuated and diffracted in different amounts according to the anatomical structure and thickness of the body. This section is focused on attenuation-based projection radiography. The incorporation of diffraction effects, which is referred to as phase-contrast imaging, will be discussed in Section 13.5.

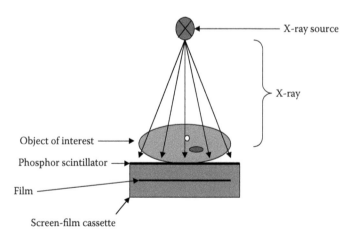

FIGURE 13.8   Schematic of the formation of a projection radiograph.

The conventional projection radiograph is a spatially modulated attenuation pattern of the anatomical structure of the object. Thus, a projection radiograph is a 2D *x-ray shadow image* of the 3D anatomy of the patient. Specifically, a projection radiograph is a 2D map of $I(x, y)$:

$$I(x, y) = I_0 \exp\left(- \int I(x, y; s) ds \right), \tag{13.19}$$

where
    I_0 is the incident x-ray intensity
    $I(x, y; s)$ is the detected intensity at position $(x, y; s)$, where s is the distance along the ray direction from the focal spot to point (x, y)

The integral in Equation 13.19 gives the projection sum of the linear attenuation coefficients along the ray path. It is important to note that this projection image is different than the images from longitudinal tomography and CT, in which an image of a tissue slice is a 2D representation of the map of tissue linear attenuation coefficients $\mu(x, y; s)$ of the slice at s. Due to space limitations, tomography will not be covered in this chapter.

X-ray detection can be provided by screen-film combinations or digital imaging detectors. Film was the first radiographic detector used in medicine, and it was widely used in medical imaging until recently. The purpose of radiographic film is not limited to detection, as it also functions as the display device and the archiving medium. Unexposed film is a thin sheet of inert plastic, which is coated with emulsion on one or both sides. Film is insensitive to the x-ray energies used in medical practice; therefore, x-ray images are typically formed through the use of a screen-film combination. The term *screen*, or *intensifying screen*, refers to a luminescent sheet that contains densely packed luminescent materials. The luminescent substances must be highly efficient for x-ray absorption and conversion of x-ray to light, and they should have light emission spectra matching the spectral sensitivity of the film. Currently, most intensifying screens use gadolinium oxysulfide (Gd_2O_2S) as the luminescent material. Gd_2O_2S-based intensifying screens are capable of converting each x-ray photon to numerous green light photons. For example, a single 30 keV x-ray photon is converted to approximately 1500 green light photons. For detection, the film is placed in direct contact with the intensifying screen in the cassette. During x-ray exposure, the x-ray photons exiting from the patient first interact with the Gd_2O_2S-based intensifying screen, which converts the x-ray to green light. Subsequently, the green light exposes the film, and through a chemical development process, the original radiographic image of the patient is captured permanently on the film.

13.4.2 Digital Radiography

In recent years, radiology has undergone a revolutionary change from screen-film-based radiology to digital radiology, which uses optoelectronic detectors to record the images. A digital image detector records the number of transmitted x-ray photons for each pixel, which is the field of a single detector element. Thus, the digital image appears as an array of pixels. Figure 13.9 provides an example representing a simple 1D image in both analog and digital format. To minimize the loss of information from discontinuities in the image due to pixel averaging, the detector element size must be significantly smaller than the important features within the image. Although the digital image can be captured with a large dynamic range, interpretation of the radiograph requires a viewing mechanism, which is either on-screen or in hard-copy format. The information in these representations of the image is typically truncated to 8-bit data from 12- or 14-bit data. This is not necessarily a problem, as the features of interest are often within a smaller grayscale range than the entire dynamic range of the detector. However, high-fidelity electronic display and hard-copy printing devices are necessary to preserve diagnostic quality.

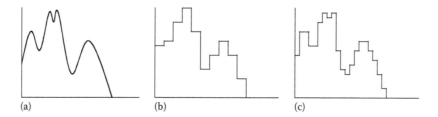

FIGURE 13.9   Analog image information is recorded as a sequence of individual pixel values, as opposed to a continually changing function. The digital value at a pixel can be thought of as the average of the analog value across the area of the pixel. The analog image (a) can lose resolution as it is converted to a digital signal (b). To improve resolution, the detector element size, that is, pixel size, can be decreased (c).

Various optoelectronic detectors have been developed and successfully applied in clinical practice. Three types of detectors are used in the majority of digital imaging systems: charge-coupled device (CCD) detector systems, flat-panel thin-film transistor (TFT) detector systems, both of which are illustrated in Figure 13.10, and photostimulable phosphor imaging plate detector systems. Each detector type possesses advantages and disadvantages and is the most effective when applied to particular tasks. Prior to describing and comparing these detectors in detail, the specification parameters for digital imaging detectors will first be presented. The primary parameters include field coverage, detector sensitivity and quantum efficiency, spatial resolution, noise factors, and dynamic range.

The first important factor in selecting a detector is the field coverage, which describes the image size requirements. For example, stereotactic breast biopsy imaging acquires relatively small images; thus, a single CCD detector including a demagnification step would be acceptable, due to the minimal amount of demagnification necessary.[10] However, larger images such as chest images require a higher degree of demagnification, which can decrease the image resolution to an unacceptable level. CCDs are therefore

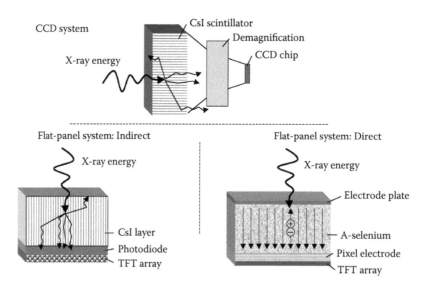

FIGURE 13.10   Two types of digital radiography detectors are detailed: the CCD system (top) and the TFT flat-panel system (bottom). The CCD system converts the x-rays to visible light with a CsI scintillator screen before the signal is demagnified and detected by the CCD. The indirect flat-panel system converts the x-ray signal to visible light before it is converted to charge by photodiodes at the detector, while the direct flat-panel system converts the x-rays directly to charge in a layer of amorphous selenium. The charges are drawn to the detector by an applied electric field.

combined into detector arrays for use in larger imaging applications. Another alternative involves the use of full-field TFT arrays, which are manufactured in standard film sizes and may have better performance potential for larger image fields.

Detector sensitivity is a measurement of the ability of the detector to convert the x-ray signal into electric charge. The efficiency of this conversion is referred to as quantum efficiency. The x-ray quanta interact with the detector material primarily according to the photoelectric effect, wherein one or more photons are produced as the x-ray quanta transmit energy to a high-Z detector atom. The quantum efficiency η is related to both the attenuation properties of the detector material and the detector thickness.[11] The attenuation properties influence the effectiveness of the x-ray in transmitting energy to a detector atom, and the thickness determines the likelihood of the x-ray to encounter a detector atom for the energy transmission. The attenuation properties are determined by the composition of the detector material, as well as the energy of the incident x-rays. In general, high-energy x-rays can penetrate farther into the detector material due to a smaller attenuation coefficient, whereas low-energy x-rays cannot penetrate as far because of a larger attenuation coefficient. Another factor affecting quantum efficiency is the *fill factor* of the detector, which is the ratio of the active detector material area to the total detector element area. As the fill factor approaches 100%, less undetected radiation is generated for an image of adequate intensity, and thus, the total radiation dose is minimized.

The spatial resolution of the detector plate is dependent on characteristics of the detector as well as external factors. Significant detector characteristics affecting resolution are the size of the active portion of each detector element, or the effective aperture size, the distance between detector elements, or the spatial sampling interval, and lateral spreading effects, which are due to limitations of the detector material or transfer of information from the detector to the computer. External factors influencing spatial resolution include relative motion between the detector and the x-ray source or the patient and image unsharpness resulting from magnification due to the spreading of the x-ray beam.[11] Different resolutions are necessary for different types of imaging, depending upon the size and spacing of significant features.

Another factor affecting the sharpness of an image is noise. X-ray images are statistical in nature; therefore, since x-rays arrive at the detector in quantum packets of energy, the image will inherently contain some degree of graininess or quantum noise. Ideal image acquisition systems are denoted as quantum noise limited due to the absence of other sources of noise. The x-ray image signal must be significantly stronger than the noise to create a discernable image. The signal-to-noise ratio (SNR) is a quantity that defines the relationship between the useful signal and the noise in the image. The detective quantum efficiency (DQE) describes the effectiveness of transferring the SNR of the incoming x-ray signal to the output digital image. The mathematical formula for the DQE, as well as a detailed DQE analysis, will be presented in the next subsection. Ideally, the DQE is equal to the quantum efficiency, but detectors add noise from different sources due to their particular characteristics. For example, some detectors are sensitive to visible light as well as x-rays, and light leakage into the detector casing increases noise. Other detectors are very sensitive to heat and must be operated at low temperatures to reduce thermal noise. Background noise can often become insignificant if the incident image signal is intensified; however, a challenging balance exists between minimizing radiation dose and achieving reasonable output SNR.

The dynamic range of a detector describes the range of signal levels at which the detector can accurately record an image, considering intrinsic noise factors. The range must provide the ability to measure values encompassing the least to the most radio-opaque regions of the image. The dynamic range is limited at low levels because the signal can become consumed by noise. At high levels, the detector elements can become saturated and leak onto adjacent elements, blurring the final image. Although most digital detectors are capable of acquiring images with a significantly reduced x-ray dose as compared to their screen-film counterparts, the noise sources must be controlled in order to maintain adequate imaging ability.

The first detector system category is the CCD, which is illustrated in Figure 13.10. Systems utilizing the CCD as the detector element have had a few variants in the decades since its advent. The CCD is manufactured as a 2–5 cm^2 chip comprised of 256 by 256 to 2048 by 2048 sensitive detectors, which correspond to pixels in the digital image. CCD detectors utilize an indirect conversion system incorporating a conversion step before the detection step, in which incident x-rays are converted to visible light by the scintillation screen. Although both unstructured and structured scintillators are used, structured scintillators such as crystalline cesium iodide (CsI) have better resolution capabilities. CsI forms needlelike crystals that act as optical fibers by directing scattered light to the photodiode to improve the spatial resolution.[12] Although other scintillator materials are used, light produced by phosphor materials in unstructured screens is more likely to spread to adjacent pixels and reduce the resolution properties. The CCD is too small for most imaging applications; thus, a step involving a type of detector field expansion or image demagnification must be performed. The detector field can be expanded by combining several CCDs into a detector array to obtain an image with a single exposure or by scanning a single CCD or a smaller CCD array throughout the image field to obtain piecewise images, which are combined at the end of the imaging process.[10] Image demagnification can be accomplished with a system of lenses or tapered optical fibers, as illustrated in Figure 13.11. The efficiency of the lens coupling is limited by the sampled light signal incident on the collecting optics, and the image is susceptible to distortion due to lens defects.[11] Consequently, only a fraction of the signal emitted by the phosphor plate is transmitted through the lens system to reach the detector. The SNR of this type of system is highest for minimal demagnification. Optical fiber tapers also suffer from efficiency and distortion issues, as shown in Figure 13.11. Visible-light output from the phosphor plate can leak from the optical fibers due to the changing reflection angle within the optical column, and bundling multiple tapered fibers can also produce image distortion. The inefficiencies of the lens and fiber-optic systems produce lower DQE values for CCD detectors than for systems not requiring demagnification, and typically, systems that require very little demagnification have the highest DQE values. An advantage of CCD detectors involves their extremely low intrinsic noise factor, which allows them to achieve a high degree of detector capability despite demagnification inefficiencies. In addition, the CCD has a broad dynamic range and a highly linear response to the incident signal.[11]

The second detector system category is the flat-panel system, which utilizes a TFT array as the detector, and is shown in Figure 13.10. Within this category, there are two types: direct conversion systems, which convert the x-rays directly to electric charge that can be read out by a computer as a digital signal, and indirect conversion systems, which require an intermediate conversion from x-ray photons to visible-light photons. Both systems are illustrated in Figure 13.13.

As depicted in Figure 13.13a, the indirect conversion detector performs signal modification steps before the analog image is converted to a digital image. First, a phosphor at the scintillation screen, which is typically crystalline cesium iodide (CsI), absorbs the x-rays and reemits energy in the visible spectrum according to the photoelectric effect. High-energy x-ray quanta incident on the plate are each

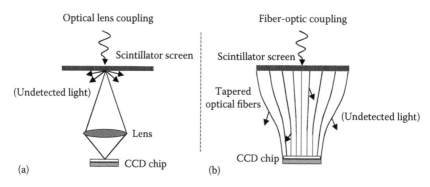

FIGURE 13.11 The CCD detector receives the visible-light image after demagnification by a lens system (a) or a tapered optical fiber system (b). The lens system only transmits a portion of the light from the CsI screen, leading to a reduced SNR at the detector and thus a reduced DQE value. The tapered optical fiber system is also inefficient, as it leaks light as the reflection angle changes along the length of the fiber.

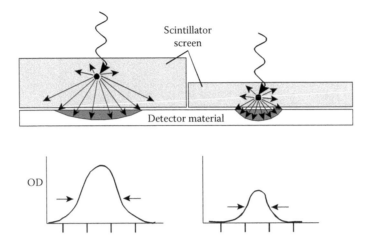

FIGURE 13.12 The ideal scintillator screen would maximize intensity with increased thickness while minimizing image distortion due to scattering with decreased thickness.

converted to several visible-light quanta, resulting in an intensification of the signal known as quantum gain.[11] Increasing the thickness of the phosphor layer increases the likelihood of the x-rays to interact with the phosphor to create photons and maximize the quantum gain. However, the light emitted from the phosphor is not necessarily emitted in the same direction as the incident x-ray. Consequently, this conversion adds a scattering, or blurring, effect to the original signal, which is directly related to the distance the light photons must travel before detection, that is, the thickness of the phosphor. Thus, the thickness of the layer must be determined by compromising these effects. As detailed in Figure 13.12, the ideal thickness would maximize the intensity while minimizing the distortion of the output signal.[11] CsI crystals are grown on the surface of the microelectronic detector plates, in an effort to improve the spatial resolution and efficiency of the detector. At the exit face of the scintillator screen, the visible light is detected by an array of amorphous silicon photodiodes that transmits a proportion of the charge to the transistors, where it is stored until readout.

As illustrated in Figure 13.13b, the direct conversion system is constructed of a layer of amorphous selenium between a single electrode plate at the entry face and pixel-sized TFTs at the exit face. A voltage applied to the electrode plate during image acquisition creates an electric field within the selenium

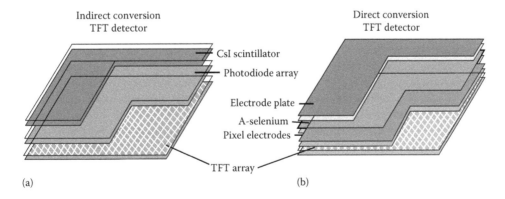

FIGURE 13.13 The indirect conversion flat-panel detector (a) has three layers: a CsI scintillator plate, an array of pixel-sized photodiodes, and a layer of amorphous Silicon (a-Si) TFTs. The direct conversion flat-panel detector (b) has four layers: an electrode plate, an amorphous selenium semiconductor layer, an array of pixel electrodes, and a layer of a-silicon TFTs.

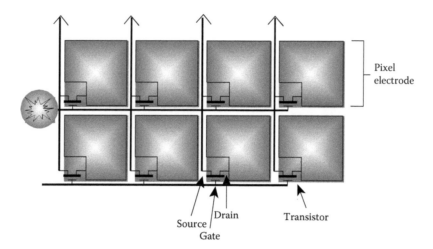

FIGURE 13.14 Information is read from the detector through an active matrix readout method. An electric pulse called a starburst is sent along a row, allowing the stored charge to be retrieved at each pixel column location, as indicated by the arrows at the top. The entire array is read one row at a time and multiplexed into a digital image file.

that maximizes the image quality. The incident x-ray signal passes unaltered through the electrode plate and is absorbed in the selenium layer, where electrons are liberated by the x-ray energy. These electrons are drawn by the electric field directly to the pixel electrodes at the exit face. This design results in very little image scatter and a fill factor that theoretically approaches 100%, because the electric field funnels the charge into the transistors. Therefore, a minimal amount of the signal from the area between active portions of detector elements is lost.

For both direct and indirect conversion systems, the information is retrieved through an active matrix readout method, which is depicted in Figure 13.14. An electric pulse is applied to the gate of the transistors one row at a time, allowing the charge stored at the drain to be measured at the source. For each row, the charge at each column location is amplified and multiplexed. Once the information has been retrieved from the transistors, it is compiled into a complete digital image file.[13] Each pixel in the image is stored in the file as an indexed 12- or 14-bit numerical value in base-10 format, which supports numbers from zero to several thousand.

The third detector system category is computed radiography (CR), which is actually a misnomer, due to the fact that the method actually utilizes photostimulable phosphor imaging plates for detection. Also known as storage phosphors, they are currently the most popular large-area electronically readable detectors. Photostimulable phosphors are comprised of barium fluorohalide family compounds, which are denoted BaFX, where X represents I, Br, or Cl, doped with bivalent europium ions that provide the luminescence centers. Incident x-ray produces electron–hole pairs in the crystal. The halogen ion vacancies trap electrons to create the metastable F-centers, and the trapped electrons form a latent image[14] that is retrieved through the process demonstrated in Figure 13.15. First, the exposed phosphor plate must be placed in a laser scanner. A red He–Ne laser beam raster scans the exposed phosphor, which releases the trapped electrons. Undertaking atomic energy-level transitions, these released electrons migrate to the europium ions to release the stored energy as luminescence blue light. A photomultiplier tube collects the emitted blue light as the signals forming the image. The storage plate is exposed to intensive illumination after erasure to ensure reusability. The spatial resolution depends on the spatial sampling frequency of the laser scanner.

The major advantage of CR is that the storage plates are used exactly as conventional portable cassettes, with the latent image stored in a reusable material instead of film. The storage plates are available in different sizes matching the standard field of view (FOV) sizes, and they have adequate dynamic ranges for radiography. For these reasons, storage plates have been widely used since their debut in the early 1990s,

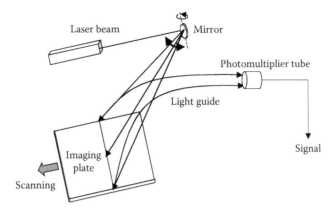

FIGURE 13.15 Schematic of the laser scanner utilized for reading exposed photostimulable phosphor plates.

and more than 10,000 CR units have been installed in the United States. However, this technology also faces several disadvantages. First, the laser light scattering in the phosphor reduces the spatial resolution. Spatial resolutions are approximately 1.5 lp/mm at 50% of the modulation transfer function (MTF), which is the normalized value of the system transfer function; the limiting resolution is approximately 3.5 lp/mm. Secondly, CR systems typically produce low DQE(f) values due to the low efficiency of collecting the signal light, as well as the granularity noise involved in the process, especially at high spatial frequencies. The DQE value is approximately 15% for low spatial frequencies and decreases rapidly with increasing spatial frequency. Thus, the CR DQE is lower than that of the screen-film-based radiography, and the radiation doses are therefore more than 50% higher than those with conventional radiography. Third, the work throughput of radiography with phosphors is lower than that of the conventional radiography.

13.4.3 Image Intensifier TV Chain and Fluoroscopy

Another important modality of projection x-ray imaging is fluoroscopy, in which the x-ray exposures are continuous and acquired images are displayed on a TV monitor, typically at a rate of 30 fps. Therefore, fluoroscopy effectively provides real-time imaging capabilities, which have established it as an extremely useful modality for diagnostic imaging, image guidance for surgical procedures, and therapeutic imaging, which includes cardiac angioplasty and interventional procedures.

The key device for fluoroscopy is the II-TV chain. A flowchart detailing fluoroscopic image formation is shown in Figure 13.16. A continuous x-ray exposure is projected on the desired area of the body, and the transmitted x-ray is detected by an II. The II is comprised of a vacuum bottle with an x-ray

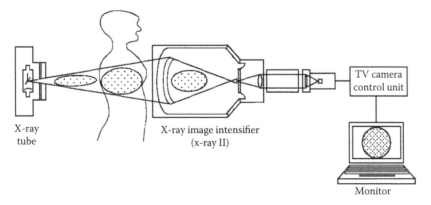

FIGURE 13.16 The flowchart for fluoroscopic image formation.

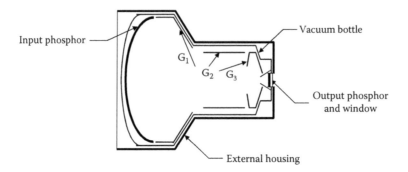

FIGURE 13.17   Schematic of the II.

transparent input window and a glass or fiber-optic output window through which the image is displayed. Figure 13.17 provides a schematic of an II. The transmitted x-ray is incident upon a scintillation layer, which is commonly composed of CsI:Na. The x-ray photons are then absorbed via the photoelectric effect, which was detailed in Section 13.2. The absorbed energy is converted to low-energy secondary electrons, which recombine under the emission of light. The wavelengths of the light depend on the scintillator and the doping material used in the II. For the CsI:Na scintillator, the peak wavelength of the emitted light is approximately 420 nm, which corresponds to an absorbed x-ray photon of 30 keV producing approximately 1500 light photons. The light photons travel to the semitransparent photocathode, which is comprised of antimony and various alkali metals such as cesium. For example, cesium antimonide (Cs_3Sb) is commonly used for the photocathode. In order to increase the efficiency of the II, the light sensitivity of the photocathode corresponds to the wavelength of the scintillation light. Through the photoelectric effect, the light photons emit electrons from the photocathode, and the detected x-ray has now completed the conversion to photoelectrons. The spatial distribution of the photoelectrons is merely a *contact print* of the light image in the input phosphor of the II. As the thickness of the input phosphor (e.g., the CsI scintillation layer) increases, more light is generated and, hence, more electrons are converted. However, the increase in thickness also leads to an increase in the lateral diffusion of light inside the layer, which consequently reduces the spatial resolution. Typically, the thickness of the CsI layer varies from 300 to 450 μm, which results in an x-ray photon of 30 keV generating approximately 200 electrons.[15] Thus, the x-ray attenuation-based image detected by the input phosphor is converted to a photoelectronic image, which is not convenient for projection on a television camera for display, although it is relatively easily *intensified*. Therefore, the photoelectronic image must first be amplified, and then it can be converted into a visible image for display on the TV camera. This amplification is accomplished through electron acceleration by an applied high voltage. An output phosphor, or output screen, is employed to convert the amplified photoelectronic image into a visible image, which is an intensified version of the original x-ray attenuation-based image. For the amplification, a high voltage is applied between the photocathode ($V = 0$) and the output phosphor ($V = 25–35$ kV; see Figure 13.17). Through this method, each electron gains in energy by approximately 30 keV.

A common output phosphor is the P20 phosphor, which is a mixture of zinc cadmium sulfide doped with silver ($Zn_{0.6}Cd_{0.4}S:Ag$)[15,16] that emits green light at a wavelength of 520 and 540 nm. Striking the output phosphor, each of the accelerated electrons causes the emission of approximately 1000 green light photons. As mentioned previously, an absorbed x-ray photon of 30 keV generates approximately 200 electrons from the photocathode; therefore, each photon generates 2×10^5 green light photons at the output window. Comparing this figure to the Gd_2O_2S-based intensifying screens used in conventional radiography, which were presented in Section 13.4, the light photon gain from an II is approximately 100–200 times larger. To further increase the light output luminance, or flux intensity, a demagnification technique is also employed. The ratio of the input phosphor size to the output phosphor size is called the demagnification ratio. The diameter of the output phosphor is approximately 1.5–3.5 cm, which is much smaller than the 15–40 cm diameter of the II entrance fields. The luminance of the output phosphor is the light flux density; thus, the luminance is proportional to the square of the demagnification ratio. Therefore, demagnification produces a 100-fold increase in the output light luminance. Combining the II intrinsic gain and the demagnification gain, the overall gain of an II can be defined as the conversion factor, which expresses the amount of output light luminance per unit exposure rate in units of mR/s. A modern 12″ II delivers a conversion factor that is greater than 200 Nit/(mR/s). When the conversion factor degrades to a value less than 100, the II should be replaced to avoid poor image quality and high radiation doses to the patient and the operator.

In addition to image intensification, another requirement for an II involves providing images without much blurring or distortion. The electron optics ensure that the photoelectrons emitted by the photocathode are focused on the output phosphor with a tolerable level of distortion. Three additional electrodes, referred to as G_1, G_2, and G_3 in Figure 13.17, are inserted between the photocathode and the output screen to implement the electron optics, and these five pieces form the pentrode structure of the electron optics. First, the G_3 electrode provides the ability to zoom the image, by reducing the portion of the input screen currently projected onto the output phosphor. For example, by increasing the G_3 voltage, a smaller portion of the input phosphor is projected onto the output phosphor, which reduces the demagnification ratio. Since the size of the output phosphor is fixed during the adjustment of the G_3 voltage, the reduction of the demagnification ratio magnifies the images. IIs of a specific size provide magnification modes corresponding to smaller entrance sizes. For example, a typical 12″ II also provides magnification modes for 9″ and 6″ sizes. Secondly, the G_2 electrode is the focusing electrode. When the spatial resolution in the fluoroscopy images decreases to a value less than 1 lp/mm for a 12″ II, it is typically recommended to test the G_2 voltage, as well as the TV camera focusing. Finally, the G_1 electrode adjusts the resolution uniformity.

Once the x-ray attenuation images have been converted to visible-light images at the output phosphor, a TV camera is used to generate the video signals for display on a TV monitor, as illustrated in Figure 13.16. The TV camera is optically coupled to the output screen of the II by the conjugate lens. The CCD device discussed previously is generally a good choice for a TV camera. However, the vacuum camera tube is commonly used instead. This is a vacuum tube of approximately 1″ in external diameter, which consists of a target plate composed of light-sensitive photoconductive materials such as antimony trisulfide (Sb_2S_3), an electron gun, electron scanning, and focusing coils. A green light image from the II output phosphor is projected by the lens onto the target of the camera tube. The target is photoconductive; thus, one light photon creates a mobile electron–hole pair. Therefore, the local electric resistances of the target vary according to the illumination intensities received. Larger intensity values result in lower local resistance. The projected image therefore forms a map of the resistance changes on the target. When an electron beam scans each line of the target, which is either 512 or 1024 lines, it detects the resistance changes and converts them into electric current changes. The signal current, which is also known as the displacement current, ranges from approximately 100 nA for an average image brightness to 2000 nA for a very bright image. The signal current I_s changes with the illumination intensity according to the following formula:

$$I_s = cE^\gamma + I_d, \tag{13.20}$$

where
   c is a constant
   E is the illumination intensity
   γ describes the rate at which the signal current changes with the illumination intensity
   I_d is the dark current

Therefore, the value of γ determines the signal transfer characteristics and consequently influences the image contrast scale and the dynamical range as well. While the beam scans each line of the target, the video signal updates accordingly. The camera tube functions as a signal current source for the video amplifier. The video signal, or voltage signal, is combined with the TV synchronization signals to form the composite video signal, which is then amplified and transmitted to a TV monitor for display.

The most commonly used TV camera is the vidicon tube, which uses antimony trisulfide (Sb_2S_3) as the target photoconductive material. The vidicon tube has a γ value of 0.7, which corresponds to a good dynamic range. The video amplifier for fluoroscopy is linear, and the TV monitor has a γ value of approximately 2; thus, the overall system γ value is approximately 1.4. In addition to γ, other important parameters of a TV camera are the lag, sensitivity, noise, resolution, and burn resistance. Lag is the inertia defined by the residual signal percentage after 20 scans. It is the most important parameter, as it essentially determines whether the camera device can be used for an imaging task. For example, vidicon has a relatively large lag of 8%–16%; thus, it cannot be used for angiography and image-guided interventional procedures. However, it has the advantage of noise reduction for fluoroscopy, which is accomplished through the integration of image frames. The target material is the primary factor determining the lag of a camera tube. For example, a plumbicon (PbO) target delivers a lag of 1%, while the lag for a saticon (SeAsTe) target is 6%.[16] In addition, the CCD camera yields a very low lag value. Thus, these camera tubes can be used in angiography and interventional procedures. With the exception of vidicon, all TV cameras, including CCD, deliver unit gamma.

Another important aspect of fluoroscopy is AEC. Due to the fact that anatomical structures have varying attenuation values, the x-ray factors of tube energy (kVp) and tube current (mA) must be adjusted accordingly during the exposure, in an effort to maintain comparable image brightness and minimize radiation exposure to the patient. AEC achieves this by detecting the exposure rate of x-rays incident on the II entrance during fluoroscopy and adjusting the kVp and mA values through a feedback control of the x-ray generator. The target II entrance exposure value should be determined as a balance of acceptable image quality and minimized radiation dose to the patient and the medical staff. In clinical applications, the target II entrance exposure rates are typically specified to achieve a low contrast resolution, which will be detailed in the next subsection in terms of the SNR, of 2.5%–3.5% for features approximately 1 cm in diameter. This corresponds to a 12″ II entrance exposure rate of approximately 1.2–2.4 mR/min. These values must be scaled inversely with the square of the ratio of the II sizes. For example, the 9″ II entrance exposure rate should be approximately 2.4–4.8 mR/min. The II photocathode current and the video signal from a TV camera can both be used as the sensing signal for the AEC used in fluoroscopy. With AEC, low kVp and mA values are used for imaging small and easily penetrable areas of the body; consequently, the x-ray exposure rate is also relatively low in these cases. As the attenuation in the areas of the body being imaged increases, AEC automatically raises the kVp and mA values accordingly to maintain comparable image brightness. Through this method, constant average image brightness is achieved and unnecessary radiation exposure to the patient and the medical staff is avoided. For the sake of radiation protection, the exposure rate is limited to a specified maximum value. As increasing attenuation drives the AEC towards this maximum, the gain of the video amplifier must be increased to maintain approximately constant image brightness. This video gain adjustment is implemented by the automatic gain control (AGC) circuitry. According to US federal regulations, the maximum exposure rate at the patient skin entrance must not exceed 10 R/min, unless the x-ray system provides a high-level control and special means for its activation. In this case, the maximum exposure rate at the patient skin entrance must not exceed 20 R/min during activation of the high-level control.

13.4.4 Signal-to-Noise Ratio Analysis

In radiological imaging, the x-ray quantum efficiency and corresponding imaging characteristics such as SNR, noise power spectrum (NPS), and DQE are crucial to design considerations and performance evaluations, including lesion detectability and patient radiation dose. The following modeling of SNR,

NPS, and DQE will provide a comprehensive summary of the theoretical and practical aspects of a radiological imaging apparatus. For analysis purposes, the optically coupled CCD system described in the previous subsection will be utilized as an example, although the concept can be applied to many other radiological imaging systems. In an optically coupled CCD x-ray imaging system without an II in the imaging chain, the transfer of light from the x-ray intensifying screen to the CCD imager can be accomplished by direct contact between these components. However, currently available CCD systems require a demagnifying optical coupling component, which is typically either a lens or fiber taper, between the intensifying screen and the detector to provide an imaging area larger than the size of the detector. In the quantum transfer of the image data between the intensifying screen and the imager, the optical coupling component represents a weak link in the cascaded imaging chain. Thus, in the 1960s and 1970s, IIs were considered integral components for achieving quantum noise limitation in electronic imaging systems. To determine whether this assumption holds for newer electronic detectors, the equation detailed in the following was derived for analyzing the SNR provided by a system.

The noise in an optically coupled CCD system is a combination of quantum noise and additive noise. Quantum noise includes x-ray quantum noise as well as secondary quantum noise generated through the cascaded process, and additive noise refers to noise related to the detector or the detector electronics. Although each noise component can be analyzed separately using existing mathematical methods,[17] the equation for the combined SNR was derived to include the effects of both quantum and additive noise.[18] The equation is based on the principle of cascaded imaging analysis and other SNR models.[17] Although it can be applied to many imaging systems, it is particularly convenient for analyzing performance or optimizing design trade-offs for optically coupled CCD x-ray imaging systems. The details and derivation of the following equation can be found in Ref. [18]:

$$\text{SNR} = C(\eta N_i)^{1/2} \left[1 + \frac{1}{g_1 g_2} + \frac{1}{g_1 g_2 g_3} + \frac{N_a^2}{(g_1 g_2 g_3)^2 \eta N_i} \right]^{-1/2}, \qquad (13.21)$$

where

η is the quantum efficiency of the intensifying screen or other scintillator used in the imaging chain

N_i is the x-ray photon flux, which is the number of x-ray photons per pixel at the entrance of the intensifying screen

N_a is the total additive noise of the overall imaging chain

g_1 is the x-ray-to-light conversion ratio or quantum gain of the intensifying screen

g_2 is the optical coupling efficiency of the lens, fiber taper, or other coupling component

g_3 is the quantum efficiency of the CCD or other electronic detector

C is the SC

It is assumed that the statistical processes of absorption, photon transmission through the screen, and photoemission can all be described and characterized by the quantum efficiency η. In addition, the product of $g_1 g_2 g_3$ is the overall quantum efficiency or total quantum gain of the system, which is the number of electrons produced in the CCD per x-ray photon absorbed in the scintillator.

The quantum efficiency of a Min-R medium mammographic screen has been estimated as $\eta = 0.65$.[19] Assuming a typical mammographic screen entrance exposure of 12 mR and an average x-ray photon energy of 20 keV, the number of x-ray photons per pixel at the entrance of the intensifying screen for a detector with a pixel size of 0.048 mm × 0.048 mm is $\eta N_i = 1600$ x-ray photons/pixel. Therefore, the number of absorbed x-ray photons per pixel is $\eta N_i = 1040$. For this analysis, a contrast C of 1 is assumed. The total additive noise N_a is typically less than 15 electrons for a system using a cooled CCD, while it is usually larger than 500 electrons for a TV tube. The x-ray-to-light conversion ratio g_1 of a high-resolution mammography intensifying screen has been reported to be 400–600 in the forward direction.[20]

Conservative estimates of g_3 are 0.35 for a front-illuminated CCD, 0.60 for a back-illuminated CCD such as the Tektronix (TK2048EB), and 0.20 for a TV tube. In a previous work,[21] the optical coupling efficiency of a lens was estimated as follows:

$$g_2 = \frac{0.75}{4F^2(1+M)^2 + 1}, \tag{13.22}$$

where
   F is the F-number of the lens, which is the ratio of the focal length to the effective diameter
   M is the demagnification ratio

For example, an $F/0.8$, or $F = 0.8$, lens providing a demagnification factor of 2 corresponds to a g_2 value of 3.1%. Equation 13.21 can then be utilized to identify the dominant noise component in a cascaded electronic imaging system. If the total quantum gain of the imaging chain, which is represented by the $g_1 g_2 g_3$ factor, is small or the additive noise N_a is large, the resulting value of the denominator will be larger than 1. In this case, the SNR of the system is dominated by one of the cascaded stages or additive noise. While $g_1 g_2 g_3$ is small, the value of N_a significantly affects the performance of the system. As $g_1 g_2 g_3$ increases, the value of the denominator approaches 1 and the equation reduces to SNR = $C/\eta N_i$, which represents a perfect x-ray quantum noise-limited imaging system without additive noise.

Typical parameters for lens-coupled TV camera systems, which were extensively investigated in the 1960s and 1970s, will now be utilized to illustrate an application of Equation 13.21. Substituting $g_1 g_2 g_3 = (500)(0.031)(0.2) = 3.1$ and $N_a = 500$ into Equation 13.21 gives

$$\text{SNR} = \frac{C(\eta N_i)^{1/2}}{(1.32+25)^{1/2}} = 0.2 C(\eta N_i)^{1/2}. \tag{13.23}$$

This example illustrates that the lens-coupled TV system is not x-ray quantum noise limited. In fact, the additive noise N_a dominates the SNR instead of the total quantum gain $g_1 g_2 g_3$.

The introduction of the II, which was discussed previously, provided a solution to the additive noise issue by boosting the image signal and increasing the quantum gain. The value of $g_1 g_2 g_3$ may therefore approach 400, and the corresponding SNR of an II-TV system can be expressed as follows:

$$\text{SNR} = \frac{C(\eta N_i)^{1/2}}{(1+0.004)^{1/2}} = 0.99 C(\eta N_i)^{1/2}, \tag{13.24}$$

which indicates that the II-TV system is x-ray quantum noise limited. For this reason, analog and digital II-TV systems are both used currently in many clinical procedures. However, electro-optical devices such as IIs have limitations that reduce spatial resolution and contrast sensitivity. Therefore, modalities such as mammography that require both high spatial resolution and high contrast sensitivity cannot be performed with a conventional II-TV system.

Examining Equations 13.21 through 13.24 more closely, it is theoretically intuitive that x-ray quantum noise limitation might be achieved *without* an II if the additive noise level could be greatly reduced. Modern CCD receptors, which can have an additive noise level as low as 15 electrons, are therefore suitable detector candidates. For current CCD devices, a typical total quantum gain can be expressed as $g_1 g_2 g_3 = (500)(0.031)(0.6) = 9.3$ electrons per x-ray photon. Using Equation 13.21, the corresponding SNR can be calculated as follows:

$$\text{SNR} = \frac{C(\eta N_i)^{1/2}}{(1.1+0.002)^{1/2}} = 0.95 C(\eta N_i)^{1/2}. \tag{13.25}$$

TABLE 13.3 Impact of Total Quantum Gain and Additive Noise on the SNR

	Lens TV	II-TV	Lens CCD
Additive noise, N_a	500 electrons	500 electrons	15 electrons
Quantum gain, $g_1g_2g_3$	3.1 electrons/x-ray	400 electrons/x-ray	9.3 electrons/x-ray
SNR	$0.2C(\eta N_i)^{1/2}$	$0.99C(\eta N_i)^{1/2}$	$0.95C(\eta N_i)^{1/2}$

Therefore, the degradation in the SNR as a result of the cascaded stages and the additive noise is nearly negligible for a cooled CCD system, which illustrates that it is possible for an optically coupled CCD imaging system to be x-ray quantum noise limited.

Assuming a contrast value of 1 and a constant phosphor noise level for the three systems, the preceding analyses can be summarized as shown in Table 13.3. For this table, the value of $g_1g_2g_3$ for the lens TV was calculated under the assumption that the quantum efficiency of the TV tube has a value of 0.2. Similarly, the calculation of $g_1g_2g_3$ for the lens CCD assumed that the quantum efficiency of a back-illuminated CCD has a value of 0.6. Figure 13.18 demonstrates the relationships of the SNR values to the total quantum gain and the total additive noise for the three detector systems. The figure illustrates that a total quantum gain value of 10 electrons per absorbed x-ray photon allows a CCD imaging system to be x-ray quantum noise limited within the low-frequency range. According to our calculations and experiments, it is feasible to design a lens-coupled or a fiber optically coupled CCD x-ray imaging system to meet these requirements under clinical conditions. In comparison, other electronic detectors have noise levels of a few hundred or even a thousand electrons.[22] To achieve x-ray quantum noise limitation under these conditions, a total quantum gain value of 100–200 electrons per absorbed x-ray photon is necessary.

The NPS analysis of image noise and noise transfer provides a complete description of noise. When experimentally characterizing the noise properties of real or proposed digital mammographic systems, the NPS is calculated directly from the noise fluctuations using the fast Fourier transform (FFT):

$$NPS(f_x, f_y) = FFT_{2D}[N(x, y)], \qquad (13.26)$$

where
FFT_{2D} represents the FFT
$N(x, y)$ is a 2D data array of noise fluctuation, which is referred to as the noise-only image

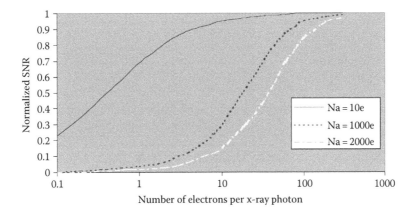

FIGURE 13.18 Normalized SNR curves plotted as functions of total quantum gain (electrons/x-ray) and additive noise (electrons).

1. Acquire images $A(x, y)$ and $B_1(x, y)$, ..., $B_{50}(x, y)$ under identical conditions simulating clinical mammography procedures. A Lucite slab of 4.5 cm in thickness is used, and the entire imaging field is uniformly irradiated.
2. Determine the *noiseless* image as an average of the 50 images as follows:

$$\langle B(x, y) \rangle = \frac{\sum B_n(x, y)}{50}. \tag{13.27}$$

This averaging process is typically necessary to avoid statistical uncertainty.

3. Calculate the noise-only image $N(x, y) = A(x, y) - B(x, y)$ as the difference between the single image $A(x, y)$ and the noiseless image $B(x, y)$ determined in step 2.
4. NPS(f_x, f_y) is a 2D data array in the frequency domain. The proposed CCD imaging system is assumed to be symmetric in the x and y directions; thus, a slice of the data, NPS(f_x), can be utilized to evaluate the noise properties of the entire image.

Repeating this procedure 20 times generates 20 NPS(f_x) curves. Each NPS(f_x) curve is normalized with respect to its value at zero frequency, in order to facilitate a zero frequency value equal to 1. The normalized NPS is then given by the following:

$$NPS'(f_x) = \frac{1}{20} \sum \frac{NPS(f_x)}{NPS(0)}. \tag{13.28}$$

The preceding discussion on the NPS provides an important foundation for understanding the concept of noise propagation in a cascaded imaging chain, as well as its relationship to the SNR and the DQE. The measured NPS curves of various optically coupled CCD x-ray imaging systems can be found in the literature.[23,24]

The DQE describes the SNR transfer characteristics of an imaging system as a function of the spatial frequency[23,25]:

$$DQE(f) = \frac{SNR_{out}^2(f)}{SNR_{in}^2(f)}, \tag{13.29}$$

where
   $SNR_{out}(f)$ is the output SNR
   $SNR_{in}(f)$ is the input SNR

The DQE(f) therefore provides a measurement of the efficiency of the imaging system in terms of the spatial frequency. In order to determine DQE(f), the following derivation was conducted:

$$SNR_{out}^2(f) = \frac{S_{out}^2(f)}{NPS(f)} = \frac{S_{out}^2(0)MTF^2(f)}{NPS(0)nps(f)} = \frac{SNR_{out}^2(0)MTF^2(f)}{nps(f)}, \tag{13.30}$$

where
   $S_{out}(f)$ is the output signal, which can be expressed as the product of its zero frequency value $S_{out}(0)$
   MTF(f) is the normalized value of the system transfer function[26]

Similarly, NPS(f) can be simplified to the product of its normalized form nps(f) and the normalization factor NPS(0). Assuming the input x-ray quanta obey Poisson statistics and produce a flat noise spectrum within the range of the spatial frequency of practical interest, the following holds:

$$\text{SNR}_{\text{in}}^2(f) = CN_i, \tag{13.31}$$

where N_i is the incident x-ray photon flux, which is the number of x-ray photons per pixel at the entrance of the intensifying screen. Thus, the DQE can be represented as follows:

$$\text{DQE}(f) = \frac{\text{DQE}(0)\text{MTF}^2(f)}{\text{nps}(f)}, \tag{13.32}$$

where the ratio of $\text{MTF}^2(f)$ to nps(f) provides a spatial frequency modulation term for the DQE.

To determine the value of DQE(0), recall that Equation 13.21 can be simplified as follows for zero frequency:

$$\text{SNR}_{\text{out}}(f) = C(\eta N_i)^{1/2} \left[1 + \frac{1}{g_1 g_2} + \frac{1}{g_1 g_2 g_3} + \frac{N_a^2}{(g_1 g_2 g_3)^2 \eta N_i} \right]^{-1/2}, \tag{13.33}$$

$$\text{SNR}_{\text{in}}(f) \equiv CN_i^{1/2}.$$

Therefore,

$$\text{DQE}(0) = \frac{\text{SNR}_{\text{out}}^2(0)}{\text{SNR}_{\text{in}}^2(0)} = \frac{\eta}{[1 + (1/g_1 g_2) + (1/g_1 g_2 g_3) + (N_a^2/(g_1 g_2 g_3)^2 \eta N_i)]}. \tag{13.34}$$

Analyses of DQE(0) and SNR at low frequencies both provide useful tools for evaluating the design trade-offs for electronic x-ray imaging systems, such as scintillator selection, optical coupling techniques, and electronic imager selection.

Using Equation 13.34, the DQE(0) values for several electronic x-ray imaging systems were calculated as functions of the total quantum gain $g_1 g_2 g_3$ and the additive noise N_a, the results of which are given in Figure 13.19. For a low additive noise system such as the optically coupled CCD, a total quantum gain of 10 electrons per x-ray photon corresponds to a DQE value that is close to its maximum value. Further increasing the total gain will not significantly improve the DQE. The preceding analysis applies to the low-frequency range. In order to preserve the value of the DQE in the HF range, as well as ensure that the system is x-ray quantum noise limited at high frequencies, a total quantum gain of 10 electrons per x-ray photon is again necessary.[23] These guidelines have been used in the development of both fiber optically and lens-coupled CCD systems. For a lens-coupled prototype, a large aperture lens has been custom designed and utilized with a back-illuminated CCD with a quantum efficiency value nearly twice that of a front-illuminated CCD. The prototype was verified to provide a total quantum gain value meeting the specification of 10 electrons per x-ray photon. A fiber optically coupled CCD could be designed with a total quantum gain value much greater than 10 electrons per x-ray photon, due to the high efficiency of optical fiber.[27] However, in a practical design trade-off, an optical fiber component with a heavy extramural absorption material was selected, despite the fact that it provides only moderate efficiency in return for improved contrast and lower cost.[28] The curves presented in Figure 13.19 also demonstrate that 100–200 electrons per x-ray photon are required in order to maximize the DQE for electronic imaging systems with higher detector noise.

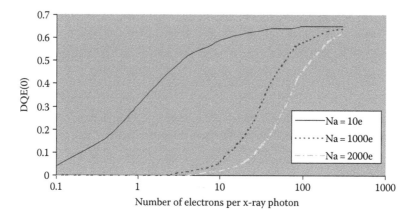

FIGURE 13.19 DQE curves plotted as functions of total quantum gain (electrons/x-ray) and additive noise (electrons). The quantum efficiency of the scintillating screen was assumed to be $\eta = 0.65$. The DQE values presented in this figure are the maximum achievable values.

The quantum efficiency η of the scintillating screen is a significant influence on the DQE and the radiation efficiency. According to Equation 13.34, the maximum achievable DQE of an x-ray quantum noise-limited system is limited primarily by the value of η. In practice, a variety of scintillating screens are used in radiological imaging. Early optically coupled CCD spot mammography systems[28] utilized Min-R screens with a quantum efficiency of 55%–65%, which corresponds to $\eta = 0.55$–0.65. Recently developed crystalline cesium iodide (CsI) screens offer an efficiency of $\eta = 0.90$ or higher, which also produces a higher system DQE.[29] In Figure 13.20, the DQE(0) curves of two optically coupled CCD mammographic systems are given as a function of the total quantum gain and the quantum efficiency of the scintillating screen. The DQE values presented in this figure represent the maximum achievable values. This figure demonstrates that the scintillating screen significantly affects the DQE of the overall system. Based on the DQE analysis, we have developed a high-resolution digital imaging system, and Figure 13.21 depicts a bone image acquired with this system.[29]

It must be emphasized that the SNR analyses performed in this chapter are based on single-pixel values (i.e., x-ray photons per pixel and electrons per pixel). Single-pixel analysis is useful and convenient

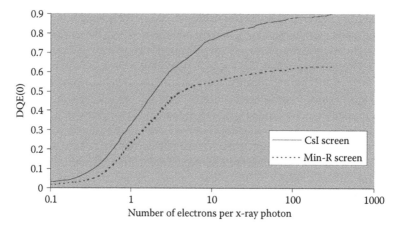

FIGURE 13.20 The effect of the quantum efficiency of the scintillating screen (η) on the x-ray quantum efficiency of the overall system. In this figure, DQE(0) curves of two optically coupled CCD systems with different scintillators are plotted as a function of the quantum efficiency of the scintillator screen (η) and the total quantum gain (electronics/x-ray). The DQE values presented in this figure represent the maximum achievable values.

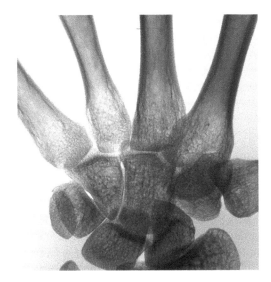

FIGURE 13.21   Image of bones acquired by a prototype high-resolution digital x-ray imaging system.

for determining whether an imaging system is x-ray quantum noise limited. However, it is not valid for lesion detectability evaluations, which are more appropriately analyzed with the Rose model[30] or quasi-ideal SNR.[31,32] In addition, the methods presented in this section can also be applied to other optoelectronic x-ray imaging systems.

13.5 Phase-Contrast X-Ray Imaging

As introduced in Section 13.2, in-line phase-contrast imaging directly measures the Laplacian of the phase $\nabla^2\phi$, while x-ray interferometry and diffraction-enhanced imaging directly measure the phase ϕ and the phase gradient $\nabla\phi$, respectively. In-line phase-contrast imaging is currently the only method that can be performed with an x-ray tube as the x-ray source; therefore, this imaging modality holds great potential for clinical applications. Although in-line phase-contrast imaging is still in its infancy, it will be presented in detail in this section, due to its potential in biomedical diagnostic imaging.

The configuration of in-line phase-contrast imaging is similar to conventional radiography, with the exception of a larger object-to-detector distance. For the discussion of the theory behind phase-contrast imaging, consider a plane wave x-ray source. If the x-ray projection is in the z-axis direction, the phase shift and attenuation effects of a body part can be modeled as a 2D transmission function $q(x, y)$ in the x–y plane:

$$q(x,y) = \exp\left(i\phi(x,y) - \frac{\mu(x,y)}{2} \right), \tag{13.35}$$

where $\phi(x, y)$ and $\mu(x, y)$ are the z-projections of the object phase and linear attenuation coefficient, respectively. More specifically, if the object has 3D distributions of the refractive index decrement $\delta(x, y, z)$ and linear attenuation coefficients $\mu(x, y, z)$, then the projected phase and attenuation values, respectively, are as follows:

$$\phi(x,y) = \frac{2\pi}{\lambda} \int \delta(x,y,z) dz$$

and

$$\mu(x,y) = \int \mu(x,y,z) dz. \tag{13.36}$$

TABLE 13.4 Maximum Object Thickness Allowing Valid Projection
Approximation for Different Resolutions and X-Ray Photon Energies

X-Ray Energy (keV)	Object's Finest Feature (mm)	Object Thickness Maximum (m)
20	1.00E−02	8.06E−01
20	1.00E−03	8.06E−03
50	1.00E−02	2.02E+00
50	1.00E−03	2.02E−02
100	1.00E−02	4.03E+00
100	1.00E−03	4.03E−02

For example, assume that the object is illuminated at $z = 0$ by a plane wave x-ray $\exp(-ikz)$ with a wavelength of λ, where $k = 2\pi/\lambda$ is referred to as the wave number. The thickness of the object T is assumed to meet the requirements of the projection approximation. It can be shown that the approximation holds as long as the size of the finest feature in the object is larger than $\sqrt{\lambda}\sqrt{T}$. Table 13.4 presents the maximum object thickness facilitating a valid projection approximation for different resolutions and x-ray photon energies. The table verifies that human body parts can be treated as thin objects for resolutions of 10 μm and photon energies from 10 to 150 keV. In general, the incident x-ray is both refracted and diffracted by the object. For diagnostic x-ray, the wavelength is much smaller than the features of the object being imaged. The diffraction angles are very small, typically on the order of milliradians (mR), due to the tissue structure. Therefore, the diffracted x-ray wave field can be described by the small angle (i.e., paraxial) approximation of the Fresnel diffraction theory[33]:

$$f(x,z) = \left(\frac{i}{\lambda z}\right)^{1/2} \exp(-ikz) \int q(X)\exp\left(-ik\frac{(x-X)^2}{2z}\right) dX,$$
(13.37)

where
  z is the distance in wave propagation from the object (i.e., the body part)
  X is the coordinate in the transverse plane

For the sake of concise notation, the y-dimension can be omitted without loss of generality. The object transmission function can be utilized to calculate the integral in Equation 13.37, in order to determine the transmitted x-ray wave field $f(x, z)$ at z. The x-ray detector used for the imaging process is x-ray phase insensitive; therefore, only the intensity of the transmitted x-ray at z is detected:

$$I(x,z) = ff^* = |f(x,z)|^2 .$$
(13.38)

In conventional x-ray imaging, the diffraction effects are negligible; thus, $f(x, z) = q(x)\exp(-ikz)$. Using Equation 13.35, the following formula can be derived:

$$I(x,z) = |f(x,z)|^2 = |q(x)|^2 = \exp(-\mu(x)).$$
(13.39)

In this equation, $I(x, z)$ represents the conventional radiographic image of the object $q(x)$. The object actually diffracts the x-ray, and the diffracted wave $f(x, z)$ is different than $q(x)$ in general. Therefore, the detected $I(x, z)$ at z can be considered to be an in-line hologram, and $I(x, z)$ is a complicated function of $q(x)$. Thus, $I(x, z)$ represents the phase-contrast image of the object.

In order to explore the general features of phase-contrast imaging, the Fresnel diffraction process can be applied through linear filtration of the object transmission function.[33] The concept of linear filtering is not new to x-ray imaging. In fact, a conventional x-ray image is a tissue attenuation map filtered by the optical transfer function of the imaging system (e.g., MTF analysis). In this case, a phase-contrast image is a map of the object transmission function filtered by a linear filter corresponding to the Fresnel diffraction process. In fact, the Fresnel integral for the diffracted x-ray wave field $f(x, z)$ is a convolution. The Fourier transform (FT) of $f(x, z)$ with respect to x from Equation 13.37 is calculated as follows:

$$F(u,z) = \exp(-ikz)Q(u)\exp(i\pi\lambda zu^2), \tag{13.40}$$

where
   u is the spatial frequency in the object plane
   $F(u, z)$ and $Q(u)$ are the FTs of the x-ray wave field $f(x, z)$ and the object transmission function $q(x)$, respectively

Equation 13.40 demonstrates that the linear filter $\exp\{i\pi\lambda zu^2\}$, which is applied to the transmitted frequencies, accounts for the Fresnel diffraction in in-line phase-contrast imaging. To explore the effects of this filter, consider a pure phase object with small phase $\phi(x)$. In this case, the object transmission function can be approximated with Equation 13.35 as follows:

$$q(x) \approx 1 + i\phi(x), \tag{13.41}$$

and the FT of $q(x)$ is

$$Q(u) \approx \delta(u) + i\Phi(u), \tag{13.42}$$

where
   $\delta(u)$ is the δ-function
   $\Phi(u)$ is the FT of the object phase $\phi(x)$

Substituting Equation 13.42 into 13.40 gives the FT of the diffracted x-ray wave field:

$$F(u) \approx \exp(-ikz)\{\delta(u) + i\Phi(u)\}\exp(i\pi\lambda zu^2), \tag{13.43}$$

and $F(u)$ can be further simplified as follows:

$$F(u) \approx \exp(-ikz)\{\delta(u) - \Phi(u)\sin(\pi\lambda zu^2) + i\Phi(u)\cos(\pi\lambda zu^2)\}. \tag{13.44}$$

In x-ray diagnostic imaging, the energy of the x-ray photons ranges from 10 to 150 keV, and the corresponding x-ray wavelengths vary from 0.124 to 0.0083 nm, as calculated with Equation 13.1. For clinical applications, the object-to-detector distance z is typically not larger than 1 m, and the maximum spatial resolution is approximately 20 lp/mm. The phase transfer factor $\sin \chi$ has been calculated for a plane wave x-ray source as a function of x-ray photon energy, object-to-detector distance, and target spatial frequency. The calculations are applicable for cases relevant to clinical imaging, and the results are provided in Table 13.5. Thus, $\sin(\pi\lambda zu^2) \approx \pi\lambda zu^2$, $\cos(\pi\lambda zu^2) \approx 1$, and the FT of the diffracted x-ray wave from Equation 13.44 can be updated accordingly:

$$F(u) \approx \exp(-ikz)\{\delta(u) - \pi\lambda zu^2\Phi(u) + i\Phi(u)\}. \tag{13.45}$$

Applying the inverse FT, the diffracted x-ray wave field at z can then be determined:

$$f(x,z) \approx \exp(-ikz)\left\{1 + \frac{\lambda z}{4\pi}\nabla^2\phi(x) + i\phi(x)\right\}. \tag{13.46}$$

TABLE 13.5   Phase Transfer Parameter as a Function of X-Ray Photon Energy, Object-to-Detector Distance, and Target Spatial Frequency with a Plane Wave X-Ray Source

X-Ray (keV)	X-Ray Wavelength, λ (nm)	Object-to-Detector Distance, Z (m)	Target Freq. (1 p/mm)	$\chi = \pi\lambda z u^2$	At Target Frequency, $\sin(\chi)$
10	1.24E–01	0.5	20.0	7.79E–02	7.78E–02
20	6.20E–02	0.5	20.0	3.90E–02	3.89E–02
50	2.48E–02	0.5	20.0	1.56E–02	1.56E–02
150	8.27E–03	0.5	20.0	5.19E–03	5.19E–03

Equation 13.38 is then utilized to calculate the phase image intensity for a pure phase object with small phase to the first order in $\phi(x)$:

$$I(x,z) = |f(x,z)|^2 = 1 + \frac{\lambda z}{2\pi}\nabla^2\phi(x). \tag{13.47}$$

This result demonstrates that the detected image contrast will be proportional to $\nabla^2\phi$, which is the Laplacian, or second derivative, of the projected phase ϕ of the object. Recall that ϕ is related to the tissue refractive index decrement δ by Equation 13.36, as well as to tissue composition by Equations 13.9 and 13.10. With the exception of the x-ray absorption edge of tissue, the object phase $\phi(x)$ is proportional to the tissue electron density, and the phase contrast of the image is proportional to the Laplacian of the tissue electron density. Therefore, the boundary between areas with different tissue electron densities will be greatly enhanced, as if the images have been edge enhanced with digital processing.

In addition, the preceding equation indicates that the phase-contrast amount is proportional to the object-to-detector distance. Thus, if this distance $z = 0$, the phase contrast will not be evident. Moreover, Equation 13.47 reveals that this technique is possible with polychromatic x-ray sources such as x-ray tubes. Section 13.3 detailed the fact that x-rays from an x-ray tube consist of both Bremsstrahlung and characteristic radiation. Bremsstrahlung is a broadband x-ray; however, since in-line phase contrast is proportional to the Laplacian of the tissue electron densities, the phase contrast generated by photons of different wavelengths is combined, provided that the photons propagate along approximately the same path. Although temporal coherence (monochromaticity) is not required, spatial coherence is critical for phase imaging. In practice, a plane wave source emits a bundle of plane waves with a divergent angle α. The spatial coherence of a plane wave x-ray beam is characterized by the lateral coherence width $2\lambda/\alpha$. Optimizing this value is essential; otherwise, the diffraction patterns generated by plane waves from different tissues can combine to produce blur instead of improved edges. Larger lateral coherence width values produce improved phase image resolution. A quantitative analysis of phase image resolution can found in the literature.[33]

For clinical imaging applications, an x-ray tube is more likely to be used. For a point x-ray source, the x-ray wave field from the source is spherical. Assume that the SOD is R_1 and the SDD is $R_1 + R_2$. In this case, the Fresnel diffraction wave field formula is the same as that of a plane wave, as defined in Equation 13.37, with the exception that z is replaced with R_2/M and x is replaced with x/M, where $M = (R_1 + R_2)/R_1$ represents the geometric magnification factor. For a point-like source such as an x-ray tube, the spatial coherence criterion for phase imaging necessitates a very small focal spot size, on the order of tens of microns or smaller. As discussed in Section 13.3, conventional x-ray tubes have focal spot sizes ranging from 0.1 to 1.5 mm. In addition, an x-ray tube with a tiny focal spot is limited by a reduced operating tube current and the resulting low output exposure rates. These challenges are the focus of current active research in the field of phase-contrast imaging.

In the theoretical analysis of phase-contrast imaging, the phase image intensity formula in Equation 13.47 was derived under a weak phase assumption ($\phi(x) \ll 1$). A similar formula can be derived with the assumption of $\phi(x) \ll 1$ and $\mu(x) \ll 1$. However, these assumptions will be grossly violated for body parts

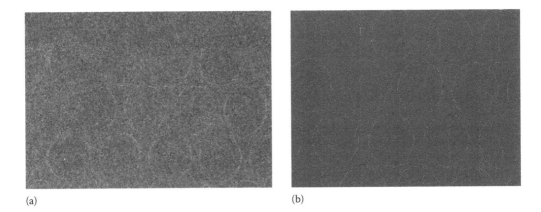

(a)   (b)

FIGURE 13.22 A comparison between a conventional attenuation-only image (a) and a phase-contrast image (b) of a piece of small bubble wrap. The phase-contrast image clearly demonstrates the edge enhancement of very fine structures, which is a characteristic feature of phase-contrast imaging.

in possible clinical applications. From the discussion of tissue attenuation in Section 13.2, the average $\mu(x)$ value for an anterior–posterior projection of an abdomen for an x-ray energy as high as 120 kVp will be approximately 4–6. For x-rays in mammography, a phase change of 2π can result from a few tens of microns in breast tissue thickness. Therefore, the phase image intensity formula in Equation 13.47 is invalid for these cases. With the goal of analyzing phase contrast in clinical imaging, a phase image intensity formula for a point-like x-ray source has recently been derived. This formula is valid for both strong and weak object phase $\phi(x)$ and attenuation $\mu(x)$.[34] Figure 13.22 provides a comparison between a conventional attenuation-only image (a) and a phase-contrast image (b) of a piece of small bubble wrap. The phase-contrast image clearly demonstrates the edge enhancement of very fine structures, which is a characteristic feature of phase-contrast imaging. Recent studies have conducted preliminary investigations of the clinical feasibility of phase-contrast imaging.[35–37]

References

1. Hubbel, J.H., Photon mass attenuation and energy-absorption coefficients from 1 keV to 20 MeV, *Int. J. Appl. Radiat. Isot.*, 33, 1269–1290, 1982.
2. Dyson, N., *X-Rays in Atomic and Nuclear Physics*, Logman Group Limited, London, U.K., 1973.
3. Piestrup, M.A., Wu, X., Kaplan, V.V., Uglov, S.R., Cremer, J.T., Rule, D.W., and Fiorito, D.B., A design of mammography units using a quasi-monochromatic x-ray source, *Rev. Sci. Instrum.*, 27, 2159–2170, 2001.
4. Wilkins, S.W., Gureyev, T.E., Gao, D., Pogany, A., and Stevenson, A.W., Phase-contrast imaging using polychromatic hard x-rays, *Nature*, 384, 335–338, 1996.
5. Momose, A. and Fukuda, J., Phase-contrast radiograph of nonstained rat cerebellar specimen, *Med. Phys.*, 22, 375–379, 1995.
6. Chapman, D., Thomlinson, W., Johnston, R.E., Washburn, D., Pisano, E., Gmür, N., Zhong, Z., Menk, R., Arfelli, F., and Sayers, D., Diffraction enhanced x-ray imaging, *Phys. Med. Biol.*, 42, 2015–2025, 1997.
7. Wu, X., Barnes, G.T., and Tucker, D.M., Effect of filtration and kilovolt peak on image contrast and radiation dose in mammography, *Radiology*, 177, 244, 1990.
8. Wu, X., Gingold, E., Barnes, G.T., and Tucker, D.M., Normalized average glandular dose in molybdenum target-rhodium filter and rhodium target-rhodium filter mammography, *Radiology*, 193, 83–89, 1994.
9. Gingold, E.L., Wu, X., and Barnes, G.T., Contrast and dose in Mo/Mo, Mo/Rh and Rh/Rh target/filter mammography, *Radiology*, 195, 639–644, 1995.

10. Kimme-Smith, C., New digital mammography systems may require different x-ray spectra and, therefore, more general normalized glandular dose values, *Radiology*, 213, 7–10, 1999.

11. Yaffe, M.J. and Rowlands, J.A., X-ray detectors for digital radiography, *Phys. Med. Biol.*, 42, 1–39, 1997.

12. Chotas, H.G., Dobbins III, J.T., and Ravin, C.E., Principles of digital radiography with large-area, electronically readable detectors: A review of basics, *Radiology*, 210, 595–599, 1999.

13. Matsuura, N., Zhao, W., Huang, Z., and Rowlands, J.A., Digital radiography using active matrix readout: Amplified pixel detector array for fluoroscopy, *Med. Phys.*, 26, 672–681, 1999.

14. Kato, H., Photostimulable phosphor radiography design considerations, in Seibert, J., Barnes, G., and Gould, R. (eds.), *Specification, Acceptance Testing and Quality Control of Diagnostic X-Ray Imaging Equipment*, AAPM, Washington, DC, 1994.

15. De Groot, P., Image intensifier design and specifications, in Seibert, J., Barnes, G., and Gould, R. (eds.), *Specification, Acceptance Testing and Quality Control of Diagnostic X-Ray Imaging Equipment*, AAPM, Washington, DC, 1994.

16. Krestel, E., *Imaging Systems for Medical Diagnostics*, Siemens Aktieng, Berlin, Germany, 1990.

17. Macovski, A., *Medical Imaging Systems*, Prentice-Hall, Inc., Englewood Cliffs, NJ, 1983.

18. Liu, H., Digital fluoroscopy with an optically coupled charge-coupled device, PhD dissertation, Worcester Polytechnic Institute, Worcester, MA, 1992.

19. Barnes, G.T. and Chakraborty, D.P., Radiographic mottle and patient exposure in mammography, *Radiology*, 145, 815–821, 1982.

20. Dick, C.E. and Motz, J.W., Utilization of monoenergetic x-ray beams to examine the properties of radiographic intensifying screen, *IEEE Trans. Nucl. Sci.*, Ns-28, 1554–1558, 1981.

21. Liu, H., Karellas, A., Moore, S.C., Harris, L.J., and D'Orsi, C.J., Lesion detectability considerations for an optically coupled CCD x-ray imaging system, *IEEE Trans. Nucl. Sci.*, 41, 1506–1509, 1994.

22. Gruner, S.M., CCD and vidicon x-ray detectors: Theory and practice (invited), *Rev. Sci. Instrum.*, 60, 1545, 1989.

23. Maidment, A.D.A. and Yaffe, M.J., Analysis of the spatial-frequency-dependent DQE of the optically coupled digital mammography detectors, *Med. Phys.*, 21, 721–729, 1994.

24. Roehrig, H., Fajardo, L.L., Tong, Y., and Schempp, W.V., Signal, noise and detective quantum efficiency in CCD based x-ray imaging systems for use in mammography, *Proc. SPIE*, 2163, 320–329, 1994.

25. Nishikawa, R.M. and Yaffe, M.J., Model of the spatial-frequency-dependent detective quantum efficiency of phosphor screens, *Med. Phys.*, 17, 894–904, 1990.

26. Dainty, J.C. and Shaw, R., *Image Science*, Academic Press, Boston, MA, 1974, p. 312.

27. Liu, H., Karellas, A., Harris, L., and D'Orsi, C., Optical properties of fiber tapers and their impact on the performance of a fiber optically coupled CCD x-ray imaging system, *SPIE Proc.*, 1894, 136–147, 1993.

28. Liu, H., Fajardo, L.L., Buchanan, M., McAdoo, J., Halama, G., and Jalink, A., CCD-scanning techniques for full-size digital mammography, *Radiology*, 197, 291, 1995.

29. Liu, H., Fajardo, L.L., Barrett, J.R., Williams, M.B., and Baxter, R.A., Contrast-detail detectability analysis: Comparison of a digital spot mammography system and an analog screen-film mammography system, *Acad. Radiol.*, 4, 197–203, 1996.

30. Rose, A., The sensitivity performance of the human eye on an absolute scale, *J. Opt. Soc. Am.*, 38, 196, 1948.

31. Wagner, R. and Brown, D., Unified SNR analysis of medical imaging systems. *Phys. Med. Biol.*, 30, 489–518, 1985.

32. Liu, H., Karellas, A., and Harris, L., Methods to calculate lens efficiency in optically coupled CCD x-ray imaging systems, *Med. Phys.*, 21, 1193–1195, 1994.

33. Pogany, A., Gao, D., and Wilkins, S.W., Contrast and resolution in imaging with a microfocus x-ray source, *Rev. Sci. Instrum.*, 68, 2774–2782, 1997.

34. Wu, X. and Liu, H., A general theoretical formalism for x-ray phase-contrast imaging, *J. X-Ray Sci. Technol.*, 11, 33–42, 2003.

35. Wu, X. and Liu, H., Clinical implementation of x-ray phase-contrast imaging: Theoretical foundations and design considerations, *Med. Phys.*, 30, 2169–2179, 2003.

36. Tanaka, T., Honda, C., Matsuo, S., Noma, K., Oohara, H., Nitta, N., Ota, S. et al., The first trial of phase contrast imaging for digital full-field mammography using a practical molybdenum x-ray tube, *Invest. Radiol.*, 40, 385–396, 2005.

37. Zhang, D., Donovan, M., Fajardo, L., Archer, A., Wu, X., and Liu, H., Preliminary feasibility study of an in-line phase contrast x-ray imaging prototype, *IEEE Trans. Biomed. Eng.*, 55, 2249–2257, 2008.

14

Optical Pumping and MRI of Hyperpolarized Spins

Xizeng Wu
*University of Alabama
at Birmingham*

Thomas Nishino
*University of Texas
Medical Branch*

Hong Liu
University of Oklahoma

14.1 Introduction

Nuclear spins and their interaction with the electromagnetic field form the basis of nuclear magnetic resonance (NMR). Based on NMR, magnetic resonance imaging (MRI) is one of the two most powerful clinical imaging modalities. To perform MRI, the targeted nuclear spins need to be placed in a strong magnetic field to become polarized. The polarization is proportional to the magnetic field strength in conventional MRI, as is the signal-to-noise-ratio (SNR). The ever-increasing demand on high SNR drives magnetic field strengths of MRI scanners ever higher. Presently, the standard high field strength is 1.5 T (1 tesla [T] = 10^4 gauss [G]), and a new trend in this new century is redefining the standard to 3 T. Needless to say, the higher the field strength, the more expensive the MRI scanner. Currently, a 3 T MRI scanner costs at least $1 million more than a 1.5 T scanner. Moreover, high field strengths make scanners bulky and aggravate problems such as magnetic susceptibility artifacts and lengthening of the spin–lattice relaxation time.

Ironically, the nuclear spin polarizations at these high magnetic fields are really tiny because thermal spin polarizations are determined by the Boltzmann factor $e^{-h\nu/k_BT}$, where T is the temperature and ν the magnetic transition frequency. Here h (6.6266×10^{-34} J/s) is Planck's constant and k_B (1.38×10^{-23} J/K) is Boltzmann's constant. The magnetic transition frequencies are radio frequencies (RF) and range from 10^8 to 10^9 Hz in MRI. The resulting polarizations are approximately 10^{-6} to 10^{-5} only.

On the other hand, the optical photons are much more energetic than the RF quanta in MRI. The optical transition frequencies are much higher ($v \sim 10^{14}$ to 10^{15} Hz), and the thermal polarizations for optical transitions are of the order of unity. Optical pumping uses light photons to polarize the atomic electron spins first, and then the nuclear spins of noble gases are polarized through the spin exchange between atomic electron spins and nuclear spins. Using optical pumping, nuclear spins of noble gases such as ^{3}He and ^{129}Xe can be polarized to 50% or higher—100,000 times higher than the proton polarization in conventional MRI. A powerful imaging technique developed in the mid-1990s,[1] MRI of hyperpolarized ^{3}He and ^{129}Xe shows great potential for clinical applications. Moreover, as we will show in this chapter, the SNR of MRI with hyperpolarized spins is almost independent of the magnetic field strength of the scanner. Therefore, relatively inexpensive low field scanners will benefit greatly from this SNR characteristic.

We discuss optical pumping from a biomedical photonics perspective in detail in Section 14.3. The special features of hyperpolarized spin MRI, such as the signal intensity estimates, the RF flip angle optimization, and diffusion-associated signal attenuation, are covered in Section 14.4. This relatively short chapter is not intended to present a comprehensive review of the field; rather, the emphasis is placed on working principles, analytical methods, and general techniques of optical pumping and MRI of hyperpolarized spins. A brief introduction to MRI is also presented in Section 14.2.

14.2 MRI Basics

14.2.1 Nuclear Magnetism

All atoms are composed of protons, neutrons, and electrons. The nucleus of an atom consists of protons and neutrons. Nuclei with an odd number of protons or neutrons possess a net nuclear spin-angular momentum. These nuclei have a magnetic moment μ that characterizes the magnetic field localized around the nucleus. This magnetic field is analogous to the magnetic field generated by a bar magnet.

In free space at room temperature, these magnetic moments (dipoles) are randomly oriented in space due to thermal fluctuations. However, in the presence of an external static magnetic field, these dipoles are inclined to align with the magnetic field. For hydrogen protons, the nuclear spin quantum number $I = 1/2$. The external magnetic field, denoted by B_0, creates two different energy states for hydrogen protons. Each energy state is identified by the magnetic quantum number $m_s = \pm 1/2$. The energy state $m_s = +1/2$ has a component parallel to the external magnetic field and has a lower energy than the energy state $m_s = -1/2$, which has a component antiparallel to B_0.

The phases of the magnetic moments are randomly distributed for both energy states with each ensemble of spins forming the surface of a cone. The net magnetization is the vector sum of all the individual magnetic moments. At room temperature, both energy states have approximately the same number of spins, which results in zero net longitudinal magnetization along the z-axis. Furthermore, because of the lack of phase coherence, no net transverse magnetization exists in the x–y plane.

On the other hand, in the presence of a strong external magnetic field (e.g., 1.5 T = 15,000 G, which is about 20,000 times the Earth's magnetic field), the populations in the two energy states are no longer equal. In fact, the lower energy state will have an excess population of about 3 spins per million at 1.0 T. A more general formula for the thermal equilibrium polarization will be given in Equation 14.37. Thus, in 1 cm³ of water at 1.0 T there are roughly 10^{15} excess spins in the lower energy level. The number of excess spins in the lower energy state is directly related to the external magnetic field strength. This imbalance of spins in the two energy states gives rise to a net magnetization along the external magnetic field. Of course, thermal noise will cause spins to go from one energy state to the other, but as time passes, an equilibrium longitudinal magnetization, M_0 (along the z-axis), will be produced. Because the human body is composed primarily of water (H_2O), hydrogen (protons) is the preferred imaging isotope because of its relative abundance and sensitivity compared with other atomic nuclei found in the human body.

14.2.2 Magnetic Resonance

Resonance is a phenomenon through which energy can be transferred between objects or systems. In MRI, resonance refers to the induction of transitions between different energy states ($I = \pm 1/2$ for protons) by an RF wave with its magnetic field perpendicular to the static magnetic field B_0. The frequency of the RF wave must be such that the energy of the resonant RF quanta is equal to the difference in energy between the levels, which is given by

$$\Delta E = \gamma \hbar B_0 \tag{14.1}$$

where $h = h/2\pi$ is the reduced Planck's constant. The resonance frequency, the so-called Larmor frequency f_L, is

$$f_L = \frac{\gamma}{2\pi} B_0 \tag{14.2}$$

where γ is the gyromagnetic ratio specific to the nuclear isotope, for hydrogen, $(\gamma/2\pi) = 42.58$ MHz/T. This energy will cause the proton magnetic moments to "flip" from the lower energy state ($m = +1/2$, parallel to B_0) to their higher energy state ($m = -1/2$, antiparallel to B_0). By doing so, the net longitudinal magnetization can be diminished, reduced to zero, or even reversed entirely, depending on the amount of energy deposited to the protons.

The RF energy, in addition to causing spins to flip energy states, also forces the protons to precess in phase with each other at the resonant frequency. This phase coherence generates a transverse net magnetization, which is the only magnetization that we can physically measure, because the transverse magnetization precesses around the B_0-field and generates the inductive voltage in the receiver coil (Figure 14.1). The precession angular frequency ω_L is

$$\omega_L = 2\pi f_L = \gamma B_0 \tag{14.3}$$

Because f_L is the Larmor frequency, ω_L is called the angular Larmor frequency, or simply the Larmor frequency in the literature. Obviously, the Larmor frequency increases with the magnetic field B_0.

The resonance process can also be viewed as exerting a torque generated by a resonance RF field (an RF wave with the resonant frequency) on the magnetization vector. This is like Earth's magnetic

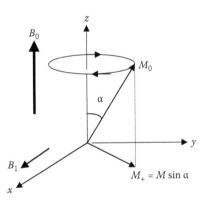

FIGURE 14.1 The magnetization vector M_0 is precessing about the static magnetic field B_0. The magnetic field B_1 of the RF pulse flips magnetization vector M_0 by an angle α. The projection of magnetization vector M_0 onto x–y plane is the transverse magnetization M_+.

field exerting a torque on the magnetic needle of a compass. This is especially convenient to view the RF wave in the so-called rotating frame, a reference frame rotating about B_0 with Larmor frequency. In this frame the effect of a resonant RF wave is represented by a stationary magnetic field in the rotating frame. This field is also called the flip field, B_1, because it flips magnetization. This torque exerted by the flip field B_1 is equal to the vector product of the flip field and magnetization. As we know from mechanics, the effect of a torque is to change the angular momentum, and the speed of change of angular momentum is equal to the torque. Nuclear magnetization is proportional to nuclear spin angular momentum; hence,

$$\frac{d\vec{M}}{dt} = \gamma \vec{M} \times \vec{B}_1 \tag{14.4}$$

From this torque equation it is clear that the flip angle, α by which a magnetization vector is flipped away from B_0 field direction by the torque, is proportional to the resonant RF field strength B_1 and lasting time (the width) of the RF pulse:

$$\alpha = \gamma B_1 t_p \tag{14.5}$$

If magnetization M_0 is originally in the z-direction (B_0 field direction), then the longitudinal magnetization $M_z = M_0$. After the application of an RF pulse of B_1, and the transverse magnetization M_+ in the x–y plane and longitudinal magnetization M_z are (see Figure 14.1)

$$M_+ = M_0 \sin\alpha, \quad M_z = M_0 \cos\alpha \tag{14.6}$$

From these equations it is obvious that a 90° RF pulse tips the equilibrium magnetization vector into the x–y plane, yielding zero net longitudinal magnetization and maximum net transverse magnetization M_+.

When RF energy is no longer applied to the protons, the net magnetization continues to precess around the external magnetic field at the Larmor frequency. This precessing magnetization can be detected as a time-varying electrical signal across the leads of a coil of wire that can be represented as a complex number with real and imaginary parts. The net magnetization also decays exponentially, having a time constant T_2. Hence, because the induced voltage can be characterized by a decaying cosine function, it is often referred to as the free-induction decay, or FID.

14.2.3 Spin Relaxation, Tissue Characteristics, and Bloch Equation

The precessing protons interact with the surrounding tissue as well as with other protons that cause them to dephase. Each proton experiences a different local magnetic field depending on the orientation of other nearby protons. The fact that each proton feels a different local magnetic field leads to each proton having a different Larmor frequency. Consequently, because protons are now precessing at different frequencies, the phase coherence created by the RF pulse is slowly destroyed. Subsequently, the transverse magnetization decays because of the individual magnetic moments interacting with other magnetic moments causing them to dephase. This process is known as T_2 (or spin–spin) relaxation. The value of T_2 is different for various tissues and characterizes the rate at which the transverse magnetization decays to zero. The transverse magnetization decays according to the following relationship:

$$M_+(t) = M_+(0)e^{-t/T_2} \tag{14.7}$$

Note that this equation represents the decay of the transverse magnetization in a perfectly homogeneous static external magnetic field. Of course, it is impossible to create a perfectly uniform magnetic field. Pockets of tiny, but nonetheless significant, magnetic field inhomogeneities that affect the decay of the transverse magnetization always exist. When magnetic field inhomogeneities exist, the T_2 relaxation of the tissue speeds up, yielding T_2^* relaxation.

When a short RF pulse is applied to the ensemble of protons with a flip angle of 90°, the longitudinal magnetization is tipped into the x–y plane, resulting in zero longitudinal magnetization. Once the RF pulse is removed from the system, the spins in the higher state will return to the lower state, in the process giving off energy to the surrounding tissue (lattice). As more spins return to the lower energy state, the longitudinal magnetization will grow back to its original value, M_0. The rate at which the longitudinal magnetization recovers is given by the T_1 (or spin–lattice) relaxation rate of the tissue and obeys

$$M_z(t) = M_{eq} + [M_z(t = 0) - M_{eq}]\exp\left(\frac{-t}{T_1}\right) \tag{14.8}$$

where M_{eq} is the thermal equilibrium magnetization in magnetic field B_0.

The value of T_1 depends on the dissipation of absorbed energy into the surrounding molecular lattice. Energy is most easily transferred if the proton precession frequency overlaps with the "vibrational frequencies" of the lattice. The more overlap, the easier it is to transfer energy, yielding shorter T_1 values. The less overlap, the harder it is to transfer energy, yielding longer T_1 values. It is important to note that the two processes, T_1 and T_2 relaxation, are independent of each other and often quite different from one another for the same tissue. Furthermore, T_1 is greatly dependent on external magnetic field strength, but T_2 is relatively independent of the field strength. Finally, in general, $T_1 > T_2 > T_2^*$.

Figure 14.2 shows two brain images of a patient at the same brain slice. The image shown in Figure 14.2a is T_1 weighted, that is, the image reflects the T_1 relaxation difference of different brain tissues. The longer the T_1, the lower the signal for that tissue. The image shown in Figure 14.2b is T_2 weighted, that is, the T_2 relaxation difference of different brain tissues is weighted in the image. In contrast to Figure 14.2a, in Figure 14.2b the longer the T_2, the higher the signal for that tissue.

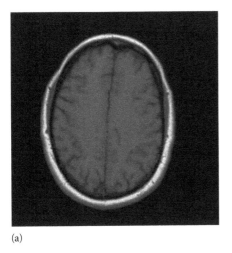
(a)

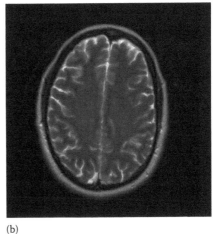
(b)

FIGURE 14.2 (a) The T_1 weighted brain image of a patient. (b) The T_2 weighted brain image of the same patient.

Combining the torque equation with the spin relaxation effects as described previously, one can write the magnetization change rate due to the flip field and relaxation as the so-called Bloch equation

$$\frac{d\vec{M}}{dt} = \gamma \vec{M} \times \vec{B}_1 - \frac{1}{T_1}(M_z - M_{eq})\vec{k} - \frac{1}{T_2}(M_x\vec{i} + M_y\vec{j}) \tag{14.9}$$

where the vectors $\vec{i}, \vec{j}$, and $\vec{k}$ are the unit vectors of the x-, y-, and z-axes, respectively. The Bloch equation is the most fundamental equation of NMR and MRI.

14.2.4 Mapping Spatial Distribution of Spins

In MRI the spatial distribution of spins is mapped by applying magnetic field gradients and performing the Fourier transform. Consider a magnetic field gradient, G_x, in the x-direction superimposing on the B_0 field of an MRI scanner's magnet. The magnetic field gradient specifies magnetic field change per unit length. For example, if $B_0 = 1.5$ T, and $G_x = 10$ mT/m, then the resulting magnetic field is 1.5 T at $x = 0$ and 1.501 T at $x = 10$ cm. Therefore, spins at different position x will experience slightly different magnetic fields. From Equation 14.3 it is clear that the spins at x will have a precessing frequency $\omega(x)$ when the spin is flipped to the transverse plan by an RF pulse:

$$\omega(x) = \gamma \cdot B_0 + \gamma G_x x \tag{14.10}$$

Therefore the MRI signal intensity at time t generated by these spins at x will be

$$s(x,t) = CM_+(x)e^{(-i\omega(x)t)} = (Ce^{-i\omega_L t})M_+(x)e^{-i\gamma G_x xt} \tag{14.11}$$

where C is a calibration constant for converting precessing M_+ to the signal. The receiver coil detects the total signal from spins all over the scan volume; hence, the total signal at time t is

$$s(\gamma G_x t) = (Ce^{-i\omega_L t})\int M_+(x)e^{-i\gamma G_x xt}\,dx \tag{14.12}$$

Using Equation 14.6, the total signal can be related to the spin magnetizations as

$$s(\gamma G_x t) = (Ce^{-i\omega_L t})\sin\alpha \int M_z(x)e^{-i\gamma G_x xt}\,dx \tag{14.13}$$

Note that the integral

$$\int M_z(x)e^{-i\gamma G_x xt}\,dx \tag{14.14}$$

is a Fourier transform of the magnetization at x. Therefore, Equation 14.13 tells in words that the signal intensity received by the receiver coil essentially is a Fourier transform of spin's spatial distribution. This being so, collecting the coil signal as a function of time t and performing an inverse Fourier transformation of the signal, we reconstruct the spin spatial distribution: the image of the spin along the x-axis. The field gradient G_x is thus called the x-encoding field gradient. Using the magnetic field gradients G_y and G_z along the y- and z-axes and applying the same strategy to the other two dimensions (y and z), we can reconstruct a three-dimensional spatial distribution of spins, i.e., a three-dimensional MRI image. In MRI, G_x is also called the frequency encoding gradient, and G_y the phase-encoding gradient. The encoding gradients used in the new generation MRI scanner can go as high as 40–50 mT/m.

From the MRI point of view, the spin spatial distribution $M_z(x)$ and the MRI signal $s(\gamma G_x t)$ form a Fourier pair; they are really two incarnations of the same identity. $M_z(x)$ represents an image characterized in the real space, and the signal $s(\gamma G_x t)$ represents the same image characterized in the k space (Fourier space or the spatial frequency space) with $k_x = \gamma G_x t$. As we collect the signal data $s(\gamma G_x t)$ for different times such as t_1, t_2, etc., one is really sampling the image at k space positions (also called encoding steps) $k_{x1} = \gamma G_x t_1$, $k_{x2} = \gamma G_x t_2$, etc. Simply stated, MRI is a technique to reconstruct M_z by sampling it in the k space through detecting NMR signals $s(k)$.

In order to sample an image in the k space, one applies a sequence of RF pulses and field gradients. Figure 14.3 shows a typical gradient echo pulse sequence. Note that the label FEG denotes the frequency encoding gradient $G_x(t)$, PEG denotes the phase encoding gradient $G_y(t)$, PEG denotes the phase encoding gradient $G_y(t)$, and SEG denotes the slice encoding gradient $G_z(t)$. In this sequence an RF pulse of flip angle α establishes a transverse magnetization M_+ first, and then spins start to precess in the x–y plane with the Larmor frequency. Meanwhile, a negative field $-G_{x1}$ gradient is applied for a short period δt, followed by a second positive field gradient G_{x2}, as shown in Figure 14.3. The data acquisition starts during the positive gradient period, which lasts for a sampling period of T_s (from a few to 10 ms). From Equation 14.14, the coil detects a time-varying signal proportional to

$$\int M_z(x)e^{-i\gamma(-G_{x1}\delta t + G_{x2}t)x}dx, \quad 0 \leq t \leq T_s \tag{14.15}$$

Again, as discussed previously, the signal detected during $0 < t < T_s$ samples magnetization $M_z(x)$ in the k space from a negative value $-\gamma G_{x1}\delta t$ to a positive value $\gamma(G_{x2T_s} - G_{x1}\delta t)$. In this way a k space line is completed. Note that, at $t = G_{x1}\delta t/G_{x2}$, the phase $(-G_{x1}\delta t + G_{x2}t)$ in the above equation becomes zero. This means all spins are precessing in the same phase at this moment; hence, the signal reaches the maximum, i.e., an echo is formed at this moment. That is why this type of pulse sequence is called the gradient echo pulse sequence. The gradients G_y shown in Figure 14.3 encode the spin's y-position on the same principle. Each G_y step encodes spins such that each k_x-line corresponds to different k_y. When the next spin-flipping RF pulse is applied, the same k_x sampling repeats but with a different G_y step. In this way, by repeating RF excitations (pulses) and using different G_y steps after each pulse (RF excitation), one samples magnetization through the k space line by line (Figure 14.4).

In MRI one often views a three-dimensional image by slices. The slice-selecting gradient G_z in Figure 14.3 encodes the z-position of spins. For a detailed introduction to MRI, refer to Smith and Lange[2] and Chen

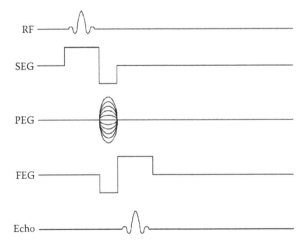

FIGURE 14.3 A typical gradient echo pulse sequence.

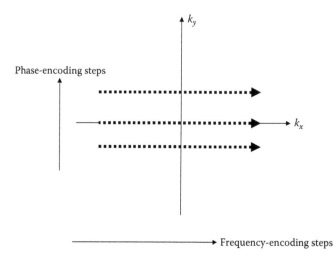

FIGURE 14.4 The *k*-space sampling process for a gradient echo pulse sequence. Each dot line represents the k_x sampling process during a signal read-out. Each dot represents a k_x point for which the signal is acquired. After the next RF excitation (RF pulse) the k_x sampling process repeats but with a new phase-encoding step (new k_y step).

and Hoult.[3] The higher the G_z, the thinner the resulting slice. It should be noted that the popular spin-echo pulse sequences of conventional MRI are not suitable for MRI with hyperpolarized spins (see Section 14.4.2).

14.3 Nuclear Spin Hyperpolarization by Optical Pumping

In the optical pumping and spin exchange approach for nuclear spin hyperpolarization, one shines a glass pumping cell (several hundred cubic centimeters in volume) containing alkali-metal vapors such as rubidium (Rb) vapor and noble gas (^{3}He or ^{129}Xe) with a circularly polarized infrared light. The cell is heated to 80°C–150°C to maintain the desired Rb vapor density. ^{3}He or ^{129}Xe gas is kept at a pressure of several atmospheres in the cell, and approximately 100 Torr of N_2 is also added to the cell for buffering. The circularly polarized infrared light polarizes the valence electrons of Rb atoms as explained later, and the polarized Rb atoms transfer their electronic spin polarization to nuclear spins of ^{3}He or ^{129}Xe by the spin-exchange collisions (Figure 14.5). In this way nuclear spin polarization of ^{3}He or ^{129}Xe can be as high as 50% or more.

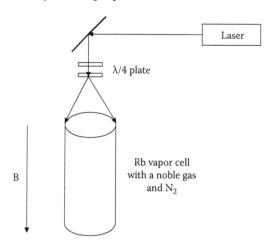

FIGURE 14.5 Schematic of the optical pumping setup. The $\lambda/4$ plates are used to generate a circular polarization of the light.

It should be noted that ³He may also be polarized by the optical pumping and metastability exchange. Using 1.083 μm circularly polarized laser light, one can polarize the metastable ³He* (the 2^3S_1 state) atoms in a ³He plasma at 1 mbar by optical pumping. Through the metastable exchange collisions between ³He* and ³He, the angular momentum is transferred from polarized ³He* to ³He nuclear spins of the ground state (the 1^1S_0 state).[4] However, the metastability exchange polarization of ¹²⁹Xe does not work so far. In this section we will discuss the optical pumping and spin exchange approach in detail.

14.3.1 Optical Depopulation Pumping of Alkali-Metal Atoms

In order to hyperpolarize nuclear spins, the first step is to use light to polarize the valence electronic spins of atoms of alkali-metal vapors such as rubidium (Rb), potassium (K), and cesium (Cs) vapors. This electron polarization process is based on the idea of depopulation pumping.[5] As is well known, an electron carries spin $s = 1/2$, just as the proton (hydrogen nucleus) carries spin $I = 1/2$. A spin-1/2 particle has two spin states, one up and one down, as discussed previously. Therefore, in ground state the valence electron of an alkali metal atom has two different spin states, one up, one down. In a weak magnetic field (the holding field) of about 10–150 G, these two states have slightly different energy levels. In other words, the ground state has two sublevels (Figure 14.6).

Ordinarily these two spin states are almost equally populated; thus, the valence electron is not polarized. The idea of depopulation pumping is as follows. Shine light on the atoms. If one ground sublevel absorbs light much more strongly than the other, then atoms are pumped out more rapidly from the strongly absorbing sublevel. The populations of the two sublevels will not be equal any more as a result of the processes of the selective light absorption, atom excitation, and transition from the excited state to ground state via the spontaneous emission. Obviously the weakly absorbing sublevel will gain excess population and electron polarization results. In order to understand the factors affecting the yield of electron polarization, let us consider the optical pumping of rubidium atoms in detail.

14.3.2 Atomic States of Rubidium

For optical pumping, one places the rubidium vapor glass chamber in a weak magnetic field (e.g., 10–150 G), as shown in Figure 14.5. In order to understand the optical pumping of Rb atoms, one should know the atomic states and energy levels. Rubidium has two isotopes: ⁸⁵Rb has a natural abundance of 72.17% and ⁸⁷Rb a natural abundance of 27.83%. First, we assume that the nuclear spins of Rb ($I = 5/2$ for ⁸⁵Rb and $I = 3/2$ for ⁸⁷Rb) are not involved in the optical pumping process. This assumption will be justified later. With this assumption, the atomic states are labeled by conventional spectroscopic notation. A letter symbol indicates the total orbital angular momentum L of the valence electrons. For example, symbols S, P, and D indicate $L = 0$, 1, and 2, respectively. A right subscript attached to the letter

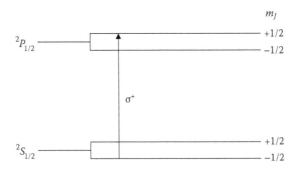

FIGURE 14.6 Energy level diagram for Rb ground state and the lowest excited state. The energy differences between the sublevels are tiny because of the weakness of the magnetic holding field.

indicates the total angular momentum J (the sum of orbital and spin angular momenta) of the state. A left superscript attached to the letter indicates the spin multiplicity $2s + 1$, where s is the total spin of valence electron. Rubidium has only one valence electron; its ground state has zero orbital angular momentum, hence $L = 0$, $s = 1/2$, and $J = s = 1/2$, indicated as $^2S_{1/2}$ (more exactly, $5^2S_{1/2}$).

Note that the ground state has two spin states; one is the spin-up state of $m_J = m_s = 1/2$, and the other is the spin-down state of $m_J = m_s = -1/2$. Here the number m_J denotes the projection of the total angular momentum along the applied holding magnetic field. Therefore the ground state has two subenergy levels. Although their energy levels are approximately the same due to the weakness of the holding field, they differ in electron spin orientations (Figure 14.6). The lowest excited state of Rb is $^2P_{1/2}$ (more exactly, $5^2P_{1/2}$). This state has two sublevels with $m_J = 1/2$ and $m_J = -1/2$ as well. (Note that, for the $^2P_{1/2}$ state, m_J is a good quantum number and m_s is not.) The energy difference between the ground state $^2S_{1/2}$ and the excited state $^2P_{1/2}$ is 1.56 eV, which corresponds to rubidium D1 absorption line at 794.8 nm.

14.3.3 Selective Absorption of Circularly Polarized Light

When a light with wavelength of approximately 794.8 nm shines on the glass cell of Rb vapor, the light propagates along the holding-field direction. The oscillating electric field of the light will induce the electric dipole and cause transitions between the ground state and the excited state. Remember that each has two sublevels with different m_J. At first glance it seems true that the valence electron from any ground state sublevel ($m_J = 1/2, -1/2$) could be promoted to any sublevels of the state $^2P_{1/2}$ just by photon absorption; however, this is not true. In fact, the angular momentum conservation imposes the selection rules on what transitions are allowed.

Suppose that the input light is a left-hand circularly polarized light (i.e., a σ^+-polarized light). A circularly polarized light can be thought of as generated by two waves whose electric field components are orthogonal and 90° out of phase. This phase difference between these two waves causes an effective rotation of the total electric field vector about an axis in direction of propagation. For a left-hand circularly polarized light, the electric field vector is perpendicular to and rotating about the holding magnetic field direction in the left-hand sense.

As is well known, a photon carries a spin $s = 1$. A σ^+-polarized photon carries a spin pointing along the magnetic field and thus the spin projection $m_s = 1$. The angular momentum conservation dictates that a σ^+-polarized light can be absorbed by the $m_J = -1/2$ sublevel of ground state $^2S_{1/2}$ to induce a transition to the $m_J = 1/2$ sublevel of excited state $^2P_{1/2}$. This is because the total change of m_J with the transition is $\Delta m_J = 1$, and this change can be compensated by absorption of a σ^+-polarized photon. By the same reason of angular momentum conservation, a σ^+-polarized light cannot be absorbed by the electron in the $m_J = 1/2$ sublevel of the ground state. In this way the σ^+-polarized light is absorbed only by the spin-down sublevel ($m_J = -1/2$) of ground state; the spin-up sublevel ($m_J = 1/2$) is "left in dark." Absorbing a light photon, the valence electron from the spin-down sublevel ($m_J = -1/2$) is promoted to the $m_J = 1/2$ sublevel of the excited state $^2P_{1/2}$ (Figure 14.7).

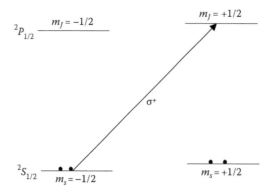

FIGURE 14.7 Schematic of the ground state excitation by optical pumping using a σ^+-polarized light.

14.3.4 De-Excitation of Rb Atoms and Ground State Polarization

The atom cannot stay in the $m_J = 1/2$ sublevel of the excited state $^2P_{1/2}$ for long because of radiative decay via the spontaneous emission of light. When the excited state decays back to the ground state by spontaneous emission, it can decay to either of the two ground state sublevels. For an isolated atom, the probability of decay back to the $m_J = -1/2$ sublevel of ground state is twice that for returning to the $m_J = 1/2$ sublevel. From depopulation pumping point of view, this, of course, is not desirable, because it is against depopulation efforts. Fortunately, one can use the buffer gas to improve this problem.

In the Rb vapor cell there are usually noble gas atoms such as He and Xe gas for the spin exchange polarization (see below). If this gas has high enough density in the cell, the excited Rb atom will collide with these noble gas atoms many times during its lifetime. These collisions will redistribute the sublevel populations of the excited state. In other words, the sublevels of $m_J = 1/2$ and $m_J = -1/2$ are to be equally populated. In this way, when these excited state sublevels undergo radiative decay via spontaneous emission, the probabilities for returning to each of the ground state sublevels become the same (Figure 14.8). This process of collisional mixing of excited state sublevel populations ensures that the spin-up or spin-down sublevels will be repopulated at the same rate during the atomic de-excitation. In this way, because the spin-down sublevel of ground state is continuously pumped into the excited state by light absorption, eventually the spin-down sublevel is completely depopulated, and the valence electron is polarized to the spin-up state eventually.

In optical pumping practice, N_2 gas is added as the quenching gas into the Rb vapor cell to eliminate the radiation trapping problem (Figure 14.8). The remitted light (spontaneous decay) from the excited state is unpolarized and propagates in any direction. Once reabsorbed by Rb atoms, these remitted unpolarized photons can depolarize the atoms. Thus, if the mean free path of these photons is much less than the cell dimension, these unpolarized photons are trapped inside the cell and reduce the yield of electron polarization from optical pumping. The added N_2 gas allows the excited Rb atoms to decay nonradiatively (without emission of photons) from the excited state $^2P_{1/2}$ back to the ground state by collisions with the N_2.[6] Therefore the N_2 gas eliminates radiation trapping as a source of depolarization. The required N_2 densities are of 0.1 amagat or more.[5] Note that the density of an ideal gas is 1 amagat = 2.69×10^{19} cm^{-3}. With adding N_2 gas to the Rb cell, the N_2 quenching becomes the main source of de-excitation.

14.3.5 Optical Pumping Dynamics and the Generalized Bloch Equation

The yield of rubidium ground state polarization depends obviously on the input light intensity, light spectral profile, and the lifetime of excited state. In order to understand the effects of these factors on polarization yield, one should find the equation of motion of ground state polarization.

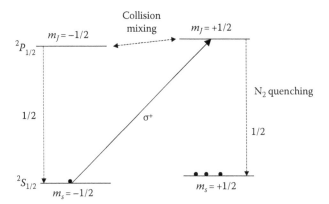

FIGURE 14.8 Schematic of the state transitions via optical pumping, collision mixing, and N_2 gas quenching.

Similar to the longitudinal (along the magnetic field B_0) magnetization in NMR discussed earlier, the ground state polarization $S_z = [P(1/2) - P(-1/2)]/2$ specifies ground state polarization, where $P(1/2)$ and $P(-1/2)$ are the occupation probability of the $m_J = 1/2$ sublevel and the $m_J = -1/2$ sublevel, respectively.

There may exist transverse (perpendicular to B) magnetizations S_x and S_y as well, since these transverse magnetizations may result from the coherence between ground state sublevel. Different from that in NMR, the pressing frequency of S_x and S_y about the magnetic field direction is faster than the Larmor frequency defined previously. The amount of difference, the so-called light shift, is proportional to the optical pumping rate and the light detuning (the amount of off-resonance of the light from the rubidium D1 line).[7] Fortunately, for typical cases where rubidium is in thermal equilibrium when the laser light is turned on, no transverse magnetization (S_x, S_y) will be generated by optical pumping. Therefore, for these cases optical pumping generates polarization S_z only.

Similar to M_z in NMR, the dynamics of S_z can be described by a generalized Bloch equation. This is no surprise because the laser–atom interactions can be described very well by the optical Bloch equation.[8] Merging the optical Bloch equations and the magnetic resonance Bloch equation for spins (electron spins), we have a generalized Bloch equation of optical pumping:

$$\frac{dS_z}{dt} = -\frac{1}{T_{eff}}(S_z - S_{op-eq}) \tag{14.16}$$

where S_{op-eq} is the equilibrium achieved using optical pumping and is given by

$$S_{op-eq} = \frac{1}{2}\frac{P_+(\Delta)}{\Gamma_{SD} + P_+(\Delta)} \tag{14.17}$$

where Γ_{SD} is the S_z-destroying (spin-destruction) relaxation rate. The most important contribution to Γ_{SD} is from collision between Rb atoms themselves. $P_+(\Delta)$ is called the optical pumping rate:

$$P_+(\Delta) = \frac{\Omega_1^2 \Gamma_2^2}{4\Gamma_2(\Gamma_2^2 + \Delta^2)} \tag{14.18}$$

Here Δ is the offset of the laser frequency from the resonance frequency (D1 line) ω_{D1}, $\Delta = (\omega - \omega_{D1})$. Γ_2 is the optical coherence decay rate and equal to one half of the Rb D1 absorption linewidth broadened by collisions. Obviously, the optical pumping rate $P_+(\Delta)$ is a function of the frequency offset. Ω_1 is the so-called optical Rabi frequency,

$$\hbar\Omega_1 = -\vec{E} \cdot \vec{D}_{ge} \tag{14.19}$$

The Rabi frequency is the scalar product of electric field E and the induced atomic dipole D_{ge} of the transition from the ground state to the excited state. Optical Rabi frequency characterizes the strength of the coupling between the incident light and Rb atoms. Because light is an electromagnetic wave, the light intensity is proportional to the square of the electric field. Therefore, squared Rabi frequency is proportional to the light intensity, and the optical pumping rate P_+ is proportional to light intensity as well.

Equations 14.16 through 14.18 determine the optical pumping dynamics. The spin polarization grows as

$$S_z(t) = S_{op-eq}(1 - e^{-t/T_{eff}}) \tag{14.20}$$

With optical pumping, the spin polarization increases with time exponentially according to this equation. Eventually spin polarization S_z reaches the maximal value S_{op-eq}. The speed with which the maximal value is reached is determined by the effective relaxation rate $1/T_{eff}$:

$$\frac{1}{T_{eff}} = \Gamma_{SD} + P_+ \tag{14.21}$$

It is important to note that the maximal spin polarization S_{op-eq} is not proportional to light intensity, as is shown by Equation 14.17. If we want to achieve 100% polarization ($S_{op-eq} = 1/2$), we should have $P_+ \gg \Gamma_{SD}$. For Rb vapor, $\Gamma_{SD} = k$ [Rb], where $k = 7.8 \times 10^{-13}$ cm³/s, and [Rb] is the Rb density. Obviously Γ_{SD} is proportional to the Rb density. As shown later, in order to get more hyperpolarized He or Xe nuclear spins, the Rb densities used must be high enough. This requires even higher P_+, since $P_+ \gg \Gamma_{SD}$ must be kept for high Rb spin polarization. In order to see the effect of the frequency offset on the optical pumping rate of a narrow band laser light, we can rewrite Equation 14.18 as

$$P_+(\Delta) = \frac{\Gamma_2^2}{(\Gamma_2^2 + \Delta^2)} P_+(0) = \frac{\Gamma_2^2}{(\Gamma_2^2 + \Delta^2)} \sigma_0 I_0 \tag{14.22}$$

Here we use the fact that $P_+(0)$ is proportional to photon number intensity (photons per unit area per unit time), and σ_0 is the on-resonance photon scattering cross section that depends on the induced dipole of Rb atom and its $D1$ linewidth. Using the above equations, we can rewrite σ_0 in terms of the spontaneous emission rate and the $D1$ line wavelength:

$$\sigma_0 = \frac{\lambda_0^2 \Gamma_{nat}}{4\pi \Gamma_2} \tag{14.23}$$

where
  λ_0 is the $D1$ line wavelength
  Γ_{nat} is the natural linewidth of Rb $D1$ line

Note that Rb has a small natural width Γ_{nat} of 5.66 MHz for the $D1$ line because, for the excited state $5^2P_{1/2}$, $n = 5$ and the natural linewidth is $n^{-4.5}$ for alkali metals. Thus, σ_0 depends on total pressure in the pumping cell due to the $D1$ line pressure broadening (see below).

This equation shows that $P_+(\Delta)$ decreases with increasing offset Δ (or detuning) showing a Lorentz line shape. It is interesting to note that the NMR spectral line shapes for nuclear spins in liquid and many biological tissues are Lorentzian as well. This is no surprise; the similarity can be traced back to the underlying dynamics described by similar Bloch equations, i.e., by the optical Bloch equation for optical pumping and by the magnetization Bloch equation for NMR spectroscopy. Again, as in NMR, the full width of half-maximum (FWHM) of $P_+(\Delta)$ is given by the optical coherence decay rate; hence, FWHM of $P_+(\Delta)$ is equal to $2\Gamma_2$. Remember that Γ_2 is the optical coherence decay rate and equal to one half of the Rb $D1$ absorption linewidth. Note that Rb $D1$ absorption linewidth increases with pressure. The Rb $D1$ line is broadened by about 18 GHz per amagat of ³He.

14.3.6 Spin Exchange and Hyperpolarized Nuclear Spins

Once Rb atomic electrons are polarized, the Rb electronic polarization is transferred to nuclear spins of He and Xe by atomic collisions. The key process is the collision transfer. During collisions, the electronic spin S of a polarized Rb atom interacts with nuclear spin I_{ng} of a noble gas atom through the hyperfine interaction

$$A(R)\vec{I}_{ng} \cdot \vec{S} \tag{14.24}$$

The hyperfine interaction arises from the magnetic field inside the nucleus of noble gas atom, and the magnetic field interacts with Rb electron spins. The factor $A(R)$ represents the coupling strength and strongly depends on the interatomic distance separation R. Because the hyperfine coupling is a scalar coupling, it is well known in NMR that a scalar coupling between spins causes mutual spin flipping. That is, during the collision the Rb electron spin and the nuclear spin of noble gas atoms are likely to flip in opposite directions. For example, an Rb electron spin flips from up to down during the collision, while the nuclear spin of the noble gas atom flips from down to up. Rb atoms have already been polarized via optical pumping; hence, certain polarization is transferred from Rb atoms to nuclear spins of noble gas during collision. That is, the polarization loss for Rb atoms is the polarization gain for nuclear spins of noble gas. Fortunately, the polarization of Rb can be constantly replenished by optical pumping. In this sense it is the angular momenta of circular polarized light that have been transferred to nuclear spins of noble gas.

The spin exchange rate equation is

$$\frac{dP_K}{dt} = \gamma_{SE}(2S_z - P_K) - \Gamma_K P_K \tag{14.25}$$

In the steady state, the noble gas nuclear spin polarization is

$$P_K = 2S_z \frac{\gamma_{SE}}{\gamma_{SE} + \Gamma_K} \tag{14.26}$$

where
    P_K is the noble gas nuclear spin polarization
    Γ_K is its relaxation rate

The relaxation is often dominated by wall collision, although dipole–dipole coupling and impurities contribute as well. Obviously, the portion of Rb electron polarization transferred to noble gas nuclear spin is determined by $\gamma_{SE}/(\gamma_{SE} + \Gamma_K)$. If the light intensity is high enough and light reaches all parts of the pumping cell, this can reach the maximal value $S_{op-eq} \sim 1/2$, so $2S_z = 2S_{op-eq} \sim 1$. In order to achieve high polarization for noble gas nuclei, one must achieve a high Rb electron polarization and suppress Γ_K such that $\gamma_{SE} \gg \Gamma_K$. Since γ_{SE} is proportional to [Rb] (the Rb number density of the Rb vapor), one needs to increase the temperature of the cell (the oven temperature) to vaporize more rubidium. Then a higher light intensity is needed to maintain high Rb polarization such that $2S_{op-eq} \sim 1$. Therefore, the practical limitation is the light intensity achievable, i.e., the cost and complexity of the laser power employed.

14.3.7 Laser Source Considerations

From the previous discussion it is clear that a laser source with high output near the Rb $D1$ line is needed for optical pumping. However, we should also decide the bandwidth requirement for lasers. For example, we can use a narrow band laser source such as the Ti:Sapphire laser, or a broadband laser source such as the laser diode arrays (LDA) with power of a few tens of watts. A titanium-doped sapphire laser (Ti:Sapphire laser) is a narrow band laser; in fact, the lasing medium $Ti^{3+}:Al_2O_3$ has a very broad (about 300 nm) emission band with the peak emission at 790 nm.

However, laser source bandwidth will have important effects on the yield nuclear spin polarization of the noble gas. At first glance, it seems that a narrow band laser with output close to the Rb $D1$ line is better than a broadband laser, because the optical pumping rate $P_+(\Delta)$ decreases with increasing light detuning (offset). However, we must consider the light attenuation along propagation, since optical pumping needs to absorb those left circularly polarized photons. Let us denote the optical pumping rate at z as $P_+(\Delta, z)$; then, similar to Equation 14.22, we have

$$P_+(\Delta,z) = \frac{\Gamma_2^2}{(\Gamma_2^2 + \Delta^2)} \sigma_0 I(z) \tag{14.27}$$

$I(z)$ is the laser photon flux as z. Hence, the optical pumping rate $P_+(\Delta, z)$ is, in fact, decreasing with $I(z)$ due to light absorption. Traveling a very small distance dz, the laser photon flux decreases by

$$\frac{dI(z)}{dz} = -[\text{Rb}]P_+(\Delta,z)\frac{\Gamma_{SD}}{P_+(\Delta,z)+\Gamma_{SD}} \tag{14.28}$$

Note that the fraction at the right in this equation is the equilibrium occupation probability of the sublevel $m_s = -1/2$ of Rb ground state, since only that sublevel absorbs left-circularly polarized photons. It is clear from this equation that photon flux attenuation along propagation decreases with increasing light detuning. Therefore, we need to balance two things for optimal results of pumping. On the one hand, for increasing the polarization yield, we want to use high Rb density and have high optical pumping rate $P_+(\Delta, z)$. On the other hand, we want to have penetrating laser light to pump more volume fraction of Rb vapor in the cell. To find out if a narrow or broadband laser source is better, we must use the above equations to calculate optical pumping yield averaged for the whole cell. Of course, in the calculations the optical pumping rate should be summed over the line shape of a broadband laser source. That is, if the photon flux at a frequency ν and position z is $\Phi(\nu, z)$, then the spectrum-summed optical pumping rate $P_+(z)$ at z is

$$P_+(z) = \int \Phi(\nu,z)P_+(\Delta,z)dz \tag{14.29}$$

With an 8 W Ti:Sapphire laser (with a linewidth of approximately 0.1 nm) the light penetration is approximately 6 cm for He gas of 5 amagat and the average Rb polarization is approximately 95%. For a 15 W laser diode array of 1.9 nm FWHM linewidth, the Rb polarization decreases from approximately 100% at $z = 0$ to approximately 25% at $z = 15$ cm.[9] These results show that, because the Rb D1 linewidth is very much broadened by the high-density He gas (45–75 GHz), the achieved Rb electron spin polarization averaged over the whole volume is about the same for the two laser sources. However, compared to the Ti:Sapphire laser, the laser diode array costs much less. A Ti:Sapphire laser pumped by an argon ion laser costs approximately \$20 K per watt; a laser diode array laser costs approximately \$200 per Watt.

The laser diode is a semiconductor device with the p–n junctions. The band structures of the semiconductor substrates largely determine the wavelength that a laser diode emits. Semiconductors have energy band structures consisting of the valence band and conducting band. GaAs, a III–V compound semiconductor, has a direct energy band structure such that the top of the valence band is directly below the bottom of the conducting band in the reciprocal space. Therefore, when an electron from the conducting band is recombined with a hole in the valence band, the energy released can be almost completely converted into that of the photon without energy loss to the crystal lattice. Doped with aluminum, gallium–aluminum arsenide [(GaAl)As] has an energy band structure such that a recombination of an electron–hole pair inside the p–n junction of (GaAl)As diode emits from 750 to 880 nm.

To cause an amplification of the light by the stimulated emission, the (GaAl)As is "pumped" up to the population inversion state by injecting sufficient minority carriers (electrons) into the p–n junction. The laser outputs are at wavelengths that satisfy two conditions. First, the wavelength must be within the bandwidth of the laser gain medium ([GaAl]As). Second, the wavelength must be in the passband of the laser resonator. The emitted light in laser diode is guided in the active zone (Figure 14.9). The common

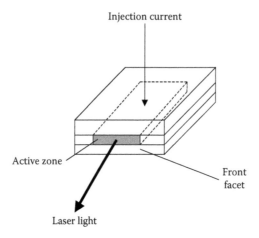

FIGURE 14.9   Schematic of the laser diode.

guiding provides a horizontal resonator structure. The guiding is realized by the built-in refractive index profiles (the index guiding) or by the concentration of the stimulating electric field.

A common type of resonator structure is the Fabry–Perot resonator. Using this resonator the emitted light will be selected and amplified by reflecting back and forth from the end-facet mirrors. For wavelengths for which the resonator length is an integral multiple of half the wavelength, all these light waves are transmitted in phase. As a result of in-phase addition, these waves are amplified greatly. Once the combination of amplification gain and end-facet reflectivity is larger than the loss, the device laser out light at these wavelengths. All these matched lasing wavelengths are called the longitudinal modes of the laser diode. The wavelengths satisfy

$$\lambda = \frac{2l}{k} \tag{14.30}$$

where
    l is the laser resonator length
    k an integer

so the spacing between these mode frequencies (Figure 14.10) is

$$\delta f = \frac{c}{2nl} \tag{14.31}$$

where *n* is the refractive index of the resonator.

Obviously, the shorter the resonator, the larger the spacing of laser modes. For example, if a laser diode's cavity length is 1 mm, then the mode spacing is approximately 150 GHz. Combined with the 1–2 THz gain bandwidth, a laser diode's output spectrum consists of 150 GHz spaced peaks modulated by the gain frequency curve (Figure 14.10). It should be noted that laser diodes are formed in arrays. A typical 40 W array of 795 nm consists of 19 diodes with emitting area 200 × 1 μm equally spaced along a 1 cm long stripe.[10] The arrays can also be coupled via the optical fiber for higher output power. External cavity effects from fiber coupling may perturb the output spectrum as well.

One important feature of LDAs is that the emitted wavelengths strongly depend on the operating temperature and injection current. Therefore, setting up the operating point in terms of the temperature and injection current is important. The temperature tuning is approximately 0.2–0.4 nm/K, and

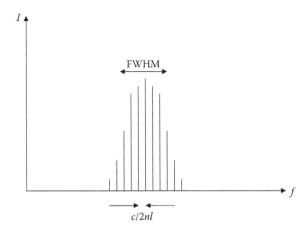

FIGURE 14.10 Schematic of the multiple longitudinal modes of a laser diode array. The laser cavity length is l, and its refractive index is n. The mode spacing is $c/2nl$.

the current tuning coefficients obviously depend on the total number of diodes in LADs. For example, it was found that the current tuning is 0.18–0.42 nm/A for LDAs of 15 W power.[11] The total output power is approximately linear with the current; however, the wavelength tuning and the power saturate at large current.

As Equation 14.27 shows, the large spectral width of LADs (2–4 nm) limits the laser power absorbed by Rb vapor. Although one may increase the absorption by adding high-pressure buffer gas to increase the Rb *D*1 line broadening, mechanical constraints from cell strength and collision-induced polarization destruction limit the maximal buffer gas pressure to approximately 10 atm. At this pressure, the *D*1 line may be broadened to 0.4 nm only. Currently, some research efforts are directed to narrowing the LDA linewidth for increasing light absorption by Rb vapor. An approach that reduced the LDA linewidth by a factor of 2 with only 6% power loss by using the etalon reflection has been reported recently.[10]

14.4 MRI of Hyperpolarized ³He and ¹²⁹Xe

In the last section we discussed how to hyperpolarize ³He and ¹²⁹Xe nuclear spins. Because these nuclei have nuclear spin $I = 1/2$—the same as a proton—the basic approaches of proton MRI can still be applied to these nuclear spins. However, there are many differences in imaging techniques as well. In this section we discuss special features of MRI with these hyperpolarized spins.

14.4.1 Signal Intensities

As mentioned in Section 14.2, in MRI the signal S from the precessing transverse magnetization M_+ is proportional to

$$S = \gamma B_0 M_+ f(T_2, TE) \tag{14.32}$$

where
    γ is the gyromagnetic ratio of the nuclei
    B_0 is the field strength of the scanner magnet
    M_+ is the transverse magnetization
    $f(T_2, TE)$ is a factor depending on scan parameters such as TE and tissue relaxation times T_2

Compared to the proton, ^{3}He and ^{129}Xe have smaller gyromagnetic ratios. While the proton's Larmor frequency is 63.9 MHz at 1.5 T, ^{3}He's Larmor frequency is 48.6 MHz (76% of the proton's) at the same field strength, ^{129}Xe's Larmor frequency is only 17.8 MHz (28% of the proton's). The signal is proportional to Larmor frequency γB_0 because it is the Larmor frequency with which the transverse magnetization precesses about the B_0 direction (see Section 14.2). The different Larmor frequencies of ^{3}He and ^{129}Xe require broadband RF systems for excitation and signal reception. Many installed MRI systems are already equipped with broadband capabilities for P-31, Na-23, and C-13 MRI, and they can be used for ^{3}He and ^{129}Xe as well. The RF coils should be tunable to the appropriate Larmor frequencies. Usually these are manually tuned surface coils[12] or Helmholtz coils.[13]

To compare signal intensities, we rewrite the longitudinal magnetization M_z before spin flipping by an RF pulse:

$$M_z = N\gamma\hbar\langle I_z\rangle \tag{14.33}$$

where
    N is the nuclear spin density
    $\langle I_z\rangle$ is the average nuclear spin along the B_0-axis before flipping

Because M_+ is determined by the flip angle α (defined in Section 14.2) and M_z:

$$M_+ = M_z\sin\alpha = N\gamma\hbar\langle I_z\rangle\sin\alpha \tag{14.34}$$

Using these equations, we find that the signal intensity S is

$$S = \gamma^2 B_0 N\hbar\langle I_z\rangle\sin\alpha f(T_2, TE) \tag{14.35}$$

We can then compare the signal intensities from MRI of protons and hyperpolarized spins to determine their signal intensity ratio, assuming the same magnetic field, the same flip angle, and the same f-factor:

$$\frac{S_{\text{He}}}{S_{\text{H}}} = \frac{\gamma^2_{\text{He}}N_{\text{He}}\langle I_z\rangle_{\text{He}}}{\gamma^2_{\text{H}}N_{\text{H}}\langle I_z\rangle_{\text{H}}} \tag{14.36}$$

For thermally polarized spins such as protons, the value of average nuclear spin $\langle I_z\rangle$ depends on the particular pulse sequence used in the scan, but it never exceeds the thermal equilibrium value $\langle I_z\rangle_{eq}$:

$$\langle I_z\rangle_{eq} = \frac{1}{4}\frac{\hbar\omega_L}{k_B T} \tag{14.37}$$

Using Equation 14.33, we obtain the equilibrium magnetization M_0

$$M_0 = \frac{N\gamma^2\hbar^2 B_0}{4k_B T} \tag{14.38}$$

where
    $k_B = 1.38 \times 10^{-23}$
    J/K is Boltzmann's constant
    T is the absolute temperature
    ω_L is the Larmor frequency of the nuclear spin

At T = 310 K and 1.5 T field strength, the proton's maximal $\langle I_z \rangle_{\mathrm{H}} = \langle I_z \rangle_{eq} = 2.47 \times 10^{-6}$. Although the proton's spin polarization $\langle I_z \rangle_{eq}$ is tiny, proton spin density N_{H} is high in tissue water, $N_{\mathrm{H}} = 6.69 \times 10^{22}$ cm^{-3}. On the other hand, for hyperpolarized ^{3}He, the polarization from the optical pumping and spin exchange can be as high as 50% or more. At 50% polarization, $\langle I_z \rangle_{\mathrm{He}} = 1/4$. Hence the optically pumped helium's spin polarization $\langle I_z \rangle_{\mathrm{He}}$ is 1.01×10^5 times higher than the proton spin polarization $\langle I_z \rangle_{\mathrm{H}}$. However, the spin density of ^{3}He in the human body is much lower than the spin density of proton in human tissue water.

Suppose ^{3}He is administered by inhalation in MRI, and at 1 bar pressure with dilution of 1/8 and body temperature (T = 310 K), the ^{3}He spin density is 2.92×10^{18}/cm^3, assuming an ideal gas state equation. Using the signal ratio formula of Equation 14.36, we find the signal intensity ratio $S_{\mathrm{He}}/S_{\mathrm{H}} = 2.56$. It should also be noted that this calculation of $S_{\mathrm{He}}/S_{\mathrm{H}}$ assumes use of the same flip angle for both ^{3}He and proton. We will see that the flip angle for ^{3}He is usually smaller than that used for proton MRI. Use of a smaller flip angle tends to reduce the ^{3}He signal. In any case, the small spin density of ^{3}He is more than compensated for by its hyperpolarization to generate higher MRI signal intensity than that in proton MRI.

It should be noted that, in some organs such as the lung, proton MRI lung imaging encounters many difficulties. First of all, proton density is low in the lungs. Second, the differences of proton bulk magnetic susceptibilities between pulmonary tissue and air generate changes of local Larmor frequencies. This causes shot T_2^* relaxation times and gross reduction of proton MRI signals by a factor $\exp(-TE / T_2^*)$, as pointed out in Section 14.2. Therefore, for lung imaging, the signal intensity turns more favorably to ^{3}He MRI. It should also be noted that, in the above comparison, we have assumed proton spin polarization is the thermal equilibrium value. This is the maximum the spin polarization can reach for protons. However, in many cases, especially with short pulse sequence repeating time TR, the spin polarization is much lower than $\langle I_z \rangle_{eq} = 2.47 \times 10^{-6}$ because, if TR is short compared to the longitudinal relaxation time T_1, the spin polarization does not have enough time to be restored to the equilibrium value $\langle I_z \rangle_{eq}$. As for ^{129}Xe, the signal intensity ratio $S_{\mathrm{Xe}}/S_{\mathrm{H}}$ is reduced to 13.4% of $S_{\mathrm{Xe}}/S_{\mathrm{H}}$ if all other conditions are the same because of the small gyromagnetic ratio of ^{129}Xe.

14.4.2 General Considerations for ^{3}He and ^{129}Xe as MRI Contrast Media

The above calculations are based on the inhalation administration of the noble gases. Note that helium is an inert and nontoxic gas. It is widely used in other cases such as in deep-sea diving, where helium is inhaled in quite a high amount and concentration (80% helium and 20% oxygen) without severe adverse effects.[14] As shown in Table 14.1, ^{3}He has a tiny natural abundance (0.014%) produced from tritium radioactive decays and generated mainly in production of nuclear weapon material. Unpolarized ^{3}He costs approximately \$100/L and recovery after exhalation is necessary. Currently ^{3}He can be polarized as high as 50% or more.

^{129}Xe has a natural abundance (26.4%). It is an inert and nontoxic gas used as an inhalation anesthetic (70% xenon and 30% oxygen). Xenon has a long history of use in medical imaging. As an inhalative contrast media, radioactive xenon isotope (^{133}Xe and ^{135}Xe) imaging has been used for the γ-ray scintigraphy in nuclear medicine, and nonradioactive xenon (^{131}Xe) for CT brain perfusion studies using its high attenuation to x-ray.

One advantage of using xenon is its relatively high solubility in water and lipid; compared to helium, it is more than 10 times more soluble in water and 100 times more soluble in fatty tissue. This also makes xenon more suitable for preparation of ^{129}Xe carriers for injection. Moreover, among all NMR-sensitive nuclei, ^{129}Xe presents the largest chemical shift range; its chemical hift in tissue can be

TABLE 14.1 Physical Parameters for ^{1}H, ^{3}He, and ^{129}Xe

Isotope	^{1}H	^{3}He	^{129}Xe
Natural abundance (%)	99.9	0.014	26.4
Nuclear spin	1/2	1/2	1/2
Larmor frequency at 1.5 T (MHz)	63.9	48.6	17.8

as high as a few hundred parts per million, making ^{129}Xe very sensitive to its chemical environment. Additionally, the chemical shift disperses from gas to blood and tissue, allowing selective imaging of xenon in blood, brain, and gas.[15] Xenon with natural abundance costs approximately a few dollars per liter. Compared to ^{3}He, ^{129}Xe can only be polarized to approximately 20% because the rate of Rb electron spin depolarization in the spin–rotation collisions with ^{129}Xe is higher. (The spin–rotation interaction is the coupling between electron spin and the rotational angular momentum of an Rb^{129}Xe pair.[16]) However, spin polarization up to 60% has been theoretically predicted, and the spin–exchange efficiency can be improved to increase polarization.[17] Compounded with its low gyromagnetic ratio, the signal intensity from ^{129}Xe will be much lower than that from hyperpolarized ^{3}He.

14.4.3 Signal-to-Noise Ratio and Magnetic Field Strength

SNR is a key imaging performance measure. In MRI it is very important to find out the SNR's dependence on magnetic field strength. Looking at just the B_0-dependence of signal intensity, Equation 14.35 states that

$$S \propto B_0 \langle I_z \rangle \tag{14.39}$$

For thermally polarized spins like protons, its nuclear spin along the B_0-axis is, at most, $\langle I_z \rangle_{eq}$. Using Equation 14.37, we find that

$$S_{\mathrm{H}} \propto B_0^2 \tag{14.40}$$

since the equilibrium polarization is proportional to the field strength B_0 as well. But for hyperpolarized helium and xenon, their nuclear spin $\langle I_z \rangle$ is achieved by optical pumping and spin exchange and is independent of field strength B_0; hence, the signal from hyperpolarized ^{3}He or ^{129}Xe is

$$S_{\mathrm{He/Xe}} \propto B_0 \tag{14.41}$$

It differs from the quadratic dependence of the proton signal intensity on B_0. On the other hand, the Johnson noise voltage V_{noise} in the RF receiver coil is equal to[3]

$$V_{\mathrm{noise}} = \sqrt{4k_B T \Delta f (R_c + R_b)} \tag{14.42}$$

where
   Δf is the signal frequency bandwidth
   R_c is the coil resistance
   R_b is the effective resistance caused by RF dissipation by the body parts
   Δf is the frequency bandwidth of the MRI signals

Roughly speaking, all spins would generate signals in Larmor frequency. However, during the data acquisition period, spins at different locations actually experience slightly different Larmor frequencies due to the applied magnetic field gradient for position encoding. Therefore, the frequency bandwidth Δf is given by

$$\Delta f = \frac{\gamma}{2\pi} G_x d_{\mathrm{FOV}} \tag{14.43}$$

where

G_x is the magnetic field gradient in the x direction

d_{FOV} is the dimension of image field of view

Hence, Δf is independent of the field strength B_0.

However, the resistances R_c and R_b are field strength B_0 dependent. R_c increases with Larmor frequency, due to the skin-depth effect, because the high-frequency current tends to stay in the skin layer of the coil's wire. This skin-depth effect effectively makes the coil's resistance increase. It turns out that R_c is proportional to $B_0^{1/2}$. The RF dissipation-caused resistance R_b increases with B_0 as B_0^2. For $B_0 > 0.2$ T, R_b dominates over R_c. Therefore, for $B_0 > 0.2$ T, the noise varies with B_0 according to

$$V_{noise} \propto \sqrt{R_b} \propto B_0 \tag{14.44}$$

Using Equations 14.40 through 14.43, we find that the SNRs for proton and hyperpolarized He/Xe are

$$\text{SNR}_H \propto \frac{B_0^2}{\sqrt{B_0^2}} \propto B_0, \quad \text{SNR}_{He/Xe} \propto \frac{B_0}{\sqrt{B_0^2}} \propto 1 \tag{14.45}$$

This result shows that, although the SNR of conventional MRI is proportional to B_0, the SNR of MRI with hyperpolarized spins is independent of B_0. As we mentioned at the beginning of this chapter, the ever-increasing demand on high SNR drives the magnetic field strengths employed in conventional MRI higher. The higher the field strength, however, the more expensive and bulky the MRI scanner. The high field strength aggravates problems such as magnetic susceptibility artifacts and spin–lattice relaxation time lengthening. Fortunately, the SNR for hyperpolarized spins is independent of B_0. A study of MRI using hyperpolarized ^{3}He at 0.1 T has been reported in the literature.[18] Moreover, MRI images were obtained using MRI using hyperpolarized ^{3}He at 21 G.[19] These efforts open doors for many potential applications such as portable MRI scanners for lung imaging.

Another advantage of low field imaging is the reduction of magnetic susceptibility artifacts. Consequently, the apparent spin–spin relaxation time T_2^* can be greatly extended from a few to hundreds of milliseconds.

14.4.4 Pulse Sequence Considerations

Hyperpolarization is a spin state that is far away from the thermal equilibrium state, which has an important consequence for flip angle selection. Suppose one flips spin by 90° for maximal signal, since sin 90° = 1. We also suppose the transverse magnetization becomes dephased after forming echo. After the flip, the longitudinal magnetization $M_z = 0$ and spins experience spin–lattice relaxation, regardless of whether the spins are thermally polarized, such as water protons, or hyperpolarized spins generated by optical pumping. As shown in Equation 14.8, the longitudinal magnetization M_z evolves as a function of time t

$$M_z(t) = M_{eq} + (M_z(t=0) - M_{eq})\exp\left(\frac{-t}{T_1}\right) \tag{14.46}$$

where

T_1 is the so-called spin–lattice relaxation time, as mentioned in Section 14.2

M_{eq} is the thermal equilibrium magnetization

More specifically, after a 90° flip, $M_z(t = 0) = 0$, $M_z(t)$ recovers according to

$$M_z(t) = M_{eq}(1 - e^{-t/T_1})$$

(14.47)

Therefore, for proton, M_z can be restored to its equilibrium M_{eq} after a long enough time (approximately 95% of M_{eq} at $3T_1$). This is true for hyperpolarized ^{3}He and ^{129}Xe as well. The difference is clear here: for proton, M_{eq} is the maximum of M_z; hence the spin–lattice relaxation restores M_z. However, for hyperpolarized ^{3}He and ^{129}Xe, the equilibrium magnetization M_{eq} for ^{3}He and ^{129}Xe are approximately 10^5 times smaller than their initial M_z before the flipping. Therefore, the RF pulses really destroy hyperpolarization irreversibly, and spin–lattice relaxation cannot restore it. With thermal equilibrium magnetizations, we cannot get strong enough signals because of the low concentration of noble gas spins. Due to this difference, we should avoid applying the conventional "pre-scan" calibration procedures to hyperpolarized ^{3}He and ^{129}Xe for preventing destroying hyperpolarization before the scan.

If we apply RF excitations of flip angle α to hyperpolarized ^{3}He or ^{129}Xe by n times, and if all transverse magnetization after each RF excitation gets completely dephased, then the remaining longitudinal magnetization is

$$M_z(n) = M_z(0)\cos^n \alpha$$

(14.48)

Here we also assume that T_1 relaxation times for ^{3}He and ^{129}Xe are long compared to the scan duration. The signal-generating transverse magnetization M_+ is

$$M_+(n) = M_z(0)\cos^{n-1} \alpha \sin \alpha$$

(14.49)

Hence, the signal intensity gets weaker by a factor of $\cos \alpha$ for each RF pulse. Because RF excitations are applied one by one for acquiring scan data in phase-encoding direction or, equivalently, for sampling the data in the k space line by line, then the later sampled lines get reduced signal due to the "consumption" of the initial hyperpolarization. Consequently, this results in nonuniform weighting of k-space scan data.

Depending on the k-space sampling order, this nonuniform weighting can cause some loss of image resolutions. As for selection of α, Equation 14.49 suggests that we must balance two needs: we want a larger flip angle for a larger signal and we must ensure that enough M_z is left for phase-encoding steps with large n. Image quality is determined largely by the data from the center of the k space; therefore, we may want to ensure optimal signal intensity there. If sequential phase encoding is adopted, and n_c is the phase-encoding step corresponding to the k-space center, then transverse magnetization M_+ at this phase-encoding step is

$$M_+(n_c) = M_z(0)\cos^{n_c-1} \alpha \sin \alpha$$

(14.50)

From the stationary point of $M_+(n_c)$ with respect to flip angle α, we find the optimal α_0 that maximizes the signal:

$$\alpha_0 = a\tan\left(\frac{1}{\sqrt{n_c - 1}}\right)$$

(14.51)

For example, if $n_c = 64$, the optical flip angle $\alpha_0 = 7.2°$. It is interesting to note that, with this flip angle, after the 127th RF pulse the remaining longitudinal magnetization is approximately 37% of the starting M_+.

To try to get constant signal as the RF excitation progresses, we must increase the flip angle to compensate the loss of hyperpolarization from previous excitation.[20] Note that if the flip angle varies as the RF-excitation progresses, then after n pulses M_z becomes

$$M_z(n) = M_z(0)\cos\alpha_1 \cos\alpha_2 \ldots \cos\alpha_{n-1}\cos\alpha_n \tag{14.52}$$

and the signal $M_+(n)$ after the nth RF pulse is

$$M_+(n) = M_z(0)\cos\alpha_1 \cos\alpha_2 \ldots \cos\alpha_{n-1}\sin\alpha_n$$

The signal $M_+(n + 1)$ after the $(n + 1)$th RF pulse is

$$M_+(n+1) = M_z(0)\cos\alpha_1 \cos\alpha_2 \ldots \cos\alpha_{n-1}\cos\alpha_n \sin\alpha_{n+1} \tag{14.53}$$

Comparing these two equations, we get the condition for a constant signal; on the other hand, in order to get a constant signal for all phase-encoding steps, we should require that

$$\tan\alpha_n = \sin\alpha_{n+1} \tag{14.54}$$

Let us suppose that we apply a 90° flip angle at the last phase-encoding step N. In this way we maximize the signal from what is left in M_z and we need not save M_z for later steps any more. From the above equation the flip angle for the $(N - 1)$th pulse should be

$$\tan\alpha_{N-1} = \sin\alpha_N = 1 \tag{14.55}$$

so the flip angle for the $(N - 1)$th pulse should be 45°. Using Equation 14.54 we find the flip angle for the nth pulse is

$$\alpha_n = a\tan\left(\frac{1}{\sqrt{N-n}}\right) \tag{14.56}$$

So if $N = 128$, we start the sequence with a flip angle of 5.1° for the 1st pulse, and end the sequence with the 128th pulse of 90°. The variable flip angle approach can provide uniform k-space sampling and more efficient use of hyperpolarization.

Most studies performed with hyperpolarized spins, however, use a constant flip angle approach because it is difficult to implement the variable flip angles accurately, and the approach's performance is sensitive to variable flip angle errors from RF-B_1 field inhomogeneity and RF transmitter calibration errors. The variable flip angle technique can also be used in NMR spectroscopy. For example, to measure hyperpolarized xenon's T_1 relaxation times in blood, one usually applies multiple excitations to measure the relaxation-induced signal decay. With variable flip angle technique, the signal decay is truly contributed by the T_1 relaxation with the RF-induced loss of magnetization being compensated.[21] So if a variable flip angle sequence with eight pulses is used, then, according to Equation 14.56, we should start with a flip angle of 21° and end with a flip angle of 90°.

The self-diffusion coefficient of He gas is high: $D_{He} = 1.8$ cm²/s at 1 atm and 20°C; self-diffusion coefficients of Xe gas are much lower: $D_{Xe} = 0.06$ cm²/s at 1 atm and 20°C.[22] In the data acquisition period, the frequency-encoding gradient is applied. In a magnetic field gradient diffusion creates additional random and position-dependent phases to the transverse magnetizations of spins, since diffusion is a random translation. The coherence between transverse magnetizations of spins at different locations has been partially destroyed by the random phases. When these transverse magnetizations are summed over all the spins at different locations, the total dephasing effect of these random phases is to attenuate the total transverse magnetization by a factor:

$$\exp\left(-\frac{\gamma^2 G^2 D T_g^3}{12}\right) \tag{14.57}$$

where

G is the field gradient strength of a bipolar rectangular gradient waveform
T_g is the time period of the transverse magnetization under field gradient

For a gradient echo sequence, G is the frequency-encoding gradient and $T_g = T_s$, the data sampling time. Because higher resolution corresponds to higher G, Equation 14.57 means that the diffusion-associated signal attenuation mainly affects the imaging of fine details. In fact, this equation can be equivalently written as

$$\exp\left(-\frac{\pi^2 D T_s}{3d^2}\right) \tag{14.58}$$

where d is the size of detail (one line pair) resolved. Consequently, the signal reduction is resolution-dependent.

The signal decreases rapidly with decreasing d. For example, for He gas and with $T_s = 6$ ms, 97% of the signal will be attenuated for $d = 1$ mm, but only 80% of the signal will be attenuated for $d = 1.5$ mm, and 33% of the signal will be attenuated for $d = 3$ mm. Reducing sampling time improves resolution rapidly as well. In the previous example, if T_s is reduced to 4 ms, 90.7% of the signal will be attenuated for $d = 1$ mm, but only 65% of the signal will be attenuated for $d = 1.5$ mm, and 23% of the signal attenuated will be for $d = 3$ mm. Xe's self-diffusion coefficient is much smaller; hence the diffusion-associated signal intensity reductions are mild. For Xe gas and with $T_s = 6$ ms, 11% of the signal will be attenuated for $d = 1$ mm, but only 5% of the signal will be attenuated for $d = 1.5$ mm, and 1.2% of the signal will be attenuated for $d = 3$ mm. These results show the diffusion-associated signal attenuation as function of feature size. As for the minimal resolvable size, it depends on the feature's contrast as well. It should also be noted that the slower Xe diffusion allows one to use larger sampling time T_s. This means a smaller frequency bandwidth Δf of the signals, and hence less noise (Equation 14.42). This helps improve the SNR for Xe imaging.

This analysis is based on pure He or Xe. Diluting He with heavier gases such as N_2 reduces helium's diffusion coefficient, thus reducing diffusion-associated signal attenuation. Furthermore, helium's apparent diffusion coefficient in lung parenchyma is further reduced due to the restricted diffusion imposed by the bronchial and alveolar walls. Some studies have reported that the apparent diffusion coefficient (ADC) of helium diluted with N_2 in lung parenchyma is reduced by an order of magnitude compared to self-diffusion coefficient.

On the flip side of the diffusion problem, one may very well use diffusion to help examine the lungs by performing diffusion-weighted MRI.[23] Using ^{3}He-MRI it was determined that He gas diffusion in the lungs is anisotropic, because the diffusion restrictions are much less along the airway axis than perpendicular to it.[24] This technique is useful for emphysema studies. In emphysema the restrictions to diffusion are reduced because of expansion of the alveoli and airway and tissue destruction. It was found that the ADCs of lungs of patients with severe emphysema are increased by a factor of 2.7 compared to the normal lung, and all the transverse and longitudinal ADCs are elevated.[24]

14.4.5 Hyperpolarized Spin Relaxation

As noted earlier, the spin–lattice relaxation (T_1 relaxation) and spin–spin relaxation (T_2 relaxation) are the basis of tissue contrast in conventional MRI. This is true for hyperpolarized spins as well; however, spin–lattice relaxation becomes more important for hyperpolarized spins. This is because in proton MRI spin–lattice relaxation restores magnetization, but in ^{3}He or ^{129}Xe MRI spin–lattice relaxation destroys the magnetization of hyperpolarized spins. If the hyperpolarization is generated at $t = 0$, using Equation 14.8 for spin–lattice relaxation and the condition $M_z \gg M_{eq}$, the magnetization of hyperpolarized spins relaxes as

$$M_z(t) \approx M_z(t=0)\exp\left(\frac{-t}{T_1}\right) \tag{14.59}$$

After $5T_1$ hyperpolarization is reduced to 0.6% of the initial hyperpolarization, and MRI signals from that much relaxed polarization will be diminished. Obviously, an MRI scan should be completed before the polarization consumed by relaxation. Relaxation time T_1 varies with the state and environment of hyperpolarized spins. Tables 14.2 and 14.3 show relaxation time T_1 for ^{3}He and ^{129}Xe in different conditions, respectively. Pure ^{3}He and ^{129}Xe would have long T_1 if there were no interaction with other impurities because the electrons of noble gases are in the filled orbitals. These electrons produce neither an electric field gradient nor a magnetic field at their nucleus. Also, noble gases are monoatomic, thus there is no intramolecular dipole–dipole coupling. That is why ^{3}He has a T_1 of several days in a clean glass container as listed in Table 14.2. The listed T_1 in glass container is obtained with a holding magnetic field of 10–20 G to fend off the stray magnetic field gradients. The holding field can be provided by a permanent magnet or battery-powered coils. For ^{129}Xe the distribution task is far more labored because ^{129}Xe should be stored at low temperatures, as shown in Table 14.3. In fact, ^{129}Xe's relaxation time T_1 increases with higher B/T for a holding field up to 1 kG.

The dominated relaxation mechanism for ^{3}He and ^{129}Xe in the human body is the relaxation by paramagnetic molecules and ions. Of clinical significance is the relaxation induced by paramagnetic molecular oxygen and by paramagnetic deoxyhemoglobin. Molecular oxygen has an atomic electronic

TABLE 14.2   Spin–Lattice Relaxation Times for ^{3}He

^{3}He Condition	T_1
Clean uncoated glass container	Several days
In a polyethylene bag	4900 s
In the lungs	28 s

TABLE 14.3   Spin–Lattice Relaxation Times for ^{129}Xe

^{129}Xe Conditions	T_1	Reference
Stored at liquid N_2 temperature	8500 s	[37]
Stored at liquid He temperature	500 h	[37]
In a polyethylene bag	120–350 s	
In the lungs	31 s	
Artery blood, at 1.5 T, 37°C	6.4 s	[21]
Venous blood, at 1.5 T, 37°C	4 s	[21]
Saline: $\lambda_{solv} = 0.079$ at 37°C	66 s	[28]
Perfluorocarbon emulsion: $\lambda_{solv} = 0.6$ at 37°C	100 s	[28]

spin $S = 1$. The intermolecular dipole–dipole coupling between the oxygen electronic spin and noble gas nuclear spins dominates the relaxation. T_1 of ^{3}He in the presence of oxygen has been measured[25]:

$$\frac{1}{T_1} = 0.45[O_2]\left(\frac{299}{T}\right)^{0.42} \text{ s}^{-1}/\text{amagat} \tag{14.60}$$

where
    T is the temperature in Kelvin
    $[O_2]$ is the oxygen concentration

This equation provides the quantitative basis for measuring $[O_2]$ using ^{3}He MRI. For human subject imaging, at the airway T is approximately 37.5°C, so

$$\frac{1}{T_1} = \frac{1}{2.27}[O_2] \text{ s}^{-1}/\text{amagat} \tag{14.61}$$

Another important aspect of noble gases MRI is the relaxation of noble gas hyperpolarization during vascular transport. The vascular transport is necessary for noble gases reaching other tissue such as brain tissues. Xe has much higher solubility in blood than He, so ^{129}Xe is more suitable than ^{3}He for brain imaging. Table 14.3 shows the spin–lattice relaxation times of ^{129}Xe in blood reported in Wolber et al.[21] At a temperature of 37°C and a field strength of 1.5 T, $T_1 = 6.4$ s for arterial blood and $T_1 = 4$ for venous blood. This is because deoxyhemoglobin in blood is paramagnetic, while oxyhemoglobin is diamagnetic. The increased relaxation of ^{129}Xe for deoxygenated blood may originate from Xe interaction with paramagnetic Fe ions in the heme group of deoxygenated hemoglobin.[21] In fact, there are four iron atoms in each hemoglobin molecule, which can bind four oxygen atoms. However, this difference of relaxation times in oxygenated and deoxygenated blood could be used for functional MRI as well. The deoxygenated hemoglobin exposes their paramagnetic iron ions to Xe causing Xe spin relaxation. Therefore Xe's spin–lattice relaxation time T_1 increases with the blood oxygenation saturation sO_2 as measured by Wolber et al.[26] Note that the physiological oxygenation range from s$O_2 = 0.6$ for the venous blood to s$O_2 = 0.98$ for the arterial blood. These measurements of T_1 as a function of sO_2 also provide a quantitative basis for measuring blood and tissue oxygenation by using ^{129}Xe MRI.

    To see the great potential of this capability of ^{129}Xe MRI, consider the functional proton MRI of the human brain, which has undergone explosive development in recent years. This functional proton MRI technique is based on the blood oxygenation level dependent (BOLD) effect. This BOLD effect is sensitive to changes in oxygenation and blood flow in response to neural stimulation. However, BOLD effect does not provide a direct measurement of blood oxygenation because blood flow changes are blended in as well. So ^{129}Xe MRI might be able to elucidate the relative contributions of perfusion and oxygenation to the BOLD effect. Finally, it should be noted that relative shift of intra- and extracellular 29Xe spectral peak is also sensitive to the blood oxygenation level.[27]

    From this discussion it is also clear that delivery of hyperpolarized ^{129}Xe from inhalation to other organs such as the brain is critically limited by loss of polarization during vascular transport. This calls for development of intravenous injection of hyperpolarized spins in biocompatible media. These media should allow much longer T_1 for ^{129}Xe and high solubility. As listed in Table 14.3, T_1 for ^{129}Xe has been increased to 66 s in saline and 100 s in perfluorocarbon emulsion.[28] However, perfluorocarbon emulsion has much higher Ostwald solubility λ_{solv} than saline does, as shown in Table 14.3. (The Ostwald solubility is defined as the volume of gas dissolved per unit volume of solvent at equilibrium.) The search of biocompatible media for ^{129}Xe and ^{3}He is just beginning.[29]

    For ^{129}Xe dissolved in liquid, dipole–dipole coupling between xenon nuclear spins and dipole–dipole coupling between xenon nuclear spins and solution nuclear spins (e.g., protons) play an important role in determining xenon's T_1. Among these spins the spin polarization transfer from hyperpolarized xenon to solution nuclear spin is observed and called SPINOE, the spin–polarization-induced nuclear Overhauser effect.[30] The mechanism underlining the polarization transfer is the nuclear Overhauser effect generated by the cross-relaxation between Xe and solution nuclear spins. Therefore, through SPINOE, hyperpolarized Xe can "light up" solution nuclear spins by enhancing their polarization. In addition, differential SPINOE enhancements in solution should provide information of selective binding of xenon to biomolecules in solution.[31]

So far, all the spin–lattice relaxation is based on the assumption that hyperpolarized Xe relaxes in the same way as the thermally polarized Xe. In fact, some data of Xe T_1 in blood are measured by using thermally polarized Xe. We note that this assumption is not completely true.[32] First, the conventional relaxation laws are derived from the assumption of weak polarization near the thermal equilibrium. Second, we find that hyperpolarization and spin dipole–dipole coupling result in multipole spin orders for hyperpolarized spins. In another words, a hyperpolarized spin state may include not only the magnetization (the dipole spin order $\langle I_z \rangle$), but also other multipole order, such as the quadrupole spin order. These multipole spin orders cross-relax each other. The longitudinal magnetization relaxation of hyperpolarized spins is, in general, bi-exponential decay, although the ordinary T_1 component dominates in many but not all cases. These findings have potential applications in quantifying the paramagnetic source in lung and other tissue and in modeling hyperpolarized xenon spin auto-relaxation and cross relaxation in biocompatible media.[33]

14.4.6 MRI of Hyperpolarized ^{3}He and ^{129}Xe for Human Subjects

Hyperpolarized spin MRI has already been applied to human subjects in recent years. Here we discuss several examples in accordance with the scope of this chapter. Hyperpolarized ^{3}He has been used to image human pulmonary morphology. This is done usually in a period of one breath after inhalation of ^{3}He gas. The pulse sequences are usually the low-flip angle-spoiled gradient echo sequences. The spatial resolution of ^{3}He MRI depends on the sampling time, T_s, used because, as shown by Equation 14.58, T_s controls the adverse effect of the He diffusive movement in air space on the resolution. In any case, the image resolution is definitely better than that of ventilation scintigraphy.[34,35] Figure 14.11 shows ^{3}He-MRI images of the lungs from a healthy volunteer and a smoker. The lung image of the smoker presented patchy and wedge-shaped signal defects due to reduced or absent entry of ^{3}He.

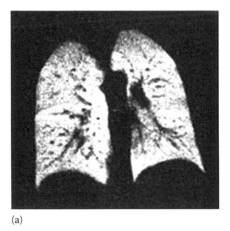
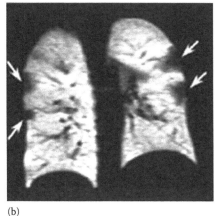

(a) (b)

FIGURE 14.11 (a) A ^{3}He MRI image of the lungs of a healthy volunteer. (b) A ^{3}He MRI image of the lungs of a smoker. (Images courtesy of Drs. W. Schreiber and R. Surkau, University of Mainz, Mainz, Germany.)

In addition to morphological study, ^{3}He gas can be used to measure the regional alveolar partial pressure of oxygen (pO$_2$). It is well known that, in the air space of the lungs, the partial pressure of oxygen varies regionally and temporally. These variations reflect the differences in ventilation-dependent oxygen delivery and perfusion-dependent oxygen uptake. Currently, there is no noninvasive means to measure pO$_2$ within occluded pulmonary segments, and the intrapulmonary pO$_2$ beyond the bronchi could not be measured even by invasive methods. However, as we pointed out earlier, the T_1 relaxation rate of He gas is proportional to the oxygen concentration [O$_2$], as shown in Equation 14.61, because molecular oxygen is paramagnetic ($S = 1$).

Therefore, using ^{3}He MRI one can derive the local alveolar pO$_2$ from the ^{3}He signal decay curve generated from a series of images acquired at a series of times.[36] Briefly speaking, this can be done as follows. Suppose one acquires N images, each is separated by a period Δt, and one uses a constant flip angle α. Equation 14.49 gives the signal intensity with the RF depolarization effect, but without T_1 relaxation during the acquisitions. On the other hand, Equation 14.59 gives the relaxation law of the hyperpolarized magnetization of ^{3}He. Compared to signal intensity of the nth image, the signal intensity of the $(n + 1)$th image should be reduced by the relaxation and the RF depolarization effects. Therefore, combining these two effects by using Equations 14.49 and 14.59, we can find the signal ratio of the two images:

$$q = \frac{S_{n+1}}{S_n} = \cos^{N_p - 1}\alpha \exp\left(-\frac{\Delta t}{T_1}\right) = \cos^{N_p - 1}\alpha \exp\left(-\frac{pO_2 \Delta t}{2.27}\right) \tag{14.62}$$

where N_p is the total number of the phase-encoding steps per image, and the partial pressure of oxygen pO$_2$ is expressed in amagats. Once the ratio q of a local region is found, then pO$_2$ can be calculated from the above equation. For further details of the technique, see Ref. [36]. This approach provides a quick and noninvasive way to assess ventilation–perfusion matching, since the local alveolar pO$_2$ manifests the local ventilation–perfusion ratio.

Acknowledgment

We are grateful to Drs. W. Schreiber, R. Surkau, and J. Schmiedeskamp for providing ^{3}He MRI images.

References

1. Albert, M., Gates, G.D., Driehuys, B., Happer, W., Saam, B., Springer, C.S., and Wishinia, A., Biological magnetic resonance imaging using laser-polarized ^{129}Xe, *Nature*, 370, 199, 1994.
2. Smith, R.C. and Lange, R.C. (eds.), *Understanding Magnetic Resonance Imaging*, CRC Press, Boca Raton, FL, 1998.
3. Chen, C. and Hoult, D., *Biomedical Magnetic Resonance Technology*, Institute of Physics, London, U.K., 1989.
4. Surkau, R., Becker, J., Ebert, M., Grossman, T., Heil, W., Hofmann, D., Homblot, H. et al., Realization of a broad band neutron spin filter with compressed, polarized ^{3}He gas, *Nucl. Instrum. Meth. Phys. Res.*, A384, 444, 1997.
5. Happer, W., Optical pumping, *Rev. Mod. Phys.*, 44, 169, 1972.
6. Wagshul, M. and Chupp, T., Optical pumping of high density Rb with a broad-band dye-laser and GaAlAs diode-laser arrays: Applications to ^{3}He polarization, *Phys. Rev.*, A24, 4447, 1989.
7. Suter, D. and Mlynek, J., Laser excitation and detection of magnetic resonance, *Adv. Magn. Opt. Reson.*, 16, 1, 1991.
8. Cohen-Tannoudji, C., Dupont-Roc, J., and Grynberg, G., *Atom–Photon Interactions: Basic Processes and Applications*, John Wiley & Sons, New York, 1998.

9. Cummings, W., Haesser, O., Lorenzon, W., Swenson, D.R., and Larson, B., Optical pumping of Rb vapor using high-power GaAlAs diode laser arrays, *Phys. Rev.*, A51, 4842, 1995.

10. Romalis, M., Narrowing of high power diode laser arrays using reflection feedback from an etalon, *Appl. Phys. Lett.*, 77, 1080, 2000.

11. Phillips, D., Wong, G.P., Bear, D., Stoner, R.E., and Walsworth, R.L., Characterization and stabilization of fiber-coupled laser diode arrays, *Rev. Sci. Instrum.*, 70, 2905, 1999.

12. MacFall, J., Charles, H.C., Black, R.D., Middleton, H., Swartz, J.C., Saam, B., Driehuys, B. et al., Human lung air spaces: Potential for MR imaging with hyperpolarized ^{3}He, *Radiology*, 200, 553, 1996.

13. Kauzor, H., Hofmann, D., Kreitner, K.F., Niljens, H., Surkay, R., Heil, W., Potthast, A., Knopp, M.V., Oten, E.W., and Thelen, M., Normal and abnormal pulmonary ventilation: Visualization at hyperpolarized ^{3}He MR imaging, *Radiology*, 201, 564, 1996.

14. Brauer, R., Hogan, P., Hugon, M., Macdonald, A., and Miller, K., Patterns of interaction of effects of light metabolically inert gases with those of hydrostatic pressure as such: A review, *Undersea Biomed. Res.*, 9, 353, 1982.

15. Swanson, S., Rosen, M.S., Coulter, K.P., Welsh, R.C., and Chupp, T.E., Distribution and dynamics of laser-polarized ^{129}Xe magnetization *in vivo*, *Magn. Reson. Med.*, 42, 1137, 1999.

16. Walker, T. and Happer, W., Spin-exchange optical pumping of noble-gas nuclei, *Rev. Mod. Phys.*, 69, 629, 1997.

17. Driehuys, B., Cates, G.D., Miron, E., Sauer, K., Wlater, D.K., and Haper, W., High-volume production of laser polarized ^{129}Xe, *Appl. Phys. Lett.*, 69, 1668, 1996.

18. Durand, E., Guillot, G., Darrasse, L., Tastevin, G., Nacher, P.J., Vignaud, A., Vattolo, D., and Bittoun, J., CPMG measurements and ultrafast imaging in human lungs with hyperpolarized ^{3}He at low field (0.1 T), *Magn. Reson. Med.*, 47, 75, 2002.

19. Tseng, C., Wong, G.P., Pomeroy, V.R., Mair, R.W., Hinton, D.P., Hoffmann, D., Stoner, R.E., Hersman, F.W., Cory, D.G., and Walsworth, R.L., Low-field MRI of laser polarized noble gas, *Phys. Rev. Lett.*, 81, 3785, 1998.

20. Zhao, L., Mulkern, R., Tseng, C., Williamson, D., Patz, S., Kraft, R., Walsworth, R., Jolez, F., and Albert, M., Pulse sequence considerations for biomedical imaging with hyperpolarized noble gas MRI, *J. Magn. Res.*, 113, 179, 1996.

21. Wolber, J., Cherubini, A., Dzik-Jurasz, A., Leach, M.O., and Bifone, A., Spin–lattice relaxation of laser-polarized xenon in human blood, *Proc. Natl. Acad. Sci. USA*, 96, 3664, 1999.

22. Patyal, B.R., Gao, J.-H., Williams, R.F., Roby, J., Saam, R., Rockwell, B.A., Thomas, R.J., Stolarski, D.J., and Fox, P.T., Longitudinal and diffusion measurements using magnetic resonance signals from laser-hyperpolarized ^{129}Xe nuclei, *J. Magn. Res.*, 126, 58, 1997.

23. Brookeman, J., Mugler, J.R., III, Knight-Scott, J., Munger, T.M., de Lange, E.E., and Bogorad, P.L., Studies of ^{3}He diffusion coefficients in the human lung: Age-related distribution patterns, *Eur. Radiol.*, 9, B21, 1999.

24. Yablonskiy, D., Sukstanskii, A.L., Leawoods, J.C., Gierada, D.S., Bretthorst, L., Lefrak, S.S., Cooper, J.D., and Conradi, M.S., Quantitative in vivo assessment of lung microstructure at the alveolar level with hyperpolarized ^{3}He diffusion MRI, *Proc. Natl. Acad. Sci. USA*, 99, 3111, 2002.

25. Saam, B., Happer, W., and Middleton, H., Nuclear relaxation of ^{3}He in the presence of O_2, *Phys. Rev.*, A52, 862, 1995.

26. Wolber, J., Cherubini, A., Leach, M.O., and Bifone, A., On the oxygenation-dependent ^{129}Xe T_1 in blood, *NMR Biomed.*, 13, 234, 2000.

27. Wolber, J., Cherubini, A., Leach, M.O., and Bifone, A., Hyperpolarized ^{129}Xe NMR as a probe for blood oxygenation, *Magn. Res. Med.*, 43, 491, 2000.

28. Lavini, C., Payne, G.S., Leach, M.O., and Bifone, A., Intravenous delivery of hyperpolarized ^{129}Xe: A compartment model, *NMR Biomed.*, 13, 238, 2000.

29. Goodson, B., Song, Y.Q., Taylor, R.E., Schepkin, V.D., Brennan, K.M., Chingas, G.C., Budinger, T.F., Navon, G., and Pines, A., In vivo NMR and MRI using injection delivery of laser-polarized xenon, *Proc. Natl. Acad. Sci. USA*, 94, 14725, 1997.

30. Navon, G., Song, Y.Q., Room, T., Appelt, S., Taylor, R.E., and Pines, A., Enhancement of solution NMR and MRI with laser-polarized xenon, *Science*, 271, 1848, 1996.

31. Luhmer, M., Godson, B., Song, Y.Q., Laws, D., Kaiser, L., Cyrier, M., and Pines, A., Study of xenon binding in cryptophane-a using laser-induced NMR polarization enhancement, *J. Am. Chem. Soc.*, 121, 3502, 1999.

32. Wu, X., Spin relaxation for laser-pumped hyperpolarized spins, *Proc. SPIE*, 3548, 67, 1998.

33. Wu, X., Autorelaxation and cross relaxation of hyperpolarized spins, *Radiology*, 221(P), 513, 2001.

34. Kauczor, H., Ebert, M., Kreitner, K.F., Nilgens, H., Surkau, R., Heil, W., Hofmann, D., Otten, E.W., and Thelen, M., Imaging of lung using ^{3}He MRI: Preliminary clinical experience in 18 patients with and without lung disease, *J. Magn. Reson. Imag.*, 7, 538, 1997.

35. Donnelly, L., MacFall, J.R., McAdams, H.P., Majure, J.M., Smith, J., Frush, D.P., Bogonad, P., Charles, H.C., and Ravin, C.E., Cystic fibrosis: Combined hyperpolarized ^{3}He-enhanced and conventional proton MR imaging in the lung—Preliminary observations, *Radiology*, 212, 885, 1999.

36. Deninger, A., Eberle, B., Ebert, M., Grossmann, T., Hanisch, G., Heil, W., Kauczor, H.U. et al., ^{3}He-MRI-based measurements of intrapulmonary pO_2 and its time course during apnea in healthy volunteers: First results, reproducibility, and technical limitations, *NMR Biomed.*, 13, 194, 2000.

37. Gatzke, M., Cates, G.D., Driehuys, B., Fox, D., Happer, W., and Saam, B., Extraordinary slow nuclear spin relaxation in frozen laser polarized ^{129}Xe, *Phys. Rev. Lett.*, 70, 690, 1993.

II

Biomedical Diagnostics and Optical Biopsy

15

Fluorescence Spectroscopy for Biomedical Diagnostics

Tuan Vo-Dinh
Duke University

Brian M. Cullum
*University of Maryland,
Baltimore County*

15.1 Introduction

In the past several decades, fluorescence spectroscopy has had a dramatic effect on many different fields of research. One such field that has seen significant advancements is that of biomedical diagnostics. Within this field, fluorescence spectroscopy has been applied to the analysis of many different types of samples, ranging from individual biochemical species (e.g., nicotinamide adenine dinucleotide [NADH], tryptophan) to organs of living people. These studies have given rise to new methods for the early or noninvasive diagnosis of various medical conditions, including tooth decay, atherosclerosis, heart arrhythmia, cancer, and many others.

The medical condition that has seen the largest effort toward fluorescence-based analyses and truly demonstrates the potential of fluorescence-based diagnoses is cancer. Fluorescence spectroscopy and/ or imaging have been investigated for the diagnosis of almost every type of cancer and early neoplastic difference found in humans. The detection of early neoplastic changes is important from an outcome viewpoint, since once invasive carcinoma and metastases have occurred, treatment is difficult. At present, excisional biopsy followed by histology is considered to be the *gold standard* for the diagnosis of early neoplastic changes and carcinoma. In some cases, cytology rather than excisional biopsy is performed. These techniques are powerful diagnostic tools because they provide high-resolution spatial and morphological information of the cellular and subcellular structures of tissues. The use of staining and processing can enhance contrast and specificity of histopathology. However, both of these diagnostic procedures require physical removal of specimens, followed by tissue processing in a laboratory. These procedures incur a relatively high cost because specimen handling is required; more importantly, diagnostic information is not available in real time. Moreover, in the context of detecting early neoplastic changes, both excisional biopsy and cytology can have unacceptable false-negative (FN) rates often arising from sampling errors.

Fluorescence techniques have the potential for performing in vivo diagnosis on tissue without the need for sample excision and processing. Another advantage of fluorescence-based diagnoses is that the resulting information can be available in real time. In addition, since removal of tissue is not required for optical diagnoses, a more complete examination of the organ of interest can be achieved than with excisional biopsy or cytology.

This chapter provides an overview of fluorescence spectroscopy and its basic principles as well as its biomedical applications. Because biomedical fluorescence spectroscopy represents an extremely large and growing field of research, we have attempted to classify the ongoing research and clinical studies into several different categories: (1) biochemical analyses of individual compounds, (2) in vitro analyses (cellular and tissue systems), and (3) in vivo analyses (animal and human studies).

15.2 Principles of Fluorescence Spectroscopy

15.2.1 Fluorescence Techniques

Luminescence is a branch of spectroscopy that deals primarily with the electronic states of an atom or molecule, as opposed to the vibrational, rotational, or nuclear energy states. Fluorescence and phosphorescence are the two sister techniques covered by the umbrella known as *luminescence spectroscopy*. These techniques involve the optical detection and spectral analysis of light emitted by a substance undergoing a transition from an excited electronic state to a lower electronic state. Most luminescence-based medical diagnoses involve fluorescence spectroscopy because organic compounds fluoresce and do not phosphoresce at room temperature. In most phosphorescence studies, the measurements have to be performed using low-temperature frozen solvents to minimize collisional quenching. A unique technique called room temperature phosphorescence (RTP) uses various solid substrates to adsorb analytes into rigid matrices (e.g., cellulose, silica gel, alumina) in order to allow phosphorescence measurements.[1] Since the vast majority of medical applications involve fluorescence analysis, this chapter will focus mainly on the theory of fluorescence. However, since phosphorescence is involved in the field of photodynamic therapy (PDT), we will also describe the relationship between fluorescence and phosphorescence.

Fluorescence diagnostic methods can be grouped into two main categories:

1. Methods that detect endogenous fluorophores in tissues
2. Methods that detect or use exogenous fluorophores or fluorophore precursors (such as 5-aminolevulinic acid [ALA])

Fluorescence that originates from native fluorescent chromophores already present in the tissue is often referred to as *autofluorescence*. Fluorescence could also originate from administered exogenous chromophores that have been synthesized to target specific tissues (e.g., dysplastic vs. normal) or may be activated by functional changes in the tissue. In a fluorescence analysis, excitation light at some specific wavelength (typically near ultraviolet [UV] or visible) excites the tissue or exogenous fluorophore molecules and induces fluorescence emission. Then some measure of the fluorescent emission is obtained, typically an emission spectrum (fluorescence emission intensity vs. wavelength).

15.2.2 Photophysical Basis of Luminescence

Most organic molecules contain an even number of electrons. In the ground state, the electrons fill the various atomic orbitals with the lowest energies in pairs. By the Pauli exclusion principle, two electrons in one given orbital must have spins in opposite directions, and the total spin S must equal 0. For this reason, the ground state has no net electron spin. Such a state is called a *singlet* state.

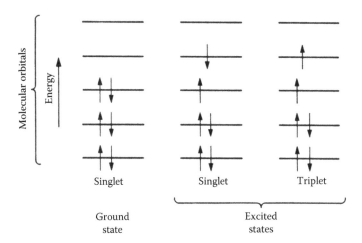

FIGURE 15.1 Schematic diagram of typical spin arrangements in MOs for the ground, excited singlet, and triplet states.

Excitation of a molecule usually results in the promotion of one electron from the highest occupied orbital to a previously unoccupied orbital (also referred to as a *virtual* orbital). Whereas the ground state is generally a singlet, the excited state can be either a singlet or a triplet, depending on the final spin state of the electron promoted to the higher orbital. For illustration, Figure 15.1 shows one ground-state and two excited-state configurations. The spins of the two electrons in the unoccupied orbitals are no longer restricted by the Pauli exclusion principle. The singlet state has two antiparallel spins, whereas the triplet state has two parallel spins and a net spin, S, of 1. In the general case, the configuration is not so easily visualized by schematic diagrams.[2]

The nature of the orbitals involved in an electronic transition is an important factor in determining the luminescence characteristics of the molecule. Organic compounds that are known to be strongly luminescent are molecules with extensive π electron systems. These compounds include aromatic molecules and a few unsaturated aliphatics. For molecules with no heteroatom, electronic transitions generally involve promotion of an electron from a bonding π orbital to an antibonding π^* orbital. Such a transition is known as a π–π^* transition, and the resulting electronic state is called the $\pi\pi^*$ excited state. For conjugated systems with heteroatoms (N, O, or S) in the conjugated system, or with substituents containing the N, O, or S atoms, an electronic state may result from the promotion of an electron from a bonding n orbital to an antibonding π^* orbital; this electronic state is called an $n\pi^*$ excited state.

15.2.2.1 Molecular Electronic Energies

In the study of luminescence, we are first concerned with the determination of the electronic states between which luminescence and other related processes such as intersystem crossing (ISC), vibrational relaxation (VR), and internal conversion (IC) occur. The basic approach for studying the luminescence behavior of molecules is to calculate the stationary-state electronic energies by solving the time-independent Schrödinger equation. A suitable wave function, Ψ, chosen to describe the properties of various molecular orbitals (MOs) involved in the photophysical processes is given by the Schrödinger equation:

$$H(q, Q)\, \Psi(q, Q) = E\, \Psi(q, Q), \tag{15.1}$$

where
    H is the Hamiltonian operator of the molecule
    q is the electronic spatial coordinates
    Q is the nuclear spatial coordinates
    E is the energy eigenvalue

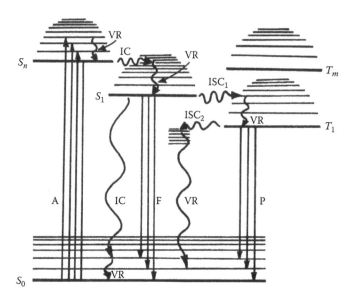

FIGURE 15.2 Jablonski diagram showing the different radiative and nonradiative transitions in a molecule upon excitation into a singlet state S_n: A (absorption), F (fluorescence), IC (internal conversion), ISC (intersystem crossing), P (phosphorescence), and VR (vibrational relaxation).

The exact solutions for the Schrödinger equation are impossible to calculate for any molecular system except H^+. Therefore, calculations of electronic energies for excited singlet and triplet states of larger systems usually involve some method of approximation. The most commonly used method is the MO method, which utilizes one-electron orbitals to form MOs. One of the simplest of these MO-based methods for calculating, or rather estimating, molecular electronic energies is the Hückel molecular orbital (HMO) method, which treats certain integrals as parameters and selects these parameters such that calculated values are in agreement with physical observables. This approach has been quite successful in describing bonding in aromatic and highly conjugated molecules.

Figure 15.2, known as the Jablonski diagram, shows energy levels for an organic molecule. In this figure, $S_0,...,S_n$ and $T_1, ..., T_m$ represent the discrete electronic energy levels of a molecule. The electronic state having the lowest energy, S_0, is known as the ground state. $S_0, ..., S_n$ and $T_1, ..., T_m$ are the excited singlet and triplet states, respectively. Each electronic state has its own set of vibrational levels. Superimposed on each vibrational level is a series of closely spaced rotational levels not shown in Figure 15.2.

15.2.2.2 Population of the Excited Electronic States

The main photophysical processes involved in the population and deactivation of excited electronic states, both singlet and triplet, are shown in Figure 15.2. These processes—absorption (A), VR, IC, fluorescence (F), ISC, and phosphorescence (P)—and related photophysical processes are discussed in the following text.

15.2.2.2.1 Absorption

At equilibrium, a group of molecules has a thermal distribution at the lowest vibrational and rotational levels of the ground state, S_0. When a molecule absorbs excitation energy, it is elevated from S_0 to some vibrational level of one of the excited singlet states, S_n, in the manifold $S_1, ..., S_n$. As postulated by the Franck–Condon principle, the time for an electronic transition (on the order of 10^{-15} s) is shorter than the time for nuclear rearrangement (on the order of 10^{-13} to 10^{-14} s). As a consequence, the molecular configuration following absorption is often a nonequilibrium nuclear configuration because the electronic absorption process is so rapid that the atomic nuclei do not have time to change positions or moments.

Thus, the adiabatic (Born–Oppenheimer) approximation is often applied to solve the Schrödinger equation (Equation 15.1) and partially separates the eigenstates of the electronic (*fast*) and nuclear (*slow*) subsystems. The intensity of the absorption (i.e., fraction of ground-state molecules promoted to the electronic excited state) depends on the intensity of the excitation radiation (i.e., number of photons) and the probability of the transition with photons of the particular energy being used. A term often used to characterize the intensity of an absorption (or induced emission) band is the oscillator strength, *f*, which may be defined from the integrated absorption spectrum by the relationship

$$f = 4.315 \times 10^{-9} \int \varepsilon_v \, dv \qquad (15.2)$$

where ε_v is the molar extinction coefficient at the frequency v.

Oscillator strengths of unity or near unity correspond to strongly allowed transitions, whereas smaller values of *f* indicate smaller transition dipole matrix elements of forbidden transitions.

15.2.2.2.2 Vibrational Relaxation

In condensed media, the molecules in the S_n state deactivate rapidly, within 10^{-13} to 10^{-11} s via VR processes, ensuring that they are in the lowest vibrational levels of S_n possible as described by the thermal Boltzmann distribution. Since the VR process is faster than electronic transitions, any excess vibrational energy is rapidly lost as the molecules are deactivated to lower vibronic levels of the corresponding excited electronic state. This excess VR energy is released as thermal energy to the surrounding medium.

Only under special circumstances—for example, in the gas phase at very low pressures ($<10^{-6}$ torr)—may emission be observed from higher vibrational levels of the excited state. These emission mechanisms, known as single-vibronic-level (SVL) luminescence processes, do not generally occur in condensed media such as tissues.

15.2.2.2.3 Internal Conversion

From the S_n state, the molecule deactivates rapidly to the isoenergetic vibrational level of a lower electronic state such as S_{n-1} via an IC process. IC processes are transitions between states of the same multiplicity. The molecule subsequently deactivates to the lowest vibronic levels of S_{n-1} via a VR process. By a succession of IC processes immediately followed by VR processes, the molecule deactivates rapidly to S_1. As a result, a molecule may be excited to S_1 or higher excited states, S_n, depending on the excitation energy being used, but the emission takes place only from the lowest excited electronic state, S_1. This is known as Kasha's rule. Fluorescence emission from upper electronic states (above S_1 or T_1) of polyatomic molecules, however, is a rare phenomenon in the condensed phase.

After VR or IC, the thermal population at a given electronic state is determined by the Boltzmann distribution, which gives the relative population of species in a given electronic or vibronic state, as compared with those in all other states. The Boltzmann distribution is expressed by

$$\frac{n_i}{\sum_j n_j} = \frac{g_i \exp\left(-E_i/kT\right)}{\sum_j g_j \exp\left(-E_i/kT\right)}$$

where
n_i is the number of molecules in electronic or vibronic state *i*
g_i is the statistical weight of state of that state
E_i is the energy of state *i*
k is the Boltzmann constant
T is the temperature

15.2.2.2.4 Fluorescence

Relaxation of the molecule from the S_1 state may occur by one of several different processes, including (1) further deactivation to S_0 in a radiationless fashion via IC and VR processes or (2) emission of a photon without a change in spin multiplicity. The latter $S_1 \rightarrow S_0$ transition is known as fluorescence. The energy of the resulting photon corresponds to the difference in energy between the lowest vibrational level of the excited state and the vibrational level of the ground state. Thus, the fluorescence spectrum primarily provides information about the vibrational structure of the ground state.

These radiative transitions are electric dipole in nature. The probability of a radiative transition $(S_i \rightarrow S_j)$ is proportional to the square of the matrix element, $\left|(\mathbf{M})_{ij}\right|^2$, where $\mathbf{M}$ is the electric dipole moment defined by

$$\mathbf{M}\left(S_i \rightarrow S_j\right) = \left\langle \psi\left(S_i\right) \left| \sum_q e\,\mathbf{r}_q \right| \psi\left(S_j\right) \right\rangle$$

where

    e is the electronic charge
    $\mathbf{r}_q$ is the position vector of electron q
    $\psi(S_i)$ is the wave function of electronic state S_i

For fluorescence ($i = 0, j = 1$), the electronic transition corresponds to $\left|M_{1,0}\right|^2$.

15.2.2.2.5 Intersystem Crossing

Another process through which molecules in the S_i state may relax is through a transition to some vibrational level of the triplet manifold via a mechanism known as an ISC process (ISC_1 transition shown in Figure 15.2). The ISC process involves a change in spin multiplicity. The molecule then relaxes to the lowest vibrational level of T_1 via successive IC and VR processes.

From this T_1 state, the molecule may return to the ground state S_0 either by a radiationless deactivation path (ISC_2 process shown in Figure 15.2) or by the emission of a photon. This latter radiative transition is known as phosphorescence.

The radiationless deactivation that quite often competes with phosphorescence is the reverse ISC process (ISC_2). This process, which is often dominant, determines the observed phosphorescence lifetime. The nonradiative rate constant corresponding to the ISC process $T_1 \rightarrow S_0$ is strongly dependent on the magnitude of the energy gap $\Delta E(T_1 \rightarrow S_0)$. The rate constant decreases exponentially with increasing ΔE; this feature is known as the energy gap law. The energy gap law is not specific only to ISC but also applies to other nonradiative transitions such as IC.

15.2.2.2.6 Phosphorescence and the Triplet State

The triplet-state manifold consists of states T_1, T_2, ..., T_n, which have energy levels lower than the corresponding singlet states S_1, S_2, ..., S_n. This is a consequence of Hund's rule, which states that the energy associated with a state having parallel spins is always lower than that of the corresponding one with antiparallel spins. Qualitatively, Hund's rule may be explained by the tendency for electrons with parallel spins to be further separated in space (i.e., to lie in different MOs) and consequently experience less coulombic interaction. As a result of Hund's rule, phosphorescence occurs at longer wavelengths than does fluorescence.[1,2]

Properties of singlet and triplet states are significantly different. The singlet state is diamagnetic, whereas the triplet state is paramagnetic. The nomenclatures *singlet* and *triplet* are derived from multiplicity considerations of the energy level splitting that occurs when the molecule is exposed to a magnetic field. Under the application of an external magnetic field, the triplet state with a spin magnetic momentum splits into three Zeeman levels. The singlet state, which has no magnetic momentum, is unchanged.

15.2.2.2.7 Spin–Orbit Coupling

Production of the triplet state in some compounds is important to photosensitization in certain biomedical applications, such as PDT. A process that leads to the production of the triplet state is spin–orbit (S-O) coupling. Transitions between different excited singlet states of the same multiplicity ($S_n \rightarrow S_m$ or $T_n \rightarrow T_m$) may occur easily, but transitions between pure-spin states of different multiplicities ($S_n \rightarrow T_n$) are forbidden by quantum mechanics under the spin selection rule ($\Delta S = 0$). Spin-forbidden transitions, however, do occur under certain conditions. If the spin and orbital motions of the electrons are independent of one another, triplet–singlet transitions do not give rise to electric dipole radiation because of the spin selection rule. However, the spin and orbital motions are actually not independent. Basically, the occurrence of spin-forbidden transitions—for example, singlet–triplet transitions—is made possible by the coupling of the electron spin with the orbital angular momentum, a nonclassical phenomenon that produces a quantum mechanical mixing of states of different multiplicities. Qualitatively, this mechanism may be explained by the fact that the orbital motion of the electron induces a magnetic field that interacts with its spin magnetic moment. This interaction results in a change of the direction of the spin angular momentum of the electron.[2] This phenomenon is known as S-O coupling.

The S-O coupling mechanism actually mixes some singlet character into triplet states and vice versa. This process therefore removes the spin-forbidden nature of the transitions between pure-spin states. Because of the importance of S-O coupling in understanding the phosphorescence process, it is essential to consider briefly the theoretical treatment of S-O coupling.

15.2.2.2.8 General Considerations for Nonradiative Properties

The VR, IC, and ISC processes are known as *radiationless transitions*. In the framework of the Born–Oppenheimer approximation, in which the nuclear and electronic motions are assumed to be independent of each other, the probability of W_{mn} of a radiationless transition between two electronic states n and m can be treated by perturbation theory and is given by the following expression[1,2]:

$$W_{mn} = \frac{8\pi^2 \tau}{h^2} \prod_{ij} \left\langle \theta_{mi} | \theta_{nj} \right\rangle^2 \left\langle \Phi_m | H' | \Phi_n \right\rangle^2$$

where
h is Planck's constant
θ_{mi} is the vibrational wave function i of the electronic state m
Φ_m is the electronic wave function of the electronic state m
τ is the relaxation time of the vibronic levels
H' is the perturbing Hamiltonian
Π_{ij} is the product over all vibronic states i and j

For radiationless transitions between states of similar multiplicity—for example, VR and IC processes—H' may be the electron–electron repulsion term and/or the vibronic interaction term. For radiationless transitions between states of different multiplicities—for example, ISC processes—H' is the S-O coupling term.

A common expression that describes the probability W_{mn} is the so-called Fermi golden rule for the statistical limit of a dense manifold for the final states. In this case, W_{mn} is given by

$$W_m = \frac{2\pi}{h} V_{mn} \cdot \rho$$

where

V_{mn} is the matrix element of the perturbation between the initial state m and final states n
ρ is the density of the final state
h is Planck's constant

15.2.2.2.9 Delayed Fluorescence

Fluorescence and phosphorescence are the two most common luminescence processes. A less common emission process is delayed fluorescence (DF). With some chemical systems, the molecule in the triplet state T_1 reverts back to the excited singlet state manifold. Since T_1 is always of lower energy than $S_1, \ldots, S_n$, this transition requires some additional activation energy. DF may occur from the S_1 state, exhibiting a spectrum identical to conventional fluorescence (often called *prompt fluorescence*) but having a longer lifetime due to the additional stay in the triplet state. Two types of DF processes can be differentiated: (1) an eosin-type (E-type) DF that is produced by repopulation of S_1 from the triplet state by thermal activation and (2) a pyrene-type (p-type) DF that is produced when pairs of triplet-state molecules interact, providing an activation energy greater than or equal to the S_1 energy. At room temperature, E-type DF can be an important mechanism and has been observed for many organic compounds adsorbed on solid substrates.

15.3 Characterization of Luminescence

Several physical observables may be used to characterize fluorescence and/or phosphorescence. These include the following:

1. Emission, excitation, and synchronous spectra
2. Quantum yields
3. Lifetimes
4. Polarization

15.3.1 Emission, Excitation, and Synchronous Spectra

It is first important to determine the positions and nature of the energy levels of the electronic states involved in the luminescence excitation and emission processes because these energy levels are characteristic properties of the compounds of interest. In general, the simplest method of studying the energy levels of the excited state is absorption spectroscopy. An alternative method for investigating the absorption process for luminescent compounds is excitation spectroscopy.

The general relationship between the absorption and emission spectra and the vibrational levels of the electronic states is illustrated in Figure 15.3. Since a fluorescence emission spectrum is due to radiative decay from S_1 to different levels of S_0, the emission spectrum exhibits the vibrational frequencies that correspond to the vibrations of the molecule in its ground state, whereas the absorption spectrum exhibits frequencies of the excited state. The intensities of the vibrational bands are determined in quantum theory by the magnitude of the wave-function overlap (Franck–Condon coefficients) for the various vibrational levels in the ground and excited states (Figure 15.3b and c). The overlap coefficients are the Franck–Condon factors. Figure 15.3a shows the potential energy curves of the excited and ground states and the transitions corresponding to excitation (or absorption) and emission processes. Figure 15.3b and c shows two typical cases of electronic states with their potential minima at different relative positions on the internuclear distance coordinate R. In Figure 15.3b, the strongest transition is the 0–0 transition, at which the overlap is the largest. In Figure 15.3c, the most probable transition is the 0–4 transition involving the vibrational level $v' = 4$ of the ground state and the vibrational level $v' = 0$ of the excited state. The envelopes of the vibrational progressions illustrated in Figure 15.3b and c depend on the relative displacement δR between the potential minima of the excited and ground states; for the simple case in which the ground vibrational level is thermally populated, the shape of the envelopes is determined by the Pekarian formula. For $\delta R = 0$, there is no vibrational progression; for large δR, the Pekarian distribution becomes a Gaussian distribution. Examination of the vibronic structure of the fluorescence, or phosphorescence, spectrum can therefore yield important information about the potential curves of the singlet and ground states or triplet and ground states, respectively.

With conventional emission (excitation) spectra, the excitation (emission) wavelength is fixed while the emission wavelength is scanned over the spectral region of interest. With synchronous spectra, both excitation and emission wavelengths are scanned synchronously while maintaining a constant wavelength interval between them.[3,4] More recently, the synchronous scanning technique, also referred to as synchronous luminescence (SL) or synchronous fluorescence (SF), has received increasing interest for biomedical diagnostics[5] (see Section 15.4.4). The SF method offers a simple way to rapidly measure fluorescence signals and spectral fingerprints of complex mixtures such as tissue. While conventional fluorescence spectroscopy uses either a fixed-wavelength excitation (λ_{exc}) to produce an emission spectrum or a fixed-wavelength emission (λ_{em}) to record an excitation spectrum, with SF method, the fluorescence signal is recorded while both λ_{em} and λ_{exc} are simultaneously scanned. A constant wavelength interval ($\Delta\lambda = \lambda_{em} - \lambda_{exc}$) is maintained between the excitation and

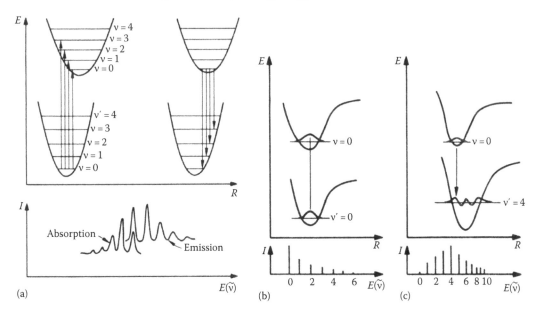

FIGURE 15.3 (a) Diagrams of the potential energy curves of two electronic states showing the absorption and emission transitions between these two states and the typical intensity distribution of the corresponding spectra. (b) Potential energy curves with unchanged potential minima. The most intense transition is 0–0 (maximum overlap of the vibronic wave functions). (c) Potential energy curves with potential minima shifted with respect to each other. In this example, the most intense transition is 0–4.

(continued)

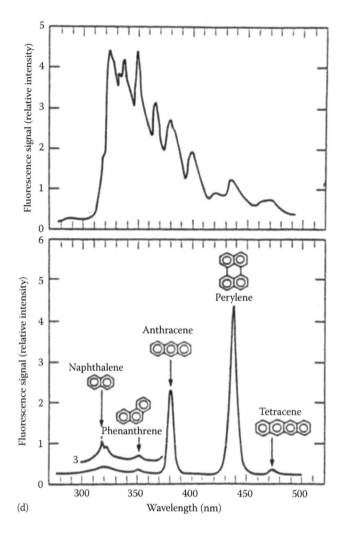

(d)

FIGURE 15.3 (continued)   (d) Top curve: conventional fluorescence spectrum of naphthalene, phenanthrene, anthracene, perylene, and tetracene using fixed excitation. Bottom curve: SF spectrum of the mixture. (Adapted from Vo-Dinh, T., *Anal. Chem.*, 50(3), 396, 1978.)

the emission wavelengths throughout the spectrum. As a result, the intensity of the synchronous signal I_s can be written as the product of three functions as follows[3,4]:

$$I_s\left(\lambda_{exc}, \lambda_{em}\right) = kc E_X\left(\lambda_{exc}\right) E_M\left(\lambda_{em}\right)$$

where
   k is a constant accounting for the measurement geometry and quantum yield
   c is a concentration of the fluorophore
   E_X is an excitation spectrum of the fluorophore
   E_M is an emission spectrum of the fluorophore

When the wavelength interval $\Delta\lambda$ between λ_{exc} and λ_{em} is chosen properly, the resulting spectrum will show one or a few features that are much more resolvable than those in the conventional fluorescence emission spectrum. For example, if the wavelength interval is chosen to be the difference between the wavelength of the maximum absorption peak (or excitation peak) and the wavelength of the maximum emission peak for a single fluorophore, the synchronous spectrum of a sample containing this fluorophore would show a single sharp peak associated with this fluorophore. This feature can significantly reduce spectral overlap in multicomponent mixtures. This can be illustrated in the SL spectrum of a mixture consisting of naphthalene, phenanthrene, anthracene, perylene, and tetracene (Figure 15.3d). Whereas the conventional fixed-excitation fluorescence spectrum exhibits overlapping peaks (Figure 15.3d, top curve), the SL spectrum shows a series of single nonoverlapping peaks for easing chemical identification.[3] The SL methodology could provide a simple way to rapidly measure the luminescence signal and spectral fingerprints of complex biological samples such as tissues. For a single molecular species, the observed intensity I_s is simplified (often to a single peak), and the bandwidth is narrower than for the conventional emission spectrum. The SL technique can also be used for biological analysis and in vivo diagnostics.[5]

15.3.2 Quantum Yields

The emission quantum efficiencies, also known as quantum yields, determine the sensitivity of the luminescence measurements. Quantum efficiencies are intrinsic molecular parameters of a compound under given conditions of temperature, solvent, and other environmental factors.

The fluorescence quantum efficiency Φ_F is defined as

$$\Phi_F = \frac{\text{Number of luminescence photons}}{\text{Number of photons absorbed}}$$

The phosphorescence quantum efficiency Φ_P is defined in a similar manner. Quantum efficiencies can also be defined for processes other than emission and are used to define the fraction of molecules that undergoes a specific process.

15.3.3 Lifetimes

Another means for characterizing a luminescence emission process is the determination of its lifetime. The luminescence lifetime, τ, is defined as the time required for the emission to decrease to $1/e$ of its original intensity following a δ-pulse excitation.

If $I(t)$ is the luminescence intensity at time t and I_0 is the intensity at $t = 0$, then is given by

$$I_L(t) = I_0 \exp\left(\frac{-t}{\tau}\right)$$

It is important to differentiate the intrinsic natural lifetime, τ^*, from the observed lifetime, τ, for a given radiative process. The intrinsic natural lifetime, τ^*, is measured only when there is no radiationless deactivation process competing with the emission—that is, when $\Phi_L = 1$ for the resulting luminescence.

Experimentally, fluorescence can be differentiated from phosphorescence by its shorter lifetime. Fluorescence lifetimes of organic molecules are on the order of 10^{-9} to 10^{-7} s, while phosphorescence lifetimes range from 10^{-3} s to several seconds. Table 15.1 gives a comparison between the oscillator strengths and radiative lifetimes of fluorescence ($S_1 \rightarrow S_0$) and phosphorescence ($T_1 \rightarrow S_0$) emission and absorption of different origins.

15.3.4 Polarization

Polarization is another physically observable characteristic of luminescence. Polarization is caused by unique symmetries and orientations of electric moments vectors and wave functions involved in electronic transitions. The electric dipole moment determines the direction along which charge is displaced in a molecule undergoing an electronic transition. It is possible to study the polarization of the transition using polarized light in to excite and detect luminescence.

TABLE 15.1 Radiative Lifetimes and Oscillator Strengths in the Electronic Transitions for Polynuclear Aromatic Compounds

Origin of Transitions	Radiative Lifetime (s)	Oscillator Strength
$S_1 \rightarrow S_0$ transitions		
$\pi\pi^*$	10^{-7}–10^{-9}	10^{-3}–1
π or π^*	$>10^{-6}$	$<10^{-2}$
$n\pi^*$	$\sim 10^{-6}$	$\sim 10^{-6}$
$T_1 \rightarrow T_0$ transitions		
$n\pi^*$ (or π^* or π^*)	10^{-2}–10^{-4}	10^{-7}–10^{-5}
$\pi\pi^*$ in haloaromatic	1–10^{-3}	10^{-9}–10^{-6}
$\pi\pi^*$ in unsaturated hydrocarbons	$\sim 10^2$	10^{-11}

A common method for determining the degree of polarization, P, is photoselection. In this method, one excites the sample with polarized light and measures the luminescence intensity along two perpendicular directions. The degree of polarization is defined as

$$P = \frac{I_{EE} - I_{EB}}{I_{EE} + I_{EB}}$$

where

I_{EE} and I_{EB} are the luminescence intensities measured along the direction parallel and perpendicular to the excitation electric vector, E, respectively

P is related to the angle, θ, between the absorption vector and the emission vector by the relationship

$$P = \frac{3\cos^2 \theta}{\cos^2 \theta + 3}$$

If the absorption and emission vectors are parallel ($\theta = 0°$), $P = 0.5$. If these vectors are perpendicular ($\theta = 90°$), $P = -0.33$. In practice, P has a value between these two limiting cases.

15.4 Biomedical Applications

Biomedical fluorescence spectroscopy is an extremely large and growing field of research. In an attempt to classify the various types of research and clinical studies that are being performed, we have grouped this field into three categories:

1. Biochemical analyses of individual compounds
2. In vitro analyses
3. In vivo analyses

Biochemical analyses are the basis for the fundamental or general studies of individual biochemical compounds that form the basic constituents of biological samples (i.e., tryptophan, NAD, NADH, hemoglobin). It is from these studies that the basic fluorescence properties of common fluorophores are generally determined and characterized. The second category, in vitro analysis, is further divided into two subcategories: cellular measurement and tissue measurement. These analyses typically provide additional information associated with complex systems such as cells and tissues. The third classification category, in vivo analyses, can also be subdivided into two more subcategories: animal studies and human clinical studies. These experiments are generally performed only for fluorescence analysis techniques that are meant to be used for optical diagnostic procedures. In addition to classification based upon the type of analysis that is performed, it is also possible to subcategorize based upon the type of analyte that is measured, whether it is an endogenous species or an exogenous fluorophore (e.g., used as a label or marker for the tissue area of interest).

15.4.1 Biochemical Analysis of Individual Species

Fluorescence analyses of a wide variety of biochemical species that have been applied to and extracted from biological samples have been performed for quite a long time. These analyses are generally classified based upon whether or not the fluorescent species is an endogenous (naturally occurring) or exogenous (externally administered) fluorophore.

15.4.1.1 Endogenous Fluorophores

A large number of endogenous fluorophores, autofluorescent species, exist within biological samples.[5–7] The majority of these species are typically associated with either the structural matrix of tissues (e.g., collagen[8] and elastin[9]) or with various cellular metabolic pathways (e.g., NAD and NADH).[10] In the case of the structural matrices, the most common fluorophores are the previously mentioned collagen and elastin. The resulting fluorescence from these compounds is due primarily to the cross-linking of various amino acids in their structure. This cross-linking typically provides the conjugated systems that are generally found in most fluorescent molecules. In addition, because of the various degrees of cross-linking that can occur in these species, the resulting fluorescence emission spectrum is typically very broad and featureless, ranging anywhere from about 325 to 600 nm.

Some of the most intense endogenous fluorophores that exist in humans and animals are involved in cellular metabolism. The predominant species in this category include the reduced form of NADH,[11] the various flavins (e.g., flavin adenine dinucleotide [FAD]),[12] and the strongly fluorescent lipopigments (e.g., lipofuscin and ceroids).[13,14] In addition to these species, there exist many other endogenous fluorophores exhibiting emission of various strengths and covering various spectral ranges in the UV and visible regions of the electromagnetic spectrum. These fluorophores include aromatics; amino acids such as tryptophan, tyrosine, and phenylalanine[6]; various porphyrins (hemoglobin, myoglobin, etc.)[6]; and in certain cases and locations, red porphyrin fluorescence due to bacteria.[10] Figure 15.4 shows the absorption and fluorescence spectra of various tissue fluorophores.

Because these biochemical species are generally either structural or metabolic, they can provide a significant amount of information about differences in tissues. One of the most common reasons for investigating these fluorescent species is the possibility for diagnosis of various diseases (e.g., cancer) without requiring exogenous fluorescent markers or tags. Since cells that are in various disease states often undergo different rates of metabolism, or have different structures, there are often distinct differences in their fluorescent emission spectra. These differences in fluorescence emission generally depend on at least one of the following parameters: fluorophore concentration or spatial distribution throughout the tissue, local microenvironment surrounding the fluorophores, the particular tissue architecture that is being interrogated, and a wavelength-dependent light attenuation due to differences in the amount of nonfluorescing chromophores. The first of these reasons, change in fluorophore concentration, can be attributed to many different events. In certain cases, various chemicals may not be produced in a diseased tissue. In other cases, the distribution or form of the fluorophore may vary throughout the tissue. For instance, NADH is an extremely fluorescent molecule in its reduced form but is nonfluorescent in the oxidized form. Therefore, depending on the specific phase of a particular metabolic reaction that may be occurring, the relative faction of NADH in the reduced and oxidized forms may vary greatly. Another reason for differences in the fluorescence emission from various tissue types is the difference in the local environment surrounding the fluorophore.

Change in the microstructure (the local environment) surrounding a particular fluorophore can have significant effects on its fluorescence properties. Fluorescence properties that are often affected by such changes include the fluorescence quantum yield, the spectral position of its fluorescence emission maximum, its spectral line width, and its fluorescence lifetime. All these factors can have a significant impact on the overall fluorescence emission of the entire tissue sample. In addition to the local environment surrounding the fluorophore, the larger macro tissue structure or architecture also plays a significant role in the resulting fluorescence because of its specific optical properties (e.g., refractive index, scattering cross sections). These are described in greater detail in the tissue optics chapters of this handbook.

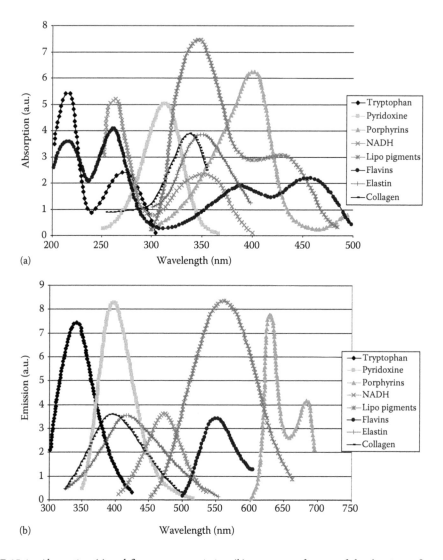

FIGURE 15.4 Absorption (a) and fluorescence emission (b) spectrum of many of the dominant fluorophores present in common tissue components. (Adapted from Wagnières, G.A.S. et al., *Photochem. Photobiol.*, 68, 603, 1998.)

An important factor that often plays a significant role in the differences associated with various disease states of tissue is the presence of nonfluorescing chromophores (hemoglobin, etc.). These chromophores, which can vary in concentration depending upon the state of the tissue, can absorb various wavelengths of fluorescent light emitted from the tissue or even absorb specific wavelengths of the excitation light being used for the analysis. One example of this case is in the fluorescence diagnosis of tumor tissue, which typically has an increase in vascularization over normal tissues due to angiogenesis. Because of this increase in vascularization, the increased presence of hemoglobin often causes increased absorption of light in the visible region of the electromagnetic spectrum.

Due to this complex nature of biological tissues, extensive studies have been performed on individual species at the fundamental biochemical level. These fundamental studies of the absorption and fluorescence properties of various biochemical fluorophores give us a better understanding of the complex interactions that may be occurring in tissue samples.

In addition to conventional spectrally resolved fluorescence analyses, which are capable of providing a significant amount of information about the various fluorophores that are present as well as some information about their local environment, there has also been some work in the field of time-resolved fluorescence analyses. An in-depth analysis of this subject can be found in the chapter on fluorescence lifetime imaging techniques. Time-resolved spectroscopic analyses can provide information about molecular interactions and motions that occur in the picosecond–nanosecond timescale range. Understanding these interactions can be especially useful in the analysis of biomolecular structure and dynamics. Recent advances in time-resolved fluorescence spectroscopy in the field of biological analyses have led to a better understanding of the origin of nonexponential fluorescence decay in proteins, the use of tryptophan analogs as unique spectroscopic probes of protein–protein interactions, the detailed characterization of protein-folding processes and intermediates, the development of new approaches to the study of DNA–protein interactions,[15] and the analysis of subdomains in proteins.[16,17]

15.4.1.2 Exogenous Fluorophores and Molecular Markers

In addition to the large number of endogenous fluorophores that have been used for biological diagnostics, many different exogenous fluorophores have been created and studied as well. These exogenous fluorophores have been created for many different purposes and applications in the field of biological monitoring, ranging from the monitoring of cellular function using fluorescent reporter dyes or molecules for various biochemical species (Ca^{+2}, Mg^{+2}, pH, nucleic acid sequences, etc.) to the demarcation of tumors with a relatively recent class of exogenous fluorophores. In the case of the monitoring of cellular function and chemical distribution, a large number of dyes with varying fluorescence properties for most of the more common cellular species can be obtained commercially from companies such as Molecular Probes. These fluorescent reporter dyes are typically used to monitor the distribution of important chemical species throughout a cell by obtaining fluorescence microscopy images after injecting it with the dye. In addition to simply monitoring the distribution of certain chemicals, several dyes can be used to determine the viability of the cells or the permeability of their membranes. A more detailed description of these dyes and the types of analyses they are capable of is presented in Section 15.4.2.

A second type of fluorescent reporter dye that has been developed recently is known as a molecular beacon.[18–21] These molecular beacons are constructed by attaching a fluorescent dye (e.g., fluorescein) to one end of an oligonucleotide sequence and a quencher molecule (e.g., DABSYL) to the other end of the oligonucleotide sequence. The particular oligonucleotide sequence that is chosen for the molecular beacon is comprised of the complementary sequence to the RNA or DNA sequence that is to be measured. For the molecular beacon to function properly, the last several nucleic acids on either end of the oligonucleotide strand must be complementary to each other. This forces the molecule to assume a hairpin form in its native state that brings the quencher molecule in close proximity to the fluorophore of the other end. The proximity of the quencher molecule to the fluorophore prevents the fluorophore from emitting any fluorescent light. However, when the molecular beacon is in the presence of its complementary sequence to the remainder of the oligonucleotide, the beacon is opened up, thus separating the quencher and fluorophore molecules and allowing the fluorescent dye to emit. This feature is described in more detail in "Novel Fluorescent Molecular Beacon DNA Probes for Biomolecular Recognition" in this handbook.

In addition to fluorescent reporter dyes and molecular beacons, a third major area of research in biologically useful exogenous fluorophores has been in the area of tumor demarcation or sensitization. The most common of these tumor markers also act as sensitizers, or tumor-killing agents, for a unique scheme of cancer treatment known as PDT. A much more detailed description of PDT is offered in Chapter 1 of *The Biomedical Photonics Handbook: Therapeutic and Advanced Biophotonics* in this handbook. Some of the most commonly used and best characterized of these photosensitizers are hematoporphyrin (Hp) derivatives (HpDs),[22,23] pheophorbide-a (Ph-a),[24] *m*THPC,[25] benzoporphyrin derivatives (BPDs),[26,27] tin etiopurpurin ($SnET_2$),[28] hypericin,[29,30] and ALA.[31–35] The best studied of these compounds are the HpDs (i.e., Photofrin). HpDs were derived from the functionalization of Hps with hydrophobic substituents that would allow these compounds to be taken up more readily in the tumor tissues than the unsubstituted Hps.[36] After these compounds had been developed, it was found that they could also serve as photosensitizers, since they are capable of being excited and activated by the absorption of visible light. While HpDs are still used quite extensively today for PDT treatments, many other compounds or classes of compounds with more appropriate characteristics for clinical drugs (such as those listed earlier) have been developed.

The most desirable optical properties of PDT sensitizers are strong absorptivity in the red or near-infrared (NIR) region of the electromagnetic spectrum and a high triplet-state quantum yield. The first of these two properties is important for several reasons. One of these reasons is that the use of red or NIR wavelengths of light for excitation of the sensitizer causes much less damage to nearby healthy tissue. At red and NIR wavelengths, naturally occurring chromophores in the tissue absorb little light. In addition, because the absorption of these wavelengths by natural chromophores is minimal, the resulting background fluorescence from nearby healthy tissue is minimized, providing a much more accurate tumor marker as well as sensitizer. A third potential benefit gained by having photosensitizers with strong absorption spectra in the red and NIR is the ability to destroy tumors under thin layers of normal tissue. When photosensitizers that are activated with visible or UV light are used, the absorption cross section of the healthy overlaying tissue is too great to allow a significant fraction of the light to penetrate deeper than approximately 100 μm. However, lower-energy photons, such as those in the red or NIR, penetrate significantly and could allow for the activation of sensitizers in tumors below healthy overlaying tissue. In addition to the desire to develop new sensitizers and markers with red-shifted absorption profiles, it is also important to obtain a high triplet-state conversion rate in these molecules. Triplet-state conversion is very important to the formation of the reactive oxygen species that are responsible for the drug's activity.[10]

15.4.2 In Vitro Analyses and Diagnostics

In vitro analyses can typically be classified in two different categories: cellular analyses and tissue analyses. In vitro analyses are important for gaining a greater understanding of basic fundamental biological processes that are occurring and understanding any potential interferences or problems that may be present when investigating more complex biological systems (i.e., living animals).

In addition to gaining a better fundamental biochemical understanding, in vitro fluorescence analyses are often performed to better understand the interactions or interferences that often take place in complex systems as opposed to individual chemicals. By investigating these effects on in vitro samples such as cells or tissues, investigators can determine potential diagnostic procedures that could be performed in vivo or identify problems with potential diagnostic procedures prior to involving live subjects. When performing analyses on neat biochemical systems, it is not possible to investigate the interactions of the various biochemicals with the others that are present in functional systems (i.e., cells, tissues). In addition, the effect of the local environment on the optical properties of the various fluorophores can be investigated much more accurately by the use of in vitro systems as compared to biochemical analyses alone.

15.4.2.1 Cellular Analyses

Cells represent one of the most basic of biological systems capable of performing chemical reactions. Monitoring of endogenous as well as exogenous fluorophores on the cellular level had provided a great deal of information about many different processes. Several different fluorescence techniques have been developed for the performance of such analyses. These techniques include probing with chemical or biochemical sensors as well as obtaining fluorescence images using any of several different forms of fluorescence microscopy. In this section, we provide a brief review of the various types of cellular processes that have been investigated using fluorescence spectroscopy.

Several other chapters in this handbook provide a more detailed description of the techniques and their applications. Chapter 15 of Volume III of this handbook provides a general review of various optical methods used for analyzing living cells; Chapters 1, 22, and 23 of Volume III provide detailed descriptions of chemical and biochemical sensors used for cellular analyses; and Chapters 10, 11, and 12 of Volume I provide a detailed review of the theory and application of fluorescence microscopy.

15.4.2.1.1 Autofluorescence of Cells

While the vast majority of fluorescence microscopy is performed with the use of exogenous reporter dyes, there has been a growing field of fluorescence microscopy that relies on autofluorescent species inside the cells themselves for diagnostic information. Such autofluorescence measurements provide an important tool for biomedical diagnostics. Much of the research in autofluorescence microscopy is performed either as preliminary research prior to testing in vivo diagnostic procedures, or as a medical diagnostic procedure itself. Some recent examples of this are described in the following.

15.4.2.1.1.1 Cell Proliferation and Cell Analysis   One of the most sought-after applications of fluorescence spectroscopy in biomedical optics is the ability to distinguish normal tissue from cancerous or even precancerous tissue in a real-time clinical setting, without the administering of any drugs. In order to determine the potential of such technique, several researchers have sought to answer the questions of whether or not unique fluorescence spectral patterns were associated with cell proliferation and whether differences between rapidly growing and slowly growing cells be identified. Native cellular fluorescence was used to identify terminal squamous differentiation of normal oral epithelial cells in culture (Figure 15.5).[37] In one such analysis, fluorescence excitation spectra were capable of distinguishing between slow and rapidly growing cells in three different types of cells. To perform the analyses, excitation spectra were obtained by scanning over the spectral range of 240–430 nm while monitoring the fluorescence emission at 450 nm. By taking the ratio of the intensity of the major broadband peak at 320–350 nm to a point on the downslope of the curve at 370 nm, investigators found that there was a statistical difference between slow and rapidly growing cells. In addition, it was also possible to distinguish the slow-growing cells from the rapidly growing cells by obtaining fluorescence emission spectra of the various cells with an excitation wavelength at 340 nm and an emission wavelength range of 360–660 nm. These results demonstrate a great potential for the discrimination of proliferating and nonproliferating cell populations in vivo.[38]

In a similar study, laser-induced fluorescence (LIF), with excitation by the 488 nm laser emission line of an argon-ion laser, was used to differentiate between normal and tumor human urothelial cells. Experiments were performed using a confocal microspectrofluorimeter, allowing individual cells to be probed; and the broadband autofluorescence emission between 550 and 560 nm, corresponding to oxidized flavoproteins, was monitored. An analysis of the data showed that the maximum autofluorescence intensity of normal urothelial cells was much higher, approximately 10 times, than that of any of the tumor cell types tested, thereby suggesting that the concentration of an oxidized flavoprotein in tumor urothelial cells is significantly less than in a normal urothelial cell. Not only could this observation lead to the development of a clinical diagnostic procedure for the real-time differentiation between normal, cancerous, and potentially precancerous urothelial tissues, but it also provides a better understanding of the biochemical differences between normal and cancerous tissues.[39]

SL is a unique approach that could improve the selectivity of fluorescence techniques for cancer diagnostics. As discussed previously, autofluorescence of neoplastic and normal tissues have been observed using fixed-wavelength laser excitation. However, the use of fixed excitation might not be sufficiently selective in some diagnostic applications due to strong overlap of the emission spectra from different fluorophores. An alternative approach is the SL method, which involves scanning both excitation and emission wavelength simultaneously while keeping a constant wavelength interval between them (58, 59). This method, also referred to as SF, has been developed for multicomponent analysis and has been used to obtain fingerprints

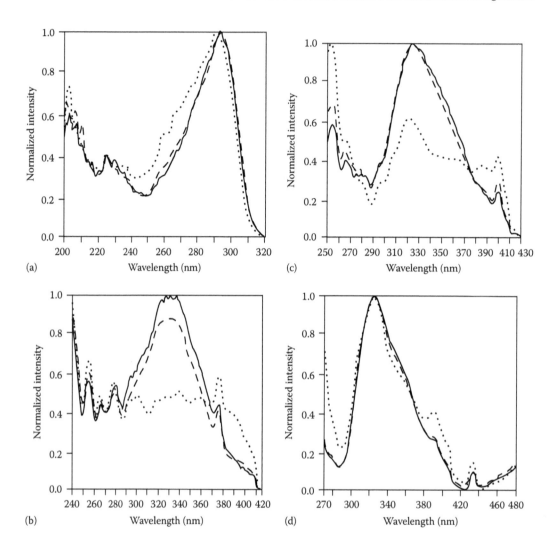

FIGURE 15.5 Native cellular fluorescence of normal oral epithelial cells in culture. This figure shows several normalized fluorescence excitation spectra of normal oral epithelial cells that have been grown in several different media: KGM (dashed line), DMEM/F12/FCS (solid line), and DMEM/F12/NaCl (dotted line). The various culturing media were used to induce different stages of squamous differentiation in the cells, with KGM providing a medium for normal growth without differentiation, DMEM/F12/FCS providing a medium known to cause cell stratification within keratinocytes, and DMEM/F12/NaCl providing a medium capable of inducing the terminal stage of squamous cell differentiation in keratinocytes. The fluorescence excitation scans were taken under the following conditions: (a) λ_{exc} 200–360 nm, λ_{em} 380 nm; (b) λ_{exc} 240–415 nm, λ_{em} 450 nm; (c) λ_{exc} 250–420 nm, λ_{em} 480 nm; (d) λ_{exc} 270–480 nm, λ_{em} 520 nm. From such spectra, it is possible to differentiate between the various states of the cells in vitro. (From Sacks, P.G. et al., *Cancer Lett.*, 104(2), 171, 1996.)

of real-life samples and for enhancing selectivity in the assay of complex systems. This SF procedure has been shown to simplify the emission spectrum and provides for greater selectivity when measuring the fluorescence or phosphorescence from mixtures of compounds.[3,4,40,41] Spectral differences in SF emission profiles are related to the specific macromolecule(s) that differed between neoplastic and normal cells. The SF technique has been shown to improve spectral selectivity in detecting normal and cancer cells for potential use in biomedical diagnostics.[41] Whereas conventional fixed-excitation fluorescence could not show any differentiation between normal and cancerous cell lines, spectral difference between the fluorescence spectra of the normal rat liver epithelial (RLE) and neoplastic rat hepatoma McA cell lines were detected using SF. The results demonstrated the great potential of SF as an improved screening tool for cancer diagnosis in specific cases where conventional fixed-excitation methods are not sufficiently effective.

15.4.2.1.1.2 Biological Fluids, Semen, Seminal Plasma, and Spermatozoa In addition to being used for the study of cancer, autofluorescence microscopy is also being investigated for its potential in many other forms of biomedical diagnostics. One potential application involves the determination of sperm viability and motility for real-time fertility diagnoses. In one such study, fluorescence emission spectra of human semen, seminal plasma, and spermatozoa, excited at 488 nm, were obtained over the range of 500–700 nm. Under these conditions, emission peaks from each component were observed at 622 nm. The intensity of the emission peaks from spermatozoa at 622 nm was strongly correlated with the concentration of spermatozoa ($r = 0.837$, $p = 0.0001$). In addition, sperm motility could also be correlated significantly, although to a poorer extent, with the intensity of the fluorescence emission peaks from spermatozoa ($r = 0.369$, $p = 0.019$) and semen plasma ($r = 0.356$, $p = 0.024$).[42] The SF method has been investigated as a rapid screening tool for monitoring DNA damage (DNA adduct metabolites) in monitoring biological fluids in animal studies, thus providing a technique for early cancer prescreening at the DNA level.[40]

15.4.2.1.2 Cellular Fluorescence Using Exogenous Dyes

Fluorescence analyses of living cells by means of exogenous reporter molecules represent the vast majority of the spectroscopic analyses performed on cells. Such analyses can generally be classified into one of two categories, optical sensor–based analyses or fluorescence imaging–based analyses. Both of these techniques have their advantages and disadvantages for measurement of individual chemical species inside a single living cell. Optical sensors allow for accurate determination of chemical concentrations at individual points in the cell, while imaging-based analyses provide a means of monitoring the spatial distribution of the analyte throughout the cell. Several types of optical sensors have been developed for minimally invasive fluorescence monitoring of individual chemical species inside a single cell.[43-50] These sensors are based on the same principles and concepts as those discussed in Chapter 1, but their dimensions are much smaller. Usually, an exogenous fluorescent dye whose properties (i.e., quantum yield, emission maximum) change in the presence of the analyte of interest is attached to the probing end of the sensor. Such sensors have been used to measure many analytes within living cells, providing information about many different biological processes. These analytes include calcium ions, magnesium ions, nitric oxide, glutamate, lactate, glucose, benzo[a]pyrene tetrol, and even oligonucleotides (i.e., DNA, RNA).[43-50] Because this relatively new field of sensors is described in greater detail in Chapters 22 and 23 in Volume III in this handbook, this chapter will not go into any further detail on the subject.

Fluorescence microscopy is the most common technique for monitoring the spatial distribution of a particular analyte at many different locations simultaneously throughout a cell. In such analyses, one or several different exogenous fluorescent dyes are introduced into the cell and allowed to disperse. After dispersing throughout the cell, they begin to interact with the analyte of interest; this interaction, in turn, causes some change in the fluorescence properties (intensity, spectral shift, etc.) of the dye. Therefore, by obtaining a fluorescence image of the cell at a specific wavelength, corresponding to the maximum emission wavelength of the dye, one can determine the relative concentrations of the analyte at specific locations. The great amount of information derived from such analyses has allowed researchers and companies (e.g., Molecular Probes) to develop many different fluorescent dyes for a wide variety of compounds. These dyes are available with many different excitation and emission maxima for most analytes, allowing the experimenter to choose the best dye for the particular application. The dyes most commonly used today for fluorescence microscopy have red or NIR excitation profiles, thus allowing the dye to be excited without providing the energy necessary to excite any of the autofluorescent species present inside the cell. In addition, the lower-energy light also causes less damage to the living cells than would visible or UV wavelengths, which are capable of cross-linking DNA or proteins.

15.4.2.1.2.1 Cell Proliferation   Cell proliferation analyses are one of the many types of analyses that are often performed using exogenous dyes. Learning about the part of the cell cycle that a particular cell or group of cells is in, or about the way in which it died (e.g., necrosis vs. apoptosis), can provide a great deal of biomedically useful information. For instance, the determination of apoptotic cell death is of particular importance in the study of chemical carcinogenesis as well as in the development of novel PDT drugs. For this reason, many different types of fluorescence analyses have been developed to determine the extent of apoptosis in cells or tissues. One such method employs a commercially available ApopTag kit and automated fluorescence image analysis to quantify the distribution of apoptosis in formalin-fixed, paraffin-embedded liver tumor sections from rats whose tumors were induced by 2-acetylaminofluorene. In this work, specific treatments of tissue sections were developed for quenching the autofluorescence background from the cells of the tissue sample. Once the autofluorescence had been quenched, propidium iodide was used as a counterstain for the nuclei. Automated statistical evaluation of the percentage of nuclei stained positively for apoptosis was determined by using dual fluorescence detection and optical microscopy. The quantitative results indicated that the staining index for apoptosis in normal rat liver cells was 0.14% ± 0.04%, whereas well and poorly differentiated tumor cells showed increases of 3.48% ± 0.59% and 7.41% ± 0.81%, respectively.[51]

15.4.2.1.2.2 Cellular Response   Another important application of fluorescence microscopy using exogenous fluorophores is in elucidating the role of particular chemicals in cellular biology and determining the associated kinetic constants for those processes. One chemical and cellular process that has been investigated using fluorescence microscopy and exogenous fluorophores is protein kinase C (PKC) and its role in signal transduction of many bioactive substances. In this study, phorbol-13-acetate-12-*N*-methyl-*N*-4-(*N*,*N*′-di(2-hydroxyethyl)amino)-7-nitrobenz-2-oxa-1,3-diazole-aminododecanoate [*N*-C12-Ac(13)], the fluorescent derivative of 12-*O*-tetradecanoylphorbol-13-acetate (TPA), was synthesized to monitor the location of phorbol ester binding sites and evaluate its potential use as a probe for PKC in viable cells. The maximum excitation wavelength of *N*-C12-Ac(13) is close to 488 nm, making possible the use of an argon-ion laser for excitation of the dye molecule. When incubated with 100 nM *N*-C12-Ac(13), P3HR-1 Burkitt lymphoma cells accumulated in the dye rapidly, reaching a maximum fluorescence (20-fold above the autofluorescence background) within 25 min. The subsequent addition of unlabeled TPA significantly decreased the fluorescence of *N*-C12-Ac(13) in the cells, in a dose-dependent manner, indicating specific displacement of the bound fluoroprobe. Using this same competitive displacement technique, researchers displaced [3*H*]-phorbol-12,13-dibutyrate ([3*H*]-PBu2) from rat brain cytosol with *N*-C12-Ac(13), which was found to exhibit an apparent dissociation constant and biological activity similar to that of TPA. In addition, like TPA, *N*-C12-Ac(13) also induced the expression of Epstein–Barr viral glycoprotein in P3HR-1 cells and differentiation of promyelocytic HL60 cells and caused predicted changes in the mitotic cycle of histiocytic DD cells. Microscopic fluorometric images of single cells for such analyses verified that the bound dye *N*-C12-Ac(13) showed bright fluorescence in the cytoplasm and a dim fluorescence in the nuclear region, a phenomenon consistent with dye binding mainly to cytoplasmic structures and/or organelles.[52]

15.4.2.1.2.3 Immunocytofluorometric Analyses   In addition to using exogenous fluorescent dyes to monitor the concentration or distribution of various chemicals or ions within a cell, investigators have found useful applications for fluorescence spectroscopy in the identification of specific types of cells in immunocytofluorometric analyses. In such analyses, fluorescent molecules are attached to a monoclonal or polyclonal antibody that is specific to a surface protein or a class of surface proteins on a particular type of cell. The cells to be analyzed are then exposed to these fluorescently labeled antibodies. Once the antibodies have attached to the cells with the appropriate surface proteins, a fluorescence analysis system (e.g., a flow cytometer) can distinguish the cells of interest from the other cells that are present on the basis of some fluorescent property (e.g., spectral band) of the dye molecule attached to the antibody. In a recent example, a time-resolved LIF measurement system was used in conjunction with pyrene-derivatized molecules to perform immunocytofluorometric analyses. By using these pyrene-derivatized molecules [*N*-(1-pyrene)maleimide, 1-pyrenesulfonyl chloride and 1-pyreneisothiocyanate], fluorescent lifetimes for the labeled antimouse IgG were in the range of 20–55 ns. Due to this long lifetime, it was possible to easily distinguish these cells from other nonlabeled cells whose fluorescence lifetimes were much shorter.[53]

15.4.2.2 Tissue Analyses and Diagnostics

Many studies have been performed on tissue samples[7,54–62] to help us understand the interaction between cells and to bring us closer to the much more complex area of in vivo analyses. Tissue studies provide a platform that is much closer to true in vivo analyses in terms of structural architecture on both the microscopic and macroscopic scales than do cellular analyses. Ex vivo tissues provide an excellent starting point for the development of many in vivo diagnostic procedures (e.g., optical biopsy). In addition, when compared with in vivo systems, ex vivo tissue samples are much easier to handle, as well as manipulate.

Over the last two decades, many different types of fluorescent tissue analyses have been performed on a wide variety of samples. The types of tissues range from mouse and rat tumors[59] to human teeth.[60] Instrumentation has ranged from commercially available fluorescence microscopes to laboratory-built research instruments for specialized measurements. The development of fiber-optic instrumentation has made it possible to perform analyses in any area accessible to an endoscope.

15.4.2.2.1 Autofluorescence of Tissues

Many fluorescent species are present in biological tissues, and we want to develop diagnostic techniques that do not require chemical pretreatment of tissues. Therefore, analyses based on autofluorescence represent a large portion of the fluorescence diagnostic procedures that are being developed. Some of the more promising autofluorescent diagnostic results as well as their state of development are described in the following sections.

15.4.2.2.1.1 Cancer Diagnostics
Recently, there has been a great deal of interest in and research in the development of rapid, fluorescence-based clinical oncology.[6,10] Many different techniques have been developed for such analyses in different types of tissues and have shown a great deal of promise. These techniques and the instrumentation used for these measurements are described in greater detail in the following sections of this chapter. The effectiveness of these techniques is often determined by comparing their results with histological data, which is considered the *gold standard*. Based upon the results of these comparisons, we can calculate three quantitative values to provide an objective comparison of various techniques. Calculation of these three quantities (sensitivity, specificity, and accuracy) depends upon classifying a particular analysis as either a true positive (TP), which represents classification by both techniques as malignant; a false positive (FP), which corresponds to a classification as malignant by fluorescence spectroscopy and normal by histology; a FN, which corresponds to a normal classification by fluorescence and a malignant classification by histology; or a true negative (TN), which corresponds to classification by both techniques as normal. Once the appropriate classifications have been performed, sensitivity, specificity, and accuracy are calculated as follows:

$$\text{Sensitivity} = \frac{\text{TP}}{\left(\text{TP} + \text{FN}\right)}$$

$$\text{Specificity} = \frac{\text{TN}}{\left(\text{TN} + \text{FP}\right)}$$

and

$$\text{Accuracy} = \frac{\left(\text{TP} + \text{TN}\right)}{\left(\text{TP} + \text{TN} + \text{FP} + \text{FN}\right)}$$

An example of a laboratory-constructed instrument for tissue analyses is given by Alfano and coworkers, who developed a system for the differentiation of cancerous and normal human breast tissues and lung tissues.[61,62] In this work, they developed a system that uses either a pulsed or continuous-wave (cw) excitation source for the differentiation of normal and cancerous tissues. The fluorescence emission spectrum for normal tissue caused by excitation with 488 nm light from an argon-ion laser was found to be quite different than that for tumor tissue. The resulting spectra from tumor tissues had smooth emission curves with a maximum at approximately 530 nm. The resulting emission spectra from normal tissues appeared to have three peaks, at 530, 550, and 590 nm. In another study, Feld and coworkers attempted to determine the optimal excitation wavelength for distinguishing between normal and tumor tissues based upon their biochemical and histomorphological (architectural) components. They found that the most marked differences occurred when an excitation wavelength of 410 nm was used. Using this wavelength, they correctly diagnosed 20 of 22 samples studied.[63] This optimal wavelength, determined with in vitro studies, is consistent with results obtained by Vo-Dinh and coworkers from in vivo clinical studies of gastrointestinal (GI) cancer diagnostics using LIF.[64,65]

15.4.2.2.1.2 Cervical Cancer   In the field of in vitro fluorescence diagnostics for the detection of cervical cancer, there is a relatively small amount of information. However, the results that have been published forecast a promising future for this technique. In one such study, Richards-Kortum and coworkers investigated fluorescence excitation–emission matrices (EEMs) to analyze 18 cervical biopsies from 10 patients.[55] At all excitation–emission maxima, most prominently at 330 nm excitation and 385 nm emission, the average normalized fluorescence intensity of histologically normal tissue was significantly greater than that of histologically abnormal tissue. A diagnostic algorithm based upon this relative intensity difference was developed to differentiate between histologically normal and abnormal biopsies with a higher sensitivity but a lower positive predictive value and specificity than colposcopy. However, when comparisons of histologically normal and abnormal biopsies from the same patient were performed, sensitivity results of 75%, positive predictive value results of 86%, and specificity results of 88% were achieved for the spectroscopic identification of histological abnormality. These results compare favorably with colposcopy results. Based on these results, in vivo studies of cervical tissue fluorescence have also been conducted.[66]

In addition to the research demonstrating the ability to distinguish between normal cervical tissues and invasive carcinomas in cervical tissue, research has also been performed in an attempt to distinguish between dysplasia and invasive carcinomas. To this end, a technique developed recently for the in situ detection of melanomas has been applied for determining in vitro dysplasia and invasive carcinomas in the cervix uteri. The cervix uteri exhibit a fluorescence band with a peak at about 475 nm upon excitation with 365 nm light. At a fluorescence intensity of 475 nm, the fluorescence intensity increases concomitantly with the degree of dysplasia, ranging from 30 counts/100 ms (healthy) to approximately 200 counts/100 ms (carcinoma in situ [CIS] 3). At the rim of a malignancy, the intensity is 250 counts/100 ms and higher. The excitation and emission spectra of the tissue suggest that the endogenous chromophore responsible for the observed fluorescence is NADH.[67]

15.4.2.2.1.3 Colon Cancer   Another major form of cancer that has seen a significant amount of research and advancement in terms of in vitro fluorescence diagnosis is colon cancer. In one study, unstained frozen sections of colon were studied by fluorescence microscopy to determine which structures fluoresce and to what extent they fluoresce in normal colon tissue and colonic adenomas. Tissues were excited by the 351–364 nm emission from an argon-ion laser. The resulting fluorescence signals from various locations in the tissue samples were correlated to the tissue morphology at those locations via histological analyses with conventional stains (hematoxylin and eosin [H&E], Movat pentachrome, mucicarmine, and oil red O dye). In normal colon tissues, the measured fluorescence signals correlated morphologically with connective tissue fibers (mainly collagen) in all layers of the bowel wall and with cytoplasmic granules within eosinophils present between the crypts in the lamina propria of the mucosa. In addition, fluorescent signals from the crypts of normal cells were very faint. However, a significant fluorescence emission was observed in the cytoplasms of dysplastic epithelial cells in the crypts of colonic adenomas. In the lamina propria of colonic adenomas, a decrease in fluorescence intensity compared to that of normal colon tissue was found to exist. The decrease could be correlated to fewer fluorescent connective tissue fibers in the case of the adenomas. Finally, it was found that a larger number of fluorescent eosino-phils exist in adenomas colonic tissue than in normal colon tissue.[68] Similar results were also found in another study, in which a confocal fluorescence microscope was used.[69]

In an additional study, also aimed at determining the biochemical differences between the fluorescence signals from normal and adenoma colonic tissues, it was found that the fluorescent signals from plasma-soluble melanins derived from various sources were related to the overall autofluorescence signal of adenomatous tissue samples. It was also determined in this study that the fluorescence component of melanins derived from 3-hydroxyanthranilic acid, excited by 324 nm light and measured at 413 nm, was less than the fluorescence caused by melanins derived from other sources (i.e., dopa, catecholamines, catechol, and 3-hydroxykynurenine), with fluorescence excitation and emission maxima at 345 and 445 nm.[70]

In a quantitative determination of the efficacy of fluorescence spectroscopy to classify colonic tissues as adenoma, adenocarcinoma, or nonneoplastic, a series of analyses have been performed on 83 biopsy specimens from several patients. In these tests, fluorescence emission spectra covering a spectral range of 450–800 nm were measured. From these measurements, it was found that the spectral properties were significantly different for the three different tissue classifications. In fact, the results of these analyses had a sensitivity of 80.6% and 88.2% and a specificity of 90.5% and 95.2% in discriminating neoplastic from nonneoplastic mucosa and adenoma from nonneoplastic mucosa, respectively.[71]

With preliminary fluorescence analyses of colon tissues providing promise for a minimally invasive real-time classification procedure for colon cancer, a significant deal of effort is being devoted toward the optimization of this procedure, both experimentally and through data analysis methods. In one such study, fluorescence EEMs were obtained to determine the optimal excitation regions for obtaining fluorescence emission spectra that can be used to differentiate normal and pathologic tissues. In the case of normal and adenomatous colon tissue, the optimal excitation wavelengths were found to be 330, 370, and 430 nm ± 10 nm. These excitation wavelengths were used with simple difference techniques as well as ratiometric analyses to determine the optimal emission wavelengths. Based upon these results, the optimal excitation wavelength for discrimination between normal and adenomas colon tissues in vitro was found to be 370 nm, and the optimal emission wavelengths for analysis based upon this excitation were found to be 404, 480, and 680 nm.[72] In a second study, in which the optimization was based upon data analysis algorithms, 35 resected colonic tissue samples were excited by the 325 nm line of a helium cadmium laser and the resulting fluorescence spectra were measured over the spectral range of 350–600 nm. Scores were derived from these analyses by a multivariate linear regression (MVLR) analysis that accounted for six wavelengths in the emission spectra. Normal tissue samples, adenomatous tissue samples, and hyperplastic tissue samples were classified by using the resulting scores with accuracies of 100%, 100%, and 94%, respectively.[73]

15.4.2.2.1.4 Gastric Cancer Application of fluorescence spectroscopy to in vitro detection of gastric cancers has also been performed. In this work, fluorescence was measured following tissue excitation with the 325 nm light from a helium cadmium laser.[63] Fluorescence images of 72 surface areas of 21 resected tissue samples were recorded in six regions of the visible spectrum by a cooled charge-coupled device (CCD) camera. The fluorescence emission intensities measured at 440 and 395 nm, both normalized to the intensity measured at 590 nm, differed significantly for malignant tissues, premalig-nant tissues, and normal gastric tissues. When these differences were used as a diagnostic parameter, classification of malignant tumor tissues with a sensitivity of 96% and a predictive value of 42% was possible. Additionally, the same approach applied to the diagnosis of abnormal (but nontumor) stomach tissues gave values of 80% and 98%, respectively.[74]

15.4.2.2.1.5 Oral Cancer Biopsy specimens from clinically suspicious lesions and normal-appearing oral mucosa were obtained from patients, and fluorescence EEMs were measured.[54] From these EEMs, it was determined that the optimal excitation wavelength for differentiation between normal and dysplastic tissues was 410 nm. Based upon the fluorescence emission spectra produced by this wavelength for excitation, the 22 different resected samples, 12 histologically normal and 10 abnormal (dysplastic or malignant), were analyzed. From this analysis, 20 of the 22 samples were correctly classified as either normal or abnormal tissues.[63]

15.4.2.2.1.6 Atherosclerosis LIF has been used for the differentiation of calcified and noncalcified plaques in arterial tissues.[64] In this work, 248 nm laser light from a krypton–fluorine excimer laser was used to irradiate normal and severely atherosclerotic segments of human postmortem femoral arteries. In order to analyze deeper layers of the tissue, while measuring the resulting fluorescence from each layer, 16 ns laser pulses were used, each having a fluence of 5 J/cm^2. Pulse powers of this magnitude were sufficient to ablate as well as excite the tissue. By synchronizing the detector with each of the laser pulses, it was possible to determine the characteristic composition of the tissue layer that was ablated. Normal tissue layers provided fluorescence spectra exhibiting a broad-continuum emission between 300 and 700 nm with peak fluorescence of equal intensity at wavelengths of 370–460 nm. Fluorescence maxima of atheromas without calcification occurred at the same wavelengths but with significantly reduced intensity at 460 nm. In contrast to these broad-continuum fluorescence signals from normal and noncalcified atheromas, calcified plaques displayed multiple-line atomic fluorescence (atomic emission) with the most prominent peaks at wavelengths of 397, 442, 450, 461, 528, and 558 nm. These fluorescence/emission criteria identified the histologically classified target tissue precisely. Comparison of this technique to histological examination of the corresponding arterial layers indicated an extremely accurate characterization. These results demonstrated the potential for simultaneous real-time tissue identification and the feasibility of ablation by laser irradiation under strict laboratory conditions.[75]

To diagnose the arterial tissue before ablation, many researchers have attempted to use less powerful and less energetic lasers for fluorescence excitation alone and have had a great deal of success. In one such study, UV-excited LIF using excitation wavelengths ranging from 306 to 310 nm was used to distinguish between normal and atherosclerotic arteries.[65] In this study, two distinct fluorescence emission bands were observed in the LIF spectra of both normal and pathologic aorta, a short-wavelength band peaking at 340 nm (attributed to tryptophan) and a long-wavelength band peaking at 380 nm (attributed to a combination of collagen and elastin). In addition, the intensity of the short-wavelength band was found to be very sensitive to the choice of excitation wavelength while the long-wavelength band remained unchanged; this feature allowed for the relative contributions of each band to be controlled precisely by choice of excitation wavelength. It was found that by using 308 nm excitation to simultaneously observe emissions from both the short- and long-wavelength bands, two ratios could be determined and that from them it was possible to distinguish between normal and atherosclerotic aortic tissue. These two ratios characterized both the relative tryptophan fluorescence content and the ratio of elastin to collagen. In addition, normal and atherosclerotic aortas were correctly distinguished in 56 of 60 total cases by a binary classification scheme in which these parameters were combined. Furthermore, atherosclerotic plaques, atheromatous plaques, and exposed calcifications could be classified individually with sensitivities and predictive values of 90% and 90%, 100% and 75%, and 82% and 82%, respectively.[76]

In another study, even less energetic light was used to excite autofluorescent species in blood vessels for the differentiation of normal tissue and atherosclerotic lesions. The use of longer wavelengths of light for excitation not only caused less photodamage to the irradiated tissue but also allowed better transmission through optical fibers, which were necessary for in vivo light delivery. In this work, 325 nm light was used for excitation of the sample, and a ratio of the fluorescence intensity at 480 nm to the fluorescence intensity at 420 nm was determined for each of the different types of tissues. Based upon these ratios, a clear differentiation between normal and mild as well as between normal and severe atherosclerotic lesions was observed. In the case of normal tissue, there was an increased intensity in the range from 420 to 540 nm, whereas atherosclerotic lesions had no or only a small peak at 480 nm. In addition, the spectroscopic results showed no differences between the samples taken from different types of vessels.[77]

Further studies have extended the wavelengths used for excitation of atherosclerotic tissue samples to 458 nm[78] and even 476 nm.[79] In both cases, even though the autofluorescent tissue components responsible for the fluorescence emission were different from those excited by UV light, good differentiation between normal arterial tissue, noncalcified arterial plaques, and calcified arterial plaques was demonstrated. When these longer wavelengths are used for excitation, differentiation is based upon the ratio of the fluorescence signals from structural proteins (elastin and collagen) and ceroid, which can be correlated to the concentration of these various components.

Several other studies have been performed to correlate LIF signals to the histochemical composition of human arteries and veins.[80,81] In one such study, unstained frozen sections of normal and atherosclerotic human aorta and coronary artery were examined by histochemical and fluorescence microscopy techniques to identify the species responsible for autofluorescence following excitation with light ranging from 351 to 364 nm. The species investigated included the structural proteins elastin and collagen in normal and atherosclerotic specimens, calcium deposits in calcified plaques, and granular or ring-shaped deposits histochemically identified as ceroid found in both calcified and noncalcified plaques. Both the emission wavelength and intensity of ceroid autofluorescence differed greatly from that of elastin or collagen, with the ceroid emission being red shifted and showing a much greater resistance to photobleaching than the structural proteins, thus making it a prime candidate for investigation in the classification of arterial plaques.[80]

In another study aimed at determining the relationship between the histochemical and morphological characteristics of atherosclerotic tissue and their LIF spectra, unstained frozen sections of 47 normal and atherosclerotic human aortas and coronary arteries were excited by 476 nm laser light. The resulting fluorescence images were measured with a bright-field epifluorescence microscope. The samples were then stained with various dyes (including H&E, Movat pentachrome, and oil red O) for histological analysis. In the case of normal artery autofluorescence, the signals correlated with the structural proteins elastin and collagen in the intima, media, and the adventitia. In atherosclerotic plaque, autofluorescence correlated morphologically with lipid or calcific deposits in the atheroma core. The autofluorescence of these deposits was different from that of elastin and collagen in distribution, intensity, and wavelength and increased with the severity of the plaque.

Such excellent correlation both qualitatively and quantitatively suggests that 476 nm excitation-based LIF analyses of arterial tissues would be useful.[81] However, it has recently been found that 476-nm induced autofluorescence in arterial tissues suffers from changes in two prominent spectral characteristics of the emission spectrum. The changes related to alterations in the individual tissue chromophores being excited are a permanent decrease in the peak fluorescence intensity and a reversible change in the fluorescence emission profile (line shape). The permanent changes in absolute fluorescence intensity are due to irreversible photodamage to the tissue fluorophores; the reversible changes in fluorescence line shape are due to some type of alterations in tissue absorbers. An attempt has been made to minimize these effects; excitation intensity levels and exposure times have been investigated to establish the thresholds that these alterations are minimized.[82,83]

To develop a fluorescence guidance system for the laser ablation of arterial plaques in femoral arteries, Gaffney and coworkers have developed a technique that employs dual excitation wavelengths. Information about the fatty plaque content could be obtained from 325 nm excited fluorescence; information about structural proteins and calcific content could be obtained from fluorescence following 476 nm excitation. The fluorescence emission spectra obtained from each of the excitation wavelengths were used to perform ratiometric analyses. For 325 nm excited fluorescence spectra, 78 ratios were determined based upon 13 different wavelengths, and for 476 nm excited spectra, 55 ratios were determined based upon 11 different wavelengths. From these analyses, atherosclerotic lesions in human coronary arteries were characterized by an increase in normalized fluorescence intensity at longer wavelengths when excited with either UV or visible light. Calcific plaque content greater than 10% in lesions more than 1 mm thick was identified by increased normalized fluorescence intensity at 443 nm produced by excitation at 325 nm, and fatty plaque content was found to correlate with fluorescence intensity ratios produced by 325 nm excitation, whereas fibrous and calcific content correlated well with fluorescence ratios during 458 nm excitation.[78]

In addition to using multiple-excitation wavelengths to increase the accuracy and sensitivity of prediction of atherosclerotic tissue, there has also been a recent investigation into the use of time-resolved fluorescence detection rather than spectral-based detection for the differentiation of atherosclerotic tissue from normal tissue. Based upon the temporal differences in the fluorescence emission from atherosclerotic plaques and normal blood vessels, an enhanced differentiation between the two tissue types was reported.[84]

15.4.2.2.1.7 Heart Arrhythmia Autofluorescence spectral properties of tissue have also been used in the diagnosis of heart-related illnesses. Heart arrhythmias are often caused by the formation of nodal conductive tissues. In severe cases of arrhythmia that cannot be treated through conventional medical therapies, transcatheter ablation of the nodal conductive tissue can be performed. Therefore, prior to any tissue ablation, it is important to be able to classify the tissue of interest as nodal conductive tissue, atrial endocardium, or ventricular endocardium. To perform this diagnosis, Lucas and coworkers have studied the fluorescence emission of in vitro heart tissue samples excited by the 308 nm laser line of a XeCl excimer laser (1.5 mJ/pulse, 10 Hz). Following excitation at 308 nm, the nodal tissue could clearly be distinguished from atrial endomyocardial tissue by a visible decrease in fluorescence emission intensity between 440 and 500 nm, peak area between 440 and 500 nm, and peak width. Nodal conduction tissue could also be distinguished from ventricular endocardium by its relative increase in fluorescence emission between 430 and 550 nm. Specificities of 73% and 88% and sensitivities of 73% and 60% were possible for sinus nodal and atrioventricular nodal conduction tissue identification, respectively.[85]

15.4.2.2.1.8 Tooth Decay The field of dentistry has also seen a recent growth of research in the use of fluorescence spectroscopy. In work involving the use of a confocal scanning laser microscope (CLSM), autofluorescence spectra were taken of teeth with demineralized dentin on the root surfaces. The resulting spectra were then compared with spectra taken at other locations on the tooth with minimal to no demineralization in the dentin. When observed in CLSM images, demineralized dentin (excited at 488 nm) exhibited an increased fluorescence emission at 529 nm when compared with the spectra of healthy dentin. This difference in fluorescence intensity decreased deeper into the root, as the healthy dentin underneath the lesion was beginning to be excited. In contrast, when fluorescence spectrophotometry was used with excitation around 460 and 488 nm, it yielded a lower fluorescence emission intensity, about 520 nm, for demineralized dentin than for healthy dentin, but in a more pronounced peak. From excitation spectra obtained by a fixed emission wavelength of 520 nm, it could be seen that in demineralized dentin the contribution of excitation between 480 and 520 nm was more important than in healthy dentin. Because of the small sampling volume used in CLSM image acquisition, the recorded fluorescence was not affected by demineralization-induced changes in scattering and absorption properties. Thus, the increased fluorescence for demineralized dentin implies an increased quantum yield. However, in fluorescence spectrophotometry, where the measurement volume is large relative to the lesions, changes in scattering and absorption properties do have an influence on the fluorescence signal. Therefore, increased absorption by nonfluorescing chromophores and increased reabsorption around the emission wavelength may compensate for the increase in quantum yield and absorption around the excitation wavelength by the fluorophores.[86]

15.4.2.2.1.9 Eosinophils Eosinophils are rare granulocytes that are typically associated with allergic diseases or responses to various parasitic infections. Many types of human cancers, however, are also associated with extensive eosinophilia, either within the tumor itself, in the peripheral blood, or in both locations. Special techniques such as autofluorescence or immunohistochemistry are sometimes needed to detect the presence of intact and degranulating eosinophils within the tumors. With the help of these techniques, extensive amounts of eosinophilia have been found in hematologic tumors such as Hodgkin's disease and certain lymphomas. However, many other types of cancer, such as cancer of the colon, cervix, lung, breast, and ovary, also contain eosinophilia, and it can be identified if diligently sought. Although the presence or absence of eosinophilia within these tumors does not appear to have a major influence on the prognosis of the disease, eosinophils may play an important role in the host interaction with the tumor, perhaps by promoting angiogenesis and connective tissue formation adjacent to the cancer. In addition, tumor-related eosinophilia provides some interesting clues into tumor biology, particularly with regard to production of cytokines by the tumor cells.[87] Characterization of the fluorescence properties of human eosinophils isolated from peripheral blood of normal donors has been performed by measuring EEMs over a wide range of wavelengths. Circulating eosinophils possess three fluorescence emission maxima: one at 330 nm following excitation at 280 nm, which can be attributed to tryptophan, a second peak at 440 nm following excitation at 360 nm, and the last at 415 nm following excitation with 380 nm light. Fluorescence microscopy studies also showed that the fluorescence of eosinophils appears to be site dependent. For instance, when observed following excitation by 365 nm light, circulating eosinophils fluoresce blue violet, while tissue-dwelling eosinophils fluoresce amber gold. Therefore, when fluorescence spectroscopy is used to develop optical biopsy techniques based upon eosinophils in human tissue, the differences in their local environments may have a significant impact on fluorescence spectra.[88]

15.4.2.2.2 *Tissue Analysis Using Exogenous Dyes*

Due to the significant differences in tissue uptake and storage of various exogenous fluorophores between in vitro specimens and in vivo specimens, relatively few studies have been performed in this area in terms of developing diagnostic procedures. In most cases where exogenous fluorophores are used, it is the actual location and kinetics of tissue uptake that are important. Therefore, since in vitro tissues differ in these properties, such studies generally do not provide any useful information. However, properties such as tissue reactivity to a specific chemical can be studied by using in vitro systems to provide a better understanding of the mechanism by which specific reactions take place.

15.4.2.2.2.1 Lipid Peroxidation   One system that has been studied by using fluorescence CLSM is the well-established experimental model of lipid peroxidation induced by haloalkane intoxication in liver tissues. In this study, the fluorescent reagent 3-hydroxy-2-naphtholic acid hydrazide was used to derivatize the carbonyl functional groups originating from the lipoperoxidative process in liver cryostat sections from in vivo intoxicated rats, as well as isolated hepatocytes that were exposed in vitro to the haloalkanes. The resulting CLSM images were able to visualize the tissue areas and the subcellular sites first involved in oxidative stress and lipid peroxidation. The images obtained also showed that haloalkane-induced lipid peroxidation in hepatocytes primarily involves the perinuclear endoplasmic reticulum, whereas the plasma membrane and the nuclear compartment are unaffected, and that lipid peroxidation also induces an increase of liver autofluorescence.[89]

15.4.3 In Vivo Analyses and Diagnostics

While in vitro studies can reduce the complexity of the biological system analyzed and provide useful information about basic biological functions or reactions, there is a critical need to develop in vivo analysis techniques for medical diagnosis of diseases. The range of fluorescence-based in vivo diagnostic techniques spans from the monitoring of atherosclerosis[90] to the detection of tooth decay.[60,91] One of the most common biomedical diagnostic procedures that is performed using fluorescence spectroscopy is known as *optical biopsy*.[10,24,92–102] In this procedure, some form of optical spectroscopy, typically fluorescence spectroscopy, is used to identify differences between healthy, malignant, and premalignant tissues of various organs. Over the past two decades, a great deal of research has been performed in this field for the diagnosis of many different forms of cancer.[6,59,61,64,65,99,103–118] In order to ensure that the various diagnostic procedures will work in complex living systems, two types of analyses are generally performed: animal studies and clinical human trials.

15.4.3.1 Animal Studies

Animals typically provide an excellent test system for many different types of disease diagnoses prior to clinical studies. The key in choosing an animal for these studies is to ensure that the biochemical structure of the particular organ or location of the animal that is being used is comparable to that of a human. In addition, the animal should be relatively easy to care for and should match any other criterion for the particular type of analysis that is to be performed. Mice and rats are often used as a suitable alternative for humans in many preliminary studies because of their 98% genetic compatibility with humans and because they are relatively easy to handle; however, many other animal models have also been investigated (e.g., hamster and pigs).

In the case of *optical biopsy* work or PDT, transgenic mice with transplantable tumors are the most common model system. These transgenic mice have been genetically altered to prevent the mice from providing an immune response to the tumors that are induced in them. By using these mice with transplantable tumors, valuable information useful to later clinical trials can be obtained. However, the use of animal models could have artifacts as well. For instance, when using mice with transplantable tumors for tumor detection diagnostics, the tumor tissue that is implanted generally comes from a different type of tissue and therefore may not have the same biochemistry, architecture, and vasculature as the tissue into which it is being placed. In addition, unlike spontaneous tumors in humans, transplanted tumors often remain mostly separated from the normal tissue. When exogenous fluorophores are used as contrast agents in fluorescence diagnostics, there is also an issue of species-dependent chemical distribution or pharmacokinetics. These problems also begin to become convoluted by the fact that drug pharmacokinetics are often very different between early stages and more advanced stages of cancer or transplanted tumors because vascularization differs.[119,120] One way to minimize these problems in tumor studies is to induce the tumor chemically or radiologically. This will allow the tumor to be integrated into the tissue as well as ensure that the tumor being investigated came from the same type of tissue in which it is growing.

One well-established tumor model procedure is to use dimethylbenzanthracene (DMBA) to induce lesions in the cheek pouches of hamsters. This particular model is useful as it progresses through many different stages of cancer development: normal tissue to hyperplastic tissue to dysplastic tissue to CIS and finally to invasive carcinoma.[121] Both endogenous and exogenous fluorophores have been used for in vivo diagnostics based on this model. In the case of the autofluorescence diagnostics, it has been reported that 76% sensitivity and 86% specificity have been obtained in the detection of early neoplastic tissue. In addition, by intravenously administering the photosensitizer Photofrin™ 24 h prior to analysis, both the sensitivity and the specificity could be increased to 100%.

15.4.3.1.1 Animal Studies Using Autofluorescence

With analyses on living animals, it is possible to gain a much more accurate picture in most cases than can be achieved in vitro. For instance, one of the strongest chromophores present in tissues is hemoglobin (oxy- and deoxy), in in vitro studies, there is no blood flow present, and the ratio of oxygenated hemoglobin to deoxygenated hemoglobin is very different than in live animal studies. This factor alone could have a significant effect on the autofluorescence spectrum of the tissue, either by absorbing the fluorescent light or by changing the oxidative state of some of the autofluorescent chemicals that are present.

15.4.3.1.1.1 Cancer Diagnostics

Esophageal cancer: The capacity to identify subclinical neoplastic diseases of the upper aerodigestive tract using tissue autofluorescence spectroscopy has significantly contributed to the field of fluorescence cancer screening. In 1993, the applicability of tissue autofluorescence for the early diagnosis of precancerous states in esophageal mucosa was studied through various model systems.[122] In an *N*-nitroso-*N*-methylbenzylamine (NMBA)-induced rat esophageal cancer model, alteration of the fluorescence emission pattern at 380 nm was found to correspond to disease progression from normal mucosa through dysplasia to invasive cancer. While gross assessment of the tissue was indistinguishable from the saline-treated controls, histopathologic evaluation revealed NMBA-induced preneoplastic changes in the epithelium.[123] In addition, a multicellular tumor spheroid model, induced by trans-retinoic acid (RA), was also found to alter autofluorescence intensities at multiple wavelengths including 340, 450, and 520 nm. Such RA-induced alterations corresponded to changes in the state of spheroid differentiation.[122]

Brain cancer: Brain tumors are one of the more difficult forms of cancer to treat. Unlike many other forms of cancer, where tumor margining can be less important, and healthy tissue surrounding the tumor can be removed to ensure that no malignant cells are left behind, the removal of excess brain tissue during tumor removal can have dramatic adverse effects. Because of this important requirement, a technique capable of providing an accurate demarcation between malignant cells and normal brain cells is extremely important. One method that is being developed to address this issue is autofluorescence-based optical biopsy. In initial animal studies, EEMs of rat gliomas revealed three distinct regions of decreased autofluorescence emission with respect to the normal rat brain tissue. These differences in the fluorescence emission spectra of the two different types of tissue samples occurred at 470, 520, and 630 nm, with corresponding excitation wavelengths of 360, 440, and 490 nm. The fluorescence emission at 470 nm corresponds to NAD(P)H, while the emissions of 520 and 630 nm correspond to various flavins and porphyrins, respectively. Due to the nature of the chemical differences between the normal tissue and the glioma tissue, this finding suggests that there is a relationship between brain tissue autofluorescence and metabolic activity. This is in contrast to in vitro brain tissue studies, which also found that NAD(P)H fluorescence was lower in all measured human brain tumors, but, depending on their nature, flavin and porphyrin autofluorescence in neoplastic tissues was not always lower than in normal tissue.[124]

Atherosclerosis: Due to the high occurrence rate of atherosclerosis in adults, and the preliminary success of LIF in diagnosing the disease in its various stages in vitro, animal studies have been performed to ensure that the same fluorescence phenomena occur in living systems. In one such study, a XeCl excimer laser operating at 308 nm was used to excite proteins of human aortas containing early lipid-rich noncollagenous lesions. The emitted fluorescence exhibited significant red shifts and spectral broadening compared with spectra from nonatherosclerotic human aortas. Similar red-shifted and spectrally broadened autofluorescence profiles were observed from oxidatively modified low-density lipoproteins excited by 308 nm illumination. However, in the case of native low-density lipoproteins, neither the red shift nor the spectral broadening was found to exist. In order to compare these tissue results to the autofluorescence emission from live animals, LIF studies were performed on hypercholesterolemic rabbits with early foam cell lesions. The resulting autofluorescence spectra were similar to those of oxidized beta low-density lipoprotein, the major lipoprotein accumulating in arteries of rabbits fed cholesterol, and an early indicator of atherosclerosis.[125]

15.4.3.1.2 Animal Studies Using Exogenous Dyes

The study of exogenous fluorophores in living animals can provide a great deal of information. In addition to being a model system that more closely resembles human when testing fluorescence-based diagnostic systems prior to clinical trials, they also play a large part in the field of pharmacokinetics. Using living animals with functioning circulatory systems, it is possible to watch the real-time distribution of various drugs throughout the body as well as study their uptake into various tissues and finally their excretion from the body. This is an extremely important field or research, as it ensures that drugs are delivered timely to the target tissue areas of interest.

Cancer Diagnostics: Some of the more commonly studied exogenous fluorophores in biomedical analyses are used for cancer diagnosis or treatment or both. These fluorophores, known as photolabels in the case of the former and photosensitizers in the case of the latter, represent an extensive class of compounds whose pharmacokinetics properties as well as their tumor demarcation abilities need to be studied prior to use in human trials. These studies are generally performed on animal subjects, with several of the more common ones described in the following sections.

Pharmacokinetics of photosensitizers: Photosensitizers represent a unique class of compounds, which upon being activated by the absorption of a specific wavelength of light are capable of killing the surrounding tissues. A detailed description of the mechanism of action of these photosensitizers is described in Volume III, Chapter 1 this handbook. Therefore, only salient features are briefly described here. The concept behind these photosensitizers is to develop drugs that are preferentially taken up or localized in malignant tissues and can then be photoactivated. After the drug is administered and a specific amount of time has passed for optimal uptake, light is shown on the tissue area of interest and absorbed by the sensitizer. The sensitizer then kills the surrounding tumor tissue, leaving the healthy tissue undamaged.

While the number of available photosensitizers approved for clinical use is relatively small, a large number of new potential candidates are continually being developed. These new agents are then compared with the better characterized sensitizers based upon many parameters, including tissue localization ability, effectiveness in promoting cell death, toxicity, and several other parameters. In a study to determine the most effective photosensitizer of five commonly used drugs, their tissue localization properties were studied in vivo using *sandwich* observation chambers and tumors that were growing in thigh muscle. Several common dyes that were studied include HpD, Photofrin II, aluminum phthalocyanine tetrasulfonate, uroporphyrin I, and acridine red. Of the photodynamically active dyes (the first three), aluminum phthalocyanine tetrasulfonate was found to exhibit the best in vivo tumor localization properties as determined by fluorescence spectroscopy.[126]

LIF studies have also been used to investigate the pharmacokinetic properties of ALA-induced protoporphyrin IX (PpIX). These analyses were performed in normal and tumor tissues of rats following intravenous (i.v.) injection of ALA. The aim of the study was to investigate ALA-induced (PpIX) formation and its accumulation in different types of rat tissues after the systemic administration of ALA. Tissue types investigated included a malignant rat tumor and normal tissue from 13 different organs in 8 rats. The various rats were injected with two different doses of ALA (30 and 90 mg/kg body weight), and fluorescence analyses were performed 10, 30, and 240 min after injection. Fluorescence analyses were performed by exciting the sample with 405 nm light and monitoring the resulting fluorescence with a fiber-optic probe over the spectral region of 400–750 nm. The fluorescence signal consisted of a broadband autofluorescence background with a maximum at approximately 500 nm and a characteristic dual-peak emission from the PpIX at 635 and 705 nm. From this work, it was found that the maximum tumor buildup of PpIX was achieved in less than 1 h after ALA injection, that the fluorescence demarcation between tumor and surrounding tissue was between 7:1 and 8:1 after 30 min, and that it decreased with longer retention times. Of the 13 different organs that were investigated in this study, PpIX buildup was found to be particularly high in the stomach and the intestine.[127]

Another class of exogenous dyes that have been used for tumor demarcation are Hps and HpDs. In a pharmacokinetic study of Hp, rats were administered i.v. injections of the dye, followed by immediate and continuous analysis by LIF. Excitation of the Hps was provided by the 337 nm output of a nitrogen laser, and the signal was collected by an optical multichannel analyzer (OMA), which allowed for acquisition of the entire fluorescence spectrum for each laser shot. Upon analysis of the data from several of the rat's organs, it was found that the fluorescence emission from the Hp, at 630 nm, exhibited an initial peak intensity as well as a delayed peak intensity. The DF peak was described as being due to the chemical components of intracellularly transformed HpDs. In addition, it was also discovered that by dividing the background-free 630 nm signal by the autofluorescence intensity at shorter (blue) wavelengths, a ratio exhibiting a larger contrast between tumor and surrounding tissue could be obtained that would greatly aid in tumor demarcation.[128]

A third and relatively recent photosensitizer that has been used for the demarcation of tumor tissues is benzoporphyrin derivative monoacid (BPD-MA). In LIF studies designed to provide pharmacokinetic information about this compound, 337 nm light from a nitrogen laser was used to excite the BPD-MA in rats that had been administered via i.v. The fluorescence emission, over the spectral range of 380–750 nm, was then monitored with a spectrometer equipped with a diode array detector. Three hours after the injection period, the fluorescence signals were measured from many different types of rat tissue, including malignant tumors that had been experimentally induced. These results were then compared with results from several other common sensitizers, such as Hp, polyhematoporphyrin ester (PHE), tetrasulfonated phthalocyanine (TSPc), and the commercially available Photofrin. After 3 h, the demarcation potential between tumor and surrounding tissue in terms of fluorescence signal for the tumor model used was 2:1 for BPD-MA. When compared with the other drugs such as HP, it shows about the same demarcation potential, whereas Photofrin and PHE exhibit about 3 times better and TSPc about 1.5 times better demarcation. It was also found that by employing the endogenous tissue fluorescence signature, the contrast was enhanced by a factor of about two for each of the five drugs.[129]

In work by Nilsson et al., the biodistribution of two recently developed tumor markers, trimethylated (CP(Me)3) and trimethoxylated (CP(OMe)3) carotenoporphyrin (CP), was investigated by means of LIF. In this study, 38 tumor-bearing (MS-2 fibrosarcoma) female Balb/c mice were administered the drugs through i.v. injection. At 3, 24, 48, or 96 h after administration, the CP fluorescence was measured in tumoral and peritumoral tissue, as well as in the abdominal, thoracic, and cranial cavities. Excitation of the exogenous dye was performed by using the 425 nm emission of a nitrogen-pumped dye laser and was measured by a spectrometer equipped with an intensified CCD (ICCD) at 490, 655, and 720 nm. The emission bands at 655 and 720 nm correspond to CP, whereas the band at 490 nm represents a location near the maximum of the autofluorescence emission of the tissue. The tissues that showed the greatest extent of CP-related fluorescence were the tumors and the liver tissues, whereas the cerebral cortex and muscle tissues consistently exhibited weak CP-related fluorescence. Additionally, while the fluorescence intensity of most tissue types decreased over time, it was found that the fluorescence intensity in the liver remained constant over the full 96 h that it was investigated.[130]

Oral cancer: Apart from pharmacokinetic analyses of various sensitizers, animal studies with these compounds have also been performed to verify and quantify the ability of these drugs for tumor demarcation in different types of tissues. One such study investigated the effectiveness of porfimer-sodium-derived drugs for the detection of early neoplastic changes in the oral cavity of hamsters. Neoplasia was induced in the hamsters' cheek pouches by the application of 9,10-dimethyl-1,2-benzanthracene. Following formation of neoplastic tissue in the hamster cheek pouch, autofluorescence analyses as well as fluorescence analyses using porfimer sodium as an exogenous tumor demarcation drug were performed and were compared with histological results of the same tissue sites. When the two fluorescence diagnostic techniques were compared with the histological results, it was found that the autofluorescence analysis was capable of 76% sensitivity and 83% specificity, whereas the porfimer-sodium-based fluorescence technique provided 100% sensitivity and specificity for the samples investigated.[131]

Pancreatic cancer: Ph-a represents another of the many different types of tumor demarcation drugs that have been used for optical differentiation of normal tissues and tumor tissues. To test its viability for the detection pancreatic tumors, LIF analyses of Ph-a were used to image six intrapancreatic tumors and six healthy pancreases in vivo in rats. Ph-a was intravenously administered to the rats at a concentration of 9 mg/kg body weight, and fluorescence images were acquired up to 48 h after injection of the drug. Excitation of the blue tissue autofluorescence was performed by using 355 nm light from a frequency-tripled Nd:YAG laser, while excitation of the dye was performed by the 610 nm output from an Nd:YAG pumped dye laser. Fluorescence images were obtained at three different wavelengths; band-pass filters were used for wavelength selection. Images at 470 and 640 nm were used to monitor the autofluorescence of the tissue, while images at 680 nm were taken to obtain composite images of the dye and autofluorescence emissions together. In order to achieve a good contrast between the normal pancreatic tissue and the tumor tissue, the autofluorescence intensity of the 640 nm image was normalized to the background fluorescence intensity in the 680 nm image prior to being subtracted from the 680 nm image. Following this subtraction, the differential image was divided by the autofluorescence image at 470 nm. The resulting ratiometric images allowed for safe diagnoses to be made by providing well-contrasted tumor images.[24]

Brain tumors: Animal models have also been used in studies in which HpD was used for the diagnosis of brain tumors. In this study, adult Wistar rats had C6 glioma cells implanted into their brains to act as a cerebral glioma model. After the tumors had developed to a size of 7–12 mm in diameter, they were injected intravenously with 5 mg/kg body weight of HpD, and continuous fluorescence analyses were performed for 24 h using a fiber-optic-based fluorimeter. Sixty minutes after injection, the fluorescence intensity of the normal brain tissue reached a plateau, while the glioma region reached a plateau 80 min after injection. Fluorescence analyses of glioma, brain tissue adjacent to the tumor (BTAT), and normal brain tissue 24 h after injection revealed that the fluorescence intensity of the glioma was 6.1 times greater than that of normal brain tissue; the BTAT also was 3.9 times greater than the normal tissue.[132]

Liver cancer: Testing of the efficacy of PDT using ALA-induced PpIX sensitization for the treatment of hepatic tumors was performed with rat models. Liver tumors were induced in the rats by either local inoculation of tumors cells or by administration of the tumor cells through the portal vein. Following tumor formation, 60 mg/kg body weight of ALA was administered intravenously. After 60 min, the PpIX in the heptic tumor tissue was excited, initiating the PDT treatment as well as allowing the PpIX to be excited. The resulting fluorescence emission was monitored at 635 nm. Fluorescence analyses revealed that large accumulations of the PpIX occurred in the heptic tumor as well as in the normal liver tissue but not in the abdominal wall muscles. In addition to fluorescence analyses, laser Doppler imaging was used to determine changes in the superficial blood flow in connection with PDT. Histopathological examinations were also performed to evaluate the PDT effects on the tumor and the surrounding liver tissue, including pathological features in the microvascular system. Laser Doppler imaging results indicated that there was an effect on the vascular system in the tumor as well as the surrounding tissue following PDT treatment, as determined by a decreased blood flow in the treated area. In addition, the tumor growth rate decreased significantly when evaluated 3 and 6 days after the treatment, showing that ALA-induced PDT holds promise for the treatment of heptic tumors.[133]

15.4.3.2 Human Studies and Clinical Diagnostics

The most common type of fluorescence-based biomedical diagnostic procedure used in clinical studies is by far the optical detection of malignant or premalignant tissues in various organs. Among the more common types of tumors that have been investigated with this technique are skin, urinary bladder, bronchus, GI, head and neck, gynecological, breast, and brain cancers. Currently, two very different approaches to these fluorescence-based optical biopsy techniques are employed. The first of these techniques relies on the subtle differences in the tissue composition and morphology between normal, dysplastic, and malignant tissues and their effect on the autofluorescence properties for differentiation. Examples of this type of diagnoses will be discussed in Section 15.4.3.2.1. The second type of fluorescence-based diagnostic technique that is employed relies on the presence of exogenous fluorophores, such as PDT photosensitizers, for the tissue differentiation.

15.4.3.2.1 Clinical Studies and Diagnostics Using Autofluorescence

Autofluorescence-based optical biopsy techniques represent the ideal form of fluorescence-based diagnostic procedure. In these analyses, laser light is used to excite the naturally occurring fluorophores in the tissue, and the differences in chemical composition between the various types of tissue will allow for real-time diagnoses without removal of a tissue sample or treatment with a contrast-enhancing drug. Because of this and the great deal of promise that initial studies have shown, research in this field is currently experiencing a large growth.

15.4.3.2.1.1 Cancer Diagnostics (Optical Biopsy)

Cervical cancer: Cervical cancer is the second most common malignancy in women worldwide and remains a significant health problem. Despite the widely used Papanicolaou smear (Pap smear) screening procedure, and costly treatments, the overall survival rate remains 40%. Because of these reasons, efforts to strengthen screening and prevention are needed.[134] Autofluorescence optical biopsy techniques offer just such a screening technique with automated diagnosis in real time and comparable sensitivity and specificity to colposcopy.[135] Feld and coworkers demonstrated the ability to distinguish between various types of tissues, in vivo, based upon multicomponent analysis (Figure 15.6).[37]

Richards-Kortum and coworkers have used LIF, employing 337 nm excitation to differentiate in vivo cervical intraepithelial neoplasia (CIN), nonneoplastic abnormal, and normal cervical tissues from one another.[136] In this work, a colposcope was used to identify normal and abnormal sites on the cervix. These sites were then interrogated via fluorescence spectroscopy with an optical fiber probe. Based upon the results from the fluorescence analyses, two algorithms were developed for the diagnosis of CIN. The first of these algorithms allowed for the differentiation of histologically abnormal tissues from colposcopically normal tissues with a sensitivity, specificity, and a positive predictive value of 92%, 90%, and 88%, respectively. The second algorithm then allows for the differentiation of preneoplastic and neoplastic tissues from nonneoplastic abnormal tissues with a sensitivity, specificity, and positive predictive value of 87%, 73%, and 74%, respectively. These results found that as the tissue progresses from a normal state to an abnormal state in the same patient, it is accompanied by a decrease in the absolute fluorescence contribution of collagen, an increase in the absolute attenuation by oxyhemoglobin, and an increase in the relative contribution from reduced nicotinamide dinucleotide phosphate [NAD(P)H]. Differentiation of the various tissues is then determined by the extent of each of these factors. Such results provide a great deal of hope to the future of in vivo fluorescence spectroscopy for the diagnosis of CIN at colposcopy.[136,137]

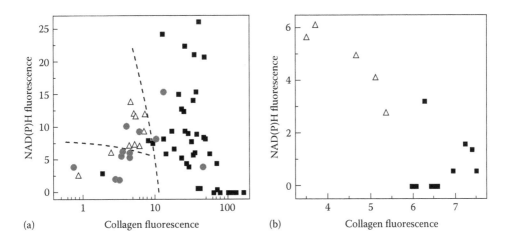

FIGURE 15.6 Study of in vivo quantitative fluorescent biomarkers of epithelial precancerous changes. This figure demonstrates the ability to distinguish between various types of tissues, in vivo, based upon a multicomponent fluorescence analysis. (a) Demonstrates the ability to differentiate between normal ectocervical tissue (n), squamous metaplasia sites (·), and high-grade squamous intraepithelial lesions based upon this 2D analysis procedure. The dashed lines represent the boundary between the different tissues, based upon logistic regression analysis. (b) Demonstrates the ability to differentiate between nondysplastic tissues (n) and high-grade dysplastic tissue sites. (From Renkoski, T.E. et al., *J. Biomed. Opt.*, 18(1), 016005, 2013.)

Esophageal cancer: Esophageal cancers, like most other cancers, generally progress through a series of stages. Barrett's esophagus (BE), named after the physician who first identified the condition,[138] is an abnormality resulting from long-term acid reflux and is associated with an increased occurrence of mucosal dysplasia and adenocarcinoma in the specialized glandular mucosa.[139–141] In addition, individuals with BE have a tendency to develop cancer of the esophagus, with a 30- to 52-fold increase over individuals without this condition.[142,143] In esophageal cancer, the mucosa progresses from *normal* through low-grade dysplasia (LGD) to high-grade dysplasia (HGD) and finally cancer. If detected early, endoscopic treatment of dysplasia with PDT or thermal ablation can be effective, thereby eliminating the need for surgical esophagectomy.

Vo-Dinh and coworkers have developed a LIF diagnostic procedure for in vivo detection of GI cancer that uses 410 nm laser light from a nitrogen-pumped dye laser passed through a fiber-optic probe to excite the tissue.[104,105,118] After the tissue is excited, the resulting fluorescence emission is collected by the same fiber-optic probe and is recorded on an OMA in 600 ms. Based upon the resulting fluorescence spectra, a diagnostic technique known as differential normalized fluorescence (DNF) was employed to enhance the slight spectral differences between normal and malignant tissues.[64,65] This technique greatly improves the accuracy of diagnosis, as compared to direct intensity measurements, since each spectrum is normalized with respect to its total integrated intensity and therefore becomes independent of the intensity factor. This in turn enhances small spectral features in weak fluorescence signals, making classification much easier. The sensitivity of the DNF method in classifying normal tissue and malignant tumors is 98%.[65,118] The LIF methodology was also employed in clinical studies of over 100 patients, in which Barrett's mucosa without dysplasia was diagnosed with a specificity of 96% (208 of 216 data points) and HGD was diagnosed with a sensitivity of 90% (9 of 10).[104,105] Figure 15.7 shows the instrument setup for GI cancer diagnostics.[64]

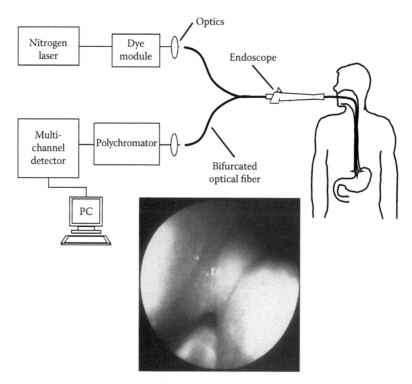

FIGURE 15.7 LIF instrument for in vivo GI cancer diagnostics. This figure shows a typical fluorescence-based optical biopsy system in which a fiber-optic probe is transmitted down a biopsy channel of an endoscope for point-by-point types of analyses. Insert photograph of the optical fiber inside the GI tract. (From Vo-Dinh, T. et al., *Appl. Spectrosc.*, 51(1), 58, 1997.)

A photograph of the optical fiber inside the GI tract is shown in the insert of this figure. Figure 15.8 shows clinical data demonstrating the capability of LIF to differentiate normal tissues from malignant tissues.[64]

Bladder cancer: Bladder cancer has also shown a significant amount of promise for being clinically diagnosed by autofluorescence analyses. In one such study, a quartz fiber-optic probe, which is placed in the working channel of a cystoscope, was used to deliver 337 nm laser light from a nitrogen laser to the tissue area of interest. Following excitation, the resulting fluorescent light was collected by a second fiber and was then spectrally dispersed before being detected by an OMA. Resulting fluorescence emission spectra were then analyzed by taking a ratio of the intensity of the fluorescent light at 385 nm to the fluorescence intensity at 455 nm. This ratiometric analysis was used to analyze 114 lesions, and it was possible to clearly differentiate between malignant and nonmalignant bladder tissues with a sensitivity of 98%.[144]

In another study, the ability of laser-induced autofluorescence spectroscopy to distinguish between neoplastic urothelial bladder lesions and normal or nonspecific inflammatory mucosa was investigated. In this study, three different pulsed-laser wavelengths were used successively for excitation: 308 nm (XeCl laser),

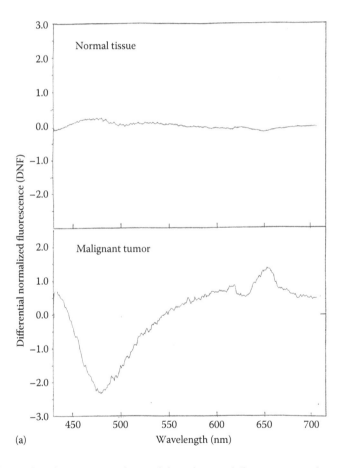

(a)

FIGURE 15.8 Clinical data demonstrating the capability of LIF to differentiate normal tissues from malignant tissues. (a) DNF emission spectra of both normal tissue (top) and malignant tissue (bottom). These DNF spectra were obtained by normalizing the fluorescence intensity at every point in the spectrum to the overall area under the curve, thus emphasizing small differences between the two types of tissues. By subtracting the DNF spectrum of a particular sample from an average DNF normal tissue spectrum, a single index value at each wavelength can be determined. (From Vo-Dinh, T. et al., *Appl. Spectrosc.*, 51(1), 58, 1997.)

(continued)

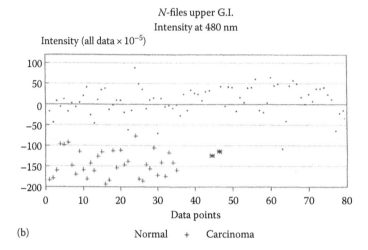

(b)   Normal   +   Carcinoma

FIGURE 15.8 (continued) Clinical data demonstrating the capability of LIF to differentiate normal tissues from malignant tissues. (b) Plot of DNF indices at 480 nm for different tissue samples using in vivo LIF measurements (taken prior to biopsy). These tissue samples were then characterized via histology as either normal (·) or carcinoma (+). As expected, the normal tissue results are scattered about the index value of zero, while the carcinoma values are significantly lower due to a decrease in fluorescence intensity at this wavelength. The samples denoted by (∗) represent points initially classified by histology as normal but were later reclassified as malignant. The sensitivity of the DNF method in classifying normal tissue and malignant tumors for GI cancer is 98%.[65,118] (From Vo-Dinh, T. et al., *Appl. Spectrosc.*, 51(1), 58, 1997.)

337 nm (N_2 laser), and 480 nm (coumarin dye laser). The excitation beam was delivered through optical fibers placed in the working channel of a standard cystoscope, and the resulting fluorescence was detected using an OMA. When 337 and 480 nm excitation wavelengths were used, the overall fluorescence intensity of bladder tumors was clearly decreased compared with normal urothelial mucosa regardless of tumor stage and grade. However, when 308 nm excitation was employed, the shape of the tumor spectra, including CIS, was markedly different from that of normal or nonspecific inflammatory mucosa.[145]

Colon cancer: Autofluorescence diagnostic procedures are used extensively to investigate colon cancers. In one such study, 337 nm light from a nitrogen laser was launched into a fiber-optic probe that was placed in the working channel of a colonoscope and was used for excitation of colon tissues, both in vivo and in vitro. The fluorescence spectra were then measured and analyzed. In all cases, the spectra exhibited peaks at 390 and 460 nm, which are believed to arise from collagen and NADH, as well as a minimum at 425 nm, consistent with absorption attributable to hemoglobin. Despite the presence of these bands in both the in vivo and in vitro samples, the relative intensity of each was quite different, especially for the NADH component, whose intensity was found to decay exponentially with time after resection. Differentiation of normal colonic tissue from hyperplastic or adenomatous tissues of the same type (i.e., in vivo vs. in vitro) could be accomplished based upon a decrease in the collagen component of the autofluorescence and an increase in hemoglobin reabsorption. When an MVLR analysis based upon these differences was used, neoplastic tissues could be distinguished from nonneoplastic tissues with a sensitivity, specificity, positive predictive value, and negative predictive value toward neoplastic tissue of 80%, 92%, 82%, and 91%, respectively. However, when this same MVLR technique was used to distinguish neoplastic polyps from nonneoplastic polyps, values of 86%, 77%, 86%, and 77%, respectively, were obtained, suggesting that the LIF measurements sense changes in polyp morphology rather than changes in fluorophores specific to polyps, and it is this change in morphology that leads indirectly to polyp discrimination.[146]

Laser-induced autofluorescence spectroscopy has been investigated to detect colonic dysplasia in vivo using an excitation wavelength of 370 nm.[139] In this work, fluorescence emission data were used to devise an algorithm to classify colonic tissue as either normal, hyperplastic, or adenomatous based on probability distributions of the fluorescence intensity at 460 nm and the ratio of the intensity at 680 nm to that at 600 nm. Fluorescence spectra were then collected from normal mucosa and colonic polyps during routine colonoscopy exams, and the predictive abilities of the diagnostic algorithm were tested in a blinded fashion, with histology results being the standard against which they were measured. Results revealed that the algorithm correctly determined the tissue type in 88% of cases, equal to the agreement of independent pathologists. In addition, the sensitivity, specificity, and positive predictive value for the detection of dysplasia was 90%, 95%, and 90%, respectively.[147]

In additional studies, by Feld and coworkers, LIF studies were performed on 20 different patients, providing analyses on 31 colonic adenomas, 4 hyperplastic polyps, and 32 samples of normal mucosa. From these studies, it was found that classification of the tissue as either adenomatous or normal colonic mucosa/hyperplastic polyp was correct, based upon an automated probabilistic algorithm, 97% of the time. The sensitivity, specificity, and positive predictive value of the technique was 100%, 97%, and 94%, respectively, once again showing a great deal of promise for this technique in the future.[148]

Lung cancer: Lung cancer accounts for 25% of all cancer deaths and is currently the most common cause of cancer death among both men and women in the United States. Currently, patients are diagnosed only when the cancer is already in a severe state, as there is no rapid, practical, and effective screening test available for lung cancer. In lung cancer, premalignant epithelium usually progresses to a malignant tumor through the development of dysplasia, starting from LGD and progressing to HGD, which is then typically followed by carcinoma.[149,150] While this well-known stepwise progression could provide the basis to survey premalignant epithelium by random biopsies, histology analyses from expert to expert typically have poor agreement, particularly for the most severe and highest-risk samples such as HGD or CIS.[151] Based on such results, it appears that optical biopsies could eventually be well suited for early diagnosis of lung cancer and could greatly increase the survival rate of this disease.

In one study determining the potential of fluorescence spectroscopy for the diagnosis of dysplastic tissues and CIS, fluorescence bronchoscopy was performed on 82 volunteers: 25 nonsmokers, 40 ex-smokers, and 17 current smokers with mean ages of 52, 55, and 49 years, respectively. Excitation of the tissue was performed using the 325 nm emission of a HeCd laser, and the ratiometric analyses of the resulting fluorescence emission wavelengths were determined. Upon analysis of the results, it was found that the sensitivity of the autofluorescence bronchoscopy was 86%, which is 50% better than conventional white-light bronchoscopy, for the detection of dysplasia and CIS.[93,113]

Upper aerodigestive tract cancers: In order to determine the potential of laser-induced autofluorescence for the diagnosis of dysplastic tissues in the upper aerodigestive tract, many different research groups have developed many types of analyses. In one study, various fluorescence excitation and emission scans were employed for the differentiation of normal mucosa from neoplastic tissues. One spectral difference was the disappearance of an excitation peak at 330 nm in tumor tissue that existed in normal tissue when an emission wavelength of 380 nm was used for fluorescence monitoring. Therefore, by ratioing the excitation scan intensity at 290 nm to that of 330 nm, the resulting value could be directly correlated to increases epithelial thickness resulting from carcinogenesis. In addition to changes in the excitation spectrum between tumor and normal tissue, it was also found that the fluorescence emission intensity at 390 nm, upon excitation with 340 nm light, was also decreased in tumor tissue relative to normal tissue. A ratio of the fluorescence emission intensity at 390 and 450 nm correlated negatively with the mean epithelial thickness, again providing an indication of the stage of dysplasia.[152] In a similar study, the same autofluorescence ratios were used to differentiate between normal and neoplastic tissues in the oral cavity and pharynx of patients with previously untreated mucosal neoplasias. Using the same ratios, researchers found that significant differences existed between the neoplastic tissue and the contralateral normal sites, leading to the thought that this technique could represent a noninvasive screening method for head and neck squamous cell cancers.[153]

In another study, autofluorescence spectral characteristics of untreated oral and oropharyngeal lesions in patients were studied with excitation wavelengths of 370 and 410 nm generated by a nitrogen-pumped dye laser. Upon examining the resulting fluorescence emission of normal and neoplastic tissues, differences in the spectral profile were noted in two regions of the spectrum for both excitation sources. However, it was found that these differences were more significant when 410 nm light is used for excitation. By ratioing the fluorescence maximum intensity of dysplastic tissue to that of normal mucosa, a quantitative means of differentiation has been developed for the differentiation of the two types of tissue.[154]

In addition to being able to determine the presence of a cancerous or precancerous lesion in a patient, it is also important to be able to determine the point or margin where the tumor ends and the healthy tissue begins. Bohle and coworker have used autofluorescence spectroscopy of tumor connective tissue to accurately determine where the tumor ends and the healthy skin begins. In this work, 365 nm light was used for the excitation of the tissue, and the resulting fluorescence either from the elastic fibers of a tumor or the keratinization of precancerous lesions was used for delineation of the tissue. Contrary to previous results in the literature, no homogeneous fluorescence gradient could be proved between darker marginal epithelium and the brighter tumor connective fibers. While the greatest differentiation between tumor and nontumor tissues was exhibited in tissues from the same patient, comparisons between different patients also showed promise for the margining of lesions using autofluorescence.[155]

Laryngeal and oral cancer: Like other cancers involving mucosal membranes, oral and laryngeal carcinomas have also been studied by autofluorescence. Fluorescence spectroscopy has been used to differentiate normal tissue from dysplastic or cancerous tissue with a sensitivity of 90% and a specificity of 88% in a training set and a sensitivity of 100% and a specificity of 98% in a validation set (Figure 15.9).[156] A study of laryngeal cancer employed a HeCd laser operating at 325 nm for excitation of the sample and an ICCD for fluorescence image collection. Images were obtained at various wavelengths with optical filters for wavelength discrimination and were analyzed to provide diagnostic fluorescence images of the area of interest. Thirty patients were evaluated with this technique, of whom 18 had suspect malignancies that were confirmed via histopathological findings.[157]

15.4.3.2.1.2 Skin Diagnostics To better understand the role of various tissue components in the autofluorescence of skin, Gratton and coworkers have employed multiphoton fluorescence microscopy for the analysis of skin tissue in vivo. In this work, multiphoton fluorescence microscopy using excitation wavelengths of 730 and 960 nm was used to image in vivo human skin cells from the surface to a depth of approximately 200 μm. Details on multiphoton techniques are described in Chapter 12 of *The Biomedical Photonics Handbook: Fundamentals, Devices, and Techniques* in this handbook. Fluorescence emission spectra and fluorescence lifetime images were obtained at selected locations near the surface (0–50 μm) and at deeper depths (100–150 μm) for both excitation wavelengths. The resulting spectroscopic data suggest that reduced pyridine nucleotides and NADH are the primary source of the skin autofluorescence when using 730 nm excitation. With 960 nm excitation, a two-photon fluorescence emission at 520 nm indicates the presence of a variable, position-dependent intensity component caused by flavoproteins. In addition, a second fluorescence emission component, which starts at 425 nm, is observed when using 960 nm excitation. Such fluorescence emission at wavelengths less than half the excitation wavelength suggests an excitation process involving three or more photons. This is further confirmed by the observation of a superquadratic dependence of the fluorescence intensity on the excitation power. Further work is still required to spectroscopically identify these emitting species; however, this study demonstrates the use of multiphoton fluorescence microscopy for functional imaging of the metabolic states of in vivo human skin cells.[158]

In addition to microscopic analyses, macroscopic autofluorescence-based analyses have also provided useful information about the tissue state of skin as well. One such property that autofluorescence

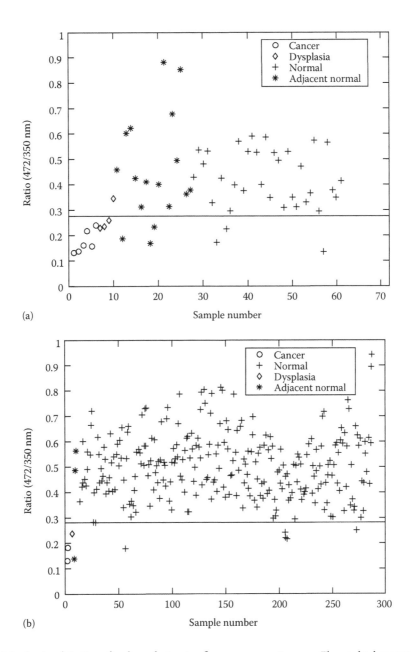

(a)

(b)

FIGURE 15.9 In vivo detection of oral neoplasia using fluorescence spectroscopy. The results demonstrate the ability of automated data analysis algorithms to classify tissues as normal (+), dysplastic (◊), cancerous (○), or normal tissue adjacent to cancerous based upon ratios of fluorescence emission data at multiple wavelengths following excitation of the oral tissue at 350 nm. Data in plot (a) represent the training set for automated analyses, while (b) represents the validation set. The solid line at 0.28 represents the threshold for separation of normal and dysplastic and/or cancerous tissue. Based upon these results, differentiation of normal tissue from dysplastic or cancerous tissue can be achieved with a sensitivity of 90% and a specificity of 88% in the training set and a sensitivity of 100% and a specificity of 98% in the validation data set. (From Heintzelman, D.L. et al., *Photochem. Photobiol.*, 72(1), 103, 2000.)

analyses of skin can provide information about is the extent of photoaging that an individual's skin has undergone. Two of the more common fluorescent components in the dermis of skin are the structural proteins, elastin and collagen, both of which are altered by age and photoexposure. Based upon in vivo fluorescence analyses of skin from 28 volunteers, it was found that fluorimetry could provide a marker for the extent of photoaging that has occurred in that person. In this study, it was found that by monitoring the fluorescence emission from UV-irradiated skin, it was possible to determine the extent of photoaging in a way that was independent of the age, pigmentation, and skin thickness of the individual. Such a marker could lead to the development of a technique capable of determining an individual's risk of cancer due to UV exposure from the sun.[159]

15.4.3.2.2 Clinical Studies and Diagnostics Using Exogenous Dyes

Exogenous fluorophores are used for many reasons in clinical applications. The most common reason for the use of these compounds is to provide a contrasting agent, which will make medical diagnoses easier, much like radionucleotides are sometimes used as contrast agents in circulation studies. However, due to the limited penetration of optical wavelengths into biological tissues, the most common type fluorescence analyses performed in vivo are cancer diagnoses of optically accessible tissues. It is for this reason that the majority clinical fluorescence diagnoses using exogenous fluorophores is in the area of cancer visualization. The most common of the exogenous fluorophores used for these studies are photosensitizers that have been developed for PDT treatments. These drugs generally exhibit strong fluorescence properties and preferentially locate in malignant tissues. Figure 15.10 illustrates the use of a fluorescence method for the monitoring the production of PDT products produced in vivo during treatment.[160] The development and applications of PDT drugs are described in Volume III, Chapters 1 and 2 of this handbook.

15.4.3.2.2.1 Photosensitizers
Investigation of the optimal photosensitizer to use for various types of tumors is a continuous field of investigation. In one such study, fluorescence analyses of the HpD-type photosensitizer Photogem™ were tested in 22 patients with tumors of the lungs, larynx, and skin; gastric and esophageal carcinoma; and cancer of the gynecological organs. Retention of the drug in the various types of tumors and tissues was monitored by fluorescence spectroscopy after excitation of the drug with 510 nm light. The results demonstrated that tumor detection by fluorescence spectroscopy when using Photogem as a contrast agent was possible even in low selectivity of drug accumulation, which appeared to be dependent on the stage and type of the disease and the organ involved.[161]

15.4.3.2.2.2 Cancer Diagnostics
Liver cancer: Monitoring and comparison of the results of ALA-induced PpIX tumor demarcation in chemically induced adenocarcinoma in the liver of rats and in an aggressive basal cell carcinoma (BCC) in a patient were studied using LIF. In this study, in vivo point monitoring and fluorescence microscopy incorporating a CCD camera were used to study the fluorescence distribution of ALA-induced PpIX in tumors. Fluorescence analyses were performed after i.v. injection of 30 mg/kg body weight of ALA. From these analyses, it was found that in the rat, there was a slightly larger concentration of PpIX in the tumor than in the surrounding healthy liver tissue or abdominal muscles. In the aggressive BCC of the human, a much greater concentration of PpIX was found in the visible regions of the BCC than in the necrotic regions and the surrounding normal skin, thereby demonstrating selective uptake/retention of PpIX in the carcinoma.[162]

Oral cancer: Diagnosis of neoplastic lesions in the oral mucosa of 11 patients was investigated using ALA-induced PpIX as a contrast agent. In this work, semiquantitative fluorescence measurements were performed at regular intervals of 3 h, following 15 min of continuous topical application of 0.4% ALA solution to the lesions. Excitation of the PpIX was performed using violet light from a xenon lamp (375–440 nm), and fluorescence images in the red region of the visible spectrum were recorded with a CCD

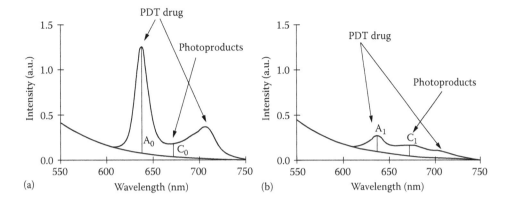

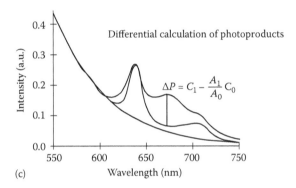

FIGURE 15.10 Fluorescence method for the monitoring the production of PDT photoproducts produced in vivo during treatment. Immediately prior to activation of the PDT drug, a fluorescence emission spectrum is measured (a). Then immediately following treatment, a second fluorescence spectrum is obtained (b). The fluorescent signal due to the PDT drug is designated A_0 for measurements prior to irradiation and A_1 for measurements following irradiation, while C_0 represents the fluorescence intensity of the photoproducts prior to irradiation and C_1 the fluorescence intensity of the photoproducts after irradiation. In order to determine the change in fluorescence intensity due to the formation of photoproducts during PDT treatment, the fluorescence intensity, at the appropriate wavelength, of the irradiated tissue is subtracted from the fluorescence intensity of the nonirradiated tissue, as shown in (c). (From Klinteberg, C. et al., *J. Photochem. Photobiol. B*, 49, 120, 1999.)

while quantitative spectral analyses were performed with an OMA. From these analyses, it was found that PpIX accumulated earlier in the necrotic tissue than in surrounding normal tissue and that a contrast ratio of 10:1 was found for the tumor tissue relative to the normal tissue 1–2 h after application of ALA.[163]

Esophageal cancer: Investigation of Photofrin-enhanced LIF differentiation of Barrett's metaplastic epithelium and esophageal adenocarcinoma in five patients has been performed, following low-dose i.v. injections (0.35 mg/kg body weight). In this work, LIF measurements were performed on tissue specimens of normal mucosa, Barrett's epithelium, and tumor tissue that had been treated with Photofrin. Based upon fluorescence measurement ratios of the Photofrin intensity divided by the autofluorescence intensity, quantitative values demonstrating the differentiation ability for the various degrees of dysplasia were determined. The mean ratio ± standard deviation for each of the types of tissue was found to be 0.10 ± 0.058 for normal esophageal mucosa, 0.16 ± 0.073 for normal gastric mucosa, 0.205 ± 0.17 for Barrett's epithelium with moderate dysplasia, 0.79 ± 0.54 for severe dysplasia, and 0.78 ± 0.56 for adenocarcinoma.[164]

Bladder cancer: Diagnosis of bladder cancer based upon the LIF of exogenous fluorophores has also been performed. In this study, a point-monitoring fluorescence diagnostic system based on a low-energy pulsed laser, fiber transmission optics, and an OMA was used for the diagnosis of 24 patients with bladder malignancies. Malignancies ranged from bladder carcinoma, CIS, and/or dysplasia. In order to provide a better contrast than can be achieved using autofluorescence, the HpD Photofrin was injected into the tissue at a concentration of either 0.35 or 0.5 mg/kg body weight. Forty-eight hours after injection, fluorescence measurements were taken and a ratio of the red photosensitizer fluorescence to the blue autofluorescence of the tissue was calculated. Based upon this ratio, excellent demarcation between papillary tumors and normal bladder wall tissue was achieved. In addition, these ratios also allowed for the objective differentiation of certain cases of dysplasia from normal mucosa and benign exophytic lesions such as malakoplakia from malignant tumors.[165]

Skin cancer: Due to the great success in using fluorescence spectroscopy for the diagnosis of many other types of malignancies, LIF has also been suggested for the noninvasive diagnosis of malignant melanomas. In one study, LIF was used for real-time monitoring of the PpIX distribution in tumor tissues and in the normal surrounding skin, before and after treatment in all patients. Based upon the comparison of fluorescence intensities from normal and tumor tissue of the same pigmentation from the same individual, PpIX distribution demonstrated excellent demarcation between tumor and normal skin of about 15:1 for BCC and Bowen's disease and 5:1 for T-cell lymphomas.[166] However, the reliability of such measurements can be seriously compromised by spatial variations in the optical properties of the tissue that are not related to malignancy (e.g., pigmentation). One approach to fluorescence-based analyses that minimizes this problem employs a double ratiometric analysis procedure and the use of the photosensitizer ALA. In this technique, two types of fluorescence ratios were calculated. The first of these ratios is the ratio of the skin's fluorescence emission between 660 and 750 nm to the emission between 550 and 600 nm following 405 nm excitation. The second ratio was calculated by dividing the fluorescence emission between 660 and 750 nm by the emission between 550 and 600 nm following excitation with 435 nm. These two excitation wavelengths were chosen to be close to the fluorescence emission wavelength of ALA-induced PpIX, but some distance from the Soret excitation band of the porphyrins. Analysis of either of the two single ratios showed a significant correlation to not only the presence of a lesion but also the color of the skin tissue. However, when the 405 nm excited ratio is divided by the 435 nm excited ratio, a value can be determined that is independent of skin coloration and can be based primarily on the presence of the ALA-induced photosensitizer. Such a technique will enable the in vivo studies of the pharmacokinetics of tumor-localizing agents in pigmented lesions and may significantly contribute to the development of a noninvasive diagnostic tool for malignant melanoma.[167]

Colon cancer: Another class of compounds that are beginning to be tested for in vivo tumor demarcation is fluorescently labeled antibodies. Based on previous experiments performed using nude mice, a feasibility study was performed to determine whether or not LIF of fluoresceinated monoclonal antibodies against carcinoembryonic antigens localized specifically in human carcinoma xenografts could be used for clinical colon cancer diagnoses. In this study, six patients with known primary colorectal carcinoma were given an i.v. injection of 4.5 or 9 mg of mouse–human chimeric anticarcinoembryonic antigen monoclonal antibody labeled with 0.10–0.28 mg of fluorescein. In addition, the monoclonal antibody was also labeled with 0.2–0.4 mCi of [125]I. Photodetection of the tumor was done ex vivo on surgically resected tissues from all six patients and in vivo by fluorescence rectosigmoidoscopy for one of the six patients. Fluorescence analyses revealed that the dye-labeled antibody localized preferentially in the tumor tissue at concentrations up to 0.059% of the injected dose per gram of tumor. This was 10 times greater than in the normal tissue, which exhibited a concentration of 0.006% of the injected dose per gram of normal mucosa. Such immunophotodiagnoses may prove very useful in the clinical setting for rapid tumor diagnoses in the colon and potentially other organs.[168]

15.4.4 Recent Advances in Instrumentation, Methodologies, and Applications

Recent advances in instrumentation and method development have led to significant improvement in fluorescence-based diagnostic modalities. Traditional screening techniques for colon cancer generally use white-light endoscopy. While most abnormal lesions can detected by this method, some could be missed during colonoscopy, potentially leading to further disease progression. A prototype UV spectral imager monitoring autofluorescence and reflectance has been developed and applied in a study of 21 fresh human colon surgical specimens.[169] This device used six excitation wavelengths from 280 to 440 nm and utilized a ratio imaging method, which caused neoplasms to appear bright compared to normal tissue. The results indicated that the contrast may be due to increased levels of reduced NADH, increased hemoglobin absorption, and reduced signal from submucosal collagen.

Advanced techniques in optical imaging offer a high potential for noninvasive detection of cancer in humans. Recent advances in instrumentation for diffuse optical imaging have led to new capabilities for the detection of cancer in highly scattering tissue such as the female breast. A time-gated method for fluorescence imaging and spectroscopy with strong suppression of tissue autofluorescence was investigated for the detection of BE and with colitis ulcerosa.[170]

Changes in fluorescence from certain amino acids, structural proteins, and enzymatic cofactors in tissue were investigated in order to predict a diagnosis of malignancy and to estimate the risk of developing ovarian cancer.[171] Ovarian biopsies were interrogated using 270–550 nm excitation and fluorescence was recorded from 290 to 700 nm. Measurements were performed on 49 patients undergoing oophorectomy. Data were analyzed using parallel factor analysis to determine excitation and emission spectra of the underlying fluorophores that contribute to the total detected fluorescence intensity. The results showed that performance of high-risk versus low-risk classification decreased when normal samples include both pre- and postmenopausal women. The best diagnostic performance for cancer detection and risk-status assessment were obtained using excitation over 270–400 and 380–560 nm, respectively. The study indicates that analysis of endogenous fluorescence could be useful in screening women at increased risk of developing ovarian cancer.

A clinical study was conducted using intraoperative confocal endomicroscopy for early detection and resection of squamous cell carcinoma (SCC) of the head and neck.[172] Diagnostic and therapeutic procedures used a prototype of a rigid laser endoscope in combination with autofluorescence detection. The study involved 15 patients with SCC of the oral cavity, hypopharynx, and larynx. Real-time visualization of cellular and subcellular details were collected during endoscopy. Diagnostic scores were applied to differentiate dysplastic and malignant mucosal changes of SCC of the head and neck from normal squamous cell mucosa using this method. Results were correlated with the histological analysis and demonstrated the potential of a virtual real-time histological analysis, which will have quicker intraoperative diagnosis, less need for multiple frozen sections, and more precise resection margins.

A clinical study was conducted to compare the accuracy of PpIX fluorescence and autofluorescence-normalized PpIX fluorescence detection systems for the localization nonmelanoma skin cancers (NMSCs).[173] The clinical study involved 30 patients, 14 females and16 males, having skin type I–III and being suspected of having one or more NMSC. The patients were investigated using a fluorescence detection system capable of both normalized and nonnormalized PpIX fluorescence measurements. Liposomal encapsulated ALA was used as the photosensitizer. For each area being investigated, the associated normalized and nonnormalized fluorescence measurements were directly compared. The results of the analysis were confirmed by clinical investigation using a dermatoscope. The results showed that the use of autofluorescence in PpIX fluorescence detection of NMSC is more accurate than PpIX fluorescence detection alone.

Multiphoton tomography was investigated for early detection of skin cancer based on noninvasive optical sectioning of skin by two-photon autofluorescence and second harmonic generation.[174] Deep-tissue pigmented lesions—nevi—were imaged with intracellular resolution using NIR femtosecond laser radiation. The study involved over 250 patients. Cancerous tissues exhibited significant morphological differences compared to normal skin layers. Luminescence from melanocytes was detected in malignant melanoma. The results indicated the potential of multiphoton tomography as a noninvasive method to obtain high-resolution 3D optical biopsies for early cancer detection, treatment control, and in situ drug screening.

A compact point-detection fluorescence spectroscopy system and data analysis methods to quantify the intrinsic fluorescence redox ratio were developed to diagnose brain cancer in an orthotopic brain tumor rat model.[175] The system employed one compact cw diode laser (407 nm) to excite two primary endogenous fluorophores, reduced NADH and FAD. The spectra were first analyzed using a spectral filtering modulation method to derive the intrinsic fluorescence redox ratio, which has the advantages of insensitivity to optical coupling and rapid data acquisition and analysis. This method represents a convenient and rapid alternative for achieving intrinsic fluorescence-based redox measurements as compared to those complicated model-based methods. The method can also extract total hemoglobin concentration at the same time if the emission path length of fluorescence light is long enough so that the effect of absorption on fluorescence intensity due to hemoglobin is significant. Then a multivariate method was used to statistically classify normal tissues and tumors. While the first method offers quantitative tissue metabolism information, the second method provides high overall classification accuracy. The two methods provide complementary capabilities for understanding cancer development and noninvasively diagnosing brain cancer. The results of this study demonstrated that this portable system can be used to demarcate the elusive boundary between a brain tumor and the surrounding normal tissue during surgical resection.

LIF spectroscopy has already been reported to distinguish HGD from nondysplastic BE.[64,65,103-107] Active inflammatory features detected microscopically in nondysplastic BE may result in an FP classification as HGD. A study was conducted to determine whether LIF spectroscopy using a DNF index is adversely affected by active inflammatory changes in nondysplastic BE resulting in FP readings as HGD.[176] A 410 nm laser light was used to induce autofluorescence of Barrett's mucosa in 49 patients. The clinical study included 37 males and 12 females. The spectra were analyzed using the DNF index technique at 480 nm. Each spectrum was classified as either positive or negative using the criteria previously developed for detecting HGD. Using DNF at 480 nm technique, 92.6% of nondysplastic samples with active inflammation were classified correctly (162/175), and 92.2% of nondysplastic samples without active inflammatory features were classified correctly (118/128). Comparing the ratios of FPs among the two sample groups, there was not a statistically significant difference between the two groups. Therefore, LIF spectroscopy using the DNF technique for classification of nondysplastic Barrett's mucosa did not result in FPs due to active inflammatory features within Barrett's mucosa.

The effectiveness of PDT for ablation of HGD in BE is typically reported histologically. Tumor markers may provide evidence of decreased cancer risk at a molecular level. A study was performed to determine whether PDT for BE/HGD would decrease the mutant p53 protein expression in the treated area in addition to its replacement with squamous (neosquamous) mucosa.[177] Patients were divided into two groups. Group I patients ($n = 12$) were those who had been treated with PDT for HGD and provided 23 biopsy samples of neosquamous mucosa. Group II patients ($n = 10$) were those who had not received any ablative therapies for their BE. Fourteen HGD samples were obtained from Group II patients. Group II patients also provided 17 biopsy samples from normal squamous mucosa, 22 samples of nondysplastic Barrett's, and 21 samples of LGD. Immunohistochemical staining for mutant p53 protein was performed using mouse antihuman monoclonal antibody DO-1. The degree of p53 protein expression in the cell nuclei was scored using an established immunohistochemical scoring (IHC) system (0 for negative samples and range of 2–8 for positive samples). Expression of p53 was significantly increased in specimens from Group II patients as the dysplasia grade progressed in severity. The results of this study show a significant reduction in mutant p53 protein expression was detected in neosquamous mucosa of patients who had received PDT for HGD in BE, suggesting a decreased cancer risk after treatment.

Hemoglobin concentration and oxygenation in tissue are important biomarkers that are useful in both clinical and biological applications. A simple two-step ratiometric method was proposed to estimate total hemoglobin concentration and oxygen saturation in tissue based on a single fluorescence emission spectrum.[178] In the first step, total hemoglobin concentration was estimated by comparing a ratio of fluorescence intensities at two emission wavelengths to a calibration curve. The second step was to estimate oxygen saturation by comparing a double ratio that involved three emission wavelengths to another calibration curve that was a function of oxygen saturation for a known total hemoglobin concentration. Theoretical derivation and tissue phantom experiments showed that those calibration curves were insensitive to the scattering property of the tissue model for the chosen probe geometry. Compared to existing optical methods for hemoglobin measurements in tissue, this method offers the following advantages. This method is immune to the variation in system throughput caused by inconsistent optical coupling because of its ratiometric nature. Moreover, only fluorescence intensities at a few wavelengths in a single fluorescence emission spectrum are needed in this method, which minimizes the amount of required data and potentially reduces the size of the required equipment. The fact that this method does not use nonlinear regression can significantly reduce computation time in data processing. The ratiometric nature of this method makes it resistant to the variation in optical coupling. Simple calibration curves are established for estimating total hemoglobin concentration and oxygen saturation. It is found that these curves are insensitive to the scattering coefficient for chosen probe geometry. These features are highly desirable in clinical measurements.

Recently, SF spectroscopy, an underexploited methodology, has gained interest in cancer detection. Based on the idea of wavelength synchronous scanning introduced by Lloyd,[179] Vo-Dinh further developed the method and provided the basic theory and fundamental operating principle for multicomponent analysis and medical applications.[3–5,180–183] Traditionally, most cancer diagnostic investigations used fixed-wavelength excitation. However, the use of fixed excitation might not be sufficiently selective in some diagnostic applications due to strong overlap of the emission spectra from different fluorophores. An alternative approach is the SL method, which involves scanning both excitation and emission wavelength simultaneously while keeping a constant wavelength interval between them. The operating principle of the SF method is discussed previously in Section 15.3.1. The SF modality was initially developed by for multicomponent analysis[3,4] and used for chemical and biological analysis.[40,41,180–190] The SF technique has been used to detect biomarkers in cells,[41,188] bodily fluids of animal samples,[40] and in tissue diagnosis.[36–38] Recently, the SF approach has been applied to both in vitro and in vivo tissue imaging for cancer detection and medical diagnostics.[190–196] An SF imaging system has been developed to combine the great diagnostic potential of synchronous scanning spectroscopy and the large field of view of imaging for cancer diagnosis.[189,190] This system has been tested in a mouse skin model to capture SF images. A simple discriminant analysis method and a more sophisticated multivariate statistical method have been developed to generate a single diagnostic image from a large number of raw fluorescence images. Moreover, it was demonstrated that the diagnostic image generated from synchronous data is comparable to that generated from full spectral data in classification accuracy. Three-dimensional total SF spectroscopy (TSFS) was investigated for discrimination between normal and malignant breast tissues.[191] Data from TSFS measurements of normal and malignant breast tissue samples are introduced in supervised self-organizing maps, a type of artificial neural network (ANN), to obtain diagnosis.[192] SF spectroscopy has been used for the detection and characterization of cervical cancers.[195,196] The resurgence of the SF method indicates that this unique technique can offer a simple way to rapidly measure fluorescence signals and spectral fingerprints of complex mixtures such as tissue for medical diagnostics.

15.5 Conclusion

This chapter illustrates the usefulness of fluorescence spectroscopy in a wide variety of medical applications spanning from cellular screening to tissue analysis and in vivo diagnostics. The major advantage of fluorescence (as well as of other techniques such as Raman scattering, diffuse scattering, elastic scattering, and NIR absorption) is that biochemical and morphological information about the native tissue state can be obtained without the need for physical removal of tissues. In addition, because tissue removal is not needed for diagnostics, a more comprehensive examination of the organ of interest can be achieved than is possible with excised tissue. Fluorescence techniques can also be combined with imaging so that images of diseased tissue sites versus normal sites can be constructed. Thus, these diagnostic techniques inherently provide superior coverage and do not suffer from sampling errors, which often occur with biopsy or cytology. Real-time diagnostic information is a significant added benefit.

At the early stage of development, fluorescence diagnostic techniques have to be verified by comparison with pathology, the current *gold standard*, which itself varies in reliability. Thus, the sensitivity and specificity of spectroscopic diagnostics depends upon the reliability of pathology in each specific desired application. If *optical biopsy* is going to have a role in clinical diagnosis, the problem becomes what gold standard we are going to use for calibrating the optical measurements. Using pathology as the gold standard for intraepithelial neoplasia (preinvasive cancer) has its own difficulties, since pathologists often disagree on their interpretation of these lesions, with the level of consistency varying for different organs. Therefore, building decision-making boundaries using optical measurements that are based on conventional pathology is problematic. Since both under- and overdiagnosis are undesirable, it is imperative to establish objective and standardized pathological classification systems for grading preinvasive lesions for each separate organ area where these new optical technologies may be applied.

Another important application for optical diagnostic technologies such as fluorescence is the possible use of these techniques for guidance of surgical intervention and treatment. In such surgical-assist applications, the ability of fluorescence diagnostic technologies to provide real-time information would be critically useful. Fluorescence techniques may also be used to provide real-time assessment of tissue response to therapy—as in the assessment of tissue viability and necrosis in thermal, laser interstitial therapy, or PDT.

Fluorescence technologies could also be used for noninvasive measurement of the concentrations of various drugs and biological species in tissues. This capability would provide a variety of benefits in medical research. One example of such a benefit is in the case of chemotherapy drugs used for the treatment of various cancers. The therapeutic benefit is determined by the concentration of the drug in the tissues of the targeted organ or site; currently, the only minimally invasive check available to the oncologist is to track the blood serum concentration and to assume a relationship between the amount of drugs at the target organs and the tissue concentration. More generally, the ability to track concentrations of compounds in tissue noninvasively would be a tremendous advantage. Optical methods such as fluorescence could bypass many of the tedious and time-consuming trials that attempt to relate dosage to metabolic rates and target organ concentrations. Using the synchronous scanning method, the SF technique can further improve spectral selectivity for improved diagnostics. Because of all of these desirable features, it is evident that fluorescence spectroscopy can be a powerful tool both for the medical researcher to obtain a better understanding of the disease process and for the physician to perform real-time in vivo diagnoses and, ultimately, provide treatment at the point of care.

Acknowledgments

This work was sponsored by the National Institutes of Health (RO1 CA88787-01) and by the US Department of Energy (DOE) Office of Biological and Environmental Research, under contract DEAC05-00OR22725 with UT-Battelle, LLC, and the Duke University Exploratory Research Project. T.V.D. acknowledges contributions from Bergein F. Overholt and Masoud Panjehpour at the Thompson Cancer Survival Center.

References

1. Vo-Dinh, T., *Room Temperature Phosphorimetry for Chemical Analysis*, Wiley, New York, 1984.
2. McGlynn, S. P., Azumi, T., and Kinoshita, M., *Molecular Spectroscopy of the Triplet State*, Prentice-Hall, Englewood Cliffs, NJ, 1969.

3. Vo-Dinh, T., Multicomponent analysis by synchronous luminescence spectrometry, *Analytical Chemistry* 50(3), 396–401, 1978.
4. Vo-Dinh, T., Synchronous luminescence spectroscopy—Methodology and applicability, *Applied Spectroscopy* 36(5), 576–581, 1982.
5. Vo-Dinh, T., Principle of synchronous luminescence (SL) technique for biomedical diagnostics, in *Biomedical Diagnostic, Guidance, and Surgical-Assist Systems II*, Vo-Dinh, T., Grundfest, W. S., and Benaron, D. A. (eds.), *Proceedings of the SPIE* 3911, SPIE Publishers, Bellingham, WA, pp. 42–49, 2000.
6. Richards-Kortum, R. and Sevick-Muraca, E., Quantitative optical spectroscopy for tissue diagnosis, *Annual Review of Physical Chemistry* 47, 555–606, 1996.
7. Bottiroli, G. C., Croce, A. C., Locatelli, D., Marchesini, R., Pignoli, E., Tomatis, S., Cuzzoni, C., Dipalma, S., Dalfante, M., and Spinelli, P, Natural fluorescence of normal and neoplastic human colon: A comprehensive ex vivo study, *Lasers in Surgery and Medicine* 16, 48–60, 1995.
8. Fujimoto, D., Akiba, K. Y., and Nakamura, N., Isolation and characterization of a fluorescent material in bovine achilles-tendon collagen, *Biochemical and Biophysical Research Communications* 76(4), 1124–1129, 1977.
9. Richards-Kortum, R. R., Rava, R. P., Baraga, J., Fitzmaurice, M., Kramer, J., and Feld, M. S., Survey of the UV and visible spectroscopic properties of normal and atherosclerotic human artery using fluorescence EEMs, in *Optronic Techniques in Diagnostic and Therapeutic Medicine*, Pratesi, R. (Ed.), Plenum Press, New York, 1990.
10. Wagnières, G. A., Star, W. M., and Wilson, B. C., In vivo fluorescence spectroscopy and imaging for oncological applications, *Photochemical Photobiology* 68, 603–632, 1998.
11. Lakowicz, J. R., *Principles of Fluorescence Spectroscopy*, Plenum Press, New York, 1985.
12. Masters, B. R. and Chance, B., Redox confocal imaging: Intrinsic fluorescent probes of cellular metabolism, in *Fluorescent and Luminescent Probes for Biological Activity*, Maon, W. T. (Ed.), Academic Press, London, U.K., 1993, pp. 44–56.
13. Tsuchida, M., Miura, T., and Aibara, K., Lipofuscin and lipofuscin-like substances, *Chemistry and Physics of Lipids* 44(2–4), 297–325, 1987.
14. Eldred, G. E., Miller, G. V., Stark, W. S., and Feeneyburns, L., Lipofuscin—Resolution of discrepant fluorescence data, *Science* 216(4547), 757–759, 1982.
15. Millar, D. P., Time-resolved fluorescence spectroscopy, *Current Opinion in Structural Biology* 6(5), 637–642, 1996.
16. Viallet, P. M., Vo-Dinh, V., Bunde, T., Ribou, A. C., Vigo, J., and Salmon, J. M., Fluorescent molecular reporter for the 3-D conformation of protein subdomains: The Mag-Indo system, *Journal of Fluorescence* 9(3), 153–161, 1999.
17. Viallet, P. M., Vo-Dinh, T., Ribou, A. C., Vigo, J., and Salmon, J. M., Native fluorescence and Mag-indo-1-protein interaction as tools for probing unfolding and refolding sequences of the bovine serum albumin subdomain in the presence of guanidine hydrochloride, *Journal of Protein Chemistry* 19(6), 431–439, 2000.
18. Tyagi, S. and Kramer, F. R., Molecular beacons: Probes that fluoresce upon hybridization, *Nature Biotechnology* 14(3), 303–308, 1996.
19. Gao, W. W., Tyagi, S., Kramer, F. R., and Goldman, E., Messenger RNA release from ribosomes during 5′-translational blockage by consecutive low-usage arginine but not leucine codons in *Escherichia coli, Molecular Microbiology* 25(4), 707–716, 1997.
20. Tyagi, S., Bratu, D. P., and Kramer, F. R., Multicolor molecular beacons for allele discrimination, *Nature Biotechnology* 16(1), 49–53, 1998.
21. Tyagi, S., Marras, S. A. E., and Kramer, F. R., Wavelength-shifting molecular beacons, *Nature Biotechnology* 18(11), 1191–1196, 2000.
22. Protio, A. E. and Sarnaik, J., Fluorescence of HpD for tumor detection and dosimetry in photoradiation therapy, in *Porphyrin Localization and Treatment of Tumors*, Doiron, D. R., Gomer, C. J., and Liss, A. R. (Eds.), Liss, New York, 1984, pp. 163–175.

23. Lam, S. H., Hung, J., and Palcic, B., Detection of lung cancer by ratio fluorometry with and without photofrin II, *Proceedings of SPIE* 1201, 561–568, 1990.

24. Tassetti, V., Hajri, A., Sowinska, M., Evrard S., Heisel, F., Cheng, L. Q., Miehe, J. A., Marescaux, J., and Aprahamian, M., In vivo laser-induced fluorescence imaging of a rat pancreatic cancer with pheophorbide-a, *Photochemical Photobiology* 65, 997–1006, 1997.

25. Kim, R. Y., Hu, L. K., Flotte, T. J., Gragoudas, E. S., and Young, L. H. Y., Digital angiography of experimental choroidal melanomas using benzoporphyrin derivative, *American Journal of Ophthalmology* 123, 810–816, 1997.

26. Kollias, N., Lui, H., Wimberly, J., and Anderson, R. R., Monitoring of benzoporphyrin derivative monoacid ring A (BPD-MA) in skin tumors by fluorescence during photodynamic therapy, *Proceedings of SPIE* 1881, 41–47, 1993.

27. Peyman, G. A., Moshfeghi, D. M., Moshfeghi, A., Khoobehi, B., Doiron, D. R., Primbs, G. B., and Crean, D. H., Photodynamic therapy for choriocapillaris using tin ethyl etiopurprin (SnET2), *Ophthalmic Surgery Lasers* 28, 409–417, 1997.

28. Koren, H., Schenk, G. M., Jindra, R. H., Alth, G., Ebermann, R., Kubin, A., Koderhold, G., and Kreitner, M., Hypericin in phototherapy, *Journal of Photochemical and Photobiology B* 36, 113–119, 1996.

29. Diwu, Z., Novel therapeutic and diagnostic applications of hypocrellins and hypericins, *Photochemistry and Photobiology* 61, 529–539, 1995.

30. Dets, S. M., Buryi, A. N., Melnik, I. S., Joffe, A. Y., and Rusina, T. V., Laser-induced fluorescence detection of stomach cancer using hypericin, *Proceedings of SPIE* 2926, 51–56, 1996.

31. Peng, Q., Berg, K., Moan, J., Kongshaug, M., and Nesland, J. M., 5-Aminolevulinic acid-based photodynamic therapy—Principles and experimental research, *Photochemical and Photobiology* 65, 235–251, 1997.

32. Battle, C. and Dell, A. M., Phorophyrins, phorphyrias, cancer and photodynamic therapy: A model of carcinogenesis, *Journal of Photochemical and Photobiology B* 20, 5–22, 1993.

33. Cox, G. S., Bobillier, C., and Whitten, D. G., Photooxidation and singlet oxygen sensitization by photophyrin IX and its photooxidation products, *Photochemical and Photobiology* 36, 401–407, 1982.

34. Peng, Q., Warloe, T., Berg, K., Moan, J., Kongshaug, M., Giercksky, K. E., and Nesland, J. M., 5-Aminolevunic acid based photodynamic therapy. Clinical research and future challenges, *Cancer* 79, 2282–2308, 1997.

35. Marcus, S. L., Sobel, R. S., Golub, A. L., Carroll, R. L., Lundahl, S., and Shulman, D. G., Photodynamic therapy (PDT) and photodiagnosis (PD) using endogenous photosensitization induced by 5-aminolevulinic acid (ALA): Current clinical and developmental status, *Laser Medicine Surgery* 14, 59–66, 1996.

36. Schwartz, S., Historical perspectives, in *Photodynamic Therapy: Basic Principles and Clinical Applications*, Henderson, B. W. and Dougherty, T. J. (Eds.), Marcel Dekker, New York, 1992, pp. 1–8.

37. Sacks, P. G., Savage, H. E., Levine, J., Kolli, V. R., Alfano, R. R., and Schantz, S. P., Native cellular fluorescence identifies terminal squamous differentiation of normal oral epithelial cells in culture: A potential chemoprevention biomarker, *Cancer Letters* 104(2), 171–181, 1996.

38. Zhang, J. C., Savage, H. E., Sacks, P. G., Delohery, T., Alfano, R. R., Katz, A., and Schantz, S. P., Innate cellular fluorescence reflects alterations in cellular proliferation, *Lasers in Surgery and Medicine* 20(3), 319–331, 1997.

39. Anidjar, M., Cussenot, O., Blais, J., Bourdon, O., Avrillier, S., Ettori, D., Villette, J. M., Fiet, J., Teillac, P., and LeDuc, A., Argon laser induced autofluorescence may distinguish between normal and tumor human urothelial cells: A microspectrofluorimetric study, *Journal of Urology* 155(5), 1771–1774, 1996.

40. Uziel, M., Ward, R. J., and Vo-Dinh, T., Synchronous fluorescence measurement of BaP metabolites in human and animal urine, *Analytical Letters* 20(5), 761–776, 1987.

41. Watts, W. E., Isola, N. R., Frazier, D., and Vo-Dinh, T., Differentiation of normal and neoplastic cells by synchronous fluorescence: Rat liver epithelial and rat hepatoma cell models, *Analytical Letters* 32(13), 2583–2594, 1999.

42. Amano, T., Kunimi, K., and Ohkawa, M., Fluorescence spectra from human semen and their relationship with sperm parameters, *Archives of Andrology* 36(1), 9–15, 1996.

43. Xu, H., Aylott, J., and Kopelman, R., Sol-gel pebble sensors for biochemical analysis inside living cells, *Abstracts of Papers of the American Chemical Society* 219, 97-ANYL, 2000.

44. Tan, W. H., Thorsrud, B. A., Harris, C., and Kopelman, R., Real time pH measurements in the intact rat conceptus using ultramicrofiber-optic sensors, in *Polymers in Sensors*, American Chemical Society, Washington, DC, 1998, pp. 266–272.

45. Clark, H. A., Hoyer, M., Philbert, M. A., and Kopelman, R., Optical nanosensors for chemical analysis inside single living cells. 1. Fabrication, characterization, and methods for intracellular delivery of PEBBLE sensors, *Analytical Chemistry* 71(21), 4831–4836, 1999.

46. Clark, H. A., Kopelman, R., Tjalkens, R., and Philbert, M. A., Optical nanosensors for chemical analysis inside single living cells. 2. Sensors for pH and calcium and the intracellular application of PEBBLE sensors, *Analytical Chemistry* 71(21), 4837–4843, 1999.

47. Tan, W. H., Kopelman, R., Barker, S. L. R., and Miller, M. T., Ultrasmall for cellular, *Analytical Chemistry* 71(17), 606A–612A, 1999.

48. Cullum, B. M., Griffin, G. D., Miller, G. H., and Vo-Dinh, T., Intracellular measurements in mammary carcinoma cells using fiber-optic nanosensors, *Analytical Biochemistry* 277(1), 25–32, 2000.

49. Cullum, B. M. and Vo-Dinh, T., The development of optical nanosensors for biological measurements, *Trends in Biotechnology* 18(9), 388–393, 2000.

50. Vo-Dinh, T., Alarie, J. P., Cullum, B. M., and Griffin, G. D., Antibody-based nanoprobe for measurement of a fluorescent analyte in a single cell, *Nature Biotechnology* 18(7), 764–767, 2000.

51. Kong, J. and Ringer, D. P., Quantitative in situ image analysis of apoptosis in well and poorly differentiated tumors from rat liver, *American Journal of Pathology* 147(6), 1626–1632, 1995.

52. Balazs, M., Szöllösi, J., Lee, W. C., Haugland, R. P., Guzikowski, A. P., Fulwyler, M. J., Damjanovich, S., Feurstein, B. G., and Pershadsingh, H. A., Fluorescent tetradecanoylphorbol acetate: A novel probe of phorbol ester binding domains, *Journal of Cellular Biochemistry* 46(3), 266–276, 1991.

53. Andeoni, A., Bottiroli, G., Colasanti, A., Giangare, M. C., Riccio, P., Roberti, G., and Vaghi, P., Fluorochromes with long-lived fluorescence as potential labels for pulsed laser immunocyto-fluorometry: Photophysical characterization of pyrene derivatives, *Journal of Biochemical and Biophysical Methods* 29(2), 157–172, 1994.

54. Fritsch, C., Batz, J., Bolsen, K., Schulte, K. W., Zumdick, M., Ruzicka, T., and Goerz, G., Ex vivo application of delta-aminolevulinic acid induces high and specific porphyrin levels in human skin tumors: Possible basis for selective photodynamic therapy, *Photochemistry and Photobiology* 66(1), 114–118, 1997.

55. DaCosta, R. S. L., Andersson, H. M. S., Cirocco, M., Kandel, G., Kortan, P., Haber, G., Marcon, N. E., and Wilson, B. C., Correlation of autofluorescence (AF) & ultrastructures of ex vivo colorectal tissues & isolated living epithelial cells from primary cell cultures (PCC) of normal colon & hyperplastic & dysplastic polyps: Implications for early diagnosis, altered cell metabolism, & cytopathology, *Gastroenterology* 116(4), G1721, 1999.

56. Han, I., Saito, H., Fukatsu, K., Inoue, T., Yasuhara, H., Furukawa, S., Matsuda, T., Lin, M. T., and Ikeda, S., Ex vivo fluorescence microscopy provides simple and accurate assessment of neutrophil-endothelial adhesion in the rat lung, *Shock* 16(2), 143–147, 2001.

57. Sculean, A., Auschill, T. M., Donos, N., Brecx, M., and Arweiler, N. B., Effect of an enamel matrix protein (Emdogain®) on ex vivo dental plaque vitality, *Journal of Clinical Periodontology* 28(11), 1074–1078, 2001.

58. Harth, R., Gerlach, M., Riederer, P., and Gotz, M. E., A highly sensitive method for the determination of protein bound 3,4-dihydroxyphenylalanine as a marker for post-translational protein hydroxylation in human tissues ex vivo, *Free Radical Research* 35(2), 167–174, 2001.

59. Alfano, R. R., Tata, D. B., Cordero, J., Tomashefsky, P., Longo, F. W., and Alfano, M. A., Laser-induced fluorescence spectroscopy from native cancerous and normal tissue, *IEEE Journal of Quantum Electronics* 20(12), 1507–1511, 1984.

60. Alfano, R. R., Lam, W., Zarrabi, H. J., Alfano, M. A., Cordero, J., Tata, D. B., and Swenberg, C. E., Human-teeth with and without caries studied by laser scattering, fluorescence, and absorption-spectroscopy, *IEEE Journal of Quantum Electronics* 20(12), 1512–1516, 1984.

61. Alfano, R. R., Tang, G. C., Pradhan, A., Lam, W., Choy, D. S. J., and Opher, E., Fluorescence-spectra from cancerous and normal human-breast and lung tissues, *IEEE Journal of Quantum Electronics* 23(10), 1806–1811, 1987.

62. Tang, G. C., Pradhan, A., Sha, W., Chen, J., Liu, C. H., Wahl, S. J., and Alfano, R. R., Pulsed and Cw laser fluorescence-spectra from cancerous, normal, and chemically treated normal human-breast and lung tissues, *Applied Optics* 28(12), 2337–2342, 1989.

63. Ingrams, D. R., Dhingra, J. K., Roy, K., Perrault, D. F., Bottrill, I. D., Kabani, S., Rebeiz, E. E. et al., Autofluorescence characteristics of oral mucosa, *Head and Neck* 19(1), 27–32, 1997.

64. Vo-Dinh, T., Panjehpour, M., Overholt, B. F., and Buckley, P., Laser-induced differential fluorescence for cancer diagnosis without biopsy, *Applied Spectroscopy* 51(1), 58–63, 1997.

65. Vo-Dinh, T., Panjehpour, M., and Overholt, B. F., Laser-induced fluorescence for esophageal cancer and dysplasia diagnosis, in *Advances in Optical Biopsy and Optical Mammography*, New York Academy of Sciences, New York, 1998, pp. 116–122.

66. Richards-Kortum, R., Mitchell, M. F., Ramanujam, N., Mahadevan, A., and Thomsen, S., In vivo fluorescence spectroscopy: Potential for non-invasive, automated diagnosis of cervical intraepithelial neoplasia and use as a surrogate endpoint biomarker, *Journal of Cellular Biochemistry Supplement* 19, 111–119, 1994.

67. Lohmann, W., Mußmann, J., Lohmann, C., and Kunzel, W., Native fluorescence of cervix uteri as a marker for dysplasia and invasive carcinoma, *European Journal of Obstetrics, Gynecology, and Reproductive Biology* 31(3), 249–253, 1989.

68. Romer, T. J., Fitzmaurice, M., Cothren, R. M., Richardskortum, R., Petras, R., Sivak, M. V., and Kramer, J. R., Laser-induced fluorescence microscopy of normal colon and dysplasia in colonic adenomas—Implications for spectroscopic diagnosis, *American Journal of Gastroenterology* 90(1), 81–87, 1995.

69. Fiarman, G. S., Nathanson, M. H., West, A. B., Deckelbaum, L. I., Kelly, L., and Kapadia, C. R., Differences in laser-induced autofluorescence between adenomatous and hyperplastic polyps and normal colonic mucosa by confocal microscopy, *Digestive Diseases and Sciences* 40(6), 1261–1268, 1995.

70. Hegedus, Z. L. and Nayak, U., Relative fluorescence intensities of human plasma soluble melanins in normal adults, *Archives Internationales de Physiologie, de Biochimie et de Biophysique* 102(6), 311–313, 1994.

71. Marchesini, R., Brambilla, M., Pignoli, E., Bottiroli, G., Croce, A. C., Dal Fante, M., Spinelli, P., and diPalma, S., Light-induced fluorescence spectroscopy of adenomas, adenocarcinomas and non-neoplastic mucosa in human colon I. In vitro measurements, *Journal of Photochemistry and Photobiology B* 14(3), 219–230, 1992.

72. Richards-Kortum, R., Rava, R. P., Petras, R. E., Fitzmaurice, M., Sivak, M., and Feld, M. S., Spectroscopic diagnosis of colonic dysplasia, *Photochemistry and Photobiology* 53(6), 777–786, 1991.

73. Kapadia, C. R., Cutruzzola, F. W., O'Brien, K. M., Stetz, M. L., Enriquez, R., and Deckelbaum, L. I., Laser-induced fluorescence spectroscopy of human colonic mucosa, *Gastroenterology* 99(1), 150–157, 1990.

74. Chwirot, B. W., Chwirot, S., Jedrzejczyk, W., Jackowski, M., Raczynska, A. M., Winczakiewicz, J., and Dobber, J., Ultraviolet laser-induced fluorescence of human stomach tissues: Detection of cancer tissues by imaging techniques, *Lasers in Surgery and Medicine* 21(2), 149–158, 1997.

75. Laufer, G., Wollenek, G., Hohla, K., Horvat, R., Henke, K. H., Buchelt, M., Wutzl, G., and Wolner, E., Excimer laser-induced simultaneous ablation and spectral identification of normal and atherosclerotic arterial tissue layers, *Circulation* 78(4), 1031–1039, 1988.

76. Baraga, J. J. R., Rava, R. P., Taroni, P., Kittrell, C., Fitzmaurice, M., and Feld, M. S., Laser induced fluorescence spectroscopy of normal and atherosclerotic human aorta using 306–310 nm excitation, *Lasers in Surgery and Medicine* 10(3), 245–261, 1990.

77. Bosshart, F., Utzinger, U., Hess, O. M., Wyser, J., Mueller, A., Schneider, J., Niederer, P., Anliker, M., and Krayenbuehl, H. P., Fluorescence spectroscopy for identification of atherosclerotic tissue, *Cardiovascular Research* 26(6), 620–625, 1992.

78. Lucas, A. R., Radosavljevic, M. J., Lu, E., and Gaffney, E. J., Characterization of human coronary artery atherosclerotic plaque fluorescence emission, *Canadian Journal of Cardiology* 6(6), 219–228, 1990.

79. Richards-Kortum, R., Rava, R. P., Fitzmaurice, M., Kramer, J. R., and Feld, M. S., 476 nm excited laser-induced fluorescence spectroscopy of human coronary-arteries—Applications in cardiology, *American Heart Journal* 122(4), 1141–1150, 1991.

80. Verbunt, R., Fitzmaurice, M. A., Kramer, J. R., Ratliff, N. B., Kittrell, C., Taroni, P., Cothren, R. M., Baraga, J., and Feld, M., Characterization of ultraviolet laser-induced autofluorescence of ceroid deposits and other structures in atherosclerotic plaques as a potential diagnostic for laser angiosurgery, *American Heart Journal* 123(1), 208–216, 1992.

81. Fitzmaurice, M., Bordagaray, J. O., Engelmann, G. L., Richards-Kortum, R., Kolubayev, T., Feld, M. S., Ratliff, N. B., and Kramer, J. R., Argon ion laser-excited autofluorescence in normal and atherosclerotic aorta and coronary arteries: Morphologic studies, *American Heart Journal* 118(5 pt 1), 1028–1038, 1989.

82. Chaudhry, H. W., Rebecca, R.-K., Kolubayev, T., Kittrell, C., Partovi, F., Kramer, J. R., and Feld, M. S., Alteration of spectral characteristics of human artery wall caused by 476-nm laser irradiation, *Lasers in Surgery and Medicine* 9(6), 572–580, 1989.

83. Andersson-Engels, S., Johansson, J., Svanberg, K., and Svanberg, S., Fluorescence imaging and point measurements of tissue: Applications to the demarcation of malignant tumors and atherosclerotic lesions from normal tissue, *Photochemistry and Photobiology* 53(6), 807–814, 1991.

84. Andersson-Engels, S., Johansson, J., Stenram, U., Svanberg, K., and Svanberg, S., Time-resolved laser-induced fluorescence spectroscopy for enhanced demarcation of human atherosclerotic plaques, *Journal of Photochemistry and Photobiology B* 4(4), 363–369, 1990.

85. Perk, M. F., Flynn, G. J., Gulamhusein, S., Wen, Y., Smith, C., Bathgate, B., Tulip, J., Parfrey, N. A., and Lucas, A., Laser induced fluorescence identification of sinoatrial and atrioventricular nodal conduction tissue, *Pacing and Clinical Electrophysiology* 16(8), 1701–1712, 1993.

86. van der Veen, M. H. and ten Bosch, J. J., Autofluorescence of bulk sound and in vitro demineralized human root dentin, *European Journal of Oral Sciences* 103(6), 375–381, 1995.

87. Samoszuk, M., Eosinophils and human cancer, *Histology and Histopathology* 12(3), 807–812, 1997.

88. Barnes, D., Aggarwal, S., Thomsen, S., Fitzmaurice, M., and Richards-Kortum, R., A characterization of the fluorescent properties of circulating human eosinophils, *Photochemistry and Photobiology* 58(2), 297–303, 1993.

89. Pompella, A. and Comporti, M., Imaging of oxidative stress at subcellular level by confocal laser scanning microscopy after fluorescent derivatization of cellular carbonyls, *American Journal of Pathology* 142(5), 1353–1357, 1993.

90. Richards-Kortum, R., Mehta, A., Hayes, G., Cothren, R., Kolubayev, T., Kittrell, C., Ratliff, N. B., Kramer, J. R., and Feld, M. S., Spectral diagnosis of atherosclerosis using an optical fiber laser catheter, *American Heart Journal* 118(2), 381–391, 1989.

91. Alfano, R. R. and Yao, S. S., Human-teeth with and without dental-caries studied by visible luminescent spectroscopy, *Journal of Dental Research* 60(2), 120–122, 1981.

92. Zellweger, M., Goujon, D., Conde, R., Forrer, M., van den Bergh, H., and Wagnieres, G., Absolute autofluorescence spectra of human healthy, metaplastic, and early cancerous bronchial tissue in vivo, *Applied Optics* 40(22), 3784–3791, 2001.

93. Zellweger, M., Grosjean, P., Goujon, D., Monnier, P., van den Bergh, H., and Wagnieres, G., In vivo autofluorescence spectroscopy of human bronchial tissue to optimize the detection and imaging of early cancers, *Journal of Biomedical Optics* 6(1), 41–51, 2001.

94. Wang, T. D., Crawford, J. M., Feld, M. S., Wang, Y., Itzkan, I., and Van Dam, J., In vivo identification of colonic dysplasia using fluorescence endoscopic imaging, *Gastrointestinal Endoscopy* 49(4), 447–455, 1999.

95. Wennberg, A. M., Gudmundson, F., Stenquist, B., Ternesten, A., Molne, L., Rosen, A., and Larko, O., In vivo detection of basal cell carcinoma using imaging spectroscopy, *Acta Dermato-Venereologica* 79(1), 54–61, 1999.

96. Schantz, S. P., Kolli, V., Savage, H. E., Yu, G. P., Shah, J. P., Harris, D. E., Katz, A., Alfano, R. R., and Huvos, A. G., In vivo native cellular fluorescence and histological characteristics of head and neck cancer, *Clinical Cancer Research* 4(5), 1177–1182, 1998.

97. Major, A. L., Rose, G. S., Chapman, C. F., Hiserodt, J. C., Tromberg, B. J., Krasieva, T. B., Tadir, Y., Haller, U., DiSaia, P. J., and Berns, M. W., In vivo fluorescence detection of ovarian cancer in the NuTu-19 epithelial ovarian cancer animal model using 5-aminolevulinic acid (ALA), *Gynecologic Oncology* 66(1), 122–132, 1997.

98. Andersson Engels, S., afKlinteberg, C., Svanberg, K., and Svanberg, S., In vivo fluorescence imaging for tissue diagnostics, *Physics in Medicine and Biology* 42(5), 815–824, 1997.

99. Ramanujam, N., Chen, J. X., Gossage, K., Richards-Kortum, R., and Chance, B., Fast and noninvasive fluorescence imaging of biological tissues in vivo using a flying-spot scanner, *IEEE Transactions on Biomedical Engineering* 48(9), 1034–1041, 2001.

100. Brancaleon, L., Durkin, A. J., Tu, J. H., Menaker, G., Fallon, J. D., and Kollias, N., In vivo fluorescence spectroscopy of nonmelanoma skin cancer, *Photochemistry and Photobiology* 73(2), 178–183, 2001.

101. Koenig, F., Knittel, J., and Stepp, H., Diagnosing cancer in vivo, *Science* 292(5520), 1401–1403, 2001.

102. Brewer, M., Utzinger, U., Silva, E., Gershenson, D., Bast, R. C., Follen, M., and Richards-Kortum, R., Fluorescence spectroscopy for in vivo characterization of ovarian tissue, *Lasers in Surgery and Medicine* 29(2), 128–135, 2001.

103. Panjehpour, M., Overholt, B. F., Vodinh, T., Farris, C., and Sneed, R., Fluorescence spectroscopy for detection of malignant-tissue in the esophagus, *Gastroenterology* 104(4), A439, 1993.

104. Panjehpour, M., Overholt, B. F., Schmidhammer, J. L., Farris, C., Buckley, P. F., and Vodinh, T., Spectroscopic diagnosis of esophageal cancer—New classification model, improved measurement system, *Gastrointestinal Endoscopy* 41(6), 577–581, 1995.

105. Panjehpour, M., Overholt, B. F., VoDinh, T., Haggitt, R. C., Edwards, D. H., and Buckley, F. P., Endoscopic fluorescence detection of high-grade dysplasia in Barrett's esophagus, *Gastroenterology* 111(1), 93–101, 1996.

106. Panjehpour, M., Overholt, B. F., VoDinh, T., Haggitt, R. C., Edwards, D. H., Buckley, F. P., and Decosta, J. F., Fluorescence spectroscopy for detection of dysplasia in Barrett's esophagus, *Gastroenterology* 110(4), A574, 1996.

107. Overholt, B. F., Panjehpour, M., VoDinh, T., Farris, C., Schmidhammer, J. L., Sneed, R. E., and Buckley, P. F., Spectroscopic diagnosis of esophageal cancer—Improved technique, *Gastroenterology* 106(4), A425, 1994.

108. Ramanujam, N., Fluorescence spectroscopy of neoplastic and non-neoplastic tissues, *Neoplasia* 2(1–2), 89–117, 2000.

109. Ramanujam, N., Mitchell, M. F., Mahadevan-Jansen, A., Thomsen, S. L., Staerkel, G., Malpica, A., Wright, T., Atkinson, N., and Richards-Kortum, R., Cervical precancer detection using a multivariate statistical algorithm based on laser-induced fluorescence spectra at multiple excitation wavelengths, *Photochemistry and Photobiology* 64(4), 720–735, 1996.

110. Lam, S. and Shibuya, H., Early diagnosis of lung cancer, *Clinics in Chest Medicine* 20(1), 53–61, 1999.

111. Lam, S. and Palcic, B., Autofluorescence bronchoscopy in the detection of squamous metaplasia and dysplasia in current and former smokers, *Journal of the National Cancer Institute* 91(6), 561–562, 1999.

112. Lam, S., Macaulay, C., Hung, J., Leriche, J., Profio, A. E., and Palcic, B., Detection of dysplasia and carcinoma in situ with a lung imaging fluorescence endoscope device, *Journal of Thoracic and Cardiovascular Surgery* 105(6), 1035–1040, 1993.

113. Lam, S., Hung, J. Y. C., Kennedy, S. M., Leriche, J. C., Vedal, S., Nelems, B., Macaulay, C. E., and Palcic, B., Detection of dysplasia and carcinoma in situ by ratio fluorometry, *American Review of Respiratory Disease* 146(6), 1458–1461, 1992.

114. Alfano, R. R. and Alfano, M. A., Medical diagnostics—A new optical frontier, *Photonics Spectra* 19(12), 55–60, 1985.

115. Alfano, R. R., Tang, G. C., Pradhan, A., and Wenling, S., Investigation of optical spectroscopy of cancerous and normal human-tissues, *Journal of the Electrochemical Society* 135(8), C387, 1988.

116. Alfano, R. R., Tomaselli, V. P., Beuthan, J., Feld, M. S., Flotte, T. J., Fujimoto, J. G., and Thomsen, S., Advances in optical biopsy and optical mammography—Panel discussion—Review and summary of presentations, in *Advances in Optical Biopsy and Optical Mammography*, Annals of the New York Academy of Sciences, Vol. 838, New York Academy of Sciences, New York, 1998, pp. 194–196.

117. Alfano, R. R., Advances in optical biopsy and optical mammography—Closing remarks, in *Advances in Optical Biopsy and Optical Mammography*, Annals of the New York Academy of Sciences, Vol. 838, New York Academy of Sciences, New York, 1998, p. 197.

118. Vo-Dinh, T., Panjehpour, M., Overholt, B. F., Farris, C., Buckley, F. P., and Sneed, R., In-vivo cancer-diagnosis of the esophagus using differential normalized fluorescence (DNF) indexes, *Lasers in Surgery and Medicine* 16(1), 41–47, 1995.

119. Braichotte, D., Savary, J. F., Glanzmann, T., Westermann, P., Folli, S., Wagnieres, G., Monnier, P., and Vandenbergh, H., Clinical pharmacokinetic studies of tetra(meta-hydroxyphenyl)chlorin in squamous-cell carcinoma by fluorescence spectroscopy at 2 wavelengths, *International Journal of Cancer* 63(2), 198–204, 1995.

120. Braichotte, D. R., Wagnieres, G. A., Bays, R., Monnier, P., and Vandenbergh, H. E., Clinical pharmacokinetic studies of photofrin by fluorescence spectroscopy in the oral cavity, the esophagus, and the bronchi, *Cancer* 75(11), 2768–2778, 1995.

121. Andrejevic, S., Savary, J.-F., Fontolliet, C., Monnier, P., and van den Bergh, H. E., 7,12-Dimethylbenz(a) anthracene-induced early squamous-cell carcinoma in the golden Syrian hamster: Evaluation of an animal model and comparison with early forms of human squamous-cell carcinoma in the upper aerodigestive tract, *International Journal of Experimental Pathology* 77, 7–14, 1996.

122. Schantz, S. P. and Alfano, R. R., Tissue autofluorescence as an intermediate end-point in cancer chemoprevention trials, *Journal of Cellular Biochemistry* 17F, 199–204, 1993.

123. Glasgold, R., Glasgold, M., Savage, H., Pinto, J., Alfano, R., and Schantz, S., Tissue autofluorescence as an intermediate end-point in NMBA-induced esophageal carcinogenesis, *Cancer Letters* 82(1), 33–41, 1994.

124. Chung, Y. G., Schwartz, J. A., Gardner, C. M., Sawaya, R. E., and Jacques, S. L., Diagnostic potential of laser-induced autofluorescence emission in brain tissue, *Journal of Korean Medical Science* 12(2), 135–142, 1997.

125. Oraevsky, A. A., Jacques, S. L., Pettit, G. H., Sauerbrey, R. A., Tittel, F. K., Nguy, J. H., and Henry, P. D., XeCl laser-induced fluorescence of atherosclerotic arteries. Spectral similarities between lipid-rich lesions and peroxidized lipoproteins, *Circulation Research* 72(1), 84–90, 1993.

126. van Leengoed, E., Versteeg, J., van der Veen, N., van der Berg-Blok, A., Marijnissen, H., and Star, W., Tissue-localizing properties of some photosensitizers studied by in vivo fluorescence imaging, *Journal of Photochemistry and Photobiology B* 6(1–2), 111–119, 1990.

127. Johansson, J., Berg, R., Svanberg, K., and Svanberg, S., Laser-induced fluorescence studies of normal and malignant tumour tissue of rat following intravenous injection of delta-amino levulinic acid, *Lasers in Surgery and Medicine* 20(3), 272–279, 1997.

128. Svanberg, K., Kjellen, E., Ankerst, J., Montan, S., Sjoholm, E., and Svanberg, S., Fluorescence studies of hematoporphyrin derivative in normal and malignant rat-tissue, *Cancer Research* 46(8), 3803–3808, 1986.

129. Andersson-Engels, S., Ankerst, J., Johansson, J., Svanberg, K., and Svanberg, S., Laser-induced fluorescence in malignant and normal tissue of rats injected with benzoporphyrin derivative, *Photochemistry and Photobiology* 57(6), 978–983, 1993.

130. Nilsson, H., Johansson, J., Svanberg, K., Svanberg, S., Jori, G., Reddi, E., Segalla, A., Gust, D., Moore, A. L., and Moore, T. A., Laser-induced fluorescence studies of the biodistribution of carotenoporphyrins in mice, *British Journal of Cancer* 76(3), 355–364, 1997.

131. Pathak, I., Davis, N. L., Hsiang, Y. N., Quenville, N. F., and Palcic, B., Detection of squamous neoplasia by fluorescence imaging comparing porfimer sodium fluorescence to tissue autofluorescence in the hamster cheek pouch model, *American Journal of Surgery* 170, 423–426, 1995.

132. Tsai, J. C., Kao, M. C., and Hsiao, Y. Y., Fluorospectral study of the rat brain and glioma in vivo, *Lasers in Surgery and Medicine* 13(3), 321–331, 1993.

133. Svanberg, K., Liu, D. L., Wang, I., Andersson-Engels, S., Stenram, U., and Svanberg, S., Photodynamic therapy using intravenous delta-aminolaevulinic acid-induced protoporphyrin IX sensitisation in experimental hepatic tumours in rats, *British Journal of Cancer* 74(10), 1526–1533, 1996.

134. Mitchell, M. F., Tortolero-Luna, G., Wright, T., Sarkar, A., Richards-Kortum, R., Hong, W. K., and Schottenfeld, D., Cervical human papillomavirus infection and intraepithelial neoplasia: A review, *Journal of the National Cancer Institute Monographs* 21, 17–25, 1996.

135. Mitchell, M. F., Hittelman, W. N., Lotan, R., Nishioka, K., Tortolero-Luna, G., Richards-Kortum, R., and Hong, W. K., Chemoprevention trials in the cervix: Design, feasibility, and recruitment, *Journal of Cellular Biochemistry Supplement* 23, 104–112, 1995.

136. Ramanujam, N., Mitchell, M. F., Mahadevan, A., Warren, S., Thomsen, S., Silva, E., and Richards-Kortum, R., In vivo diagnosis of cervical intra epithelial neoplasia using 337-nm-excited laser-induced fluorescence, *Proceedings of the National Academy of Sciences of the United States of America* 91(21), 10193–10197, 1994.

137. Ramanujam, N., Mitchell, M. F., Mahadevan, A., Thomsen, S., Silva, E., Richards-Kortum, R., Fluorescence spectroscopy: A diagnostic tool for cervical intra epithelial neoplasia (CIN), *Gynecologic Oncology* 52(1), 31–38, 1994.

138. Barrett, N., Chronic peptic ulcer of the oesophagus, *British Journal of Surgery* 38, 175–182, 1950.

139. Spechler, S. J. and Goyal, R. K., Barrett's esophagus, *New England Journal of Medicine* 315, 362–371, 1987.

140. Burbige, E. J. and Radigan, J. J., Characteristics of the columnar-lined (Barrett's) esophagus, *Gastrointestinal Endoscopy* 24, 133–136, 1979.

141. Cameron, A. J., Zinsmeister, A. R., and Ballard, D. J., Prevalence of columnar-lined (Barrett's) esophagus: Comparison of population-based and autopsy findings, *Gastroenterology* 99, 918–922, 1990.

142. Spechler, S. J., Robbins, A. H., Rubins, H. B., Vincent, M. E., Heeren, T., Doos, W. G., Colton, T., and Schimmel, E. M., Adenocarcinoma and Barrett's esophagus, an overrated risk, *Gastroenterology* 87, 927–933, 1984.

143. Polopalle, S. C. and McCallum, R. W., Barrett's esophagus: Current assessment and future perspectives, *Gastroenterology Clinics of North America* 19, 733–744, 1990.

144. Koenig, F., McGovern, F. J., Althausen, A. F., Deutsch, T. F., and Schomacker, K. T., Laser induced autofluorescence diagnosis of bladder cancer, *Journal of Urology* 156(5), 1597–1601, 1996.

145. Anidjar, M., Ettori, D., Cussenot, O., Meria, P., Desgrandchamps, F., Cortesse, A., Teillac, P., LeDuc, A., and Avrillier, S., Laser induced autofluorescence diagnosis of bladder tumors: Dependence on the excitation wavelength, *Journal of Urology* 156(5), 1590–1596, 1996.

146. Schomacker, K. T., Frisoli, J. K., Compton, C. C., Flotte, T. J., Richter, J. M., Nishioka, N. S., and Deutsch, T. F., Ultraviolet laser-induced fluorescence of colonic tissue: Basic biology and diagnostic potential, *Lasers in Surgery and Medicine* 12(1), 63–78, 1992.

147. Cothren, R. M., Sivak, M. V., VanDam, J., Petras, R. E., Fitzmaurice, M., Crawford, J. M., Wu, J. et al., Detection of dysplasia at colonoscopy using laser-induced fluorescence: A blinded study, *Gastrointestinal Endoscopy* 44(2), 168–176, 1996.

148. Cothren, R. M., Richardskortum, R., Sivak, M. V., Fitzmaurice, M., Rava, R. P., Boyce, G. A., Doxtader, M. et al., Gastrointestinal tissue diagnosis by laser-induced fluorescence spectroscopy at endoscopy, *Gastrointestinal Endoscopy* 36(2), 105–111, 1990.

149. Lashner, B. A. and Brzezinski, A., Cancer mortality-rates in ulcerative-colitis surveillance programs, *Gastroenterology* 106(1), 278, 1994.

150. Lashner, B. A., Provencher, K. S., Bozdech, J. M., and Brzezinski, A., Worsening risk for the development of dysplasia or cancer in patients with chronic ulcerative-colitis, *Gastroenterology* 106(4), A718, 1994.

151. Jensen, P., Krogsgaard, M. R., Christiansen, J., Braendstrup, O., Johansen, A., and Olsen, J., Observer variability in the assessment of type and dysplasia of colorectal adenomas, analyzed using kappa-statistics, *Diseases of the Colon & Rectum* 38(2), 195–198, 1995.

152. Kolli, V. R., Shaha, A. R., Savage, H. E., Sacks, P. G., Casale, M. A., and Schantz, S. P., Native cellular fluorescence can identify changes in epithelial thickness in-vivo in the upper aerodigestive tract, *American Journal of Surgery* 170(5), 495–498, 1995.

153. Kolli, V. R., Savage, H. E., Yao, T. J., and Schantz, S. P., Native cellular fluorescence of neoplastic upper aerodigestive mucosa, *Archives of Otolaryngology: Head & Neck Surgery* 121(11), 1287–1292, 1995.

154. Dhingra, J. K., Perrault, D. F., McMillan, K., Rebeiz, E. E., Kabani, S., Manoharan, R., Itzkan, I., Feld, M. S., and Shapshay, S. M., Early diagnosis of upper aerodigestive tract cancer by autofluorescence, *Archives of Otolaryngology: Head & Neck Surgery* 122(11), 1181–1186, 1996.

155. Fryen, A., Glanz, H., Lohmann, W., Dreyer, T., and Bohle, R. M., Significance of autofluorescence for the optical demarcation of field cancerization in the upper aerodigestive tract, *Acta Otolaryngologica (Stockholm)* 117(2), 316–319, 1997.

156. Heintzelman, D. L., Utzinger, U., Fuchs, H., Zuluaga, A., Gossage, K., Gillenwater, A. M., Jacob, R., Kemp, B., and Richards-Kortum, R. R., Optimal excitation wavelengths for in vivo detection of oral neoplasia using fluorescence spectroscopy, *Photochemistry and Photobiology* 72(1), 103–113, 2000.

157. Zargi, M., Šmid, L., Fajdiga, I., Bubnic, B., Lenarcic, J., and Oblak, P., Detection and localization of early laryngeal cancer with laser-induced fluorescence: Preliminary report, *European Archives of Otorhinolaryngology* 254 (Suppl. 1), S113–S116, 1997.

158. Masters, B. R., So, P. T., and Gratton, E., Multiphoton excitation fluorescence microscopy and spectroscopy of in vivo human skin, *Biophysical Journal* 72(6), 2405–2412, 1997.

159. Leffell, D. J., Stetz, M. L., Milstone, L. M., and Deckelbaum, L. I., In vivo fluorescence of human skin. A potential marker of photoaging, *Archives of Dermatology* 124(10), 1514–1518, 1988.

160. Klinteberg, C., Enejder, A. M. K., Wang, I., Andersson, E., Svanberg, S., and Svanberg, K., Kinetic fluorescence studies of 5-aminolaevulinic acid-induced protoporphyrin IX accumulation in basal cell carcinomas, *Journal of Photochemistry and Photobiology B* 49, 120–128, 1999.

161. Chissov, V. I. Sokolov, V. V., Filonenko, E. V., Menenkov, V. D., Zharkova, N. N., Kozlov, D. N., Polivanov, I. N., Prokhorov, A. M., Pyhov, R. L., and Smirnov, V. V., Clinical fluorescent diagnosis of tumors using photosensitizer photogem, *Khirurgiia (Mosk)* 5, 37–41, 1995.

162. Heyerdahl, H., Wang, I., Liu, D. L., Berg, R., AnderssonEngels, S., Peng, Q., Moan, J., Svanberg, S., and Svanberg, K., Pharmacokinetic studies on 5-aminolevulinic acid-induced protoporphyrin IX accumulation in tumours and normal tissues, *Cancer Letters* 112(2), 225–231, 1997.

163. Leunig, A., Rick, K., Stepp, H., Goetz, A., Baumgartner, R., and Feyh, J., Fluorescence photodetection of neoplastic lesions in the oral cavity following topical application of 5-aminolevulinic acid, *Laryngo-Rhino-Otologie* 75(8), 459–464, 1996.

164. von Holstein, C. S., Nilsson, A. M., Andersson-Engels, S., Willen, R., Walther, B., and Svanberg K., Detection of adenocarcinoma in Barrett's oesophagus by means of laser induced fluorescence, *Gut* 39(5), 711–716, 1996.

165. Baert, L., Berg, R., Vandamme, B., Dhallewin, M. A., Johansson, J., Svanberg, K., and Svanberg, S., Clinical fluorescence diagnosis of human bladder-carcinoma following low-dose photofrin injection, *Urology* 41(4), 322–330, 1993.

166. Svanberg, K., Andersson, T., Killander, D., Wang, I., Stenram, U., Anderssonengels, S., Berg, R., Johansson, J., and Svanberg, S., Photodynamic therapy of nonmelanoma malignant-tumors of the skin using topical delta-amino levulinic acid sensitization and laser irradiation, *British Journal of Dermatology* 130(6), 743–751, 1994.

167. Sterenborg, H., Saarnak, A. E., Frank, R., and Motamedi, M., Evaluation of spectral correction techniques for fluorescence measurements on pigmented lesions in vivo, *Journal of Photochemistry and Photobiology B, Biology* 35(3), 159–165, 1996.

168. Folli, S., Wagnieres, G., Pelegrin, A., Calmes, J. M., Braichotte, D., Buchegger, F., Chalandon, Y. et al., Immunophotodiagnosis of colon carcinomas in patients injected with fluoresceinated chimeric antibodies against carcinoembryonic antigen, *Proceedings of the National Academy of Sciences of the United States of America* 89(17), 7973–7977, 1992.

169. Renkoski, T. E., Banerjee, B., Graves, L. R., Rial, N. S., Reid, S. A. H., Tsikitis, V. L., Nfonsam, V. N., Tiwari, P., Gavini, H., and Utzinger, U., Ratio images and ultraviolet C excitation in autofluorescence imaging of neoplasms of the human colon, *Journal of Biomedical Optics* 18(1), 016005, 2013.

170. Ebert, B. and Grosenick, D., Optical imaging of breast tumors and of gastrointestinal cancer by laser-induced fluorescence, *Recent Results in Cancer Research* 187, 331–350, 2013.

171. George, R., Michaelides, M., Brewer, M. A., and Utzinger, U., Parallel factor analysis of ovarian autofluorescence as a cancer diagnostic, *Lasers in Surgery and Medicine* 44, 282–295, 2012.

172. Pogorzelski, B., Hanenkamp, U., Goetz, M., Kiesslich, R., and Gosepath, J., Systematic intraoperative application of confocal endomicroscopy for early detection and resection of squamous cell carcinoma of the head and neck, a preliminary report, *Archives of Otolaryngology: Head & Neck Surgery* 138(4), 404–411, 2012.

173. Van der Beek, N., de Leeuw, J., Demmendal, C., Bjerring, P., Neumann, H. A. M., PpIX fluorescence combined with auto-fluorescence is more accurate than PpIX fluorescence alone in fluorescence detection of non-melanoma skin cancer: An intra-patient direct comparison study, *Lasers in Surgery and Medicine* 44, 271–276, 2012.

174. Koenig, K., Riemann, I., Ehlers, A., Bueckle, R., Dimitrow, E., Kaatz, M., Fluhr, J., and Elsner, P., In vivo multiphoton tomography of skin cancer, in *Multiphoton Microscopy in the Biomedical Sciences VI*, Periasamy, A. and So, P. T. C. (Eds.), *Proceedings of the SPIE* 6089, SPIE Publishers, Bellingham, WA, p. R890, 2006.

175. Liu, G., Grant, G., Li, L., Zhang, Y., Hu, F., Li, S., Wilson, C., Chen, K., Bigner, D., and Vo-Dinh, T., Compact point-detection fluorescence spectroscopy system for quantifying intrinsic fluorescence redox ratio in brain cancer diagnostics, *Journal of Biomedical Optics* 16, 037004, 2011.

176. Panjehpour, M., Overholt, B. F., Vo-Dinh, T., and Coppola, D., The effect of reactive atypia/inflammation on the laser-induced fluorescence diagnosis of non-dysplastic Barrett's esophagus, *Lasers in Surgery and Medicine* 44, 390–396, 2012.

177. Panjehpour, M., Coppola, D., Overholt, B. F., Vo-Dinh, T., and Overholt, S., Photodynamic therapy of Barrett's esophagus: Ablation of Barrett's mucosa and reduction in P53 protein expression after treatment, *Anticancer Research* 28, 485–489, 2008.

178. Liu, Q. and Vo-Dinh, T., Spectral filtering modulation method for estimation of hemoglobin concentration and oxygenation based on a single fluorescence emission spectrum in tissue phantoms, *Medical Physics* 36, 4819–4829, 2009.

179. Lloyd, J. B. F., Synchronized excitation of fluorescence emission spectra, *Nature Physical Science* 231, 64, 1971.

180. Vo-Dinh, T., Gammage, R. B., and Martinez, P. R., Analysis of a workplace air particulate sample by synchronous luminescence and room temperature phosphorescence, *Analytical Chemistry* 53, 253–258, 1981.

181. Alarie, J. P., Vo-Dinh, T., Miller, G., Ericson, M. N., Maddox, S. R., Watts, W., Eastwood, D., Lidberg, R., and Dominguez, M., Development of a battery-operated portable synchronous luminescence spectrofluorometer, *Review of Scientific Instruments* 64, 2541–2546, 1993.

182. Hueber, D. M., Stevenson, C. L., and Vo-Dinh, T., Fast scanning synchronous luminescence spectrometer based on acousto-optic tunable filters, *Applied Spectroscopy* 49, 1624–1631, 1995.

183. Stevenson, C. L. and Vo-Dinh, T., Laser-excited synchronous luminescence spectroscopy, *Applied Spectroscopy* 47, 430, 1993.

184. Stevenson, C. L., Johnson, R. W., and Vo-Dinh, T., Synchronous luminescence: A new detection technique for multiple fluorescent probes used for DNA sequencing, *Biotechniques* 16, 1104, 1994.

185. Vo-Dinh, T., Viallet, P., Del Olmo, I. M., Hueber, D., Stevenson, C. L., and Campiglia, A. D., Laser-excited synchronous fluorescence system for the analysis of polycyclic aromatic compounds, *Polycyclic Aromatic Compounds* 9, 265–272, 1996.

186. Askari, M., Miller, G., and Vo-Dinh, T., Synchronous luminescence: A simple technique for the analysis of hydrolysis activity of the fragile histidine triad protein, *Biotechnology Letters* 23, 1697–1702, 2001.

187. Viallet, P. M., Vo-Dinh, T., Vigo, J., and Salmon, J. M., Investigation of lysozyme-chitobioside interactions using synchronous luminescence and lifetime measurements, *Journal of Fluorescence* 12, 57–63, 2002.

188. Askari, M. D. and Vo-Dinh, T., Implication of mitochondrial involvement in apoptotic activity of fragile histidine triad gene: Application of synchronous luminescence spectroscopy, *Biopolymers* 73, 510–523, 2004.

189. Liu, Q., Chen, K., Martin, M., Wintenberg, A., Lenarduzzi, R., Panjehpour, M., Overholt, B. F., and Vo-Dinh, T., Development of a synchronous fluorescence imaging system and data analysis methods, *Optics Express* 15, 12583–12594, 2007.

190. Liu, Q. and Vo-Dinh, T., Investigation of synchronous fluorescence method in multi-component analysis in tissue, *IEEE Journal of Selected Topics in Quantum Electronic* 16, 927–940, 2010.

191. Dramicanin, T., Dramicanin, M. D., Jokanovic, V., Nikolic-Vukosavljevic, D., and Dimitrijevic, B., Three-dimensional total synchronous luminescence spectroscopy criteria for discrimination between normal and malignant breast tissues, *Photochemistry and Photobiology* 81, 1554–1558, 2005.

192. Dramicanin, T., Dimitrijevic, B., and Dramicanin, M. D., Application of supervised self-organizing maps in breast cancer diagnosis by total synchronous fluorescence spectroscopy, *Applied Spectroscopy* 65(3), 293–297, 2011.

193. Diagaradjane, P., Yaseen, M. A., Jie, Y., Wong, M. S., and Anvari, B., Synchronous fluorescence spectroscopic characterization of DMBA-TPA induced squamous cell carcinoma in mice, *Journal of Biomedical Optics* 11, 14012, 2006.

194. Patra, D. and Mishra, A. K., Recent developments in multi-component synchronous fluorescence scan analysis, *TrAC—Trends in Analytical Chemistry* 21, 787–798, 2002.

195. Vengadesan, N., Anbupalam, T., Hemamalini, S., Ebenezar, J., Muthvelu, K., Koteeswaran, D., Aruna, P. R., and Ganesan, S., Characterization of cervical normal and abnormal tissues by synchronous luminescence spectroscopy, *Proceedings of the SPIE* 4613, 13–17, 2002.

196. Ebenezar, J., Aruna, P., and Ganesan, S., Synchronous fluorescence spectroscopy for the detection and characterization of cervical cancers in vitro, *Photochemistry and Photobiology* 86, 77–86, 2010.

16

Elastic-Scattering Spectroscopy and Diffuse Reflectance

Judith R. Mourant
Los Alamos National Laboratory

Irving J. Bigio
Boston University

16.1 Basic Concepts

Wavelength-dependent spectral measurements of elastically scattered light from tissue, performed in a manner that is sensitive to scattering and absorption properties, may be used to detect and diagnose tissue pathologies. Many tissue pathologies, including a majority of cancers, exhibit significant architectural changes at the cellular and subcellular level. In making a diagnosis, pathologists determine some of these architectural changes by examining surgically removed samples called biopsies. Microscopic assessment, often referred to as histopathology, is performed on the biopsy samples to determine cell and tissue architecture, including the sizes and shapes of cells, the ratio of nuclear to cellular volume, the form of the bilipid membrane, cell clustering patterns, etc. The properties of light elastically scattered in tissue also depend on architectural features. For example, the size of the structures in tissue responsible for the scattering of light determines how much more strongly a short wavelength, for example, blue light, is scattered than a long wavelength, for example, red light.

This concept is illustrated in Figure 16.1, where the likelihood of scattering is plotted as a function of wavelength for suspensions of two different sizes of spheres. If the scattering structures are much smaller than the measurement light wavelengths, the scattering probability decreases as $1/\lambda^4$, where λ is wavelength. If the particles are of a size near that of the measurement light wavelengths or larger, scattering will not decrease nearly as rapidly with wavelength. Light is scattered by structures with a variety of shapes and sizes in tissue. Properties of light that has scattered inside tissue, such as the wavelength-dependent intensity, can provide information on cell and tissue structure.

The full range of information available and its relationship to traditional histopathology are still under investigation. Most likely, noninvasive light scattering methods will provide a subset of traditional histopathologic characterization as well as some information not traditionally available. The propagation

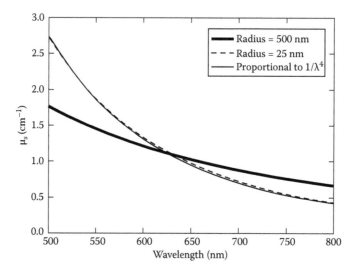

FIGURE 16.1 The wavelength dependence of the scattering coefficient, μ_s, for two sizes of spheres. The scattering coefficient, typically denoted by μ_s, is the inverse of the mean free path between scattering events. The spheres had an index of refraction of 1.39 and were immersed in a medium of index 1.35. The concentration of spheres with a radius of 25 nm was 300 times greater than the concentration of spheres with a radius of 500 nm. All calculations were performed using a solution to Maxwell's equations for a plane wave incident on an object, in this case a sphere called Mie theory. (For a discussion of Mie theory, see Bohren, C.F. and Huffman, D.R., *Absorption and Scattering of Light by Small Particles*, Wiley-Interscience, New York, 1983.)

of light through tissue depends on absorption as well as scattering properties. The three primary light absorbing compounds in healthy, nonskin tissue are oxygenated hemoglobin, deoxygenated hemoglobin, and water. Absorption spectra of these chromophores are shown in Figure 16.2. Concentrations of these compounds can serve as important diagnostic criteria. The importance of hemoglobin oxygenation and the ability of optical systems to provide quantitative information have already been demonstrated by the pulsed oximeter, which is in widespread use.[1]

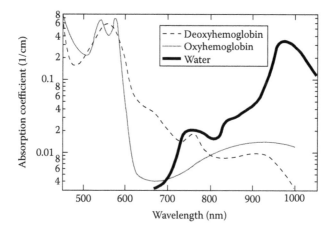

FIGURE 16.2 Absorption spectra of oxyhemoglobin, deoxyhemoglobin, and water. The concentration of heme groups is taken to be 20 mM. (The hemoglobin spectra are a combination of data taken by the authors and from van Assendelft, O.W., *Spectrophotometry of Haemoglobin Derivatives*, Royal Vangorcum Ltd., Assen, the Netherlands, 1970; Wray, S. et al., *Biochim. Biophys. Acta*, 933, 184, 1988.) The absorption of water has been scaled by a factor of 0.7 to be consistent with the idea that tissue is about 70% water. (The water spectra data are from Kou, L. et al., *Appl. Opt.*, 32, 3531, 1993.)

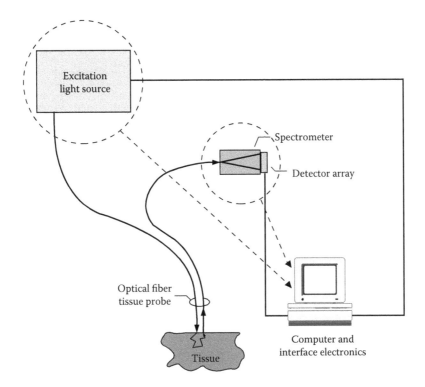

FIGURE 16.3 A schematic of a system for measuring elastic scattering and diffuse reflectance. The excitation light source is typically a tungsten bulb or a mercury arc-lamp. The optical fibers are multimode, often with diameters of 200 μm, although larger diameter fibers are sometimes used. The spectrometer is commonly a CCD (charge-coupled device), although diode arrays have also been used.

The basic geometry of the measurements described in this chapter is shown in Figure 16.3. Broad band-width light is incident on the tissue, typically through a flexible optical fiber with a diameter of 0.2–0.4 mm. This light travels into the tissue and can be absorbed and scattered. The absorption depends strongly on wavelength; it is greatest at visible wavelengths for which hemoglobin absorbs and much lower at near-infrared wavelengths between the hemoglobin and water absorption bands. Tissue is highly scattering, and the average distance between scattering events is on the order of 100 μm (0.1 mm). A small fraction of the light that is not absorbed will be scattered such that it can be collected by a probe on the surface near the original delivery location. Thus, the light collected and transmitted to the analyzing spectrometer has typically undergone several scattering events through a small volume of the tissue. No light is collected from surface reflection. The measurements typically take a fraction of a second and cause no damage to the tissue.

Systems that use light levels meeting FDA guidelines have been designed. The components of the optical system in Figure 16.3 have an intrinsic wavelength dependence; for example, silicon CCD detectors are more efficient at some wavelengths than at others. Consequently, the spectral dependence of the measurement system must be determined. Commonly, this is accomplished using a control sample that reflects equally at all wavelengths. An example of the elastic-scatter spectrum of tissue (from the esophagus), corrected for the wavelength dependence of the measurement system, is shown in Figure 16.4. The dips at 419, 543, and 577 nm are due to absorption by hemoglobin. Past 650 nm and before water absorption becomes significant, the decreasing intensity is due to the decreased scattering probability with increasing wavelength. The distance the collected photons travel in the tissue is several times greater than the separation of the light delivery and detection points. Consequently, in addition to the scattering spectral sensitivity to microscopic tissue morphology, this type of system can have good sensitivity to the optical absorption bands of the tissue components.

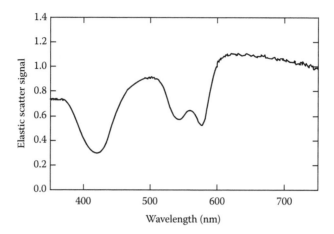

FIGURE 16.4   In vivo elastic scatter spectra of Barrett's esophagus. Light was delivered to the tissue with a 400 μm diameter optical fiber and collected with an adjacent 200 μm diameter optical fiber.

Sensitivity to absorption increases as the source and detector are separated. Quantitative measurements of the compounds in Figure 16.2 as well as possibly other absorbing compounds, such as fat and melanin, may be made at the same time tissue structural properties are determined. The intensity and wavelength dependence of the elastic-scatter spectrum depend on several light transport properties. The likelihood of scattering is generally quantified as the scattering coefficient, μ_s, which has units of inverse length. The scattering coefficient is the inverse of the average distance light travels between scattering events.

In addition to the scattering coefficient, μ_s, a complete description of the scattering properties of a tissue requires knowledge of the angular scattering probability distribution, often written as $P(\theta)$, where the deflection angle, θ, ranges from 0 to π. Physically, $P(\theta)$ is the probability that when a photon is scattered it is deflected by an angle θ. Using $P(\theta)$ as the angular scattering probability distribution is a simplification of the physics of light scattering in tissue that assumes the scattering centers are spherical in shape. In tissue, the scattering structures are not spherically symmetric and the angular scattering probability is, in principle $P(\theta,\phi)$, where ϕ is the azimuthal angle, ranging from 0 to 2π. To complete the description of the light transport properties of a medium, the absorption coefficient, μ_a, must be known. The absorption coefficient quantifies the decrease in light intensity when light is absorbed. If light with an initial intensity I_0 travels a distance L through an absorbing medium, the resultant intensity, I, is given by

$$I = I_0 \exp(-\mu_a L) \tag{16.1}$$

When the scattering coefficient, μ_s, absorption coefficient, μ_a, and angular scattering probability, $P(\theta,\phi)$ are all known, the transport of light through tissue can be calculated using the "transport equation."[2-4] (This equation can be derived from conservation of photons traveling into and out of a small volume.[2]) However, it can only be solved analytically for special geometries and consequently approximations are often used.

The most common approximation is the diffusion equation, which holds when the light collection is well separated from light delivery—typically a few centimeters.[5,6] (This approximation assumes that $P(\theta,\phi)$ and the light source term can be expanded in Legendre polynomials and only terms with $\ell \leq 1$ kept.) In this approximation, the light transport properties can be described by μ_a and the reduced scattering coefficient, $\mu_s' = \mu_s(1 - g)$, where $g = \langle \cos \theta \rangle$. The anisotropy parameter, g, is 0 when scattering from an object is equally likely in the forward and backward directions and is near 1 when scattering is primarily forward directed. The reduced scattering coefficient, μ_s', is quite intuitive; it is greater for a substance that appears more scattering, such as whole milk compared to skim milk. In contrast, two scattering suspensions with the same scattering coefficients may appear quite different. A suspension in

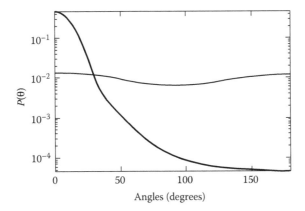

FIGURE 16.5 The probability of scattering s to s', where s is the incoming direction of propagation, s' is the direction of propagation after scattering, and $\cos \theta = s \times s'$. The thin line was calculated for spheres of 25 nm diameter with an index of 1.39 immersed in a medium of index 1.35 at 600 nm, $g = 0.025$. The thick line was calculated for spheres of 500 nm diameters with all other parameters the same, $g = 0.948$.

which scattering is forward directed will not appear to scatter light as strongly as a scattering medium in which scattering is equally likely in the forward and backward directions. In tissue, most light scattering is forward directed; in other words the deflection angle, θ, is on average quite small.

The identity of the morphological features that scatter light is not known with certainty and is an active area of research. Several structures have been proposed, including the cell membrane, the nucleus, mitochondria, and features within these and other organelles. The size, shape, and refractive index of tissue and cellular structural features determine how light is scattered. Figure 16.1 demonstrated how size affects the wavelength dependence of the scattering coefficient, μ_s. The size shape and refractive index also strongly influence the angular dependence of scattering at each wavelength. For example, as shown in Figure 16.5, particles much smaller than the measurement wavelength scatter light equally in the forward and backward directions, while light scattering from particles with dimensions on the order of the measurement wavelength is primarily in the forward direction.

The intensity of the collected light depends strongly on $P(\theta)$ and consequently on details of tissue structure. When the light source and collection areas are adjacent[7] and especially if they overlap,[8] the intensity of collected light correlates with the probability of high angle scattering events. For these measurement geometries, the details of $P(\theta)$ are quite important. As the separation between the small area of light delivery and the small area of light collection is increased, the dependencies of the collected light on the probability of large angle scattering events and on the details of $P(\theta)$ decreases. In fact, at larger separations (centimeters), only μ_s' and μ_a are needed to predict light collection and the diffusion approximation becomes valid. In this chapter, we are only interested in measurements with small source–detector separations because that geometry provides the greatest sensitivity to details of light-scattering properties. A further advantage of small distances between light delivery and detection is that the measurements can be made using fiber optics through the working channel of an endoscope. This feature enables access to many of the epithelial layers of tissue where most adult cancers arise.

16.2 Clinical Studies

Several small-scale, in vivo clinical trials have demonstrated the potential of elastically scattered light to diagnose tissue pathologies. Results of these trials are commonly presented in terms of the sensitivity and specificity for detecting a specified abnormality. Sensitivity is defined as the percentage of abnormal samples that the test found to be abnormal, whereas specificity is the percentage of normal samples that the test found to be normal. These two metrics can sometimes provide a quantitative method for comparing studies; however, the numbers should be interpreted with care. In many of the early studies, separate training and testing data sets were not used. Consequently, the reported sensitivity and specificity may be higher than they would be if determined with an independent data set. Furthermore, the gold standard used for these studies, histopathology, is not perfect; therefore, a sensitivity of 100% means that the test agrees with the pathologists, not that 100% of the abnormal samples were detected.

The measurement methods used in the following studies varied significantly. Methods for optimizing sensitivity to tissue pathology based on a detailed understanding of the physics and biology of light scattering in tissue are discussed in subsequent sections. The clinical studies described here will hopefully motivate that discussion by demonstrating the potential of light transport to provide clinically relevant information.

Skin is the most accessible organ for testing light-scattering methods for cancer diagnosis. Consequently, the earliest work examined lesions of the skin. Research in this area is still motivated by a need for noninvasive methods to distinguish melanoma from benign pigmented lesions (nevi). The earliest work involved only a small number of in vivo measurements[9] and concentrated on the absorption properties of skin due to melanin and hemoglobin.[10,11] Attempts to understand these spectra have led to a detailed understanding of the optical properties of skin.[12–14] In studies with a greater number of patients, statistical methods were applied to determine the significance of the results. Measurements of 31 primary melanomas and 31 benign nevi were made using a modified integrating sphere with a standard ultraviolet–visible spectrophotometer over the spectral range of 420–780 nm. The data were used to develop discriminant functions. A sensitivity of 90.3% and a specificity of 77.4% were obtained for distinguishing the melanomas from nevi with leave-one-out cross validation.[15]

More recently, wavelength-dependent reflectance images of skin have been obtained.[16] Light that entered the tissue and was scattered back to the surface as well as reflection off of the tissue surface was measured, making interpretation of the multispectral images difficult. It was noted that images of benign lesions fade faster with increasing wavelength than do images of cutaneous melanoma. The analysis of the data, however, did not make use of the wavelength dependence of any features, but rather used properties of individual images, such as lesion size and border irregularity. A sensitivity of 80% and a specificity of only 51% were obtained on the training data set.

A recent study by Wallace et al. measured the diffuse-reflectance spectra of skin over the spectral range of 300–1100 nm without any artifacts due to surface reflectance.[17] These data were analyzed using multivariate discriminant analysis and artificial neural networks.[18] The best results were obtained with the artificial neural network and yielded a sensitivity of 83.6% and specificity of 85.3% for diagnosing melanoma compared to compound nevi for the training set. When the artificial neural network was applied to new cases, the sensitivity and specificity changed to 90.9% and 58.8%, respectively.

As with most cancers, the survival rate for bladder cancer increases with early detection. While most frank tumors can be detected by a clinician, some flat (early) cancerous lesions are indistinguishable from inflammation. One of the earliest endoscopic clinical studies of elastic-scattering spectroscopy involved 10 patients undergoing examination for bladder cancer. Light was delivered using fiber optics with a center-to-center separation of about 350 μm at the distal end of the probe, which was placed in contact with the tissue. With knowledge of the pathology for each measured spectra, the slope from 330 to 370 nm found to be a diagnostic criteria with a sensitivity of 100% and a specificity of 97%.[19] Koenig et al.[20] have also tested scattering spectroscopy for sensing bladder cancer, but with distributed illumination of the tissue. They sensed the changes in hemoglobin absorption due to increased perfusion in neoplastic areas, but did not sense the spectral differences associated with structural changes. Consequently, the sensitivity was good (91%) but the specificity was poor (60%), because simple inflammation also causes increased perfusion. As with the previous study, the method has not been tested on a separate data set.

Several diseases of the gastrointestinal tract have been correlated with increased risk for the development of adenocarcinoma, including Barrett's esophagus, Crohn's disease (in the colon), and chronic ulcerative colitis of the colon. Consequently, clinical tests for diagnosis of cancer in the gastrointestinal tract have been performed. In an early study of 60 sites in the colon and rectum of 16 patients, a spectral metric was developed based on the regions of the hemoglobin absorption bands (400–440 nm and 540–580 nm). Eight sites diagnosed under histopathology as being dysplasia (a potentially premalignant condition), adenoma (premalignant growth), or adenocarcinoma were differentiated from sites of normal mucosa or more benign conditions such as hyperplastic polyps or quiescent colitis. The sensitivity of this metric on the set of data used to generate the metric was 100% with a specificity of 98%.[21]

A very clinically relevant study of the colon with both training and testing data sets has been published by Ge et al.[22] in which adenomatous polyps, which must be removed, and hyperplastic polyps, which do not need to be surgically resected, were distinguished. Three methods for spectral classification were tried: multiple linear regression, linear discriminant analysis, and neural network pattern recognition. The best predictive sensitivity and specificity were 89% and 75%, respectively, obtained using multiple linear regression. In a third study of the colon, diffuse reflectance spectra of 13 patients were measured and analyzed to obtain information on specific morphological and biochemical features.[23] These data were analyzed by applying the diffusion approximation to the transport equation in order to separate the effects of scattering and absorption. While the use of the diffusion approximation is possibly inappropriate because of the close proximity of the light detection and delivery fibers and may lead to systematic errors, this approach does have the advantage of yielding quantitative results. Hemoglobin concentration was significantly increased in the adenomatous polyps as compared to the normal mucosa, while hemoglobin oxygenation was essentially unchanged. Effective scatter density was decreased and effective scatterer size increased in the adenomatous polyps.

A few studies of light scattering for the diagnosis of dysplasia in patients with Barrett's esophagus have also been performed. Wallace et al. measured spectra at 76 sites in 13 patients.[24] These data were analyzed by a model assuming two components to the scattered light. One component is light that has been diffusely reflected and has an intensity that decreases monotonically with wavelength; the other is assumed to be an oscillatory component due to scattering from epithelial nuclei. After using eight samples to define the criteria for classifying the samples, the spectra were prospectively analyzed resulting in a sensitivity of 90% and a specificity of 90% for detecting dysplasia.

Bigio et al. measured spectra at 67 sites in 39 patients with Barrett's esophagus.[25] These data were analyzed using artificial neural networks and hierarchical cluster analysis. Sensitivity and specificity were calculated using 80% of the data for training, 20% for testing, and repeating this method five times until the sensitivity and specificity were determined for all of the data. The best results were obtained with hierarchical cluster analysis and resulted in an average sensitivity of 82% and an average specificity of 80%.

Light-scattering methods have also been combined with fluorescence to increase the accuracy of diagnosis of dysplasia in patients with Barrett's esophagus. In a study of 15 patients, the combined methods were able to separate dysplasia from nondysplastic Barrett's with a sensitivity and a specificity of 100% using leave-one-out cross validation.[26]

The advantages of early detection for cervical cancer have been demonstrated by the Papanicolaou (Pap) smear. However, the Pap smear has limitations such as sampling errors and a low sensitivity.[27] Nordstrom et al. have studied the ability of reflectance spectra to identify the stages of cervical intraepithelial neoplasia (CIN) in 41 patients.[28] Their measurements used flood illumination in a geometry that did not block the surface reflectance and consequently caused reduced sensitivity to the spectral differences associated with structural changes. They obtained a predictive sensitivity and specificity of 77% and 76%, respectively, for distinguishing CIN II/III from metaplasia.

Georgakoudi et al. demonstrated that when light-scattering methods are combined with fluorescence, the sensitivity and specificity for detecting squamous intraepithelial lesions increases substantially. Using pathology as the gold standard, and leave-one-out cross validation, their method had a sensitivity of 92% and a specificity of 71% for detecting squamous intraepithelial lesions versus mature squamous epithelium or squamous metaplasia.[29] Richards-Kortum's group has investigated the application of reflectance spectroscopy to additional gynecological cancers. In an exploratory study of ovarian cancer with 18 patients, Utzinger et al. were able to separate ovarian cancers retrospectively from normal ovary and benign neoplasms with a sensitivity of 86% and specificity of 80%.[30]

Clinical studies have also addressed applications to assist in the diagnosis and management of breast cancer. If a reliable method of diagnosing lesions through a needle could be developed, thousands of lumpectomies could be avoided each year in the United States alone. In the surgical arena, elastic-scattering spectroscopy could potentially assist the surgeon in determining tumor margins. An in vivo study of 72 biopsy sites in 24 patients has been performed; 80% of the data was used for training and 20% for testing of an artificial neural network. This procedure was repeated five times with disjoint testing sets and the average sensitivity and specificity for separating cancerous breast tissue from noncancerous breast were calculated to be 69% and 85%, respectively.[31] Another important diagnostic criterion in the evaluation of breast cancer is the involvement of the sentinel node, which is the first lymph node that drains the part of the breast containing the tumor. In the same breast cancer study cited above, hierarchical cluster analysis was used to separate involved from noninvolved sentinel nodes with a sensitivity of 91% and a specificity of 77%.

Another potential clinical benefit of optical light-scattering measurements using small probes is identification of tissues during brain surgery. Johns et al.[32] investigated the use of scattering spectroscopy to distinguish gray matter from white matter in vivo. This identification is important for surgeries such as pallidotomy, a treatment for Parkinson's patients. For this treatment the boundary of the globus pallidus, a structure composed of gray matter surrounded by white matter, must be accurately determined. The ability of reflectance spectroscopy in combination with fluorescence spectroscopy to identify brain tumors and infiltrating margins in vivo has been investigated by Mahadevan-Jansen and co-workers.[33] Using a two-step empirical discrimination algorithm, they obtained a retrospective sensitivity of 100% and a specificity of 76%.

16.3 Increasing Sensitivity to Structures of Interest

The details of the measurement geometries employed in the studies described above varied. This variation is likely to have influenced the reported sensitivities and specificities. An active area of research has been, and continues to be, the development of measurement methods to enhance the ability of elastic light scattering to detect cancerous and precancerous changes. Most cancers originate in the epithelium, which is typically 100–300 μm thick. Consequently, methods that only probe this top layer of tissue are desired. The separation of the source and detector is one controlling factor for sampling the top layer. As the source and detector are moved closer together a more superficial region is probed. If the illumination and detection areas overlap, the sensitivity will be further restricted to the epithelium.

Some of the probes designed by the biomedical spectroscopy group at MIT have this quality. By placing a quartz wedge on the probe surface, they were able to have overlapping light delivery and collection without interference from surface reflectance.[23] The use of a single fiber with a beveled tip for light delivery and detection can also increase sensitivity to the top surface. Measurements with linearly polarized light can be used to reject some of the multiply scattered light from deeper than the tissue layer of interest. An example of linearly polarized light is light propagating perpendicular to and toward the tissue surface while the electric field is oscillating in a direction parallel to the tissue surface (such as parallel to a line connecting the source and detector fibers). If polarized light incident on tissue returns to the surface after only a few scattering events, the polarization is likely to be very similar to the incident light polarization. If light penetrates more deeply into the tissue, the polarization will be randomized.

Measurement systems can be set up for which the light incident on the tissue is linearly polarized and the intensities of light returning to the surface with the same polarization or a perpendicular polarization are separately collected. Subtraction of these two light intensities is a measure of scattering near the tissue surface. Jacques et al. have demonstrated that when imaging with polarized light, they could obtain images that only pertained to approximately the top 265 μm of skin.[34] Backman et al. used broad-wavelength, polarized light scattering to isolate light scattered from near the tissue surface. Measurements were made individually of the light intensities scattered with polarizations parallel to or perpendicular to the incident light polarization, and the two intensities were subtracted.[35] Sokolov et al. have also made measurements of the diffuse reflectance of polarized light that are particularly sensitive to scattering near the surface.[36] In addition to localizing the measurement volume to the epithelium, these techniques are reported to provide quantitative characteristics of nuclei and are discussed in more detail in Section 16.6.

A third way to focus measurements primarily on the epithelium and not the underlying tissue is to make measurements of tissue morphology using wavelengths of light that do not penetrate deeply into tissue. When diffuse reflectance measurements are made at wavelengths that strongly absorb light, a shallower region of tissue is probed and the distance traveled in tissue is reduced. These results are illustrated in Figure 16.6, which shows typical trajectories for collected photons, as calculated by a Monte Carlo simulation. (This technique is described later in the chapter.) Representative trajectories for light transport with absorption are plotted on the left, while trajectories with no absorption are plotted on the right. For the case of absorption, the trajectories are quite short. In the case of no absorption, there are very few short trajectories; most are medium to long in length. By keeping the statistics on a large number of collected photons, the average pathlength for the case of no absorption was found to be 0.30 cm, and when absorption was present the pathlength was 0.17 cm. Similarly the median depth of scattering interactions changed from 0.062 to 0.037 cm. Light cannot penetrate deeply into tissue at wavelengths for which hemoglobin absorbs strongly. Therefore, if methods can be developed for measuring tissue morphology and architecture with only a single wavelength, then measurements that probe different tissue depths can be potentially achieved by using different wavelengths.

Techniques that use linearly polarized light, in a geometry different from that described above, are being developed to quantify the effective size and concentration of scattering centers in cells. This work will be described in more detail in Section 16.6. The basic physics of polarized light propagation in scattering media is still under active investigation. Yao and Wang have presented time-resolved movies of polarized light propagation in turbid media.[37] The preservation of polarization in lipid, myocardium, and polystyrene spheres has been studied in detail,[38,39] and methods for examining light scattered from tissues in the exact backscattering direction have also been developed.[40]

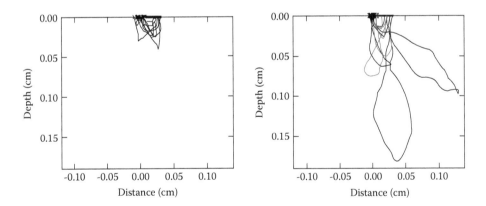

FIGURE 16.6 Trajectories for light transport through tissue calculated using Monte Carlo simulations. For both simulations, the scatterers were 500 nm radii spheres at a concentration such that the scattering coefficient was 245 cm^{-1} leading to a reduced scattering coefficient of 12.4 cm^{-1} at 600 nm. For the graph on the left, there was no absorption; for the graph on the right absorption was 1 cm^{-1}. The entry points for all trajectories are marked with crosses that lie between −0.01 and 0.01 cm; a black bar marks the position of the collection fiber, 0.01–0.03 cm. The trajectories have been projected onto the plane containing the delivery and detection fibers. Many more photons were run in the Monte Carlo simulation. The average trajectory length for the case of no absorption was found to be 0.30 cm; when absorption was present, the average trajectory length was 0.17 cm.

16.4 Understanding the Origins of Light Scattering in Tissue

The development of measurement systems to sense small changes in tissue and cellular architecture can be facilitated by an understanding of what structures in tissue are responsible for the scattering of light. In particular, the development of measurement systems may be improved with knowledge of the properties of light scattered from specific structures. Furthermore, the analysis of diffuse reflectance measurements, in terms of particular tissue or cellular structures, requires an understanding of scattering properties for specific architectural features.

Light scattering occurs at refractive index boundaries. As examples, light will scatter off an interface between two media of different indices, or from a sphere with an index of refraction different from its surrounding medium. Tissue is composed of materials with different refractive indices. For example, membranes have a higher index than water and will scatter light. Similarly high concentrations of DNA or protein can also scatter light. A wide variety of physical structures contain high concentrations of lipid, protein, or DNA within mammalian cells. Nuclei are on the order of 5–10 μm in diameter[41]; mitochondria, lysosomes, and peroxisomes have dimensions on the order of 0.2–2 μm.[42] Ribosomes are on the order of 20 nm in diameter[43] and structures within various organelles can have dimensions up to a few hundred nanometers. Refractive indices for some of these organelles have been compiled.[44] In liver tissue, mitochondria have been demonstrated to be a significant source of scattering.[45,46] Also for liver tissue, Schmitt and Kumar demonstrated that the spectrum of index variations exhibits a power-law behavior for a wide range of spatial frequencies.[47]

Models of tissue having a broad range of discrete particle sizes have been proposed; calculated scattering properties compared well with those available in the literature.[48] Further evidence for a broad size range of architectural features contributing to tissue light scattering comes from experimental measurements of light scattering from epithelial cells. Because the epithelium is primarily a cellular structure without much intracellular material, studying scattering from only the cells is quite relevant. The size distribution of refractive-index structure variations in epithelial cells was found to include particles with effective radii from smaller than a few hundred nanometers to ~2 μm. There are orders of magnitude more structures the size of macromolecules than there are particles the size of organelles scattering light.[49] Consistent with results that most scatterers are small, cell shape and cell–cell contact were found to have only very minor effects on light scattering.[50] Furthermore, the result that much of the light scattering occurs from structures a few hundred nanometers or less in radius implies that light scattering is likely to be sensitive to some structures smaller than those commonly investigated by standard pathology methods.

As discussed earlier, the importance of high angle scattering events for determining the intensity of collected light is increased when the separation between the illumination and light collection locations is reduced. Therefore, changing the source–detector separation may change the contribution of different structures to the elastic-scatter signal, if the contribution of various structure sizes to light scattering varies with scattering angle. There is evidence that different physical structures within cells are responsible for scattering at different angles. Cell size can be determined by measurements of scattering in the angle range of $\theta = 0.5°$–$1.5°$.[51] Scattering at angles between about 2° and 25° has been attributed to scattering from the nuclei. Measurements of Chinese hamster ovary (CHO) cells showed a fine structure between $\theta = 2.5°$ and 25° that could be modeled as a coated sphere, that is, a nucleus surrounded by cytoplasm, although for HeLa cells no fine structure was observed.[52]

Both experimental and modeling work indicate that small internal structures have a strong influence on the scattering pattern at angles greater than 40°.[44,53] Consequently, a decreased source–detector separation may increase the relative contribution of small structures to the measured diffuse reflectance. The contribution of the nucleus to light scattering from biological cells has been a topic of investigation by several groups because of the known changes in the nucleus accompanying carcinogenesis, including an increased nuclear-to-cytoplasmic ratio and changes in nuclear structure, one of which is apparent in histopathology as hyperchromaticity (dark irregular staining of DNA). For fibroblast cells, less than 40% of the scattered light at any angle was determined to have been scattered from the nucleus.[53]

Finite difference time-domain methods, which can calculate scattering from objects with very inhomogeneous index of refraction structures, have been used to study potential contributions of nuclei to light scattering.[44,54] Consistent with the idea that the nuclei contribute significantly to scattering at angles less than 25°, increasing the size of the nucleus increased the forward scattering.

If the nucleus is heterogeneous, high angle scattering also increases with nuclear size.[44] There is experimental evidence for nuclear heterogeneity. A determination of the size distribution of scattering centers within nuclei isolated from epithelial cells found that the size of scattering structures ranged from less than a few hundred nanometers to 2 μm.[49] Not only is the physical composition of biological cells very heterogeneous, but so also is the composition of the nuclei within them. A correlation between DNA content and light-scattering properties has been observed. When cells are growing exponentially, their DNA content is increased compared to cells in the plateau phase of growth. Light scattering measurements of cells harvested in the exponential phase of growth showed stronger backscattering and a steeper decrease in scattering as a function of wavelength than did cells harvested in the plateau phase of growth.[53] Both these scattering changes are indicative of an increased concentration of small scattering centers.

Nearly all of the research described here focused on understanding scattering from cells. Scattering from tissue layers underlying the epithelium has not been as well studied. Mechanical support for most epithelial layers is provided by the lamina propria, a thin layer of connective tissue with a large collagen content. Muscle tissue commonly underlies the lamina propria. Studies of skin provide a small amount of information relevant to the lamina propria because skin also contains a large amount of collagen, although the organization of collagen fibers in the lamina propria varies with the organ studied and, therefore, may be different from the organization of collagen fibers in skin. The large collagen fibers from the dermis of the skin can be one of the primary sources of scattering from skin; microscopic changes in collagen fibers have been correlated with macroscopically observed light-scattering changes.[14] Collagen fibers can also cause an anisotropy in the macroscopically measured light scattering. The measured reduced scattering coefficient of the skin can vary by a factor of 2 depending on the measurement orientation.[55] Muscle also demonstrates large scale anisotropy, particularly with polarized light.[56]

Several microscopic methods for examining the spatial variations of the angular scattering probability, $P(\theta)$, are under development. A microscope-based, light-scattering instrument that can measure the angular dependent scattering of an 80 μm spot from 0° to 60° has been developed.[57] The ratio of wide angle to narrow angle scatter can be examined at microscopic resolution[58]; an interferometric method for measuring of scattering at angles near 180° has been demonstrated[59] and could potentially be integrated into a microscopic imaging system.

16.5 Monte Carlo Methods

An important tool for developing and understanding elastic-scattering spectroscopy has been Monte Carlo simulation of light transport.[60,61] In a Monte Carlo simulation, a photon is injected into a scattering medium and then propagated through the medium based on knowledge of μ_s, μ_a, and $P(\theta,\phi)$ for the scattering medium. Photon propagation is then simulated, typically, for millions of photons. A common assumption is that the scattering centers are spherical. In this case, all ϕ are equally likely and $P(\theta)$ can be calculated using a solution to Maxwell's equations for a plane wave incident on a sphere, called Mie theory.[62] Henyey–Greenstein phase functions, which resemble phase functions computed by Mie theory, are sometimes used.[63] The advantage of Henyey–Greenstein phase functions is their simple analytical form; however, they cannot be used in simulations of polarized light scattering or to simulate scattering from nonspherical particles. In principle, the scattering centers could be ellipsoids of revolution or other particles because computational codes for calculating scattering parameters from these shapes are now available.[64] In fact, the evidence is that, when polarized light propagation in tissue is simulated, a model using spherical particles will not be adequate. Ellipsoids of revolution or other nonspherical particles must be used because the physical structures in epithelial cells do not scatter light like spherical scatterers.[49]

Monte Carlo simulations are particularly useful for determining features of light transport that are not easily measured, such as the depth to which light penetrates into tissue before being collected, the length of the path the light travels in tissue, and the polarization of light within the tissue. The degree of polarization in a scattering medium as a function of depth and lateral distance from the delivery point can be seen in simulations by Yao and Wang.[37] The depth probed as a function of the incident and detected light polarization for fixed source–detector separations has also been examined using Monte Carlo simulations.[65] The depth probed depends on the collected polarization relative to the incident polarization. As expected from the discussion in Section 16.3, a deeper depth can be probed when the collected light is polarized perpendicular to the incident light polarization. A less intuitive result is that the depth probed when the incident and collected polarizations are the same depends on the measurement geometry.

Consider two collection fibers, each 550 μm from the light delivery fiber, such that a line connecting the first collection fiber to the delivery fiber and a line connecting the second collection fiber to the delivery fiber form a right angle. If the polarization for delivery and collection is oriented along one of the lines, then the depth probed by the fiber connected by that line will be greater. For example, for $\mu_s' = 15$ cm^{-1}, $\mu_a = 2$ cm^{-1}, and $g = 0.61$, the median depth probed is 230 μm for one of the collection fibers and ~300 μm for the other. Regardless of polarization, the depth probed decreases with fiber separation. The depth probed when using a single fiber-optic for delivery and for detection of unpolarized light is 170 μm for a similar highly scattering medium with $\mu_s' = 15$ cm^{-1}, $\mu_a = 2$ cm^{-1}, and $g = 0.83$.[8] (There is an error in Table 2 of Ref. [8]: cm^{-1} should be mm^{-1}.)

Monte Carlo simulations indicate that, with a fiber optic probe separation of 250 μm, primarily the epidermal layer and papillary dermis of skin are probed.[66] Monte Carlo simulations also make clear that the distance photons travel in tissue is much greater than the depth they probe. When the mean path length within myocardium for diffusely reflected light is 1.3 mm, the depth examined is only ~365 μm.[67] Measurements of the average distance traveled by light in tissue between the delivery and collection fiber have been calculated for a few different sets of light transport parameters.[68] For example, when the source and detector are separated by 1.75 mm and the absorption is 0.01 mm^{-1}, the distance traveled by light in the tissue is about 10 mm. As discussed in Section 16.7, at this fiber separation, the distance light travels between the source and detector does not depend strongly on the scattering properties. Finally, the distribution of scattering angles of the scattering events undergone by light that reaches the collection fiber can be calculated using Monte Carlo simulations. When the source and detector are in close proximity, for example, 200 or 250 μm apart, the collected photons undergo significantly more high angle scattering events than do photons that entered the tissue, but were not collected.[7,69] Monte Carlo methods are also used for the determination of quantitative optical properties from experimental measurements as described in Section 16.6.

16.6 Quantification of Morphological and Biochemical Properties

An ultimate goal of several research groups is to provide quantitative biochemical and morphological information from noninvasive optical measurements of tissue. Georgakoudi et al. provide a review of much of the work in this area using a wide variety of techniques (see Chapter 31 of this handbook). Here, we discuss methods aimed at obtaining quantitative information from wavelength-dependent, light-scattering measurements.

In order to develop methods for quantifying optical properties or specific morphological parameters, it is necessary to have well-characterized media for which the optical and morphological properties are known. Tissue is much too complicated to use and requires special handling procedures. Consequently, tissue phantoms are frequently used. Two common phantoms are intralipid and suspensions of polystyrene spheres. Intralipid is a fat emulsion consisting of soybean oil, glycerin, lecithin, and water.[70,71] Small vesicles formed primarily of soybean oil scatter light; polystyrene spheres can be used to make tissue phantoms with precisely known properties. Measurements of these phantoms can be compared directly to theory. The disadvantages of phantoms made with polystyrene spheres are that the relative index of polystyrene in water is very different from that of biological materials in water and the broad distribution of structure sizes found in tissue is hard to reproduce with polystyrene spheres. Absorbing materials, such as oxy- or deoxyhemoglobin can be added to intralipid of polystyrene sphere suspensions and both types of phantoms have proven very useful in the development of quantitative methods.

When the source and detector are sufficiently separated, the diffusion approximation to the transport equation can be applied and the absorption coefficient, μ_a, and reduced scattering coefficient, μ_s', calculated. Initially, this method was demonstrated to measure the absorption of methemoglobin[72] using a frequency-domain system—a more intricate measurement system that oscillates the incident light.[73,74] The addition of broad-wavelength, steady-state techniques to frequency-domain measurements performed only at a few wavelengths can improve the accuracy of absorption measurements.[75] Steady-state illumination alone can be used[76-80] and the concentration of cytochrome and hemoglobin quantified in scattering suspensions containing mitochondria and red blood cells.[80] A probe with an oblique angle of light incidence has also been developed for separately measuring absorption and the reduced scattering coefficient using a steady-state source.[81,82]

When the source–detector separation, ρ, and the reduced scattering coefficient, μ_s', have values such that their product, $\rho\mu_s'$ is less than about 2, the diffusion approximation is no longer valid.[7] This limit of applicability of the diffusion solution depends on several additional factors such as absorption, numerical aperture of the fiber, and details of $P(\theta)$.[83] Consequently, different researchers have found different limits for the validity of the diffusion approximation. The value of 2 stated above for the source–detector separation is smaller than values obtained and discussed by Bevilacqua and Depeursinge.[84]

Modifications to diffusion equation solutions have been made in order to increase their accuracy.[85] Venugoplan et al. have presented an extension of the standard diffusion approximation that shows improved agreement with experimental results at small fiber separations and high absorption.[86] A different improvement on the diffusion approximation is the P_3 approximation. For the diffusion approximation, the radiance and source term of the Boltzmann transport equation are expanded in spherical harmonics and terms up to $\ell = 1$ are kept. The P_3 solution keeps terms up to $\ell = 3$. This solution demonstrates significantly improved results for the determination of optical properties, particularly for the determination of large absorption coefficients (>0.25 mm^{-1}) when light transport is measured with relatively small (<1 cm) source–detector separations.[87]

Multiple polynomial regression methods[88] and an iterative Monte Carlo method[89] have been proposed as methods to more accurately determine tissue optical properties using source–detector separations less than 1 cm. An iterative Monte Carlo method has been applied to hyperspectral data. When reflectance data measured over the range of 0.5–2.5 mm from the source location were used, the accuracy of calculated μ_a and μ_s' were ±12% and ±4%, respectively.[90] A fast perturbative Monte Carlo method can accurately quantify changes in μ_a or μ_s'. In test cases using layered media with a top layer thickness of only 0.5 mm and detectors up to 3 mm from the source, excellent results were obtained for μ_a and μ_s' perturbations in each layer.[91]

Many of the papers cited in the previous paragraph used Henyey–Greenstein phase functions. When $\rho\mu_s'$ is small enough that the diffusion approximation does not hold, the intensity of collected light will depend on details of the phase function. For example, with $\rho\mu_s' = 2.4$, Monte Carlo simulations of photon transport demonstrate that the intensity of light collected can be 60% greater when a Mie phase function is used rather than a Henyey–Greenstein phase function, assuming the other scattering parameters, g, μ_s, and μ_a, are held constant.[69] Bevilacqua and Depeursinge[84] have determined the effect of the moments of $P(\theta)$ on light transport. The first moment is g; the second moment is given by

$$g_2 = \int_0^\pi \frac{1}{2}(3\cos^2\theta - 1)P(\theta)\sin\theta\, d\theta \qquad (16.2)$$

An important result from their work is that, from $\rho\mu_s' > 0.5$ up to values for which the diffusion equation holds, light transport can be described by three parameters: μ_s', μ_a, and $\gamma = (1 - g_2)/(1 - g_1)$.[84] A procedure to determine μ_s', μ_a, and γ from diffuse reflectance data, taken at several fiber separations from 0.3 to 1.4 mm, resulted in values of μ_s' with errors <10% and values of μ_a accurate to approximately 0.01 mm^{-1}.[92]

So far the quantification of morphological and biochemical properties has been stated as the quantification of light transport properties. As an alternative to quantifying μ_s' or μ_a and the properties of the angular dependent scattering function, it may be useful to determine the effective size of scattering structures and their concentrations directly. Methods using polarized light are being developed to quantify morphological properties directly. At least two separate approaches are being taken. One method is based on the observation of interesting optical patterns generated by the propagation of polarized light many years ago. A crosslike pattern was observed over the macular area of the eye when the macula was photographed using crossed polarizers as early as 1978.[93] The physical origin of pattern features is well understood[94–98] and methods for obtaining effective scatterer size and concentration from polarized backscattering images of polystyrene sphere suspensions have been described.[99] Recently a fiber-optic method for measuring polarized light scattering that can determine average scatterer size and density of polystyrene spheres was demonstrated.[65] Polarized fiber-optic and imaging measurements of cell suspensions also provide information about scattering structures.[65,100,101] For example, the apparent size of scattering centers in tumorigenic MR1 rat fibroblast cells is greater than the apparent size of scattering centers in nontumorigenic M1 rat fibroblast cells as determined by polarization images obtained with circularly polarized light.[101]

The other method, mentioned in Section 16.3, subtracts measurements of light returning to the same location on the surface with polarizations parallel and perpendicular to the incident light polarization. When the subtraction is performed as a function of wavelength, the resulting spectrum can be fit to a theoretical expression for scattering from spheres. Backman et al. have assumed that this spectrum is due to backscattering from nuclei, and they report that the distribution of cell-nucleus sizes obtained agrees with microscopic measurements of nuclear size.[35] This technique has also been implemented in an imaging geometry, for which the analyses to determine nuclear size and refractive index are performed for each 25 µm × 25 µm pixel.[102]

Sokolov et al.[36] have also made measurements of the diffuse reflectance of polarized light. Specifically, they measured the depolarization ratio,

$$\frac{\left[I_\parallel(\lambda) - I\perp(\lambda) \right]}{\left[I_\parallel(\lambda) + I\perp(\lambda) \right]}$$

for epithelial cells in phosphate buffered saline above a highly scattering medium. They assumed a cell in phosphate buffer consisted of two independent scatterers: a spherical nucleus in an environment with the refractive index of cytoplasm and a spherical cytoplasm in an environment with the refractive index of water. Additionally, their model assumes that the wavelength-dependent scattering is a linear sum of forward and backward scattering from these spheres. With this model they were able to obtain wavelength-dependent fits to the data using sphere sizes similar to those obtained for the cells and nuclei by phase-contrast microscopy.

16.7 Other Applications

In addition to the diagnosis and detection of cancer, elastic-scattering spectroscopy may be used for diagnosing other tissue pathologies, for tissue identification, and for monitoring changes to tissue. Freezing of tissue is used in cancer treatment (cryosurgery) and in tissue preservation and transplantation. For these applications, it is important to know the location of the ice-front boundaries. Benaron and co-workers found that there is a large overall intensity change in the transmitted light upon freezing.[103] The opposite of cryosurgery, thermotherapy, also affects the optical properties of tissue. There is an increase in absorption, probably due to accumulation of erythrocytes and a decrease in the size of scattering centers.[104]

Applications of reflectance spectrometry have also been developed for measurement of bilirubin concentration[105,106] and a small hand-held device is currently on the market. One of the difficulties with measuring absorption in tissue is that the distance traveled by light between the source and detector is not known and depends on the scattering properties, which are generally also not known. In order to mitigate this problem, an illumination–detection separation can be chosen for which the effect of scattering variations on the pathlength is weak. Mourant et al. have demonstrated that, for a source–detection separation of ~1.7 mm, the variation in pathlength for a large range of scattering properties found in tissue (5–20 cm^{-1}) is less than about 20%.[68] This result is being further developed to measure the pharmacokinetics of investigational drugs. The basis of the technique is a simple manipulation of Equation 16.1, given by

$$\log\left[\frac{I(t)}{I_0}\right] = \mu_a L \tag{16.3}$$

where

$I(t)$ is the intensity of light measured at time t after a drug was administered
I_0 is the intensity of light measured before the drug was administered
μ_a is the absorption coefficient
L is the distance light travels through the tissue

By measuring with a geometry (shown in Figure 16.3) using a distance of ~1.7 mm between the illuminating and collecting fibers, the dependence of pathlength on variations in scattering coefficient can be substantially ignored. However, as mentioned in Section 16.3, the path-length will still depend on absorption. The dependence of L on μ_a can be parameterized as $L = x_0 + x_1 \exp(-x_2\mu_a)$, where x_0, x_1, and x_2 are parameters that depend on details of the measurement probe, such as the exact fiber separation and the numerical aperture of the fibers.

The measurement of drug concentrations in tissue as a function of time using the principles described previously has been named "optical pharmacokinetics" and a proof of principle demonstration of optical pharmacokinetics has been published.[107] The concentration of mitoxantrone (a chemotherapy drug) was followed as a function of time in subcutaneous human cancer tumors grown in nude (immune-suppressed) mice. The conventional method used for pharmacokinetics studies during drug development is animal sacrifice followed by tissue assay. This method is time- and labor-intensive as well as quite costly in terms of laboratory animals required—statistically significant studies require hundreds of animals (multiple animals for each time-point for each dose tested). An alternative method of measuring pharmacokinetics sometimes used in hospitals, microdialysis, is also invasive and utilizes a needle with a semipermeable membrane that may irritate surrounding tissue. Another drawback of microdialysis is that intracellular concentrations cannot be determined. Intracellular concentrations are more significant for understanding the therapeutic dose of a drug than the intercellular concentration.

Single photon emission computed tomography and positron emission tomography have been used to quantify in vivo imaging of radiolabeled drugs.[108–110] These techniques do not depend on the optical properties of tissue; however, they do require handling radioactive compounds and using expensive equipment. Also, the spatial resolution of the imaging is limited and subsecond imaging of fast drug dynamics is likely to be difficult. In contrast to animal sacrifice/tissue assay or microdialysis, optical pharmacokinetics is noninvasive and can provide real-time, site-specific measurements of absolute drug concentrations in vivo. Measurements over time can determine the entire pharmacokinetic time history (for a given dosage) of a drug at specific tissue sites with just one laboratory animal.

Optical measurements can also be used to assess properties of tumor neovasculature. A fast sequence of measurements made immediately following intravenous administration of a short bolus of optical contrast agent can be used to determine important parameters of angiogenesis. Because tumor capillaries (particularly those that are still immature) in the angiogenesis process are leaky,[111] macromolecules that do not leak from normal capillaries will often pass through the permeable walls of angiogenic microvessels and can be used to quantify the leakiness of these capillaries and, therefore, the angiogenesis process.[112] Very rapid sequences of optical pharmacokinetics measurements (>2 measurements/s) would permit tracking the fast dynamics of the first-pass kinetics of compounds in neovascularized tissue, and the leakage into the extracellular fluid space, following administration of a short bolus of an optical contrast agent with a known leakage rate.

Thus, possible clinical applications of optical pharmacokinetics include monitoring photodynamic therapy drug concentrations so that the drug can be activated by light at the optimum time, measuring blood pooling, and using first-pass kinetics to monitor neovasculature and assess the response to treatment by antiangiogenic drugs.

16.8 Summary

Elastic-scattering spectroscopy and diffuse reflectance are two terms for noninvasive methods of measuring the propagation of light through tissue to obtain biochemical and morphological information that can be used in diagnosing tissue pathologies. Light is incident on a small area, typically a spot 200–400 μm diameter, and enters the tissue where it is scattered or absorbed. Some of the light will return to the surface where properties such as intensity versus wavelength and polarization can be measured. The properties of the light returning to the surface will depend on some of the structural and biochemical properties of the tissue. Clinical trials using elastic scattering and diffuse reflectance have demonstrated the potential of light scattering to diagnose cancerous and precancerous lesions. For many of these trials, the same set of data was used to calculate the sensitivity and specificity as was used to develop the distinguishing metrics. More prospective clinical studies that have independent testing data sets are now needed to prove the diagnostic accuracy.

The full power of elastic scattering and diffuse reflectance, however, has not yet been realized, partly because the relationship between the biology of the tissue and the physics of light propagation is not completely understood. Such an understanding will facilitate optimization of measurement methods and analysis to provide the most accurate and clinically relevant information possible. Significant progress has been made towards understanding which structural features in tissue are responsible for light scattering and the contribution of light scattering from these structural features to the properties of the detected light intensity.

New methods for quantifying physical scattering properties and biomedically important properties, such as nuclear characteristics or drug metabolism, are being developed. At present few of the methods have been implemented by more than one or two research groups and there are some apparent contradictions in results. For example, the idea that nuclear size can be determined from backscattering measurements may appear to be at odds with evidence that backscattering occurs primarily from structures much smaller than the nucleus and that the nucleus contributes primarily to forward scattering. It is important that published work include the details of measurements and analysis so that other research groups can validate, reconcile, and expand on results. The development of new analysis and measurement methods, along with new technical developments and ideas, will enable diffuse reflectance and elastic-scattering spectroscopy to reach their potentials as tools for the noninvasive characterization of tissue. Information about tissue presently only available by biopsy and histopathology, as well as new information not available via traditional methods, may be provided by light-scattering methods. We hope that in the coming years elastic scattering and diffuse reflectance will be developed into accurate, real-time, noninvasive, and, possibly, hand-held tools for measuring diagnostically relevant characteristics of tissue.

Acknowledgments

Support for researching and writing this chapter was provided by NIH CA17898 and CA82104. The authors thank James P. Freyer, Paul W. Fenimore, and Toru Aida for comments on the manuscript.

References

1. Sinex, J.E., Pulse oximetry: Principles and limitations, *Am. J. Emerg. Med.*, 17, 59, 1999.
2. Case, K.M. and Zweifel, P.F., *Linear Transport Theory*, Addison-Wesley, Reading, MA, 1967, Chap. 1.
3. Ishimaru, A., *Wave Propagation and Scattering in Random Media*, Oxford University Press, Oxford, U.K., 1997, Chap. 2.
4. Groenhuis, R.A.J., Ferwerda, H.A., and Ten Bosch, J.J., Scattering and absorption of turbid materials determined from reflection measurements. 1. Theory, *Appl. Opt.*, 22, 2456, 1983.
5. Farrell, T.J. and Patterson, M.S., A diffusion theory model of spatially resolved, steady-state diffuse reflectance for the noninvasive determination of tissue optical properties, *Med. Phys.*, 19, 8798, 1992.
6. Haskell, R.C., Svaasand, L.O., Tsay, T.-T., Feng, T.-C., McAdams, M.S., and Tromberg, B.J., Boundary condition for the diffusion equation in radiative transfer, *J. Opt. Soc. Am.*, 2727, 1994.
7. Canpolat, M. and Mourant, J.R., High-angle scattering events strongly affect light collection in clinically relavent measurement geometries for light transport through tissue, *Phys. Med. Biol.*, 45, 1127, 2000.
8. Canpolat, M. and Mourant, J.R., Particle size analysis of turbid media with a single optical fiber in contact with the medium to deliver and detect white light, *Appl. Opt.*, 40, 3792, 2001.
9. Kollias, N. and Baqer, A.H., Quantitative assessment of UV-induced pigmentation and erythema, *Photodermatology*, 5, 53, 1988.
10. Dawson, J.B., Barker, D.J., Ellis, D.J., Grassam, E., Cotteril, J.A., Fisher, G.W., and Feather, J.W., A theoretical and experimental study of light absorption and scattering by in vivo skin, *Phys. Med. Biol.*, 25, 6969, 1980.
11. Feather, J.W., Hajizadeh-Saffar, M., Leslie, G., and Dawson, J.B., A portable scanning reflectance spectrophotometer using visible wavelengths for the rapid measurement of skin pigments, *Phys. Med. Biol.*, 34, 807, 1989.
12. Anderson, R.R. and Parrish, J.A., The optics of human skin, *J. Invest. Dermatol.*, 77, 13, 1981.
13. Hajizadeh-Saffar, M., Feather, J.W., and Dawson, J.B., An investigation of factors affecting the accuracy of measurements of skin pigments by reflectance spectrophotometry, *Phys. Med. Biol.*, 35, 1301, 1990.
14. Saidi, I.S., Jacques, S.L., and Tittel, F.K., Mie and Rayleigh modeling of visible-light scattering in neonatal skin, *Appl. Opt.*, 34, 7410, 1995.
15. Marchesini, R., Cascinelli, N., Brambilla, M., Clemente, C., Mascheroni, L., Pignoli, E., Testori, A., and Ventroli, D.R., In vivo spectrophotometric evaluation of neoplastic and non-neoplastic skin pigmented lesions. II. Discriminant analysis between nevus and melanoma, *Photochem. Photobiol.*, 55, 515, 1992.
16. Farina, B., Bartoli, C., Bono, A., Colombo, A., Lualdi, M., Tragni, G., and Marchesini, R., Multispectral imaging approach in the diagnosis of cutaneous melanoma: Potentiality and limits, *Phys. Med. Biol.*, 45, 1243, 2000.
17. Wallace, V.P., Crawford, D.C., Mortimer, P.S., Ott, R.J., and Bamber, J.C., Spectrophotometric assessment of pigmented skin lesions: Methods and feature selection for evaluation of diagnostic performance, *Phys. Med. Biol.*, 45, 735, 2000.
18. Wallace, V.P., Banber, J.C., Crawford, D.C., Ott, R.J., and Mortimer, P.S., Classification of reflectance spectra from pigmented skin lesions, a comparison of multivariate discriminant analysis and artificial neural networks, *Phys. Med. Biol.*, 45, 2859, 2000.
19. Mourant, J.R., Bigio, I.J., Boyer, J., Conn, R.L., Johnson, T., and Shimada, T., Spectroscopic diagnosis of bladder cancer with elastic light scattering, *Lasers Surg. Med.*, 17, 350, 1995.
20. Koenig, F., Larne, R., Enquist, H., McGovern, F.J., Schomacker, K.T., Kollias, N., and Deutsch, T.F., Spectroscopic measurement of diffuse reflectance for enhanced detection of bladder carcinoma, *Urology*, 51, 342, 1998.
21. Mourant, J.R., Bigio, I.J., Boyer, J., Johnson, T.M., and Lacey, J., Elastic scattering spectroscopy as a diagnostic for differentiating pathologies in the gastrointestinal tract: Preliminary testing, *J. Biomed. Opt.*, 1, 1, 1996.

22. Ge, Z., Schomacker, K.T., and Nishioka, N.S., Identification of colonic dysplasia and neoplasia by diffuse reflectance spectroscopy and pattern recognition techniques, *Appl. Spectrosc.*, 52, 833, 1998.

23. Zonios, G., Perelman, L.T., Backman, V., Manahoran, R., Fitzmaurice, M., Van Dam, J., and Feld, M., Diffuse reflectance spectroscopy of human adenomatous colon polyps *in vivo*, *Appl. Opt.*, 38, 6628, 1999.

24. Wallace, M.B., Perelman, L.T., Backman, V., Crawford, J.M., Fitzmaurice, M., Seiler, M., Badizadigan, K. et al., Endoscopic detection of dysplasia in patients with Barrett's esophagus using light-scattering spectroscopy, *Gastroenterology*, 119, 677, 2000.

25. Bigio, I.J., Bown, S.G., Kelly, C., Lovat, L., Pickarde, D., and Ripley, P.M., Developments in endoscopic technology for oesophageal cancer, *J. R. Coll. Surg. Edinb.*, 25, 267, 2000.

26. Georgakoudi, I., Jacobson, B.C., van Dam, J., Backman, V., Wallace, M.B., Muller, M.G., Zhanv, Q. et al., Fluorescence, reflectance, and light-scattering spectroscopy for evaluating dysplasia in patients with Barrett's esophagus, *Gastroenterology*, 120, 1620, 2001.

27. Wall, J.M.E., Cervical cancer: Developments in screening and evaluation of the abnormal smear, *West. J. Med.*, 169, 304, 1998.

28. Nordstrom, R.J., Burke, L., Niloff, J.M., and Myrtle, J.F., Identification of cervical intraepithelial neoplasia (CIN) using UV-excited fluorescence and diffuse-reflectance spectroscopy, *Lasers Surg. Med.*, 29, 118, 2001.

29. Georgakoudi, I., Sheets, E.E., Muller, M.G., Backman, V., Crum, C.P., Badizadegan, K., Dasarim, R.R., and Feld, M.S., Tri-modal spectroscopy for the detection and characterization of cervical pre-cancers *in vivo*, *Am. J. Obstet.*, 186, 374, 2001.

30. Utzinger, U., Brewer, M., Silvio, E., Gershenson, D., Blast, R.C., Follen, M., and Richards-Kortum, R., Reflectance spectroscopy for in vivo characterization of ovarian tissue, *Lasers Surg. Med.*, 28, 56, 2001.

31. Bigio, I.J., Bown, S.G., Briggs, G., Kelley, C., Lakhani, S., Pickard, D., Ripley, P.M., Rose, I.G., and Saunders, C., Diagnosis of breast cancer using elastic-scattering spectroscopy: Preliminary clinical results, *J. Biomed. Opt.*, 5, 221, 2000.

32. Johns, M., Giller, C., and Liu, H., Computational and in-vivo investigation of optical reflectance from human brain to assist neurosurgery, *J. Biomed. Opt.*, 3, 437, 1998.

33. Lin, W.-C., Toms, S.A., Jonson, M., Jansen, E.D., and Mahadaven-Jansen, A., In vivo brain tumor demarcation using optical spectroscopy, *Photochem. Photobiol.*, 73, 396, 2001.

34. Jacques, S.L., Roman, J.R., and Lee, K., Imaging superficial tissue with polarized light, *Lasers Surg. Med.*, 26, 119, 2000.

35. Backman, V., Gurjar, R., Badizadegan, K., Itzkan, I., Dasari, R.R., Perelman, T., and Feld, M.S., Polarized light scattering spectroscopy for quantitative measurement of epithelial structures *in situ*, *IEEE J. Sel. Top. Quant. Electron.*, 5, 1019, 1999.

36. Sokolov, K., Drezek, R., Gossage, K., and Richards-Kortum, R., Reflectance spectroscopy with polarized light: Is it sensitive to cellular and nuclear morphology, *Opt. Express*, 5, 302, 1999.

37. Yao, G. and Wang, L.V., Propagation of polarized light in turbid media: Simulated animation sequences, *Opt. Express*, 7, 1983, 2000.

38. Vanitha, S., Everett, M.J., Maitland, D.J., and Walsh, J.T., Comparison of polarized-light propagation in biological tissue and phantoms, *Opt. Lett.*, 24, 1044, 1999.

39. Sankaran, V., Walsh, J.T., and Maitland, C.J., Polarized light propagation through tissue phantoms containing densely packed scatterers, *Opt. Lett.*, 25, 239, 2000.

40. Studinski, R.C.N. and Vitkin, I.A., Methodology for examining polarized light interactions with tissues and tissuelike media in the exact backscattering direction, *J. Biomed. Opt.*, 5, 330, 2000.

41. Junqueiram, L.C., Carneiro, J., and Kelley, R.O., *Basic Histology*, Appleton and Lange, Norwalk, CT, 1992.

42. Lodish, H., Baltimore, D., Berk, A., Zipursky, S.L., Matsudaira, P., and Darnell, J., *Molecular Cell Biology*, 3rd edn., Scientific American Books, New York, 1995, pp. 173 and 847.

43. Stryer, L., *Biochemistry*, 3rd edn., W.H. Freeman, New York, 1988, p. 760.

44. Drezek, R., Dunn, A., and Richards-Kortum, R., Light scattering from cells: Finite-difference time-domain simulations and goniometric measurements, *Appl. Opt.*, 38, 3651, 1999.

45. Beauvoit, B., Kitai, T., and Chance, B., Contribution of the mitochondrial compartment to the optical propertires of the rat liver: A theoretical and practical approach, *Biophys. J.*, 67, 2501, 1994.

46. Beauvoit, B. and Chance, B., Time-resolved spectroscopy of mitochondira, cells and tissues under normal and pathological conditions, *Mol. Cell. Biochem.*, 184, 445, 1998.

47. Schmitt, J.M. and Kumar, G., Turbulent nature of refractive-index variations in biological tissue, *Opt. Lett.*, 21, 1310, 1996.

48. Schmitt, J.M. and Kumar, G., Optical scattering properties of soft tissue: A discrete particle model, *Appl. Opt.*, 37, 2788, 1998.

49. Mourant, J.R., Johnson, T.M., Carpenter, S., Guerra, A., and Freyer, J.P., Polarized angular-dependent spectroscopy of epithelial cells and epithelial cell nuclei to determine the size scale of scattering structures, *J. Biomed. Opt.*, 7, 378, 2001.

50. Mourant, J.R., Johnson, T.M., and Freyer, J.P., Angular dependent light scattering from multicellular spheroids, *J. Biomed. Opt.*, 7, 93, 2002.

51. Watson, J.V., *Introduction to Flow Cytometry*, Cambridge University Press, Cambridge, U.K., 1991, Chap. 10.

52. Brunsting, A. and Mullaney, P.F., Differential light scattering from spherical mammalian cells, *Biophys. J.*, 14, 439, 1974.

53. Mourant, J.R., Canpolat, M., Brocker, C., Esponda-Ramos, O., Johnson, T., Matanock, A., Stetter, K., and Freyer, J.P., Light scattering from cells: The contribution of the nucleus and the effects of proliferative status, *J. Biomed. Opt.*, 5, 131, 2000.

54. Drezek, R., Dunn, A., and Richards-Kortum, R., A pulsed finite-difference time-domain (FDTD) method for calculating light scattering from biological cells over broad wavelength ranges, *Opt. Express*, 6, 147, 2000.

55. Nickell, S., Hermann, M., Essenpreis, M., Farrell, T.J., Kramer, U., and Patterson, M.S., Anisotropy of light propagation in human skin, *Phys. Med. Biol.*, 45, 2873, 2000.

56. Jarry, G., Henry, F., and Kaiser, R., Anisotropy and multiple scattering in thick mammalian tissues, *J. Opt. Soc. Am. A*, 17, 149, 2000.

57. Valentine, M.T., Popp, A.K., Weitz, D.A., and Kaplan, P.D., Microscope-based light-scattering instrument, *Opt. Lett.*, 26, 890, 2001.

58. Boustany, N.N., Kuo, S.C., and Thakor, N.V., Optical scatter imaging, subcellular morphometry in situ with Fourier filtering, *Opt. Lett.*, 1063, 2001.

59. Wax, A., Yang, C., Dasari, R.R., and Feld, M.S., Measurement of angular distributions by use of low-coherence interferometry for light-scattering spectroscopy, *Opt. Lett.*, 26, 322, 2001.

60. Jacques, S.L. and Wang, L., Monte Carlo modeling of light transport in tissues, in *Optical-Thermal Response of Laser Irradiated Tissue*, Welch, A.J. and van Gemert, M.J.C., eds., Plenum Press, New York, 1995, p. 73.

61. Wang, L., Jacques, S.L., and Zheng, L., MCML—Monte Carlo modeling of light transport in multi-layered tissues, *Comput. Methods Programs Biomed.*, 47, 131, 1995.

62. Bohren, C.F. and Huffman, D.R., *Absorption and Scattering of Light by Small Particles*, Wiley-Interscience, New York, 1983.

63. Henyey, L.G. and Greenstein, J.L., Diffuse radiation in the galaxy, *Astrophys. J.*, 93, 70, 1941.

64. Mishchenko, M.I., Hovenier, J.W., and Travis, L.D., *Light Scattering by Nonspherical Particles. Theory, Measurements and Applications*, Academic Press, San Diego, CA, 2000.

65. Mourant, J.R., Johnson, T.M., and Freyer, J.P., Characterizing mammalian cells and cell phantoms by polarized backscattering fiber-optic measurements, *Appl. Opt.*, 40, 5114, 2001.

66. Meglinsky, I.V. and Matcher, S.J., Modeling the sampling volume for skin blood oxygenation measruements, *Med. Biol. Eng. Comput.*, 39, 4, 2001.

67. Gandjbakhche, A.H., Bonner, R.F., Arai, A.E., and Balaban, R.S., Visible-light photon migration through myocardium in vivo, *Am. J. Physiol. Heart Circ. Physiol.*, 46, H698, 1999.

68. Mourant, J.R., Bigio, I.J., Jack, D.A., Johnson, T.M., and Miller, H.D., Measuring absorption coefficients in small volumes of highly scattering media: Source–detector separations for which path lengths do not depend on scattering properties, *Appl. Opt.*, 36, 5655, 1997.

69. Mourant, J.R., Boyer, J., Hielscher, A.H., and Bigio, I.J., Influence of the scattering phase function on light transport measurements in turbid media performed with small source–detector separations, *Opt. Lett.*, 21, 546, 1996.

70. van Staveran, H.J., Moes, C.J.M., van Marle, J., Prahl, S., and van Gemert, M.J.C., Light scattering in Intralipid 10% in the wavelength range of 400 to 1100 nm, *Appl. Opt.*, 30, 4507, 1991.

71. Flock, S.T., Jacques, S.L., Wilson, B.C., Star, W.M., and van Gemert, M.J.C., Optical properties of intralipids: A phantom medium for light propagation studies, *Lasers Surg. Med.*, 12, 510, 1992.

72. Fishkin, J.B., So, P.T.C., Cerussi, A.E., Fantini, S., Franceschini, M.A., and Gratton, E., Frequency-domain method for measuring spectral properties in multiple-scattering media: Methemoglobin absorption spectrum in a tissue-like phantom, *Appl. Opt.*, 34, 1143, 1995.

73. Tuchin, V., *Tissue Optics Light Scattering Methods and Intruments for Medical Diagnosis*, SPIE Press, Bellingham, WA, 2000.

74. Mahadevan-Jansen, A., Patil, C.A., and Pence, I.J., Raman spectroscopy: From benchtop to bedside, in *The Biomedical Photonics Handbook, Second Edition: Biomedical Diagnostics*, Vo-Dinh, T., ed., Taylor & Francis Group, Abingdon, U.K., 2014.

75. Bevilacqua, F., Berger, A.J., Cerussi, A.E., Jakubowski, D., and Tromberg, J., Broadband absorption spectroscopy in turbid media by combined frequency-domain and steady state methods, *Appl. Opt.*, 39, 6498, 2000.

76. Nichols, M.G., Hull, E.L., and Foster, T.H., Design and testing of a white-light, steady-state diffuse reflectance spectrometer for determination of optical properties of highly scattering systems, *Appl. Opt.*, 36, 93, 1997.

77. Mourant, J.R., Fuselier, T., Boyer, J., Johnson, T.M., and Bigio, I., Predictions and measurements of scattering and absorption over broad wavelength ranges in tissue phantoms, *Appl. Opt.*, 36, 949, 1997.

78. Hull, E.L., Nichols, M.G., and Foster, T.H., Quantitative broadband near-infrared spectroscopy of tissue-simulating phantoms containing erythrocytes, *Phys. Med. Biol.*, 43, 3381, 1998.

79. Ghosh, N., Mohanty, S.K., Majumder, S.K., and Gupta, P.K., Measurement of optical transport properties of normal and malignant human breast tissue, *Appl. Opt.*, 40, 176, 2001.

80. Hull, E.L. and Foster, T.H., Cytochrome spectroscopy in scattering suspensions containing mitochondria and red blood cells, *Appl. Opt.*, 55, 149, 2001.

81. Wang, L. and Jacques, S.L., Use of laser beam with an oblique angle of incidence to measure the reduced scattering coefficient of a turbid media, *Appl. Opt.*, 34, 2362, 1995.

82. Lin, S.-P., Wang, L., Jacques, S.L., and Tittel, F.K., Measurements of tissue optical properties by use of oblique-incidence optical fiber reflectometry, *Appl. Opt.*, 136, 1997.

83. Keinle, A., Forster, F.K., and Hibst, R., Influence of the phase function on determination of the optical properties of biological tissue by spatially resolved reflectance, *Opt. Lett.*, 26, 1571, 2001.

84. Bevilacqua, F. and Depeursinge, C., Monte Carlo study of diffuse reflectance at source–detector separations close to one transport mean free path, *J. Opt. Soc. Am. A*, 16, 2935, 1999.

85. Keinle, A. and Patterson, M.S., Improved solutions of the steady-state and the time-resolved diffusion equations for reflectance from a semi-infinite turbid medium, *J. Opt. Soc. Am. A*, 14, 246, 1997.

86. Venugoplan, V., You, J.S., and Tromberg, B.J., Relative transport in the diffusion approximation: An extension for highly absorbing media and small source–detector separations, *Phys. Rev. E*, 58, 2395, 1998.

87. Hull, E.L. and Foster, T.H., Steady-state reflectance spectroscopy in the P_3 approximation, *J. Opt. Soc. Am. A*, 18, 584, 2001.

88. Dam, J.S., Pederson, C.B., Dalgaard, T., Fabricius, P.E., Aruna, P., and Andersson-Engels, S., Fiber-optics probe for noninvasive real-time determination of tissue optical properties at multiple wavelengths, *Appl. Opt.*, 40, 1155, 2001.

89. Pifferi, A., Taroni, P., Valentini, G., and Andersson-Engels, S., Real-time method for fitting time-resolved reflectance and transmittance measurements of a Monte Carlo model, *Appl. Opt.*, 37, 2774, 1998.

90. Pham, T.H., Bevilacqua, F., Spott, T., Dam, J.S., and Tromberg, B.J., Quantifying the absorption and reduced scattering coefficients of tissue-like turbid media over a broad spectral range with noncontact Fourier-transform hyperspectral imaging, *Appl. Opt.*, 39, 6487, 2000.

91. Hayakawa, C.K., Spanier, J., Bevilacqua, F., Dunn, A.K., You, J.S., Tromberg, B.J., and Venugoplan, V., Perturbation Monte Carlo methods to solve inverse photon migration problems in heterogeneous tissues, *Opt. Lett.*, 26, 1335, 2001.

92. Bevilacqua, F., Piguet, D., Marquet, P., Gross, J.D., Tromberg, B.J., and Depeusinge, C., In vivo local determination of tissue optical properties: Applications to human brain, *Appl. Opt.*, 38, 4939, 1999.

93. Hochheimer, B.F., Polarized light retinal photography of a monkey eye, *Vision Res.*, 18, 19, 1978.

94. Johnson, T.M. and Mourant, J.R., Polarized wavelength-dependent measurements of turbid media, *Opt. Express*, 4, 200, 1997.

95. Pal, S.R. and Carswell, A.I., Polarization anisotropy in lidar multiple scattering from atmospheric clouds, *Appl. Opt.*, 24, 3464, 1985.

96. Dogariu, A., Dogariu, M., Richardson, K., Jacobs, S.D., and Boreman, G.D., Polarization asymmetry in waves backscattering from highly absorbance random media, *Appl. Opt.*, 36, 8159, 1997.

97. Dogariu, M. and Asakura, A., Polarization-dependent backscattering patterns from weakly scattering media, *J. Opt. (Paris)*, 24, 271, 1993.

98. Rakovic, M.J. and Kattawar, G.W., Theoretical analysis of polarization patterns from incoherent backscattering of light, *Appl. Opt.*, 37, 3333, 1998.

99. Hielscher, A.H., Mourant, J.R., and Bigio, I.J., Influence of particle size and concentration on the diffuse backscattering of polarized light from tissue phantoms and biological cell suspensions, *Appl. Opt.*, 36, 125, 1997.

100. Hielscher, A.H., Eick, A.A., Mourant, J.R., Shen, D., Freyer, J.P., and Bigio, I.J., Diffuse backscattering Mueller matrices of highly scattering medium, *Opt. Express*, 1, 441, 1997.

101. Mourant, J.R., Hielscher, A.H., Eick, A.A., Johnson, T.M., and Freyer, J.P., Evidence of intrinsic differences in the light scattering properties of tumorigenic and nontumorigenic cells, *Cancer Cytopathol.*, 84, 366, 1998.

102. Gurjar, R.S., Backman, V., Perelman, L.T., Georgakoudi, I., Badizadegan, K., Itzkan, I., Dasari, R.R., and Feld, M.S., Imaging human epithelial properties with polarized light-scattering spectroscopy, *Nat. Med.*, 7, 1245, 2001.

103. Ottne, D.M., Rubinsky, B., Cheong, W.-F., and Benaron, D.A., Ice-front propagation monitoring in tissue by the use of visible-light spectroscopy, *Appl. Opt.*, 37, 6006, 1998.

104. Nilsson, A.M.K., Sturesson, C., Liu, D.K., and Andersson-Engels, S., Changes in spectral shape of tissue optical properties in conjunction with laser-induced thermotherapy, *Appl. Opt.*, 37, 1256, 1998.

105. Optical transcutaneous bilirubin detector, U.S. patent 5,259,382, 1991.

106. Saidi, I.S., Transcutaneous optical measurements of hyperbilirubinemia in neonates, PhD thesis, Rice University, Houston, TX, 1992.

107. Mourant, J.R., Johnson, T.M., Los, G., and Bigio, I.J., Non-invasive measurement of chemotherapy drug concentrations in tissue: Preliminary demonstrations of in vivo measurements, *Phys. Med. Biol.*, 44, 1397, 1999.

108. Firnau, G., Maass, D., Wilson, B.C., and Jeeves, W.P., ^{64}Cu labeling of hematoporphyrin derivative for non-invasive *in-vivo* measurements of tumour uptake, *Prog. Clin. Biol. Res.*, 170, 629, 1984.

109. Jeeves, W.P., Wilson, B.C., Firnau, G., and Brown, K., *Methods in Porphyrin Photosensitization*, Plenum Press, New York, 1985, p. 51.

110. Scasnar, V. and van Lier, J.E., Biological activities of phthalocyanines. XV. Radiolabeling of the dif-ferently sulfonated ^{67}Ga-phthalocyanines for photodynamic therapy and tumor imaging, *Nucl. Med. Biol.*, 20, 257, 1993.

111. Schwickert, H.C., Stiskal, M., Roberts, T.P., van Dijke, C.F., Mann, J., Muhler, A., Shames, D.M., Demsar, F., Disston, A., and Brasch, R.C., Contrast-enhanced MR imaging assessment of tumor capillary permeability: Effect of irradiation on delivery of chemotherapy, *Radiology*, 198, 893, 1996.

112. Turetschek, K., Huber, S., Floyd, E., Helbich, T., Roberts, T.P., Shames, D.M., Tarlo, K.S., Wendland, M.F., and Brasch, R.C., MR imaging characterization of microvessels in experimental breast tumors by using a particulate contrast agent with histopathologic correlation, *Radiology*, 1218, 562, 2000.

113. van Assendelft, O.W., *Spectrophotometry of Haemoglobin Derivatives*, Royal Vangorcum Ltd., Assen, the Netherlands, 1970.

114. Wray, S., Cope, M., Delpy, D.T., Wyatt, J.S., and Reynolds, E.O.R., *Biochim. Biophys. Acta*, 933, 184, 1988.

115. Kou, L., Labrie, D., and Chylek, P., *Appl. Opt.*, 32, 3531, 1993.

17

Quantitative Diffuse Reflectance Imaging of Tumor Margins

Bing Yu
University of Akron

Nirmala Ramanujam
Duke University

17.1 Introduction

Quantitative diffuse reflectance imaging (QDRI) is an emerging modality that collects and analyzes reflectance spectra produced as ultraviolet–visible (UV–VIS) light propagated through a turbid medium to determine the absorption and scattering properties of the medium. From the absorption spectra, tissue composition maps, such as the concentrations of oxyhemoglobin (HbO_2) and deoxyhemoglobin (Hb), can be extracted, while the scattering map reflects the tissue morphological information, such as nuclear size and density. Both tissue compositions and morphological information have been identified as useful biomarkers for cancer diagnostics. QDRI has attracted growing interest for noninvasive tissue characterization in the last decade. One, and maybe the most important, application of this technology is for noninvasive detection of tumor margins during surgeries, such as breast-conserving surgery (BCS) and brain surgery, where maximal preservation of normal tissue or functionality is critical.

This chapter provides an overview of various QDRI techniques that have been developed for intraoperative detection of tumor margins in the last several years. We start with (Section 17.2) a description of BCS procedures to explain the need for intraoperative margin assessment and the available techniques. Although the technologies discussed in this chapter are generally applicable to or can be readily modified for many other tumor types, we focus on breast tumors for ease of discussion in this chapter. Section 17.3 briefly introduces the basic principles of UV–VIS diffuse reflectance spectroscopy (UV–VIS DRS) that QDRI is based on. Section 17.4 presents the general requirements for intraoperative imaging of breast tumor margins. Section 17.5 reviews several noncontact and contact QDRI systems and their clinical applications. Finally, the main features of current QDRI techniques are summarized and the challenges and future directions for QDRI are discussed in Section 17.6.

17.2 Intraoperative Tumor Margin Detection

The American Cancer Society estimates that there will be a total of 1,665,540 new cancer cases diagnosed in the United States in 2014 and about 585,720 cancer-related deaths, corresponding to over 1,605 deaths per day [1]. Among all cancer types, breast cancer is the second leading cause of cancer death in women and about one in eight women in the United States will develop invasive breast cancer during their lifetime [1]. As for many other solid tumors, breast tumors are most commonly treated by surgery, followed by radiation therapy and/or chemotherapy. The chemotherapy and radiation are often utilized to shrink the tumor size prior to surgery or to kill cancer cells left behind after surgery, with an objective to increase the cure rate.

The American Cancer Society estimates that 232,340 new invasive breast cancers and 64,640 new in situ breast cancers were diagnosed in 2013 [2]. For patients who are diagnosed with early-stage breast cancer, one treatment option is BCS or lumpectomy. The goal of BCS is to completely remove the tumor while preserving as much of the normal tissue as possible. After the tumor is removed from the breast, it undergoes x-ray examination to ensure that the correct location is excised and to look at how close the tumor is to the margin (or surface). On average, between 50% and 75% of patients with breast cancer undergo BCS [3,4].

The tumor margins are then evaluated pathologically. As shown in Figure 17.1, a margin is considered positive if there are tumor cells at the margin or close if tumor cells are within ~2 mm of the margin. If there is at least 2 mm of normal tissue, the margin is considered negative. If the margin is close or positive, the woman undergoes re-excision to reduce the risk of the cancer from locally recurring. Approximately 20%–70% of women undergo re-excision surgery because the cancer was incompletely removed during the first BCS [5]. Ductal carcinoma in situ (DCIS) accounts for a significant proportion of residual disease [6–8]. The pathologic margin status is an important predictor of local recurrence of an invasive or in situ cancer after BCS [9,10]. It has been shown that one death is averted for every four women in which local recurrence of breast cancer is avoided [11]. Thus, reducing the occurrence of positive margins in cancer surgery is a tractable problem that would have significant health and financial benefits to patients, surgeons, and payers.

Currently, there is no widely accepted tool for intraoperative margin assessment and only a few hospitals actually use intraoperative assessment, such as frozen section and touch prep. Intraoperative frozen section is an involved technique for margin assessment, which performs poorly on fatty breast tissue and typically samples only a very small portion of the surgical margin [12,13]. Only a handful of high-volume breast centers in the United States, such as MD Anderson, use routine frozen section analysis. Intraoperative touch prep cytology is less labor intensive than frozen section; however, it can only detect cancer on the surface of the margin [14,15]. Both techniques require a pathologist on site and 30 min of operation room (OR) time, while very small area of a margin is examined. However, a significant number of patients undergoing BCS have their surgery at an ambulatory surgery center without on-site pathology. Thus, there is a critical need for an efficient and effective intraoperative margin tool to help surgeons to reduce the re-excision rates and the risk of recurrence for patients for whom intraoperative assessment is not available.

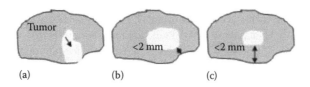

(a)   (b)   (c)

FIGURE 17.1   A cartoon of cross-sectional images of (a) positive, (b) close, and (c) negative tumor margins.

A number of academic [14,16–29] and commercial [30–35] groups have worked on or are developing tools for intraoperative assessment of breast tumors. Dune Medical, an Israeli company, has developed a pen-like probe called the MarginProbe, which uses radio waves to measure the electromagnetic properties of breast tissue over a 7 mm diameter area and 1 mm deep volume. A sensitivity and specificity of 70% was reported in 2010 based on 869 tissue measurement sites (165 cancerous and 588 nonmalignant sites) in 76 patients from three medical centers [36]. The device sensitivity was found to change from 56% to 97% as the cancer feature size increased from 0.7 to 6.6 mm [36]. The MarginProbe System received an FDA approval in January 2013 based on a 664-patient prospective, multicenter, randomized, double-arm study [37].

Pioneering optical studies to detect breast tumor margins was carried out by Bigio et al. [27] where elastic scattering spectroscopy in the UV–VIS range was used to look at sites within the tumor bed in 24 patients (13 cancer and 59 normal sites). This work was important in that it represented initial evidence of absorption and/or scattering contrast in residual breast cancer. Keller et al. [38] employed diffuse reflectance and fluorescence spectroscopy to detect cancerous sites on excised breast tumor margins in 32 patients (145 normal and 34 individual tumor sites) and reported a sensitivity and specificity of 85% and 96%, respectively, for classifying individual sites (not margins). Raman spectroscopy was used by Haka et al. [28] on freshly sliced lumpectomy specimens in 21 patients (123 benign and 6 malignant tissue sites) to achieve a sensitivity and specificity of 83% and 93%, respectively, for classifying individual sites. Nguyen et al. [17] demonstrated that optical coherence tomography (OCT) detects ex vivo margin positivity in 20 patients (11 positive/close margins and 9 negative margins), with sensitivity and specificity of 100% and 82%, respectively, by exploiting scattering associated with increased cell density. All these studies have shown excellent sensitivity or/and specificity in detection of positive tumor margins, but the devices used are mostly a single-point device and restricted to sampling a very small area of the margin.

Recently, several groups have reported the development of a number of new imaging systems based on quantitative UV–VIS DRS for intraoperative margin detection. Gebhart et al. designed a spectral imaging system to perform diffuse reflectance imaging of brain tumor margins using a liquid-crystal tunable filter (LCTF), and Keller et al. [38] tested this device for breast surgical margin analysis. Lue et al. [39] developed a margin scanner that can cover a 10 cm × 10 cm at high spatial resolution. Wilke et al. [40], Brown et al. [41], and Bydlon et al. [42] have multiplexed a single-point fiber-optic probe into a 4 × 2 imaging array and conducted a clinical study at Duke University Medical Center on over 100 patients. Brown et al. [43] reported a 49-channel QDRI system that can image a 4.2 cm × 4.2 cm tumor margin in less than 5 s. Fu et al. [44] and Dhar et al. [45] also proposed a photodiode (PD) array-based spectral imaging system for margin assessment. This chapter focuses on these different approaches of using UV–VIS DRS as an intraoperative tool for ex vivo margin imaging.

17.3 UV–VIS DRS

UV–VIS DRS is a nondestructive technique that is very sensitive to the absorption and scattering properties of biological tissue. This technology launches a broadband light into a tissue and then detects the diffusely reflected photons, through either free-space optics or a fiber-optic probe that is in contact with the tissue, as shown in Figure 17.2. By analyzing the collected reflectance spectrum using a Monte Carlo [46–49] or diffusion-based model [50–52], this approach provides quantitative information; specifically, the wavelength-dependent absorption and scattering properties from which the underlying tissue physiological and morphological information can be derived. The principle of DRS has been described in detail in Chapter 29 (1st edition).

UV–VIS DRS has recently been investigated for precancer detection and cancer diagnostics [47,50,53–63], intraoperative tumor margin assessment [19,41,64], monitoring of tumor response to therapy [19,65–67], and tissue oximetry [68]. An overview of recent progress in UV–VIS DRS for diagnosis, prognosis, and treatment of various cancers can be found in two review articles by Brown et al. [69] and Liu [70].

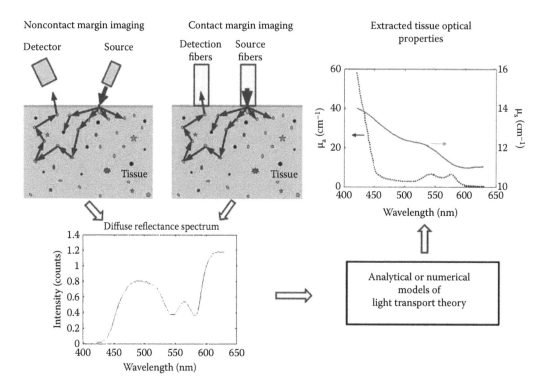

FIGURE 17.2 Illustration of contact vs. noncontact DRS. The spectrum represents diffuse reflectance measured from a single pixel in a noncontact imaging system or a single channel in a contact imaging system. μ_a represents the absorption coefficient and μ_s' represents the reduced scattering coefficient of the tissue.

Endpoints of the quantitative DRS analysis that solely reflect *tissue* characteristics can be compared across different patient studies measured with different instruments. This quantitative DRS approach will facilitate consensus on methods for validation and translation and widen the acceptance of this technique for biomedical applications. DRS in the UV–VIS range has a penetration depth from hundreds of micrometers to several millimeters in tissue and thus is suitable for tumor margin assessment.

17.4 Margin Imaging Considerations

Several important criteria and aspects that have to be considered when designing an effective and efficient intraoperative margin assessment tool for BCS are described in the following text:

Sensitivity and specificity: A margin imaging device with sensitivity comparable to that of frozen section or touch prep but without an on-site pathologist and radiologist would enable many more patients than just those at high-volume breast centers to benefit from lower re-excision rates. As a frame of reference, the sensitivity of frozen section ranges from 59% to 91% [12,26,71–75] and that of touch prep varies from 75% to 100% [14,76–79]. The specificity of imaging device should be such that it does not adversely affect the cosmesis of the breast. In other words, normal tissue should not be unnecessarily removed to achieve clear margins. At the minimum, the device should improve upon surgeon specificity. Although this number is not readily available in the literature, our own experience at Duke University Medical Center on more than 150 margins shows that approximately 75% of the negative primary margins received unnecessary additional shavings, reflecting a surgeon specificity of 25%.

Sensing depth: Currently, there is no accepted standard definition of a *clear margin* that will reduce the risk of local recurrence. It is important to note, however, that the majority of pathologists use 2 mm as

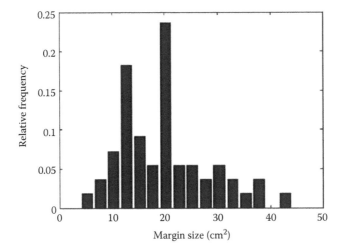

FIGURE 17.3 Distribution of single-margin areas observed in 120 BCS patients at Duke University Medical Center. (From Brown, J.Q. et al., *IEEE J. Sel. Top. Quant. Electron.*, 16, 530, 2010.)

the pathologic criterion for clear margins [8,80–84]. In addition, long-term data have shown a reduced risk of local recurrence associated with a 1–3 mm clear margin [15,85].

Time constraints: In cases of invasive malignancy (75% of new breast cancers), the surgeon performs sentinel node mapping during surgery to determine if the malignancy has spread to lymph nodes. Sentinel node mapping is performed prior to the lumpectomy and is then sent to the pathologist for frozen section to determine if the patient needs a complete axillary node dissection. The lumpectomy is performed during this 20–40 min window [42]. There is currently no published data on the time needed to remove the primary tumor as it varies by breast and tumor size and extent of disease in the lymph nodes. However, the time required for intraoperative assessment should be well within this time window and ideally allow the surgeon to do other tasks while the tumor margin is being assessed.

Sampling area and resolution: The two most commonly observed sizes of breast tumor margins reported by Brown et al. [41] were 4.5 cm × 4.5 cm (~20 cm²) and 3.2 cm × 3.2 cm (~10 cm²), and the vast majority of the margins had an area that was in between, as shown in Figure 17.3. This reflects the large area of tumor margins within which residual disease might be found [86]. Margins can contain multiple, small foci of positivity that is common in breast cancers that have rootlike borders [87]. Thus, an intraoperative assessment device must provide rapid and comprehensive coverage of the entire specimen margin in order to identify focal disease [88,89]. The sampling resolution of pathology is directly related to the thickness of each bread-loafed section, which is around 3 mm, but varies between hospitals. Although the higher the spatial resolution, lesser the chance that a positive site will be missed, it is challenging to achieve complete coverage of large (~20 cm²) tumor margins with extremely high resolution in a clinically reasonable time.

In vivo or ex vivo samples: Margin assessment can be implemented either by examining the resection cavity in vivo or looking at the margins of the excised tumor mass. While it is ideal to be able to map out the tumor margins inside the cavity after the tumor is removed, there have been only a few studies aimed at examining breast margins in vivo [16,27], which were performed on a small number of patients and these technologies evaluated only a small portion of the tumor cavity. In contrast, all of the very recent studies reporting on optical technologies have been carried out on resected tumor margins [17,28,38,40,90]. There are several issues that make in vivo breast margin assessment extremely challenging to implement. One issue is limited visibility and access to all parts of the cavity since the cavity is not planar and in some instances will need to be accessed through tunnels in the tissue. For in vivo margin assessment, a probe must be small enough to maneuver around the cavity, but at the same time, it must provide sufficient coverage to examine areas of varying sizes. Pathologic validation of in vivo margin images will require additional and unnecessary tissue shavings in a procedure that aims to conserve the breast and thus is a more invasive approach to validate the technology. More importantly, in vivo margin assessment requires probe sterilization and has higher risk of infection to the patient.

Contact vs. noncontact imaging: Diffuse reflectance spectrum may be obtained through either contact or noncontact imaging. The noncontact imaging method relays the light to and from the tissue via free-space optics, while the contact imaging employs an optical probe directly in contact with the tissue for light delivery and detection, as illustrated in Figure 17.2. The noncontact imaging features large and flexible margin coverage, very high spatial resolution, high speed, and ease of use. The major drawbacks are that it does not provide a well-defined sensing depth and suffers from cross talk between adjacent tissue pixels due to tissue scattering. Also, the spectral information obtained with these systems are generally displayed as intensity maps at a few discrete wavelengths and, thus, do not fully exploit the spectral information content in the data and also do not provide any quantitative molecular composition information underlying the measured diffuse reflectance intensities. On the other hand, contact imaging has a sensing depth defined by the probe geometry and tissue optical properties that can be tuned to meet the current requirement for a *clear margin*. Most contact imaging systems can provide quantitative molecular information from the diffuse reflectance spectral measurements. This is important in providing quantitative endpoints that are independent of the instrument used, such that the underlying molecular composition can be compared across different instruments. In addition, the imaging geometry of a contact probe can also be designed to minimize cross talk between adjacent channels.

17.5 Quantitative Diffuse Reflectance Imaging

This section describes the five most advanced QDRI margin imaging systems.

17.5.1 Vanderbilt Noncontact Spectral Imaging

Gebhart et al. [21] at Vanderbilt University designed and characterized a noncontact imaging system for the detection of brain tumor margins. The spectral imaging system employs a 200 W halogen lamp as the broadband light source. The light is delivered to the tissue through a 10 mm core liquid light guide and free-space optics. A CCD camera coupled with an LCTF collects a 2D reflectance image, from a tumor mass 180 mm below the camera, at each wavelength from 400 to 720 nm in 10 nm increments, forming an image cube. The system can acquire the entire spectral data cube from a 25 mm field of view (FOV) with spatial resolution of 49.6 μm within 15 s. The spectral data cube from a margin is presented either as an overall intensity map (a summation of the measured spectral intensities at each pixel) or as a full spectrum for a pixel or a group of pixels (binned pixels). A fluorescence imaging channel is also included in the spectral imaging system. Using this noncontact spectral imaging system, Keller et al. [38] collected both DRS and fluorescence images from a single BCS specimen and observed clear difference between a normal and a calcified lesion only in the fluorescence image.

17.5.2 MIT Margin Scanner

Lue et al. at MIT [39] developed a portable, quantitative, spectroscopic tissue scanner, as shown in Figure 17.4, for intraoperative diagnostic imaging of surgical margins. The margin scanner includes two single-point optical fiber probes: one for DRS and the other for intrinsic fluorescence spectroscopy (IFS). The DRS probe, with a 75 W Xenon arc lamp as the source and an Ocean Optics USB2000+ spectrometer for spectrum detection, collects full reflectance between 350 and 700 nm with a 2 nm spectral resolution. The collagen and NADH fluorescence is excited with a 7 mW Q-switched solid-state laser at 355 nm. The two probes are 7.5 mm apart to minimize cross talk between the two probes. During a scan, the tissue specimen was rested on a 1.6 mm thick glass plate, and the probes were mechanically scanned

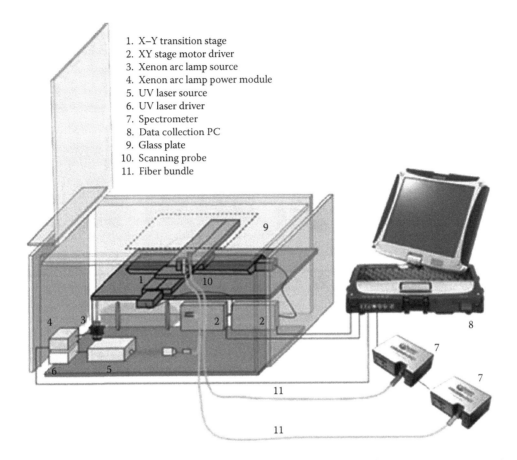

1. X–Y transition stage
2. XY stage motor driver
3. Xenon arc lamp source
4. Xenon arc lamp power module
5. UV laser source
6. UV laser driver
7. Spectrometer
8. Data collection PC
9. Glass plate
10. Scanning probe
11. Fiber bundle

FIGURE 17.4 Schematic diagram of the MIT margin scanner. (From Lue, N. et al., *PLoS One*, 7, e30887, 2012.)

under the plate across the whole tumor margin using a motorized XY stage. Full DRS and fluorescence spectra were recorded from each pixel scanned. The scanner can image an 8 cm × 8 cm margin area with 0.25 mm resolution in less than 20 min and has a maximum margin coverage of 10 cm × 10 cm. Typically, only one of the six tumor margins can be imaged within the 20 min window. The DRS spectra were analyzed using a diffusion approximation model to generate the parameter maps for scattering, Hb, and β-carotene. The IFS spectra (corrected for tissue absorption and scattering) were analyzed using a linear combination model based on multivariate curve resolution (MCR) to obtain the parameter map for collagen. The whole system was controlled by a custom LabVIEW program. The tissue scanner was tested in tissue phantoms and less than 5% error in measuring phantom optical properties was obtained. A proof-of-concept study was performed on a paired set of unfixed, frozen breast tissues that contains one cancerous and a normal breast tissue containing multiple foci of DCIS from the same patient as shown in Figure 17.5a and b. Figure 17.5 shows the DRS intensity at 545 nm (c) and the extracted parameter maps for tissue scattering (d–f), Hb (g), and β-carotene (h) concentrations. The authors also demonstrated that the margin scanner can detect small foci of breast cancer in a background of normal breast tissue.

17.5.3 Duke 8-Channel QDRI

Bydlon et al. [42] and Brown et al. [41] at Duke University multiplexed a single-point UV–VIS DRS probe that has been extensively validated in multiple phantom and clinical studies [58,91–95] into a 4 × 2 array for intraoperative assessment of tumor margins during BCS. The distance between adjacent probes in the array is fixed at 10 mm to minimize the cross talk between neighboring channels. The probe array

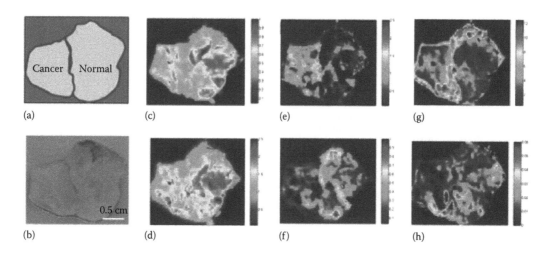

(a)   (c)   (e)   (g)

(b)   (d)   (f)   (h)

FIGURE 17.5 **(See color insert.)** Breast tissue images obtained with the MIT margin scanner. (a) Diagram of normal and breast cancer tissues placed on glass plate during scanning; (b) gross photograph of breast tissues; (c) DRS spectral intensity map of normal and cancer tissues at 545 nm; (d–f) scattering parameters a (related to the amount of Mie scatterers), b (related to the size of the scatterers), and c (related to the amount of Rayleigh scatterers); (g) Hb concentration (mg/mL) map; and (h) β-carotene concentration (mg/mL) map. (From Lue, N. et al., *PLoS One*, 7, e30887, 2012.)

is interfaced with the lumpectomy specimen in a plexiglass container through holes on the container, as shown in Figure 17.6. The holes on the container box are 5 mm apart that determines the minimal spatial resolution of the device. The specimen container also functions to maintain the orientation of the tumor mass so that the spectroscopic images can be easily coregistered with pathology diagnosis.

The 8-channel QDRI instrument employs a 450 W Xe arc lamp as the broadband light source and an imaging spectrograph with a cooled 512 × 512 CCD for spectrum detection, both from HORIBA Scientific Ltd. in Edison, NJ. Each probe of the imaging array has 19 closely packed illumination fibers and 4 detection fibers around them at the common end (200 μm in core diameter). At the source end, the illumination fibers from all eight probes are bundled together. At the collection end, the four detection fibers in each probe are packed as a 2 × 2 array, and the eight 2 × 2 arrays are aligned with the spectrograph slit with another 2 × 2 array of inactive fibers between adjacent channels for spacing to minimize the cross talk on the CCD. A spatial resolution of 5 mm can be achieved by multiple probe placements on each tumor margin. The number of manual placements depends on the size of the margin to be imaged.

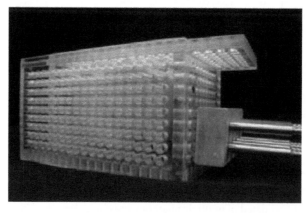

FIGURE 17.6 The Duke 8-channel QDRI device interfaced with a lumpectomy specimen inside a plexiglass container.

The time required to image a typical margin (~20 cm²) with a 5 mm resolution is around 7–8 min, and about 1–3 margins may be imaged for each lumpectomy specimen within the available time window. A custom LabVIEW program with MATLAB® scripts is used to control the data acquisition, tracking the pixels or tissue sites imaged, and data analysis immediately following the collection of DRS spectra from all sites. The diffuse reflectance spectra per site were analyzed with a feature extraction algorithm based on a fast, scalable Monte Carlo model developed by Palmer et al. [46,91] to quantitatively determine absorption spectrum ($\mu_a(\lambda)$) and reduced scattering spectrum ($\mu_s'(\lambda)$) in the breast tissue, as illustrated in Figure 17.2. The dominant absorbers in the breast are β-carotene and hemoglobin. Scattering primarily reflects the size and density of the cells and subcellular organelles. These sources of contrast are used to create tissue composition maps that are used in a decision-tree model to differentiate positive from negative margins.

Bydlon et al. [42] characterized the performance matrices of the 8-channel QDRI system, including an average signal to noise ratio (SNR) (>100), error in the extraction of optical properties (<15%), probe sensing depth over the wavelength range of 450–600 nm (0.5–2.2 mm), cross talk between adjacent channels of the multichannel probe (<1% on the tissue end), and measurement reproducibility (coefficient of variation <0.11). Brown et al. [41] reported the study results from 55 resection margins from 48 BCS patients (from portion of a larger patient study) at Duke University Medical Center. The samples were imaged within 18 ± 5 min of resection. Several tissue sites imaged by the QDRI device were randomly selected and inked for pathology diagnosis. The device identified that the concentrations of β-carotene and total hemoglobin normalized by the wavelength-averaged reduced scattering coefficient ($\langle\mu_s'\rangle$) exhibited the greatest differences between positive and negative margins. An overall accuracy of 75% in detecting positive margins was calculated based on those two tissue parameters.

17.5.4 Duke 49-Channel QDRI

Building upon the same principle as the Duke 8-channel QDRI device, a 49-channel QDRI was developed by Yu et al. to achieve the goal of imaging all six breast tumor margins within a time period of 15 min [43]. A schematic diagram of the system is shown in Figure 17.7. The 49-channel system consists of a 300 W Xe light source, an imaging spectrograph with a back-illuminated 512 × 512 CCD camera for

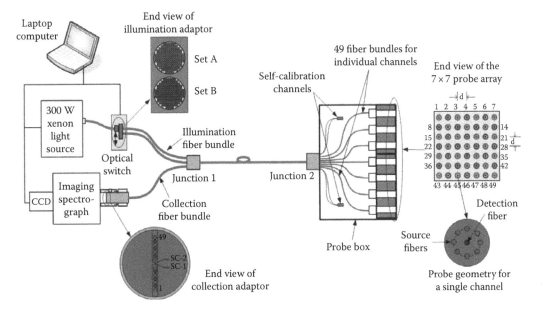

FIGURE 17.7 Schematic diagram of the Duke 49-channel QDRI system and imaging probe for tumor margin detection.

multitrack spectra detection, and a 49-channel fiber-optic probe to interface the instrument to a tumor specimen. The 49 channels are arranged as a 7 × 7 array with a channel spacing of d = 6 mm and can cover a ~20 cm² margin in a single placement. Each channel consists of eight 200 μm fibers forming an illumination ring around a single 200 μm detection fiber with a source-detector separation of 600 μm, resulting in a simulated sensing depth of 0.8–2.5 mm in typical breast tissues.

On the tissue end, the 49 pixels are divided into two sets: the odd and even sets. In the illumination adaptor, the source fibers in the odd and even channels are combined into two different bundles (Set A and Set B in Figure 17.7), respectively. The illumination bundles are mounted on a custom-built optical switch and can be selectively connected to a quartz light guide that is connected to the Xe light source. In the collection adaptor, the detection fibers from the odd and even pixels are alternated, forming a linear array of 12.24 mm in length, and aligned to the slit of the spectrograph. Two self-calibration (SC) channels were also added, one for each channel set to correct for the wavelength-dependent instrument response and to remove real-time system fluctuations [96,97]. In the 8-channel QDRI system and previous single-point systems, such a calibration measurement was performed after all tissue images were collected and the probe was cleaned, which is time-consuming and less accurate. The odd and even pixels are turned on and off sequentially using the optical switch to increase the effective channel spacing to 8.5 mm, thus reducing the cross talk between adjacent channels both on the tissue end and on the CCD. Figure 17.8 shows a photograph of the QDRI console and 49-channel imaging probe. The system is automated by a custom LabVIEW software with built-in MATLAB scripts that acquire and analyze a margin image and display the tissue parameter maps on the computer screen in less than 30 s.

Figure 17.9 shows three images acquired with the 49-channel QDRI system under different illumination conditions, where each horizontal track corresponds to a spectrum from one detection fiber and the vertical waveforms on the left are the intensity profiles of the columns at the cursor. Figure 17.9a shows all channels (1–49, from bottom to top), except the two SC channels, illuminated by the fluorescence room light, showing that all 51 detection fibers can be imaged onto the 0.5 in. CCD chip with minimum *smile* (distortion) at the edges in the vertical direction. The dark area between two tracks is due to the clad of the fibers. The double peaks of the fluorescence lamp spectrum at 542.4 and 546.5 nm can be resolved, indicating that the spectral resolution is around 3–4 nm. Figure 17.9b and c shows the spectroscopic images acquired from a white target with all odd channels on (25 tissue channels plus an SC channel SC-1 at the center) or all even channels on (24 tissue channels plus an SC channel SC-2 at the center), respectively.

The cross talk between the adjacent pixels on the probe end due to tissue scattering was simulated using the probe geometry shown in Figure 17.10 and a forward Monte Carlo model developed by Wang et al. [98]. The cross talk for the central pixels is expected to be the highest cross talk and

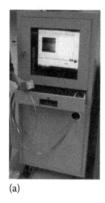
(a)

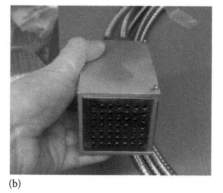
(b)

FIGURE 17.8 Photograph of (a) the QDRI console and (b) 49-channel imaging probe.

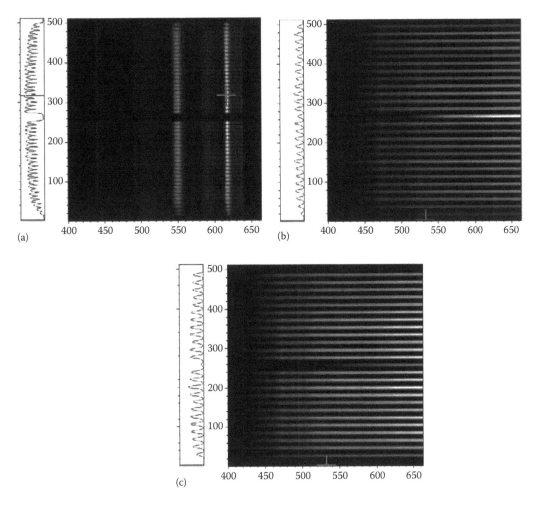

(a) (b) (c)

FIGURE 17.9 Images of (a) all channels (1–49, from bottom to top), except the two SC channels in the middle, illuminated by fluorescence room light (the wavelength calibration was a few nanometers off when these images were taken, but was recalibrated later); (b) reflectance image acquired with all odd channels on (25 tissue channels plus SC channel 1); and (c) diffuse reflectance image acquired with all even channels on (24 tissue channels plus SC channel 2). The x-axis represents the wavelengths and the y-axis represents the position of the detection fibers (tracks).

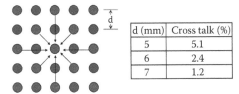

d (mm)	Cross talk (%)
5	5.1
6	2.4
7	1.2

FIGURE 17.10 The multichannel probe model used to simulate the probe cross talk due to tissue scattering.

was determined for adipose tissue at 600 nm (the lightest breast tissue type according to Bydlon et al. [42]) to be less than 2.4% at a channel spacing of 6 mm. The CCD cross talk between the adjacent tracks was measured experimentally by lighting up only every other four detection fibers and measuring the counts in the center channel (inactive) between two adjacent active fibers. This number was calculated to be below 1%.

TABLE 17.1 Summary of the Phantom metHb Concentration and Wavelength-Averaged
Optical Properties between 420 and 630 nm

Phantom #	Expected $\langle \mu_s' \rangle$ (cm^{-1})	Expected $\langle \mu_a \rangle$ (cm^{-1})	metHb Concentration (µM)
1	10.40	0.69	5.19
2	9.95	1.31	9.95
3	9.55	1.89	14.31
4	9.17	2.42	18.33
5	8.83	2.91	22.05
6	8.51	3.37	25.50
7	8.21	3.79	28.71
8	7.93	4.19	31.70
9	7.67	4.56	34.49
10	7.43	4.90	37.10
11	7.20	5.23	39.56
12	6.98	5.53	41.87

Twelve tissue-simulating liquid phantoms with known optical properties were utilized to evaluate the performance of the 49-channel QDRI system for measuring tissue optical properties. The phantoms contained variable concentrations of methemoglobin (metHb) as the absorber and 1 µm polystyrene microspheres as the scatterer. The μ_a of the phantoms was determined from a spectrophotometer measurement of a diluted metHb stock solution, and μ_s' was calculated using the Mie theory [99] for known size, density, and refractive index of the scatterers. A summary of the phantom metHb concentrations and wavelength-averaged optical properties between 420 and 630 nm is provided in Table 17.1.

Diffuse reflectance images were taken from each phantom with all channels. An SC spectrum was also taken concurrently for each probe set (odd and even) for each phantom. For comparison with tradition calibration, a separate calibration spectrum was also measured from a 99% Spectralon reflectance standard for each probe set immediately after the collection of all phantom images. The phantom reflectance spectra were either normalized to the SC spectrum taken concurrently or the Spectralon calibration spectrum. The calibrated spectra were analyzed using the same approach as described by Yu et al. [96,97] to extract the phantom $\mu_a(\lambda)$ and $\mu_s'(\lambda)$ between 420 and 630 nm, and the results are shown in Figure 17.11. The SC significantly reduced the errors for extraction of the

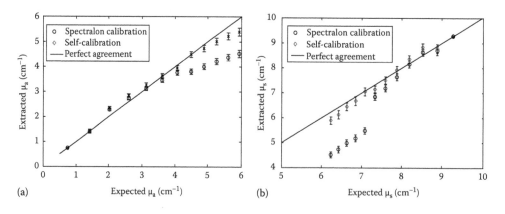

FIGURE 17.11 Extracted vs. expected wavelength-averaged phantom (a) absorption and (b) reduced scattering coefficients obtained using Spectralon and SC methods. The error bar represents the standard deviation across all 49 channels.

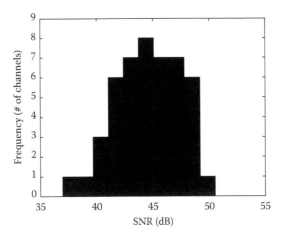

FIGURE 17.12 Distribution of measured SNR for all 49 channels.

phantom μ_a (from 11.2% ± 1.1% to 5.3% ± 0.7%) and μ_s' (from 13.2% ± 1.2% to 4.5% ± 0.7%). The SNR was also calculated for the darkest phantom (phantom #12) from 20 repeated measurements, and Figure 17.12 shows the SNR distribution across all 49 channels with a mean of 44.5 dB. In general, most channels approached the SNR of the Xe lamp (~50 dB), and those close to the bottom and top edges of the CCD have the lowest SNR due to the relatively higher loss of the spectrograph and lower sensitivity of the CCD pixels.

To investigate the capability of the device to quantitatively image a heterogeneous target, 49 holes matching the probe geometry were drilled in a uniform solid phantom, as shown in Figure 17.13a. The holes were filled with liquid phantoms. The red holes have higher concentrations of metHb and scatterers than the blue ones. The optical properties of the solid and the liquid phantoms are also included in Figure 17.13a. Figure 17.13b shows the extracted metHb concentration map and Figure 17.13c shows the extracted reduced scattering map. The patterns in both parameter maps are very clear although a few pixels are blurred in the scattering map that is attributed to the overflow of the liquid phantom to adjacent pixels.

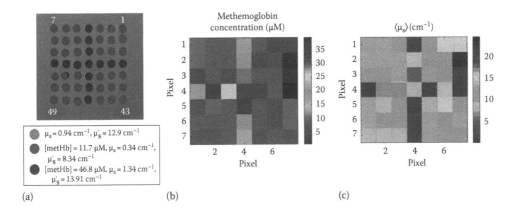

FIGURE 17.13 **(See color insert.)** Quantitative image of a heterogeneous phantom target. (a) Forty-nine holes matching the probe geometry were drilled in a homogeneous solid phantom. The holes were filled with liquid phantoms. The red holes have higher concentrations of metHb and microspheres than the blue ones. (b) Extracted metHb concentration. (c) Extracted scattering coefficient.

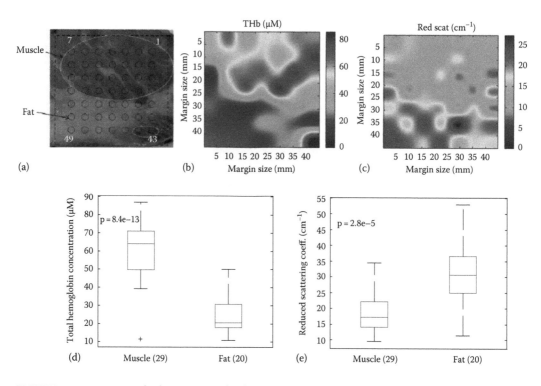

FIGURE 17.14 Imaging of a heterogeneous beef target. (a) Photograph of the beef target, (b) extracted THb, (c) extracted wavelength-averaged reduced scattering coefficient, and boxplots of THb (d) and reduced scattering coefficient (e).

A heterogeneous biological sample, a piece of beef with clear boundary between the muscles and fatty tissues as shown in Figure 17.14a, has also been imaged by the 49-channel probe. The area covered by the whole imaging probe is outlined by the dashed black lines and the tissue sites imaged are outlined by the dotted black circles. The tissue contents were then visually examined. The tissue sites inside the yellow ellipses were assigned to the muscle group, while the remaining sites were treated as fatty tissues. Figure 17.14b and c shows the contour maps of the beef total hemoglobin concentration (THb) and $\langle \mu_s'(\lambda) \rangle$. Apparently, the fatty tissues show much lower THb, but higher scattering than the muscles. The differences can also be clearly seen on the boxplots shown in Figure 17.14d and e. These results agree with those found by Xia et al. [100] and Bashkatov et al. [101] and explain why fatty tissues appear much whiter than muscles. The 49-channel QSI system is currently under clinical evaluation for margin detection in 200 patients undergoing BCS at the Duke University Ambulatory Surgery Center.

17.5.5 Duke Miniature QDRI

In a series of efforts to build a miniature and cost-effective imaging device for intraoperative tumor margin detection, Yu et al. [102], Lo et al. [103], Fu et al. [44], and Dhar et al. [45] have reported some preliminary results on a new QDRI device based on PDs. Yu et al. [102] and Lo et al. [103] investigated the feasibility of replacing the spectrograph and CCD camera used in traditional UV–VIS DRS or QDRI system with a silicon (Si) PD and the detection efficiency of two different probe geometries (an optical fiber next to the PD or in the center of the PD with a drilled through hole). Fu et al. [44] multiplexed the second probe geometry to a 3 × 3 array, as shown in Figure 17.15a, and demonstrated a good SNR and accuracy in characterization of phantom optical properties. As shown in Figure 17.15b and c, the illumination light from a wavelength tunable Xe light source is delivered through the optical fibers at

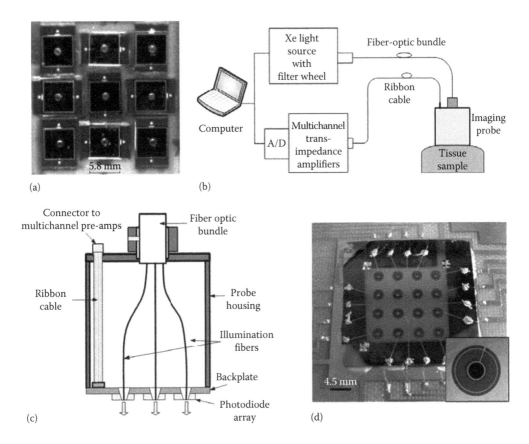

FIGURE 17.15 Duke miniature QDRI margin imaging device. (a) Nine-pixel probe made of drilled Si PDs for fiber-based illumination, (b) proof-of-concept miniature spectral imaging system, (c) fiber-based light delivery, and (d) photograph of a custom-made thin-film Si-PD arrays for free-space, back illumination. ([a, b] are from Fu, H.L. et al., *Opt. Express*, 18, 12630, 2010; [d] from Dhar, S. et al., *Biomed. Opt. Express*, 3, 3211, 2012.)

the center of each PD that is in direct contact with tissue. The diffuse reflectance signals detected by the PDs are amplified by a multichannel trans-impedance amplifier (TIA) and acquired by the laptop computer with a data acquisition card (A/D). Dhar et al. [45] reported a custom-made thin-film Si-PD array consisting of 16 ring-shaped detectors, each has a clear aperture at the center, as shown in Figure 17.15d. Free-space, back illumination of the tissue under the thin-film Si-PD array is used. The wavelength tunable Xe light source may be replaced by more compact and less expensive LEDs for illumination.

17.6 Discussions

BCS is a less radical treatment modality than mastectomy that causes less physical disfigurement and psychological trauma to the patient and has been widely performed in the treatment of early-stage breast tumors. The pathologic margin status is an important predictor of local recurrence of an invasive or in situ cancer after the BCS. However, a significant percentage of BCS patients have to undergo a second surgery because the cancer has not been completely removed during the first BCS. Currently, there is no widely accepted tool available for breast surgeons to evaluate the margin status during surgery.

QDRI is very sensitive to intrinsic tissue absorption and scattering and thus provides quantitative information about tissue compositions and morphology. This technology is noninvasive and has a great potential in intraoperative imaging of tumor margins. QDRI techniques based on a contact fiber-optic probe that are designed for ex vivo measurements have a number of advantages, including a well-defined

TABLE 17.2 Main Features of the MIT Margin Scanner and the Duke 8-Channel and 49-Channel QDRI Systems

Systems	Coverage/ Scan	Spatial Resolution (mm)	Time to Image a 20 cm² Margin	Sensing Depth (mm)	Cross Talk (%)	Sensitivity	Specificity
MIT scanning probe [39]	Single point	0.25	~5 min[a]	<1	0	NA	NA
Duke 8-channel [41,42]	~3.8 cm²	5	~8 min	0.5–2.2	>10[b]	79.4%	66.7%
Duke 49-channel [97]	17 cm²	6	~5 s	0.8–2.5	2.4[c]	N/A	N/A

[a] Calculated based on the time required to image an 8 × 8 cm margin.
[b] Dominated by the cross talk on the CCD end.
[c] Dominated by the cross talk due to tissue scattering.

sensing depth that is compatible with current pathology, minimal pixel to pixel cross talk, model-based algorithms that extract quantitative tissue physiological and morphological parameters, and low risk to patients. Various phantom and clinical studies by several research groups have demonstrated the capability of QDRI for margin imaging. Table 17.2 summarized the main features of three of these systems discussed in this chapter.

The MIT scanning probe provides very high spatial resolution and do not suffer from any cross talk limit and thus may be able to catch small foci of breast cancer. The major limitation to this scanning probe is the relatively long scan time that makes it difficult to image all six margins of a lumpectomy specimen within the available time window, usually 15–20 min. So far, no clinical studies with the scanning probe have been reported. The Duke 8-channel QDRI device is the only QDRI that has been used in a completed clinical study, though the achieved sensitivity and specificity are both below 80%. The major challenges facing the 8-channel QDRI device are manual re-placement of the probe, which is slow and has difficulty in tracking the sites imaged, small coverage in a scan shot, and relatively high cross talk on the CCD. The recently developed Duke 49-channel QDRI imaging array features large margin coverage in a single scan, superfast imaging speed, and relatively low cross talk. The resolution of the 49-channel QDRI is limited to 6 mm but can be improved by multiple placements of the probe. The 49-channel device is yet to be fully tested in a clinical study to evaluate the sensitivity and specificity in detection of positive tumor margins.

In addition to the trade-offs between margin coverage, spatial resolution, and imaging speed, QDRI is also facing some other challenges for intraoperative margin imaging. Bydlon et al. [104] have found that postexcision kinetics of ex vivo tissue and the presence of cautery and patent blue dye may play an important role in modifying the tissue reflectance spectra, thus affecting the extracted tissue composition and morphological properties. Although the available time window is around 20 min for margin imaging in the OR, postexcision change of the tissue optical properties could significantly reduce the intrinsic optical contrast, which requires a very short sample transition time between the surgeon and the engineer and even faster imaging speed. Accurate coregistration between optical measurement and pathology is another challenge to validate the accuracy of the optical measurements. While QDRI surveys tens or even hundreds of tissue sites on each tumor margin, pathologic examination usually diagnoses only a few inked sites due to the labor and time involved. This makes it very difficult to calculate the site-level sensitivity and specificity of a new margin imaging device.

While the current applications have been focused on breast tumor margin imaging, QDRI may be easily modified to study other cancer types, such as brain, head and neck, and prostate tumors, where preserving normal tissue and accurate detection of tumor margins are critical. However, different probe geometry and data analysis models may be needed for each cancer type due to the difference in the tissue optical properties and compositions. Clinical validation of these QDRI techniques is also important before wide hospital acceptance can happen.

References

1. American Cancer Society, Cancer facts & figures 2013, American Cancer Society, Atlanta, GA, http://www.cancer.org/research/cancerfactsstatistics/cancerfactsfigures2014/index (accessed April 4, 2013).
2. American Cancer Society, Breast cancer facts & figures 2013–2014, American Cancer Society, Atlanta, GA, http://www.cancer.org/acs/groups/content/@research/documents/document/acspc-040951.pdf (accessed April 4, 2013).
3. Lee, M. C., Rogers, K., Griffith, K., Diehl, K. A., Breslin, T. M., Cimmino, V. M., Chang, A. E., Newman, L. A., and Sabel, M. S., Determinants of breast conservation rates: Reasons for mastectomy at a comprehensive cancer center, *Breast J*, **15**(1): 34–40 (2009).
4. Morrow, M., Jagsi, R., Alderman, A. K., Griggs, J. J., Hawley, S. T., Hamilton, A. S., Graff, J. J., and Katz, S. J., Surgeon recommendations and receipt of mastectomy for treatment of breast cancer, *JAMA*, **302**(14): 1551–156 (2009).
5. Jacobs, L., Positive margins: The challenge continues for breast surgeons, *Ann Surg Oncol*, **15**(5): 1271–1272 (2008).
6. Vicini, F. A., Kestin, L. L., Goldstein, N. S., Baglan, K. L., Pettinga, J. E., and Martinez, A. A., Relationship between excision volume, margin status, and tumor size with the development of local recurrence in patients with ductal carcinoma-in-situ treated with breast-conserving therapy, *J Surg Oncol*, **76**(4): 245–254 (2001).
7. O'Sullivan, M. J., Li, T., Freedman, G., and Morrow, M., The effect of multiple reexcisions on the risk of local recurrence after breast conserving surgery, *Ann Surg Oncol*, **14**(11): 3133–3140 (2007).
8. Dillon, M. F., Mc Dermott, E. W., O'Doherty, A., Quinn, C. M., Hill, A. D., and O'Higgins, N., Factors affecting successful breast conservation for ductal carcinoma in situ, *Ann Surg Oncol*, **14**(5): 1618–1628 (2007).
9. Kunos, C., Latson, L., Overmoyer, B., Silverman, P., Shenk, R., Kinsella, T., and Lyons, J., Breast conservation surgery achieving > or = 2 mm tumor-free margins results in decreased local-regional recurrence rates, *Breast J*, **12**(1): 28–36 (2006).
10. Elkhuizen, P. H., van de Vijver, M. J., Hermans, J., Zonderland, H. M., van de Velde, C. J., and Leer, J. W., Local recurrence after breast-conserving therapy for invasive breast cancer: High incidence in young patients and association with poor survival, *Int J Radiat Oncol Biol Phys*, **40**(4): 859–867 (1998).
11. Clarke, M., Collins, R., Darby, S., Davies, C., Elphinstone, P., Evans, E., Godwin, J. et al., Effects of radiotherapy and of differences in the extent of surgery for early breast cancer on local recurrence and 15-year survival: An overview of the randomised trials, *Lancet*, **366**(9503): 2087–2106 (2005).
12. Olson, T. P., Harter, J., Munoz, A., Mahvi, D. M., and Breslin, T., Frozen section analysis for intraoperative margin assessment during breast-conserving surgery results in low rates of re-excision and local recurrence, *Ann Surg Oncol*, **14**(10): 2953–2960 (2007).
13. Camp, E. R., McAuliffe, P. F., Gilroy, J. S., Morris, C. G., Lind, D. S., Mendenhall, N. P., and Copeland, E. M., 3rd, Minimizing local recurrence after breast conserving therapy using intraoperative shaved margins to determine pathologic tumor clearance, *J Am Coll Surg*, **201**(6): 855–861 (2005).
14. Valdes, E. K., Boolbol, S. K., Ali, I., Feldman, S. M., and Cohen, J. M., Intraoperative touch preparation cytology for margin assessment in breast-conservation surgery: Does it work for lobular carcinoma? *Ann Surg Oncol*, **14**(10): 2940–2945 (2007).
15. Singletary, S. E., Surgical margins in patients with early-stage breast cancer treated with breast conservation therapy, *Am J Surg*, **184**(5): 383–393 (2002).
16. Haka, A., Volynskaya, Z., Gardecki, J., Nazemi, J., Lyons, J., Hicks, D., Fitzmaurice, M., Dasari, R., Crowe, J., and Feld, M., In vivo margin assessment during partial mastectomy breast surgery using Raman spectroscopy, *Cancer Res*, **66**(6): 3317–3322 (2006).

17. Nguyen, F. T., Zysk, A. M., Chaney, E. J., Kotynek, J. G., Oliphant, U. J., Bellafiore, F. J., Rowland, K. M., Johnson, P. A., and Boppart, S. A., Intraoperative evaluation of breast tumor margins with optical coherence tomography, *Cancer Res*, **69**(22): 8790–8796 (2009).

18. Giuliano, A., Intraoperative assessment of surgical lumpectomy margins, DoD Breast Cancer Research Program (online database) (2006), http://www.cbcrp.org/RESEARCH/PageGrant.asp?grant_id=4845 (accessed January 21, 2010).

19. Bigio, I. J. and Bown, S. G., Spectroscopic sensing of cancer and cancer therapy: Current status of translational research, *Cancer Biol Ther*, **3**(3): 259–267 (2004).

20. Zysk, A. M. and Boppart, S. A., Computational methods for analysis of human breast tumor tissue in optical coherence tomography images, *J Biomed Opt*, **11**(5): 054015 (2006).

21. Gebhart, S. C., Thompson, R. C., and Mahadevan-Jansen, A., Liquid-crystal tunable filter spectral imaging for brain tumor demarcation, *Appl Opt*, **46**(10): 1896–1910 (2007).

22. D'Halluin, F., Tas, P., Rouquette, S., Bendavid, C., Foucher, F., Meshba, H., Blanchot, J., Coue, O., and Leveque, J., Intra-operative touch preparation cytology following lumpectomy for breast cancer: A series of 400 procedures, *Breast*, **18**(4): 248–253 (2009).

23. Wang, C., Chen, H.-b., Du, D.-l., Xiao, Y.-s., and Sun, H.-j., Electrode structure optimum for impedance measurement of intraoperative breast cancer focus, *IEEE Comput Soc.* **2**: 425–429 (2008).

24. Muttalib, M., Tai, C. C., Briant-Evans, T., Maheswaran, I., Livni, N., Shousha, S., and Sinnett, H. D., Intra-operative assessment of excision margins using breast imprint and scrape cytology, *Breast*, **14**(1): 42–50 (2005).

25. Tohnosu, N., Nabeya, Y., Matsuda, M., Akutsu, N., Watanabe, Y., Sato, H., Kato, T., Uehara, T., Ishii, S., and Yamazaki, E., Rapid intraoperative scrape cytology assessment of surgical margins in breast conservation surgery, *Breast Cancer*, **5**(2): 165–169 (1998).

26. Cabioglu, N., Hunt, K. K., Sahin, A. A., Kuerer, H. M., Babiera, G. V., Singletary, S. E., Whitman, G. J. et al., Role for intraoperative margin assessment in patients undergoing breast-conserving surgery, *Ann Surg Oncol*, **14**(4): 1458–1471 (2007).

27. Bigio, I. J., Bown, S. G., Briggs, G., Kelley, C., Lakhani, S., Pickard, D., Ripley, P. M., Rose, I. G., and Saunders, C., Diagnosis of breast cancer using elastic-scattering spectroscopy: Preliminary clinical results, *J Biomed Opt*, **5**(2): 221–228 (2000).

28. Haka, A. S., Volynskaya, Z., Gardecki, J. A., Nazemi, J., Shenk, R., Wang, N., Dasari, R. R., Fitzmaurice, M., and Feld, M. S., Diagnosing breast cancer using Raman spectroscopy: Prospective analysis, *J Biomed Opt*, **14**(5): 054023 (2009).

29. Keller, M. D., Majumder, S. K., and Mahadevan-Lansen, A., Spatially offset Raman spectroscopy of layered soft tissues, *Opt Lett*, **34**(7): 926–928 (2009).

30. Uzgiris, E. E., Sood, A., Bove, K., Grimmond, B., Lee, D., and Lomnes, S., A multimodal contrast agent for preoperative MR imaging and intraoperative tumor margin delineation, *Technol Cancer Res Treat*, **5**(4): 301–309 (2006).

31. Toker, E., Intra-operative radiographic margin assessment tool for breast-conserving surgery, NIH Small Business Innovative Research Awards (Online database), (2007), http://silk.nih.gov/public/cbz2zoz.@www.sbirsttr.fy2008.txt (accessed April 4, 2013).

32. Black, R., MRI-compatible fiber-optically sensorized surgical tools for precision removal of solid tumors, DoD STTR Program Phase I Selections for FY08 (2008), http://www.dodsbir.net/selections/sttr1_08.htm (accessed April 4, 2013).

33. Allweis, T. M., Kaufman, Z., Lelcuk, S., Pappo, I., Karni, T., Schneebaum, S., Spector, R. et al., A prospective, randomized, controlled, multicenter study of a real-time, intraoperative probe for positive margin detection in breast-conserving surgery, *Am J Surg*, **196**(4): 483–489 (2008).

34. Tafra, L., Karni, T., and Cheng, Z., Handheld intraoperative margin assessment device for partial mastectomy specimens, Paper presented at *7th Annual Meeting of the American Society of Breast Surgeons*, Baltimore, MD, April 5–9, 2006.

35. Karni, T., Pappo, I., Sandbank, J., Lavon, O., Kent, V., Spector, R., Morgenstern, S., and Lelcuk, S., A device for real-time, intraoperative margin assessment in breast-conservation surgery, *Am J Surg*, **194**(4): 467–473 (2007).

36. Pappo, I., Spector, R., Schindel, A., Morgenstern, S., Sandbank, J., Leider, L. T., Schneebaum, S., Lelcuk, S., and Karni, T., Diagnostic performance of a novel device for real-time margin assessment in lumpectomy specimens, *J Surg Res*, **160**(2): 277–281 (2010).

37. Graffeo, M. and Muscara, K., Dune medical devices receives FDA approval for breakthrough advancement in breast cancer surgery [cited April 3, 2013], http://www.multivu.com/mnr/58891-dune-medical-devices-fda-approval-marginprobe-system-breast-cancer-surgery (2013).

38. Keller, M. D., Majumder, S. K., Kelley, M. C., Meszoely, I. M., Boulos, F. I., Olivares, G. M., and Mahadevan-Jansen, A., Autofluorescence and diffuse reflectance spectroscopy and spectral imaging for breast surgical margin analysis, *Lasers Surg Med*, **42**(1): 15–23 (2010).

39. Lue, N., Kang, J. W., Yu, C. C., Barman, I., Dingari, N. C., Feld, M. S., Dasari, R. R., and Fitzmaurice, M., Portable optical fiber probe-based spectroscopic scanner for rapid cancer diagnosis: A new tool for intraoperative margin assessment, *PLoS One*, **7**(1): e30887 (2012).

40. Wilke, L. G., Brown, J. Q., Bydlon, T. M., Kennedy, S. A., Richards, L. M., Junker, M. K., Gallagher, J., Barry, W. T., Geradts, J., and Ramanujam, N., Rapid noninvasive optical imaging of tissue composition in breast tumor margins, *Am J Surg*, **198**(4): 566–574 (2009).

41. Brown, J. Q., Bydlon, T. M., Richards, L. M., Yu, B., Kennedy, S. A., Geradts, J., Wilke, L. G., Junker, M., Gallagher, J., and Ramanujam, N., Optical assessment of tumor resection margins in the breast, *IEEE J Sel Top Quantum Electron*, **16**: 530–544 (2010).

42. Bydlon, T. M., Kennedy, S. A., Richards, L. M., Brown, J. Q., Yu, B., Junker, M. K., Gallagher, J., Geradts, J., Wilke, L. G., and Ramanujam, N., Performance metrics of an optical spectral imaging system for intra-operative assessment of breast tumor margins, *Opt Express*, **18**(8): 8058–8076 (2010).

43. Brown, B. Y. J. Q., Junker, M., Lo, J. Y., Fu, H. L., Bydlon, T. M., Kennedy, S. A., Kuech, T. F., Geradts, J., Wilke, L. G., and Ramanujam, N., Quantitative spectral imaging for intraoperative breast tumor margin assessment, *European Conferences on Biomedical Optics*, Munich, Germany, May 22–26, 2011.

44. Fu, H. L., Yu, B., Lo, J. Y., Palmer, G. M., Kuech, T. F., and Ramanujam, N., A low-cost, portable, and quantitative spectral imaging system for application to biological tissues, *Opt Express*, **18**(12): 12630–12645 (2010).

45. Dhar, S., Lo, J. Y., Palmer, G. M., Brooke, M. A., Nichols, B. S., Yu, B., Ramanujam, N., and Jokerst, N. M., A diffuse reflectance spectral imaging system for tumor margin assessment using custom annular photodiode arrays, *Biomed Opt Express*, **3**(12): 3211–3222 (2012).

46. Palmer, G. M. and Ramanujam, N., Monte Carlo-based inverse model for calculating tissue optical properties. Part I: Theory and validation on synthetic phantoms, *Appl Opt*, **45**(5): 1062–1071 (2006).

47. Arifler, D., Schwarz, R. A., Chang, S. K., and Richards-Kortum, R., Reflectance spectroscopy for diagnosis of epithelial precancer: Model-based analysis of fiber-optic probe designs to resolve spectral information from epithelium and stroma, *Appl Opt*, **44**(20): 4291–4305 (2005).

48. Thueler, P., Charvet, I., Bevilacqua, F., St Ghislain, M., Ory, G., Marquet, P., Meda, P., Vermeulen, B., and Depeursinge, C., In vivo endoscopic tissue diagnostics based on spectroscopic absorption, scattering, and phase function properties, *J Biomed Opt*, **8**(3): 495–503 (2003).

49. Wang, Q., Yang, H., Agrawal, A., Wang, N. S., and Pfefer, T. J., Measurement of internal tissue optical properties at ultraviolet and visible wavelengths: Development and implementation of a fiberoptic-based system, *Opt Express*, **16**(12): 8685–8703 (2008).

50. Zonios, G., Perelman, L. T., Backman, V., Manoharan, R., Fitzmaurice, M., Van Dam, J., and Feld, M. S., Diffuse reflectance spectroscopy of human adenomatous colon polyps in vivo, *Appl Opt*, **38**(31): 6628–6637 (1999).

51. Farrell, T. J., Patterson, M. S., and Wilson, B., A diffusion theory model of spatially resolved, steady-state diffuse reflectance for the noninvasive determination of tissue optical properties in vivo, *Med Phys*, **19**(4): 879–888 (1992).

52. Volynskaya, Z., Haka, A. S., Bechtel, K. L., Fitzmaurice, M., Shenk, R., Wang, N., Nazemi, J., Dasari, R. R., and Feld, M. S., Diagnosing breast cancer using diffuse reflectance spectroscopy and intrinsic fluorescence spectroscopy, *J Biomed Opt*, **13**(2): 024012 (2008).

53. Utzinger, U., Brewer, M., Silva, E., Gershenson, D., Blast, R. C., Jr., Follen, M., and Richards-Kortum, R., Reflectance spectroscopy for in vivo characterization of ovarian tissue, *Lasers Surg Med*, **28**(1): 56–66 (2001).

54. Mirabal, Y. N., Chang, S. K., Atkinson, E. N., Malpica, A., Follen, M., and Richards-Kortum, R., Reflectance spectroscopy for in vivo detection of cervical precancer, *J Biomed Opt*, **7**(4): 587–594 (2002).

55. Badizadegan, K., Backman, V., Boone, C. W., Crum, C. P., Dasari, R. R., Georgakoudi, I., Keefe, K. et al., Spectroscopic diagnosis and imaging of invisible pre-cancer, *Faraday Discuss*, **126**: 265–279; discussion 303–311 (2004).

56. Schwarz, R. A., Gao, W., Daye, D., Williams, M. D., Richards-Kortum, R., and Gillenwater, A. M., Autofluorescence and diffuse reflectance spectroscopy of oral epithelial tissue using a depth-sensitive fiber-optic probe, *Appl Opt*, **47**(6): 825–834 (2008).

57. Marin, N. M., Milbourne, A., Rhodes, H., Ehlen, T., Miller, D., Benedet, L., Richards-Kortum, R., and Follen, M., Diffuse reflectance patterns in cervical spectroscopy, *Gynecol Oncol*, **99**(3 Suppl 1): S116–S120 (2005).

58. Zhu, C., Palmer, G. M., Breslin, T. M., Harter, J., and Ramanujam, N., Diagnosis of breast cancer using diffuse reflectance spectroscopy: Comparison of a Monte Carlo versus partial least squares analysis based feature extraction technique, *Lasers Surg Med*, **38**(7): 714–724 (2006).

59. Skala, M. C., Palmer, G. M., Vrotsos, K. M., Gendron-Fitzpatrick, A., and Ramanujam, N., Comparison of a physical model and principal component analysis for the diagnosis of epithelial neoplasias in vivo using diffuse reflectance spectroscopy, *Opt Express*, **15**(12): 7863–7875 (2007).

60. Sharwani, A., Jerjes, W., Salih, V., Swinson, B., Bigio, I. J., El-Maaytah, M., and Hopper, C., Assessment of oral premalignancy using elastic scattering spectroscopy, *Oral Oncol*, **42**(4): 343–349 (2006).

61. Muller, M. G., Valdez, T. A., Georgakoudi, I., Backman, V., Fuentes, C., Kabani, S., Laver, N. et al., Spectroscopic detection and evaluation of morphologic and biochemical changes in early human oral carcinoma, *Cancer*, **97**(7): 1681–1692 (2003).

62. Amelink, A., Kaspers, O. P., Sterenborg, H. J., van der Wal, J. E., Roodenburg, J. L., and Witjes, M. J., Non-invasive measurement of the morphology and physiology of oral mucosa by use of optical spectroscopy, *Oral Oncol*, **44**(1): 65–71 (2008).

63. Nieman, L. T., Kan, C. W., Gillenwater, A., Markey, M. K., and Sokolov, K., Probing local tissue changes in the oral cavity for early detection of cancer using oblique polarized reflectance spectroscopy: A pilot clinical trial, *J Biomed Opt*, **13**(2): 024011 (2008).

64. Lin, W. C., Toms, S. A., Motamedi, M., Jansen, E. D., and Mahadevan-Jansen, A., Brain tumor demarcation using optical spectroscopy; an in vitro study, *J Biomed Opt*, **5**(2): 214–220 (2000).

65. Sunar, U., Quon, H., Durduran, T., Zhang, J., Du, J., Zhou, C., Yu, G. et al., Noninvasive diffuse optical measurement of blood flow and blood oxygenation for monitoring radiation therapy in patients with head and neck tumors: A pilot study, *J Biomed Opt*, **11**(6): 064021 (2006).

66. Wang, H. W., Zhu, T. C., Putt, M. E., Solonenko, M., Metz, J., Dimofte, A., Miles, J. et al., Broadband reflectance measurements of light penetration, blood oxygenation, hemoglobin concentration, and drug concentration in human intraperitoneal tissues before and after photodynamic therapy, *J Biomed Opt*, **10**(1): 14004 (2005).

67. Amelink, A., van der Ploeg van den Heuvel, A., de Wolf, W. J., Robinson, D. J., and Sterenborg, H. J., Monitoring PDT by means of superficial reflectance spectroscopy, *J Photochem Photobiol B*, **79**(3): 243–251 (2005).

68. Maxim, P. G., Carson, J. J., Benaron, D. A., Loo, B. W., Jr., Xing, L., Boyer, A. L., and Friedland, S., Optical detection of tumors in vivo by visible light tissue oximetry, *Technol Cancer Res Treat*, **4**(3): 227–234 (2005).

69. Brown, J. Q., Vishwanath, K., Palmer, G. M., and Ramanujam, N., Advances in quantitative UV–visible spectroscopy for clinical and pre-clinical application in cancer, *Curr Opin Biotechnol*, **20**(1): 119–131 (2009).

70. Liu, Q., Role of optical spectroscopy using endogenous contrasts in clinical cancer diagnosis, *World J Clin Oncol*, **2**(1): 50–63 (2011).

71. Cendan, J. C., Coco, D., and Copeland, E. M., 3rd, Accuracy of intraoperative frozen-section analysis of breast cancer lumpectomy-bed margins, *J Am Coll Surg*, **201**(2): 194–198 (2005).

72. Sauter, E. R., Hoffman, J. P., Ottery, F. D., Kowalyshyn, M. J., Litwin, S., and Eisenberg, B. L., Is frozen section analysis of reexcision lumpectomy margins worthwhile? Margin analysis in breast reexcisions, *Cancer*, **73**(10): 2607–2612 (1994).

73. Weber, S., Storm, F. K., Stitt, J., and Mahvi, D. M., The role of frozen section analysis of margins during breast conservation surgery, *Cancer J Sci Am*, **3**(5): 273–277 (1997).

74. Noguchi, M., Minami, M., Earashi, M., Taniya, T., Miyazaki, I. I., Mizukami, Y., Nonomura, A. et al., Pathologic assessment of surgical margins on frozen and permanent sections in breast conserving surgery, *Breast Cancer*, **2**(1): 27–33 (1995).

75. Pleijhuis, R. G., Graafland, M., de Vries, J., Bart, J., de Jong, J. S., and van Dam, G. M., Obtaining adequate surgical margins in breast-conserving therapy for patients with early-stage breast cancer: Current modalities and future directions, *Ann Surg Oncol*, **16**(10): 2717–2730 (2009).

76. Cox, C. E., Ku, N. N., Reintgen, D. S., Greenberg, H. M., Nicosia, S. V., and Wangensteen, S., Touch preparation cytology of breast lumpectomy margins with histologic correlation, *Arch Surg*, **126**(4): 490–493 (1991).

77. Creager, A. J., Shaw, J. A., Young, P. R., and Geisinger, K. R., Intraoperative evaluation of lumpectomy margins by imprint cytology with histologic correlation: A community hospital experience, *Arch Pathol Lab Med*, **126**(7): 846–848 (2002).

78. Johnson, A. T., Henry-Tillman, R., and Klimberg, V. S., Breast conserving surgery: Optimizing local control in the breast with the assessment of margins, *Breast Dis*, **12**: 35–41 (2001).

79. Rubio, I. T., Korourian, S., Cowan, C., Krag, D. N., Colvert, M., and Klimberg, V. S., Use of touch preps for intraoperative diagnosis of sentinel lymph node metastases in breast cancer, *Ann Surg Oncol*, **5**(8): 689–694 (1998).

80. Huston, T. L., Pigalarga, R., Osborne, M. P., and Tousimis, E., The influence of additional surgical margins on the total specimen volume excised and the reoperative rate after breast-conserving surgery, *Am J Surg*, **192**(4): 509–512 (2006).

81. Mendez, J. E., Lamorte, W. W., de Las Morenas, A., Cerda, S., Pistey, R., King, T., Kavanah, M., Hirsch, E., and Stone, M. D., Influence of breast cancer margin assessment method on the rates of positive margins and residual carcinoma, *Am J Surg*, **192**(4): 538–540 (2006).

82. Menes, T. S., Tartter, P. I., Bleiweiss, I., Godbold, J. H., Estabrook, A., and Smith, S. R., The consequence of multiple re-excisions to obtain clear lumpectomy margins in breast cancer patients, *Ann Surg Oncol*, **12**(11): 881–885 (2005).

83. Kurniawan, E. D., Wong, M. H., Windle, I., Rose, A., Mou, A., Buchanan, M., Collins, J. P., Miller, J. A., Gruen, R. L., and Mann, G. B., Predictors of surgical margin status in breast-conserving surgery within a breast screening program, *Ann Surg Oncol*, **15**(9): 2542–2549 (2008).

84. Bani, M. R., Lux, M. P., Heusinger, K., Wenkel, E., Magener, A., Schulz-Wendtland, R., Beckmann, M. W., and Fasching, P. A., Factors correlating with reexcision after breast-conserving therapy, *Eur J Surg Oncol*, **35**(1): 32–37 (2009).

85. Azu, M., Abrahamse, P., Katz, S. J., Jagsi, R., and Morrow, M., What is an adequate margin for breast-conserving surgery? Surgeon attitudes and correlates, *Ann Surg Oncol*, 17(2): 558–563 (2010).

86. Fisher, E., Lumpectomy margins and much more, *Cancer*, **79**(8): 1453–1458 (1996).
87. Carter, D., Margins of "lumpectomy" for breast cancer, *Hum Pathol*, **17**(4): 330–332 (1986).
88. Schnitt, S. J., Abner, A., Gelman, R., Connolly, J. L., Recht, A., Duda, R. B., Eberlein, T. J., Mayzel, K., Silver, B., and Harris, J. R., The relationship between microscopic margins of resection and the risk of local recurrence in patients with breast cancer treated with breast-conserving surgery and radiation therapy, *Cancer*, **74**(6): 1746–1751 (1994).
89. Gage, I., Schnitt, S. J., Nixon, A. J., Silver, B., Recht, A., Troyan, S. L., Eberlein, T. et al., Pathologic margin involvement and the risk of recurrence in patients treated with breast-conserving therapy, *Cancer*, **78**(9): 1921–1928 (1996).
90. Brown, J. Q., Wilke, L. G., Geradts, J., Kennedy, S. A., Palmer, G. M., and Ramanujam, N., Quantitative optical spectroscopy: A robust tool for direct measurement of breast cancer vascular oxygenation and total hemoglobin content in vivo, *Cancer Res*, **69**(7): 2919–2926 (2009).
91. Palmer, G. M., Zhu, C., Breslin, T. M., Xu, F., Gilchrist, K. W., and Ramanujam, N., Monte Carlo-based inverse model for calculating tissue optical properties. Part II: Application to breast cancer diagnosis, *Appl Opt*, **45**(5): 1072–1078 (2006).
92. Bender, J. E., Vishwanath, K., Moore, L. K., Brown, J. Q., Chang, V., Palmer, G. M., and Ramanujam, N., A robust Monte Carlo model for the extraction of biological absorption and scattering in vivo, *IEEE Trans Biomed Eng*, **56**(4): 960–968 (2009).
93. Bender, J. E., Shang, A. B., Moretti, E. W., Yu, B., Richards, L. M., and Ramanujam, N., Noninvasive monitoring of tissue hemoglobin using UV–VIS diffuse reflectance spectroscopy: A pilot study, *Opt Lett*, **17**(26): 23396–23409 (2009).
94. Zhu, C., Palmer, G. M., Breslin, T. M., Xu, F., and Ramanujam, N., Use of a multiseparation fiber optic probe for the optical diagnosis of breast cancer, *J Biomed Opt*, **10**(2): 024032 (2005).
95. Chang, V. T., Cartwright, P. S., Bean, S. M., Palmer, G. M., Bentley, R. C., and Ramanujam, N., Quantitative physiology of the precancerous cervix in vivo through optical spectroscopy, *Neoplasia*, **11**(4): 325–332 (2009).
96. Yu, B., Fu, H., Bydlon, T., Bender, J. E., and Ramanujam, N., Diffuse reflectance spectroscopy with a self-calibrating fiber optic probe, *Opt Lett*, **33**(16): 1783–1785 (2008).
97. Yu, B., Fu, H. L., and Ramanujam, N., Instrument independent diffuse reflectance spectroscopy, *J Biomed Opt*, **16**(1): 011010 (2011).
98. Wang, L.-H., Jacques, S. L., and Zheng, L.-Q., MCML—Monte Carlo modeling of photon transport in multi-layered tissues, *Comput Methods Programs Biomed*, **47**: 131–146 (1995).
99. Prahl, S., Oregon medical laser center, http://omlc.ogi.edu/software/mie/index.html (2005) (accessed April 4, 2013).
100. Xia, J. J., Berg, E. P., Lee, J. W., and Yao, G., Characterizing beef muscles with optical scattering and absorption coefficients in VIS-NIR region, *Meat Sci*, **75**(1): 78–83 (2007).
101. Bashkatov, A. N., Genina, É. A., Kochubey, V. I., and Tuchin, V. V., Optical properties of the subcutaneous adipose tissue in the spectral range 400–2500 nm, *Opt Spectrosc*, **99**(5): 836–842 (2005).
102. Yu, B., Lo, J. Y., Kuech, T. F., Palmer, G. M., Bender, J. E., and Ramanujam, N., Cost-effective diffuse reflectance spectroscopy device for quantifying tissue absorption and scattering in vivo, *J Biomed Opt Lett*, **13**: 060505 (2008).
103. Lo, J. Y., Yu, B., Fu, H. L., Bender, J. E., Palmer, G. M., Kuech, T. F., and Ramanujam, N., A strategy for quantitative spectral imaging of tissue absorption and scattering using light emitting diodes and photodiodes, *Opt Express*, **17**(3): 1372–1384 (2009).
104. Bydlon, T. M., Barry, W. T., Kennedy, S. A., Brown, J. Q., Gallagher, J. E., Wilke, L. G., Geradts, J., and Ramanujam, N., Advancing optical imaging for breast margin assessment: An analysis of excisional time, cautery, and patent blue dye on underlying sources of contrast, *PLoS One*, **7**(12): e51418 (2012).

18

Near-Infrared Fluorescence Imaging and Spectroscopy in Random Media and Tissues

E.M. Sevick-Muraca
Texas A&M University

E. Kuwana
Texas A&M University

A. Godavarty
Texas A&M University

J.P. Houston
Texas A&M University

A.B. Thompson
Texas A&M University

R. Roy
Texas A&M University

18.1 Introduction

Most radiation-based spectroscopic and imaging techniques are typically dependent upon evaluating a nonscattered or singly scattered signal for retrieval of quantitative information. For example, absorption spectroscopy depends upon the survival of unscattered light across a known path length, L; dynamic light scattering or photon correlation spectroscopy requires the fluctuation of light intensity owing to its scatter by Brownian motion out of the optical path; x-ray and computed x-ray tomography depend upon the straight-line path of nonabsorbed x-rays, and so forth. Yet most systems of interest multiply scatter radiation of low energy and, in particular, require diluted suspensions or nonscattering media when dealing with optical interrogation. Hence, optical techniques developed for imaging and spectroscopy are usually plagued by the influence of scatter. In order to expand the quantitative applicability of optical techniques to these real systems, new techniques have been developed that focus on coherence properties, temporal and spatial correlation, and other properties in order to extract the nonscattered or singly scattered light from a multiply scattered signal. Yet these approaches neglect the largest portion of the signal, the scattered signal, in favor of that portion that possesses the smallest signal to noise ratio (SNR).

In this chapter, we first review continuous wave (CW) and time-resolved techniques along with the associated diffusion equation for quantitative absorption, scattering, and fluorescence spectroscopy using multiply scattered light. In addition, since in the wavelength window of 600–900 nm light is multiply scattered by most biological tissues, we next focus upon the development of these optical techniques for biomedical spectroscopy and imaging, namely, optical tomography. Owing to the limitation of endogenous chromophores in tissues in this wavelength regime, we provide a comprehensive review on the methods of fluorescence-enhanced optical spectroscopy and imaging, including measurement methods, solutions to the forward and inverse imaging problems, and attributes for clinical and sensing fluorophore development.

18.2 Background: Probing Random Media with Multiply Scattered Light

Before presenting the measurement methods and analysis for probing random media with multiply scattered light, it is instructive to first consider traditional light spectroscopy techniques that depend upon monitoring the light transmitted across a known path length, L.

18.2.1 Beer–Lambert Relation for Absorption and Turbidity Spectroscopy

Absorption and turbidity measurements consist of monitoring the attenuation of light intensity $I(\lambda)$ at wavelength λ, given incident light intensity, $I_o(\lambda)$, in order to determine the absorption or scattering coefficients (μ_a [cm^{-1}] or μ_s [cm^{-1}], respectively):

$$\log \frac{I(\lambda)}{I_o(\lambda)} = -\mu_a(\lambda)L \text{ or } -\mu_s(\lambda)L \tag{18.1}$$

where the absorption coefficient is provided by the product of the concentration of light-absorbing species, $[C_i]$ (mM), and its extinction coefficient at wavelength λ, ε_i^λ (cm^{-1} mM^{-1}):

$$\mu_a(\lambda) = 2.303 \sum_{i=1}^{N} \varepsilon_i^\lambda [C_i] \tag{18.2}$$

and the scattering coefficient can be predicted from

$$\mu_s(\lambda) = \int\limits_0^\pi \frac{12\phi}{k^2} \int\limits_0^\infty \frac{f(x_i)}{x_i^3} \int\limits_0^\infty \frac{f(x_j)}{x_j^3} F_{i,j}(n, x_i, x_j, \lambda, \theta) \cdot S_{i,j}(x_i, x_j, q, \phi) \sin\theta \, dx_j \, dx_i \, d\theta \tag{18.3}$$

where

$F_{i,j}$ is the binary form factor between the particles with different sizes x_i and x_j

$S_{i,j}$ is the corresponding partial structure factor, which describes the correction factor of coherent scattering due to particle interactions of particles i and j

n is the relative refractive index of the particles to the medium

λ is the wavelength

θ is the scattering angle

ϕ is the volume fraction of particles in the suspension

$f(x)$ is the particle size distribution

q is the magnitude of the wave vector, $q = 2k \sin(\theta/2)$, where k is given by $2\pi m/\lambda$ and m is the refractive index of the medium

The structure factor is a direct measure of the local ordering of colloidal particles, and the values of $S_{i,j}$ are equal to unity in the absence of particle interactions (e.g., in a dilute suspension).

Determination of absorption and scattering coefficients through the Beer–Lambert relationship in Equation 18.1 assumes that light is absorbed or scattered *out of the path* and that there is no light scattered back *into the path*. Absorption and scattering mechanisms can be considered simultaneously in dilute suspension terms of an effective absorption cross section:

$$\mu_{eff} = \mu_a + \mu_s \tag{18.4}$$

18.2.2 Fluorescence Spectroscopy and Fluorescence Lifetime Spectroscopy

Fluorescence spectroscopy, whether measured using time-resolved or CW techniques, is based upon the absorption of excitation light at λ_x across a path length, L, by fluorophores of concentration $[C_i]$. The quantum efficiency, α, describes the fraction number of emission photons at fluorescence wavelength λ_m, emitted for each excitation photon absorbed by the fluorophore and is typically described as the rate of radiative decay, Γ, relative to the sum of radiative and nonradiative decay rates ($\Gamma + k_{nr}$). In other words, $\alpha = \Gamma/(\Gamma + k_{nr})$. The intensity of detected fluorescence light, I_m, in response to a constant intensity of incident excitation light, $I_o^{\lambda_x}$, can be provided by the expression [1]

$$I_m \propto I_o^{\lambda_x} \alpha \left[\varepsilon_i^{\lambda_x} [C_i] \right] \cdot \int\limits_0^\infty g(t) dt \tag{18.5}$$

Here, $g(t)$ represents the time-dependent fluorescence decay that describes the process of radiative and non-radiative relaxation of the activated fluorophore, elevated to an excited state by absorption of excitation light. For most laser dyes, the relaxation is a first-order process described by a mean lifetime, τ, of the activated state. Consequently, the time-invariant emission intensity predicted by Equation 18.5 can be rewritten as

$$I_m \propto I_o^{\lambda_x} \alpha \left[\varepsilon_i^{\lambda_x} [C_i] \right] \cdot \int\limits_0^\infty \exp\left[-\frac{t}{\tau} \right] dt \propto I_o^{\lambda_x} \alpha \left[\varepsilon_i^{\lambda_x} [C_i] \right] \tau \tag{18.6}$$

where the fluorescence lifetime, τ, is influenced by the relative rates of radiative and nonradiative decay (i.e., $\tau = 1/(\Gamma + k_{nr})$).

Ratiometric fluorescent probes in which reemission is monitored across two or more wavelengths (such as bis-carboxyethyl carboxyfluorescein [BCECF] or seminaphthofluorescein [SNAFL]) also provide a means to monitor changes in the decay kinetics using CW methods. The ratio of the emission intensities at λ_{m1} and λ_{m2} following excitation at a single excitation wavelength is independent of the concentration of fluorophore available and dependent only upon the decay kinetics probed at the two emission wavelengths:

$$\frac{I_m(\lambda_{m1})}{I_m(\lambda_{m2})} = \frac{I_o^{\lambda_x}\alpha^{\lambda_{m1}}\left[\varepsilon_i^{\lambda_x}[C_i]\right]\tau^{\lambda_{m1}}}{I_o^{\lambda_x}\alpha^{\lambda_{m2}}\left[\varepsilon_i^{\lambda_x}[C_i]\right]\tau^{\lambda_{m2}}} = \frac{\alpha^{\lambda_{m1}}}{\alpha^{\lambda_{m2}}} \cdot \frac{\tau^{\lambda_{m1}}}{\tau^{\lambda_{m2}}} \tag{18.7}$$

In time-domain measurements where an incident impulse of excitation light is used to excite the sample, the resulting time-dependent emission intensity can be predicted by

$$I_m(t) \propto I_o^{\lambda_x}(\delta)\alpha\left[\varepsilon_i^{\lambda_x}[C_i]\right] \cdot \int_0^t \exp\left[-\frac{t'}{\tau}\right]dt' \tag{18.8}$$

Thus, upon exciting a dilute fluorescence sample with an impulse of excitation light and monitoring the emission intensity as a function of time, the lifetime or decay kinetics that govern the relaxation of the activated state to the ground state can be quantitated independently of the concentration of fluorophore present. The measurement of the time-dependent emission light following activation in a diluted, non-scattering suspension with an incident impulse of excitation light is also the basis of the time-domain measurements described below for random media.

Earlier, CW and time-domain analyses were presented for fluorophores exhibiting first-order decay kinetics, whereby the form of the decay kinetics, $g(t)$, is given by

$$g(t) = \exp\left(-\frac{t}{\tau}\right) \tag{18.9}$$

However, most analyte fluorophores exhibit more complex decay kinetics such as multiexponential decays:

$$g(t) = \sum_{j=1}^N a_j \exp\left[\frac{-t}{\tau_j}\right] \tag{18.10}$$

or stretched exponential decay kinetics, which indicates collisional quenching between species j:

$$g(t) = \sum_{j=1}^N a_j \exp\left[-\alpha_j \cdot t - \beta_j\sqrt{t}\right] \tag{18.11}$$

By monitoring the time dependence of the emitted fluorescence light as a function of time following excitation, the decay kinetics can be best ascertained and correlated with the local environment that impacts the relaxation process. For example, the Stern–Volmer equation relates the quencher concentration, [Q], and fluorescence intensity measurements made in the absence and presence of the quencher, I_m^o and I_m, respectively:

$$\frac{I_m^o}{I_m} = 1 + K[Q] = 1 + \left(k_q \tau_o\right)[Q] \tag{18.12}$$

where
K is the Stern–Volmer constant
k_q and τ_o are the bimolecular quenching constant and the lifetime of the fluorophore in the absence of quencher

The decay kinetics of many analyte-sensing fluorophores can be used to assess concentrations of analytes such as H^+ and Ca^{2+}, which may have no appreciable absorption cross section at the emission and excitation wavelengths used. Consequently, fluorescence lifetime spectroscopy broadens the applicability of absorption spectroscopy, given that a fluorophore with analyte-sensitive decay kinetics can be identified.

While time-dependent techniques provide the best means for assessing fluorescence decay kinetics, their need for Dirac pulse of excitation light complicates instrumentation and/or limits quantitation. Frequency-domain approaches provide an alternative approach to the impulse function by exciting with an intensity-modulated excitation light modulated at MHz–GHz modulation frequencies, ω. Activation of the fluorophore creates isotropic, intensity-modulated fluorescent light that is both phase-delayed and amplitude-attenuated relative to the incident light owing to the kinetics of the relaxation process. For a simple, first-order system, the decay kinetics; the phase delay, $\theta(\omega)$; and the modulation ratio, $M(\omega)$, at modulation frequency ω can be predicted from

$$M(\omega)\exp\left(-i\theta(\omega)\right) = \int_0^\infty g(t)\exp\left[-i\omega t\right] dt = \int_0^\infty \exp\left[-\frac{t}{\tau}\right]\exp\left[-i\omega t\right] dt \tag{18.13}$$

$$M(\omega) = \frac{I_{AC}(\omega)}{I_{DC}(\omega)} = \frac{\mu_a \alpha}{\sqrt{1+(\omega\tau)^2}}; \quad \theta(\omega) = \tan^{-1}\left[\omega\tau\right]$$

where the amplitude and average of the modulated emission light is given by $I_{AC}(\omega)$ and $I_{DC}(\omega)$. In dilute, nonscattering media, the fluorescent emission is collected at right angles to the excitation illumination in order to avoid inadvertently collecting excitation light.

As a means of introduction, the concept of absorption and scattering spectroscopy employing the Beer–Lambert relationship as well as the CW, time-domain, and frequency-domain fluorescence spectroscopy approaches for quantitative spectroscopy when scatter back into the optical path does not corrupt attenuation or intensity measurements has been put forward. However, most systems of interest are comprised of random media, that is, that which absorb, multiply scatter, as well as fluoresce. In the following, we outline the techniques of CW, time-domain, frequency-domain, and associated approaches to perform quantitative spectroscopy and imaging in random media.

18.2.3 Measurement Approaches for Quantitative Spectroscopy and Imaging in Random Media

Herein, we restrict our discussion of quantitative spectroscopy and imaging in random media in which the diffusion approximation to the radiative transport equation holds. Those conditions are the following: (1) the source of incident (excitation) light is isotropic; (2) the scattering capacity of the tissue exceeds that of its absorption capacity, that is, $\mu_a \ll (1 - g)\mu_s$, where g is the mean cosine of angular scatter of the medium; and (3) the light that is collected has been multiply scattered. When referring to measurements of multiply scattered light, that is, light that has traveled a distribution of path lengths or of *times of flight*, we term the measurements as ones of *photon migration* measurements.

18.2.3.1 CW and Time-Resolved Measurement Approaches

CW measurements employ a light source whose intensity nominally does not vary with time. The constant power, isotropic source illuminates the random medium with light whose intensity becomes exponentially attenuated with increasing distance from the tissue surface. Increased absorption or scattering properties of the medium result in increased light attenuation as it propagates deeper into the random medium. In CW measurements, the time-invariant intensity is measured as a function of distance away from the incident source and is primarily a function of the product $\mu_a \mu_s'$. The amount of generated fluorescent light at any position $\bar{r}$ is proportional to the product of the concentration of fluorophore, $[C_i]$, and the local excitation fluence, $\Phi_x(r)$, which is effectively the concentration of excitation photons times the speed of light within the medium. Thus, the origin of emission light predominates from the region in which the excitation fluence, Φ_x, is greatest. For time-invariant CW measurements, the region with the greatest excitation fluence always remains close to the point of incident excitation illumination. Consequently, the origin of fluorescence is predominantly from the surface or subsurface regions. Fluorescence spectroscopy for determination of fluorescent optical properties in a uniform medium with CW techniques may not be impacted by the confinement of the origin of emission light, if the random medium is indeed homogeneous. However, in imaging scenarios whereby the concentration of fluorophore is nonuniform, CW techniques will undoubtedly emphasize surface and subsurface regions. In imaging cases whereby the fluorescent dye acts as a contrast agent and has *perfect uptake* (i.e., partitioning of the dye occurs exclusively in the tissue of interest without any residual dye in the intervening tissues between the target and the surface), then CW techniques may be appropriate. However, the elusive *holy grail* of contrast-based imaging for all medical imaging modalities is to develop agents that maximize their partitioning in the target region of interest. It is unlikely that near-infrared (NIR) techniques involving fluorescent contrast agents for clinical imaging will involve CW measurement despite the simplicity of its instrumentation.

Time-domain photon migration (TDPM) measurements employ a light source that delivers a pulse of excitation light that broadens and attenuates as it propagates through the random medium as shown in Figure 18.1. TDPM techniques employ single photon counting (sometimes called time-correlated counting) or gated integration measurements to acquire the emitted pulse broadened by as much as several nanoseconds of photon *time of flight*. As the absorption properties of the random media increase, the broadening of the excitation pulse lessens and greater attenuation occurs. In the case of increased scattering properties, the excitation pulse increasingly broadens and attenuates during its propagation away from the incident point source. Clearly, the impact of absorption and scattering has differing effects on the photon *time of flight*: increased absorption decreases the path and travel time of migrating photons, while increased scattering enhances it. When exciting fluorophores within the random medium, a propagating excitation pulse generates a propagating emission pulse that is further broadened owing to the decay kinetics of the dye.

Since the region of highest excitation fluence is not stationary and propagates away from its incidence with time following delivery to the surface, the origin of fluorescent signals activated by the propagating excitation pulse may not be restricted to surface or subsurface tissues as in the case of CW measurements. If the time constant of the dye's decay kinetics is less than or comparable to the detected excitation photon *time of flight*, then the fluorescence measured at a distance away from the incident excitation source may originate deeply within the random media. On the other hand, if the time constant of the dye's decay kinetics is greater than the detected excitation photon *times of flight*, then the fluorescence will originate from shallow locations within the random medium [2].

The phenomenon can be explained in the following manner: at the medium surface, the position of maximum excitation fluence travels from its point of incidence to deep within the medium and exponentially attenuates as it penetrates. Consider a fluorophore that has an instantaneous rate of radiative relaxation. The maximum emission fluence will likewise follow the trend of the propagating excitation pulse: At time $t = 0$, when the excitation pulse is launched, the emission fluence will be greatest at the point of incidence, and as time progresses, the point of greatest emission fluence will propagate into the medium and will attenuate as it does so. The emission light that reaches the surface will initially

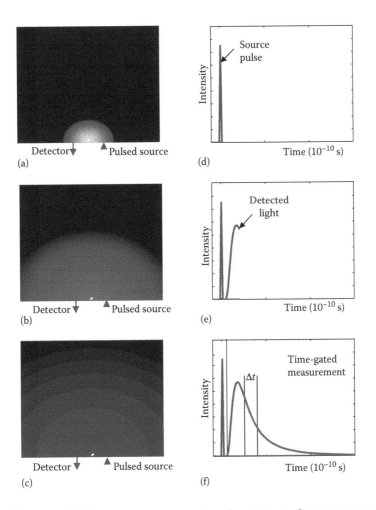

FIGURE 18.1 Schematic of TDPM measurement approach used in NIR optical spectroscopy and tomography. TDPM imaging approaches utilize an incident impulse of light that results in the propagation of the pulse that attenuates as a function of distance from the source and time following its delivery. The detected pulse is measured as intensity versus time that represents the photon *time of flight*. Panel (a) illustrates the light distribution in tissue from a pulse point source after 1×10^{-10} s, (b) 25×10^{-10} s, and (c) 150×10^{-10} s following the incident impulse. The corresponding recorded data during the time intervals at the detector are illustrated in Panels (d–f). A time-gated illumination measurement is shown in Panel (f) in which the integrated intensity measured within a specified window is measured. (Reproduced from Hawrysz, D.J. and Sevick-Muraca, E.M., *Neoplasia*, 2, 388, 2000. With permission.)

originate from regions closest to the incident source and then from deeper within the random medium with increased time after the initial impulse of excitation light. However, consider the case of a phosphorescent agent that possesses a slow radiative relaxation rate and has an effective lifetime on the order of milliseconds—much larger than the measured photon migration *time of flights*. In this case, the greatest concentration of activated fluorophore will reside close to the incidence point of excitation illumination, and while the pulse of excitation fluence transits deeper within the random media, the slow decay of the activated fluorophore closest to the point of incident of excitation will result in a pulse of emission fluence that does not propagate spatially with time into the random media and away from the point of the incident excitation illumination. Consequently, for imaging and spectroscopic imaging applications whereby information from within the random media is desired, long-lived fluorophores cannot be employed.

Earlier, the qualitative CW and TDPM measurements for fluorescence spectroscopy and imaging are described. Quantitative prediction is also possible with the radiative transport equation, Monte Carlo, and diffusion equations, given the proper model for fluorescent decay is incorporated. Herein, we restrict our analysis to media in which the diffusion approximation to the radiative transfer equation applies. The photon diffusion equation may be written to predict CW and TDPM measurements of excitation (subscript x) and emission (subscript m) fluence, $\Phi_{x,m}(\vec{r})$ and $\Phi_{x,m}(\vec{r},t)$, respectively [3,4]:

$$\vec{\nabla} \cdot \left(D_{x,m} \vec{\nabla} \Phi_{x,m}(\vec{r},t) \right) - \mu_{ax,m} \Phi_{x,m}(\vec{r},t) = \frac{1}{c} \frac{\partial \Phi_{x,m}(\vec{r},t)}{\partial t} - S_{x,m}(\vec{r},t) \tag{18.14}$$

where $D_{x,m}$ is the optical diffusion coefficient at the excitation or emission wavelength, (cm) given by

$$D_{x,m} = \frac{1}{3 \left[\mu_{a_{x,m}} + \mu'_{s_{x,m}} \right]} \tag{18.15}$$

and $\mu'_{s_{x,m}}$ is the isotropic scattering coefficient given by $(1-g)\mu_{s_{x,m}}$. The excitation or emission fluence, $\Phi_{x,m}(\vec{r},t)$ [W/m²], is the angle-integrated, scalar flux of photons and is defined as the power incident on an infinitesimally small sphere divided by its area. Again, it can also be thought of as the local concentration of photons times the speed of light, c, at a given position $\vec{r}$ and (for time-dependent cases) time t. For CW spectroscopy or imaging, there is no time dependence and the source term, $S_x(\vec{r},t)$, becomes time invariant. Assuming the source is isotropic, this term is equivalent to the power deposited over its area. For TDPM measurements, the source $S_x(\vec{r},0)$ is assumed to be a Dirac delta function assuming a finite value at time zero, but zero at all other times. For both CW and TDPM measurements, Equation 18.14 can be solved to predict the excitation fluence, $\Phi_x(\vec{r})$ or $\Phi_x(\vec{r},t)$, in response to the known spatial distribution of absorption and scattering properties, $\mu_{a_x}(\vec{r})$ and $\mu'_{s_x}(\vec{r})$, of the media volume at the excitation wavelength. Here, the absorption coefficient at the excitation wavelength is comprised of contributions from the endogenous chromophores ($\mu_{a_{x \rightarrow}}(\vec{r})$) as well as the exogenous fluorophores ($\mu_{a_{x \rightarrow m}}(\vec{r})$).

Since a closed form solution for $\Phi_x(\vec{r},t)$ exists only for the simple geometries such as infinite and semi-infinite media of uniform optical properties, the solutions are otherwise developed numerically, using finite difference or finite element methods.

Of the three boundary conditions commonly used, the partial current condition is the most rigorous [5,6]. It states that a photon leaving the tissue never returns and uses a reflectance parameter to account for Fresnel reflection at the tissue–air surface. If the boundary condition is perfectly transmitting (thereby exhibiting no Fresnel reflection), then the fluence evaluated at the boundary must fall to zero creating a discontinuity that violates the diffusion approximation that assumes isotropic radiance. By considering the Fresnel reflection at the boundary, this violation is eased by modeling a portion of the photons to be reflected back into the medium. The partial current boundary condition can be expressed in terms of the fluence and its gradient normal to the boundary:

$$\Phi_{x,m}(\vec{r},t) = 2 \cdot \frac{1+R_{eff_{x,m}}}{1+R_{eff_{x,m}}} \cdot D_{x,m} \vec{\nabla}_n \Phi_{x,m}(\vec{r},t) \tag{18.16}$$

where R_{eff} is the effective reflection coefficient whose quantity predicts the amount of light reflection and degree of anisotropy at the boundary.

A slightly simpler condition, the extrapolated boundary condition, is an approximation of the partial current condition and yields similar solutions to the diffusion equation [7,8]. In this case, the fluence is set to zero at an extrapolated boundary located at a specified distance outside of the medium in order to account for Fresnel reflection at the surface.

The third boundary condition, the zero condition, merely sets the fluence to zero on the boundary and is used for its simplicity. In a homogeneous scattering medium, the zero boundary condition results in an analytical solution to the diffusion equation in terms of the absorption and scattering coefficients [8,9].

The measured flux or photon current in CW or TDPM measurements, $J_{x,m}(\vec{r})$ or $J_{x,m}(\vec{r},t)$, is then determined by the gradient of fluence, $\vec{\nabla}\Phi_{x,m}(\vec{r})$ and $\vec{\nabla}\Phi_{x,m}(\vec{r},t)$, at the surface (also known as Fick's law):

$$J_{x,m}(\vec{r},t) = -D_{x,m}\vec{\nabla}\Phi_{x,m}(\vec{r},t) \tag{18.17}$$

The combination of Fick's law and the partial current or extrapolated boundary conditions results in the measured flux or photon density to be simply proportional to the fluence at the surface.

Since red light multiply scatters as it transits tissues, it has the opportunity to excite exogenous fluorescent agents that in turn act as uniformly distributed sources of fluorescent light. The fluence at the emission wavelength, $\Phi_m(\vec{r})$ or $\Phi_m(\vec{r},t)$, is generated and propagates within the multiple scattering medium and can also be described by Equation 18.14, provided that its source emission kinetics is properly modeled in the source term, $S_m(\vec{r})$ or $S_m(\vec{r},t)$. The isotropic scattering coefficient at the emission wavelength, μ'_{sm}, may be considered to be different than that at the excitation wavelength. The absorption coefficient at the emission wavelength, $\mu_{a_m}(\vec{r})$, is owing to endogenous chromophores and, if reabsorption of the emission light from the fluorophore occurs, owing to the reabsorption of fluorescent light by the exogenous agent. While it is relatively straightforward to include secondary reabsorption and photobleaching effects, for the case in which the excitation and emission spectra are well separated and the fluorophore is in dilute concentrations, we neglect this contribution to absorption at the emission wavelength. The general form for the emission source, $S_m(\vec{r},t)$, is

$$S_m = \mu_{a_{x\to m}}(\vec{r})\alpha\Xi_m\int_0^t \Phi_x(\vec{r},t')\cdot g(t')\mathrm{d}t' \tag{18.18}$$

where $\Phi_x(\vec{r},t)$, α, and Ξ_m are the excitation photon density, quantum efficiency of the fluorophore, and the detection efficiency factor of the system at the emission wavelength (which contains the system spectral response and the fluorophore spectral emission efficiency [10]). The time-invariant source for CW measurements, $S_m(\vec{r})$, is described with the earlier equation with the upper limit of the time integral equal to infinity. The source of emission light from a mixture of fluorophores undergoing various decay kinetics is simply a combination of the earlier expressions.

Provided that the solution for the excitation fluence, $\Phi_x(\vec{r})$ or $\Phi_x(\vec{r},t)$, is first obtained, the emission fluence, $\Phi_m(\vec{r})$ or $\Phi_m(\vec{r},t)$, can then be solved using one of the three commonly used boundary conditions described earlier and given the decay kinetics and optical properties at the emission wavelength. The measured flux or photon current in CW or TDPM measurements is then determined from the gradient of the emission fluence.

While CW measurements can be limited in information content regarding decay kinetics and spatial discrimination, TDPM measurements are tedious in that they require an incident Dirac pulse or convolution/deconvolution of the pulse, suffer from low SNR, and mathematically require the solution of an integral–differential equation for spectroscopy and imaging application. Indeed, the large dynamic range of SNR over the entire distribution of photon times of flight in TDPM approaches can require significant data acquisition times to resolve or reduce uncertainty in the resulting images. However, some developers prefer to employ TDPM measurements to construct optical property maps since its information content is the wealthiest [11]. Frequency-domain approaches sidestep these issues with the use of a sinusoidally modulated light source that is easily achievable, measurements possessing high SNR, and, as shown in the next section, a more tractable set of equations for solution of the spectroscopy and imaging inverse problems.

18.2.3.2 Frequency-Domain Measurement Approaches

Frequency-domain measurements in random media are similar to those described in the earlier section. An intensity-modulated point source of excitation light is launched into a scattering media, and the propagating *photon density wave* is attenuated and phase-delayed relative to the incident source as it propagates through the random medium as shown in Figure 18.2. The detected phase delay and amplitude attenuation measured at the excitation wavelength can be used to determine the optical properties of the random medium, whether they are uniform (for solution of the inverse spectroscopy problem) or nonuniform (for solution of the inverse imaging problem). The diffusion equation for solution of the forward problem of predicting measurements also applies, with the difference that the equation is cast in the frequency domain, rather than in the time domain:

$$\vec{\nabla} \cdot \left(D_{x,m} \vec{\nabla} \Phi_{x,m}(\vec{r}, \omega) \right) - \left[\mu_{a_{x \to m}} + \frac{i\omega}{c} \right] \Phi_{x,m}(\vec{r}, \omega) + S_{x,m}(\vec{r}, \omega) = 0 \qquad (18.19)$$

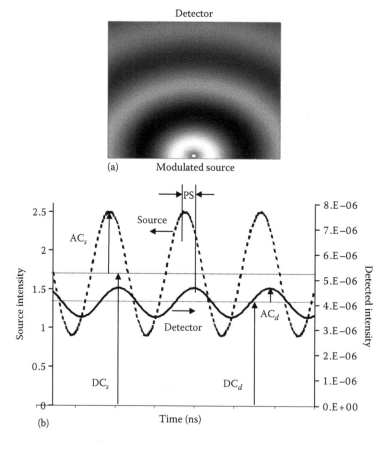

FIGURE 18.2 Schematic of the FDPM measurements used in NIR optical spectroscopy and tomography. FDPM traditionally consists of an incident, intensity-modulated light source that creates a *photon density wave* that spherically propagates continuously throughout the tissue. Panel (a) is a depiction of light distribution in tissue due to a modulated source (exaggerated for purposes of illustration) and Panel (b) illustrates the detected signal (in *solid line*) in response to the source illumination (in *dotted line*). The typical frequency-domain data, where the measurable quantities are the phase shift θ, the amplitude of each wave I_{AC}, and the average value I_{DC} of intensity. As shown in panel (b), the intensity wave that is detected some distance away from the source is amplitude attenuated and phase-delayed relative to the source. (Reproduced from Hawrysz, D.J. and Sevick-Muraca, E.M., *Neoplasia*, 2, 388, 2000. With permission.)

where the fluence, $\Phi_{x,m}(\vec{r},\omega)$, is now a complex number describing the characteristics of the photon density wave at position $\vec{r}$ and modulated at angular frequency ω. Moreover, the fluence is comprised of alternating, $\Phi_{AC_{x,m}}(\vec{r},\omega)$, and nonalternating, $\Phi_{DC_{x,m}}(\vec{r},0)$, components of which the former can provide an accurate description of the phase delay, $\theta_{x,m}$, and amplitude, $I_{AC_{x,m}}$, of the wave at position $\vec{r}$:

$$\Phi_{x,m}(\vec{r},\omega) = \Phi_{AC_{x,m}}(\vec{r},\omega) + \Phi_{DC_{x,m}}(\vec{r},0)$$
$$= I_{AC_{x,m}} \exp(i\theta_{x,m}) + I_{DC_{x,m}}(\vec{r},0) \tag{18.20}$$

The nonalternating component of the fluence, $\Phi_{DC_{x,m}}(\vec{r},0)$, is simply the fluence that is measured when using a CW source ($\omega = 0$). The preexponential factor, $I_{AC_{x,m}}$, is the amplitude of the photon density wave, and the exponential factor, $\theta_{x,m}$, is the phase delay of the wave relative to the incident source. At larger modulation frequencies, the photon density wave attenuates more rapidly during its propagation and experiences greater phase lag. Consequently, the amplitude decreases with increasing modulation frequency, while the phase delay increases with modulation frequency. Often, the amplitude or modulation ratio is reported as a measurement. The modulation ratio is simply the amplitude of the wave normalized by $I_{DC_{x,m}}(\vec{r},0)$.

For the solution of the excitation fluence via Equation 18.19, the source function is either a point source (as shown in Figure 18.2) or a plane source of modulated light:

$$S_x(\vec{r},\omega) = S(\vec{r_s},\omega)\exp(i\theta_s(\vec{r_s},\omega)) \tag{18.21}$$

where the strength (or amplitude) of the excitation source at its position of incidence $\vec{r_s}$ is $S(\vec{r_s},\omega)$ and its absolute phase is $\theta_s(\vec{r_s},\omega)$. Typically, frequency-domain photon migration (FDPM) measurements are conducted between a point source of illumination, and the amplitude and phase of the detected light (also collected at a point) are determined relative to the source. Consequently, in most cases within the literature, the source strength is designated as unity and the phase of the incident source is taken as zero. As described in the subsequent section, emission fluence in response to incident planar wave excitation can be employed and predicted by the diffusion equation provided that the spatial phase, $\theta_s(\vec{r_s},\omega)$, and amplitude, $S(\vec{r_s},\omega)$, of the source are properly accounted [12].

The boundary conditions for frequency-domain measurements in random media are identical to that described earlier for CW and TDPM techniques and the partial current boundary condition is similarly written:

$$\Phi_{x,m}(\vec{r},\omega) = 2 \cdot \frac{1+R_{eff_{x,m}}}{1+R_{eff_{x,m}}} \cdot D_{x,m}\vec{\nabla}_n\Phi_{x,m}(\vec{r},\omega) \tag{18.22}$$

The measured flux or photon current in frequency-domain measurements, $J_{x,m}(\vec{r},\omega)$, is then determined by Fick's law:

$$J_{x,m}(\vec{r},\omega) = -D_{x,m}\vec{\nabla}\Phi_{x,m}(\vec{r},\omega) \tag{18.23}$$

The combination of Fick's law and the partial current or extrapolated boundary conditions results in the measured flux or photon density of the wave (now a complex number) to be simply proportional to the fluence at the surface. Consequently, the measured phase, $\theta_{x,m}$, and amplitude, $I_{AC_{x,m}}$, are predicted from the fluence, $\Phi_{AC_{x,m}} = I_{AC_{x,m}} \exp(i\theta_{x,m})$.

As with CW and TDPM methods, the radiative relaxation of the activated fluorophore serves at a distributed source of emission light within the random media. The emission source $S_m(\vec{r},\omega)$ for single exponential decay kinetics is

$$S_m(\vec{r},\omega) = \mu_{a_{x\to m}}\left(\frac{1}{1-i\omega\tau}\right)\Phi_x(\vec{r},\omega)\alpha\,\Xi_m \tag{18.24}$$

and for any arbitrary decay kinetics expressed by $g(t)$, the source term can be generally derived from

$$S_m(\vec{r},\omega) = \mu_{a_{x\to m}}\Phi_x(\vec{r},\omega)\alpha\,\Xi_m\int_0^\infty\!\left(g(t)e^{(i\omega t)}\mathrm{d}t\right) \tag{18.25}$$

From the solution of Equation 18.19 describing the propagation of excitation light, the excitation fluence, $\Phi_x(\vec{r},\omega)$, can be directly obtained and used as input for the source term to solve Equation 18.19 for the emission fluence, $\Phi_m(\vec{r},\omega)$ [13]. Thus, the solution of the coupled equations with the specified boundary conditions and the phase and amplitude of the detected emission wave relative to the incident excitation source can be directly determined.

As with TDPM measurements, the ability to use fluorescence to interrogate within the random medium afforded by FDPM measurements when the lifetime of the fluorescent agent is small in comparison to the photon *time of flights*. Effective contrast for FDPM approaches is also limited, as are TDPM approaches, to fluorescence rather than phosphorescent or long-lived compounds. This was demonstrated in the Photon Migration Laboratory (PML) by comparing FDPM contrast offered by tris (2,2′-bipyridyl) dichloro-ruthenium (II) Ru(bpy)$_3^{2+}$ with a lifetime of 600 ns and indocyanine green (ICG) with a lifetime of 0.56 ns. In this case, the FDPM contrast was defined as the change in the phase and amplitude of the emission light as the position of the target changed relative to the position of the point of excitation illumination and emission detection. Using a single target with 100-fold greater concentration than the background in a phantom (see Figure 18.3 for measurement geometry of the phantom), the phase and amplitude modulation contrast at each of the detectors could be seen when ICG was used (Figure 18.4a), whereas no contrast was measured when ruthenium dye, Ru(bpy)$_3^{2+}$, was used as the contrast agent (Figure 18.4b). These results confirm computational predictions that effective contrast agents must possess shorter lifetimes than the *time of flight* of photon propagation [14].

Consequently, in order to develop fluorescence lifetime spectroscopy and imaging techniques, the time dependence of the photon migration process has to be accounted for in order to obtain lifetime

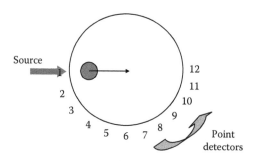

FIGURE 18.3 Schematic of the phantom tests to show the change in emission phase measurements as a fluorescent and phosphorescently tagged, 10 mm diameter target was moved from the periphery toward the center of a 100 mm diameter cylindrical vessel.

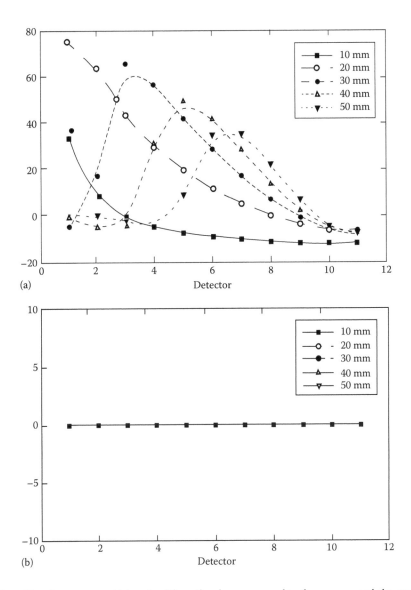

FIGURE 18.4 The phase contrast (determined from the phase measured in the presence and absence of a target) measured at the emission light for a 100:1 target to background ratio for (a) phosphorescent dye with lifetime of 1 ms and (b) fluorescent dye with lifetime of 1 ns. The phase contrast is predicted from simulation of the target moving from the perimeter (10 mm) toward the center (50 mm) of a 10 cm diameter cylinder under conditions of maximum phase contrast, that is, $\omega\tau = 1$, and uniform lifetime. The detectors are located around half of the perimeter of the cylinder as described in Figure 18.3.

information. Whether imaging or spectroscopy, the inverse problem becomes one of separating photon migration from fluorescence decay kinetics. Some investigators have sought to avoid the problem by employing phosphorescent dyes wherein the photon migration *times of flight* of picoseconds to nanoseconds are insignificant in comparison to the lifetimes on the order of micro- to milliseconds. Nonetheless, time-dependent emission measurements will not be able to interrogate beyond the surfaces or subsurfaces when long-lived dyes are employed. When used as contrast agents for imaging, these long-lived dyes certainly have utility, but only if their partitioning within the target is perfect and there is no residual dye in the background.

Finally, since the amplitude of the detected fluorescence, I_{AC_m}, is insensitive to the intensity owing to the ambient light, the frequency-domain approach has clear advantages for application in non-light-tight environments. In addition, since frequency-domain approaches offer a steady-state measurement of time-dependent light propagation processes, they have comparatively high SNR with respect to time-domain approaches and retain the signal dependency upon lifetime that is otherwise missing in CW measurements. Owing to the ease of instrumentation of frequency-domain over time-domain approaches, and owing to the superior information of time-dependent techniques over CW measurements, in the remainder of this chapter, we focus on FDPM measurements but reference works conducted using CW and TDPM techniques.

18.3 Frequency-Domain Measurement Approaches

For spectroscopy and imaging of random media, there have been two approaches employed: (1) point detection and point illumination and (2) area detection and area illumination. Point detection schemes typically employ heterodyne or I&Q mixing techniques that employ signal mixing at the photodetector following it in order to extract signals of phase and amplitude modulation at a single point. In order to conduct FDPM measurements between a number of sources and detectors, scanning of the source/detector or transmitter/receiver pair is required or replication of the receiver/transmitter circuitry is necessary. Consequently, this restricts FDPM imaging and spectroscopy to sparse data sets for solving the inverse spectroscopy and imaging problems. While sufficient for solving the inverse spectroscopy problem (as discussed in Section 18.4), the point illumination and point detection provide sparse sets for optical tomography or solution of the inverse imaging problem (as discussed in Section 18.5). The use of an incident point of excitation light delivered by a fiber optic requires a number of measurements as its position is scanned or replicated along the surface for image purposes (Figure 18.5) [15]. Since excitation fluence attenuates rapidly, each point source illumination will not necessarily probe significant volumes and may *miss* the fluorescent target region of interest. Consequently, a high density of measurements is typically required for a relatively confined volume for imaging purposes, and area illumination and

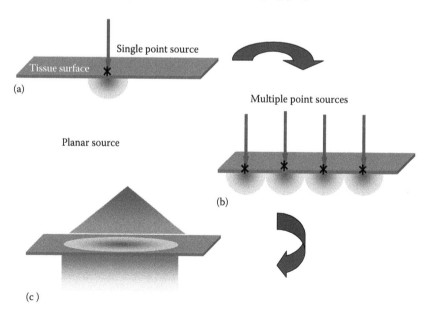

FIGURE 18.5 Illustration of different geometries for illumination of deep tissues. (a) Single point source of excitation light delivery; (b) multiple point sources that in the extreme of high density of simultaneous sources are representative of (c); and (c) planar source of excitation light with illumination spread over an area of the tissue surface.

area detection schemes may become pertinent for imaging. It should be noted, however, that for optical tomography work employing endogenous contrast, measurement geometries are necessarily restricted to point illumination and point detection. In the following, we describe the overall principles of conducting frequency-domain measurements of fluorescence in random media using heterodyne point measurements and homodyning area measurements, challenges for fluorescence spectroscopy and imaging in random media, and finally, measurement geometries.

18.3.1 Heterodyne Mixing for Frequency-Domain Photon Migration

Point illumination and point detection measurements are most common owing to their prevalence in frequency-domain spectrometers for measurement of decay kinetics in nonscattering, diluted samples. For imaging systems, the point source and point detection schemes and tomographic approaches are exclusively developed for this geometry. The heterodyned point illumination and point detection measurements consist of three parts: (1) the modulated source, (2) the detector that may also act as the mixer, and (3) the electronics to accomplish mixing. A schematic of the system is illustrated in Figure 18.6.

The modulated source can be either a coherent light source that is externally modulated via an electro-optic modulator, a laser diode that is modulated by use of RF signal via a bias tee, or, more complicated, a pulsed source with a constant and known pulse repetition rate. A master oscillator drives the source that is focused to illuminate a point on the surface of the random medium or coupled to the surface through the use of fiber optics. Typically, modulation frequencies are on the order of 30–500 MHz, and in order to detect the amplitude and phase delay of the detected photon density wave at excitation and emission wavelengths, a fast detector, either a silicon photodiode, avalanche photodiode, or fast photomultiplier, is required. In order to acquire the signal for standard data acquisition, the signal, L, of frequency ω is *mixed down* to a more manageable frequency, $\Delta\omega$, by mixing with another signal of frequency $\omega + \Delta\omega$. For example, the mixing can be accomplished through direct gain modulation of the photomultiplier

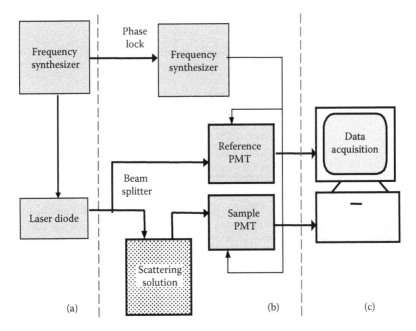

FIGURE 18.6 Schematic of heterodyned FDPM system that consists of three parts: (a) the modulated source (shown as laser diode), (b) the detector (PMT) that also acts as the mixer, and (c) the data acquisition hardware and software to accomplish mixing.

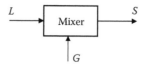

FIGURE 18.7   Schematic of mixer for heterodyne and homodyne detection of $I_{AC_{x,m}}$ and $\theta_{x,m}$ for FDPM.

tube or after the detector at the mixer (Figure 18.7). Consider the signal representing the detected light, L, which has propagated to a position and has experienced phase delay θ and has amplitude L_{AC} and average signal, L_{DC}:

$$L = L_{DC} + L_{AC} \cdot \cos\left[\omega t + \theta\right] \tag{18.26}$$

Consider the signal G generated by a slave oscillator to be in phase with the master oscillator (i.e., there is no phase delay relative to the incident light) and has amplitude G_{AC} and average signal level, G_{DC}:

$$G = G_{DC} + G_{AC} \cdot \cos\left[(\omega + \Delta\omega)t + \theta_{inst}\right] \tag{18.27}$$

whereby θ_{inst} represents the phase delay introduced into the signal owing to instrumentation aspects rather than light propagation. Upon mixing the signals, one obtains S, which consists of high- ($2\omega + \Delta\omega, \omega + \Delta\omega, \omega$) and low-frequency ($\Delta\omega$) components:

$$\begin{aligned}
S &= L \times G \\
S &= L_{DC} \cdot G_{DC} + L_{DC} \cdot G_{AC} \cdot \cos\left[(\omega + \Delta\omega)t + \theta_{inst}\right] \\
&\quad + G_{DC} \cdot L_{AC} \cdot \cos\left[\omega t + \theta\right] \\
&\quad + \frac{L_{AC} \cdot G_{AC}}{2} \cdot \cos\left[\Delta\omega t - \theta + \theta_{inst}\right] \\
&\quad + \frac{L_{AC} \cdot G_{AC}}{2} \cdot \cos\left[(2\omega + \Delta\omega)t + \theta + \theta_{inst}\right]
\end{aligned} \tag{18.28}$$

Upon filtering the mixed signal with a low band-pass filter, the final detected signal is

$$S = L_{DC} \cdot G_{DC} + \frac{L_{AC} \cdot G_{AC}}{2}\cos\left[\Delta\omega t - \theta + \theta_{inst}\right] \tag{18.29}$$

whereby the information of the signal L is preserved in the low-frequency signal whereby $\Delta\omega$ is typically 100 Hz or kHz. Following subtraction of the average of the signal, $L_{DC} \cdot G_{DC}$, Fourier analysis of the mixed signal at frequency $\Delta\omega$ yields the phase information, $[-\theta + \theta_{inst}]$, as well as the product of $L_{AC} \cdot G_{AC}$. In order to solve the inverse spectroscopy or imaging problem, accurate assessment of L_{AC} and θ must be determined using a referencing approach to eliminate θ_{inst}, G_{AC}, and G_{DC}.

When using external cavity modulation or laser diode modulation, the modulation frequencies can be swept continuously providing a frequency spectrum of $\Phi_{x,m}(\omega)$ or $\theta_{x,m}(\omega)$ and $I_{AC_{x,m}}(\omega)$. However, in the case of a pulsed light source, such as a Ti:sapphire picosecond or femtosecond laser, the master oscillator is set by the length of the laser cavity that sets the laser repetition rate, $1/\omega$, and the signal G is swept across the harmonics of the laser repetition frequency plus a small offset, $n\omega + \Delta\omega$, $n = 1,2,\dots$ Thus, pulsed sources provide a frequency spectrum of $\Phi_{x,m}(n\omega)$ or $\theta_{x,m}(n\omega)$ and $I_{AC_{x,m}}(n\omega)$ where $n = 1,2,\dots$ The reader is referred to Ref. [16] for further information of frequency-domain measurements with pulsed laser sources.

18.3.2 Homodyne Mixing for Frequency-Domain Photon Migration

The homodyne approach is similar to the heterodyne approach described in the earlier text with the exception that the signal, L, of frequency ω is *mixed down* to DC signal through mixing with another signal of identical frequency. Consider the signal G generated by the master oscillator with an introduced phase delay, η, with amplitude, G_{AC}, and average signal level, G_{DC}:

$$G = G_{DC} + G_{AC} \cdot \cos\left[\left(\omega\right)t + \theta_{inst} + \eta\right] \tag{18.30}$$

whereby θ_{inst} represents the phase delay introduced into the signal owing to instrumentation aspects rather than light propagation.

Upon mixing the signals L and G, one obtains S, which consists of a high-frequency component $(2\omega, \omega)$ and a DC component:

$$
\begin{aligned}
S &= L \times G \\
S &= L_{DC} \cdot G_{DC} + L_{DC} \cdot G_{AC} \cdot \cos\left[\left(\omega\right)t + \theta_{inst} + \eta\right] \\
&\quad + G_{DC} \cdot L_{AC} \cdot \cos\left[\omega t + \theta\right] \\
&\quad + \frac{L_{AC} \cdot G_{AC}}{2} \cdot \cos\left[-\theta + \theta_{inst} + \eta\right] \\
&\quad + \frac{L_{AC} \cdot G_{AC}}{2} \cdot \cos\left[\left(2\omega\right)t + \theta + \theta_{inst} + \eta\right]
\end{aligned}
\tag{18.31}
$$

Upon filtering the mixed signal with a low band-pass filter, the final detected DC signal is

$$S = L_{DC} \cdot G_{DC} + \frac{L_{AC} \cdot G_{AC}}{2}\cos\left[-\theta + \theta_{inst} + \eta\right] \tag{18.32}$$

By changing the phase delay η by known values, one can evaluate $L_{DC} \cdot G_{DC}$, $L_{AC} \cdot G_{AC}/2$, $[-\theta + \theta_{inst}]$ and by proper referencing can determine those quantities that define signal L and the light propagation within the random medium.

Owing to the slow time response of area detection using image intensifiers, used in area detection schemes, the homodyne approach is typically used. Figure 18.8 illustrates the image-intensified charge-coupled device (ICCD) homodyne FDPM system consisting of three major components including (1) a charge-coupled device (CCD) camera, which houses essentially a multipixel array of photosensitive detectors; (2) a gain-modulated image intensifier, which as described below acts as the mixer; and (3) oscillators that sinusoidally modulate the laser diode light source and the image intensifier's photocathode gain at the same frequency, ω. A 10 MHz reference signal between the oscillators ensures that they operate at the same frequency with a constant phase difference. Emitted light from the tissue or phantom surface is imaged via a lens onto the photocathode of the image intensifier. As before, the light (L) that reaches the photocathode of the image intensifier has a phase delay, $\theta(r)$; average intensity, $L_{DC}(r)$; and amplitude intensity, $L_{AC}(r)$, that may vary as a function of position on the sample and consequently across the photocathode face.

The gain of the image intensifier has an average, G_{DC}; a possible phase delay owing to the instrument response time, θ_{inst}; and an amplitude, G_{AC}, at the modulation frequency as the source. The modulated gain is accomplished by modulating the potential between the photocathode, which converts the NIR photons into electrons, and the multichannel plate (MCP), which multiplies the electrons before they are focused onto the phosphor screen (Figure 18.9). The resulting signal at the phosphor screen is a mixed homodyne signal (S), containing all the amplitude, DC, and phase information of the optical signal collected by the detector. Yet, since the phosphor screen has response times on the order of

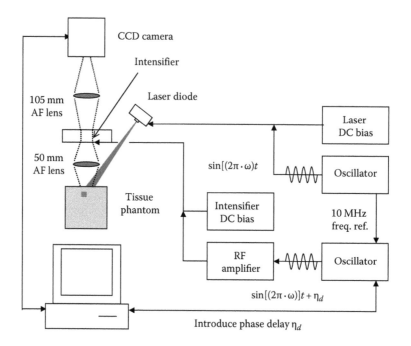

FIGURE 18.8 Schematic of the ICCD homodyne FDPM system in the PML.

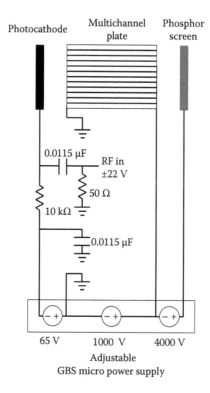

FIGURE 18.9 Schematic of the image intensifier circuit and system used in the homodyne ICCD system. (Reproduced from Thompson, A.B. and Sevick-Muraca, E.M., *J. Biomed. Opt.*, 8, 111, 2002. With permission.)

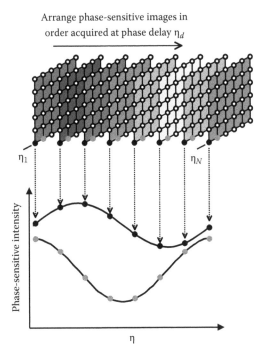

Arrange phase-sensitive images in
order acquired at phase delay η_d

η_1 η_N

Phase-sensitive intensity

η

FIGURE 18.10 The process in which the phase delay between the image intensifier and laser diode modulation is adjusted between 0° and 360° yielding phase-sensitive, yet constant intensity images at the phosphor screen. Upon compiling the intensities at each pixel, the sine wave is reconstructed and the phase and amplitude attenuation is obtained from simple FFT. (Reproduced from Thompson, A.B. and Sevick-Muraca, E.M., *J. Biomed. Opt.*, 8, 111, 2002. With permission.)

submilliseconds, it acts as a low-pass filter so that the image transferred to the CCD camera is simply the homodyne signal represented in Equation 18.32. The time-invariant, but phase-sensitive image on the phosphor screen is then imaged onto the CCD using either a lens or fiber coupling [12,17–19].

Rapid multipixel FDPM data acquisition proceeds as follows. The phase of the photocathode modulation is stepped, or delayed, at regular intervals between 0° and 360° relative to the phase of the laser diode modulation. At each phase delay η_d, the CCD camera acquires a phase-sensitive image for a given exposure time (see Figure 18.10), which is on the order of milliseconds. A computer program then arranges the phase-sensitive images in the order acquired and performs a fast Fourier transform (FFT) to calculate modulation amplitude, I_{AC}, and phase, θ, at each CCD pixel (i,j) using the following relationships:

$$I_{AC}(i,j) = \frac{\left[\left\{\mathrm{IMAG}\left[I\left(f_{max}\right)_{ij}\right]\right\}^2 + \left\{\mathrm{REAL}\left[I\left(f_{max}\right)_{ij}\right]\right\}^2\right]^{1/2}}{N/2} \tag{18.33}$$

$$\theta(i,j) = \mathrm{arc}\ \tan\left(\frac{\mathrm{IMAG}\left[I\left(f_{max}\right)_{ij}\right]}{\mathrm{REAL}\left[I\left(f_{max}\right)_{ij}\right]}\right) \tag{18.34}$$

$I(f)$ is the Fourier transform of the phase-sensitive intensity data, $I(\eta_d)$. IMAG$[I(f_{max})]$ and REAL$[I(f_{max})]$ symbolize the imaginary and real components in the digital frequency spectrum that best describe the sinusoidal data. N relates the number of phase delays between the gain modulation of the image intensifier and the incident light source.

Area illumination is accomplished simply by expanding a modulated laser diode beam onto the surface of the phantom or tissue to be imaged. To date, there has been no attempt to employ area illumination and area detection for tomographic reconstructions since all formulations are based upon the propagation of light from a point excitation source to a point on the medium's surface. Yet despite its current lack of acceptance by the tomographic community (as discussed in Section 18.5 and Table 18.1), planar wave illumination is by far the most common way to illuminate photodynamic therapy (PDT) agents for assessing therapeutic drug distribution and to provide excitation for assessing diagnostic fluorochrome distribution in subcutaneous tumor-bearing rodents. Typically, CW light from a xenon or tungsten lamp, laser, or laser diode is expanded to illuminate an entire animal or a portion of the animal. Incident powers range from $\mu W/cm^2$ to mW/cm^2, and area detection can be accomplished using a CCD with or without an image intensifier coupling and with or without a spectrograph for spectral discrimination. Typically, CW measurements are conducted in mice and rats of small tissue volumes, while the frequency-domain measurements of fluorescence-enhanced contrast have been performed in canines (Section 18.5, see Table 18.1).

In addition to the area measurements, the ICCD can be employed to rapidly conduct single-pixel measurements for tomographic reconstructions by simply using the ICCD to simultaneously measure the phase and amplitude of light collected by a number of fibers whose ends are affixed onto an interfacing plate that is focused on the photocathode of the image intensifier via a lens (Figure 18.11).

18.3.3 Homodyne I&Q

Another homodyning method for frequency-domain measurements that does not depend upon conducting successive measurements at varying phase delays, η, imposed upon signal, G, employs I and Q demodulation [20]. The technique depends upon mixing the signal L with two signals, G_1 and G_2, at the same frequency ω, but phase shifted by $90°$ (Figure 18.12):

$$G_1 = G_{AC}\cos(\omega t); \quad G_2 = G_{AC}\sin(\omega t) \tag{18.35}$$

When L is mixed with G_1, the signal output, S_1, is given by

$$S_1 = L_{DC}\cdot G_{AC}\cdot\cos(\omega t) + \frac{L_{AC}\cdot G_{AC}}{2}\cdot\left[\cos\left(2\omega t + \theta + \theta_{inst} + \frac{\pi}{2}\right) + \cos\left(\theta + \theta_{inst} + \frac{\pi}{2}\right)\right] \tag{18.36}$$

When L is mixed with G_2, the signal output, S_2, is given by

$$S_2 = L_{DC}\cdot G_{AC}\cdot\sin(\omega t) + \frac{L_{AC}\cdot G_{AC}}{2}\cdot\left[\sin\left(2\omega t + \theta + \theta_{inst} + \frac{\pi}{2}\right) - \sin\left(\theta + \theta_{inst} + \frac{\pi}{2}\right)\right] \tag{18.37}$$

Upon passing through a low-pass filter, the high-frequency components at ω and 2ω can be eliminated leaving two DC signals:

$$S_1 = \frac{L_{AC}\cdot G_{AC}}{2}\cdot\left[\cos\left(\theta + \theta_{inst} + \frac{\pi}{2}\right)\right]$$

$$S_2 = \frac{L_{AC}\cdot G_{AC}}{2}\cdot\left[-\sin\left(\theta + \theta_{inst} + \frac{\pi}{2}\right)\right] \tag{18.38}$$

Upon combining the two signals, the quantities of $L_{AC}\cdot G_{AC}/2, [-\theta + \theta_{inst}]$ can be determined, and by proper referencing, the AC and phase delay associated with signal L and with the light propagation within the random medium can be determined.

TABLE 18.1 Chronological Listing of In Vivo Imaging Studies Using Different Fluorescent Contrast Agents

Author	Imaging System (Incident Fluence)	Animal Model	Dose	Contrast Agent	λ (Excitation/ Emission)	Comments
Biolo et al. [33]	Spectrograph for point detection of fluorescence following surface illumination	Mouse	0.12 mg/kg bw ~0.24 μmol/kg bw	ZnPc (phthalocyanine) in liposomes, spectral detection of fluorescence at λ	600 nm	Study was to provide measurements for assessing pharmacokinetics of PDT agent.
Pelegrin et al. [78]	Area illumination with area (133 mW/cm²) detection using photography	Mouse, deceased	100 μg/animal ~600 pmol/kg bw	Fluorescein isothiocyanate (FITC) coupled to MoAb	488 nm Kodak Wratten filter #12 for excitation light rejection	Study the localization of dye targeted to human colon carcinoma in mice after coupling to MAb.
Straight et al. [82]	Interstitial illumination (20 mW) with area detection using CCD camera	Mouse	20 mg/kg bw ~70 μmol/kg bw	Photofrin II	514.5/spectral discrimination 585–730 nm	This study validated the CCD technology for imaging drug distribution in tumors.
Folli et al. [79]	Fiber through endoscope illumination (10 mW/cm²) with area detection using photography	Human	0.1–0.28 mg/patient ~0.1–0.28 nmol/ patient	FITC coupled to MoAb	488 nm Kodak Wratten filter #12 for excitation light rejection	Study immunophotodiagnosis in colon carcinoma patients.
Cubeddu et al. [84,85]	Area illumination (75 μW/cm²) with pulsed dye laser with gated CCD video camera	Mouse	5–25 mg/kg bw ~17–87 μmol/kg bw [84] 0.1 mg/kg ~0.35 μmol/kg bw [85]	Hematoporphyrin derivative (HpD)	405/>560 nm	Demonstrated the use of time-dependent measurements to identify HpD distinct from native fluorescence based upon long fluorescent lifetimes.
Kohl et al. [83]	Intensified CCD	Mouse	0.2–1 mg/kg bw ~0.7–3.5 μmol/kg bw	Porphyrin-based photosensitizers		Demonstrated the ability to image s.c. tumor.
Folli et al. [80]	Area illumination with area (13 mW/cm²) detection using photography	Mouse, deceased	100 μg/animal ~600 pmol/kg bw[a]	Indopentamethine-cyanine coupled to MAb directed against squamous cell carcinoma	640 nm Kodak Wratten filter 70 for excitation light rejection	Showed the ability to detect IR dye targeted to squamous cell carcinoma in the upper respiratory tract through MAb E48 without the need to remove skin as was necessary when fluorescein was employed.

(continued)

TABLE 18.1 (continued) Chronological Listing of In Vivo Imaging Studies Using Different Fluorescent Contrast Agents

Author	Imaging System (Incident Fluence)	Animal Model	Dose	Contrast Agent	λ (Excitation/ Emission)	Comments
Haglund et al. [81]	Area illumination (100-W tungsten–halogen bulb) and area detection with CCD camera	Rat	1.0 mg/kg bw 1.3 μmol/kg bw	ICG	780/830 nm	Distinguish rat gliomas from normal brain tissue through free-agent fluorophore imaging with CCD camera.
Mordon et al. [86]	Area illumination (150 W xenon lamp, 2.5 mW/cm² with area detection using intensified CCD	Mouse	5 mg/kg bw (~13 μmol)	5,6-CF carboxyfluorescein (BCECF)	465/490 and 515 nm	This study showed the use of dual-wavelength measurements of a ratiometric dye to provide a 2D pH image of tumor tissues.
Ballou et al. [87]	Area illumination with area detection using intensified video camera or cooled CCD	Mouse	10–100 μg/animal ~40 pmol to 6 nmol/ animal	Cyanine fluorochromes coupled to MAb	550–674/565–694 nm	Demonstrated the use of tumor-targeting antibodies using Cy 3.18, Cy 5.18, and Cy 5.5.18 cyanine fluorochromes.
Devoisselle et al. [88]	Area (50 mm²) illumination (Xe lamp) with point detection using fiber optics and spectrograph	Mouse	7.5 mg/kg bw ~10 μmol/kg bw	ICG emulsion	720 nm/spectra discrimination of fluorescence	Demonstrated the use of emulsion preparation to alter the pharmacokinetics of ICG.
Rokahr et al. [89]	N2 laser pulsed through fiber and detected with fiber to spectrometer	Human undergoing urinary bladder cystoscopy	50 mg/patient (ALA induces fluorescence)	Protoporphyrin IX	337 and 405/380 through 685 spectral discrimination	Discriminate malignant and normal bladder tissue with ALA-induced protoporphyrin imaging.
Haglund et al. [90]	Area illumination with photography lights and area detection with CCD camera	Human (open brain)	1 mg/kg bw ~1.3 mmol/kg bw	ICG	790/805 nm	Study detection of human glioma with ICG imaging.

Reference	Method	Model	Dose	Agent	Wavelength	Comments
Sakatani et al. [91]	Cooled CCD camera, 100 mW laser diode	Rat	554 pmol/rat	ICG–lipoprotein	790/840 nm	Cerebrospinal imaging with ICG bound to lipoprotein, injected intracranially
Neri [92]	Method similar to Folli et al. [80]; 100 W tungsten lamp for area illumination with detection via an 8-bit CCD in a light-tight box	Mouse	100 μL/mouse of a concentrated antibody solution of 1 mg/mL with dye/MAb ratio of 1:1	Fragments of human antibodies directed against B-FN and labeled with CY-7	673–748/765–855 nm	Demonstrated the use of B-FN targeting for providing diagnostic imaging and therapy of cancer targeting angiogenic vessels.
Ballou et al. [93]	Area illumination and area detection via CCD	Mouse	50 μg/animal MAb/dye (1:2) ~600 pmol/animal	Cy3, Cy5, Cy5.5, Cy7 labeled antibodies against human nucleolin and stage-specific embryonic antigen-1		Results demonstrated the ability to penetrate more deeply with Cy 7 dye.
Eker et al. [94]	Fiber for excitation and collection in a colonoscope for detection via a spectrometer	Human	5 mg/kg bw ~30 nmol/kg bw	Protoporphyrin IX, as a metabolized product of ALA (photosensitizer)	337, 405, 436 nm excitation	Demonstrated the use of ALA as a contrast agent for detecting adenomatous polyps of the colon and showed promise for distinguishing adenomatous from hyperplastic polyps.
Reynolds et al. [95]	Area illumination with laser diode (1 mW/cm^2) and area detection using intensified FDPM CCD system	Canine	1.0 mg/kg bw ~1.3 μmol/kg bw	ICG	780/830 nm	Demonstrated the ability to detect spontaneous disease of the canine mammary chain as well as reactive lymph nodes.
Becker et al. [96]	Area illumination and area detection with CCD and MRI	Mouse	2 μmol/kg bw (1:2.4 or 2 for Tf or HSA)	ITCC and ultrasmall superparamagnetic iron oxide particles coupled to Tf or HSA		Demonstrated targeting of tumors that express the Tf receptor using an optical agent as well as an MRI agent.
Weissleder et al. [23]; Mahmood et al. [97]	Area illumination and area detection using CCD in a light-tight chamber; illumination with 150 W halogen lamp with interference filters, 10–100 μW/cm^2	Mouse	10 μmol/animal (92 MEG, 11 dye molecules); 250 pmol/animal	Cy 5.5. loaded onto a polylysine and methoxypolyethylene glycol polymer backbone with cathepsin B and H cleavage sites	610–650/>700 nm	Demonstrated that tumor proteases can be used as molecular targets. SNR for 30 s exposure 173 for 200 pmol in phantom.

(continued)

TABLE 18.1 (continued) Chronological Listing of In Vivo Imaging Studies Using Different Fluorescent Contrast Agents

Author	Imaging System (Incident Fluence)	Animal Model	Dose	Contrast Agent	λ (Excitation/Emission)	Comments
Becker et al. [98]	Area illumination and area detection with CCD	Mouse	2 μmol/kg bw	Tf and HSA coupled with ITCC dye	740/780–900 nm	Demonstrating targeting to the tumors expressing Tf receptor.
Gurfinkel et al. [99]	Area illumination (1.98 and 5.5 mW/cm²) and area detection using intensified FDPM CCD system	Canine	1.1 and 1.0 mg/kg bw ~1.3 μmol/kg bw	ICG and carotene-modified PDT agent (HPPH) conjugated with carotene moiety for reduction of phototoxicity	780/830 nm (ICG) 660/710 nm (HPPH-car)	Demonstrated the use of temporal AC measurements to image pharmacokinetic parameters in order to discern diseased tissues.
Licha et al. [100]	Single point detection and point illumination (5 mW) using FDPM	Rat	0.5 μmol/kg bw	Derivatives of ICG (unclear whether fluorescence was detected in vivo)	750 and 786 nm excitation	Provided measurements of absorption at the excitation wavelength as a function of time to provide pharmacokinetic evaluation of ICG and its hydrophilic derivatives.
Yang et al. [101]; Hoffman [102]	Area illumination and detection using CCD camera	Mouse	—	GFP expressed in vivo		Demonstrated visualization of tumors and tumor metastasis by whole-body fluorescence imaging.
Ntziachristos et al. [72]	Fiber bundle to PMT using TDPM, point illumination, and point detection	Breast	0.25 mg/kg bw ~0.32 μmol/kg bw	ICG		Fluorescence was not used, but absorption provided contrast that was validated by simultaneous MRI images obtained with gadolinium contrast.
Bugaj et al. [103]; Achilefu et al. [104–106]	Area illumination (40 mW) and area detection using CCD camera	Rat	5.2–6.0 mg/kg bw ~6.7–7.7 μmol/kg bw	ICG, ICG-small-peptide conjugates (cytate and cybesin)	780/830 nm	Targeting to rat tumor lines expressing the somatostatin and bombesin receptors.
Becker et al. [107]	Area illumination and detection using CCD camera	Mouse	0.02 μmol/kg bw	Peptide–cyanine dye conjugate, IDCC, and ITCC conjugated to octreotate, an analog of somatostatin	740/780–900 nm	Targeting to mouse tumor lines expressing the somatostatin receptors.

Reference	Method	Animal	Dose	Agent	Wavelength	Description
Bremer et al. [108]	Area illumination and area detection using CCD in a light-tight chamber; illumination with 150 W halogen lamp with interference filters, 10–100 µW/cm²	Mouse	167 pmol/animal (i.v.)	Polylysine polymer coupled with mMP-2 peptide substrates holding Cy5.5	610–650/>700 nm	Measure MMP activity in vivo for directing the therapeutic use of proteinase inhibitors.
Ebert et al. [109]	Area illumination with pulsed laser and detection using CCD camera (ambient light rejection)	Rat	2 µmol/kg bw (i.v.)	SIDAG (hydrophilic derivative of cyanine dye), 1-1′-bis-(4-sulfbutyl) ITCC 5,5′-dicarboxylic acid diglucamide monosodium salt; Nd:Yag	740 nm, 3 ns FWHM, 50 Hz/750–800 nm	Demonstrated localization of tumor and presented phantom data using FDPM with contrast ratios of 6:1.
Finlay et al. [110]	Point illumination with fiber probe, point detection with fibers directed to a spectrograph and CCD	Rat	200 mg/kg bw (ALA injected)	ALA-induced porphyrin	514/676 nm emission	Photobleaching kinetics of ALA-induced protoporphyrin measured.
Rice et al. [111]	Area detection of light-emitting probes with CCD	Mouse	Bioluminescence of fluorescent proteins	Firefly luciferase	>600 nm emission	Imaging light-emitting probes.
Soukos et al. [112]	Area illumination using pumped dye laser (15 mW/cm²) and detection using room temperature CCD camera	DMBA-induced tumor in hamster cheek pouch	670 µg/animal ~3.3 nmol/kg bw[a]	Anti-EGFR MAb (C225) coupled to Cy 5.5 (1:2.1) IgG–Cy5.5 (1:2.3)	670/>700 nm	Demonstrated the targeted MAb–dye complex could be used to provide immunophotodiagnostic information thereby guiding therapeutic intervention.
Yang et al. [34]	Single-pixel FDPM using point source and point detector	Rat	1.5 mg/kg bw ~2 µmol/kg bw	ICG, DTTCI		Work toward demonstration of fluorescence imaging in vivo.
Zaheer et al. [122]	Area illumination (18 mW/cm²)	Mice (hairless)	2.6 nmol/kg (i.v.)	IR dye78 conjugated to pamidronate with hydroxyapatite binding properties	771/796 nm	Used to assess osteoblastic activity for skeletal development, osteoblastic metastasis, and coronary atherosclerosis.

[a] Molecular weight of proteins is estimated on the order of 10^5.

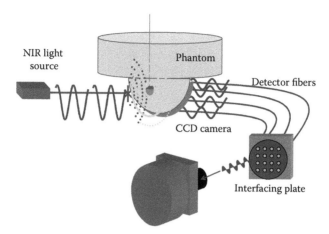

FIGURE 18.11 The adaptation of a number of single fibers collecting detected light for imaging by the ICCD system (i.e., depicted in Figure 18.9).

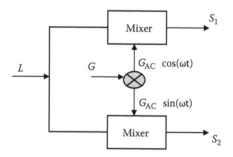

FIGURE 18.12 Illustration of the homodyne FDPM detection employing the mixing of L, G_1, and G_2, where G_2 is phase shifted by 90° relative to G_1.

18.3.4 Excitation Light Rejection Considerations

Regardless of the measurement method (i.e., CW, time domain, or frequency domain) and regardless of the measurement geometry (point or area illumination and detection), one of the greatest and largely unrecognized challenges in fluorescence spectroscopy and imaging in random media is the importance of excitation light rejection. As described in Section 18.4, in fluorescence spectroscopy of dilute, nonscattering samples, the isotropic emission light is collected at right angles to the incident excitation light to avoid corruption of excitation light in the fluorescence measurements. Yet in random media, the excitation light is propagated isotropically, potentially corrupting measurements in random media. Generally, the Stokes shift associated with many fluorophores is small and in the case of ICG, a Food and Drug Administration (FDA)-approved agent, is 50 nm. The wavelength sensitivity at the photocathode does not discriminate between excitation and emission wavelengths requiring a mechanism for excitation light rejection and passage of only emission light for accurate spectroscopy and imaging data. The excitation light reaching a detector at a location on the surface is the predominate signal and can be as little as 10^3 times greater than the emission fluence when the fluorophore concentration is high and significantly greater as the fluorophore concentration is reduced to nanomolar and femtomolar levels as might be expected in fluorescent contrast agent identification of small cancer metastases. For planar wave illumination, specularly reflected excitation light would create an even greater portion of the signal, further compounding the discrimination of the weak fluorescent signal emitted from the tissue surface (Figure 18.5). Generally, investigators employ interference filters with a rejection capability of OD 3 for excitation light, which generally sets the noise floor of the fluorescent measurement and limits the smallest amount of detectable fluorophore. Upon stacking interference and band-pass filters for emission light passage, and holographic filters for excitation light rejection, the noise floor can be reduced as much as nine orders of magnitude [21]. Clearly, the sensitivity of fluorescence spectroscopy and imaging in random media hinges upon the success for excitation light rejection.

The *forward* spectroscopy and imaging problems consist of using the diffusion model to predict light propagation, fluorescence generation, and the resulting measurements at the medium–air interface given the spatial distribution of optical properties within the entire volume. For the purposes of solving the *inverse* spectroscopy problem, we assume a uniform distribution of optical properties with the unknowns being (1) the optical properties at the excitation and emission wavelengths, (i.e., $\mu_{a_{x,m}}, \mu'_{s_{x,m}}$) and (2) the optical properties associated with the fluorescent agent (i.e., $\alpha\mu_{a_{x\to m}}, \tau$), which experiences first-order decay kinetics. In Section 18.5, we further develop the inverse solution to the imaging problem for tomographic imaging.

18.4 Fluorescence Spectroscopy in Random Media

Fluorescence lifetime spectroscopy is advantageous for quantitative spectroscopy of analytes and metabolites since the measurement of fluorescence decay kinetics (rather than the fluorescence intensity) eliminates the necessity for the knowledge of the sensing fluorophore concentration [1]. As described in Section 18.1, frequency-domain techniques provide measurement of fluorescence lifetime (τ) using simple relationships of the phase delay (θ) and modulation ratio (M) of the reemitted fluorescence as a function of the modulation frequency relative to intensity-modulated excitation light. However, the development of fluorescence lifetime spectroscopy for NIR biomedical tissue diagnostics for sensing using systematically administered dyes [22,23] or implantable devices [24,25] requires deconvolving the influence of multiple scatter upon the measured emission phase delay and amplitude attenuation. As will be shown in this section, the addition of scatter increases the sensitivity of fluorescence lifetime spectroscopy over traditional methods that focus on isotropic emission light generation across a fixed path length, L.

Approaches to appropriately model the multiple scattering of NIR excitation and fluorescence photons and to use diffusion models for quantitative spectroscopy have been previously demonstrated [10,26,27] for dyes exhibiting single exponential decay kinetics. Failure to properly account for multiply scattered excitation and emission light propagation in random media. For example, upon conducting phase-modulation measurements on a solution of Intralipid containing the NIR excitable fluorophore, ICG, Lakowicz and coworkers [28] did not incorporate the propagation of light yet attribute multiexponential decay kinetics to this dye, which typically exhibits a single exponential decay.

18.4.1 Single Exponential Decay Spectroscopy

Generally, for a uniform media of unknown optical properties containing a fluorophore exhibiting a first-order radiative relaxation process, there are six unknowns to be solved: $\mu_{a_{\lambda_x}}, \mu_{a_{\lambda_m}}, \mu'_{s_{\lambda_x}}, \mu'_{s_{\lambda_m}}, \alpha\mu_{a_{x\to m}}, \tau$ with the subscripts altered slightly from the past nomenclature to emphasize the optical properties at two separate wavelengths, λ_x and λ_m.

18.4.1.1 Optical Property Determination

For a uniform random medium, the optical property determination has been demonstrated to be accurately determined from multidistance frequency-domain measurements [29,30]. The analytical solution to the diffusion equation with point source illumination at wavelength, λ,

$$\vec{\nabla}\cdot\left(D_\lambda\vec{\nabla}\Phi_\lambda(\vec{r},\omega)\right)-\left[\mu_{a_{x,m}}+\frac{i\omega}{c}\right]\Phi_\lambda(\vec{r},\omega)+S_\lambda(\vec{r},\omega)=0 \qquad (18.39)$$

in an infinite medium provides three equations for I_{AC_λ}, θ_λ, and I_{DC_λ} as a function of modulation frequency, ω, distance away from the source, r, in terms of the optical properties, $\mu_{a_\lambda}, \mu'_{s_\lambda}$.

Upon conducting FDPM measurements as a function of modulation frequency, nonlinear regression can be performed to arrive at the optical properties of the medium. Conversely, upon referencing the measurements of I_{AC_λ}, θ_λ, and I_{DC_λ} at position r to a *reference* position r_o, linear regression of the following equations

$$DC_{rel} \equiv \frac{DC(r)}{DC(r_0)} = \frac{r_0}{r} \exp\left[-(r-r_0)\left(\frac{\mu_a}{D}\right)^{1/2}\right] \tag{18.40}$$

$$AC_{rel} \equiv \frac{AC(r)}{AC(r_0)} = \frac{r_0}{r} \exp\left\{-(r-r_0)\left(\frac{v^2\mu_a^2 + \omega^2}{v^2 D^2}\right)^{1/4} \cos\left[\frac{1}{2}\tan^{-1}\left(\frac{\omega}{v\mu_a}\right)\right]\right\} \tag{18.41}$$

$$\theta_{rel} \equiv \theta(r) - \theta(r_0) = (r-r_0)\left(\frac{v^2\mu_a^2 + \omega^2}{v^2 D^2}\right)^{1/4} \sin\left[\frac{1}{2}\tan^{-1}\left(\frac{\omega}{v\mu_a}\right)\right] \tag{18.42}$$

enables accurate estimation of the optical properties at a single modulation frequency using a single detector. Referencing of frequency-domain measurements is required to eliminate contributions of G_{AC}, G_{DC}, and θ_{inst} as denoted in Equation 18.29, before data are regressed to Equations 18.40 through 18.42 earlier.

An alternative referencing method was devised by Mayer et al. [27] that involved measurement of modulation and phase delay at two positions, r_1 and r_2, using two unmatched detectors. Unlike traditional fluorescence spectroscopy measurement across a known path length, L, the instrument response function for frequency-domain measurements in scattering media can be corrected without the use of a reference dye. The correction can be obtained by multiplexing two unmatched detectors (L_1, L_2) at two different positions in the sample (G_1, G_2) [27]. The two fibers leading to the unmatched detectors shown in Figure 18.13 are of the same length, to ensure equal optical path lengths of the two received signals, L_1, L_2.

The measured relative phase shift (RPS) between detector 1 and detector 2, $\theta_{rel,12}$, and measured modulation ratio, $M_{rel,12}$, between the two detectors reflects light propagation (and fluorescence generation, in the case of fluorescence measurements) in the sample between the incident source and the two detectors (i.e., $\theta_1, \theta_2, (L_{AC_1}/L_{DC_1}), (L_{AC_2}/L_{DC_2})$) and the instrument function ($\theta_{inst_1}, \theta_{inst_2}, (G_{AC_1}/G_{DC_1}), (G_{AC_2}/G_{DC_2})$):

$$\theta_{rel,12} = \left(-\theta_1 + \theta_{inst_1}\right) - \left(-\theta_2 + \theta_{inst_2}\right) \tag{18.43}$$

$$M_{rel,12} = \frac{L_{AC_1}G_{AC_1}}{L_{AC_2}G_{AC_2}} \cdot \frac{L_{DC_2}G_{DC_2}}{L_{DC_1}G_{DC_1}} \tag{18.44}$$

After multiplexing, the measured RPS between detector 2 and detector 1, $\theta_{rel,21}$, and measured modulation ratio, $M_{rel,21}$, between the two detectors continues to reflect light propagation (and fluorescence generation, in the case of fluorescence measurements) in the sample ($\theta_1, \theta_2, (L_{AC_1}/L_{DC_1}), (L_{AC_2}/L_{DC_2})$) as well as the instrument function ($\theta_{inst_1}, \theta_{inst_2}, (G_{AC_1}/G_{DC_1}), (G_{AC_2}/G_{DC_2})$):

$$\theta_{rel,21} = -\left(-\theta_1 + \theta_{inst_1}\right) + \left(-\theta_2 + \theta_{inst_2}\right) \tag{18.45}$$

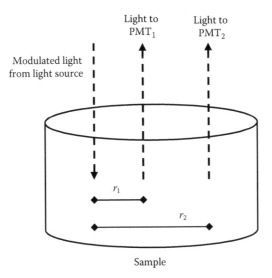

FIGURE 18.13 Schematic of fiber-optically coupled source and detector placement for fluorescence measurements in scattering media. The two detector fibers are of the same length to ensure equal optical path lengths.

$$M_{rel,21} = \frac{L_{AC_2}G_{AC_2}}{L_{AC_1}G_{AC_1}} \cdot \frac{L_{DC_1}G_{DC_1}}{L_{DC_2}G_{DC_2}} \tag{18.46}$$

where the subscript 12 denotes the relative value of the signal detected at detector 1 to the signal detected at detector 2, and the subscript 21 denotes otherwise.

Combining Equations B1 and B3 and Equations B2 and B4, one can obtain the phase shift and modulation ratio that are devoid of instrument function:

$$\Delta\theta = \theta_2 - \theta_1 = \frac{1}{2}\left(\theta_{rel,12} - \theta_{rel,12}\right) \tag{18.47}$$

$$M = \left(\frac{M_{rel,12}}{M_{rel,21}}\right)^{1/2} = \left(\frac{\dfrac{L_{AC_1}G_{AC_1}}{L_{AC_2}G_{AC_2}} \cdot \dfrac{L_{DC_2}G_{DC_2}}{L_{DC_1}G_{DC_1}}}{\dfrac{L_{AC_2}G_{AC_2}}{L_{AC_1}G_{AC_1}} \cdot \dfrac{L_{DC_1}G_{DC_1}}{L_{DC_2}G_{DC_2}}}\right)^{1/2} = \left(\frac{L_{AC_1}/L_{AC_2}}{L_{DC_2}/L_{DC_1}} \frac{G_{AC_1}/G_{AC_2}}{G_{DC_2}/G_{DC_1}}\right) \tag{18.48}$$

For matched detectors, $\left(\dfrac{G_{AC_1}/G_{AC_2}}{G_{DC_2}/G_{DC_1}}\right)$ is unity. For unmatched detectors, the ratio must be experimentally determined [31].

Figure 18.14 captures the multiplexing system for the conventional two-channel frequency-domain system developed for fluorescence lifetime spectroscopy.

The multiplexing method described earlier can be performed for measurements performed with sources at the excitation and emission wavelengths, and hence single distance (multifrequency) nonlinear regression [29] can be performed to obtain optical properties of the medium without corruption from the instrument functions. In a recent study, we showed that measurements made at multiple distances enable linear regression of parameters [29] and result in the most precise optical property estimation [30]. Regardless of whether from referenced or multiplexed frequency-domain measurements conducted with point source illumination at wavelengths λ_x and λ_m, the optical properties of $\mu_{a_{\lambda_x}}$, $\mu_{a_{\lambda_m}}$, $\mu'_{s_{\lambda_x}}$, $\mu'_{s_{\lambda_m}}$ can be accurately obtained.

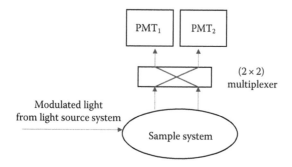

FIGURE 18.14 Illustration of multiplexing system for the two-channel frequency-domain detection apparatus.

18.4.1.2 Determination of Single Exponential Decay Lifetime

After estimating the optical properties from frequency-domain measurements employing the two wavelength sources, the emission fluence is measured in response to point source illumination at the excitation wavelength using excitation light rejection filters to reduce the noise floor. From the referenced measurement to determine $\Phi_m(\vec{r},\omega) = I_{AC_m} \exp(i\theta_m)$, the fluorescent properties of $\alpha\mu_{a_{x \to m}}$ and τ are determined from the solution to Equations 18.19 and 18.24 for an infinite medium:

$$\Phi_m(\vec{r},\omega)ac = \frac{\alpha\mu_{a_{x \to m}} \Xi_m(SA)}{4\pi v D_x D_{mr}} \frac{1}{\left[1+(\omega\tau)^2\right]} \left\{ \left[\psi - \kappa\omega\tau\right] + i\left[\kappa + \psi\omega\tau\right] \right\} \tag{18.49}$$

where
  r is the distance to the excitation point source
  SA is the complex fluence of the source describing its modulation depth and phase
  ψ and κ are functions of optical properties (μ_a and μ'_s), c, and ω [10,27]:

$$\psi(\vec{r},\omega) = \frac{\delta(\vec{r},\omega)\xi + \zeta(\vec{r},\omega)\rho(\omega)}{\xi^2 + \rho(\omega)^2} \tag{18.50}$$

$$\kappa(\vec{r},\omega) = \frac{\zeta(\vec{r},\omega)\xi - \delta(\vec{r},\omega)\rho(\omega)}{\xi^2 + \rho(\omega)^2} \tag{18.51}$$

$$\delta(\vec{r},\omega) = \exp\left[-\beta_x(\omega)r\right]\cos\left[\gamma_x(\omega)r\right] - \exp\left[-\beta_m(\omega)r\right]\cos\left[\gamma_m(\omega)r\right] \tag{18.52}$$

$$\zeta(\vec{r},\omega) = \exp\left[-\beta_x(\omega)r\right]\sin\left[\gamma_x(\omega)r\right] - \exp\left[-\beta_m(\omega)r\right]\sin\left[\gamma_m(\omega)r\right] \tag{18.53}$$

$$\xi = \frac{\mu_{am}}{D_m} - \frac{\mu_{ax}}{D_x} \tag{18.54}$$

$$\rho(\omega) = \frac{\omega}{c}\left[\frac{1}{D_x} - \frac{1}{D_m}\right] \tag{18.55}$$

Using FDPM measurements at both the excitation and emission wavelengths, the ability to measure the single exponential lifetimes of ICG and 3,3′-diethylthiatricarbocyanine iodide (DTTCI) [27], Rhodamine B [10], and mixtures ICG and DTTCI [13] in tissue-like scattering media of Intralipid has been demonstrated experimentally.

Yet most analyte-sensing fluorophores exhibit multiexponential decays or stretched exponential decay kinetics increasing the number of unknowns from two ($\alpha\mu_{a_{x \to m}}, \tau$) to 2_{j+1} for a fluorophore experience j activated states (Equation 18.10), ($\mu_{a_{x \to m}}, \tau_j, a_j$), to 3_{j+1} for a fluorophore undergoing collisional quenching (Equation 18.11), ($\mu_{a_{x \to m}}, \tau_j, a_j, \alpha_j, \beta_j$).

18.4.2 Multiexponential Decay Kinetics

In general, the solution for the emission fluence in an infinite medium of uniform optical properties is given by

$$\Phi_m(\vec{r}, \omega) = \frac{\alpha\mu_{a_{x \to m}} \Xi m(SA)}{4\pi v D_x D_{mr}} \left\{ (\psi - i\kappa) \int_0^\infty \left(g(t) e^{(i\omega t)} dt \right) \right\} \tag{18.56}$$

Generally, frequency-domain measurements are insensitive to the form of the decay kinetics used to describe the relaxation process. As an example, Figure 18.15 illustrates the phase and modulation ratio

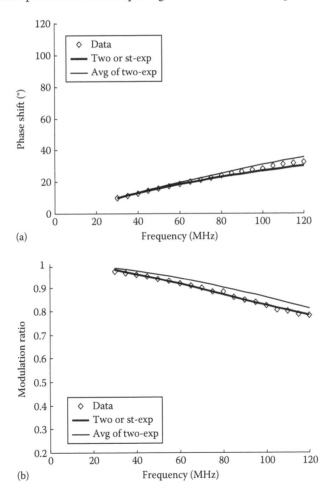

FIGURE 18.15 The plot of fluorescence phase shift (a) and modulation ratio (b) as a function of modulation frequency on ICG–DTTCI mixture (ICG/DTTCI = 0.15:0.5 mM, in a dilute nonscattering medium) for corrected experimental measurements (*black diamond*) and that predicted by incorporating two-exponential decay kinetics or stretched exponential decay kinetics (*bold black line*) and average of two-exponential decay kinetics (*thin gray line*).

measured in a dilute, nonscattering sample using traditional fluorescence lifetime spectroscopy techniques. The emitted fluorescence is owing to a combination of two dyes, ICG and DTTCI, each of which individually exhibits first-order relaxation kinetics. The frequency-domain data are equally well fit using a single exponential decay (which represents the average of the decay times), a two-exponential decay, and a stretched exponential decay model—indicating that the data are insufficient at these modulation frequencies to discern the relaxation processes. Typically, differences in decay kinetics are manifested at higher modulation frequencies, which unfortunately suffer from a small instrument response function and low SNR. However, upon predicting the phase delay and modulation ratio from the solution to the diffusion equation for infinite media employing the differing kinetic models for radiative relaxation, one can see significant differences in frequency-domain data taken at modulation frequencies below 150 MHz (Figure 18.16). In Figure 18.16, the model predictions for the two dyes within a scattering

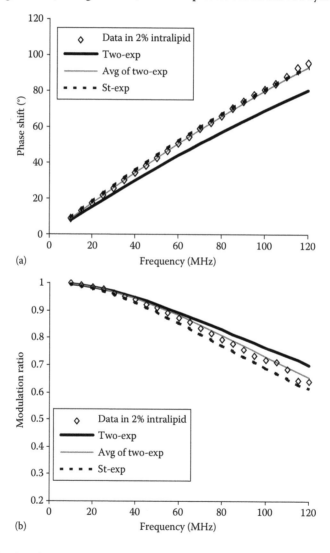

FIGURE 18.16 The plot of fluorescence phase shift (a) and modulation ratio (b) as a function of modulation frequency on ICG–DTTCI mixture (ICG/DTTCI = 0.15 mM:0.5 mM, in 2% intralipid solution) for corrected experimental measurements (*black diamond*) and that predicted by the propagation model incorporating two-exponential decay kinetics (*bold black line*), average of two-exponential decay kinetics (*thin gray line*), and the stretched exponential decay kinetics (*dotted black line*).

medium experiencing different relaxation mechanisms are shown along with the data—indicating the potential for enhanced sensitivity of fluorescence lifetime spectroscopy in random or multiply scattered media. Note that between Figures 18.15 and 18.16, the phase delay and modulation ratios span a larger range in scattering media as opposed to nonscattering media.

In summary, the challenges for solving the inverse fluorescence spectroscopy problem still remain to extract parameters that accurately predict changes in decay kinetics and therefore changes in analyte or metabolite concentrations. While there are a few studies in the literature demonstrating the ability to solve the inverse spectroscopy problem for fluorescence lifetime in random media, to date, there has been no demonstration of the solution of the inverse problem for the multiexponential decay functions that exist for analyte-sensing fluorophores. However, as long as the number of unknown remains smaller than the number of measurements, the solution to the inverse spectroscopy entails a straightforward least square minimization problem. In contrast to the inverse spectroscopy problem, the inverse imaging problem entails a smaller number of measurements than unknown parameters, necessitating optimization approaches.

18.5 Fluorescence FDPM for Optical Tomography[*]

The solution to the inverse imaging problem, called optical tomography, has been motivated over the past decade by optical mammography, that is, the use of deeply penetrating NIR light to detect breast cancer on the basis of endogenous optical property contrast between normal and diseased tissues. The optical property contrast in scattering and absorption has been postulated to be due to the increased size and density of neoplastic cells in a tumor region and the increased vascular blood supply (as a result of angiogenesis), which locally increases the hemoglobin, a primary chromophore in tissues. While there have been many accomplishments in the development of optical mammography, most notably in the application of FDPM [32], TDPM [33], and CW [7] measurements (as reviewed elsewhere [22]), the necessity of angiogenesis-mediated absorption contrast for diagnostic optical mammography limits the potential for optical mammography. Since the endogenous contrast owing to angiogenesis can be expected to be low in small lesions and nonspecific to cancer, there is certainly a limitation for NIR detection of nonpalpable disease in dense breast tissue without the addition of contrast. Hence, the capability for moderately resolved, biochemical molecular imaging within tissues using unassisted NIR optical techniques is somewhat limited and can be expanded through the use of contrast-enhancing agents.

Fluorescent contrast agents have been proposed and independently confirmed as the most efficient means for inducing optical contrast when time-dependent measurements (i.e., TDPM or FDPM) are conducted [3,26]. Furthermore, they may in the near future offer a host of opportunities for molecular imaging that is limited only by synthetic design. The basic principles behind fluorescence-enhanced NIR optical tomography are focused first upon the kinetics of the fluorescence generation. It is the kinetics of the fluorescent decay process that imparts the superior contrast of fluorescence over absorbance when TDPM or FDPM measurements are made.

Figure 18.17 provides a simple schematic describing the physics behind why fluorescent contrast is greater than that possible by absorption for FDPM imaging. Consider a tissue volume illuminated by intensity-modulated light source at source position, r_s. The propagating wave is denoted with dotted lines. As the propagating excitation wave transits through the tissue, it is attenuated and phase-delayed owing to the tissue optical properties. If the wave encounters a light-absorbing heterogeneity, such as a highly vascularized tumor, a portion of the intensity wave is reflected. The strength of the *reflected wave* (or dotted line) is dependent upon the absorption contrast and the size and depth of the heterogeneity. This *reflected wave* makes a small contribution to the wave that ultimately is detected at detector position r_d. It is this small, added contribution that is used to detect the heterogeneity when endogenous

---

[*] Adapted from Sevick-Muraca et al. [15].

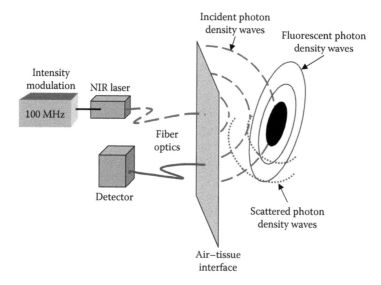

FIGURE 18.17 Schematic detailing the propagation of excitation photon density waves (*solid lines*) and their perturbation by absorbing heterogeneities (*dotted lines*) and the generation of emission photon density waves (*solid, gray lines*) within the tissues. Fluorescence contrast-enhanced optical tomography provides greater localization capability because the detected emission waves act as *beacons* providing information regarding the tagged heterogeneity.

contrast is employed. If the added contribution is not within the measurement noise, then it provides information for image recovery in one of the inversion strategies outlined below. However, if the heterogeneity were contrasted by fluorescence, then upon reaching the heterogeneity, the excitation wave generates an emission wave (solid lines). The emission wave then acts as a beacon, and upon employing appropriate filters to reject the excitation light, it can be measured to directly locate the heterogeneity. In small tissue volumes, such as the mouse or rat, inversion algorithms may not be required to detect the fluorescent heterogeneity, as shown in the literature results summarized in Table 18.1. However, in larger tissue volumes, the forward and inverse imaging problems require solution for effective image recovery. Most importantly, since there are a phase delay and amplitude attenuation between the activating excitation wave and the reemitted fluorescent wave that is associated with the fluorescence decay kinetics, the fluorescence decay increases the contrast or phase delay and amplitude attenuation change associated with the detected signal. Finally, since a fluorescent probe can be *tuned* to exhibit differing fluorescence decay characteristics dependent upon its local environment, the reemitted signal can contain diagnostic information about the tissue of interest.

There are few studies that successfully invert NIR tissue optical measurements to render images of exogenously contrasted tissues or tissue-mimicking phantoms. Table 18.2 outlines several investigations that have employed *synthetic* data sets and phantom [34–54]. Basically, the approaches are similar to those used in NIR optical tomography work with the exception of three points: (1) Owing to the low quantum yield of fluorescent dyes, the SNR for CW, TDPM, and FDPM measurements is inarguably lower, potentially making it more difficult to successfully reconstruct images; (2) owing to the fluorescence lifetime delay, both TDPM and FDPM approaches have additional contrast in the time-dependent photon migration characteristics; and finally (3) owing to the ability to directly invert the fluorescence kinetic parameters of fluorescence lifetime and quantum efficiency, the technique can be used to perform quantitative imaging via dyes that report cancer [55].

The latter characteristic of fluorescence lifetime imaging reveals its similarity to magnetic resonance imaging (MRI). In MRI, imaging is accomplished by monitoring the RF signal arising from the relaxation of a magnetic dipole perturbed from its aligned state using a pulsed magnetic field. In fluorescence

TABLE 18.2   Fluorescence-Enhanced Contrast Imaging: Literature of Imaging Reconstructions

Author	Inversion Formulation	Data Type	Noise	2D or 3D	Forward Method	Measurement Method	Contrast Agent	Uptake Ratio
O'Leary et al. [36]	Localization	Experimental phantom	Yes	2D	None	TDPM	ICG	Perfect uptake
Wu et al. [37]	Localization	Experimental phantom	Yes	3D	None	TDPM	Diethylthiatricarbocyanine	Perfect uptake
Chang et al. [38]	POCS, CGD, SART	Experimental phantom	Yes	2D	NS	CW	Rhodamine 6G dye	Perfect uptake and 1000:1
O'Leary et al. [39]	Integral (SIRT)	Synthetic data	0.1° in phase; 1% in amplitude	2D	Analytical	FDPM	ICG	Perfect uptake and 20:1
Paithankar et al. [40]	Differential (Newton–Raphson)	Synthetic data	0.1°–1° in phase; 0.01 in log AC (Gaussian)	2D	MFD	FDPM	ICG	20:1
Wu et al. [41]	Laplace transform	Experimental phantom	Yes	2D	NS	TDPM	HITCI iodide dye	Perfect uptake
Chang et al. [42]	Differential (conjugate gradient)	Synthetic data	1%–10% white noise	2D or 3D	NS	CW/FDPM	N/A	100:1
Jiang [43]	Differential (Newton's iterative method)	Synthetic data	0%–5%	2D	FEM	FDPM	N/A	2:1 contrast in ϕ, τ
Eppstein et al. [45,46]	Differential	Synthetic data	0.1° in phase; 1% in log AC (Gaussian)	2D, 3D	MFD	FDPM	N/A	Perfect uptake and 100:1, 10:1

(continued)

TABLE 18.2 (continued) Fluorescence-Enhanced Contrast Imaging: Literature of Imaging Reconstructions

Author	Inversion Formulation	Data Type	Noise	2D or 3D	Forward Method	Measurement Method	Contrast Agent	Uptake Ratio
Chenomordik et al. [35]	Random walk theory	Experimental phantom	Yes	2D, 3D	NS	CCD	Rhodamine	Perfect uptake
Roy and Sevick-Muraca [47,48]	Differential (gradient-based and truncated Newton method)	Synthetic data	0.1° in phase; 1% in log AC (Gaussian)	2D	FEM	FDPM	N/A	2.5:1, 5:1, 10:1
Yang et al. [34]	Marquardt and Tikhonov regularization	In vivo (rats)	Yes	2D images	FEM	FDPM	ICG and DTTCI	Perfect and imperfect uptake
Eppstein et al. [49]; Hawrysz et al. [50]	Differential	Experimental phantom	Yes	3D	MFD	FDPM	ICG	50:1, 100:1
Roy and Sevick-Muraca [51,52]	Differential (gradient-based optimization and truncated Newton's method)	Synthetic data	55 dB in excitation; 35 dB in emission	2D, 3D	FEM	FDPM	N/A	10:1
Ntziachristos [53]	Integral (normalized Born expansion)	Experimental phantom	2% amplitude noise in source	2D along z-planes	FD	CW	ICG in background; Cy5.5 as contrast tumor	Perfect uptake
Lee and Sevick-Muraca [54]	Integral (distorted BIM)	Experimental phantom	Yes	3D	MFD	FDPM	ICG	100:1

Abbreviations: CCD, charge-coupled device; CGD, conjugate gradient descent; CW, continuous wave imaging; FD, finite difference; FDPM, frequency-domain photon migration; FEM, finite element method; MFD, multigrid finite difference; N/A, not applicable; NS, not specified; POCS, projection onto convex sets; SART/SIRT, simultaneous algebraic reconstruction techniques; TDPM, time-domain photon migration; φ, τ, quantum efficiency and lifetime of the contrast agent.

contrast-enhanced optical tomography, imaging is accomplished by monitoring the emission signal arising from the electronic relaxation from an optically activated state to its ground state. Unfortunately, the emission light is multiply scattered; hence, the resolution afforded by MRI is unlikely to be matched by contrast-enhanced optical tomography. Unlike contrast agents for conventional imaging modalities, optical contrast owing to fluorescent agents may be imparted in two ways: (1) through increased target/ background concentration ratios and (2) through alteration in the fluorescence decay kinetics upon partitioning within tissue regions of interest [55]. Section 18.6 summarizes the literature reports of fluorescent contrast agents and their development over the past decade. In the following, the approaches for solving the inverse imaging problem are presented.

18.5.1 Approaches to the Inverse Imaging Problem

Attempts to solve the fluorescence-enhanced optical imaging problem have been made both by solving a formal inverse problem and by taking a less rigorous model-based approach. For example, localization of a fluorescent target has been demonstrated using localization techniques in which the strength of reradiating target is used to ascertain its central position within a background containing no fluorophore. Using FDPM measurements between a point source and detector as the pair was scanned over the phantom surface, the center of a single fluorescent target could be accurately identified [36]. In yet another approach, an analytical solution to the spherical propagation of emission light in uniform scattering media was used to determine the x,y,z position of the point source of fluorescence in an otherwise nonfluorescent background probed by CW measurements [35]. Using time-domain measurements, Wu and coworkers [37,41] developed a system for assessing the position of a fluorescent target in turbid media by evaluating the early-arriving photons to determine the origin of the fluorescence generation. Hull and coworkers similarly used spatially resolved CW measurements to determine the location of the fluorescent target in scattering media [44]. Unlike these studies described earlier, the presence of background signal or the goal of reporting fluorescent decay kinetics prevents localization approach and requires solution to the full inverse imaging problem.

The solution of a formal inverse problem requires the use of the appropriate mathematical models described in Section 18.2. Specifically, a guess of the interior optical or fluorescence properties is iteratively updated until the predicted measurements given by the solution of the forward problem match the actual measurements. Since the number of unknowns (or optical and/or fluorescent contrast agent properties) is greater than the number of measurements, the problem is underdetermined and especially difficult. This inverse problem is unavoidably *ill posed*, a term that generally means that the solutions are nonunique and unstable in the presence of measurement error. In addition, the optical tomography problem in general is highly nonlinear and attempts to linearize its result in solution instabilities and often intractably long computational times if the update step is to remain within the range of accuracy of the linearization. The solution of the inverse problem is an intensive area of research in itself that is motivated by several different research areas, including biomedical NIR optical tomography based upon endogenous contrast. In order to assess the performance of an inverse problem algorithm, the achieved solution must be compared to the known distribution of optical properties. As a consequence, studies to investigate the inverse optical tomography problem are performed using either (1) *synthetic* measurements, that is, measurements that are predicted by the forward problem to which artificial random *noise* is added to simulate measurement error, or (2) phantom studies in which tissue-mimicking scattering media of known optical properties are used to collect experimental CW, time, or frequency-domain measurements that are used for the inverse solution. In the following sections, we briefly review the methods to solve the fluorescence-enhanced optical tomography problems, broadly classified into the categories of integral and differential approaches and employing a number of parameter-updating schemes. Finally, example reconstructions from actual experimental data are presented.

18.5.2 Integral Formulation of the Inverse Problem

One of the more common methods of formulating the inverse problem is by way of an integral treatment. Since the emission diffusion equation is in the form of an inhomogeneous differential equation, Green's function is used to obtain the analytical solution of the emission fluence $\Phi_m(\vec{r},\omega)$. Equation 18.19 can be rewritten to account for variation in the endogenous and exogenous optical properties, including the absorption owing to fluorophore, $\mu_{a_{x\to m}}(\vec{r})$, and the optical diffusion coefficient, $D_m(\vec{r})$:

$$\vec{\nabla}^2\Phi_m(\vec{r},\omega)+k_m^2(\vec{r})\Phi_m(\vec{r},\omega)=-\frac{S_m(\vec{r})}{D_m(\vec{r})}-\frac{\vec{\nabla}D_m(\vec{r})\cdot\vec{\nabla}\Phi_m(\vec{r},\omega)}{D_m(\vec{r})} \tag{18.57}$$

where the complex diffusion wave number can be expressed as

$$k_m^2(\vec{r})=\frac{1}{D_m(\vec{r})}\left(-\mu_{a_m}(\vec{r})+i\frac{\omega}{c}\right) \tag{18.58}$$

The term $\left[\vec{\nabla}D_m(\vec{r})/D_m(\vec{r})\right]\cdot\vec{\nabla}\Phi_m(\vec{r})$ in Equation 18.57 accounts for the discontinuity in $D_m(\vec{r})$. However, since there is little or no variation of isotropic scattering coefficient, the component that constitutes the overwhelming contribution to $D_m(\vec{r})$ at the emission wavelength, λ_m, the term presented earlier is negligible. Green's function corresponding to Equation 18.57 consequently satisfies

$$\vec{\nabla}^2 G_f\left(\vec{r},\vec{r}'\right)+k_m^2(\vec{r})G_f\left(\vec{r},\vec{r}'\right)=-\delta(\vec{r}-\vec{r}') \tag{18.59}$$

By manipulating Equations 18.57 and 18.19 (at the excitation wavelength), and with the use of Green's theorem, $\int_v\left(U\vec{\nabla}^2 G-G\vec{\nabla}^2 U\right)d^3r=\oint_S\left(U\vec{\nabla}G-G\vec{\nabla}U\right)\cdot dS$, one can obtain the expression of the emission fluence measured at r_d following point excitation at r_s, $\Phi_m(r_d,r_s)$, which arises due to $S_m(r',r_s)$, the emission generation at point r' following the incident illumination of excitation light at r_s, and due to the propagation of the emission light from position r' to detector point r_d as predicted from Green's solution, $G_f(r_d,r_s)$:

$$\tilde{\Phi}_m\left(\vec{r}_d,\vec{r}_s\right)=\int_\Omega G_f\left(\vec{r}_d,\vec{r}'\right)S_m\left(\vec{r}',\vec{r}_s\right)d\Omega$$

$$=\int_\Omega G_f\left(\vec{r}_d,\vec{r}'\right)\frac{\alpha\mu_{a_{x\to m}}\left(\vec{r}'\right)}{D_m(\vec{r})(1-i\omega\tau)}\Phi_x\left(\vec{r}',\vec{r}_s\right)d\Omega \tag{18.60}$$

where
   Ω is the volume of integration
   $\vec{r}_d$ is the point detector location
   $\vec{r}_s$ is the point source location

In order to reconstruct the spatial map of $\mu_{a_{x\to m}}\left(\vec{r}\right)$ detailing the heterogeneity, Equation 18.60 is discretized into a series of equations in terms of G_f, $\Phi_x\left(\vec{r}',\vec{r}_s\right)$, and the vector of measurements of $\tilde{\Phi}_m\left(\vec{r}_d,\vec{r}_s\right)$. We consider the excitation source to be amplitude modulated by a frequency of ω. Measurements of phase shift, θ_m, and amplitude of AC component, I_{AC} (or $\Phi_m\left(\vec{r}_d,\vec{r}_s\right)=I_{AC_m}e^{i\theta_m}$), are obtained at detector positions, $\vec{r}_d$, in response to excitation source at $\vec{r}_s$. *It is important to note that it is assumed that the phase shift and the AC component are predicted relative to the incident excitation light at $\vec{r}_s$. In addition, it is important to note that it is assumed absolute measurements of I_{AC_m} and θ_m are used as inputs.* Upon discretizing Equation 18.60, one obtains

$$\tilde{\Phi}_m\left(\vec{r}_d,\vec{r}_s\right)=\sum_{j=1}^N G_f\left(\vec{r}_j,\vec{r}_d\right)\Phi_x\left(\vec{r}_j,\vec{r}_s\right)\frac{\alpha\mu_{a_{x\to m}}\left(\vec{r}_j\right)\Delta}{D_m(\vec{r})(1-i\omega\tau)} \tag{18.61}$$

where

    N is the total number of cells in the domain

    Δ is the area or volume of the pixel or voxel

If there are K sources and L detectors, then $\tilde{\Phi}_m = FX$ can be denoted as

$$
\begin{pmatrix}
\tilde{\Phi}_m\left(\vec{r}_d,\vec{r}_s\right)_1 \\
\tilde{\Phi}_m\left(\vec{r}_d,\vec{r}_s\right)_2 \\
\vdots \\
\vdots \\
\tilde{\Phi}_m\left(\vec{r}_d,\vec{r}_s\right)_M
\end{pmatrix}
=
\begin{pmatrix}
F_{11} & \cdots & F_{1N} \\
F_{21} & \cdots & F_{2N} \\
\vdots & \ddots & \vdots \\
\vdots & \ddots & \vdots \\
F_{M1} & \cdots & F_{MN}
\end{pmatrix}
\begin{pmatrix}
X\left(\vec{r}_1\right) \\
X\left(\vec{r}_2\right) \\
\vdots \\
\vdots \\
X\left(\vec{r}_N\right)
\end{pmatrix}
\tag{18.62}
$$

$$
F_{ij} = \frac{G_f\left(\vec{r}_{di},\vec{r}_j\right)\Phi_x\left(\vec{r}_{si},\vec{r}_j\right)\alpha\Delta}{D_m(\vec{r})\left(1-i\omega\tau\right)}
\tag{18.63}
$$

$$
X\left(\vec{r}_j\right) = \mu_{a_{x\to m}}\left(\vec{r}_j\right)
\tag{18.64}
$$

where $F \in C^{M\times N}, X \in \Re^N, \tilde{\Phi}_m \in C^M$, respectively, and $M = K \times L$.

    Equation 18.64 is also appropriate if imaging is performed on the basis of fluorophore absorption cross section with a constant lifetime, τ. It is noteworthy that the problem formulated in Equations 18.62 through 18.64 is nonlinear in $\mu_{a_{x\to m}}$ since the excitation fluence, $\Phi_x(\vec{r})$, is also a function of absorption.

    However, it is also noteworthy that if tomographic reconstruction on lifetime were pursued, the problem would become linear, and Equations 18.63 and 18.64 would be rewritten as

$$
F_{i,j} = \frac{G_f(\vec{r}_{di},\vec{r}_j)\Phi_x(\vec{r}_{si},\vec{r}_j)\Delta}{D_m(\vec{r})}
\tag{18.65}
$$

$$
X(\vec{r}_j) = \frac{\alpha\mu_{a_{x\to m}}(\vec{r}_j)}{(1-i\omega\tau)}
\tag{18.66}
$$

where the vector X represents the sources of fluorescence within the random media.

    The formulation of the inverse problem for lifetime is called fluorescence lifetime imaging [39,40,56] and has been the subject of tomographic reconstructions from synthetic measurements. It is noteworthy that for CW measurements ($\omega = 0$), fluorescence lifetime imaging is not possible. To date, fluorescence lifetime imaging has been accomplished using actual experimental measurements only in limited works [34], probably due to the fact that there are few contrast agents designed with *tunable* lifetimes.

    Nonetheless, the opportunity for lifetime imaging is clearly evidenced by ICCD measurements using the instrumentation depicted in Figure 18.8. Two fluorescent targets were positioned 0.5 cm from the imaged surface of a tissue-simulating phantom, which were embedded in a $10 \times 10 \times 10$ cm^3 of 0.5% Intralipid. The first target encapsulated a 1 µM solution of ICG, and the second encapsulated a 1.42 µM solution of DTTCI. These solution concentrations were chosen to equilibrate the number of fluorescent photons emitted from each target given an equivalent number of excitation photons encounter each target. Figure 18.18a and b confirms this equilibration, as it is difficult to differentiate the targets from the DC and AC measurements. However, Figure 18.18c and d plots the phase delay and the modulation ratio (I_{AC}/I_{DC}) and provides differentiation of the two volumes. The differentiation, which results from a disparity in lifetime (0.62 ns) between the two fluorescent agents, demonstrates the potential of fluorescence lifetime imaging. While these images present raw data, quantitative tomographic recovery of fluorescent lifetime is possible with solution to the inverse imaging problem.

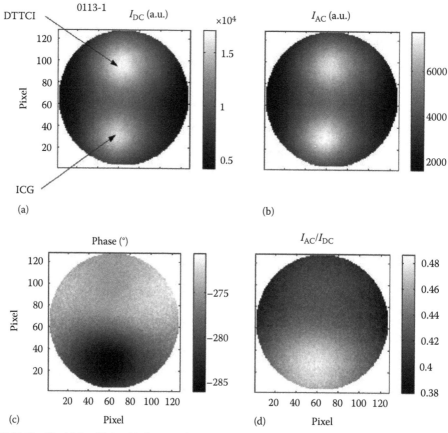

FIGURE 18.18   The (a) I_{DC}, (b) I_{AC}, (c) phase, and (d) I_{AC}/I_{DC} modulation ratio of two submerged targets of differing fluorescent lifetime showing that I_{DC} cannot distinguish the difference in fluorescence decay kinetics.

The inverse imaging problem can be approximated as linear problem and iteratively solved using Gauss–Newton method:

$$\Phi_m^{meas}(\vec{r}_d,\vec{r}_s) - \Phi_m^{comp}(\vec{r}_d,\vec{r}_s) = \mathbf{F}\cdot\Delta\mathbf{X}(\vec{r}). \tag{18.67}$$

Regardless of whether it is absorption or fluorescence lifetime imaging to be performed, parameter updating can be accomplished by noting that $\mathbf{F}$ is simply the Jacobian, $\mathbf{J}$, and the difference between measurement and model-predicted fluence, $\Phi_{meas} - \Phi_{comp} = \Delta\Phi$, can be used to update the optical property map, $\Delta X(\vec{r})$, by the relationship specified earlier or alternatively by

$$\Delta\Phi = \mathbf{J}\cdot\Delta\mathbf{X} \tag{18.68}$$

While a number of investigators report reconstructions based upon the integral approaches using frequency-domain or CW ($\omega = 0$) approaches, all assume that the measurements of phase shift and amplitude attenuation could be accurately measured relative to the incident light. Yet, in practice, it is nearly impossible to perform such a measurement. Typically, a portion of the incident light is split for simultaneous measurement at a reference detector that cannot report the source strength or the phase delay of light that is incident on the medium surface. Calibration of the source via a *reference* phantom may also be conducted if a 3D model can be used to predict the measurements and if the source strength can be accurately recovered from the measurements and model. Yet such a procedure is cumbersome, susceptible to errors, and increases the challenges for incorporation into medical imaging in clinical situations. A method to eliminate *calibration* against an external standard would eliminate the number of measurements as well as improve measurement accuracy. In the following sections, three general approaches to reference measurements for the recovery of optical properties are presented in light of image reconstruction formalisms: (1) emission measurements at detector position r_d referenced to the background emission wave, $\Phi_m^b(\vec{r}_s, \vec{r}_d)$; (2) emission measurements at detector position r_d referenced to the detected emission wave at a single reference position r_r, $\Phi_m(\vec{r}_s, \vec{r}_r)$; and (3) emission measurements at detector position r_d referenced to the detected excitation wave at a single reference position r_r, $\Phi_x(\vec{r}_s, \vec{r}_r)$.

18.5.2.1 Measurement Referenced to the Background Emission Wave, $\Phi_m^b(\vec{r}_s, \vec{r}_r)$

In this approach, the calibration of the detection system is achieved by normalizing the measurement in the presence of the heterogeneity with that measured or predicted in its absence. Typically, the *absence* case consists of a uniform medium with constant and known optical properties. In the *absence* case, the main problem associated with matching experimental data to the solution of Equation 18.57 has been the unknown source strength and the unknown phase delay from the timing characteristics of various components of the detection system and the amplitude gain or loss. The advantage of using background or a well-defined reference phantom is that it enables to eliminate the most systematic errors common to both background and actual measurement data sets. This approach has been widely employed in both frequency- [57,58] and time-domain [59,60] photon migration measurements. However, this is an unrealistic approach in clinical sense because unlike phantom studies, in clinical applications, it is impossible to have the *absence* case or to measure the *background* fluence. For contrast-enhanced imaging, the *absence* case may be achieved prior to the administration of a contrast agent or activation-induced contrast such as that owing to blood flow. Yet when the agent is fluorescent, there is no emission signal to measure the *absence* case; hence, the absence case is unrealistic in fluorescence imaging.

For heterodyne FDPM measurements, the referenced measurements enable elimination of instrument responses. For example, an emission measurement referenced to the *background* case in which the target,

$$\frac{\Phi_{AC_m}(r_d, r_s)}{\Phi_{AC_m}^b(r_d, r_s)} = \frac{L_{AC_m} G_{AC} \exp\left(i\left(-\theta_m + \theta_{instr}\right)\right)}{L_{AC_m}^b G_{AC} \exp\left(i\left(-\theta_m^b + \theta_{instr}\right)\right)} = \frac{L_{AC_m}}{L_{AC_m}^b} \exp\left[i\left(\theta_m^b - \theta_m\right)\right]$$

successfully eliminates the instrument response, and the background optical properties are known.

To illustrate the mechanics of inverting data referenced to the background *absence* case, the following equation shows the relationship between the measurement and the inversion algorithm for a source–detector pair when Born-type inversion scheme is used for fluorescent measurements, where the referenced measurement is represented by $\left.\dfrac{\Phi_{AC_m}\left(\vec{r}_s, \vec{r}_d\right)}{\Phi_{AC_m}^b\left(\vec{r}_s, \vec{r}_d\right)}\right|_{exp}$

$$\left.\frac{\Phi_{AC_m}\left(\vec{r}_s, \vec{r}_d\right)}{\Phi_{AC_m}^b\left(\vec{r}_s, \vec{r}_d\right)}\right|_{exp} = \frac{1}{\left[\Phi_{AC_m}^b\left(\vec{r}_s, \vec{r}_d\right)\right]_{a\ priori}} \int_\Omega \frac{\alpha}{D_m\left(1 - i\omega\tau\right)} G_f\left(\vec{r}_d, \vec{r}\right) \Phi_x\left(\vec{r}_s, \vec{r}\right) \mu_{ax \to m}(\vec{r})\, d\Omega \quad (18.69)$$

Here, $\left[\Phi_{AC_m}^b\left(\vec{r}_s, \vec{r}_d\right)\right]_{a\ priori}$ is the background emission wave detected at the same detector position, $\vec{r}_d$, as in the presence of heterogeneity case in response to excitation from the source position, $\vec{r}_s$. $\Phi_{AC_m}^b(\vec{r}_s, \vec{r}_r)$ is computed from the known optical properties of the assumed uniform *background* case or measured in the case of an *absent* heterogeneity.

In contrast to the absolute measurement case, where the matrix, **F**, itself is the Jacobian matrix (Equation 18.63), the problem with relative measurement schemes arises with the added complication in calculating Jacobian matrix when using the integral equation. However, in this case, the $\Phi_{AC_m}^b(\vec{r}_s, \vec{r}_d)$ stays constant throughout the iteration due to its homogeneous nature, the inversion problem remains linear, and the calculation of Jacobian matrix is straightforward. As a result, the reconstruction remains stable during iterative process, while the source strength dependency and other calibration problems are eliminated. Even though the reference to the background emission fluence approach is relatively easy to implement in phantom study and is a good benchmark to test the inversion algorithms, it would face difficulty in actual clinical application to the clinical trials where a true *absence* condition does not occur, or the spatially distributed optical properties are not known.

18.5.2.2 Measurement Referenced to the Emission Wave, $\Phi_m(\vec{r}_s, \vec{r}_r)$

The unrealistic nature of referencing to the background emission wave leads to the inversion scheme using the emission fluence at the reference point on the tissue surface. This approach involves the measurements of the emission fluence relative to one another, where the referenced measurement is

represented by $\left. \dfrac{\Phi_m(\vec{r}_s, \vec{r}_d)}{\Phi_m(\vec{r}_s, \vec{r}_r)} \right]_{exp}$ and

$$\frac{\Phi_{AC_m}(r_d, r_s)}{\Phi_{AC_m}(r_d, r_r)} = \frac{L_{AC_m}(r_d)\, G_{AC} \exp\left(i\left(-\theta_m + \theta_{instr}\right)\right)}{L_{AC_m}(r_r)\, G_{AC} \exp\left(i\left(-\theta_m(r_r) + \theta_{instr}\right)\right)} = \frac{L_{AC_m}(r_d)}{L_{AC_m}(r_r)} \exp\left[i\left(\theta_m(r_r) - \theta_m(r_d)\right)\right]$$

and Fredholm's equation to be solved is written as

$$\frac{\Phi_m(\vec{r}_s, \vec{r}_d)}{\Phi_m(\vec{r}_s, \vec{r}_r)} = \frac{1}{\Phi_m(\vec{r}_s, \vec{r}_r)} \int_\Omega \frac{\alpha}{D_m(1 - i\omega\tau)} G_f(\vec{r}_d, \vec{r}) \Phi_x(\vec{r}_s, \vec{r}) \mu_{a_{x \to m}}(\vec{r})\, d\Omega \qquad (18.70)$$

Here, $\Phi_m(\vec{r}_s, \vec{r}_r)$ is the emission wave detected at the reference position, $\vec{r}_r$, in response to excitation from the source position, $\vec{r}_s$. This referencing approach is the most reasonable method to match the actual measurement data with simulation data since it does not require the separate measurement of a homogeneous background wave. Also, this referencing approach has merit in that it uses the measurements at the same wavelength as opposed to the excitation wavelength, an approach shown in the following section.

While referencing to the emission wave, $\Phi_m(\vec{r}_s, \vec{r}_r)$, is more practical than referencing to the background emission wave, $\Phi_{AC_m}^b(\vec{r}_s, \vec{r}_d)$, the normalization by $\Phi_m(\vec{r}_s, \vec{r}_r)$ renders the inversion algorithm using the Born-type integral approach highly nonlinear. This nonlinearity is absent when referencing to the background emission wave. Consequently, the calculation of Jacobian matrix is not as straightforward as in the case with the background emission wave (for details, see Lee and Sevick-Muraca [54]).

Hence, the formulated inverse imaging problem is inherently unstable owing to its nonlinear nature. Using Marquardt–Levenberg regularization, Lee and Sevick-Muraca [54] were unable to recover optical property maps in 2D or 3D synthetic data. In contrast, using the approximate extended Kalman filter (AEKF) for nonlinear systems [61–63], 3D reconstructions were possible in a large 256 cm³ volume from sparse experimental measurements [46].

18.5.2.3 Measurement Referenced to the Excitation Wave, $\Phi_x(\vec{r}_s, \vec{r}_r)$

Another practical referencing scheme utilizes measurements of excitation fluence at the fixed reference positions to be used as the normalization factors and would in turn eliminate the source strength dependency. This approach is more realistic than the measurements referenced to the background emission case because it does not require separate and impractical measurements with and without the heterogeneity.

The relationship between the experimental measurements and the simulation for a given source and detector pair is represented by

$$\frac{\Phi_{AC_m}(r_d, r_s)}{\Phi_{AC_x}^b(r_d, r_r)} = \frac{L_{AC_m}(r_d)\, G_{AC_m} \exp\left(i\left(-\theta_m(r_d) + \theta_{instr}^m\right)\right)}{L_{AC_x}(r_r)\, G_{ACx} \exp\left(i\left(-\theta_x(r_r) + \theta_{instr}^m\right)\right)} \approx \frac{L_{AC_m}(r_d)}{L_{AC_x}(r_r)} \exp\left[i\left(\theta_x(r_r) - \theta_m(r_d)\right)\right]$$

and described by the following integral equation:

$$\left. \frac{\Phi_{AC_m}\left(\vec{r}_s,\vec{r}_d\right)}{\Phi_{AC_x}\left(\vec{r}_s,\vec{r}_r\right)} \right]_{exp} = \frac{1}{\Phi_{AC_x}\left(\vec{r}_s,\vec{r}_r\right)} \int_{\Omega} \frac{\alpha}{D_m\left(1-i\omega\tau\right)} G_f\left(\vec{r}_d,\vec{r}\right)\Phi_x\left(\vec{r}_s,\vec{r}\right)\mu_{a_{x\to m}}(\vec{r})d\Omega \tag{18.71}$$

where the referenced measurement is represented by $\left. \dfrac{\Phi_{AC_m}\left(\vec{r}_s,\vec{r}_d\right)}{\Phi_{AC_x}\left(\vec{r}_s,\vec{r}_r\right)} \right]_{exp}$.

Here, $\Phi_{AC_x}\left(\vec{r}_s,\vec{r}_r\right)$ represents the excitation fluence detected at a fixed reference position, $\vec{r}_r$, in response to excitation from the source position, $\vec{r}_s$.

Even though the excitation fluence, $\Phi_{AC_x}\left(\vec{r}_s,\vec{r}_r\right)$, is updated during the iteration, the Jacobian matrix can be directly calculated from Equation 18.71, and the change in $\Phi_x(\vec{r}_s,\vec{r}_r)$ is small compared to change in $\Phi_m(\vec{r}_s,\vec{r}_r)$. As the source term of the emission diffusion equation is modified after each iteration (Equation 18.57), changes in the emission fluence are greater than that of the excitation fluence. The same consequence can be inferred from the integral equation (Equation 18.71). Moreover, the phase of the emission fluence is greater than that of the excitation fluence and the normalized fluence, Φ_m/Φ_x, maintains a high phase contrast.

Owing to noise and the ill condition of the Jacobian matrix and for inverting the systems of equations, updating can be accomplished using Newton's method [64] with Marquardt–Levenberg parameters λ:

$$(J^T J + \lambda I)\Delta X = J^T \left[\left[\frac{\Phi_{AC_m}\left(\vec{r}_s,\vec{r}_d\right)}{\Phi_{AC_x}\left(\vec{r}_s,\vec{r}_r\right)} \right]^{meas} - \left[\frac{\Phi_{AC_m}\left(\vec{r}_s,\vec{r}_d\right)}{\Phi_{AC_x}\left(\vec{r}_s,\vec{r}_r\right)} \right]^{comp} \right] \tag{18.72}$$

Using excitation referencing at a single reference point, Lee and Sevick-Muraca [54] reconstructed an $8 \times 4 \times 8$ cm^3 phantom containing a $1 \times 1 \times 1$ cm^3 target with 100-fold greater ICG concentration, by using 8 excitation sources, 24 detection fibers for collecting excitation light, and 2 reference detection fibers (one on either side of the reflectance and transillumination measurements) for collecting excitation light. Figure 18.19a is the original map containing 2D slices that demark the heterogeneity placement, while Figure 18.19b is the 3D reconstructed image.

While the results in Figure 18.19 represent reconstructions based upon emission FDPM measurements relative to excitation FDPM measurements at a fixed reference position, Ntziachristos and Weissleder [53] successfully reconstructed two fluorescent targets in a 2.5 diameter, 2.5 cm long cylindrical vessel containing ICG and Cy 5.5 and using CW emission measurements referenced to excitation measurements at each of the 36 detector fibers as a result of point excitation at 24 source fibers. The high density of measurements for reconstruction of the small simulated tissue volume is troublesome for validity of the diffusion equation used in the forward solver, but is similar to that demonstrated by Yang and coworkers [34] who reconstructed ICG and DTTCI in similarly sized phantoms and mice, presumably from absolute FDPM measurements at the emission wavelength alone.

It is noteworthy that the studies of the reconstruction presented earlier assumed that the absorption and scattering properties were known a priori. However, using differential approaches coupled with Bayesian reconstruction approaches (see below), Eppstein and coworkers [65] were able to demonstrate the insensitivity of reconstructions to changes in endogenous optical properties. Using a synthetic 256 cm^3 volume containing 0.125 cm^3 targets with 10:1 contrast in absorption owing to the fluorophore and surrounded on four sides with 68 sources and 408 detection fibers, Eppstein was able to show that when the absorption cross section at the excitation wavelength, $\mu_{a_{xi}}$, varied as much as 90% and was unmodeled while the scattering coefficient, $\mu_{s_{xi}}$, varied 10% or less and was also unmodeled, the impact on the reconstruction was minimal, or negligible. Similar results have recently been shown by Roy et al. [66] who show unmodeled variations in all endogenous optical properties by as much as 50%, which did not impact reconstructions when emission FDPM measurements were individually self-referenced to excitation FDPM measurements,

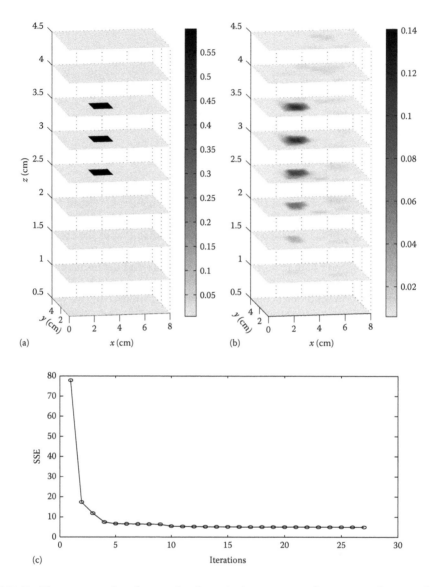

FIGURE 18.19 The reconstruction of $\mu_{a \to m}$ using the excitation wave as a reference using the integral approach and Marquardt–Levenberg reconstruction. The image was required after Figure 18.27 iterations with regularization parameters for I_{AC} ratio (ACR), $\lambda_{AC} = 1.0$, and for RPS, $\lambda_0 = 0.02$. (a) Optical property maps of true $\mu_{a \to m}$ distribution and (b) reconstructed $\mu_{a \to m}$ distribution. Peak values of $\mu_{a \to m}$ reached 0.1205 cm^{-1}. (c) Iteration versus SSE.

as were done with the CW measurements of Ntziachristos and Weissleder [53]. While it appears promising that fluorescence-enhanced optical tomography can be accomplished *without* much a priori information regarding the endogenous optical properties, these results are nonetheless on synthetic studies and need to be conducted on actual tissues of substantive and clinically relevant volumes for validation.

18.5.3 Differential Formulation of the Inverse Problem

A second approach of the full inverse imaging problem may be the differential formulation, but in reality, this time, it is rewritten for measurement $Z(\vec{r}_d, \vec{r}_s)$, whether absolute, or relative to a reference measurement at the emission or excitation wavelength, or self-referenced relative to the excitation wavelength at each detector position, $\vec{r}_d$. We term this approach the differential formulation because a small change in the predicted measurements is directly expressed in terms of a small change in the optical properties, $\Delta \mathbf{X}$, using a Jacobian matrix, $\mathbf{J}$, $\partial(\Delta Z_i)/\partial X_j$. Consider a number of detectors, M; then the error function is defined as the sum of square of errors between the measured and calculated values at detector $i = 1 \dots M$:

$$F(\mathbf{X}) = \sum_{i=1}^{M} \left[\left(Z_i \right)^{(m)} - \left(Z_i \right)^{(c)} \right]^2 = \sum_{i=1}^{M} \left[f_i(X) \right]^2 \tag{18.73}$$

We refer to each f_i as a residual and the gradients of the error function with respect to the property, $\mathbf{X}$:

$$\nabla F(\mathbf{X}) = 2\mathbf{J}^T f(X) \tag{18.74}$$

$$\nabla^2 F(\mathbf{X}) = 2\left[\mathbf{J}^T\mathbf{J} + \sum_{i=1}^{M} f_i(X)\nabla^2 f_i(X) \right] \tag{18.75}$$

Consider Taylor's expansion of function F around a small perturbation of optical properties, $\Delta \mathbf{X}$:

$$F(\mathbf{X} + \Delta\mathbf{X}) = F(\mathbf{X}) + \nabla F(\mathbf{X}) \cdot \Delta\mathbf{X} + \frac{1}{2}\Delta\mathbf{X}^T \cdot \nabla^2 F(\mathbf{X}) \cdot \Delta(\mathbf{X}) \tag{18.76}$$

which can be expressed as

$$F(\mathbf{X} + \Delta\mathbf{X}) = F(\mathbf{X}) + 2\mathbf{J}^T f(\mathbf{X}) \cdot \Delta\mathbf{X} + 2 \cdot \Delta\mathbf{X}^T \left[\mathbf{J}^T\mathbf{J} + \sum_{i=1}^{M} f_i(X)\nabla^2 f_i(X) \right] \cdot \Delta\mathbf{X} \tag{18.77}$$

and the function to be minimized, $\Phi(\Delta\mathbf{X})$, can be explicitly written as

$$\Phi(\Delta\mathbf{X}) = F(\mathbf{X} + \Delta\mathbf{X}) - F(\mathbf{X}) = 2\mathbf{J}^T f(\mathbf{X}) \cdot \Delta\mathbf{X} + 2 \cdot \Delta\mathbf{X}^T \left[\mathbf{J}^T\mathbf{J} + \sum_{i=1}^{M} f_i(X)\nabla^2 f_i(X) \right] \cdot \Delta\mathbf{X} \tag{18.78}$$

For first-order Newton's methods, the term $2 \cdot \Delta\mathbf{X}^T \left[\sum_{i=1}^{M} f_i(X)\nabla^2 f_i(X) \right] \cdot \Delta\mathbf{X}$ is neglected and the Gauss–Newton method becomes one of minimizing

$$\nabla\Phi(\Delta\mathbf{X}) \Rightarrow 0 = \mathbf{J}^T\mathbf{J} \cdot \Delta\mathbf{X} + \mathbf{J}^T f(\mathbf{X}) \tag{18.79}$$

$$\mathbf{J}^T\mathbf{J} \cdot \Delta\mathbf{X} = -\mathbf{J}^T f(\mathbf{X}) \tag{18.80}$$

The Levenberg–Marquardt method of optimization becomes

$$\left[\mathbf{J}^T\mathbf{J} + \lambda\mathbf{I} \right] \cdot \Delta X = -\mathbf{J}^T f(\mathbf{X}) \tag{18.81}$$

The gradient-based truncated Newton's method is based upon retaining the second-order terms such that Equation 18.78 becomes [47]

$$\nabla\Phi(\Delta\mathbf{X}) \Rightarrow 0 = \mathbf{J}^T f(\mathbf{X}) + \left[\mathbf{J}^T\mathbf{J} + \sum_{i=1}^{M} f_i(X)\nabla^2 f_i(X) \right] \cdot \Delta\mathbf{X} \tag{18.82}$$

or alternatively,

$$\Phi'(\Delta\mathbf{X}) \Rightarrow 0 = \nabla F(\mathbf{X}) + \nabla^2 F(\mathbf{X}) \cdot \Delta\mathbf{X} \tag{18.83}$$

Typically, first-order Newton's methods are employed with the exception of the work by Roy and Sevick-Muraca [67]. In Newton's methods, it is assumed that $\Delta\Phi = \mathbf{J} \cdot \Delta\mathbf{X}$ and the solution are found using one of the several optimization approaches. The Jacobian can be computed either directly from the stiffness matrices of the finite element formulation or simply but more computationally time consuming, from backward, forward, or central differencing approaches that compute the differences in the values of $Z(\vec{r}_d, \vec{r}_s)$ with small differences in the parameter to be updated, $X(\vec{r}_j)$. The Gauss–Newton and the Levenberg–Marquardt algorithms performed poorly in a large residual problem. Since the inverse is highly nonlinear and ill conditioned due to the error in measurement data, the residual at the solution will be large. It seems reasonable, therefore, to consider the truncated Newton method.

For the truncated Newton's method, the additional computational cost of computing the Hessian (associated with $\nabla^2 F(\mathbf{X})$) is assisted by reverse automatic differentiation [47,67]. Using synthetic data, Roy has shown the feasibility for using the technique for 3D reconstruction of lifetime, τ, and absorption coefficient $\mu_{a_{x \to m}}$ changes in frustum and slab geometries from synthetic data containing noise that mimics experimental data [51].

18.5.4 Regularization and Other Approaches for Parameter Updating

In both the integral and differential formulations of the inverse problem, the tissue to be imaged must be mathematically discretized into a series of nodes or volume elements (voxels) in order to solve these inverse problems. The unknowns of the inverse problems are then comprised of the optical properties at each node or voxel. The final image resolution is naturally related to the density nodes or voxels. However, the dimensionality of the imaging problem is directly related to the number of nodes and can easily exceed 10,000 unknowns for a 3D image. In a problem of this scale, the calculation of Jacobian matrices and matrix inversions involved in updating the optical property map is computationally intensive and contributes to the long computing times required in order to reconstruct the image. The instability arises because the measurement noise in the data or errors associated with the validity of the diffusion approximation can result in large errors in the reconstructed image. One of the greatest challenges associated with fluorescence-enhanced tomography is the propagation of error. In comparison to absorption imaging based upon measurements of excitation light, fluorescence measurements have a reduced signal level and SNR. Lee and Sevick-Muraca [68] measured the SNR for single-pixel excitation and emission frequency-domain measurements at 100 MHz to be 55 and 35 dB, respectively. In addition to the reduced signal, the noise floor of emission measurements can be expected to be elevated when excitation light leakage constitutes an increased proportion of the detected signal. Consequently, for emission tomography measurements, excitation light leakage is crucial, and interference filters that attenuate excitation light four orders of magnitude (i.e., filters of OD 4) may be clearly insufficient. Excitation light leakage will be a significant problem when emission measurements are conducted in tissue regions in which the target is absent and fluorescent contrast agents are not activated. Unfortunately, this type of error is not present in synthetic studies and is undoubtedly underestimated in the vast proportion of tomography investigations to date.

18.5.4.1 Regularization

Regularization is a mathematical tool used to stabilize the solution of Newton's inverse problem and to make it more tolerant to measurement error. Regularization approaches will play an important role in the development of suitable algorithms for actual clinical screening. For example, when discretized, the differential and integral general formulations result in a set of linear Newton's equations generally denoted by $AY = Z$, where Y are the unknown optical properties and Z are the measurements.

This system is commonly solved in the least squares sense where the object function $Q = \|AY - Z\|^2 + \lambda \|Y\|^2$ is minimized, where λ is called the regularization parameter. The minimization of this function results in $Y = (A^TA + \lambda I)^{-1}A^TZ$. The regularization parameter is generally chosen either arbitrarily or by a Levenberg–Marquardt algorithm so that the object function is minimized [69]. Thus, the choice of regularization parameter is through a priori information and adds another degree of freedom to the inverse problem solution. While this section is not meant to be a mathematical treatise of inverse algorithm and regularization approaches, we nonetheless point out that in a recent work by Pogue and coworkers [70], they presented a physically based rationale for empirically choosing a spatially varying regularization parameter in order to improve image reconstruction.

18.5.4.2 Bayesian Regularization

Eppstein and coworkers [45,46,49,65] use actual measurement error statistics to govern the choice of varying regularization parameters in their Kalman filter implementation to optical tomography. In their work, they developed the novel Bayesian reconstruction technique, called automatic progressive parameter-reducing inverse zonation and estimation (APPRIZE), specifically for groundwater problems and adapted them to fluorescence-enhanced optical tomography [61–63]. Unique components of the APPRIZE method are an AEKF, which employs measurement error and parameter uncertainty to regularize the inversion and compensate for spatial variability in SNR, and a unique approach to stabilize and accelerate convergence, called data-driven zonation (DDZ). Using the notation $(\Delta X, f(X))$ as described in Section 18.5.3, here, Newton's solution is formulated as [49]

$$\Delta \mathbf{X} = \left[\left[\mathbf{J}^T (\mathbf{Q} + \mathbf{R})^{-1} \mathbf{J} + \mathbf{P}_{xx}^{-1} \right]^{-1} \cdot \mathbf{J}^T (\mathbf{Q} + \mathbf{R})^{-1} \right] \cdot f(\mathbf{X}) \tag{18.84}$$

where
  Q is the system noise covariance that describes the inherent model mismatch between the forward model (the diffusion equation) and the actual physics of the problem
  R is the covariance of the measurement error that is actually acquired in the measurement set
  $\mathbf{P}_{xx}$ is the recursively updated error covariance of the parameters, **X**, being estimated from the measurement error, $f(\mathbf{X})$

The use of this spatially and dynamically variant covariance matrix results in the minimization of the variance of the estimated parameters taking into account the measurement and system error.

The novel Bayesian minimum-variance reconstruction algorithm compensates for the spatial variability in SNR that must be expected to occur in actual NIR contrast-enhanced diagnostic medical imaging. Figure 18.20 illustrates the image reconstruction of a 256 cm³ tissue-mimicking phantom containing none, one, or two 1 cm³ heterogeneities with 50- to 100-fold greater concentration of ICG dye over background levels. The spatial parameter estimate of absorption owing to the dye was reconstructed from only 160–296 surface reference measurements of emission light at 830 nm in response to incident 785 nm excitation light modulated at 100 MHz. Measurement error of acquired fluence at fluorescent emission wavelengths is shown to be highly variable.

Another important feature of the Bayesian APPRIZE algorithm is the use of DDZ. With DDZ, spatially adjacent voxels with similarly updated estimates are identified through cluster analysis and merged into larger stochastic parameter *zones* via random field union [71]. Thus, as the iterative process proceeds, the number of unknown parameters, **X**, decreases dramatically, and the size, shape, value, and covariance of the different *parameter zones* are simultaneously determined in a data-driven fashion. Other approaches to reduce the dimensionality of the problems involve concurrent NIR optical imaging with MRI [72–74] and ultrasound [75] to compartmentalize tissue volumes and to reduce the number of parameters to be recovered in the optical image reconstruction.

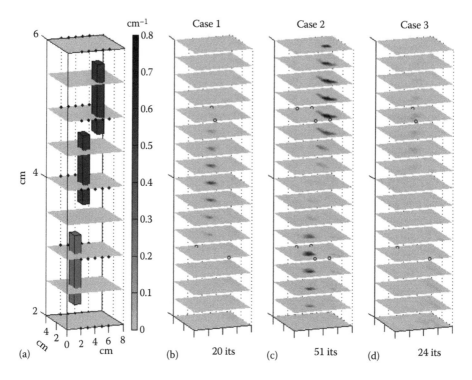

FIGURE 18.20 Image reconstruction with APPRIZE. (a) The initial homogeneous estimate discretized onto the $9 \times 17 \times 17$ grid used for the initial inversion iteration and shown with the true locations of the 3 heterogeneities and the 50 detectors (*small dots*). (b) Case 1: the reconstructed absorption due to the middle fluorescing heterogeneity, interpolated onto the $17 \times 33 \times 33$ grid used for prediction and shown with the locations of the four sources used (*open circles*). (c) Case 2: the reconstructed absorption due to the top and bottom fluorescing heterogeneities shown with the locations of the eight sources used (*open circles*). (d) Case 3: the reconstructed absorption of a homogeneous phantom shown with the locations of the four sources used (*open circles*). Although the phantoms and reconstructions were actually 8 cm in the vertical dimension, only the center four vertical cm is shown here. (Reproduced from Eppstein, M.J. et al., *Proc. Natl. Acad. Sci. USA*, 99, 9619, 2002. With permission.)

18.5.4.3 Simply Bounded Constrained Optimization

Imposing restrictions on the ill-posed problem can transform it to a well-posed problem as discussed earlier. Regularization is one method to reduce the ill posedness of the problem [76]. In the optical tomography problem, its solution, that is, the optical properties of tissue, must satisfy certain constraints, and imposing these conditions in itself can regularize or stabilize the problem. Imposing these constraints explicitly restricts the solution sets and can restore uniqueness.

Provencher and Vogel [76] have suggested two techniques: (1) prior knowledge and (2) parsimony for well posedness of the problem. The first condition requires that all prior physical knowledge about the solution be included in the model. The second condition protects against the introduction of nonphysical phenomena. Tikhonov and Arsenin [77] also suggested that, to obtain a unique and stable solution from the data, supplementary information should be used so that the inverse problem becomes well posed. The basic principle of using a priori knowledge of the properties of the inverse problem is to restrict the space of possible solutions so that the data uniquely determine a stable solution.

In his work, Roy showed that the constrained optimization technique, which places simple bounds on a physical parameter to be estimated, maybe more appropriate for solving the fluorescence-enhanced optical tomography problem [48]. Specifically, a range of fluorescent optical properties is physically defined for the problem and the recovered parameter, **X**, must always be positive. Specifically, he demonstrated the use of the bounding parameter, ε, not only as a means to regularize and accelerate convergence but also as a means to set the level of optical property contrast that is to be reconstructed using referenced emission measurements [66]. Here, the possible values of parameter estimates are stated to lie between upper and lower bounds. In the first pass of the iterative solution, the optical property map is recovered and parameter estimates that lie within the upper and lower bounds plus and minus a small bounding parameter, ε, are recovered and held constant for the next iteration. In this manner, the number of unknowns decreases with iteration. Indeed, the value of the bounding parameter can be used to set the resolution and the performance of the tomographic image. For example, if the bounding parameter is large, then the tomographic image will *filter* out artifacts not associated with the target, while if the bounding parameter is small, the tomographic image may sensitively capture artifacts and heterogeneity that is not necessarily associated with the target. Figure 18.21 illustrates the reconstruction

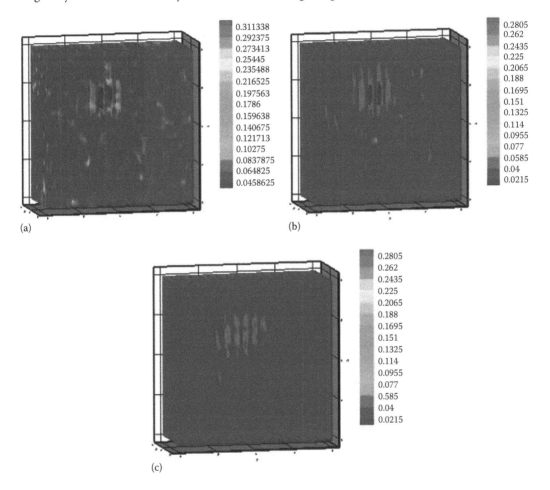

(a)   (b)

(c)

FIGURE 18.21 (See color insert.) A 3D reconstruction from simply bound truncated Newton's method. (a) Actual distribution of fluorophore absorption coefficient of background tissue variability of endogenous (50%) and exogenous (500%) properties; (b) reconstructed fluorophore absorption coefficient of background tissue variability of endogenous (50%) and exogenous (500%) properties using relative measurement of the emission fluence with respect to the excitation fluence at the same detector point, $\varepsilon = 0.0001$; (c) reconstructed fluorophore absorption coefficient of background tissue variability of endogenous (50%) and exogenous (500%) properties using relative measurement of the emission fluence with respect to the excitation fluence at the same detector point. (Reproduced from Roy, R. et al., *IEEE Trans. Med. Imaging*, 22, 824, 2003. With permission.)

using the simply bounded truncated Newton's method, which shows that, as the bounding parameter is increased, the recovered image becomes less sensitive to the background *noise*. This approach may have significant application for increasing the target to background signals, an issue with nuclear imaging that impairs tomographic reconstructions.

18.6 Fluorescent Contrast Agents for Optical Tomography*

Table 18.1 provides a chronological listing of studies reported in the literature over the past decade, which involve a number of different fluorescent contrast agents [23,33,34,72,78–112]. While the studies have progressed from using photodynamic agents; freely diffusable agents, such as ICG; fluorochromes conjugated to monoclonal antibodies (MAbs) and their fragments; small-peptide targeting agents similar to those employed in nuclear imaging; and, finally, activatable and *reporting agents*, unfortunately, the translation of these agents to human clinical studies has been limited. Furthermore, investigations have been largely confined to superficial or subcutaneous tumors where the true advantages of NIR fluorescent agents, that is, deep tissue penetration and optical tomography, cannot be aptly demonstrated. Nonetheless, the strategies for NIR fluorescent contrast agent have been impressive and have included using simple blood-pooling agents to highlight hypervascularity, employing contrast provided by pharmacokinetic model parameter estimates of uptake, and designing agents that specifically target membrane receptors of cells lining neovasculatures as well as the neoplastic cells that the vasculature feeds. Strategies that focus upon lysosomal activity and enzyme cleavage for fluorochrome activation and mediation of fluorescence decay as well as for fluorochrome accumulation specific to cancer cells have also been demonstrated. Table 18.1 outlines these fluorochromes used within in vivo studies. When available, the chronological listing also notes the excitation and emission wavelengths used, the incident illumination, measurement geometry and type, as well as the number of fluorochrome molecules used to detect a signal. The fluorophores are broadly classified into PDT agents, nontargeting blood-pooling agents, agents that *report* or sense, targeting agents based upon immunodiagnostics and small-peptide conjugation, and activatable agents.

18.6.1 PDT Agents

Starting with the area of photodynamic imaging, the early studies relating to fluorescence-enhanced imaging date back to 1991 and focused upon evaluating the spatial distribution as well as the pharmacokinetics of therapeutic photodynamic (PDT) agents for dosimetry purposes. Measurements were typically conducted in tumor-bearing mice with total agent administration between 0.1 and 90 μM/kg bw using area illumination and CCD camera detection. PDT agents are likely candidates for fluorescence-enhanced imaging, more than likely due to their existing FDA investigational new drug (IND) applications for therapeutic use. The ability to obtain an IND for a diagnostic agent previously approved for therapeutic use enhances the opportunity for fluorescence-enhanced optical imaging. Yet, despite the attractiveness for their current and pending INDs, photodynamic agents do *not* possess the excitation and emission spectra favorable for fluorescent contrast agents for imaging deep tissues. First, in order to maximize penetration depth into tissues, excitation needs to be between 750 and 800 nm, and the Stokes shift needs to be significant (~50 nm) in order to enable discrimination of the small fluorescent component from the overwhelming large component of excitation light. An insufficient Stokes shift of 10 nm or less complicates the process for rejecting multiply scattered light as the efficiency of filters cannot be guaranteed. Next, the fluorochrome for systemic administration should not experience a net lifetime or long-lived decay kinetics that exceed the photon *time of flight*, as described in Section 18.2.3. For these reasons, the usefulness of PDT agents for contrast (and for therapy) is largely limited to epithelial linings of accessible tissues and not for deep tissues. However, one notable use of a PDT agent

---

* Adapted from Sevick-Muraca et al. [15].

for contrast-enhanced surface imaging involves the use of its metabolic by-product. Using exogenous δ-aminolevulinic acid (ALA) for natural production of protoporphyrin IX, Eker et al. [94] showed the ability to detect adenomatous polyps of the colon in humans and provided evidence to suggest the ability to discriminate between hyperplastic and adenomatous polyps. While excitation at 337, 405, and 436 nm does not classify this agent as an NIR probe for deep tissue penetration, this study is nonetheless significant in that it employs a natural *reporting* mechanism in which the nonfluorescent ALA is hypermetabolized in diseased tissue to the fluorescent porphyrin form.

18.6.2 Nontargeting, Blood-Pooling Agents

ICG, with its 778/830 nm excitation/emission maxima, was an early contrast agent choice used as a blood-pooling agent for assessing hypervascularity and *leaky* angiogenic vessels of high permeability. While many advances in dye development have accelerated within the past 2 years, the majority of studies investigating NIR fluorescent contrast agents have been limited to ICG, a compound with FDA approval for systemic administration for investigating hepatic function [113] and retinal angiography [114]. ICG is excited at 780 nm and emits at 830 nm. It has an extinction coefficient of 130,000 M^{-1} cm^{-1}, a fluorescent lifetime of 0.56 ns, and a quantum efficiency of 0.016 for the 780/830 nm excitation/emission wavelengths in water [115]. It should be noted that these values are not necessarily what will be observed in vivo.

When dissolved in blood, ICG binds to proteins such as albumin and lipoproteins. The absorption maximum shifts up to 805 nm but the wavelength of maximum fluorescence is stable near 830 nm, and the fluorescent intensity is dependent upon its concentration [116,117]. ICG is a nonspecific agent and is cleared rapidly from the blood, but tends to collect in regions of dense vascularity through extravasation. Devoiselle et al. [88] demonstrated the use of ICG in an emulsion preparation at an administration of 10 μmol/kg bw in a tumor-bearing rat in order to measure its prolonged pharmacokinetics, while Reynolds et al. [95] used free ICG (1.3 μmol/kg bw) as a fluorescent agent in canines to image spontaneous mammary disease on a veterinary outpatient basis.

In a study by Reynolds et al. [95], frequency-domain approaches were employed whereby the canine mammary chain area was illuminated with intensity-modulated light and the resulting amplitude of the generated fluorescent light that propagated to the surface was imaged by a gain-modulated image-intensified camera. The approach enabled rejection of room light and provided the first demonstration of fluorescence-enhanced imaging in a spontaneous tumor as in a large animal (Figure 18.22). Since canines are the only other species to naturally encounter mammary and prostate cancer besides man [118], this is an excellent animal model in which to assess the potential of detecting diseased tissue via a contrast agent. However, penetration depths are nonetheless limited to 0.5–2 cm, still not meeting the deep imaging potential of fluorescence-enhanced optical imaging.

In their measurements of the canine mammary chain, a homodyned, gain-modulated image intensifier was employed as described in Section 18.3.2. Excitation was accomplished by illuminating the tissue surface with a 4 cm diameter expanded beam of a 20 mW, 780 nm laser, which was modulated at 100 MHz. Figure 18.23 shows the DC, amplitude, phase, and modulation ratio (I_{AC}/I_{DC}) of 830 nm wavelength emitted from the left fourth mammary gland with a palpable 1.2 cm (longitudinal) by 0.5 cm (axial) papillary adenoma located approximately 1 cm deep within the mammary tissue. The image was acquired 23 min following i.v. injection of l mg/kg ICG. The diseased region is clearly shown in the raw, unprocessed DC, amplitude, phase, and modulation images.

The use of ICG for optical tomography has already been identified by the Chance group at the University of Pennsylvania. In a combined time-domain and MRI imaging study of 11 patients, Ntziachristos et al. [72] administered 0.2 mg/kg ICG i.v. and conducted measurements in response to pulsed excitation at 780 nm. Their time-domain system involved pulsed laser diodes at 780 and 830 multiplexed into 24 source fibers and collected at 8 detection points [119]. Using the MRI images to validate their integral inversion results, they were able to reconstruct images of an infiltrating ductal carcinoma owing to the enhanced signature from the vascular blood pooling of ICG. Unfortunately,

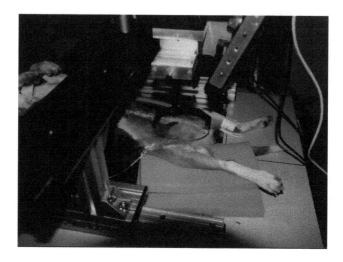

FIGURE 18.22 Photograph illustrating the use of an incident expanded beam on the mammary chain of the canine to excite systemically administered fluorophore and to collect the emission of generated light from the tissue surface. (Reproduced from Hawrysz, D.J. and Sevick-Muraca, E.M., *Neoplasia*, 2, 388, 2000. With permission.)

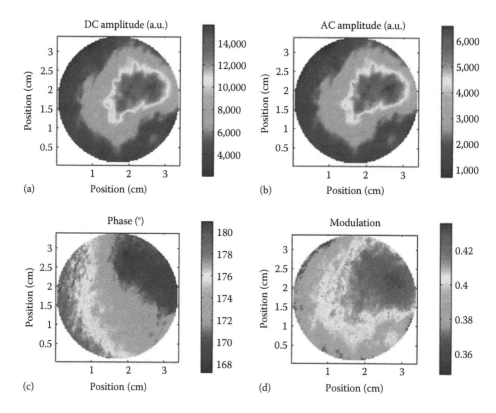

FIGURE 18.23 **(See color insert.)** The 128×128 pixel-based imaging of 830 nm fluorescence of (a) CW DC, (b) amplitude I_{AC}, (c) phase delay, and (d) modulation ratio of the detected fluorescence generated from the area cranial of the left fourth mammary gland of a canine. Illumination was accomplished with an expanded 780 nm laser diode. Modulation frequency was 100 MHz. (Reproduced from Reynolds, J.S. et al., *Photochem. Photobiol.*, 70, 87, 1999. With permission.)

fluorescence signals were not acquired, due possibly to the low SNR available with TDPM measurements, and the images were reconstructed from signals at the incident wavelength.

Later, using the modulated ICCD system, Gurfinkel et al. [99] employed FDPM measurements with ICG as a blood-pooling agent as well as with a photodynamic agent, carotene-conjugated 2-devinyl-2-(1-hexyloxyethyl) pyropheophorbide (HPPH-car), in order to provide the difference in pharmacokinetics. The time course of images was clearly able to discriminate between the nonselective uptake of the ICG blood-pooling agent, whose contrast was due mainly to the density of the microvasculature associated with the disease, and the specific uptake of the HPPH agent, whose uptake is hypothesized to be mediated with the enhanced overexpression of low-density lipoprotein (LDL) receptors on the surface of cancer cells and the association of HPPH and LDL in the blood compartment. Figure 18.24 represents the values of the AC intensity as a function of time at a single point in the area detection corresponding to the subcutaneous tumor following i.v. injection of ICG as well as HPPH-car. Upon fitting the time course of AC intensity measurements with pharmacokinetic models, a map of uptake parameters shown in Figure 18.25 shows the ability to enhance optical contrast based on pharmacokinetics as is currently done in MRI. In an effort to tune the pharmacokinetics of cyanine dyes by changing the level of hydrophobicity/philicity, Licha et al. [100] and Ebert et al. [109] showed that a hydrophilic derivative of cyanine dyes could enhance uptake and be detected using single point illumination and detection at the excitation wavelength (0.5 µmol/kg bw) and area illumination and area detection at the emission wavelength (2 µmol/kg bw).

In addition to using ICG as a means for assessing hypervascularity associated with cancer, ICG may also be used to assess lymph flow. Figure 18.26 is an in vivo ICCD image of a canine-acquired cranial to the nipple of the left fifth gland 30 min after ICG injection. While the imaged area was not associated with a palpable nodule, pathologic examination confirmed that the fluorescence was attributed to a blood vessel that bifurcated approximately 1 cm below the tissue surface in an area cranial to a regional lymph node. Figure 18.27 represents the in vivo FDPM images of the fluorescence generated from the area of the right fifth mammary gland 43 min after injection of the ICG. Pathologic examination showed that the fluorescent source in this image corresponds to the regional lymph node.

The ability to detect fluorescence signals originating from regional lymph nodes suggests that FDPM fluorescence imaging coupled with improved fluorescent dyes could provide a valuable diagnostic method for assessing regional lymph node status in breast cancer patients. Lymph node status in breast cancer patients can be a powerful predictor of recurrence and survival, and the number of lymph nodes with metastases provides crucial prognostic information regarding the choice of adjuvant therapy [120]. Currently, lymph node involvement is assessed by dissection and subsequent pathological examination, but researchers are investigating the use of other diagnostic modalities including MRI, x-ray computed tomography, and sonography [120]. More recently, nuclear imaging of a technetium-99 sulfur colloid injected into the tissue area of a known breast tumor has been used to identify the sentinel lymph nodes. With the simultaneous or sequential injection of a blue dye to visually aid in its location, the sentinel lymph node can then be surgically removed [120,121]. Moreover, with NIR fluorescent agents, sentinel lymph node mapping could possibly be achieved without the use of the radionucleotide and without the introduction of a second dye to aid in surgical incision. Furthermore, with the development of peptide-, protein-, or antibody-conjugated fluorescent dye described below, there exists the potential for nonsurgical, optical diagnosis of nodal involvement.

Using intracranial injection of ICG bound to lipoprotein, Sakatani and coworkers [91] also showed the use of the ICG to map the cerebrospinal fluid pathways in a rat. Area illumination using a 100 mW laser diode and area detection with a cooled CCD camera were sufficient to detect meaningful images of fluid pathways following injection of 554 pmol of ICG.

18.6.3 Nontargeting, Contrast Agents That Report or Sense Environment

While not employing the favorable excitation/emission characteristics, the studies of Mordon et al. [86] are especially intriguing in that they are the first studies to employ a *reporting* dye, or a dye whose emission characteristics varied with tissue milieu. Specifically, they employed the pH-sensitive dye of 5,6-CF

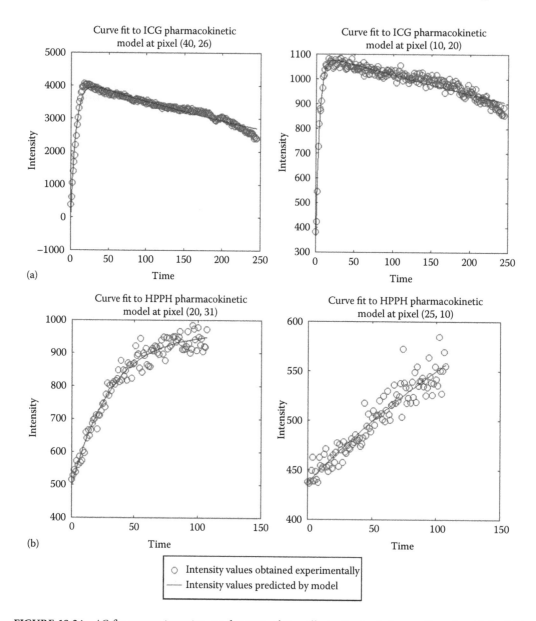

FIGURE 18.24 AC fluorescent intensity as a function of time illustrating typical curve fits using (a) the ICG pharmacokinetic model and (b) the HPPH-car pharmacokinetic model. The symbols denote actual measurements, while the solid curve denotes the model fit. (Reproduced from Gurfinkel, M. et al., *Photochem. Photobiol.*, 72, 94, 2000. With permission.)

carboxyfluorescein (BCECF), which is a ratiometric dye sensitive to pH. Using CW, spectrally resolved measurements of fluorescence resulting from area illumination with excitation light at 465 and 490 nm, they employed area detection using an intensified CCD camera, to determine changes in fluorescence with change in wavelength of the excitation light. Using an in vitro calibration of the ratiometric dye, Mordon and coworkers were able to correlate the 2D fluorescent images to provide 2D images of tumor pH in an s.c. mouse model. While CW measurements are not time-dependent methods, this study did not directly measure changes in the fluorescence decay kinetics, but rather used spectral ratiometric changes to demark the change in the radiative relaxation rates that arose owing to acidotic tissue conditions.

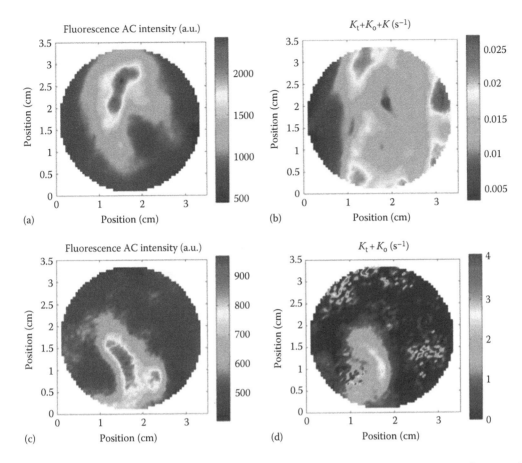

FIGURE 18.25 **(See color insert.)** (a) Fluorescence I_{AC} intensity map from ICG delineating diseased tissue and (b) map of pharmacokinetic uptake parameters obtained from fitting the time sequences of fluorescence intensity images showing no specific uptake of ICG in diseased tissue. (c) Fluorescence AC intensity map from HPPH-car delineating diseased tissue and (d) map of pharmacokinetic uptake parameters obtained from fitting the time sequences of fluorescence intensity images showing specific uptake of HPPH-car in diseased tissue. (Reproduced from Gurfinkel, M. et al., *Photochem. Photobiol.*, 72, 94, 2000. With permission.)

18.6.4 Targeting, Contrast Agents: Immunophotodiagnosis

Folli et al. [80] were the first to demonstrate the use of NIR targeting agents by coupling an indopentamethinecyanin dye coupled to a MAb E48 for targeting squamous cell carcinoma in the upper respiratory tract in mice. On the order of 600 pmol of conjugated dye molecules was injected into mice and imaged postmortem using simple planar illumination and photography. This was the first demonstration of NIR immunophotodiagnosis that followed prior work to employ non-NIR, fluorescein-labeled antibodies targeted against carcinoembryonic antigen (CEA) in mouse [78] and clinical studies [79]. The study was repeated by Neri [92] who used generated antibodies targeted to oncofetal fibronectin (B-FN), which is present in the angiogenic vessels of neoplasms, but is not so in mature vessels. Further emphasizing the use of NIR fluorochromes for deep tissue penetration for photoimmunodiagnosis, Ballou et al. [87,93] conjugated the cyanine dye class of Cy3, Cy5, Cy5.5, and Cy7 fluorochromes and not unsurprisingly found they could probe more deeply with the Cy7-conjugated MAbs in living tumor-bearing mice. They were able to image targeted delivery of fluorochromes of 40 pmol to 6 nmol/kg bw and 600 pmol/animal using area illumination and an intensified or cooled CCD camera. More recently, Soukos et al. [112] employed a 7,12-dimethylbenz(a)anthracene (DMBA)-induced tumor in the hamster

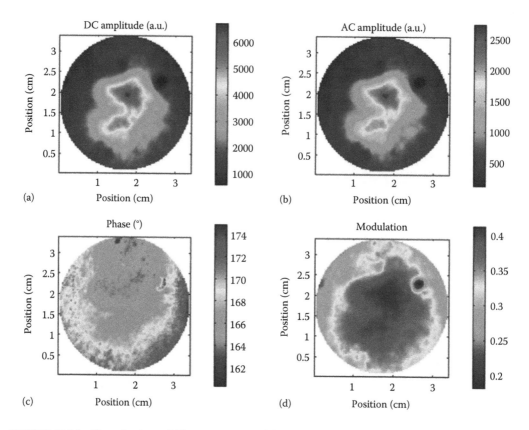

FIGURE 18.26 **(See color insert.)** The 128 × 128 pixel-based imaging of 830 nm fluorescence of (a) CW I_{DC}, (b) amplitude I_{AC}, (c) phase delay, and (d) modulation ratio of the detected fluorescence generated from the area cranial of the left fifth mammary gland of a canine. Illumination was accomplished with an expanded 780 nm laser diode. Modulation frequency was 100 MHz. (Reproduced from Reynolds, J.S. et al., *Photochem. Photobiol.*, 70, 87, 1999. With permission.)

cheek pouch model and showed the ability to target cyanine dye to express endothelial growth factor receptor (EGFR) using the anti-EGFR MAb (C225) in surface illumination and detection. Approximately 3.3 nmol of fluorochrome was employed in each animal.

18.6.5 Targeting, Contrast Agents: Small-Peptide Conjugations

A significant advancement in the design of optical contrast agents mimicked those used in other medical imaging modalities. Achilefu et al. [104–106] and Bugaj et al. [103] used area illumination and area CCD detection in tumor-bearing rats in order to detect ~6–7 µmol/kg b.w. of cyanine dye conjugated to small peptides for targeting somatostatin and bombesin receptors. One commercial nuclear diagnostic agent, namely, Octreoscan®, is based upon targeting of the somatostatin receptor that is overexpressed in neuroendocrine tumors. Bugaj and coworkers showed that the optical imaging using the derivatized and peptide-conjugated ICG, cytate, is similar to the radiolabeled peptide analog for somatostatin. Similar results were reported for using the peptide-conjugated derivative of ICG, cybesin, which is similar to the radiolabeled peptide analog for bombesin. Becker et al. [107] reported similar work in tumor-bearing mice with detection limits reduced to 0.02 µmol/kg b.w. using a similar targeting construct. In their work, they conjugated the indodicarbocyanine (IDCC) dyes and the indotricarbocyanine (ITCC) dyes with analogs of somatostatin, somatostatin-14, and

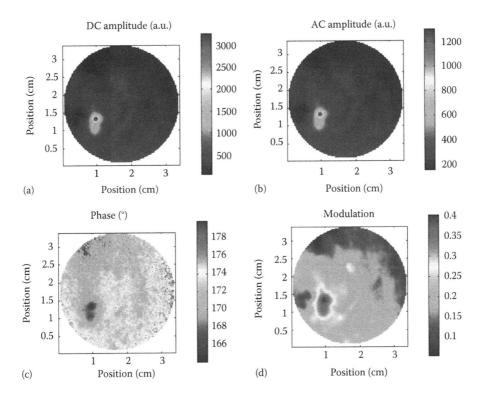

FIGURE 18.27 **(See color insert.)** The 128×128 pixel-based imaging of 830 nm fluorescence of (a) CW DC, (b) amplitude I_{AC}, (c) phase delay, and (d) modulation ratio of the detected fluorescence generated from a lymph node in the area of the right fifth mammary gland. Illumination was accomplished with an expanded 780 nm laser diode. Modulation frequency was 100 MHz. (Reproduced from Reynolds, J.S. et al., *Photochem. Photobiol.*, 70, 87, 1999. With permission.)

octreotate. In another approach, Becker and coworkers [96,98] followed the targeting approach previously employed for methotrexate and PDTs, MRI gadolinium and magnetic particle contrast by using human serum albumin (HSA), and transferrin (Tf) coupled to ITCC dyes. While Tf binds to specific cell-surface receptors, HSA binds nonspecifically. Their studies show the contrast enhancement of targeting specificity using the Tf–ITCC.

In another study involving peptide conjugation, Zaheer and coworkers [122] conjugated a bisphosphonate derivative, pamidronate, which exhibits specific binding to hydroxyapatite to an indocyanine (IR) dye to image bone structure in hairless mouse. The system may be capable of NIR detection of osteoblastic activity, enabling NIR imaging of skeletal development, coronary atherosclerosis, and other diseases.

18.6.6 Reporting or Sensing Contrast Agents

A novel *reporting* optical contrast design was reported by Weissleder and colleagues [23] who employed fluorophore Cy5.5 loaded onto a polylysine backbone with methoxypolyethylene glycol polymer. When conjugated to the polymer backbone in high concentration, the fluorochrome tends to quench itself. However, when the polymer backbone is cleaved by cathepsin B or H, lysosomal proteases whose activity may be enhanced in cancer cells, the fluorochromes become free and radiatively relax to produce fluorescence. In contrast to the small-peptide-conjugated dyes, this system requires fluorochrome internalization. The pioneering work enabled detection of 10 μmol of agent or 250 pmol of fluorochrome administered per tumor-bearing animal and represented the first time an optical contrast agent based upon an internalization construct had been demonstrated. Along the same lines, another agent that reported on the basis of protease activity was developed using the same design principles. Bremer et al. [108] coupled matrix metalloproteinase-2 (MMP-2) peptide substrates onto a polylysine polymer backbone and onto the peptides further conjugated by Cy 5.5. The fluorochromes were sufficiently packed to be quenched upon activation. Upon action of the proteinase on the peptide, the Cy 5.5 was freed and able to radiatively relax, reporting proteinase activity. MMPs are overexpressed in cancers, and MMP-2 in particular has been identified as being responsible for the collagen IV degradation, which is the major component of basement membranes. The MMP-2 activity is thought to be responsible for the pathogenesis of cancer, including spread, metastasis, and angiogenesis. Using area illumination and detection, as little as 167 pmol per animal resulted in detected fluorescence to measure MMP activity in vivo for directing the therapeutic use of proteinase activity.

18.6.7 Combined Targeting and Reporting Dyes

Finally, Licha and coworkers [123] sought to combine fluorochrome targeting using membrane receptors, such as transferrin or presumably the somatostatin and bombesin receptors with an acid-cleavable construct that would enable internalization of the fluorochromes in the lysosomal compartments and recycling of the receptors. Such constructs to augment the accumulation and therefore concentrate the signal from the targeting fluorochrome would only be enhanced if the contrast agent has a long half-life in the circulation. Coupling these cyanine dyes to different acid-cleavable hydrazone links that were bound to peptides, proteins, and antibodies, this group furthermore sought to develop a pH-sensitive contrast agent whose fluorescence is mediated by tumor acidosis.

In another innovative development, Huber et al. [124] synthesized bifunctional contrast agents containing a metal chelator for binding of a paramagnetic ion such as gadolinium and a conjugated fluorescent dye such as tetramethylrhodamine in order to combine optical imaging and MRI of experimental animals. While Rhodamine excites again within the visible with maximum absorbance at 547 nm and emission at 572 nm, the approach was successful for imaging of *Xenopus laevis* embryos. With the conjugation of an NIR excitable dye, the potential to develop bifunctional contrast agents for deep tissue medical imaging could also be realized. Again the reader should be cautious, however, in assessing contrast agent studies conducted in mice and rats. These tissue volumes are not comparable to those in humans, and it is unlikely that emission signals at these wavelengths can be detected with sufficient SNR for image reconstruction in large volumes.

18.6.8 Summary

In summary, the approaches for fluorescent contrast agent development have to date focused upon the following:

- Blood-pooling agents that are specific to increased microvessel density in neovascularized tumors
- Targeting agents based upon
  - Immunophotodiagnosis
  - Small-peptide conjugations targeting overexpressed receptors

  whose location of action is directed to
  - Membrane receptors of endothelial cells that line angiogenic vessels of tumors
  - Membrane receptors of cancer cells
- Reporting agents that change their fluorescence decay kinetics either through self-quenching or through environmental changes associated with
  - Interstitial pH
  - Membrane-associated proteases and receptors
  - Lysosomal, enzymatic degradation

In addition, from the summary of the literature reports presented in Table 18.1, one can conclude the following:

- Fluorescence-enhanced optical imaging has not been demonstrated on large tissue volumes that are scalable to the clinic.
- The minimum number of fluorochrome molecules reported detected in a mouse or rat is 167 pmol.
- Favorable excitation and emission spectra are currently achievable using only the cyanine dye family.

Table 18.1 also contains limited references to endogenous fluorescence-enhanced contrast owing to green fluorescence protein–expressing tumors. In these systems, the green fluorescent protein has been transduced into cancer cell lines to *report* tumor and metastases as well as their response to therapy. While the approach uses similar detection technology, it is not succumb to the excitation light rejection issues that can plaque fluorescence-enhanced contrast imaging. We present literature in this area for completeness.

In the following section, we summarize the theory and mathematics, which enable us to predict the success of optical imaging using CW, time-domain, and frequency-domain approaches as well as to develop the tomographic algorithms for fluorescence-enhanced optical tomography.

18.7 Challenges for NIR Fluorescence-Enhanced Imaging and Tomography

In the earlier sections, an overview of the status of fluorescence-enhanced optical imaging was presented. The opportunity to develop an emission-based tomographic imaging modality similar to that provided by nuclear imaging but without the use of radionucleotides is offered by NIR fluorescent agents. Yet the added challenge for NIR fluorescence-enhanced imaging over nuclear imaging is that, unlike nuclear techniques, an activating or excitation signal must first be delivered to the contrast agent before there is registration of the emission signal from the tissue. Preliminary data from animals (Table 18.1) and phantoms (not presented herein) suggest that penetration depth and sensitivity may very well be comparable to nuclear techniques. A side-by-side comparison of NIR fluorescence-enhanced imaging with nuclear imaging is needed before the comparative performance can be ascertained.

Another opportunity for optical imaging is the ability for tomographic reconstruction and additional diagnostic information based upon the fluorescence decay kinetics of smartly designed probes. Tomography of large tissue-simulating volume has been demonstrated from experimental data as well as synthetic data as reviewed herein (Table 18.2), albeit with the rather inconvenient point source and point detector geometries. The single point source and detector geometry is a *throwback* to NIR optical tomography from endogenous contrast studies and may not be the appropriate geometry for fluorescence-enhanced optical imaging, especially when transillumination through large tissues is required. Nonetheless, the tomographic algorithms as reviewed in Section 18.5 are already established for these systems. The challenge for the future is to develop tomographic algorithms for illumination and detection that are clinically feasible and adaptable for hybrid, nuclear imaging.

While the young area of NIR fluorescence-enhanced optical imaging is less than a decade old, the developments are apt to continue for the coming decade, hopefully resulting in an adjuvant tomographic imaging modality for nuclear imaging.

Acknowledgments

The review is supported in parts from the National Institutes of Health grants R01CA67176 and R01CA88082 and the State of Texas Advanced Research/Advanced Technology Program.

References

1. Lakowicz, J.R. *Principles of Fluorescence Spectroscopy*. Plenum Press, New York, 1983.
2. Sevick-Muraca, E.M.; Burch, C.L. Origin of phosphorescence re-emitted from tissues. *Opt. Lett.* 1994, *19*, 1928–1930.
3. Patterson, M.S.; Pogue, B.W. Mathematical model for time-resolved and frequency-domain fluorescence spectroscopy in biological tissue. *Appl. Opt.* 1994, *33*, 1963–1964.
4. Sevick, E.M.; Chance, B.; Leigh, J.; Maris, M.; Nioka, S. Quantitation of time-resolved and frequency-resolved optical-spectra for the determination of tissue oxygenation. *Anal. Biochem.* 1991, *195*(2), 330–351.
5. Haskell, R.C.; Svassand, L.O.; Tsay, T.-T.; Feng, T.-C.; McAdams, M.S.; Tromberg, B.J. Boundary conditions for the diffusion equation in radiative transfer. *J. Opt. Soc. Am. A, Opt. Image Sci. Vis.* 1994, *11*, 2727–2741.
6. Keijzer, M.; Star, W.M.; Storchi, P.R.M. Optical diffusion in layered media. *Appl. Opt.* 1988, *27*, 1820–1824.
7. Patterson, M.S.; Chance, B.; Wilson, B. Time resolved reflectance and transmittance for the non-invasive measurement of tissue optical properties. *Appl. Opt.* 1989, *28*, 2331–2336.
8. Hielscher, A.H.; Jacques, S.L.; Wang, L.; Tittel, F.K. The influence of boundary conditions on the accuracy of diffusion theory in time-resolved reflectance spectroscopy of biological tissues. *Phys. Med. Biol.* 1995, *40*, 1957–1975.
9. Farrell, T.J.; Patterson, M.S.; Wilson, B. A diffusion theory model of spatially resolved, steady-state diffuse reflectance for the noninvasive determination of tissue optical properties in vivo. *Med. Phys.* 1992, *9*, 879–888.
10. Cerussi, A.E.; Maier, J.S.; Fantini, S.; Franceschini, M.A.; Mantulin, W.W.; Gratton, E. Experimental verification of a theory for time-resolved fluorescence spectroscopy of thick tissues. *Appl. Opt.* 1997, *36*, 116–124.
11. Grosenick, D.; Wabnitz, H.; Rinnebert, H.H.; Moesta, K.T.; Schlag, P.M. Development of a time-domain optical mammography and first in vivo applications. *Appl. Opt.* 1999, *38*, 2927–2943.
12. Thompson, A.B.; Sevick-Muraca, E.M. NIR fluorescence contrast enhanced imaging with ICCD homodyne detection: Measurement precision and accuracy. *J. Biomed. Opt.* 2002, *8*, 111–120.
13. Kuwana, E.; Sevick-Muraca, E.M. Fluorescence lifetime spectroscopy in multiply scattering media with dyes exhibiting multi-exponential decays kinetics. *Biophys. J.* 2002, *83*, 1165–1176.
14. Chen, A. Effects of fluorescence and phosphorescence lifetime on frequency domain optical contrast for biomedical optical imaging. M.S. thesis, Purdue University, West Lafayette, IN, 1997.
15. Sevick-Muraca, E.M.; Godavarty, A.; Houston, J.P.; Thompson, A.B.; Roy, R. Near-infrared imaging with fluorescent contrast agents. In: *Fluorescence in Biomedicine* (eds. B. Pogue and M.-A. Mycek), Marcel Dekker, New York, 2003.
16. Alcala, J.R.; Gratton, E.; Jameson, D.M. A multifrequency phase fluorometer using the harmonic content of a mode-locked laser. *Anal. Instrum.* 1985, *14*(3–4), 225–250.
17. Reynolds, J.S.; Troy, T.L.; Sevick-Muraca, E.M. Multipixel techniques for frequency-domain photon migration imaging. *Biotechnol. Progr.* 1997, *13*(5), 669–680.
18. Lakowicz, J.R.; Berndt, K. Lifetime-sensitive fluorescence imaging using an rf phase-camera. *Rev. Sci. Instrum.* 1991, *62*, 1727–1734.
19. Sevick, E.M.; Lakowicz, J.R.; Szmacinski, H.; Nowaczyk, K.; Johnson, M. Frequency-domain imaging of obscure absorbers: Principles and applications. *J. Photochem. Photobiol.* 1992, *16*, 169–185.
20. Yang, Y.; Liu, H.; Li, X.; Chance, B. Low-cost frequency-domain photon migration instrument for tissue spectroscopy, oximetry, and imaging. *Opt. Eng.* 1997, *36*(5), 1562–1569.
21. Houston, J.P. Near-infrared fluorescence enhanced optical imaging: An analysis of penetration depth. M.S. thesis, Texas A&M University, College Station, TX, 2002.

22. Hawrysz, D.J.; Sevick-Muraca, E.M. Developments toward diagnostic breast cancer imaging using near-infrared optical measurements and fluorescent contrast agents. *Neoplasia* 2000, *2*(5), 388–417.

23. Weissleder, R.; Tung, C.H.; Mahmood, U.; Bogdanov Jr., A. In vivo imaging of tumors with protease-activated near-infrared fluorescent probes. *Nat. Biotechnol.* 1999, *17*, 375–378.

24. Qing, C.; Lakowicz, J.R.; Murtaza, Z.; Rao, G. A fluorescence lifetime-based solid sensor for water. *Anal. Chim. Acta* 1997, *350*(1–2), 97–104.

25. Russell, R.J.; Cote, G.L.; Gefrides, C.C.; McShane, M.J.; Pishko, M.V. A fluorescence-based glucose biosensor using concanavalin A and dextran encapsulated in a poly(ethylene glycol) hydrogel. *Anal. Chem.* 1999, *71*, 3126–3132.

26. Hutchinson, C.L.; Lakowicz, J.R.; Sevick-Muraca, E.M. Fluorescence lifetime-based sensing in tissues: A computational study. *Biophys. J.* 1995, *68*, 1574–1582.

27. Mayer, R.H.; Reynolds, J.S.; Sevick-Muraca, E.M. Measurement of fluorescence lifetime in scattering media using frequency-domain photon migration. *Appl. Opt.* 1999, *38*, 4930–4938.

28. Lakowicz, J.R.; Abugo, O.O. Modulation sensing of fluorophores in tissue—A new approach to drug compliance monitoring. *J. Biomed. Opt.* 1999, *4*(4), 429–442.

29. Fishkin, J.B.; Cerussi, A.E.; Fantini, S.; Franceschini, M.A.; Gratton, E.; So, P.T.C. Frequency-domain method for measuring spectral properties in multiple scattering media—Methemoglobin absorption spectrum in a tissue-like phantom. *Appl. Opt.* 1995, *34*, 1143.

30. Zhigang, S.; Yingqing, H.; Sevick-Muraca, E.M. Precise analysis of frequency domain photon migration measurement for characterization of concentrated colloidal suspensions. *Rev. Sci. Instrum.* 2002, *73*(2), 383–393.

31. Lee, J. Fluorescence-enhanced biomedical optical imaging using frequency-domain photon migration. PhD thesis, Purdue University, West Lafayette, IN, 2001.

32. Hattery, D.; Chernomordik, V.; Gannot, I.; Loew, M.; Gandjbakhche, A.H. Fluorescence measurement of localized, deeply embedded physiological processes. *Proc. SPIE* 2000, *3978*, 377–382.

33. Biolo, R.; Jori, G.; Kennedy, J.C.; Nadeau, P.; Potteir, R.; Reddi, E.; Weagle, G. A comparison of fluorescence methods used in the pharmacokinetic studies of Zn(II) phthalocyanine in mice. *Photochem. Photobiol.* 1991, *53*, 113–118.

34. Yang, Y.; Iftimia, N.; Xu, Y.; Jiang, H. Frequency-domain fluorescent diffusion tomography of turbid media and in vivo tissues. In: *Proceedings of SPIE on Optical Tomography and Spectroscopy of Tissue IV*, San Jose, CA, 2001, Vol. 4250, pp. 537–545.

35. Chenomordik, V.; Hattery, D.; Gannot, I.; Gandjbakhche, A.H. Inverse method 3-D reconstruction of localized in vivo fluorescence—Application to Sjogren syndrome. *IEEE J. Sel. Top. Quantum Electron.* 1999, *54*, 930–935.

36. O'Leary, M.A.; Boas, D.A.; Chance, B.; Yodh, A.G. Reradiation and imaging of diffuse photon density waves using fluorescent inhomogeneities. *J. Luminesc.* 1994, *60–61*, 281–286.

37. Wu, J.; Wang, Y.; Perleman, L.; Itzkan, I.; Dasari, R.R.; Feld, M.S. Time-resolved multichannel imaging of fluorescent objects embedded in turbid media. *Opt. Lett.* 1995, *20*, 489–491.

38. Chang, J.; Barbour, R.L.; Graber, H.; Aronson, R. Fluorescence optical tomography. *Proc. SPIE* 1995, *2570*, 59–72.

39. O'Leary, M.; Boas, D.A.; Li, X.D.; Chance, B.; Yodh, A.G. Fluorescence lifetime imaging in turbid media. *Opt. Lett.* 1996, *21*(2), 158–160.

40. Paithankar, D.Y.; Chen, A.U.; Pogue, B.W.; Patterson, M.S.; Sevick-Muraca, E.M. Imaging of fluorescent yield and lifetime from multiply scattered light reemitted from random media. *Appl. Opt.* 1997, *36*, 2260–2272.

41. Wu, J.; Perelman, L.; Dasari, R.R.; Feld, M.S. Fluorescence tomographic imaging in turbid media using early-arriving photons and Laplace transforms. *Proc. Natl. Acad. Sci.* 1997, *94*, 8783–8788.

42. Chang, J.; Graber, H.L.; Barbour, R.L. Improved reconstruction algorithm for luminescence when background luminophore is present. *Appl. Opt.* 1998, *37*, 3547–3552.

43. Jiang, H. Frequency-domain fluorescent diffusion tomography: A finite-element-based algorithm and simulations. *Appl. Opt.* 1998, *37*(22), 5337–5343.

44. Hull, E.L.; Nichols, M.G.; Foster, T.H. Localization of luminescent inhomogeneities in turbid media with spatially resolved measurements of cw diffuse luminescence emittance. *Appl. Opt.* 1998, *37*, 2755–2765.

45. Eppstein, M.J.; Dougherty, D.E.; Hawrysz, D.J.; Sevick-Muraca, E.M. Three-dimensional optical tomography. *Proc. SPIE* 1999, *3497*, 97–105.

46. Eppstein, M.J.; Dougherty, D.E.; Troy, T.L.; Sevick-Muraca, E.M. Biomedical optical tomography using dynamic parameterization and Bayesian conditioning on photon migration measurements. *Appl. Opt.* 1999, *38*, 2138–2150.

47. Roy, R.; Sevick-Muraca, E.M. Truncated Newton's optimization scheme for absorption and fluorescence optical tomography: Part II reconstruction from synthetic measurements. *Opt. Exp.* 1999, *4*, 372–382.

48. Roy, R.; Sevick-Muraca, E.M. Active constrained truncated Newton method for simple-bound optical tomography. *J. Opt. Soc. Am. A, Opt. Image Sci. Vis.* 2000, *17*(9), 1627–1641.

49. Eppstein, M.J.; Hawrysz, D.J.; Godavarty, A.; Sevick-Muraca, E.M. Three-dimensional, near-infrared fluorescence tomography with Bayesian methodologies for image reconstruction from sparse and noisy data sets. *Proc. Natl. Acad. Sci. USA* 2002, *99*, 9619–9624.

50. Hawrysz, D.J.; Eppstein, M.J.; Lee, J.; Sevick-Muraca, E.M. Error consideration in contrast-enhanced three-dimensional optical tomography. *Opt. Lett.* 2001, *26*(10), 704–706.

51. Roy, R.; Sevick-Muraca, E.M. Three-dimensional unconstrained and constrained image-reconstruction techniques applied to fluorescence, frequency-domain photon migration. *Appl. Opt.* 2001, *40*(13), 2206–2215.

52. Roy, R.; Sevick-Muraca, E.M. A numerical study of gradient-based nonlinear optimization methods for contrast-enhanced optical tomography. *Opt. Express* 2001, *9*(1), 49–65.

53. Ntziachristos, V.; Weissleder, R. Experimental three-dimensional fluorescence reconstruction of diffuse media by use of a normalized Born approximation. *Opt. Lett.* 2001, *26*(12), 893–895.

54. Lee, J.; Sevick-Muraca, E.M. 3-D fluorescence enhanced optical tomography using references frequency-domain photon migration measurements at emission and excitation measurements. *J. Opt. Soc. Am. A, Opt. Image Sci. Vis.* 2002, *12*, 759–771.

55. Sevick-Muraca, E.M.; Paithankar, D.Y. Fluorescence imaging system and measurement. US Patent 5,865,754, February 2, 1999.

56. Paithankar, D.Y.; Chen, A.; Sevick-Muraca, E.M. Fluorescence yield and lifetime imaging in tissues and other scattering media. *Proc. SPIE* 1996, *2679*, 162–175.

57. Pogue, B.; McBride, T.; Prewitt, J.; Osterberg, U.; Paulsen, K. Spatially varying regularization improves diffuse optical tomography. *Appl. Opt.* 1999, *38*, 2950–2961.

58. Holboke, M.J.; Yodh, A.G. Parallel three-dimensional diffuse optical tomography. In: *Biomedical Topical Meetings*, OSA, Miami Beach, FL, 2000, pp. 177–179.

59. Xu, M.; Lax, M.; Alfano, R.R. Time-resolved fourier diffuse optical tomography. In: *Biomedical Topical Meetings*, OSA, Miami Beach, FL, 2000, pp. 345–347.

60. Arridge, S.R.; Hebden, J.C.; Schweiger, M.; Schmidt, F.E.W.; Fry, M.E.; Hillman, E.M.C.; Dehghani, H.; Delpy, D.T. A method for three-dimensional time-resolved optical tomography. *Int. J. Imaging Syst. Technol.* 2000, *11*, 2–11.

61. Eppstein, M.J.; Dougherty, D.E. Optimal 3-D traveltime tomography. *Geophysics* 1998, *63*, 1053–1061.

62. Eppstein, M.J.; Dougherty, D.E. Efficient three-dimensional data inversion: Soil characterization and moisture monitoring from cross-well ground penetrating radar at a Vermont test site. *Water Resour. Res.* 1998, *34*, 1889–1900.

63. Eppstein, M.J.; Dougherty, D.E. Three-dimensional stochastic tomography with upscaling. US Patent application 09/110,506, July 9, 1998.

64. Yorkey, T.J.; Webster, J.G.; Tompkins, W.J. Comparing reconstruction algorithms for electrical impedance tomography. *IEEE Trans. Biomed. Eng.* 1987, *34*, 843–852.

65. Eppstein, M.J.; Dougherty, D.E.; Hawrysz, D.J.; Sevick-Muraca, E.M. Three-dimensional Bayesian optical image reconstruction with domain decomposition. *IEEE Trans. Med. Imaging* 2000, *20*(3), 147–163.

66. Roy, R.; Godavarty, A.; Sevick-Muraca, E.M. Fluorescence-enhanced, optical tomography using referenced measurements of heterogeneous media. *IEEE Trans. Med. Imaging* 2003, *22*, 824–836.

67. Roy, R.; Sevick-Muraca, E.M. Truncated Newton's optimization scheme for absorption and fluorescence optical tomography: Part I theory and formulation. *Opt. Exp.* 1999, *4*, 353–371.

68. Lee, J.; Sevick-Muraca, E.M. Fluorescence-enhanced absorption imaging using frequency-domain photon migration: Tolerance to measurement error. *J. Biomed. Opt.* 2000, *6*(1), 58–67.

69. Arridge, S.R. Optical tomography in medical imaging. *Inverse Probl.* 1999, *15*, R41–R93.

70. Pogue, B.W.; McBride, T.O.; Prewitt, J.; Osterberg, U.L.; Paulsen, K.D. Spatially variant regularization improves diffuse tomography. *Appl. Opt.* 1999, *38*, 2950–2961.

71. Eppstein, M.J.; Dougherty, D.E. Simultaneous estimation of transmissivity values and zonation. *Water Resour. Res.* 1996, *32*, 3321–3336.

72. Ntziachristos, V.; Yodh, A.G.; Schnall, M.; Chance, B. Concurrent MRI and diffuse optical tomography of the breast after indocyanine green enhancement. *Proc. Natl. Acad. Sci. USA* 2000, *97*, 2767–2772.

73. Pei, Y.; Lin, F.-B.; Barbour, R.L. Modeling of sensitivity and resolution to an included object in homogeneous scattering media and in MRI-derived breast maps. *J. Biomed. Opt.* 1999, *5*, 302–219.

74. Pogue, B.W.; Paulsen, K.D. High-resolution near-infrared tomographic imaging simulations of the rat cranium by use of *a priori* magnetic resonance imaging structural information. *Opt. Lett.* 1998, *23*, 1716–1718.

75. Holboke, M.J.; Tromberg, B.J.; Li, X.; Shah, N.; Fishkin, J.; Kidney, D.; Butler, J.; Chance, B.; Yodh, A.G. Three-dimensional diffuse optical mammography with ultrasound localization in a human subject. *J. Biomed. Opt.* 2000, *5*, 237–247.

76. Provencher, S.W.; Vogel, R.H. Regularization techniques for inverse problems in molecular biology. In: *Numerical Treatment of Inverse Problems in Differential and Integral Equations* (eds. P. Deuflhard and E. Hairer), Birkhauser Press, Boston, MA, 1983, pp. 304–319.

77. Tikhonov, A.N.; Arsenin, V.Y. *Solution of Ill-Posed Problems.* V.H. Winston & Sons, Washington, DC, 1977.

78. Pelegrin, A.; Folli, S.; Buchegger, F.; Mach, J.-P.; Wagnieres, G.; van den Bergh, H. Antibody-fluorescein conjugates for photoimmunodiagnosis of human colon carcinoma in nude mice. *Cancer* 1991, *67*, 2529–2537.

79. Folli, S.; Wagnieres, G.; Pelegrin, A.; Calmes, J.M.; Braichotte, D.; Buchegger, F.; Chalandon, Y. et al. Immunophotodiagnosis of colon carcinomas in patients injected with fluoresceinated chimeric antibodies against carcinoembryonic antigen. *Proc. Natl. Acad. Sci. USA* 1992, *89*, 7973–7977.

80. Folli, S.; Westermann, P.; Braichotte, D.; Pelegrin, A.; Wagnieres, G.; van den Bergh, H.; Mach, J.P. Antibody-indocyanin conjugates for immunophotodetection of human squamous cell carcinoma in nude mice. *Cancer Res.* 1994, *54*, 2643–2649.

81. Haglund, M.M.; Hochman, D.W.; Spence, A.M.; Berger, M.S. Enhanced optical imaging of rat gliomas and tumor margins. *Neurosurgery* 1994, *35*, 930–939.

82. Straight, R.C.; Benner, R.E.; McClane, R.W.; Go, P.M.N.Y.; Yoon, G.; Dixon, J.A. Application of charge-coupled device technology for measurement of laser light and fluorescence distribution in tumors for photodynamic therapy. *Photochem. Photobiol.* 1991, *53*, 787–796.

83. Kohl, M.; Sukowski, U.; Ebert, B.; Neukammer, J.; Rinneberg, H.H. Imaging of superficially growing tumors by delayed observation of laser-induced fluorescence. *Proc. SPIE* 1993, *1881*, 206–221.

84. Cubeddu, R.; Canti, G.; Taroni, P.; Valentini, G. Time-gated fluorescence imaging for the diagnosis of tumors in a murine model. *Photochem. Photobiol.* 1993, *57*, 480–485.

85. Cubeddu, R.; Canti, G.; Pifferi, A.; Taroni, P.; Valentini, G. Fluorescence lifetime imaging of experimental tumors in hematoporphyrin derivative-sensitized mice. *Photochem. Photobiol.* 1997, *66*, 229–236.

86. Mordon, S.; Devoisselle, J.M.; Maunoury, V. In vivo pH measurement and imaging of tumor tissue using a pH-sensitive fluorescent probe (5,6-carboxyfluorescein): Instrumental and experimental studies. *Photochem. Photobiol.* 1994, *60*, 274–279.

87. Ballou, B.; Fisher, G.W.; Waggoner, A.S.; Farkas, D.L.; Reiland, J.M.; Jaffe, R.; Mujumdar, R.B.; Mujumdar, S.R.; Hakala, T.R. Tumor labeling in vivo using cyanine-conjugated monoclonal antibodies. *Cancer Immunol. Immunother.* 1995, *41*, 257–263.

88. Devoisselle, J.M.; Soulie, S.; Mordon, S.R.; Mestres, G.; Desmettre, T.M.D.; Maillols, H. Effect of indocyanine green formulation on blood clearance and in vivo fluorescence kinetic profile of skin. *Proc. SPIE* 1995, *2627*, 100–108.

89. Rokahr, I.; Andersson-Engels, S.; Svanberg, S.; D'Hallewin, M.-A.; Baert, L.; Wang, I.; Svanberg, K. Optical detection of human urinary bladder carcinoma utilising tissue autofluorescence and protoporphyrin IX-induced fluorescence following low-dose ALA instillation. *Proc. SPIE* 1995, *2627*, 2–12.

90. Haglund, M.M.; Berger, M.S.; Hochman, D.W. Enhanced optical imaging of human gliomas and tumor margins. *Neurosurgery* 1996, *38*, 308–316.

91. Sakatani, K.; Kashiwasake-Jibu, M.; Taka, Y.; Wang, S.; Zuo, H.; Yamamoto, K.; Shimizu, K. Noninvasive optical imaging of the subarachnoid space and cerebrospinal fluid pathways based on near-infrared fluorescence. *J. Neurosurg.* 1997, *87*, 738–745.

92. Neri, D. Targeting by affinity-matured recombinant antibody fragments of an angiogenesis-associated fibronectin isoform. *Nat. Biotechnol.* 1997, *15*, 1271–1275.

93. Ballou, B.; Fisher, G.W.; Deng, J.-S.; Hakala, T.R.; Srivastava, M.; Farkas, D.L. Fluorochrome-labeled antibodies in vivo: Assessment of tumor imaging using Cy3, Cy5, Cy5.5, and Cy7. *Cancer Detect. Prev.* 1998, *22*(3) 251–257.

94. Eker, C.; Montan, S.; Jaramillo, E.; Koizumi, K.; Rubio, C.; Andersson-Engels, S.; Svanberg, K.; Svanberg, S.; Slezak, P. Clinical spectral characterization of colonic mucosal lesions using autofluorescence and d aminolevulinic acid sensitizations. *Gut* 1999, *44*, 511–518.

95. Reynolds, J.S.; Troy, T.L.; Mayer, R.H.; Thompson, A.B.; Waters, D.J.; Cornell, K.K.; Snyder, P.W.; Sevick-Muraca, E.M. Imaging of spontaneous canine mammary tumors using fluorescent contrast agents. *Photochem. Photobiol.* 1999, *70*, 87–94.

96. Becker, A.; Licha, K.; Kresse, M.; Riefke, B.; Sukowski, U.; Ebert, B.; Rinneberg, H.; Semmler, W. Transferrin-mediated tumor delivery of contrast media for optical imaging and magnetic resonance imaging. In: *Proceedings of SPIE on Biomedical Imaging: Reporters, Dyes, and Instrumentation*, San Jose, CA, 1999, Vol. 3600, pp. 142–150.

97. Mahmood, U.; Tung, C-H.; Bogdanov, A.; Weissleder, R. Near-infrared optical imaging of protease activity for tumor detection. *Radiology* 1999, *21*(3), 866–870.

98. Becker, A.; Riefke, B.; Ebert, B.; Sukowski, U.; Rinneberg, H.; Semmler, W.; Licha, K. Macromolecular contrast agents for optical imaging of tumors: Comparison of indotricarboyanine-labeled human serum albumin and transferrin. *Photochem. Photobiol.* 2000, *72*, 234–241.

99. Gurfinkel, M.; Thompson, A.B.; Ralston, W.; Troy, T.L.; Moore, A.L.; Moore, T.A.; Gust, J.D. et al. Pharmacokinetics of ICG and HPPH-car for the detection of normal and tumor tissue using fluorescence, near-infrared reflectance imaging: A case study. *Photochem. Photobiol.* 2000, *72*, 94–102.

100. Licha, K.; Riefke, B.; Ntziachristos, V.; Becker, A.; Chance, B.; Semmler, W. Hydrophilic cyanine dyes as contrast agents for near-infrared tumor imaging: Synthesis, photophysical properties and spectroscopic in vivo characterization. *Photochem. Photobiol.* 2000, *72*, 392–398.

101. Yang, M.; Baranov, E.; Sun, F.; Li, X.; Li, L.; Hasegawa, S.; Bouvet, M. et al. Whole-body optical imaging of green fluorescent protein-expressing tumors and metastases. *Proc. Natl. Acad. Sci. USA* 2000, *97*, 1206–1211.

102. Hoffman, R.M. Visualization of GFP-expressing tumors and metastasis in vivo. *Biotechniques* 2001, *30*, 1016–1026.

103. Bugaj, J.E.; Achilefu, S.; Dorshow, R.B.; Rajagopalan, R. Novel fluorescent contrast agents for optical imaging of in vivo tumors based on a receptor-targeted dye-peptide conjugate platform. *J. Biomed. Opt.* 2001, *6*, 122–133.

104. Achilefu, S.; Dorshow, R.B.; Bugaj, J.E.; Rajagopalan, R. Tumor specific fluorescent contrast agents. *Proc. SPIE* 2000, *3917*, 80–86.

105. Achilefu, S.; Bugaj, J.E.; Dorshow, R.B.; Jimenez, H.N.; Rajagopalan, R. New approach to optical imaging of tumors. In: *Proceedings of SPIE on Biomarkers and Biological Spectral Imaging*, San Jose, CA, 2001, Vol. 4259, pp. 110–114.

106. Achilefu, S.; Bugaj, J.E.; Dorshow, R.B.; Jimenez, H.N.; Rajagopalan, R.; Wilhelm, R.R.; Webb, E.G.; Erion, J.L. Site-specific tumor targeted fluorescent contrast agents. *Proc. SPIE* 2001, *4156*, 69–78.

107. Becker, A.; Hessenius, C.; Licha, K.; Ebert, B.; Sukowski, U.; Semmler, W.; Wiedenmann, B.; Grotzinger, C. Receptor-targeted optical imaging of tumors with near-infrared fluorescent ligands. *Nat. Biotechnol.* 2001, *19*, 327–331.

108. Bremer, C.; Tung, C.; Weissleder, R. In vivo molecular target assessment of matrix metalloproteinase inhibition. *Nat. Med.* 2001, *7*, 743–748.

109. Ebert, B.; Sukowski, U.; Grosenick, D.; Wabnitz, H.; Moesta, K.T.; Licha, K.; Becker, A.; Semmler, W.; Schlag, P.M.; Rinneberg, H. Near-infrared fluorescent dyes for enhanced contrast in optical mammography: Phantom experiments. *J. Biomed. Opt.* 2001, *6*(2), 134–140.

110. Finlay, J.C.; Conover, D.L.; Hull, E.L.; Foster, T.H. Porphyrin bleaching and PDT-induced spectral changes are irradiance dependent in ALA-sensitized normal rat skin in vivo. *Photochem. Photobiol.* 2001, *73*, 54–63.

111. Rice, B.W.; Cable, M.D.; Nelson, M.B. In vivo imaging of light-emitting probes. *J. Biomed. Opt.* 2001, *6*(4), 432–440.

112. Soukos, N.S.; Hamblin, M.R.; Keelm, S.; Fabian, R.L.; Deutsch, T.F.; Hasan, T. Epidermal growth factor receptor-targeted immunophotodiagnosis and photoimmunotherapy of oral precancer in vivo. *Cancer Res.* 2001, *61*, 4490–4496.

113. Leevy, C.M.; Smith, F.; Longueville, J. Indocyanine green clearance as a test for hepatic function. Evaluation by dichromatic ear densitometry. *JAMA* 1967, *200*, 236–240.

114. Kogure, K.; David, N.J.; Yamanouchi, U.; Choromokos, E. Infrared absorption angiography of the fundus circulation. *Arch. Ophthalmol.* 1970, *83*(2), 209–214.

115. Sevick-Muraca, E.M.; Lopez, G.; Troy, T.L.; Reynolds, J.S.; Hutchinson, C.L. Fluorescence and absorption contrast mechanisms for biomedical optical imaging using frequency-domain techniques. *Photochem. Photobiol.* 1997, *66*, 55–64.

116. Landsman, M.L.; Kwant, G.; Mook, G.; Zijlstra, W.G. Light-absorbing properties, stability, and spectral stabilization of indocyanine green. *J. Appl. Physiol.* 1976, *40*, 575–583.

117. Mordon, S.; Devoisselle, J.M.; Soulie-Begu, S.; Desmettre, T. Indocyanine green: Physiochemical factors affecting its fluorescence *in vivo*. *Microvasc. Res.* 1998, *55*, 146–152.

118. Schafer, K.A.; Kelly, G.; Schrader, R.; Griffith, W.C.; Muggenburg, B.A.; Tierney, L.A.; Lechner, J.F.; Janovitz, E.B.; Hahn, F.F. A canine model of familial mammary gland neoplasia. *Vet. Pathol.* 1998, *35*, 168–177.

119. Ntziachristos, V.; Ma, X.; Chance, B. Time-correlated single photon counting imager for simultaneous magnetic resonance and near-infrared mammography. *Rev. Sci. Instrum.* 1998, *69*, 4221–4233.

120. McMaster, K.M.; Giuliano, A.E.; Ross, M.I.; Reintgen, D.S.; Hunt, K.K.; Klimberg, V.S.; Whitworth, P.W.; Tafra, L.C.; Edwards, M.J. Sentinel lymph node biopsy for breast cancer—Not yet the standard of care. *N. Engl. J. Med.* 1998, *339*, 990–995.

121. Krag, D.; Weaver, D.; Ashikaga, T.; Moffat, F.; Klimberg, S.; Shriver, C.; Feldman, S. et al. The sentinel node in breast cancer—A multicenter validation study. *N. Engl. J. Med.* 1998, *339*, 941–946.

122. Zaheer, A.; Lenkinski, R.E.; Mahmood, A.; Jones, A.G.; Cantley, L.C.; Frangioni, J.V. In vivo near-infrared fluorescence imaging of osteoblastic activity. *Nat. Biotechnol.* 2001, *19*(12), 1148–1154.
123. Licha, K.; Becker, A.; Kratz, F.; Semmler, W. New contrast agents for optical imaging: Acid-cleavable conjugates of cyanine dyes with biomolecules. *Proc. SPIE* 1999, *3600*, 29–35.
124. Huber, M.M.; Staubili, A.B.; Kustedjo, K.; Gray, M.H.B.; Shih, J.; Fraser, S.; Jacobs, R.E.; Meade, T.J. Fluorescently detectable magnetic resonance imaging agents. *Bioconjug. Chem.* 1998, *9*, 242–249.

19

Interferometric Light Scattering Techniques for Measuring Nuclear Morphology and Detecting Dysplasia

Yizheng Zhu
Duke University

Francisco E. Robles
Duke University

Neil G. Terry
Duke University

Adam Wax
Duke University

19.1 Introduction

Elastically scattered light from biological media carries ample information about the subject that can be used for biomedical applications such as the study of cell morphology and the assessment of tissue health [1–5]. The dependence of the scattered field distribution on wavelength, angle, and polarization has been used to extract structural information such as the size of nuclei and organelles, as well as optical properties such as the refractive index and absorption spectrum of the scatterer [6–8]. Such quantitative light scattering information can be obtained by the analysis of either singly scattered photons (e.g., light scattering spectroscopy [LSS]) [1,9] or multiply scattered photons (e.g., elastic scattering spectroscopy) [3,4] and has been shown to be effective for the diagnosis of dysplasia, a precancerous state typically found in the epithelial layer of tissue where the majority of human cancers originate [1].

Light scattering techniques are highly responsive to changes in cellular morphology and optical properties because the far-field scattering intensity distribution from objects whose dimension is comparable to the probing wavelength is extremely sensitive to small changes in size or shape. In most of these techniques, however, only the intensity of the scattering signal can be measured and the phase information is lost; they are therefore noninterferometric in nature and cannot provide diagnostic analysis as a function of depth in the tissue.

In this chapter, we review two light scattering techniques that take advantage of low-coherence interferometry (LCI) to generate depth-dependent diagnostic information for measuring cell morphology and detecting dysplasia. The following section introduces Fourier-domain (FD) LCI, which combines the depth-resolved imaging capability of optical coherence tomography (OCT) with the spectroscopic analysis of light scattering. The introduction of a novel dual-window (DW) signal processing method allows for the study of local spectral oscillations with both high spatial and spectral resolutions and has been shown to be effective in determining local nucleus size in animal models. The second technique, termed angle-resolved LCI (a/LCI), detects the angular scattering distribution as a function of depth in tissue and has been clinically demonstrated for detecting dysplasia in patients with Barrett's esophagus (BE), a metaplastic transformation of the epithelial lining of the lower esophagus that is considered a premalignant condition associated with a markedly increased risk of esophageal adenocarcinoma [10]. The last part of the chapter presents a fiber-optic interferometric 2D scattering (FITS) measurement system, which is a novel extension of the 1D a/LCI technique. The FITS system enables polarization-sensitive 2D angular scattering measurement with depth resolution, providing an advanced tool for the study of light scattering by aspherical scatterers.

19.2 Fourier Domain Low Coherence Interferometry

FD LCI (fLCI) is an emerging optical technique used to quantitatively assess cell nuclear morphology in tissue as a means of detecting early cancer development. Using a similar approach to that used in spectroscopic optical coherence tomography (SOCT), fLCI measures oscillatory features in depth-resolved spectra, also known as *local oscillations*, which result from coherent fields induced by the scattering from the front and back surfaces of cell nuclei in tissue [11]. Thus, fLCI uses nuclear morphology as a biomarker of disease, making it sensitive to the earliest stages of precancerous development. In this section, we provide an in-depth description of the instrumentation and theory behind fLCI and present studies of a tissue phantom and ex vivo tissues to illustrate the potential of the fLCI method.

19.2.1 Experimental System

The fLCI method utilizes a modified Michelson interferometer with a white-light source, which yields access to the visible region of the spectrum. As illustrated in Figure 19.1, the interferometer is modified by the addition of four lenses (L2–L5), which form a 4f interferometer and are used to deliver collimated light onto the sample and reference arm [12]. The samples are placed atop a cover glass that is slightly tilted to avoid saturation from specular reflection and thus allows collection of only the scattered light. This is called *scatter-mode* imaging. The scattered light from the sample and the reflected light from the reference mirror are imaged onto the entrance slit of an imaging spectrograph. A 2D charge-coupled device (CCD) array simultaneously collects the interferometric signal (as a function of wavelength, λ) across a range of lateral positions. By taking a 1D Fourier transform with respect to wave number, $k = 2\pi/\lambda$ for the spectral data at each lateral position, this method achieves B-mode OCT images in a single exposure. This configuration is known as a parallel frequency-domain OCT (pfdOCT) system.

The 4f interferometer configuration [12] of the pfdOCT system does not only achieve parallel acquisition of multiple A-scans but it also enables effective interferometric detection using a Xe-arc lamp. To understand the properties of the 4f system, consider that the field generated by the arc lamp consists of multiple uncorrelated spatial modes, each with a different phase. Thus, if the light is focused onto the

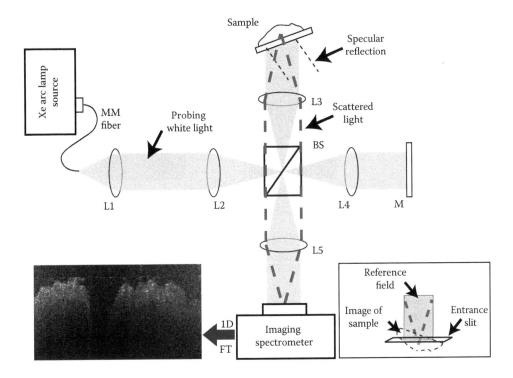

FIGURE 19.1 pfdOCT system and sample B-mode OCT image acquired by a single exposure. L1, collimating lens; L2–L5, lenses for 4F interferometer; M, reference mirror.

sample, as is commonly done in OCT, each mode will contribute to the signal; unfortunately, in an FD OCT configuration (as is the case here), the different phases are added coherently. This coherent summation causes the fringe visibility to be washed out and thus decreases the contrast in the image. On the other hand, by collimating the beam, and thus illuminating the sample with the conjugate field of the fiber output, we spatially separate each uncorrelated mode. This simple difference avoids fringe washout and allows effective detection of the interferometric signal using a white-light source [13].

19.2.2 Dual-Window Signal Processing

Depth-resolved spectroscopic information may be obtained from the interferometric data to yield functional information of the sample. This approach has been utilized in SOCT to provide information about shifts of the spectrum's center of mass, yielding a *qualitative* contrast mechanism [14]. To gain access to this information, a short-time Fourier transform (STFT) is typically implemented. This process involves sweeping a window across the interferometric data while simultaneously taking a Fourier transform at each step, thus giving a map of the spectral content confined within a spatial (or depth) region (see Figure 19.2). The maps acquired using this process are known as time-frequency distributions (TFDs); however, TFDs obtained using a single STFT suffer from an inherent trade-off between the resulting spectral and depth resolution. This trade-off has hindered the ability of SOCT to provide *quantitative* spectroscopic information about the sample, which could be used to quantify absorber concentrations or scattering cross sections in tissue. Furthermore, in order to gain access to the local oscillations using fLCI, high resolution in both dimensions must be obtained. For this purpose, we have developed the DW processing method.

The DW method is based on calculating two separate STFTs and then multiplying the results. The first STFT uses a broad spectral Gaussian window to obtain high depth resolution, while the second

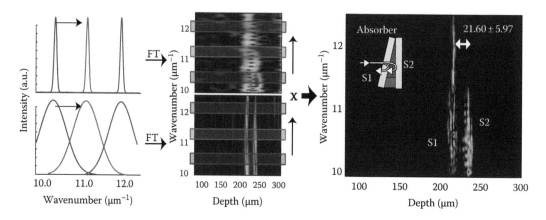

FIGURE 19.2 Procedure for calculating the DW TFD. The interferometric signal is generated from an absorbing phantom with two scattering surfaces, S1 and S2. (Adapted from Robles, F. et al., *Opt. Express*, 17, 6799, 2009; Robles, F. et al., *Biomed. Opt. Express*, 1, 736, 2010. With permission.)

STFT uses a narrow spectral window to generate high spectroscopic resolution. Therefore, the resulting DW TFD simultaneously achieves high resolution in both dimensions. Mathematically, this can be described as

$$
\mathrm{DW}(k,z) = |E_R|^2 \int 2\langle E_S \rangle \cos(\kappa_1 \times \Delta\mathrm{OPL}) e^{-\frac{(\kappa_1-k)^2}{2w_1^2}} e^{-i\kappa_1 z} d\kappa_1
$$

$$
\times \int \left(2\langle E_S \rangle \cos(\kappa_2 \times \Delta\mathrm{OPL}) e^{-\frac{(\kappa_2-k)^2}{2w_2^2}} e^{-i\kappa_2 z} \right)^* d\kappa_2,
$$

(19.1)

where
  E_S describes the sample field
  E_R is the reference field that is assumed to vary slowly with respect to wave number
  $\langle\cdots\rangle$ denotes an ensemble average
  $\Delta\mathrm{OPL}$ is the optical path length difference between the sample and reference arms
  z is the axial distance
  w_1 and w_2 are the standard deviations of the two windows

Figure 19.2 illustrates the procedure for computing the DW TFD for a signal generated by an absorbing phantom with two scattering surfaces: S1 and S2.

From the DW TFD, one can observe that the two scattering surfaces are clearly spatially resolved and that the spectrum from S2 clearly exhibits absorption. In more detail, Figure 19.3a and b shows the spectrum from the light returned from the two cover glasses, S1 and S2, respectively. Here, we note that the spectral resolution of the STFT and the DW is comparable to that of the ideal case (obtained by transmission measurement). However, the time marginals, shown in Figure 19.3d, demonstrate the superior depth resolution of the DW method compared to that of an optimized STFT. The spatial resolution of the STFT can be improved by choosing a wider spectral window; however, this process would degrade the spectral resolution.

The depth-resolved spectra from the DW TFD also contain high-frequency oscillations: these are the local oscillations that reveal structural information about the sample. By taking a Fourier transform of these oscillations (e.g., dotted line in Figure 19.3a), one obtains a correlation function, which, as seen in Figure 19.3d, contains a clear peak at a correlation distance of 21.60 ± 0.57 μm. This distance

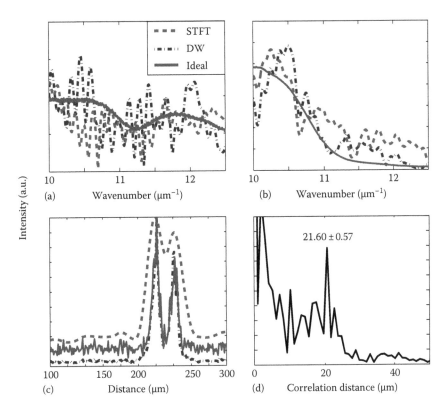

FIGURE 19.3 Depth-resolved spectra from S1 (a) and S2 (b). (c) Time marginals. (d) Correlation function calculated by the Fourier transform of the DW depth-resolved spectra from S1 (dotted line in (a)). The peak corresponds to the physical distance between S1 and S2. (Adapted from Robles, F. et al., *Opt. Express*, 17, 6799, 2009. With permission.)

corresponds to the spacing between the two scattering surfaces and can be compared to the distance obtained by imaging (see Figure 19.2 or 19.3c), which gives 21.6 ± 5.97 μm. It is worth mentioning again that by analyzing the periodicity of the local oscillations, one can precisely probe the features of scattering structures in the sample. This mechanism is exploited in fLCI to recover information about the cell nuclear diameter in tissue [15].

19.2.3 Phantom Study

The DW fLCI approach has been validated by investigating the scattering properties of a turbid medium containing different populations of scatterers. The analysis consists of processing with the DW method and then using fLCI and LSS to obtain structural information. LSS extracts the size of spherical scatterers by analyzing periodicity in the spectrum of singly scattered light [17]. The periodicities correspond to the scattering cross section of spherical structures and are well described by the van de Hulst approximation [18]. Further, the periodicities exhibit lower-frequency spectral oscillations compared to the local oscillations used in fLCI; thus, fLCI and LSS measurements can be obtained simultaneously by looking at the high- and low-frequency components of the depth-resolved spectra, respectively.

The turbid sample for this experiment consists of two layers with spherical polystyrene beads (index of refraction $n_b = 1.59$) of different sizes suspended in a mixture of agar (2% by weight) and water ($n_a = 1.35$). The bead diameter in the top layer is $d = 4.00 \pm 0.033$ μm, and in the bottom layer $d = 6.98 \pm 0.055$ μm. Figure 19.4a shows an OCT image of the phantom acquired by the pfdOCT system (note that no scanning is necessary).

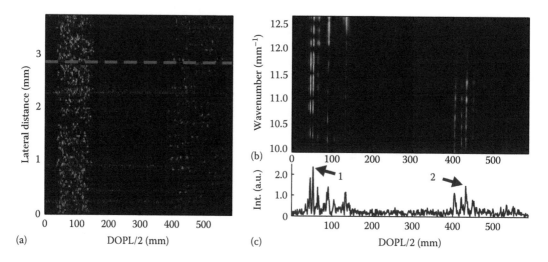

FIGURE 19.4 (a) pfdOCT image of a two-layer phantom. The top layer (OPL difference/2 [ΔOPL/2] ranging from 35 to 125 µm) contains 4.00 µm beads, while the bottom layer (400–550 µm) contains 6.98 µm beads. The dashed line corresponds to a single lateral channel or A-scan (c) from which the DW TFD is generated (b). The spectra and correlation function of points 1 and 2 are analyzed later in Figure 19.5. (Adapted from Robles, F.E. and Wax, A., *Opt. Lett.*, 35, 360, 2010. With permission.)

To process the DW TFD, five steps are taken: (1) The sample and reference arm intensities are acquired separately and subtracted from the raw interferometric signal. (2) The resulting signal is divided by the intensity of the reference field to normalize for the source spectrum and detector efficiencies. This step is of particular importance for quantitative comparison of depth-resolved spectra, since the remaining spectral dependence is assumed to arise solely from absorption of forward scattered light and scattering cross sections of backscattered light. (3) The data are resampled into a linear wave number vector, $k = 2\pi/\lambda$. (4) Chromatic dispersion is digitally corrected [19]. (Note that steps 1–4 are also performed in order to compute the OCT image.) (5) As a last step, the DW TFD is generated for each lateral line (or A-scan) with window sizes $w_1 = 0.0454$ µm^{-1} ($\Delta\lambda = 2.39$ nm) for high spectral resolution and $w_2 = 0.6670$ µm^{-1} ($\Delta\lambda = 35.1$ nm) for high depth resolution. The resulting DW TFD, computed from the A-scan delineated by the dotted red line in Figure 19.4a, is shown in Figure 19.4b. Figure 19.4c is the corresponding A-scan [20].

As stated above, the depth-resolved spectra of the DW contain two components that relay structural information of the sample. The first component, contained in the low frequencies, corresponds to the scattering cross section of the beads; thus, the van de Hulst approximation [18] can be used to determine the bead size (LSS method). To achieve this, the DW spectral profile is low-pass filtered with a hard cutoff frequency of 3.5 µm (three cycles); then, a least-squares fit is used to obtain the scatterer diameter by comparing the spectrum to the van de Hulst model. In Figure 19.5a and b, the dotted green curves show the low-pass filtered data used for fitting, which yield $d_1 = 3.97$ µm and $d_2 = 6.91$ µm for points 1 and 2 in Figure 19.4c, respectively. The results are in good agreement with the known sizes: 4.00 ± 0.033 µm and 6.98 ± 0.055 µm, respectively. The dashed red curves give the theoretical scattering cross section corresponding to the best fits: note that these are in excellent agreement with the processed signals [20].

The second component of the depth-resolved spectra is analyzed using fLCI, which consists of the local oscillations (high frequencies), which, in this case, arise from the scattering from the front and back surfaces of the beads. To compute this parameter, the spectral dependence is removed by subtracting the line of best fit from the LSS analysis above. Then, the residuals are Fourier transformed to yield a correlation function, where the maximum indicates the round-trip optical path length (ΔOPL) through the scatterer. Figure 19.5c and d plots the correlation function for points 1 and 2, from Figure 19.4c,

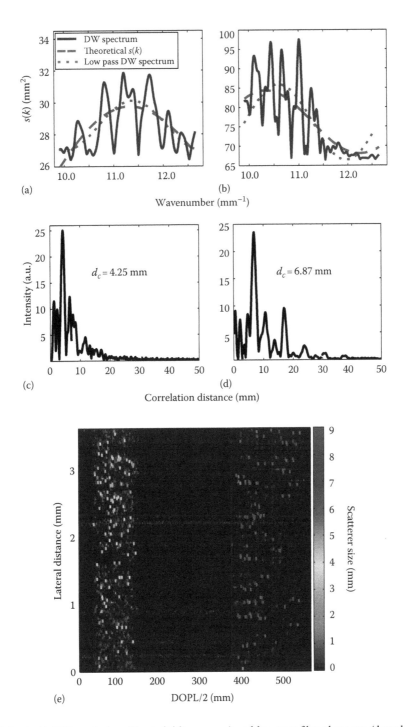

FIGURE 19.5 (a, b) DW spectral profiles (solid line curves) and low-pass filtered spectra (dotted line curves) from points 1 and 2 in Figure 19.4c, respectively. Dashed line curves are the theoretical scattering cross sections for 3.97 and 6.91 μm spherical scatterers for points 1 and 2, respectively. (c, d) Correlation function from points 1 and 2, with correlation distances (d_c) of 4.25 and 6.87 μm, respectively. (e) Overlay of the fLCI measurements with the OCT image. (Adapted from Robles, F.E. and Wax, A., *Opt. Lett.*, 35, 360, 2010. With permission.)

respectively. The correlation peaks for these points are located at $d_c = \Delta OPL/(2n_b) = 4.25$ and 6.87 μm, in good agreement with both the LSS measurements and known bead size in each layer [20].

The LSS and fLCI procedures were repeated for all A-scan and all points in the OCT image. Figure 19.5e shows the results by overlaying the fLCI measurements with the OCT image. The LSS map (not shown) yields similar results. In the top layer, the average scatterer size was 3.82 ± 0.67 μm and 3.68 ± 0.41 μm for the fLCI and LSS measurements, respectively (112 points). In the bottom layer, the average scatterer size was 6.55 ± 0.47 μm and 6.75 ± 0.42 μm for fLCI and LSS, respectively (113 points) [20].

The results from this phantom study show that the DW fLCI technique yields accurate and precise morphological measurements throughout the whole OCT image. Further, this phantom study confirms the potential for fLCI to measure enlargement of epithelial cell nuclei, which are nonabsorbing, to detect precancerous development at different depth layers within tissues.

19.2.4 Azoxymethane Rat Carcinogenesis Model Study

In this section, we utilize fLCI to measure early changes indicative of colorectal cancer (CRC) development using an analysis of ex vivo tissues drawn from the azoxymethane (AOM) rat carcinogenesis model. Further, we analyze the functional data of the ex vivo samples at three depths and along two different longitudinal sections of the left colon (LC) to demonstrate the ability of fLCI to detect areas where neoplastic development has occurred, in addition to being able to detect changes arising from the field effect of carcinogenesis. The phenomenon of the field effect of carcinogenesis describes observations that neoplastic development in one part of the colonic epithelium distorts nano- and microtissue morphology, as well as tissue function, along the entire organ. This has been a subject of much interest since it indicates that adequate screening may be achieved by only probing certain (and more readily accessible) sections of the colon [21–23], thus leading to less invasive screening for CRC.

This study used the AOM rat carcinogenesis model, a well characterized and established model for colon cancer research and drug development [24]. The cancerous progression of this model is similar to that seen in humans and is a good surrogate for human colon cancer development. In addition, the short induction period and high incidence of aberrant crypt foci (ACF), which are preneoplastic lesions [25], make this model a practical choice for testing the ability of fLCI to detect precancerous development in the colon.

All animal experimental protocols were approved by the Institutional Animal Care and Use Committee of the Hamner Institute and Duke University. Forty F344 rats were randomized into groups of 10, where 30 received intraperitoneal (IP) injections of AOM > 90% pure with a molar concentration of 13.4 M at a dose level of 15 mg/kg body weight, once per week, for 2 consecutive weeks (two doses per animal). The remaining 10 animals received saline by IP and served as the control group. At 4, 8, and 12 weeks after the completion of the dosing regimen, the animals (10 AOM-treated and 3 or 4 saline-treated rats per time point) were sacrificed by CO_2 asphyxiation. The colon tissues were harvested, opened longitudinally, and washed with saline. Then, the tissue was split into four to five different segments, each with a length of 3–4 cm, where only the two most distal segments were analyzed: the distal LC and proximal LC. Each sample was placed on a cover glass for examination with the pfdOCT system. Finally, the tissue samples were fixed in formalin and stained with methylene blue in order to be scored based on the number of ACF.

To obtain the OCT image and the DW TFDs, we followed the same procedure given in Section 19.2.3. Moreover, for this study, we achieved a lateral resolution of 10 μm by setting the focal lengths of lenses L3 and L4 to 50 mm and the rest to 100 mm. The axial resolution was experimentally determined to be ~1.1 μm, where an index of refraction of $n = 1.38$ is used to convert the OPL to physical axial distance in tissue [26]. For the generation of the DW TFDs, the window standard deviations used were $w_1 = 0.029$ μm^{-1} and $w_2 = 0.804$ μm^{-1}, resulting in TFDs with an axial resolution of 3.45 μm and spectral resolution of 1.66 nm. The spatial information provided by the OCT images is used to co-register the spectroscopic information. This allows for the spectra to be consistently analyzed at specific tissue depths. This process involves using the images to identify the contour of the tissue surfaces and calibrate the analysis relative to this *zero* depth.

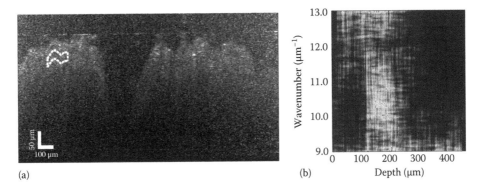

FIGURE 19.6 (a) pfdOCT image of an ex vivo rat colon sample. The white line delineates an example region that is averaged across to determine the nuclear diameter. (b) DW TFD (after alignment and averaging laterally), from laterally delineated region. (Adapted from Robles, F. et al., *Biomed. Opt. Express*, 1, 736, 2010. With permission.)

Once the spectra are properly aligned, regions of interest, both laterally and axially, are identified and averaged in order to provide sufficient fringe contrast of the local oscillations. In the lateral direction, 20 DW TFDs are averaged to yield 10 different lateral segments in each OCT image. In the axial direction, we calculate the spectral averages of 25 μm depth segments from three different sections: at the surface (surface section 0–25 μm), centered about 35 μm in depth (midsection 22.5–47.5 μm), and centered about 50 μm in depth (low section 37.5–62.5 μm). Figure 19.6a illustrates an OCT image for an AOM-treated rat tissue sample, where the dotted red line delineates a resulting averaged region for the mid-depth section. The corresponding DW TFD (after alignment and averaging laterally) is shown in Figure 19.6b.

As described previously, the spectra from the averaged regions contain two components. The first component is the low-frequency oscillations, which were previously analyzed with LSS; however, we have found that due to the lack of knowledge of the precise refractive index of the scatterer and the surrounding medium in tissue [27], the amount of useful information that can be extracted from this method is limited. Therefore, the low-frequency oscillations are isolated using a smoothing function and subsequently removed from the spectra. This process isolates the second component: the high-frequency components of the spectra, which correspond to the local oscillations resulting from coherent fields induced by the cell nuclei in the averaged region (fLCI method). Note that we assume that the cell nuclei contain a constant nuclear refractive index (RI) of $n_n = 1.395$ for this analysis [26]. Figure 19.7a illustrates the depth-resolved spectrum (gray solid line), along with the low-frequency component (dotted black line), for the average region shown in Figure 19.6a. Figure 19.7b shows the isolated local oscillations, and Figure 19.7c shows the corresponding correlation function with a peak at 7.88 μm corresponding to the average cell nuclear diameter in the region of analysis. The process is automated to analyze all segments of the image for all tissue samples.

Statistical analysis of the data (using a two-sided student *t*-test) revealed that the most significant layer for diagnosis using fLCI was the mid-depth section. Thus, the two tissue segments (proximal and distal LC) were analyzed separately only for this section. The measured cell nuclear diameters and number of ACF are summarized in Figure 19.8. We found that for all the time points, and for both segments, the measured nuclear diameters for the treated groups were significantly different from the control group (*p* values < 10^{-4} **). Furthermore, significant differences were observed for both segments after only 4 weeks posttreatment. This measured increase in the nuclear diameter, however, remained relatively constant thereafter, with the exception of the last time point in the proximal LC. Here, the nuclear diameter increased dramatically from ~6.0 to ~7.2 μm. To investigate this effect further, Figure 19.8c plots the nuclear diameter as a function of the average number of ACF, which are preneoplastic lesions.

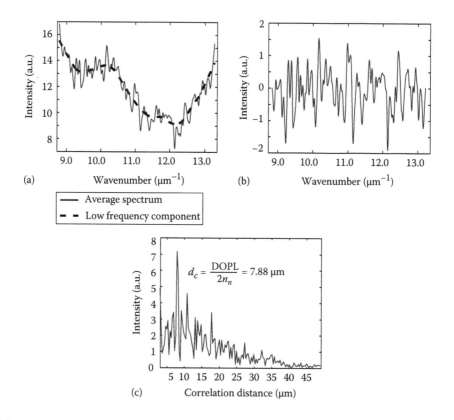

FIGURE 19.7 Average spectrum (gray solid line) from the delineated region in Figure 19.6, along with low-frequency component (black dotted line) (a). The low-frequency component is subtracted from the averaged spectrum to obtain the local oscillations (b). A Fourier transform yields a correlation function (c), where the peak corresponds to an average cell nuclear diameter of 7.88 μm in the region of analysis. (Taken from Robles, F. et al., *Biomed. Opt. Express*, 1, 736, 2010. With permission.)

For clarity, we also identify each point with its corresponding time period. Note that the formation of ACF was faster in the proximal LC compared to the distal LC and that the plot shows a region of little nuclear morphological change after the initial formation of ACF. This plateau region is present in both sections and is initially independent of the number of ACF. However, once the number of ACF increased to the maximum value observed in this study (~70), the measured increase of the nuclear diameter was specific to the region manifesting more advanced neoplastic development, in contrast to the ubiquitous and relatively constant cell nuclear diameter measurements of the plateau region [16].

In this study, fLCI detected significant changes in segments and at time points that presented early evidence of preneoplastic development, underscoring the sensitivity of the method. Further, the measured early nuclear morphological change was observed in both segments and independently of the number of ACF, which suggests a ubiquitous micromorphological change of the colonic epithelium, indicating that a field effect has been observed. This, however, was not the case when neoplastic development became more advanced (demarcated by the high number of ACF); at which point, the nuclear diameter increase was specific to the affected region. This further supports the claim that fLCI can identify specific regions where more advanced neoplastic development has occurred, which is paramount for detecting CRC development and initiating a localized therapy.

In conclusion, we have demonstrated the ability of fLCI to quantitatively distinguish between tissues that are normal and those that exhibit early precancerous development. Further, the results suggest that fLCI may be able to detect changes due to the field effect of carcinogenesis, in addition to identifying

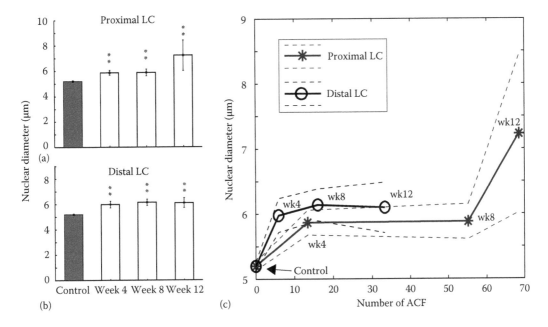

FIGURE 19.8 Results by colon length segments. Highly statistical differences (p value $< 10^{-4}$ **) were observed between the control group and treated groups for the proximal LC (a) and distal LC (b). (c) Plots the measured cell nuclear diameter as a function of the number of ACF. For clarity, the time of measurement is noted next to each point (wk, week). (Taken from Robles, F. et al., *Biomed. Opt. Express*, 1, 736, 2010. With permission.)

areas where more advanced neoplastic development has occurred locally. Lastly, this study presents strong evidence that fLCI can be used for detection of early cancer development, and we are hopeful that this will lead to a modality for in vivo, noninvasive clinical screening in the future.

19.3 Clinical FD a/LCI System Design

a/LCI is another light scattering technique that combines the ability of LSS to resolve morphological features of subcellular structure with the depth-resolving ability of OCT. Specifically, a/LCI compares the angular oscillations of backscattered light to predictions by Mie theory in order to estimate the size distributions of scatterers such as cell nuclei. In addition, it exploits LCI to separate the backscattered light from different depths of a tissue sample and generate depth-dependent diagnostic information. In the past decade, a/LCI technique has evolved over several generations from a time-domain, bench-top instrument to an FD, portable system that has been successfully demonstrated for in vivo clinical study.

19.3.1 Time-Domain a/LCI

Early a/LCI systems operated in the time domain and were based on Michelson and Mach–Zehnder interferometer geometries [28,29]. These systems achieved depth resolution, in a method analogous to time-domain OCT, by scanning a retro-reflector in the reference arm using a translation stage in order to selectively match its path length with that experienced by photons backscattered from a particular depth in the sample. By scanning an imaging field lens with a second translation stage in a direction perpendicular to the light path in the sample arm, light scattered across a range of angles was collected using a balanced photodetector for that depth. A 2D light scattering map can then be constructed with axes corresponding to sample depth and scattering angle. Depth regions of this map can be analyzed in order to determine the size distribution of the scatterers in that region.

These a/LCI systems were used to validate the technique on multiple cellular and animal models. HT29 epithelial cells were measured with subwavelength accuracy while identifying the role of long range correlations and fractal organization [29]. Time-domain a/LCI was also able to identify the presence of dysplasia retrospectively in a rat esophageal carcinogenesis model with 80% sensitivity and 100% specificity ($n = 42$) [30]. In a prospective study in the same model, dysplasia was predicted with 91% sensitivity and 97% specificity ($n = 82$) [31]. Additionally, the system was used to detect dysplasia in hamster tracheal epithelium with 78% sensitivity and 91% specificity ($n = 20$) [32].

Time-domain a/LCI is able to provide depth-resolved measurements of cellular morphology with subwavelength accuracy and precision but suffers from multiple drawbacks that preclude its use as a clinical tool appropriate for in vivo use. While the measurement time for a single location in the sample has been improved to a few minutes over these early versions [12,28], it is still two to three orders of magnitude too slow to be useful in an operating room and to overcome motion artifacts caused by natural patient processes. In addition, the free-space geometry of the system (particularly the sample arm) makes it impractical to access many tissue locations in vivo and requires an ex vivo sample to be placed on a stage rather than directing a probe to the tissue surface, as is common with typical endoscopically compatible clinical imaging tools.

19.3.2 FD a/LCI

FD a/LCI is an improved modification of the a/LCI technique that eliminates the drawbacks of the time-domain method and enables clinical measurements [33]. The approach employs an interferometric technique similar to that used in FD OCT to depth resolve the scattered light without the need to physically scan the path length of the reference arm. By spectrally resolving the detected light, FD a/LCI is able to separate contributions from various sample depths, which appear as oscillatory spectral components with frequencies that are proportional to the depths from which they originate. In addition to a significant decrease in data acquisition time due to the removal of axial scanning of the reference arm, FD methods for LCI have been shown to achieve higher signal-to-noise ratios than their time-domain counterparts [34–36].

In FD a/LCI, data acquisition speed was further improved by collecting the entire angular range simultaneously through the use of an imaging spectrometer, which can resolve detected light not only spectrally but also spatially, hence eliminating the need to physically scan the imaging lens. Additionally, by reducing the integration time of the spectrometer, the entire a/LCI scattering map can be collected in 40 msec with a single exposure, which represents a 10^4-time improvement in acquisition speed. This technique was initially validated through sizing of polystyrene microspheres with accuracy and precision comparable with time-domain a/LCI techniques [33].

In order to allow for flexibility of the sample arm and compatibility with endoscopic procedures, Pyhtila et al. presented a further modification of the system based on a coherent imaging fiber bundle [37]. In this system, the Mach–Zehnder interferometer is constructed with fiber optics such that the collimated light is delivered to the sample using a single-mode fiber and the scattered light is simultaneously collected across the face of the imaging fiber bundle. In addition, the femtosecond light source is replaced by a broadband superluminescent light-emitting diode (SLD) to allow for a significant reduction in system cost, weight, and footprint.

19.3.3 Clinical System Design

To adapt the fiber-optic FD a/LCI system for clinical use, it was modified into a portable system, as described by Zhu et al. [38]. As shown in Figure 19.9, the system employs a fiber-pigtailed broadband SLD with a center wavelength of $\lambda_0 = 830$ nm and a full-width half-maximum (FWHM) bandwidth $\Delta\lambda_{FWHM} = 19$ nm. The input light first passes through an optical isolator to prevent backreflection into the SLD cavity. A 5:95 fiber splitter then separates it into reference (5% power) and sample (95% power) arms.

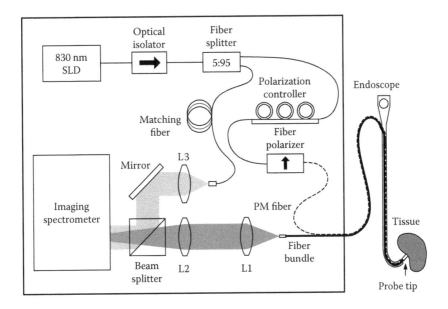

FIGURE 19.9 System configuration of clinical FD a/LCI system. (Adapted from Zhu, Y. et al., *J. Biomed. Opt.*, 16, 011003, 2011. With permission.)

In the reference arm, light is passed through a length of single-mode optical fiber, which is path length matched to the sample arm, and is collimated into free space (light gray) by lens L3. By placing the collimator on a translation stage, it is possible to perform fine adjustments to the path length of the reference arm for precise matching. The adjusted path length remains fixed during instrument operation.

In the sample arm, light is delivered to the tissue using a polarization-maintaining (PM) fiber rather than a single-mode fiber. To polarize the light, an inline fiber polarizer was used to output a linear polarization that is aligned along the slow axis of the PM fiber. The probe tip assembly collimates the light onto the sample and collects the scattered light field with the distal end of an imaging fiber bundle (2.3 m long; 1.1 mm diameter; 18,000 pixels). These sample signals are carried by the bundle back through the fiber probe to the interferometer, where it is mixed with the reference field. To preserve the spatial distribution of light, which encodes the angular scattering distribution of light from the sample, the proximal face of the fiber bundle is imaged onto the input slit of the imaging spectrometer using a 4f system created by lenses L1 and L2.

The probe tip assembly is detailed in Figure 19.10a. The endface of the PM fiber is positioned at the focal plane of a miniature drum lens. In addition to delivering collimated light to the sample, the lens collects the backscattered light (light gray). The lens is also one focal length from the face of the fiber bundle so that the angular profile of the scattered light is mapped into spatial distribution across its face. These angles are distributed with the fiber pixels closest to the PM fiber receiving the lowest scattering angles, and those at the opposite periphery of the bundle receiving light scattered at the highest angles. To protect the optical elements in the probe tip, it is covered with a protective cap consisting of a short Teflon (polytetrafluoroethylene [PTFE]) tube, a coverslip-made optical window, and a retaining ring. In order to avoid specular reflection from the protective window being collected on the fiber bundle, the window is tilted out of the incident plane.

In the interferometer, the proximal face of the fiber bundle is imaged onto the input slit of the imaging spectrometer. Consequently, only the light scattered onto the center strip of pixels of the fiber bundle is actually detected and analyzed. Figure 19.10b highlights the projection of the input slit of the spectrometer on an image of the distal face of the fiber bundle (detection area).

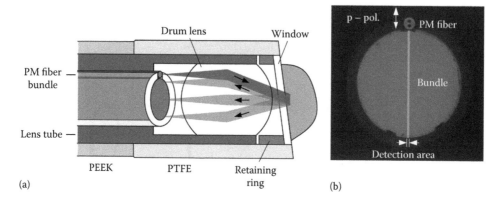

FIGURE 19.10 Design of the probe tip of the clinical a/LCI system. (a) Probe tip assembly showing sample illumination and scattering detection with fiber bundle. (b) Collection fiber bundle and delivery PM fiber with detection area highlighted. (Adapted from Zhu, Y. et al., *J. Biomed. Opt.*, 16, 011003, 2011. With permission.)

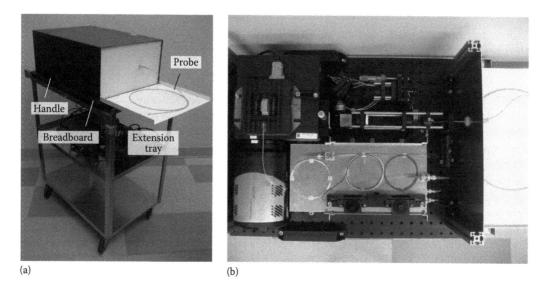

FIGURE 19.11 Clinical a/LCI system. (a) Enclosed system on the cart with the extension tray installed. (b) System detail with top cover removed. (Adapted from Zhu, Y. et al., *J. Biomed. Opt.*, 16, 011003, 2011. With permission.)

To enable in vivo measurements in the lumen of the gastrointestinal tract, the fiber probe assembly must be compatible with the accessory channel of a standard endoscope, which has a typical diameter of 2.8 mm and a working length of 105 cm. The small outer diameter (2.3 mm) of the fiber probe assembly and the low degree of friction generated between the sheath material (polyetheretherketone [PEEK]) and the inner lining of the accessory channel allow for the probe to pass through with minimal resistance.

In order for the system to be fully clinically compatible, it is built with a small footprint (24″ × 18″) and carried on a 27″ × 18″ stainless steel utility cart as pictured in Figure 19.11. During operation, the probe is placed on a detachable extension tray, also visible in Figure 19.11a. Figure 19.11b illustrates the compact design of the clinical a/LCI system, including a three-shelf rack that houses most of the fiber-optic components and minimizes footprint.

19.3.4 Signal Processing: Mie-Theory-Based Inverse Light Scattering Analysis

In order to analyze the angular scattering signal from various depths in the interrogated sample, the interferometric signal collected by the clinical a/LCI system must be processed into an angle-depth map characterizing the scattered light. Once this preprocessing technique has produced an image representative of the normalized scattering and resolved both in angle and depth, it can be segmented and postprocessed in order to correlate information regarding size distributions and indices of refraction of scatterers with various sample depths.

19.3.4.1 Preprocessing

The detected signal $I(\lambda_m, \theta_n)$ is a spectrally dispersed signal that is a function of wavelength λ and vertical position of the CCD detector n, which corresponds to a specific scattering angle θ_n. This signal can be related to the sample and reference fields (E_s, E_r) as [5]

$$I(\lambda_m, \theta_n) = \left\langle \left| E_r(\lambda_m, \theta_n) \right|^2 \right\rangle + \left\langle \left| E_s(\lambda_m, \theta_n) \right|^2 \right\rangle + 2\operatorname{Re}\left\langle E_s(\lambda_m, \theta_n) E_r^*(\lambda_m, \theta_n) \right\rangle \cos(\Delta\varphi) \qquad (19.2)$$

where

    $\Delta\varphi$ is the phase difference between the two fields
    (m, n) corresponds to a pixel location
    $\langle \cdots \rangle$ denotes an ensemble average in time

The first two terms correspond to the contributions from the reference and sample fields, respectively, while the third term represents the interferometric term of interest. To isolate this term, the sample and reference fields are measured independently and subtracted from the total intensity.

Depth-resolved information is obtained by linearly resampling the interferometric term at each scattering angle into wave number domain followed by a Fourier transform. The result represents the scattering contributions from the sample as a function of depth at that scattering angle. Prior to any postprocessing, this angle- and depth-resolved map of scattering must be corrected for dispersion, normalized by the source intensity across the input slit of the spectrometer, and squared to yield scattered intensity.

19.3.4.2 Postprocessing/Fitting

The goal of the postprocessing is to extract the angular scattering contribution from cell nuclei at each sample depth and fit it to that predicted by Mie theory in order to determine their size distribution [5,33]. It is worth noting that the angular distribution of the scattered intensity is related to the two-point spatial correlation function of the optical field through a Fourier transform [29]:

$$\Im\left[\left| E(\vec{\theta})^2 \right|\right] = \Im\left[I(\vec{\theta}) \right] = \Gamma_E(r) \qquad (19.3)$$

where r is the length scale of the spatial correlations along the transverse direction given by the angle θ.

Because of this relationship, it is possible to use a low-pass filter to remove scattering contributions by large-scale features (e.g., intercell contributions) from the total angular scattering distribution. While these scattering contributions contain information regarding organization on the cellular level, it is the contributions from subcellular organelles that are of interest in this analysis.

The nucleus is the largest of the subcellular organelles, typically having a diameter of 7–15 μm. The next largest cellular organelles are mitochondria, roughly 1 μm in size. Because the frequency of oscillations in the angular scattering pattern is proportional to scatterer size, the angular scattering contribution of all organelles smaller than the cell nuclei can be approximated as a second-order polynomial. In order to remove these contributions from the detected scattering profile, a second-order polynomial is fit to the filtered data and then subtracted from it to leave only the scattering contributions from cell nuclei.

These contributions are then compared with the predictions of Mie theory. For this purpose, a database of Mie-scattering solutions is created for a range of diameters, size distributions, and relative refractive indices.

In the fitting process, a chi-squared test is performed between the detected scattering signal and each of the candidate scattering solutions provided by the database. The theoretical solution that best fits the detected signal determines the average nuclear size distribution of the probed depth segment.

19.3.5 Detecting Dysplasia in BE

The fiber-bundle-based a/LCI system has been used to conduct three studies of tissues from patients with BE. The first two examined ex vivo resected esophageal tissues, both in laboratory and clinical settings [5,39]. The third BE study was a pilot in vivo clinical trial, in which the clinical a/LCI system was used to detect dysplasia in a population of BE patients undergoing routine surveillance [40].

19.3.5.1 Ex Vivo Study

An initial study examining resected esophageal tissue for dysplasia using the FD a/LCI system was reported by Pyhtila et al. [39]. This study utilized a version of the FD system in which the sample arm was fixed to a stage onto which the tissue sample could be placed. Tissue samples were drawn from three patients with dysplastic BE who underwent esophago-gastrectomies. The tissue was opened longitudinally and light scattering data were collected within 2 h of surgery. Following acquisition of optical biopsies, each biopsy site was marked and a corresponding traditional biopsy was taken. By examining the average nuclear size and index of refraction at each of the sampled locations and comparing to histopathological analysis, the system was able to differentiate between dysplastic tissue and gastric columnar epithelium with a sensitivity of 100% and a specificity of 100% ($n = 18$).

A further study reported by Brown et al. used a portable version of the system to examine resected segments of esophageal in a surgical setting [5]. In this study, the a/LCI system was transported to a surgical suite and used to scan tissue samples immediately following surgical resection. To facilitate ease of scanning, the system employed a fiber probe that could be manipulated by hand onto the tissue surface. The clinical a/LCI system was used to interrogate 15 tissue locations. Histopathological analysis of biopsies taken at each of these locations following optical scanning classified them as three tissue types: normal squamous mucosa (5), normal gastric mucosa (4), and BE with the presence of low-grade dysplasia (LGD) (6). By analyzing the scattering from the deep basal layer of tissue, the study was able to distinguish dysplastic tissue with 100% sensitivity and 78% specificity ($n = 15$). This result is particularly compelling, as it demonstrates the importance of isolating the scattering contributions from the basal layer of tissue to avoid the effects of inflammation and gastritis, which preferentially affect the surface layers of epithelial tissue.

19.3.5.2 In Vivo Study

The endoscopically compatible clinical a/LCI system was used to conduct an in vivo pilot study for the detection of dysplasia in BE patients [40]. In this study, the a/LCI fiber probe was inserted through the accessory channel of an endoscope during routine surveillance procedures. For each patient, three to six optical biopsies were taken at locations selected by the physician. Immediately following acquisition of the light scattering spectra at each location, the fiber probe was removed and a physical biopsy was taken at a location co-registered with the a/LCI measurement. Following the procedure, these biopsies were reviewed by a pathologist and their diagnosis was correlated to the a/LCI measurements of nucleus size and index of refraction in order to evaluate the ability of a/LCI to detect the presence of dysplasia.

Forty-six patients were scanned in this study using the clinical a/LCI system at two clinical sites. From these patients, 172 co-registered biopsies were collected. Each of these biopsies was classified as BE with high-grade dysplasia (HGD) (5), BE with LGD (8), BE indeterminate for dysplasia (14), nondysplastic BE (NDBE) (75), normal gastric tissue (31), normal squamous tissue (22), or normal squamocolumnar tissue that contained both normal and squamous tissue types (17). Tissue samples classified as dysplastic were read by a second pathologist to verify their diagnosis. In the case of disagreement, a consensus was reached by the pathologists. Samples identified as HGD and LGD were considered dysplastic, while samples identified as indeterminate for dysplasia, NDBE, normal squamous, normal columnar, and normal squamocolumnar tissue were considered negative for dysplasia. This treatment reflects the current clinical treatment protocols for physical biopsies.

For each of the optical sites, 10–30 individual data acquisitions were taken. These scans were first evaluated for sufficient signal strength and then analyzed individually and segmented into three depth segments: 0–100, 100–200, and 200–300 μm. For each depth segment, the results of the individual acquisitions were combined to reach a consensus size reading for that site. The third of these depth segments, 200–300 μm, was identified as the basal layer of tissue.

A scatterplot of the mean nuclear size and average nuclear density (ratio of average refractive index of a nucleus to that of its surroundings) for the basal layer appears in Figure 19.12. To determine the relationship between sensitivity and specificity, a receiver operating characteristic (ROC) curve was generated. When nuclear size from the basal layer was used as the distinguishing characteristic between dysplastic and nondysplastic tissues, the area under the curve (AUC) was found to be 0.91, indicating a strong correlation between dysplasia and increased nuclear size.

Using a decision line of 11.84 μm provided by the ROC curve for the basal layer, dysplastic biopsies were distinguished from nondysplastic biopsies with a sensitivity of 100% (13/13) and a specificity of 84%

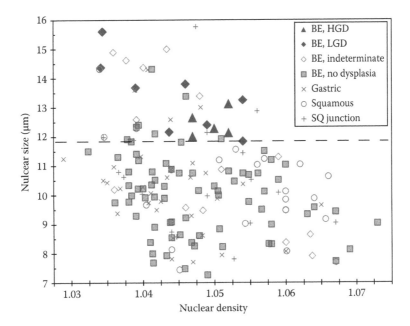

FIGURE 19.12 In vivo basal layer scatterplot for BE study. Each point represents a single optical biopsy and is color-coded by its pathological diagnosis. Dotted black line represents decision line. (From Terry, N.G. et al., *Gastroenterology*, 140, 42, 2011. With permission.)

specificity (134/159). This corresponds to a classification accuracy of 86% (147/172 biopsy sites), a positive predictive value (PPV) of 34% (13/38), and a negative predictive value (NPV) of 100% (134/134).

Statistical analyses were used to assess the association of diagnosis with morphological nuclear characteristics after adjusting for other relevant factors. Following adjustment for age and clinic site, nuclear diameter in the mucosal layer 200–300 µm beneath the surface was found to be positively associated with the presence of dysplasia at a significant level ($p = 0.0001$). In addition, increased nuclear density in the same depth segment was found to be negatively associated with the presence of dysplasia at a significant level ($p = 0.0009$).

19.3.6 Detecting Dysplasia in Colon Tissue

The clinical a/LCI was also used in a pilot study to identify the presence of dysplasia in human colon tissue segments that had been surgically resected. In this study, segments of colon tissue were scanned with the a/LCI system within 2 h of surgical resection. For each tissue sample, five to six locations were selected, scanned, and marked with India ink. Traditional biopsies were taken at each biopsy site, and their diagnosis was determined through histological analysis by a pathologist. These diagnoses were then compared to the a/LCI morphological measurements in order to evaluate the ability of a/LCI to determine the presence of dysplasia in colon tissue.

Fourteen patients were enrolled in this study, yielding a total of 72 paired biopsies. Of these patients, two were completely pathologically normal at the interrogated biopsy sites, one presented a mix of LGD and HGD, one displayed both dysplasia and adenocarcinoma, five presented only invasive adenocarcinoma, and five showed characteristics of ulcerative diseases. In this study, only biopsies that were pathologically normal or those that had a diagnosis of dysplasia (LGD or HGD) were considered. This consisted of 4 biopsies diagnosed as HGD, 5 diagnosed as LGD, and 23 from pathologically normal sites.

In this study, simple nuclear diameter alone did not appear to be predictive of dysplasia as in previous esophageal studies [5,39,40]. This is likely due to the increased complexity of the colon tissue structure when compared to the normal squamous tissue of the esophageal epithelium. Rather, two additional metrics based on the variability of the nuclear size and the calculated aspect ratio of cellular nuclei readings were used to differentiate dysplastic from nondysplastic tissue. The nuclear size variability tissue in a certain depth region of interest can be determined by averaging the absolute value of the deviations of all individual sizing measurements from the average size across that region. The aspect ratio of the spheroidal nuclei in a given depth range is recovered as the ratio of the maximum and minimum nuclear sizes (representative of spheroidal cell nuclei whose major axes are orthogonal and parallel to the delivered beam respectively) in that range.

Figure 19.13 shows scatterplots of the nuclear size variability (plotted against the maximum measured nuclear diameter) and the aspect ratio (plotted against the average measured nuclear diameter) for

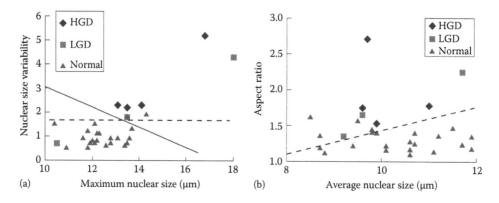

FIGURE 19.13 (a) Plot of nuclear size variability for the segment of tissue 200–400 µm below the tissue surface. Dotted black line indicates decision line. (b) Scatterplot of aspect ratio for the segment of tissue 200–400 µm below the tissue surface. Dotted black line indicates decision line.

the segment of mucosal tissue between 200 and 400 μm deep in the colon tissue samples. One normal biopsy sample and two dysplastic samples were omitted due to weak scattering from this deep mucosal layer. In the plot of the nuclear size variability, a simple decision line (dashed line) can be drawn that separates dysplastic tissue from normal tissue with a sensitivity of 86% (6/7) and a specificity of 91% (20/22). This corresponds to a PPV of 75% (6/8) and an NPV of 95% (20/21). A similar decision line uses aspect ratio to distinguish dysplastic from nondysplastic tissue with a sensitivity of 100% (7/7) and a specificity of 86% (19/22). These values correspond to a PPV of 70% (7/10) and an NPV of 100% (19/19).

These four clinical studies point to a/LCI's strong potential as a diagnostic tool for biopsy guidance in the future. Additional studies are planned to further characterize the use of a/LCI in the colon and additional epithelial tissue sites.

19.4 FITS Measurement System

Early implementations of the a/LCI technique were based on free-space optics, which in general is impractical for in vivo applications [28,33]. To address this issue, later generations utilized fiber optics, including fiber bundles and single-mode fibers, to improve system portability and reduce probe size, and have been demonstrated successfully in recent clinical study, as described in the previous section [19,38].

In these previous a/LCI systems, the scattering signal is collected along only one angular dimension (1D, in-plane), due to instrumental limitations such as the inability to adequately control the polarization of the collected scattering. Measuring scattering in two angular dimensions (2D), however, is advantageous over 1D measurement in that the additional information can help improve sizing accuracy. More importantly, it offers access to extra morphological characteristics, for example, aspect ratio and orientation of the scatterer, in addition to diameter and optical density. These parameters are unavailable in traditional a/LCI analysis, which is based on spherical approximation and comparison to Mie theory, unless the orientation of the sample can be varied across multiple measurements [41,42]. The 2D measurement allows for investigation of aspherical scatterers with unprecedented detail and the use of T-matrix-based analysis to extract comprehensive morphological information.

Motivated by these potential advantages, the latest generation of a/LCI, termed the FITS measurement system, was designed specifically to achieve these highly desired capabilities. The FITS system is built upon a novel fiber-optic Michelson–Sagnac hybrid interferometer (MSI) and is superior to previous a/LCI schemes in that it allows for accurate polarization control and hence the investigation of depth-resolved, polarization-sensitive, 2D angular scattering. In this section, we first introduce the principle behind the MSI approach and demonstrate the FITS performance with 2D scattering measurements of a double-layer microsphere phantom. We then explore 2D scattering of spheroidal scatterers with T-matrix-based analysis.

19.4.1 Principle of FITS System

Figure 19.14a shows the schematic of the FITS system. Broadband light from a Ti:sapphire laser (Coherent, Inc.: 825 nm, $\Delta\lambda = 17$ nm, 30 mW) is focused into a single-mode fiber coupler (ratio $\alpha = 0.01\%$) via a 10× objective lens. The two arms of the coupler are cleaved and their facets are placed in the focal plane of a graded index (GRIN) lens (Newport Corp.: 0.23 pitch, 1.8 mm diameter; 4.4 mm length) for illumination and collection. The GRIN lens is angled at 8° on the sample side to avoid specular reflection being back-coupled into the system. Arm 2 receives the majority of the source power and serves as the illumination fiber. Its output is collimated via the GRIN lens onto the sample. Arm 1 is the low power arm, serving as the collection fiber that receives the light scattered at angle θ. To maximize the detectable angular range, Arm 2 is positioned toward the edge of the GRIN lens, whereas Arm 1 raster-scans in 2D using a pair of motorized actuators. Both the illumination and collection fields can be tuned independently using polarization controllers (PC1&2) to be linearly polarized along any direction with extinction ratio greater than 20 dB, making it possible to measure scattering under

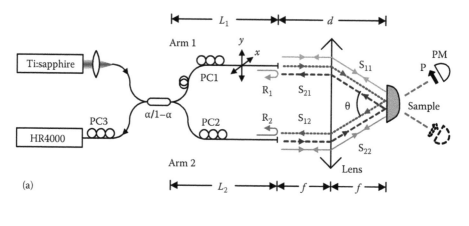

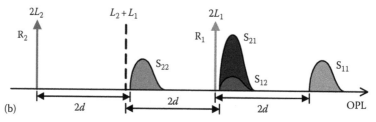

FIGURE 19.14 Principle of MSI. (a) Schematic. d—OPL from the fiber ends to the sample; θ—scattering angle; f—focal length; PC1–3—polarization controllers; P—polarizer; PM—power meter; x and y—scan directions. (b) OPL of the signals. (Taken from Zhu, Y.Z. et al., *Opt. Lett.*, 35, 1641, 2010. With permission.)

any combination of illumination and collection polarization. The spectrum of the interference signals is detected by a miniature spectrometer (Ocean Optics, Inc., HR4000).

The MSI scheme resembles a Michelson or Sagnac interferometer, but its operation relies upon coherently mixing components from both interferometers, hence the hybrid mode. Three pairs of signals are generated: (1) Michelson signals R_1 and R_2, or the fiber-end reflections, which serve as reference signals; (2) Sagnac signals S_{12} and S_{21}, or the angular scattering signals, which are the signals of interest; and (3) backscattering signals S_{11} and S_{22}, which can also be considered Michelson signals, but only represent scattering in the backscattering direction (180°). For low-coherence interferometric operation, the MSI matches the OPL of R_1 and S_{21}. To achieve this, a matching condition needs to be satisfied, where the OPL of the collection arm L_1 is set to be longer than that of the illumination arm L_2 by a specific amount. Other scattering signals will not be detected due to path length mismatch and/or attenuated intensity due to the unbalanced power splitting.

Table 19.1 lists the OPL of each signal with their relative locations illustrated in Figure 19.14b assuming $L_1 > L_2$. Note that the OPLs are entirely determined by L_1, L_2, and the lens-specific parameter d. Consequently, R_1 and S_{21} can be colocated in the OPL domain by tuning the differential of the two arms, $L_1 - L_2$, as illustrated in Figure 19.14b. Hence, depth-resolved information of S_{21} (S_{12}) can be obtained using R_1 as reference. The matching condition for hybrid operation can then be written as

$$L_1 - L_2 = 2d \quad \text{or} \quad l_1 - l_2 = \frac{2d}{n} \tag{19.4}$$

where
   n is the refractive index of the fiber
   l_1 and l_2 are the physical length of the two arms

TABLE 19.1 OPL and Intensity of MSI Signals

Signal	R_1	R_2	S_{21}	S_{12}	S_{11}	S_{22}
OPL	$2L_1$	$2L_2$	$L_1 + L_2 + 2d$	$L_1 + L_2 + 2d$	$2L_1 + 2d$	$2L_2 + 2d$
Intensity[a]	αr_1	αr_2	s_{21}	$\alpha^2 s_{12}$	αs_{11}	αs_{22}

Source: Taken from Zhu, Y.Z. et al., *Opt. Lett.*, 35, 1641, 2010. With permission.
[a] Normalized to source intensity.

With the GRIN lens, signals R_2, S_{11}, and S_{22} are far separated (ΔOPL ~$2d$) from R_1 and S_{21} (S_{12}) and will not generate detectable interference. This is attributed to a sufficiently large d (~7.3 mm) that places these high-frequency interference signals beyond the spectrometer's detection range (~4 mm).

In addition to signal selection by coherence gating, the low splitting ratio used in this scheme further attenuates undesirable scattering signals. The primary purpose of employing a small α (0.01%) is to attenuate the reference signal to achieve proper power balance with the scattering signal. The value of 0.01% is determined using intensity data from the Mach-Zehnder Interferometer (MZI) based system [8]. Table 19.1 lists simplified signal intensities with the assumption of the following: 1) $\alpha \ll 1$ and 2) the scattering coefficients and fiber-end reflectivities (all in lower case) satisfy $s_{11}, s_{22}, s_{12}, s_{21} \ll r_1, r_2 \ll 1$. Both are reasonable assumptions for reference fields generated by cleaved fibers (~3.4%) and sample fields returned by biological samples. These values indicate that a small α not only attenuates reference signals but also effectively eliminates irrelevant signals S_{11} and S_{22} by a factor of α, as well as the overlapping signal, S_{12}, by a factor of α^2. It is worth noting that the use of a small α is not a requirement for MSI operation. In contrast, path length matching is essential and by itself is sufficient to prevent detection of unwanted signals. A reduced splitting ratio, however, further isolates the signals of interest by leaving only three signals with substantial strength: sample signal S_{21}, reference signal R_1, and the noninterferometric background signal R_2 that can be frustrated by angle-polishing and antireflection coating if necessary.

The symmetry of this system points to the fact that R_2 can also serve as the reference signal from the standpoint of generating interference, provided that $L_2 > L_1$. They differ substantially, however, in that using R_1 as reference offers superior polarization control compared to that achieved with the use of R_2. If R_2 were used for reference, the signals S_{21} and R_2 would travel separate paths through Arm 1 and 2 before interfering inside the coupler. The distinct paths and ambient disturbance to the fibers would make it practically impossible to determine or control their polarization inside the coupler. As a result, no precise control is possible as to which polarization component of the scattering field is detected with this configuration. In the preferred case of using R_1 as reference, however, its mixing with S_{21} occurs at the end of Arm 1, prior to their co-propagation through the fiber. Thus, the deleterious effect of fiber disturbance is eliminated. The detected polarization component of S_{21} is determined by the direction of the linearly polarized R_1 as it exits Arm 1, which can be adjusted using a polarizer and a power meter. The illumination polarization can also be tuned in a similar way. In summary, the MSI scheme allows both the illumination and the collection to be either p- or s-polarized, offering full polarization control and hence the capability to map the full 2D angular scattering distribution.

19.4.2 Depth-Resolved 2D Scattering of Microspheres

The performance of the MSI-based FITS system is demonstrated by collecting 2D angular scattering from a double-layer polydimethylsiloxane (PDMS) phantom with embedded microspheres (Thermo Fisher Scientific, Inc.) with mean diameters of 5.990 ± 0.045 µm and 10.00 ± 0.05 µm, respectively.

In the experiment, the collection fiber (Arm 1) scans an area of 1.0 × 1.8 mm² to generate a 90 × 170 map of 2D angular scattering with an angular resolution of 0.212°. At each point of the 2D distribution, the interferometric spectrum is recorded. A Fourier transform is then taken to convert the spectrum into depth-resolved scattering intensity with a depth resolution of 17.7 µm.

For polarization-sensitive measurements, there are four possible combinations of the illumination and collection polarization: co-polarization combinations PP and SS, and cross-polarization combinations SP and PS, where the first letter indicates the polarization of the illumination field and the second letter the polarization component to be collected from the sample. For the optical configuration in Figure 19.14, theoretical calculation shows that the two cross-polarization situations PS and SP produce identical distributions, which has been confirmed by experimental results. Therefore, only three independent scattering distributions exist.

The experiment uses a fixed p-polarized illumination and measures both the PP and PS components of the field scattered by the phantom, as shown in Figure 19.15a and b, where the double-layered structure can be clearly identified. Figure 19.15c–j demonstrate good agreement between the FITS measurements and Mie-theory simulations for each layer and each polarization combination. Note that the speckle-like high-frequency fringes seen in the experimental results are likely to be the coherent scattering from adjacent microspheres in the phantom. Such information can be potentially used to estimate particle density and spacing.

To demonstrate the quantitative capability of the 2D measurements, Mie-theory fitting was performed along lines A, B, and C in Figure 19.15, producing subwavelength sizing accuracy, as shown in Figure 19.16. Data from lines A and B are typical scattering distributions as would be measured with the traditional 1D a/LCI technique. The fitting outcome for line C demonstrates that accurate sizing can also be obtained using other scattering directions and polarizations. These examples show that a single 2D data acquisition by the FITS system improves fitting accuracy to a few tens of nanometers and reduces fitting errors to less than 200 nm as compared with previous 1D a/LCI systems [19,44].

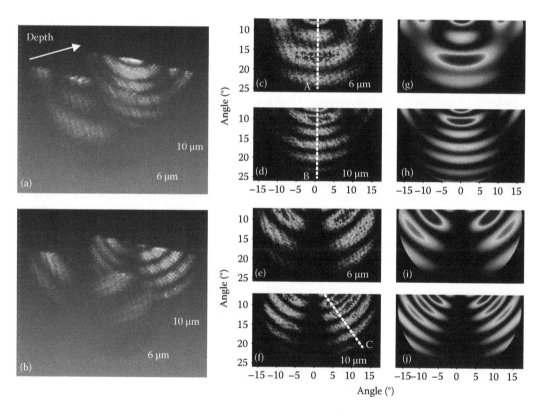

FIGURE 19.15 Scattering of the double-layer phantom under p-polarized illumination. (a, b) Depth-resolved 2D angular scattering for p- (Media 1) and s-polarized (Media 2) scattering. (c, d) p- and (e, f) s-polarized 2D scattering for 6 and 10 μm layers, respectively. (g–j) Corresponding Mie-theory simulations. A, B, and C are lines along which data fitting is executed. (From Zhu, Y.Z. et al., *Opt. Lett.*, 35, 1641, 2010. With permission.)

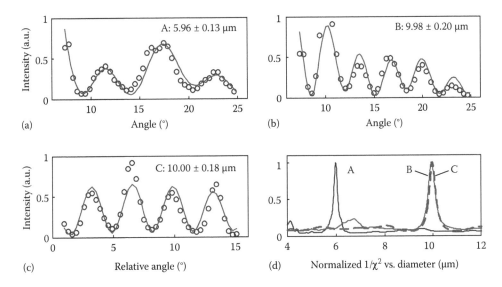

FIGURE 19.16 Mie-fitting results along (a) line A, (b) line B, and (c) line C. (d) Normalized $1/\chi^2$ values indicating best fits in diameter. (From Zhu, Y.Z. et al., *Opt. Lett.*, 35, 1641, 2010. With permission.)

19.4.3 T-Matrix Method for Scattering Analysis of Spheroids

A number of optical scattering techniques for biological samples, including a/LCI, have successfully based their analysis on Mie theory, where biological scatterers are approximated as spheres and their diameters are extracted through inverse analysis. In reality, few of these scatterers are precisely spherical; rather, they are better modeled as spheroids. Although Mie theory has shown some success in determining the diameters as well as the aspect ratio of spheroidal scatterers, such application is greatly hampered by the requirement of multiple measurements under different orientations and polarizations [41,42,45], and considerable a priori knowledge about scatterer orientation.

The T-matrix method, also known as the extended-boundary-condition method, is a superior tool for computing exact scattering field of a spheroidal scatterer [46]. Hence, direct comparison between theory and experiment is possible for accurate extraction of morphological features such as aspect ratio. Unlike Mie theory, T-matrix method can compute scattering from a variety of geometries including spheroids, Chebyshev particles, and cylinders. In principle, the method is applicable to any particle geometry, but in practice, at least one axis of symmetry is usually required for efficient computation. Furthermore, for particles much larger than the wavelength or highly aspherical, excessive rounding error may accumulate and prevents convergence. T-matrix has been used as a basis of inverse analysis that can capture details about elongation, compression, or deformation of cell nuclei [47,48].

The T-matrix method has attracted significant attention as an alternative to Mie theory for computing scattered fields. Nielson et al. modeled angular scattering from red blood cells [49], Duncan and Thomas [50] showed that variations in depolarization with wavelength were correlated with spheroidal aspect ratio [50], and Mourant et al. used spheroids as a model for scattering from both organelles and whole cells [51,52]. The multitude of parameters in T-matrix simulation allows for more comprehensive characterization of scatterer morphology; however, it also produces a much larger parameter space to search for solutions to the inverse problem. On the other hand, in all these techniques including a/LCI, the number of independent measurements that can be recorded through wavelength or 1D angular scattering is limited, giving rise to a potentially ill-conditioned inverse problem where multiple best fits may be possible and may compromise the effectiveness of the analysis. In the absence of sufficient a priori knowledge, these limited data may result in misinterpretation of the analysis results by providing numerically optimal, but physically incorrect, solutions. Given these limitations, light scattering methods have typically been focused on distinguishing a few possible tissue states over a limited range of geometries.

Two-dimensional angular scattering measurement, in contrast, provides ample information and fine details about spheroidal scattering, hence greatly facilitating the inverse analysis. Aptowicz et al. developed a 2D angular optical scattering (TAOS) system for the investigation of microdroplets [53]. Smith and Berger proposed an integrated Raman and angular scattering microscope (IRAM) that acquired detailed 2D angle-resolved and Raman scattering from single cells [7]. Both techniques base their analysis on Mie theory and no depth resolution is provided. The 2D data acquisition of FITS system, combined with T-matrix as a light scattering model, presents a new form of a/LCI inverse analysis, which effectively uses the additional knowledge obtained by 2D angular measurements for accurate characterization of spheroids.

19.4.4 2D Scattering Analysis of Spheroids Based on FITS System and T-Matrix Method

We demonstrate the accuracy and specificity of the FITS system using phantoms containing spheroidal scatterers that mimic scattering from cell nuclei, first by qualitative comparisons to the T-matrix method and then by performing quantitative inverse analysis. The resulting size and aspect ratio determinations are shown to be essentially free of multiple fits and accurate with subwavelength precision.

To fabricate spheroidal scatterers, PDMS phantoms embedded with polystyrene microspheres are stretched [41] and briefly heated past the glass transition point of polystyrene. The microspheres are hence stretched into spheroids and retain the shape after cooling. The process leaves the equal volume diameter (EVD) unchanged, but modifies the aspect ratio depending on the stretching tension applied.

Figure 19.17 presents the experimentally measured co-polarization components, PP and SS, and cross-polarization components, PS and SP (identical in theory and experiments; hence, only one is shown), of the FITS scans for spheroids with 15 µm EVD but three different aspect ratios, 1.0, 0.92, and 0.82, respectively. The aspect ratio is determined by quantitative image analysis (QIA) and used to generate T-matrix simulations, which are also shown for comparison.

Several trends are apparent in these comparisons. First, the PP and SS polarized results generally look similar for all aspect ratios, although the locations of the peaks and valleys are typically complementary between the two. In contrast, the cross-polarized SP/PS case is strikingly different, particularly for higher aspect ratios where many fewer photons are scattered in the backscattering direction (approximately the top center of each figure). These effects are observable with FITS only because of its ability to achieve full polarization control. Second, for all polarizations, the patterns appear with a high degree of azimuthal symmetry in the spherical case. In the case of a spherical scatterer (aspect ratio 1.0), the 2D scan is essentially azimuthally degenerate, as predicted by Mie theory, and FITS offers no significant advantage over conventional a/LCI scanning. However, as the scatterers are deformed, symmetry is quickly broken and the inadequacy of Mie theory becomes apparent. For the moderately deformed 0.82 aspect ratio phantom, the radial scans separated by even a few degrees of azimuth angle are nearly uncorrelated.

Inverse analysis is then performed on these 2D patterns to extract the spheroidal parameters. Since the PS/SP components do not generally guarantee high signal-to-noise ratio due to possible loss of intensity near the backscattering direction, we focus on the PP component. Figure 19.18 shows the χ^2-fitting of the experimental patterns to those generated by T-matrix simulations across a wide range of values of aspect ratio and diameter. The positions of the peak indicate the best fits, which are listed in Table 19.2 and are in excellent agreement with manufacturer data and QIA results.

The χ^2 error plots in Figure 19.7 lead to the following observations. First, FITS measurement provides a significantly better-conditioned inverse problem that is free of multiple best fits across a wide range of spheroidal parameters. Second, as aspect ratio decreases, the fitting accuracy of this parameter improves, as indicated by the narrowing width of the best fit peak. This is because aspherical particles have far more complex scattering patterns with less degeneracies than those from spherical scatterers, providing more input to the inverse analysis procedure and yielding improved accuracy and resolution.

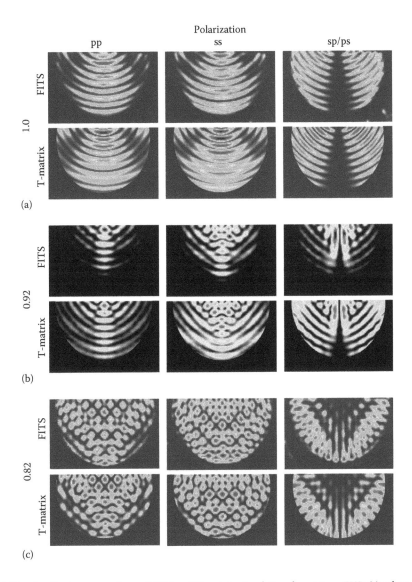

FIGURE 19.17 Qualitative comparison of FITS and T-matrix simulation for a 15 μm EVD (a) sphere, (b) prolate spheroid with aspect ratio 0.92, and (c) prolate spheroid with aspect ratio 0.82 as determined by QIA. The two cross-polarized cases are identical and thus presented as a single combined plot. The T-matrix simulations have been masked off at the GRIN lens boundaries to limit their angular extent to match the experimental range. (From Giacomelli, M. et al., *Opt. Express*, 18, 14616, 2010. With permission.)

Lastly, as scatterers elongate, an oscillatory pattern appears diagonally in the fitting plots in which the χ^2 error fluctuates above and below the mean. This corresponds to the algorithm approximately tracking a line along manifolds that keep the major scatterer axis constant. Far away from these lines, the far-field patterns are essentially uncorrelated and the χ^2 error remains nearly constant. This effect is contrasted in the 1D cross-sectional curves shown in Figure 19.18h and i.

In conclusion, we have introduced the FITS system for polarization-sensitive measurement of 2D angular scattering, as well as a T-matrix-based method for determining scatterer geometry from these measurements. Compared with previous 1D a/LCI systems, the FITS system can acquire scattering with two more degrees of freedom, that is, polarization and a second angular direction, both of which are

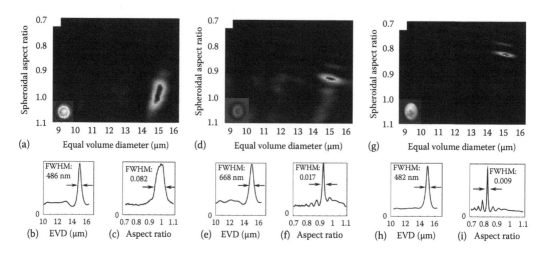

FIGURE 19.18 (a, d, g) 2D χ^2 error between scattered field of spheroids with 15 μm EVD and respective aspect ratio of 1.0, 0.92, and 0.82 and T-matrix simulated field. (b, e, h) Horizontal slice of $1/\chi^2$ error showing the FWHM EVD resolution of 0.49, 0.67, and 0.48 μm, respectively. (c, f, i) Vertical slice of $1/\chi^2$ error showing the FWHM resolution of the aspect ratio to be 0.082, 0.017, and 0.009, respectively. (Adapted from Giacomelli, M. et al., *Opt. Express*, 18, 14616, 2010. With permission.)

TABLE 19.2 FITS Measurement Results

	Spherical	Slightly Stretched	Moderately Stretched
FITS EVD (μm)	15.00 ± 0.24	14.95 ± 0.33	15.00 ± 0.24
Vendor EVD (μm)	15.02 ± 0.08	15.02 ± 0.08	15.02 ± 0.08
FITS aspect ratio	0.995 ± 0.04	0.925 ± 0.01	0.825 ± 0.005
QIA aspect ratio	1.0	0.93	0.82

Source: Adapted from Giacomelli, M. et al., *Opt. Express*, 18, 14616, 2010. With permission.

made possible by selecting R_1 as the reference signal. Preliminary results have demonstrated the system's potential as a powerful tool for advanced study of light scattering. In particular, size and shape of single and ensembles of microspheroids can be determined using T-matrix model with subwavelength accuracy and resolution over an extremely wide inverse search space.

19.5 Summary

We have reviewed development of fLCI and a/LCI, two interferometric light scattering techniques that take advantage of LCI to study scattered light as a function of depth in a sample. This ability allows for the characterization of cell morphology for a specific layer within a tissue. More significantly, it permits the identification of the tissue layer that provides the most sensitive and consistent information for the detection of dysplasia, as demonstrated by the ex vivo and in vivo studies with both techniques.

The future direction of fLCI development is to transform the free-space optical system into a compact, portable fiber-optic implementation and ultimately into a clinically viable diagnostic tool for cancer screening. For the clinical a/LCI system, pilot studies will continue on tissues of the gastrointestinal tract and possibly other organs with epithelial linings to further identify potential applications for the technique. Phantom tests on the FITS system have validated the concepts, but additional cell and tissue studies are necessary to establish its feasibility for examining biological specimens, where the focus of efforts is expected to be on the 2D processing of angular scattering distribution.

Acknowledgments

Grant support was provided by the National Institutes of Health (National Cancer Institute R01-CA138594 and R33-CA109907), US Air Force Research Laboratory (FA8650-09-C-7932), and Coulter Translational Partnership.

References

1. Backman V., M. B. Wallace, L. T. Perelman, J. T. Arendt, R. Gurjar, M. G. Muller, Q. Zhang et al., Detection of preinvasive cancer cells, *Nature* **406**, 35–36 (2000).
2. Wilson J. D. and T. H. Foster, Mie theory interpretations of light scattering from intact cells, *Opt. Lett.* **30**, 2442–2444 (2005).
3. Lovat L. B., K. Johnson, G. D. Mackenzie, B. R. Clark, M. R. Novelli, S. Davies, M. O'Donovan et al., Elastic scattering spectroscopy accurately detects high grade dysplasia and cancer in Barrett's oesophagus, *Gut* **55**, 1078–1083 (2006).
4. Nieman L. T., C. W. Kan, A. Gillenwater, M. K. Markey, and K. Sokolov, Probing local tissue changes in the oral cavity for early detection of cancer using oblique polarized reflectance spectroscopy: A pilot clinical trial, *J. Biomed. Opt.* **13**, 024011 (2008).
5. Brown W. J., J. W. Pyhtila, N. G. Terry, K. J. Chalut, T. A. D'Amico, T. A. Sporn, J. V. Obando, and A. Wax, Review and recent development of angle-resolved low-coherence interferometry for detection of precancerous cells in human esophageal epithelium, *IEEE J. Sel. Top. Quantum Electron.* **14**, 88–97 (2008).
6. Backman V., V. Gopal, M. Kalashnikov, K. Badizadegan, R. Gurjar, A. Wax, I. Georgakoudi et al., Measuring cellular structure at submicrometer scale with light scattering spectroscopy, *IEEE J. Sel. Top. Quantum Electron.* **7**, 887–893, PII S1077-260X(01)11252-9 (2001).
7. Smith Z. J. and A. J. Berger, Integrated Raman- and angular-scattering microscopy, *Opt. Lett.* **33**, 714–716 (2008).
8. Arifler D., I. Pavlova, A. Gillenwater, and R. Richards-Kortum, Light scattering from collagen fiber networks: Micro-optical properties of normal and neoplastic stroma, *Biophys. J.* **92**, 3260–3274 (2007).
9. Roy H. K., Y. Liu, R. K. Wali, Y. L. Kim, A. K. Kromine, M. J. Goldberg, and V. Backman, Four-dimensional elastic light-scattering fingerprints as preneoplastic markers in the rat model of colon carcinogenesis, *Gastroenterology* **126**, 1071–1081 (2004).
10. Shaheen N. J. and J. E. Richter, Barrett's oesophagus, *Lancet* **373**, 850–861 (2009).
11. Graf R. N., F. E. Robles, X. X. Chen, and A. Wax, Detecting precancerous lesions in the hamster cheek pouch using spectroscopic white-light optical coherence tomography to assess nuclear morphology via spectral oscillations, *J. Biomed. Opt.* **14**, 064030 (2009).
12. Wax A., C. Yang, R. R. Dasari, and M. S. Feld, Measurement of angular distributions by use of low-coherence interferometry for light-scattering spectroscopy, *Opt. Lett.* **26**, 322–324 (2001).
13. Graf R. N., W. J. Brown, and A. Wax, Parallel frequency-domain optical coherence tomography scatter-mode imaging of the hamster cheek pouch using a thermal light source, *Opt. Lett.* **33**, 1285–1287 (2008).
14. Morgner U., W. Drexler, F. X. Kartner, X. D. Li, C. Pitris, E. P. Ippen, and J. G. Fujimoto, Spectroscopic optical coherence tomography, *Opt. Lett.* **25**, 111–113 (2000).
15. Robles F., R. N. Graf, and A. Wax, Dual window method for processing spectroscopic optical coherence tomography signals with simultaneously high spectral and temporal resolution, *Opt. Express* **17**, 6799–6812 (2009).
16. Robles F., Y. Zhu, J. Lee, S. Sharma, and A. Wax, Fourier domain low coherence interferometry for detection of early colorectal cancer development in the azoxymethane rat carcinogenesis model, *Biomed. Opt. Express* **1**, 736–745 (2010).

17. Perelman L. T., V. Backman, M. Wallace, G. Zonios, R. Manoharan, A. Nusrat, S. Shields et al., Observation of periodic fine structure in reflectance from biological tissue: A new technique for measuring nuclear size distribution, *Phys. Rev. Lett.* **80**, 627–630 (1998).

18. van de Hulst H. C., *Light Scattering by Small Particles*, Dover Publications, Mineola, NY (1981).

19. Zhu Y., N. G. Terry, and A. Wax, Scanning fiber angle-resolved low coherence interferometry, *Opt. Lett.* **34**, 3196–3198 (2009).

20. Robles F. E. and A. Wax, Measuring morphological features using light-scattering spectroscopy and Fourier-domain low-coherence interferometry, *Opt. Lett.* **35**, 360–362 (2010).

21. Roy H. K., A. Gomes, V. Turzhitsky, M. J. Goldberg, J. Rogers, S. Ruderman, K. L. Young et al., Spectroscopic microvascular blood detection from the endoscopically normal colonic mucosa: Biomarker for neoplasia risk, *Gastroenterology* **135**, 1069–1078 (2008).

22. Kim Y. L., V. M. Turzhitsky, Y. Liu, H. K. Roy, R. K. Wali, H. Subramanian, P. Pradhan, and V. Backman, Low-coherence enhanced backscattering: Review of principles and applications for colon cancer screening, *J. Biomed. Opt.* **11**, 041125 (2006).

23. Braakhuis B. J. M., M. P. Tabor, J. A. Kummer, C. R. Leemans, and R. H. Brakenhoff, A genetic explanation of Slaughter's concept of field cancerization: Evidence and clinical implications, *Cancer Res.* **63**, 1727–1730 (2003).

24. Reddy B. S., Studies with the azoxymethane-rat preclinical model for assessing colon tumor development and chemoprevention, *Environ. Mol. Mutagen.* **44**, 26–35 (2004).

25. McLellan E. A. and R. P. Bird, Aberrant crypts—Potential preneoplastic lesions in the murine colon, *Cancer Res.* **48**, 6187–6192 (1988).

26. Zysk A. M., S. G. Adie, J. J. Armstrong, M. S. Leigh, A. Paduch, D. D. Sampson, F. T. Nguyen, and S. A. Boppart, Needle-based refractive index measurement using low-coherence interferometry, *Opt. Lett.* **32**, 385–387 (2007).

27. Choi W., C. Fang-Yen, K. Badizadegan, S. Oh, N. Lue, R. R. Dasari, and M. S. Feld, Tomographic phase microscopy, *Nat. Methods* **4**, 717–719 (2007).

28. Pyhtila J. W., R. N. Graf, and A. Wax, Determining nuclear morphology using an improved angle-resolved low coherence interferometry system, *Opt. Express* **11**, 3473–3484 (2003).

29. Wax A., C. H. Yang, V. Backman, K. Badizadegan, C. W. Boone, R. R. Dasari, and M. S. Feld, Cellular organization and substructure measured using angle-resolved low-coherence interferometry, *Biophys. J.* **82**, 2256–2264 (2002).

30. Wax A., C. Yang, M. G. Muller, R. Nines, C. W. Boone, V. E. Steele, G. D. Stoner, R. R. Dasari, and M. S. Feld, In situ detection of neoplastic transformation and chemopreventive effects in rat esophagus epithelium using angle-resolved low-coherence interferometry, *Cancer Res.* **63**, 3556–3559 (2003).

31. Wax A., J. W. Pyhtila, R. N. Graf, R. Nines, C. W. Boone, R. R. Dasari, M. S. Feld, V. E. Steele, and G. D. Stoner, Prospective grading of neoplastic change in rat esophagus epithelium using angle-resolved low-coherence interferometry, *J. Biomed. Opt.* **10**, 051604 (2005).

32. Chalut K. J., L. A. Kresty, J. W. Pyhtila, R. Nines, M. Baird, V. E. Steele, and A. Wax, In situ assessment of intraepithelial neoplasia in hamster trachea epithelium using angle-resolved low-coherence interferometry, *Cancer Epidemiol. Biomarkers Prev.* **16**, 223–227 (2007).

33. Pyhtila J. W. and A. Wax, Rapid, depth-resolved light scattering measurements using Fourier domain, angle-resolved low coherence interferometry, *Opt. Express* **12**, 6178–6183 (2004).

34. Choma M. A., M. V. Sarunic, C. H. Yang, and J. A. Izatt, Sensitivity advantage of swept source and Fourier domain optical coherence tomography, *Opt. Express* **11**, 2183–2189 (2003).

35. de Boer J. F., B. Cense, B. H. Park, M. C. Pierce, G. J. Tearney, and B. E. Bouma, Improved signal-to-noise ratio in spectral-domain compared with time-domain optical coherence tomography, *Opt. Lett.* **28**, 2067–2069 (2003).

36. Leitgeb R., C. K. Hitzenberger, and A. F. Fercher, Performance of Fourier domain vs. time domain optical coherence tomography, *Opt. Express* **11**, 889–894 (2003).

37. Pyhtila J. W., J. D. Boyer, K. J. Chalut, and A. Wax, Fourier-domain angle-resolved low coherence interferometry through an endoscopic fiber bundle for light-scattering spectroscopy, *Opt. Lett.* **31**, 772–774 (2006).

38. Zhu Y., N. G. Terry, J. T. Woosley, N. J. Shaheen, and A. Wax, Design and validation of an angle-resolved low coherence interferometry fiber probe for in vivo clinical measurements of depth-resolved nuclear morphology, *J. Biomed. Opt.* **16**, 011003–011010 (2011).

39. Pyhtila J. W., K. J. Chalut, J. D. Boyer, J. Keener, T. D'Amico, M. Gottfried, F. Gress, and A. Wax, In situ detection of nuclear atypia in Barrett's esophagus by using angle-resolved low-coherence interferometry, *Gastrointest. Endosc.* **65**, 487–491 (2007).

40. Terry N. G., Y. Zhu, M. T. Rinehart, W. J. Brown, S. J. Gebhart, S. D. Bright, E. Carretta et al., Detection of dysplasia in Barrett's esophagus with in vivo depth-resolved nuclear morphology measurements, *Gastroenterology* **140**, 42–50 (2011).

41. Amoozegar C., M. G. Giacomelli, J. D. Keener, K. J. Chalut, and A. Wax, Experimental verification of T-matrix-based inverse light scattering analysis for assessing structure of spheroids as models of cell nuclei, *Appl. Opt.* **48**, D20–D25 (2009).

42. Chalut K. J., S. Chen, J. D. Finan, M. G. Giacomelli, F. Guilak, K. W. Leong, and A. Wax, Label-free, high-throughput measurements of dynamic changes in cell nuclei using angle-resolved low coherence interferometry, *Biophys. J.* **94**, 4948–4956 (2008).

43. Zhu Y. Z., M. G. Giacomelli, and A. Wax, Fiber-optic interferometric two-dimensional scattering-measurement system, *Opt. Lett.* **35**, 1641–1643 (2010).

44. Pyhtila J. W. and A. Wax, Polarization effects on scatterer sizing accuracy analyzed with frequency-domain angle-resolved low-coherence interferometry, *Appl. Opt.* **46**, 1735–1741 (2007).

45. Chalut K. J., M. G. Giacomelli, and A. Wax, Application of Mie theory to assess structure of spheroidal scattering in backscattering geometries, *J. Opt. Soc. Am. A Opt. Image Sci. Vis.* **25**, 1866–1874 (2008).

46. Mishchenko M. I., J. W. Hovenier, and L. D. Travis, *Light Scattering by Nonspherical Particles: Theory, Measurements and Applications*, Academic Press, San Diego, CA (2000).

47. Chalut K. J., K. Kulangara, M. G. Giacomelli, A. Wax, and K. W. Leong, Deformation of stem cell nuclei by nanotopographical cues, *Soft Matter* **6**, 1675–1681 (2010).

48. Giacomelli M. G., K. J. Chalut, J. H. Ostrander, and A. Wax, Application of the T-matrix method to determine the structure of spheroidal cell nuclei with angle-resolved light scattering, *Opt. Lett.* **33**, 2452–2454 (2008).

49. Nilsson A. M. K., P. Alsholm, A. Karlsson, and S. Andersson-Engels, T-matrix computations of light scattering by red blood cells, *Appl. Opt.* **37**, 2735–2748 (1998).

50. Duncan D. D. and M. E. Thomas, Particle shape as revealed by spectral depolarization, *Appl. Opt.* **46**, 6185–6191 (2007).

51. Mourant J. R., T. M. Johnson, S. Carpenter, A. Guerra, T. Aida, and J. P. Freyer, Polarized angular dependent spectroscopy of epithelial cells and epithelial cell nuclei to determine the size scale of scattering structures, *J. Biomed. Opt.* **7**, 378–387 (2002).

52. Ramachandran J., T. M. Powers, S. Carpenter, A. Garcia-Lopez, J. P. Freyer, and J. R. Mourant, Light scattering and microarchitectural differences between tumorigenic and non-tumorigenic cell models of tissue, *Opt. Express* **15**, 4039–4053 (2007).

53. Aptowicz K. B., Y. L. Pan, R. K. Chang, R. G. Pinnick, S. C. Hill, R. L. Tober, A. Goyal, T. Leys, and B. V. Bronk, Two-dimensional angular optical scattering patterns of microdroplets in the mid infrared with strong and weak absorption, *Opt. Lett.* **29**, 1965–1967 (2004).

54. Giacomelli M., Y. Z. Zhu, J. Lee, and A. Wax, Size and shape determination of spheroidal scatterers using two-dimensional angle resolved scattering, *Opt. Express* **18**, 14616–14626 (2010).

20

Ultrasonically Modulated Optical Imaging

François Ramaz
Université Paris VI—Pierre et Marie Curie

Emmanuel Bossy
Université Paris VI—Pierre et Marie Curie

Michel Gross
Université Montpellier 2 and CNRS

A. Claude Boccara
Université Paris VI—Pierre et Marie Curie

20.1 Introduction

The possibility of using light for biological tissue imaging has received a lot of attention during the last two decades. Through visual observations, from a surgeon's point of view, abnormal tissues can be distinguished from normal tissues because of the differences in optical properties (optical absorption or reflection, scattering, texture). Optical imaging should therefore reveal these optical contrasts, thereby providing additional information to the routinely used imaging techniques for medical diagnosis. In addition, being noninvasive and nonionizing, light scores over x-rays. Moreover, the cost of optical imaging techniques is less than most of the usual current techniques.

Biological tissues exhibit a low absorption level in the deep red or near infrared. However, they are highly scattering media, so conventional optical tomographic methods are unable to provide good-quality images, especially in the scope to perform a resolution close to ultrasonography, which is in the mm³ range. To overcome this difficulty, a number of techniques have been proposed, such as time-resolved optical imaging [1,2] and frequency-domain optical imaging [3], to select short photon paths and, even for shallow structures, optical coherence tomography [4–8], which selects ballistic photons. These techniques have been proved to be successful in the determination of scattering and optical absorption distributions in biological tissues. Nevertheless, the standard resolution is close to 1 cm through a few-centimeters-thick samples such as breasts.

Besides these purely optical methods, hybrid techniques that combine light and ultrasounds (USs) have been proposed. These include photoacoustic imaging [9–11] and ultrasonically modulated optical tomography (UOT) [12–47]. The basic idea is to use ultrasonic waves, which scatter much less than light waves, to provide better localization information for imaging than purely optical techniques.

In ultrasonically modulated optical imaging, part of the light is modulated by an ultrasonic beam focused inside the biological tissue. Such *tagged photons* can be discriminated from the background of unmodulated photons, and their origin can be directly derived from the position of the focused ultrasonic beam. One can build 3D images by moving the focused ultrasonic beam mechanically or electronically. Several systems using a single detector were developed earlier [13–16,18,20,23,33,36]. The principal limitation of early setups was an efficient *flux* collection, which dealt with optical *etendue* (emitting surface × solid angle): according to the speckle character of the output field, the performances in terms of *signal-to-noise ratio* (*SNR*) are a priori limited to a single coherence area, thus close to λ^2.

Our laboratory had initially proposed a scheme for parallel detection using the detector array of a CCD camera, leading to a dramatic increase of *SNR* [17,19,21]. This configuration was recently improved using a digital holography approach coupled to fast CMOS cameras [28,40]. In contrast, the concept of adaptive wavefront was introduced for acousto-optic (AO) imaging using a photosensitive material (photorefractive crystal) that records a volume hologram of the *tagged photons* [34,35,37–39,41,44,45,47–49]. With such a technique it is possible to collect the interference signal of ~10^8 speckle areas efficiently using a single detector with a large area.

Here, we present the recent improvements of our ultrasonically modulated optical imaging approaches. The principle of the techniques is detailed and their performances reported. Two-dimensional AO images of phantoms with scattering properties close to biological tissues as well as thick chicken breast are shown.

A number of new approaches have been explored or used routinely, which include the use of radiation force to induce large displacements or shear waves that provide new kinds of contrasts. Future possible developments and improvements are discussed.

20.2 Principle of Acousto-Optic Imaging

The principle of AO imaging is schematically represented in Figure 20.1. The biological sample is illuminated by coherent laser light. Due to the highly scattering nature of the sample, a speckle field is generated all around it. A US beam focused in the sample induces periodic displacements of the scatterers (amplitude of a few nanometers) [14,15] and a modulation of the refractive index [26], mainly in the focal zone. As a result, the optical paths of light passing through the US focal zone are modulated. Finally, the phase of the speckle pattern is modulated at the US frequency (a few megahertz). As a consequence, new optical frequencies appear (sidebands), shifting from the laser career ω_L at $\pm \omega_{US}$ and harmonics. We will refer to tagged photons as those corresponding to one of the first sidebands $\omega_L \pm \omega_{US}$, while untagged photons correspond to those simply scattered through the medium and thus not shifted in frequency. From a simplified point of view (but somewhat wrong), one can consider that the tagged photons have crossed the ultrasonic field, whereas the untagged photons have not. The magnitude of the tagged photons is directly connected to the optical properties of the medium inside the US focal zone. This quantity remains weak (<1%) compared with the majority of untagged photons, which makes the measurement challenging. In particular, if the optical absorption in the US focal zone is high, the probability that light escapes from this zone is low, and consequently the modulation of the speckle is low. Local differences in the optical absorption and/or scattering of the sample can thus be revealed.

A simple picture to understand the principle of AO imaging is that of the *virtual modulated source*. The tissue region where both light and US are present becomes the *virtual source*, that is, the source of modulated light that can be scanned through a sample. When this source is scanned over an absorbing region, its intensity decreases. We can consider at first order the distribution of light in the medium is

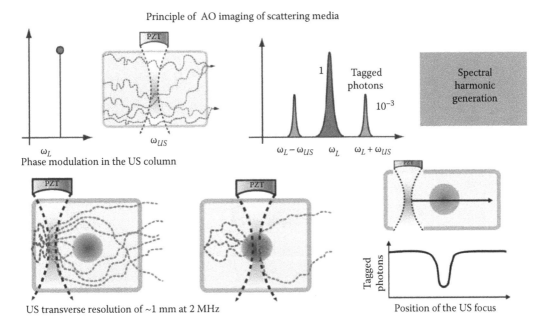

FIGURE 20.1   Schematic of AO imaging in scattering media.

uniform, so the virtual source coincides with the US beam. The spatial resolution of this imaging technique is given by the size of the US focal zone (typically a few millimeters through several-centimeters-thick samples).

20.3 Digital Off-Axis Holography/Adaptive Wavefront Holography Techniques

As mentioned by several authors earlier [15], "perhaps the most striking feature of AO imaging is the fact that the signal essentially resides in a single coherence area." Consequently, the use of parallel, multichannel detection techniques, which are able to detect simultaneously yet independently the modulations in a large number N of coherence areas (or *speckle grains*), improve the *SNR* by a factor $\sqrt{N}$. Let us describe two techniques that are able to perform parallel, multichannel detection of the tagged photon signal.

20.3.1 Experimental Setup

The experimental setups are shown in Figures 20.2 and 20.3. The first setup refers to the digital holography technique, while the second performs an adaptive wavefront holography technique. Both methods will be detailed in the following sections. The sample is immersed into a water tank (20 cm × 20 cm × 10 cm) to ensure good acoustic impedance matching with the transducer. The sample is held between lucite windows. In this configuration, the sample is slightly pressed and presents a constant thickness all over the observed region and the light paths avoid water perturbations. Indeed, an experiment performed with the light traveling in water had revealed that the speckle decorrelates very quickly due to water turbulence, inducing a poor *SNR*. The sample is then illuminated with near-infrared sources of different kinds in the 700–1100 nm region of the spectrum, corresponding to the so-called optical therapeutic window. Historically, we first used a continuous tunable titanium–sapphire of moderate power (~400 mW) with a large coherence length (>300 m). This source can be amplified with a semiconductor tapered amplifier in order to provide an output of 2.5 W at 780 nm. We recently acquired an alexandrite

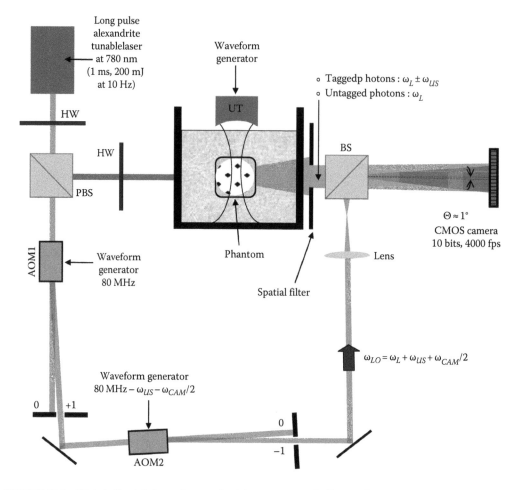

FIGURE 20.2 Digital off-axis holography setup for AO imaging. HW, half-wave plate; PBS, polarizing beam splitter; AOM, acousto-optic modulator; BS, beam splitter; UT, ultrasonic transducer. The radius of the spatial filter controls the size of the speckle grain in the plane of the CMOS camera. The reference beam and the mean direction of the scattered photons make a small angle θ to generate a sinusoidal modulation of the speckle associated with the tagged photons.

laser in a long pulse regime (1 ms at 10 Hz to 200 mJ). This source was chosen for its high-peak power (but satisfying healthcare recommendations). A reasonable coherence length (~40 cm – Δν = 750 MHz) enables to probe many optical paths due to multiple scattering within thick samples (typical 4 cm) and thus obtains a speckle pattern with a good contrast.

20.3.1.1 Digital Holography

The digital holography setup is shown in Figure 20.2. The speckle pattern formed by the emerging scattered optical field E_S contains many frequency components following the AO effect.

We will write it generically in complex notation as

$$E_S(r,t) = \sum_m E_{S,m}(r)e^{j(\omega_L + m\omega_{US})t} \tag{20.1}$$

The untagged photons correspond to the field $E_{S,0}$, while the tagged photons are related to the components $E_{S,1}$ and $E_{S,-1}$. These fields interfere with the reference local oscillator field (E_R,ω_R). This interference is then recorded on a 10-bits CMOS camera array of 1024×1024 pixels working up to some tens of kilohertz with

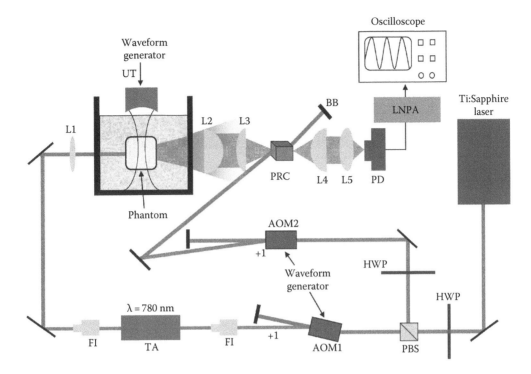

FIGURE 20.3 Wavefront-adaptive holography setup for AO imaging. PBS, polarizing beam splitter; HWP, half-wave plate; BB, beam blocker; AOM, acousto-optic modulator; FI, Faraday isolator; L_i, large aperture lens; UT, ultrasonic transducer; PRC, photorefractive crystal; PD, variable gain photodetector; TA, optical semiconductor tapered amplifier; LNPA, low-noise preamplifier.

a restricted number of pixels. In order to select the tagged photons, the local oscillator reference beam is shifted in frequency to match the tagged photon frequency ($\omega_R \cong \omega_L \pm \omega_{US}$). A simple way to operate is to put two AO modulators (AOM1 and AOM2) on the reference path. The first modulator induces a shift of +80 MHz, while the second −78 MHz. Since the bandwidth of the camera (kHz) is low compared to the US frequency ($\omega_{US} \sim 2$ MHz), the camera filters off, within the interference pattern $|E_S + E_R|^2$, the scattered versus reference fields interference ($E_{S,m=0}E_R^*$) terms, which varies at US frequency and harmonics. On the other hand, the tagged versus reference field interference ($E_{S,1}E_R^*$), which varies slowly, is selected.

As explained in the following section, the reference optical field E_R has a tilt angle of typically $\theta \sim 1°$ with the mean direction of the *tagged photons*, so that the speckle interference pattern ($E_{S,1}E_R^*$) exhibits fringes. The average diameter of a speckle grain is $\varphi_S = \lambda d/r$, where λ is the laser wavelength ($\lambda = 780$ nm), $d \sim 50$ cm is the distance between the exit face of the sample and the camera, and r is the radius of a diaphragm through which light exits the sample. To ensure a good spatial sampling of the fringes, the diameter φ_S of the speckle grains must be larger than the fringe period, which must be also larger than the pixels of the camera (18×18 μm^2). In order to fulfill these two conditions, radius r, distance d, and tilt angle θ are properly adjusted.

20.3.1.2 Adaptive Wavefront Holography

The setup used for a self-adaptive wavefront holography uses the same optical and ultrasonic sources (Figure 20.3). The difference comes from the hologram recording process and the *flux* collection. Here, the hologram coming from the interference between the speckle field and the reference is written within the volume of a photorefractive crystal. Large aperture lenses are used to collect *flux* from the sample and also to perform the conjugation between the crystal and the single detector. Depending on the frequency

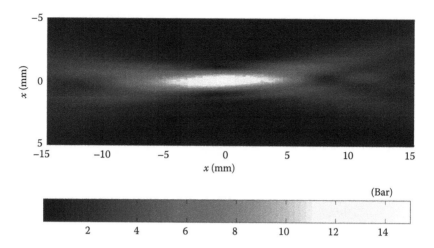

FIGURE 20.4   Map of the pressure emitted by a single-element ultrasonic transducer.

shift of the reference beam, one records the speckle associated to the tagged or the untagged photons. The AO signal comes from the interference between the selected speckle and its replica diffracted by the reference. The spatial coherence of these fields enables us to use a large-area (cm²) photodetector. A low-noise high-pass preamplifier (×50) is often used after the variable gain photodetector transimpedance amplifier. This permits us to amplify the *ac* component and cut dominant *dc* contributions.

Till now three types of crystals have been used, depending on the spectral range of interest ($Bi_{12}SiO_{20}$ at 532 nm [35,37], GaAs at 1064 nm [34,44,45,47], $Sn_2P_2S_6$:Te at 780 nm [48]). The time response of the crystal generally depends on the reference intensity (some 100 mW/mm²), and a response of about 0.3 ms has been obtained with GaAs [41]. Nevertheless, $Sn_2P_2S_6$:Te seems very promising because it exhibits a high gain (~8 cm⁻¹ in the diffusion regime—no electric field applied) in the optical therapeutic window with a relatively fast response time (<10 ms).

The focused ultrasonic beam is emitted perpendicularly to the incident light beam. We use acoustic transducers driven by an amplified sinusoidal signal (Class I power amplifier in the MHz range >10 W), having a diameter of 38 mm and a fixed focal length (69 mm). The transducer is mounted on step-by-step motorized translations in order to move the US within the scattered light volume and thus reconstructs the 3D optical properties of the medium. Replacing the single-element transducer by an echograph is of strong interest since one gets a 3D image of the acoustic properties of the sample *without the need of moving the sample or the transducer*.

By scanning a calibrated hydrophone in front of the transducer, we mapped the pressure field emitted in water (Figure 20.4). The FWHM of the focal zone is measured as 1.4 and 12.5 mm along the transverse and longitudinal directions with respect to the US propagation. Unfortunately, the US beam outside the focal zone also contributes to the speckle modulation to some extent. Consequently, while the resolution is very sharp in any transverse direction, it is somewhat lower in the longitudinal direction. Nevertheless, it is possible to retrieve a millimeter axial resolution using appropriate modulations on both US and light [32,35,45,48].

20.3.2 Principle (Lock-In Detection and Spatiotemporal Filtering)

20.3.2.1 Digital Off-Axis Holography

As explained in Section 20.3, the aim is to detect the AO modulation of the speckle at the US frequency, that is, to measure the quantity of tagged photons going onto the detection. Based on the principles presented in the previous version of this handbook [31], heterodyne off-axis holography was introduced by

Gross et al. [50–55] and brings a significant improvement compared to the camera detection described in Ref. [31]. This holographic detection, whose sensitivity is limited by shot noise [51,53,55], is tuned at the sideband frequency $\omega_L + \omega_{US}$ in order to perform a spatiotemporal filtering [54] of the wanted tagged photon signal.

We chose the 1024×1024 pixels of a CMOS array camera as the N detectors. We set the sample-to-camera spacing in order to match the coherence area of the speckle with the size of some pixels. On each pixel, we detected the magnitude of the modulation at the US frequency. We defined our signal as the sum of the N square magnitude. (*Note*: If several coherence areas were matched with one single pixel, since the relative phases of their modulations are random, the sum would cancel out on the average.)

In experiments where a single grain of speckle is detected by a single detector, the signal is usually analyzed with a lock-in amplifier. This extraction of the magnitude (and eventually of the phase*) of the modulated part of the signal can also be achieved by sampling and applying the discrete Fourier transformation in time.

When dealing with 1024×1024 individual detectors, we will of course use the second approach. Using a CCD or CMOS camera as a parallel detector raises two points of concern. First, it is an integrating detector in space (over the pixel size) and time (over the exposure time), and second, it has a limited frame rate (thus a low-sampling frequency). Time integration by the camera can be treated as a low-pass filtering process that selects the signals within a narrow frequency bandwidth centered at the sideband frequency. Proper calculations then allow us to get, on each pixel, the amplitude and phase of the *tagged photon* complex optical field $E_{S,1}$. The magnitude of the *tagged photon* signal is then obtained by summing $|E_{S,1}|^2$ over the pixels.

20.3.2.2 Holographic Spatiotemporal Filtering

20.3.2.2.1 *Temporal Filtering*

Dealing with the low-frame rate of the camera ω_{cam} (period $T_{cam} = 2\pi/\omega_{cam}$) requires a careful mixing of the acoustic modulation and the optical detection signals. The idea is to grab sequences of images $I_p(x_c, y_c)$ with $p = 0, 1, \ldots$, with a proper detuning of the reference beam frequency and to combine properly these images' data. A convenient scheme frequently used is the four-image sequence (also called four-phase acquisition) or the two-phase sequence. In the four-image method, the frequency of the local oscillator is $\omega_R = \omega_L + \omega_{US} + \omega_{cam}/4$. We thus get for the image signal I_p at time $t_p = pT_{cam}$:

$$I_{p=0,1,2,3} = I(t_p) = \frac{1}{T_{cam}} \int_{(p-1/2)T_{cam}}^{(p+1/2)T_{cam}} |E_S + E_R|^2 \, dt$$

$$= \frac{1}{T_{cam}} \int_{(p-1/2)T_{cam}}^{(p+1/2)T_{cam}} dt \begin{bmatrix} |E_S|^2 + |E_R|^2 \\ + E_{S,1}(t)E_R^*(t) + E_{S,1}^*(t)E_R(t) \\ + \sum_{m \neq 1}\left[E_{S,m}(t)E_R^*(t) + E_{S,m}^*(t)E_R(t) \right] \end{bmatrix} \tag{20.2}$$

Here, the terms $|E_S|^2$ and $|E_R|^2$ do not vary with time, and the terms $\sum_{m \neq 1}\left[E_{S,m}(t)E_R^*(t) + E_{S,m}^*(t)E_R(t) \right]$ vary fast like $\exp \pm j\,(m\omega_{US} + \omega_{cam}/4)t$; thus, the interference contributions will be restrained to the terms $E_{S,1}(t)E_R^*(t) + E_{S,1}^*(t)E_R(t)$, which vary slowly like $\exp \pm (j\omega_{camt}/4t)$.

---

* The phase of each pixel is of little interest here. It is however convenient for testing the system.

We thus have

$$I_{p=0,1,2,3} = \left|E_S\right|^2 + \left|E_R\right|^2 + C\left(p,\frac{\omega_{cam}}{4}\right)E_{S,1}(t)E_R^*(t) + C^*\left(p,\frac{\omega_{cam}}{4}\right)E_{S,1}^*(t)E_R(t)$$

(20.3)

$$\text{with,} \quad C(p,\Omega) = \frac{1}{T_{cam}}\int_{(p-1/2)T_{cam}}^{(p+1/2)T_{cam}} e^{-j\Omega t}dt = \frac{e^{+j\Omega T_{cam}/2} - e^{-j\Omega T_{cam}/2}}{j\Omega T_{cam}}e^{-jp\Omega T_{cam}} = \sin c\left(\frac{\Omega T_{cam}}{2}\right)e^{-jp\Omega T_{cam}}$$

Finally, we obtain

$$I_0 = \left|E_S\right|^2 + \left|E_R\right|^2 + C\left(0,\frac{\omega_{cam}}{4}\right)E_{S,1}E_R^* + C^*\left(0,\frac{\omega_{cam}}{4}\right)E_{S,1}^*E_R$$

$$I_1 = \left|E_S\right|^2 + \left|E_R\right|^2 - jC\left(0,\frac{\omega_{cam}}{4}\right)E_{S,1}(t)E_R^*(t) + jC^*\left(0,\frac{\omega_{cam}}{4}\right)E_{S,1}^*E_R$$

(20.4)

$$I_2 = \left|E_S\right|^2 + \left|E_R\right|^2 - C\left(0,\frac{\omega_{cam}}{4}\right)E_{S,1}E_R^* - C^*\left(0,\frac{\omega_{cam}}{4}\right)E_{S,1}^*E_R$$

$$I_3 = \left|E_S\right|^2 + \left|E_R\right|^2 + jC\left(0,\frac{\omega_{cam}}{4}\right)E_{S,1}E_R^* - jC^*\left(0,\frac{\omega_{cam}}{4}\right)E_{S,1}^*E_R$$

where $E_S(t_p)$ and $E_R(t_p)$ are written as E_S and E_R in order to simplify the notations. We then get

$$(I_0 - I_2) + j(I_1 - I_3) = 4C\left(0,\frac{\omega_{cam}}{4}\right)E_{S,1}(t)E_R^*(t) = 4\sin c\left(\frac{\pi}{4}\right)E_{S,1}(t)E_R^*(t) \cong 3.6 \times E_{S,1}(t)E_R^*(t) \quad (20.5)$$

By summing four consecutive images $I_p(x_c,y_c)$ with the proper coefficients $+1$, $+j$, -1, and $-j$, we then get the *tagged photon* complex field on the camera $E_p(x_c,y_c)$ weighted by the coefficient $4\sin c(\pi/4)e^{-j\pi/4}$, which does not depend on the pixel index.

Similarly, one can consider the two-image method. The frequency of the local oscillator is now $\omega_R = \omega_L + \omega_{US} + \omega_{cam}/2$.

In that case, one obtains

$$I_0 - I_1 = 2C\left(0,\frac{\omega_{cam}}{2}\right)E_{S,1}E_R^* = 2\sin c\left(\frac{\pi}{2}\right)E_{S,1}E_R^* + 2\sin c\left(\frac{\pi}{2}\right)E_{S,1}^*E_R \quad (20.6)$$

Here, one gets a sum of the so-called order +1 term (or true image term: $E_{S,1}E_R^*$), which is related to the field $E_{S,1}(x_c,y_c)$, while order −1 term (or twin or ghost image term: $E_{S,1}^*E_R$) is the complex conjugate of order +1. If the intensity of the laser fluctuates with time, the constant terms of Equation 20.4 slightly vary, and both four-phase and two-phase methods yield a zero-order term, which is almost uniform on all pixels. Because the AO signal is very low, this parasitic zero-order term is often much larger than the tagged photon term $E_{S,1}E_R^*$ itself and must be filtered off. As we will see, because of the off-axis geometry of the holographic setup ($\theta \sim 1°$ in Figure 20.2), it is possible to filter off both the zero- and the −1-order terms in the spatial Fourier space, as shown by Cuche et al. [56].

20.3.2.2.2 Spatial Filtering

Whatever the two- or four-image method used, one can get from a sequence of recorded images $I_{p=0,1,2,3}$ the tagged photon complex field $E_{S,1}(x_c,y_c,z_c,t_p)$ in the camera plane $z = z_c$. Since this field is recorded for all

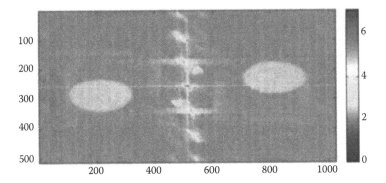

FIGURE 20.5 Reconstructed images (1024 × 512) of the circular aperture back illuminated by the tagged photon field $E_{S,1}'$. The color display corresponds to $\ln\left(\left|E_{S,1}'\right|\right)^2$.

pixels at the same time $t = t_p$, $E_{S,1}$ is a hologram (i.e. the field in the plane of the CMOS camera), from which one can reconstruct the field $E_{S,1}'$ in the plane of the spatial filter $z = z_s$, with $z_c - z_s = d$ (see Figure 20.2).

Figure 20.5 shows the reconstructed field $E_{S,1}'$ displayed in logarithmic color scale. The camera images I_p have been recorded with 2× binning over y (1204 × 512 calculation grid), and the temporal filtering is made by the two-image method. The two light blue elliptical zones correspond to the images of the circular aperture of the spatial filter. The left-hand-side zone is order +1, and the right-hand side, order −1.

Among the many usable reconstruction methods described in Ref. [57], we have used the Schnars and Jüptner method [58], which involves a single fast Fourier transform (FFT). The field $E_{S,1}'$ is

$$E_{S,1}'(x_s, y_s, z_s, t_p) = \text{FFT}\left[E_{S,1}(x_c, y_c, z_c, t_p) \times e^{jk(x_c^2 + y_c^2)/2D}\right] \tag{20.7}$$

where FFT is the 2D Fourier transform operator in (x_c, y_c) and $e^{jk(x_c^2 + y_c^2)/2D}$ is a quadratic phase factor, where $k = 2\pi/\lambda$ is the wave number and D is the length, which depends on the reconstruction distance $d = z_c - z_s$ and on the local oscillator wavefront curvature.

If the local oscillator is a plane wave, one obtains $D = z_c - z_s$ [58]. If the local oscillator is a spherical wave, whose origin is within the sample plane $z \sim z_s$ as in our experiment (see Figure 20.2), one obtains $1/D \sim 0$. In that case, each point of the aperture emits a spherical wave, which interferes with the local oscillator whose curvature is the same. One thus obtains linear Young's fringes, whose Fourier transform gives a point corresponding to the emitting point. This means that the quadratic phase factor $e^{jk(x_c^2 + y_c^2)/2D}$ reduces to 1 and that the reconstruction of the field $E_{S,1}'$ from $E_{S,1}$ is made by a simple Fourier transform. Since the order ±1 terms are complex conjugate, the Fourier transform performs the reconstruction for both orders ±1, which are located symmetrically with respect to the zero-order stray signals located in the center of the Fourier space image (red point in Figure 20.5).

If, as is generally the case, the Fourier calculation is made by FFT, the pixel sizes Δx and $\Delta'x$, respectively, in the camera and reconstructed image planes are related by

$$\sqrt{N}\,\Delta x\,\Delta x' = \frac{2\pi d}{k} \tag{20.8}$$

where $\sqrt{N}$ is the 1D number of pixel of the camera (i.e., the size of the calculation grid: $\sqrt{N} = 1024$ typically). The optical etendue $S\Omega$ corresponding to 1 pixel of the reconstructed image of the sample (area $S = |\Delta'x|^2$) emitting light toward the camera (area $N|\Delta x|^2$; viewed solid angle $\Omega = N|\Delta x|^2/d^2$) is then $S\Omega = \lambda^2$.

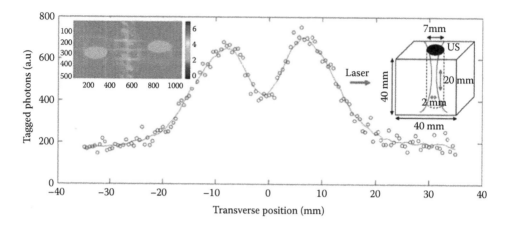

FIGURE 20.6   Transverse *AO* profile of an absorber through 4 cm of scattering gel ($\mu_s' = 10$ cm^{-1}) obtained by digital holography with a two-phase acquisition of the camera (see text for details). Area of ellipses gives the magnitude of the *tagged* photons.

The optical *etendue* for the detection of the tagged photons in λ^2 units is thus equal to the area of the circular aperture in pixel units. This number of pixels represents the number of coherent areas (spatial modes) that are detected in parallel. To optimize detection, one must play with the aperture radius *r*, with the sample set to camera distance *d*, and with the tilt angle θ in order to make the order +1 image of the aperture as big as possible without overlapping with the zero order that brings noise.

As an example, Figure 20.6 illustrates the holographic detection of tagged photons. It shows the transverse profile of an absorber made by scanning the US transducer along the transverse direction *y*. Detection is made with two phases on a scattering sample ($\mu_s' = 1/l^* = 10$ cm^{-1}) with thickness 4 cm and a continuous-wave (CW) regime for the US. The depletion of the signal reveals the presence of an absorber (a cylinder $L = 40$ mm; $\Phi = 7$ mm). The ellipses represent the magnitude of the tagged photons and the corresponding transverse profile of the signal.

20.3.2.2.3 Shot Noise

In a typical situation, the scattered field $|E_S|$ is low and does not saturate the camera. On the other hand, the reference (or local oscillator) beam is adjusted to be quite large, so we have $|E_R|^2 > |E_S|^2$. In that case, the main noise term is the shot noise on the reference field E_R, and the holographic detection is shot noise limited [51,53,55]. The noise then corresponds to the detection of a random signal with uniform energy density in all the spatial and frequency modes. This background corresponds to the uniform dark blue signal background that is seen in Figure 20.5 out of the ±1-order images of the aperture and out of the zero-order parasitics.

This noise corresponds to the detection of an equivalent signal $|E|^2$ of one photoelectron per reconstructed pixel for the two- or four-image sequence [51,53,55]. This noise also corresponds to one photon of the signal, that is, to an energy *hv* (where *h* is Planck's constant, and *v* is the optical frequency) per *mode*, where a *mode* corresponds to an *optical etendue* λ^2 per unit of time, of bandwidth.

One way to illustrate this point is to consider the high-temperature limits (i.e., $kT \gg hv$, where *T* is the temperature and *k* the Boltzmann constant) of Planck's law, where the noise is kT/hv times larger than that in the low-temperature case ($kT \ll hv$). In that case, Planck's law can be rewritten as:

$$I(v,T) = \frac{2hv^3}{c^2} \times \frac{1}{e^{hv/kT} - 1} \cong \frac{2hv^3}{c^2}\frac{kT}{hv} = \frac{2kT}{\lambda^2} \tag{20.9}$$

where *c* is the velocity of light. In Planck's law, $I(v, T)$ is a specific radiative intensity that represents the emitted power for the two polarizations per unit area of emitting surface in the normal direction, per unit solid angle, and per unit frequency. If one considers a detection time Δt, the unit of frequency becomes $\Delta v = 1/\Delta t$. For example, for the two- and four-image detection, we have $\Delta v = 1/2T_{exp}$ or $1/4T_{exp}$, where $T_{exp} < T'_{cam}$ is the camera exposure time. Planck's equation implies here that the background noise power emitted in Δt is kT (at high temperature and thus hv at low temperature) per polarization state and per *mode*, where a *mode* is a unit of optical etendue (emitting surface × solid angle) equal to λ^2 and a unit of frequency equal to $\Delta v = 1/\Delta t$.

20.3.2.2.4 *Speckle Decorrelation*

In previous sections, we considered that the scattered and tagged photon signals are delta function in frequency at ω_L and $\omega_L + \omega_{US}$. This hypothesis is by far not valid in vivo. For example, the frequency spectrum of light that travels through 4 cm of breast in vivo has an *FWHM* equal to 3 kHz [51]. This means that the motion of tissues and blood flow decorrelates the scattered and the tagged photon speckles in a time about $t_{corr} \sim 0.3$ ms. This speckle decorrelation effect, which is a huge limiting factor in vivo, is not seen in most experiments since they are carried out with phantom samples, which do not decorrelate.

Decorrelation deeply modifies holographic detection. For example, because the $E_{S,1}E_R^*$ phase is randomized from one image to the next, the $\omega_{cam}/2$ or $\omega_{cam}/4$ frequency shift that induces a π or $\pi/2$ phase shift is useless. Moreover, in the four-image detection case, one gets signal for both ±1 orders [52]. To the end, the detection sensitivity and thus *SNR* do not depend on the measurement time Δt, if $\Delta t > t_{corr}$ [54]. Because holographic detection is coherent, the detection bandwidth is $\Delta v = 1/\Delta t$, while the signal bandwidth is $\Delta v_{signal} = 1/t_{corr}$. The detected signal, which is proportional to Δt and to the ratio $\Delta v/\Delta v_{signal}$, thus does not depend on Δt [54].

20.3.3 Adaptive Wavefront Holography

The detection of *AO* signal with a single detector of a large area can bring improvements compared with the camera in terms of velocity. But, as mentioned earlier, such a scheme is a priori not possible due to an *etendue* that is limited to a single coherence area of the signal, for example, $\sim\lambda^2$. Fortunately, the use of self-developing holographic media, such as photorefractive materials [59–61], offers this possibility. These materials are photoconductive and electrooptic. A phase hologram of the interference pattern between a speckle field and a reference beam can be recorded in the volume of the crystal, with time as short as hundreds of microseconds, compatible with the speckle correlation time of living tissues. With such a time response, the crystal acts as a *low-pass* filter compared with the US modulation. A shift of the reference at the US frequency enables us to record a *time-averaged* hologram of the *tagged* photons, while an absence of shift will record a *time-averaged* hologram of the photons simply scattered by the sample. Both configurations are interesting to measure the *AO* signal. Whatever the hologram, the reference diffracts a field whose spatial wavefront is a replica of the selected speckle. The original and the diffracted speckles are spatially coherent: they can interfere coherently on a large detector and give an optimized *AO* signal. The main advantage of the technique relies on a high etendue since crystals can have optical faces of 1 cm² and thus accept coherently some 10^8 grains of speckle, while a camera can only collect some 10^6. It should be noted that at present the comparison between *SNR* of the two approaches has not been studied in detail. In principle, digital holography should perform shot-noise-limited detection of the tagged photons, but within a bandwidth Δv equal to the inverse of the camera exposure time. Another technological limitation is the data transfer rate from the camera to the computer, which renders the experiment somewhat long. This last bottleneck should be raised with the improvement of CMOS technology. The shot noise limit is more difficult to reach with photorefractive effect because the main noise contribution comes from scattering of the reference on the crystal faces, fanning effects, difficult to avoid with high-efficiency crystals. A significant advantage of the technique is the limited post-treatment and its real-time acquisition rate. For these reasons, both approaches need to be used often.

The formalism of the signal detection has been described in detail in Refs. [39,41]. It is convenient to recall here that this could have been introduced in the digital holography section. But for the sake of clarity, we consider it more appropriate to develop this in this section.

Consider the plane of the photorefractive crystal, and let $E_S(r,t)$ be the complex field that exits in the sample while $E_R(r,t)$ stands for the reference beam, eventually shifted in frequency. It is useful for detection to apply on the pressure field P (at career ω_{US}) an additional modulation, whether in amplitude $g(t)$ or in phase $f(t)$. This leads to a typical AO phase modulation of the form

$$\psi_{AO}(r,t) = \alpha(P,r)g(t)\sin[\omega_{US}t + f(t)] \qquad (20.10)$$

where $\alpha(P,r)$ is an integrated term depending on the various optical paths due to scattering within the acoustic field. According to Equation 20.10 and the scattering character of the medium, the AO modulation generates uncorrelated sidebands in the optical spectrum [39], so that the fields take the recurrent expression using a classical Bessel's development:

$$E_S(r,t) = \sum_m E_{S,m}(r,t) = \sum_{m=-\infty}^{+\infty} \sqrt{I_{S,m}(r)} e^{-j\phi_{S,m}(r)} J_m[\alpha(P,r)g(t)] e^{jmf(t)} e^{jm\omega_{US}t} e^{j\omega_L t}$$

$$E_R(t) = \sqrt{I_R} e^{-j\phi_R(r)} e^{j\Delta\omega t} e^{j\omega_L t} \qquad (20.11)$$

From a practical point of view, the pressure used in AO imaging is weak, leading to a limited number of m-sidebands. Generally speaking, a hologram is recorded within the volume of the photorefractive crystal, and according to Ref. [41], it generates along the thickness z of the crystal a local contrast of the index grating as follows:

$$\delta n(r,t) \cong \eta \left\langle \frac{E_S(r,t)E_R^*(r,t) + E_S^*(r,t)E_R(r,t)}{|E_S(r,t)|^2 + |E_R(r,t)|^2} \right\rangle_{\tau_{PR}}, \quad \text{with} \quad \eta = \gamma z \qquad (20.12)$$

where γ (cm^{-1}) is a gain factor connected to the electrooptic coefficients of the crystal (tensor-like), while $\langle\ \rangle_{\tau_{PR}}$ is classically formalized by a convolution product that reflects the low-pass filter character of the photorefractive effect:

$$\langle A \rangle_{\tau_{PR}}(t) = \frac{1}{\tau_{PR}} \int_{\tau=0}^{+\infty} A(t-\tau)e^{-\tau/\tau_{PR}} d\tau \qquad (20.13)$$

The photorefractive rate $1/\tau_{PR}$ is in general much smaller than the acoustic frequency. According to Equation 20.12, a contrast index can only be obtained for a particular sideband of the field, corresponding to an appropriate frequency shift $\Delta\omega$ of the reference beam. In general, one records the hologram of the tagged ($m = \pm 1$) or the scattered photons ($m = 0$).

To illustrate the wavefront-adaptive method, we will consider the case of a pure phase modulation $f(t)$, and thus the tagged photon $E_{S,1}$ needs to be selected, for example, with $\Delta\omega = \omega_{US}$ (Figure 20.7).

In these conditions, the index contrast reduces to

$$\delta n(r,t) \cong \eta \left\langle \frac{E_{S,1}(r,t)E_R^*(r,t) + E_{S,1}^*(r,t)E_R(r,t)}{|E_{S,1}(r,t)|^2 + |E_R(r,t)|^2} \right\rangle_{\tau_{PR}}$$

$$= \eta \frac{\sqrt{I_{S,1}(r)I_R}}{I_{S,1}(r)+I_R} J_1[\alpha(P,r)] \left\{ e^{-j[\phi_{S,1}(r)-\phi_R(r)]} \langle e^{jf(t)} \rangle_{\tau_{PR}} + e^{j[\phi_{S,1}(r)-\phi_R(r)]} \langle e^{-jf(t)} \rangle_{\tau_{PR}} \right\} \qquad (20.14)$$

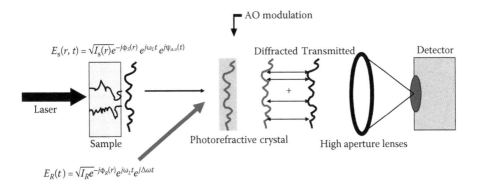

FIGURE 20.7 The principle of adaptive wavefront interferometry applied to AO imaging through scattering media.

In the following, the reference beam diffracts on the volume hologram, which has the thickness L of the crystal. For small efficiencies, the field $E_D(r,t)$ diffracted by the reference *in the direction* of the speckle field can be obtained from the first term of $\delta n(r,t)$ in a simplified manner:

$$E_D(r,t) \propto \delta n(r,t)E_R(t)$$

$$= \eta \frac{\sqrt{I_{S,1}(r)I_R}}{I_{S,1}(r)+I_R} J_1[\alpha(P,r)]e^{-j[\phi_{S,1}(r)-\phi_R(r)]}\left\langle e^{jf(t)}\right\rangle_{\tau_{PR}} \sqrt{I_R}e^{-j\phi_R(r)}e^{j\Delta\omega t}e^{j\omega_L t} \qquad (20.15)$$

$$\cong \eta\sqrt{I_{S,1}(r)}J_1[\alpha(P,r)]e^{-j\phi_{S,1}(r)}\left\langle e^{jf(t)}\right\rangle_{\tau_{PR}} e^{j\omega_{US}t}e^{j\omega_L t} \quad (I_{S,1}\ll I_R)$$

The diffracted field E_D exhibits the same wavefront as $E_{S,1}$ (wavefront adaption); it is sensitive to the low-pass property of the crystal. The modulations used in *AO* imaging are generally fast compared with τ_{PR}, so the convolution product reduces to an *averaged* value of the modulation.

The *AO* signal comes from the interference between $E_{S,1}$ and E_D, integrated on the detector surface:

$$S_{AO}(\Delta\omega = \omega\mu s,t) \propto \int_{detector} \left[E_S(r,t)E_D^*(r,t)+c.c \right]dxdy$$

$$= \eta I_{S,1}J_1^2[\alpha(P,r)]\left\langle e^{-jf(t)}\right\rangle_{\tau_{PR}} e^{jf(t)} + c.c \qquad (20.16)$$

This expression shows a phase-modulated signal proportional to the *flux* $I_{S,1}$ of the particular speckle component. In the low-pressure regime, the signal is proportional to the *square* of the peak pressure P and thus to the acoustical energy. Let us also point out that to be detectable, the phase modulation $f(t)$, introduced in Equation 20.10, must have a *nonzero* average value over τ_{PR}.

20.4 Acousto-Optic Signal: The Axial Resolution Question

As mentioned earlier, AO imaging suffers from a poor resolution along the acoustic beam because of the cumulative effect brought by the US on the optical path, even when the pressure is weak. As a consequence, a *CW regime* of the US will typically bring a resolution of 1–2 cm along the acoustic column and a few millimeters in the transverse direction, governed by the aperture of the transducer. Early techniques using a linear frequency chirp modulation of sources have been carried out either with single detectors [18,23] or cameras [32]. The chirp modulation codes an *apparent frequency* in the

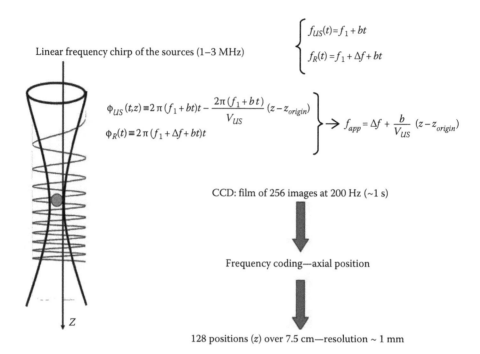

Linear frequency chirp of the sources (1–3 MHz)

$$\begin{cases} f_{US}(t) = f_1 + bt \\ f_R(t) = f_1 + \Delta f + bt \end{cases}$$

$$\phi_{US}(t,z) \equiv 2\pi\,(f_1 + bt)t - \frac{2\pi\,(f_1 + bt)}{V_{US}}(z - z_{origin})$$

$$\phi_R(t) \equiv 2\pi\,(f_1 + \Delta f + bt)t$$

$$\Bigg\} \to f_{app} = \Delta f + \frac{b}{V_{US}}(z - z_{origin})$$

CCD: film of 256 images at 200 Hz (~1 s)

Frequency coding—axial position

128 positions (z) over 7.5 cm—resolution ~ 1 mm

Z

FIGURE 20.8 Linear frequency-chirped modulation applied to AO imaging.

frequency spectrum, proportional to the position of the US along the acoustic column. A film of the chirp sequence is performed, and a Fourier transform reveals the AO signal with the axial resolution. Such a method requires the speckle to be correlated over the time of the chirp sequence and is probably difficult at present to use in real case, according to the quite slow acquisition rates of the camera (Figure 20.8).

There exist two important ways to obtain a *millimeter* axial resolution, applying on the US and light a temporal burst profile or random phase jumps.

20.4.1 Burst Method

This technique is similar to echography since a US pulse propagates through the medium (burst regime). In the camera holographic setup, one detects the *tagged* photons in shifting the reference from ω_{US}. The latter has a comparable time profile, and it is opened with a delay of τ. As the US propagates at velocity V_{US}, it means that the AO signal comes from a region centered at $z = V_{US}\tau$.

A profile of the acoustic column is then performed in measuring the signal for different delays. The spatial resolution brought by the method is determined by the width of the pulse $\Delta\tau$, which becomes $\Delta z = V_{US}\Delta\tau$. Recalling that the velocity of sound in water is 1.5 mm/µs, a burst of 2 µs exhibits a resolution of 3 mm. Such an experiment has been initially performed with a single detector [33] and has been extended to digital off-axis holography [40] and photorefractive detection [35].

In a photorefractive configuration, the US burst performs a dynamical signal [35]. In contrast to digital holography, the reference beam is *not* shifted at US frequency. In the absence of US, a hologram of the *time-averaged* scattered photons $\langle E_{S,0}\rangle$ is recorded within the crystal over the response time τ_{PR}, giving on the detector a coherent signal proportional to $\langle E_{S,0}\rangle E_{S,0}$. When the burst propagates through the illuminated zone of the medium, *tagged photons* are generated and thus $E_{S,0}$ is depleted (by conservation of energy). But the hologram built by the photorefractive effect does not follow the µs regime induced by

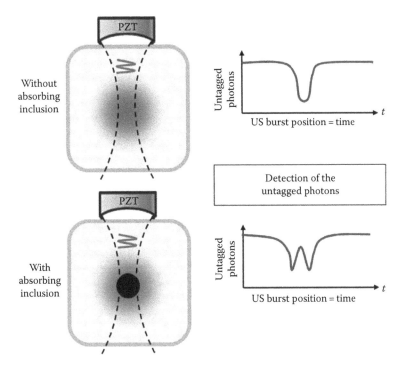

FIGURE 20.9 Schematic of the US burst method to detect an AO signal in *real time* with a photorefractive setup (see text for details).

the burst, and $\langle E_{S,0} \rangle$ keeps constant. As a consequence, the coherent signal measures a decrease of the scattered photons $E_{S,0}$. When the burst crosses an absorber, the amount of *tagged* photons is reduced and the signal recovers its initial value (see Figure 20.9).

In conclusion, the burst propagation renders a dynamical optical contrast along the US column, with a resolution determined by the width of the ultrasonic pulse, namely, $\Delta z = V_{US}\Delta\tau$. First applied with a *BSO* crystal at 532 nm [35], results have been obtained at 1064 nm [44] with GaAs and more recently at 780 nm with $Sn_2P_2S_6$:Te [48].

20.4.2 Random Phase Jumps Method

Another alternative, more favorable in terms of matching the optical and acoustical energy, consists of applying on the US and the reference (or signal beam) a phase modulation sequence $f(t)$ that contains many random jumps $(0,\pi)$ at a period τ_j, corresponding to some US periods. According to Figure 20.10, the *tagged* photons scattered from point z along the acoustic column emit a phase-*delayed* modulation $f(t - \tau_z)$, where $\tau_z = z/V_{US}$. Once the reference beam is opened at τ, the detection (camera, photodetector) records a *stationary* contribution of the heterodyne signal (Equation 20.4) if established on a characteristic timescale T_ψ small enough compared with the detection time T_d. This timescale is ruled out by a significant number of phase jumps, which ensures to $f(t)$ a good stochastic character.

If this condition is fulfilled, then the detection is sensitive to an integrated coefficient of the form

$$R_{jump}(\tau) = \int\limits_{z \in \{US\}} \int\limits_{T_d \gg T_\psi} e^{j[f(t-z/V_{US})-f(t-\tau)]} dt dz + c.c \qquad (20.17)$$

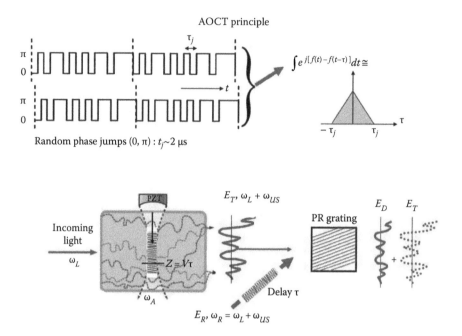

FIGURE 20.10 Principle of the *AOCT* technique. A stochastic phase sequence is applied on the US and on the reference beam with a delay τ. A hologram is recorded within the PR crystal, coming from a region located at $z = V_{US}τ$.

When dealing with a large number of phase jumps during the sequence, $f(t)$ has stochastic character, and thus $R_{jump}(τ)$ vanishes unless $τ = z/V_{US}$. In other words, a unique region is in phase with the delayed reference and contributes to the AO signal, as in the pulse method. For a large number of jumps during the phase sequence, it can be shown that digital holography acquisition leads to a spatial resolution that ideally tends to a triangle with base $Δz = 2V_{US}τ_j$, resulting from the convolution product between two jumps (*rectangle shaped*). This method is called *acousto-optical coherence tomography* (*AOCT*) [45] since the period of the jump monitors the axial resolution along the acoustic column. Of little difference is the photorefractive approach, since one measures the *square* of this apparatus function [49]. Up to now, this technique has been validated with the photorefractive setup at 1064 nm using a *GaAs* crystal in an anisotropic diffraction configuration [29,45].

20.5 Results

20.5.1 Samples

We worked mainly with two types of samples: turkey or chicken breast tissue and artificial phantoms of thickness ranging from 1 to 5 cm. The latter consists of a gelatin, in which agar grains are embedded to create small ultrasonic reflectors, and suspension of polystyrene microspheres (diameter 220 nm) or Intralipid® solution at 10%, to scatter light. We can change the scattering coefficient of the medium by adjusting the concentration of the latex. We can adjust the acoustic properties of the medium by changing the gelatin and the agar concentrations. The advantages of these artificial phantoms are their homogeneity and their well-controlled properties. However, we believe that it is necessary to study also biological tissues in order to tackle with the actual problems they will raise. Despite the absence of blood circulation in such samples, we believe they provide more realistic conditions than artificial phantoms.

20.5.2 Validation of the Principle of Simple Structures

Early experiments were performed on turkey breast tissues, in which we embedded artificial absorbing objects (dark ink or soft modeling clay) [31]. But the contrast was quite weak, with a lack of reproducibility. This forced us to go back to calibrated gels with $l^* = 1$ mm ($\mu_s' = 10$ cm^{-1}) in order to develop and test our methods.

Burst method with off-axis digital holography is illustrated in Figure 20.11 with a near-infrared light (wavelength $\lambda_L = 780$ nm) provided by a CW, single-frequency 400 mW output power Ti:sapphire laser (Coherent, MBR 110). The sample is made of an $80 \times 100 \times 25$ mm^3 jellified milk sample containing black-inked inclusions of the same material. The axial profile is extracted from a four-phase acquisition, with a camera rate of 4 kHz. The width of the US burst has been set to 3 or 5 μs in order to show the axial resolution. It must be pointed out that in such experiments, the magnitude of AO signal decreases as the square of the duty cycle since pressure is limited in time and the signal localized in space. In a random phase jump experiment, the pressure is almost uniform with time, and thus the magnitude depends on the duty cycle.

At present, the phase jumps process has been only studied in the photorefractive configuration at 1064 nm with a single GaAs crystal [45]. The laser used is a single-frequency *CW YAG:Nd* oscillator, amplified by a 5 W *Yb-doped* fiber amplifier. Figure 20.12 shows such axial-transverse images with different resolutions (in monitoring the jump period τ_j) of *millimeter* absorbing inclusions embedded within a scattering gel of 2 cm in thickness with a reduced scattering coefficient $\mu_s' = 10$ cm^{-1}. One observes a good compromise between the magnitude and resolution when the jump approaches the axial size of the inclusion, thus 3 mm in this case.

The burst method has been recently studied with the promising Sn$_2$P$_2$S$_6$:Te photorefractive crystal [48] since it exhibits a large gain in the *optical therapeutic window* (a few 10 cm^{-1}) and a reasonable time response (3 ms). Figure 20.13 demonstrates the feasibility of the method at 780 nm with a large scattering sample (thickness = 5.2 cm, $\mu_s' = 10$ cm^{-1}), bearing in mind that here peak pressure (7 MPa) and light illumination (3 W/cm^2) are still too high for clinical tests. The US burst contains two cycles at 2.3 MHz at a rate of 1 kHz (axial resolution of 1.3 mm). An absorbing cylinder of 10 mm length and 3 mm diameter is centered in the middle of the sample. As expected with this spatial resolution, the contrast of the inclusion approaches 100%. The proportion of *tagged photons* compared with the scattered ones can be measured from the *ac* and *dc* component of the signal. It corresponds to typically 0.1% of the collected

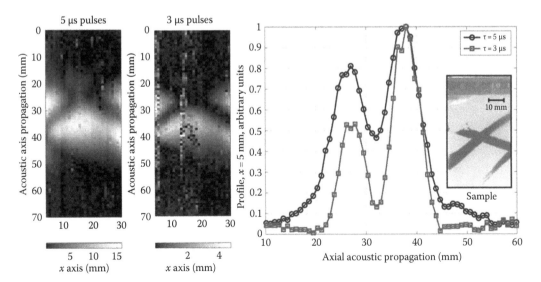

FIGURE 20.11 Longitudinal AO profiles performed with digital holography detection and the pulse method in a scattering gel containing black inclusions. The longitudinal resolution depends on the width of the acoustic burst. (Reprinted from Atlan, M. et al., *Opt. Lett.*, 30, 1360, 2005. With permission.)

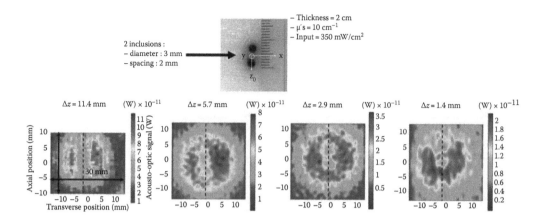

FIGURE 20.12 Illustration of the *AOCT* technique at 1064 nm with a *GaAs* massive crystal used with an aniso-tropic diffraction configuration. The axial resolution Δz is monitored by the period of the phase jump. Each image maps an *AO* signal over 30×30 mm². The plot at $\Delta z = 2.9$ mm corresponds to a phase sequence of $T = 1/2^5$ s including 2^{14} random phase jumps $(0,\pi)$.

flux. An axial profile corresponds to an 8-*bit* oscilloscope trace with 128 averaging, and the transverse position of the US is controlled with a step-by-step linear translation. In order to demonstrate a high *SNR*, this oversampled image of $(4 \times 4$ cm²) requires an acquisition time of 8 mn, but it can be reduced. Two parameters limited this acquisition: first, the ultrasonic source was a monotransducer. To avoid a transverse translation, it would be valuable to use an array of transducers. Second, the transfer of the data from the oscilloscope to the computer is not optimized and could be improved if the signal was recorded with a dedicated analog-to-digital converter.

Once the localization of objects with a strong absorption is validated, it is interesting to appreciate how the contrast changes with the local optical properties, mainly absorption and scattering variations. Some evidences are illustrated in Figure 20.14. We prepared two concentrations of ink, with absorption coefficients of 3 and 12 cm⁻¹ at 780 nm, and made identical cylinder inclusions within a scattering gel of 3 cm. Figure 20.14a shows that the contrast depends on the absorption coefficient. Assuming a *Beer–Lambert* dependence of the signal, one can check in Figure 20.14b that the depletion of the signals is in good agreement with the ratio 4 of the absorption coefficients.

Finally, a purely scattering inclusion ($l^* = 0.5$ mm) embedded within a gel ($l^* = 1.6$ mm) is also clearly localized, as shown in Figure 20.14c. Similar results have previously been observed with an indirect method [47]. This sensitivity to a scattering discrepancy is of importance for a possible use of the method to follow a high-intensity focused US therapy (*HIFU*) since local heating can affect both scattering and absorption coefficients.

All these results need further work to perform quantitative measurements, if possible at different wavelengths, in order to discriminate the nature of the absorbers.

The last example we present in Figure 20.15 is obtained through 3.8 cm of breast chicken, containing the same type of black inclusions we described earlier. The absorbers are clearly observed at a resolution of 3.5 mm (5 *cycles* at 2.3 MHz, $P_{peak} \sim 10$ MPa). These results are encouraging in the scope of in vivo imaging.

20.6 Beyond Purely Ultrasonic Modulation: The Acoustic Radiation Force

AO imaging, as discussed in the previous sections, is fundamentally based on the modulation of optical phase created by the US beam itself as a displacement and density wave. On the other hand, US beams in attenuating media may also generate displacement via the US radiation force [62]. This radiation force

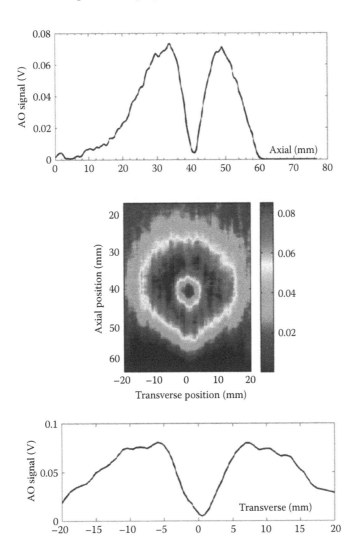

FIGURE 20.13 2D AO profile at 780 nm through a scattering gel of 5.2 cm thick, with $l^* = 1$ mm. Photorefractive crystal is $Sn_2P_2S_6$:Te, with a burst regime for the US (2 *cycles* at 2.3 MHz, 1 kHz *rate*, $P = 7$ MPa). The shape of the profile has been inverted for the sake of presentation.

corresponds to a transfer of momentum from the wave to the medium as the wave is either attenuated or is reflected by impedance mismatches. In acoustics, this property is the analog in optics of the radiation force exerted by a light impinging on a mirror or an optical absorber. In the case of soft biological tissue, which attenuates US because of absorption and/or scattering by very weak random fluctuations in acoustic impedance, the density of radiation force (unit force per unit volume) is given by the following formula [63]:

$$f = \frac{2\alpha I}{c} \tag{20.18}$$

where
α is the US attenuation coefficient (in Neper per unit distance)
I is the acoustic intensity (defined as the time-averaged US intensity over the US period)
c is the sound velocity

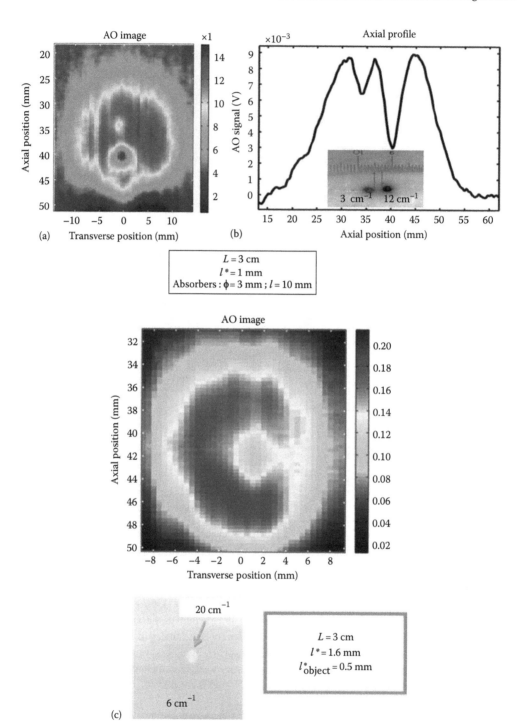

FIGURE 20.14 (a) AO images of inclusions with various optical properties.(b) The contrast of two absorbers (α = 3 and 12 cm^{-1}) and (c) the presence of an inclusion with a scattering coefficient (μ'_s = 20 cm^{-1}) that differs from the host matrix (μ'_s = 6 cm^{-1}).

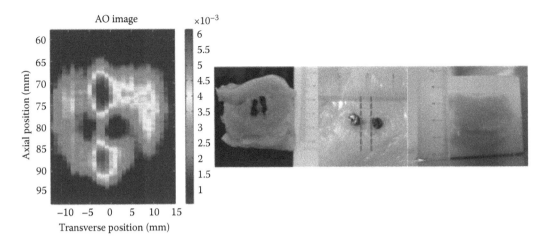

FIGURE 20.15 AO image of chicken breast with thickness 3.8 cm, containing two inclusions (3.5×10 mm^2) separated from 3.5 mm. The hot spots on the image come from a nonuniform distribution of the MOPA laser input.

As opposed to ultrasonic stresses, the direction of the radiation force is always oriented along the flow of ultrasonic energy and importantly it is defined only as a time-averaged quantity. In particular, to a pure single-frequency US wave corresponds a radiation force that is *constant* in time. In other words, only amplitude modulation of US waves can produce time-varying radiation forces.

In response to the radiation force, a soft-tissue-like medium is set into motion that involves time and amplitude scales very different from those associated with US wave. Interestingly, the radiation force generated by a focused US beam in soft tissue allows probing mechanical properties of tissue that are very different from those probed by the use of conventional US technique. While US waves used in conventional US imaging, as well as in AO imaging as described in the previous section, probe compressional properties of tissue, a focused radiation force in tissue creates a displacement field that predominantly involves shearing the tissue and therefore provides information on shear mechanical properties [64].

The measurement of such displacement is at the basis of several implementations of elastography [63–65], as the frequency response of the medium to the radiation force depends on its shear viscoelastic properties. For focused radiation forces, the displacement originating at focus subsequently propagates away through shear wave mechanisms [63,64,66]. In the context of AO imaging, such shear waves have usually been considered as detrimental to the AO modulation [67,68]. However, they may also be used to provide information complementary to that provided by AO imaging, as our group first demonstrated in the proof-of-concept experiments [69,70], described in the following paragraphs.

The experimental setup used in Ref. [70] is analogous to that of Figure 20.2. However, the pair of AO modulator in this case is only used to shift the laser frequency by half the camera rate to allow for two-phase interferometry, without shifting the frequency to detect tagged photons. In this case, the use of a reference beam is only intended to improve the SNR in the case of weak signals. But should the transmitted intensity be sufficient, simple direct speckle detection may be used, as was done in the first proof-of-concept experiment [69]. The idea in this experiment is to detect the *transient* shear waves generated by a transient millisecond radiation force. Millisecond bursts are chosen to maximize the induced shear waves while remaining shorter or of the same order of magnitude as the response time of a soft-tissue-like medium to the radiation force. Under this situation, the radiation force may be approximately considered as a delta function in time. Importantly, US is used here only to generate shear waves and not to phase modulate the light as in AO imaging [69]. The fundamental difference between the transient shear waves generated by the impulse radiation force and conventional US wave is their timescale. Transient shear waves generated by MHz-focused US beam always have a frequency content no higher than typically 1 kHz. As a consequence, a kHz frame rate camera allows taking images of speckle patterns that may be considered issued from a still medium during the exposure time. In other words, the motion induced by the shear waves may be time resolved with kHz camera. Analyzing speckle changes from the nth snapshot to the next may be performed by calculating a spatial cross-correlation coefficient, defined by the following equation:

$$c(n) = \frac{\sum_{i,j}\left(I^n_{i,j} - \overline{I^n}\right)\left(I^{n+1}_{i,j} - \overline{I^{n+1}}\right)}{\sqrt{\sum_{i,j}\left(I^n_{i,j} - \overline{I^n}\right)^2}\sqrt{\sum_{i,j}\left(I^{n+1}_{i,j} - \overline{I^{n+1}}\right)^2}} \tag{20.19}$$

where (i,j) are pixel coordinates and the bar refers to spatial averaging over all pixels. A strictly still medium will yield a correlation value of 1. In practice, measurement noise and stationary motion in the samples (such as Brownian motion and/or mechanical noise) lead to a correlation value less than 1. However, this value is stationary in time. Figure 20.16, reprinted from Ref. [69], shows the evolution of the correlation coefficient when a millisecond transient radiation force is focused into a soft-tissue-mimicking phantom. A continuous $5W$ frequency-doubled $Nd:YAG$ laser source (Verdi, Coherent) was used to illuminate the tissue-mimicking phantom. The phantom consisted of a 1% agar gel made optically diffusive by adding Intralipid. A concentration of 0.4% *Intralipid* [71] was used to obtain a reduced scattering coefficient of approximately $\mu'_s \approx 6$ cm^{-1}. The dimensions of the phantom were $40 \times 40 \times 40$ mm^3. A 5 MHz spherically focused US transducer (A307-S, GE Panametrics) was used to focus high-intensity US bursts of millisecond duration in the center of the phantom and generate transient displacements. A 1024×1024 pixel CMOS camera (HSS-4, Lavision) was used to record the optical speckle pattern with a 2 kHz frame rate and was positioned at a distance L of approximately 1 m from the phantom to match the pixel size (17 µm) to the average speckle grain dimensions. A 2 cm diameter tube was used both to hold the phantom in water and to collect light. A delay generator (BNC 565, Berkeley Nucleonics) was used to trig the camera acquisition several milliseconds before triggering the US burst.

The curve in Figure 20.16 clearly features a transient decorrelation, which lasts for several millisecond. The fact that the decorrelation continues to grow after the US burst has been turned off indicates that the detected effect is not caused by the ultrasonic oscillation of the compressional wave. Although no quantitative theory is available yet, the curve shown in Figure 20.16 is a qualitative signature of the relative displacements occurring in the medium between two consecutive images. The duration of the observed correlation drop (~7–8 ms) is due to the fact that the measurement is not only sensitive to the motion created at focus (which would yield transient effect with a typical response time of the order of 1 ms [64,72]) but also to the associated shear waves propagating away from the focal region [64].

The first experiment [69] demonstrated that it is possible to optically detect shear wave motion occurring several centimeters deep in tissue. The relevance of such a signal for tissue characterization was then demonstrated in a second proof-of-concept experiment [70]. Using tissue-mimicking phantoms

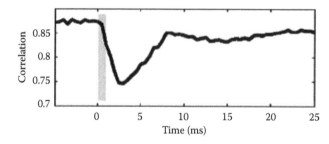

FIGURE 20.16 Correlation curve observed for a 1 ms long radiation force (gray region) in a homogeneous tissue-mimicking phantom. (Reprinted from Bossy, E. et al., *Appl. Phys. Lett.*, 90, 174111, 2007. With permission.)

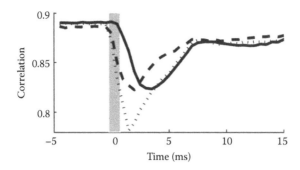

FIGURE 20.17 Correlation curves observed for a 1 ms long radiation force (gray region) in a tissue-mimicking phantom with a hard inclusion (higher Young's modulus) and a dark inclusion. The dotted line was obtained for a push centered between the two inclusions, the dashed line for a push located in the hardest inclusion, and the full line for a push located in the optically absorbing inclusion. (Reprinted from Daoudi, K. et al., *Appl. Phys. Lett.*, 94, 154103, 2009. With permission.)

with several types of inclusion, namely, optically absorbing inclusion and/or hard inclusion (with a higher Young's modulus), it was demonstrated that the correlation signal was sensitive to both optical and shear mechanical properties *at the location of the radiation force*. Moreover, the nature of an inclusion (optical or mechanical contrast) could be determined from how the correlation curve is altered compared with that obtained when pushing out of the inclusions. As shown in Figure 20.17, the presence of optical absorption at the location of the push led to a *delayed* drop in the correlation curve. This delay is caused by the fact that as long as the shear motion is confined into the dark inclusion, no effect on the transmitted speckle can occur. The observed delay simply scales as the time needed for the shear wave to exit the dark inclusion, that is, the delay is proportional to the size of the inclusion and is inversely proportional to the shear wave velocity. As also shown in Figure 20.17, pushing into a hard inclusion is revealed on the curve by a decrease of the correlation drop, while the shape of the curve remains the same. This change in amplitude reflects the fact that for a given force the amplitude of the generated shear wave depends on the shear modulus *at the location of the push*. For a harder medium, the amplitude of the shear wave is less than that for a softer medium.

By choosing appropriate parameters on the correlation curve and by scanning the radiation force step by step, it is therefore possible to reconstruct images of either optical or shear mechanical properties in a soft medium. Figure 20.18 (work submitted for publication) is an example of an image obtained by plotting the amplitude of the correlation drop as a function of push location for a tissue-mimicking phantom with two hard cylindrical inclusions, parallel to the direction of the push. While the axial resolution provided by the technique is limited to the focal depth of the ultrasonic transducer, Figure 20.18 illustrates the good lateral resolution provided by the technique for detecting hard inclusions.

While our studies described earlier have used transient radiation force to generate transient shear waves, interesting results were recently obtained by a group in Imperial College [73]. The authors observed an increase in the AO modulation signal when amplitude-modulated US is used instead of purely harmonic US. However, in this study, the AO signal was defined as a loss of speckle contrast. This signal is therefore sensitive to both pure US modulation and motion caused by the amplitude-modulated radiation force, provided that the contrast is measured over an exposure time longer than both the ultrasonic and radiation force modulations. The increase in the signal was therefore attributed to the effect of shear waves added to the purely ultrasonic modulation. The relative contribution of shear waves produced by the radiation force to the overall signal remains the subject of ongoing work.

In summary, the US radiation force provides an alternative to purely ultrasonic modulation to interact with a coherent light field in optically diffusive soft media. In particular, the response to the radiation force in a soft tissue is dictated by shear mechanical properties, while US waves used in AO imaging

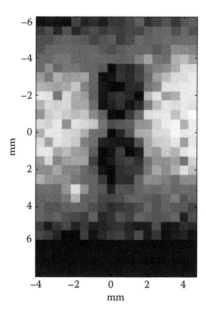

FIGURE 20.18 Optoelastic images obtained in a tissue-mimicking phantom with two cylindrical hard inclusions, 2 mm in diameter, separated by 1 mm. The radiation force is parallel to the inclusions axes. The plotted parameter is the maximum correlation drop. (Work submitted for publication.)

are only sensitive to contrast in compressional mechanical properties. As opposed to the AO modulation produced by a focused US beam, the displacement generated by the radiation force does not remain confined to the focal region where it is initially produced. Further investigations are required to quantify for each experimental situation and detection scheme which tissue volume is exactly being probed when using the acoustic radiation force.

20.7 Detection Schemes Independent of the Speckle Field Distribution: Fabry–Perot Filter, Spectral Hole Burning, and Bubble Modulation

In the preceding sections, we explained that it is of importance to record the modulation of the speckle field over a large number of speckle grains or of pixels (using megapixel cameras or gigapixel photorefractive crystals) in a time shorter than the decorrelation time of the organ under examination.

If we go back to the basic modulation scheme as shown in Figure 20.1, we see that the information to be recorded is contained in the sidebands that are shifted by a few megahertz from the laser frequency and broadened (typically by a few kilohertz) by the acoustic field and the blood flow, respectively [52]. So the ideal detection scheme would have been to get a filter centered on one of the sidebands with a good rejection of the laser frequency. With such a filter, it is possible to gather all the scattered tagged light and to measure this signal on a single detector.

To the best of our knowledge, two approaches using ultraselective filters have been proposed and validated so far.

20.7.1 Confocal Fabry–Perot

A confocal Fabry–Perot interferometer offers the double advantage of a high selectivity in frequency and large geometrical *etendue*. Indeed, typically a few tens of centimeters long interferometer offer a free

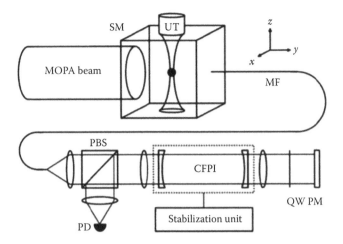

FIGURE 20.19 Confocal Fabry–Perot filtering of the tagged photons. The double-pass confocal interferometer exhibits a resolution large enough to reject efficiently untagged photon generated from the MOPA working at 1.06 micron with 10 kHz bandwidth from the tagged ones that are shifted by the ultrasonic frequency (5 MHz). (Reprinted from Rousseau, G. et al., *Opt. Lett.*, 34, 3445, 2009. With permission.)

spectral range of the order of 100 MHz, and using a finesse of 100, one can reach a typical bandwidth of 1 MHz. One knows that, at least within the paraxial approximation, a confocal Fabry–Perot exhibits a path difference between interfering *rays* that is independent of the angle of incidence of the beams impinging the interferometer, which explains the large *etendue* and the overall good efficiency in terms of light collection.

Such filters have been proposed and used by the group of J.P. Monchalin [46]. One realization of such a setup is represented in Figure 20.19: a tunable source of pulsed light (MOPA) illuminates the sample, and the emerging light is collected by a multimode fiber, collimated and selectively filtered at the *tagged photon* frequency by the double-pass (with the use of a plane mirror (PM)) confocal Fabry–Perot interferometer. This system is supposed to provide the best *etendue* used so far to detect the AO signal. It requires some expertise in the optimization and stabilization of the frequency filter, and it may be the reason of a limited use compared with photorefractive crystal filters of *tagged photons*.

20.7.2 Spectral Hole Burning

Another elegant way of building a highly selective filter is to take advantage of the spectral hole-burning phenomena. As can be seen in Figure 20.20, a highly monochromatic laser is used to saturate a two-level optical transition (at the *tagged photon* frequency) of a class of centers of an absorption band that exhibits an inhomogeneous broadening. The bandwidth of the filter is linked to the homogeneous bandwidth (small width absorption curves below the inhomogeneous broadband in the figure). The rejection of the unwanted frequencies (laser frequency) is dependent on the saturation level and on the absorbance of the sample. The absorption is larger when the doping is higher, but energy diffusion through the whole bandwidth is then more likely to appear.

This approach offers obvious advantages over the approaches that we have described before: indeed, here there is a very large etendue to collect *tagged photons* coming from a large area and filling a large solid angle. The problem is then mainly technical: crystals, mostly doped with trivalent rare earth ions, only exhibit hole burning at low temperatures, meaning that a cryostat must be used that reduces the flexibility of the experiment. For this reason, as well as the size of the crystal, this approach is still in competition with the other techniques [42,43].

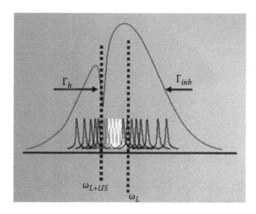

FIGURE 20.20 Spectral hole burning as a highly selective filter for the tagged photon: a sample exhibits an inhomogeneously broadened absorption line. A highly monochromatic laser is able to saturate the transition corresponding to a homogeneously broadened transition corresponding to a class of absorbing centers. If there is no diffusion, this hole exhibits a much lower absorption than the rest of the band. This is the principle that has been used in Ref. [43].

20.7.3 Bubble-Induced Transmission Modulation

It is known that bubbles are very efficient contrast agents in US in both the linear and the nonlinear regimes. They also participate in the scattering properties of the medium where they are injected (such as blood) and increase the efficiency of the AO signal by two to three orders of magnitude at a concentration of the order of 10^5 mm^{-3} compatible with medical requirements [74]. This signal amplification is valuable (modeled with an average bubble size) but still sensitive to speckle modulation characteristics and detection schemes previously mentioned.

More recently, scientists from the same university have reported that the bubble size modulation is responsible for the overall transmission variation of the sample via the variations of the scattering properties. This signal is indeed promising: whether it can be detected with a suitable bubble concentration because it does not involve any random modulation from the speckle grains but simply a transmission variation that can be obtained with an incoherent low-noise source and a large aperture collecting optics.

20.8 Prospects and Conclusions

We have explored a number of recent developments dealing with the field of US-modulated imaging in this chapter. Clearly, large improvements have been achieved in terms of SNR, speed, and resolution. Moreover, new approaches have been proposed and tested, such as the use of spectral hole burning or the use of shear waves induced by the radiation pressure field.

All these progresses have been obtained using both an ultrasonic field level and a light irradiance level lower than those imposed by the international safety requirements.

Nevertheless, as opposed to photoacoustics, AO is not yet a recognized medical tool that deserves a place in hospitals, and for this reason, improvements must be done to promote this method and push it to the place that it deserves.

One obvious part of the work will be to optimize the techniques and the instruments, in order to be more reliable and user friendly, which has been discussed in this chapter.

Another more prospective approach would be to get involved in new directions such as the very promising field of wave control of the speckle field that is at the basis of the AO effect in scattering media.

Earlier, in this chapter, we discussed the generation of rather complicated field distributions that match the speckle field of the *tagged photons* emerging from a sample submitted to both a coherent illumination and an acoustic field. This geometry was relevant to the so-called *2-waves mixing*, but one can also take advantage of the *4-waves mixing* schemes that are also obtained with the use of photorefractive crystals [75] or the wavefront control that one can realize with spatial light modulators (SLMs) over thousands and may be soon millions of pixels [76].

In the first schemes (Figure 20.21), a phase conjugate of the outgoing field (time reversal field in the case of monochromatic CW) is generated in the photorefractive crystal; this field back propagates into the sample and goes back to its initial input spatial distribution. Indeed, a clear image of a sample (S on the figure) can be recorded on the crystal through a scattering medium (beam going up toward the crystal on the figure) and read (beam going down toward the crystal) with a perfect compensation of the diffusive paths. The proposed setup is still too slow (tens of seconds) to be used in vivo (hundreds of microseconds being required).

One can think to use this scheme coupled to an acoustic field that will *destroy* the spatial coherence of the incoming beam and to use the reduction of the signal that can be detected on a single detector. This kind of detection is underway in our laboratory. Another approach has been used by the St. Louis group led by L. Wang: they phase conjugate the *tagged photon beam* that is back focused on the acoustic source. This source plays a role of an artificial star that can be placed anywhere into the scattering sample leading to improvements in contrast and tagged light level [77].

Finally, another way to manipulate the speckle field consists in using an SLM (usually a megapixel liquid crystal matrix; each pixel of the matrix can be electrically controlled in amplitude, phase, or polarization). With such systems, it is possible to monitor the wave propagation through the scattering medium by imposing, for instance, the emerging field in order to focus on a well-defined pixel [78,79]. One can think of maximizing the number of *tagged photons* along the acoustic field trajectory in order to optimize the signal that is used to construct the image and to perform an efficient detection on a single pixel grain using a single detector. The setups that have been already used (Figure 20.22) should

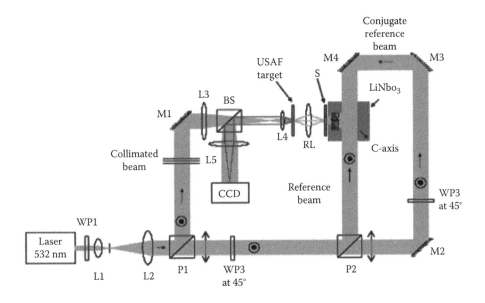

FIGURE 20.21 Four-wave mixing setup. The phase conjugation process back generates the coherent beam structure that illuminates the scattering sample here. One can break this coherence by mixing the photons paths in the scattering medium by the acoustic field that transforms untagged photons into tagged ones. (Reprinted from Yaqoob, Z. et al., *Nat. Photonics*, 2, 110, 2008. With permission.)

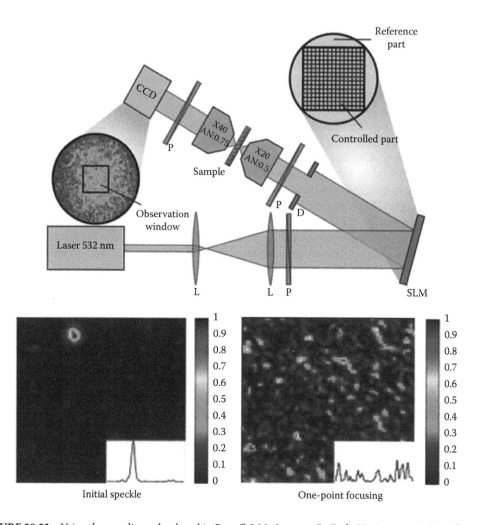

FIGURE 20.22 Using the paradigms developed in Popoff, S.M., Lerosey, G., Fink, M., Boccara, A.C., and Gigan, S., *Nat. Commun.* 1, Art. No. 81, 2010 and Popoff, S.M., Lerosey, G., Carminati, R., Fink, M., Boccara, A.C., and Gigan, S., *Phys. Rev. Lett.* 104, Art. No. 100601, 2010 (reprinted with permission), it is possible to focus efficiently the speckle field on a single grain. The local enhancement of the illumination can be increased by several orders of magnitude. In this case, the detection of the ultrasonic modulation can be simply recorded by using a single detector and a lock-in amplifier.

be adapted in the sense that, the sample being very thick, the optimization has to be done using a large number of pixels, but the main difficulty is to achieve focusing on a speckle grain in a time shorter than the decorrelation length. One can find SLM working in the kilohertz range, and there is hope that such systems would introduce a new era in the AO detection.

Acknowledgments

We would like to thank Max Lesaffre, Michaël Atlan, Salma Farahi, Emilie Benoit à la Guillaume, Khalid Daoudi, Philippe Delaye, Jean-Pierre Huignard, Germano Montemezzani, and Alexander Grabar for their contributions to the results presented here. We also wish to thank our acoustician colleagues from the Institut Langevin–ESPCI, for their collaborations, especially in characterizing the pressure field.

References

1. J.C. Hebden and D.T. Delpy, Enhanced time-resolved imaging with a diffusion model of photon transport. *Opt. Lett.* **9**, 311–313 (1994).
2. J.C. Hebden, F.E.W. Schmidt, M.E. Fry, M. Schweiger, E.M.C. Hillman, D.T. Delpy, and S.R. Arridge, Simultaneous reconstruction of absorption and scattering images using multichannel measurement of purely temporal data. *Opt. Lett.* **24**, 534–536 (1999).
3. M.A. O'Leary, D.A. Boas, B. Chance, and A.G. Yodh, Experimental images of heterogeneous turbid media by frequency-domain diffusing-photon tomography. *Opt. Lett.* **20**, 426–428 (1995).
4. D. Huang, E.A. Swanson, C.P. Lin, J.S. Schuman, W.G. Stinson, W. Chang, M.R. Hee et al., Optical coherence tomography. *Science* **254**, 1178–1181 (1991).
5. J.G. Fujimoto, M.E. Brezinski, G.J. Tearney, S.A. Boppart, B.E. Bouma, M.R. Hee, J.F. Southern, and E.A. Swanson, Optical biopsy and imaging using optical coherence tomography. *Nat. Med.* **1**, 970–972 (1995).
6. A.F. Fercher, Optical coherence tomography. *J. Biomed. Opt.* **1**, 157–173 (1996).
7. G.J. Tearney, M.E. Brezinski, B.E. Bouma, S.A. Bopart, C. Pitris, J.F. Southern, and J.G. Fujimoto, *In vivo* endoscopic optical biopsy with optical coherence tomography. *Science* **276**, 2037–2039 (1997).
8. J.A. Izatt, M.R. Hee, G.M. Owen, E.A. Swanson, and J.G. Fujimoto, Optical coherence microscopy in scattering media. *Opt. Lett.* **19**, 590–593 (1994).
9. R.A. Kruger and P. Liu, Photoacoustic ultrasound: Theory, in *Laser-Tissue Interaction V*, S.L. Jacques, ed., *Proc. SPIE* **2134A**, 114–118 (1994).
10. A.A. Oraevsky, R.O. Esenaliev, S.L. Jacques, and F.K. Tittel, Laser optic-acoustic tomography for medical diagnostics: Principles, in *Biomedical Sensing, Imaging, and Tracking Technologies I*, R.A. Lieberman, H. Podbielska, and T. Vo-Dinh, eds., *Proc. SPIE* **2676**, 22–31 (1996).
11. C.G.A. Hoelen, F.F.M. de Mul, R. Pongers, and A. Dekker, Three-dimensional photoacoustic imaging of blood vessels in tissue. *Opt. Lett.* **23**, 648–650 (1998).
12. F.A. Marks, H.W. Tomlinson, and G.W. Brooksby, A comprehensive approach to breast cancer detection using light: Photon localisation by ultrasound modulation and tissue characterization by spectral discrimination, in *Photon Migration and Imaging in Random Media and Tissues*, B. Chance and R.R. Alfa, eds., *Proc. SPIE* **1888**, 500–510 (1993).
13. L. Wang, S.L. Jacques, and X. Zhao, Continuous-wave ultrasonic modulation of scattered laser light to image objects in turbid media. *Opt. Lett.* **20**, 629–631 (1995).
14. W. Leutz and G. Maret, Ultrasonic modulation of multiply scattered light. *Physica B* **204**, 14–19 (1995).
15. M. Kempe, M. Larionov, D. Zaslavsky, and A.Z. Genack, Acousto-optic tomography with multiply scattered light. *J. Opt. Soc. Am. A* **14**, 1151–1158 (1997).
16. L. Wang and X. Zhao, Ultrasound-modulated optical tomography of absorbing objects buried in dense tissue-simulating turbid media. *Appl. Opt.* **36**, 7277–7282 (1997).
17. S. Lévêque, A.C. Boccara, M. Lebec, and H. Saint-Jalmes, A multidetector approach to ultrasonic speckle modulation imaging, in *Advances in Optical Imaging and Photon Migration*, Trends in Optics and Photonics Series, Vol. 21, paper AWA5, OSA, Washington, DC (1998).
18. L. Wang and G. Ku, Frequency-swept ultrasound-modulated optical tomography of scattering media. *Opt. Lett.* **23**, 975–977 (1998).
19. S. Lévêque, A.C. Boccara, M. Lebec, and H. Saint-Jalmes, Ultrasonic tagging of photon paths in scattering media: Parallel speckle modulation processing. *Opt. Lett.* **24**, 181–183 (1999).
20. G. Yao and L.V. Wang, Theoretical and experimental studies of ultrasound-modulated optical tomography in biological tissue. *Appl. Opt.* **39**, 659–664 (2000).
21. S. Lévêque-Fort, Three-dimensional acousto-optic imaging in biological tissues with parallel signal processing. *Appl. Opt.* **40**, 1029–1036 (2000).

22. A. Lev, Z. Kotler, and B.G. Sfev, Ultrasound tagged light imaging in turbid media in a reflectance geometry. *Opt. Lett.* **25**, 378–380 (2000).
23. G. Yao, S. Jiao, and L.V. Wang, Frequency-swept ultrasound-modulated optical tomography in biological tissue by use of parallel detection. *Opt. Lett.* **25**, 734–736 (2000).
24. S. Lévêque-Fort, J. Selb, L. Pottier, and A.C. Boccara, In situ local tissue characterization and imaging by backscattering acousto-optic imaging. *Opt. Commun.* **196**, 127–131 (2001).
25. E. Granot, A. Lev, Z. Kotler, B.G. Sfev, and H. Taitelbaum, Detection of inhomogeneities with ultrasound tagging of light. *J. Opt. Soc. Am. A* **18**, 1962–1967 (2001).
26. L.V. Wang, Mechanisms of ultrasonic modulation of multiply scattered coherent light: An analytic model. *Phys. Rev. Lett.* **87**, 043903 (2001).
27. J. Selb, Source virtuelle acousto-optique pour l'imagerie des milieux diffusants, PhD thesis, Université Paris XI, Paris, France (November 2002).
28. M. Atlan, Imagerie optique cohérente de milieux diffusants, PhD thesis, Université Paris XI, Paris, France (September 2005).
29. M. Lesaffre, Imagerie acousto-optique de milieux diffusants épais par détection photoréfractive, PhD thesis, Université Pierre et Marie Curie, Paris, France (October 2009).
30. J. Selb, L. Pottier, and A.C. Boccara, Non-linear effects in acousto-optic imaging. *Opt. Lett.* **27**(11), 918–920 (2002).
31. J. Selb, S. Lévêque-Fort, A. Dubois, B.C. Forget, L. Pottier, F. Ramaz, and C. Boccara, Chapter 35: Ultrasonically modulated optical imaging, in *Biomedical Photonics Handbook*, T. Vo-Dinh, ed., CRC Press, Boca Raton, FL.
32. B.C. Forget, F. Ramaz, M. Atlan, J. Selb, and A.C. Boccara, High-contrast fast Fourier transform acousto-optical tomography of phantom tissues with a frequency chirp modulation of the ultrasound. *Appl. Opt.* **42**(7), 1379–1383 (2003).
33. A. Lev and B.G. Sfez, Pulsed ultrasound-modulated light tomography. *Opt. Lett.* **28**(17), 1549–1551 (2003).
34. F. Ramaz, B.C. Forget, M. Atlan, AC Boccara, M. Gross, P. Delaye, and G. Roosen, Photorefractive detection of tagged photons in ultrasound modulated optical tomography of thick biological tissues. *Opt. Express* **12**(22), 5469–5474 (2004).
35. T.W. Murray, L. Sui, G. Maguluri, R.A. Roy, A. Nieva, F. Blonigen, and C.A. DiMarzio, Detection of ultrasound-modulated photons in diffuse media using the photorefractive effect. *Opt. Lett.*, **29**(21), 2509–2511 (2004).
36. A. Lev, E. Rubanov, B. Sfez, S. Shany, and A.J. Foldes, Ultrasound-modulated light tomography assessment of osteoporosis. *Opt. Lett.* **30**(13), 1692–1694 (2005).
37. E. Bossy, L. Sui, T.W. Murray, and R.A. Roy, Fusion of conventional ultrasound imaging and acousto-optic sensing by use of a standard pulsed-ultrasound scanner. *Opt. Lett.* **30**(7), 744–746 (2005).
38. L. Sui, R.A. Roy, C.A. DiMarzio, and T.W. Murray, Imaging in diffuse media with pulsed-ultrasound-modulated light and the photorefractive effect. *Appl. Opt.* **44**(19), 4041–4048 (2005).
39. M. Gross, F. Ramaz, B. Forget, M. Atlan, A. Boccara, P. Delaye, and G. Roosen. Theoretical description of the photorefractive detection of the ultrasound modulated photons in scattering media. *Opt. Express* **13**(18), 7097–7112 (2005).
40. M. Atlan, B.C. Forget, F. Ramaz, A.C. Boccara, and M. Gross, Pulsed acousto-optic imaging in dynamic scattering media with heterodyne parallel speckle detection. *Opt. Lett.* **30**(11), 1360–1362 (2005).
41. M. Lesaffre, F. Jean, F. Ramaz, A.C. Boccara, M. Gross, P. Delaye, and G. Roosen, In situ monitoring of the photorefractive response time in a self-adaptive wavefront holography setup developed for acousto-optic imaging. *Opt. Express* **15**(3), 1030–1042 (2007).
42. Y. Li, H. Zhang, C. Kim, K.H. Wagner, P. Hemmer, and L.V. Wang, Pulsed ultrasound-modulated optical tomography using spectral-hole burning as a narrowband spectral filter. *Appl. Phys. Lett.* **93**, 011111 (2008).

43. Y. Li, P. Hemmer, C. Kim, H. Zhang, and L.V. Wang, Detection of ultrasound-modulated diffuse photons using spectral-hole burning. *Opt. Express* **16**(19), 14862–14874 (2008).

44. G. Rousseau, A. Blouin, and J.P. Monchalin, Ultrasound-modulated optical imaging using a powerful long pulse laser. *Opt. Express* **16**(17), 12577–12590 (2008).

45. M. Lesaffre, S. Farahi, M. Gross, P. Delaye, C. Boccara and F. Ramaz, Acousto-optical coherence tomography using random phase jumps on ultrasound and light. *Opt. Express* **17**(20), 18211–18218 (2009).

46. G. Rousseau, A. Blouin, and J.P. Monchalin, Ultrasound-modulated optical imaging using a high-power pulsed laser and a double-pass confocal Fabry–Perot interferometer. *Opt. Lett.* **34**(21), 3445–3447 (2009).

47. L. Puxiang, R.A. Roy, and T.W. Murray, Quantitative characterization of turbid media using pressure contrast acousto-optic imaging. *Opt. Lett.* **34**(18), 2850–2852 (2009).

48. S. Farahi, G. Montemezzani, A.A. Grabar, J.P. Huignard, and F. Ramaz, Photorefractive acousto-optic imaging in thick scattering media at 790 nm with a Sn2P2S6:Te crystal. *Opt. Lett.* **35**(11), 1798–1800 (2010).

49. M. Lesaffre, S. Farahi, P. Delaye, A.C. Boccara, F. Ramaz, and M. Gross, Theoretical study of acousto-optical coherence tomography using random phase jumps on US and light. *JOSA A* **28**(7), 1436–1444 (2011).

50. F. Le Clerc, L. Collot, and M. Gross, Numerical heterodyne holography with two-dimensional photodetector arrays. *Opt. Lett.* **25**(10), 716–718 (2000).

51. M. Gross, P. Goy, and M. Al-Koussa, Shot-noise detection of ultrasound-tagged photons in ultrasound-modulated optical imaging. *Opt. Lett.* **28**(24), 2482–2484 (2003).

52. M. Gross, P. Goy, B.C. Forget, M. Atlan, F. Ramaz, A.C. Boccara, and A.K. Dunn, Heterodyne detection of multiply scattered monochromatic light with a multipixel detector. *Opt. Lett.* **30**(11), 1357–1359 (2005).

53. M. Gross and M. Atlan, Digital holography with ultimate sensitivity. *Opt. Lett.* **32**(8), 909–911 (2007).

54. M. Atlan and M. Gross, Spatiotemporal heterodyne detection. *JOSA A* **24**(9), 2701–2709 (2007).

55. F. Verpillat, F. Joud, M. Atlan, and M. Gross, Digital holography at shot noise level. *J. Display Technol.* **6**(10), 455–464 (2010).

56. E. Cuche, P. Marquet, and C. Depeursinge, Spatial filtering for zero-order and twin-image elimination in digital off-axis holography. *Appl. Opt.* **39**(23), 4070–4075 (2000).

57. P. Picart and J. Leval. General theoretical formulation of image formation in digital Fresnel holography. *JOSA A* **25**(7), 1744–1761 (2008).

58. U. Schnars and W. Jüptner, Direct recording of holograms by a CCD target and numerical reconstruction. *Appl. Opt.* **33**(2), 179–181 (1994).

59. P. Delaye, L.A. De Montmorillon, and G. Roosen, Transmission of time modulated optical signals through an absorbing photorefractive crystal. *Opt. Commun.* **118**(1–2), 154–164 (1995).

60. P. Delaye, A. Blouin, D. Drolet, L.A. de Montmorillon, G. Roosen, and J.P. Monchalin, Detection of ultrasonic motion of a scattering surface by photorefractive InP:Fe under an applied dc field. *JOSA B* **14**(7), 1723–1734 (1997).

61. L.A. De Montmorillon, P. Delaye, J.C. Launay, and G. Roosen, Novel theoretical aspects on photorefractive ultrasonic detection and implementation of a sensor with an optimum sensitivity. *J. Appl. Phys.* **82**(12), 5913–5922 (1997).

62. G.R. Torr, The acoustic radiation force. *Am. J. Phys.* **52**(5), 402–408 (1984).

63. J. Bercoff, M. Tanter, and M. Fink, Supersonic shear imaging: A new technique for soft tissue elasticity mapping. *IEEE Trans. Ultrason. Ferroelectr. Freq. Control* **51**(4), 396–409 (2004).

64. A.P. Sarvazyan, O.V. Rudenko, S.D. Swanson, J.B. Fowlkes, and S.Y. Emelianov, Shear wave elasticity imaging: A new ultrasonic technology of medical diagnostics. *Ultrasound Med. Biol.* **24**(9), 1419–1435 (1998).

65. K. Nightingale, M.S. Soo, R. Nightingale, and G. Trahey, Acoustic radiation force impulse imaging: In vivo demonstration of clinical feasibility. *Ultrasound Med. Biol.* **28**(2), 227–235 (2002).

66. J. Bercoff, M. Tanter, and M. Fink, Sonic boom in soft materials: The elastic Cerenkov effect. *Appl. Phys. Lett.* **84**(12), 2202–2204 (2004).

67. C. Kim, R.J. Zemp, and L.H.V. Wang, Intense acoustic bursts as a signal-enhancement mechanism in ultrasound-modulated optical tomography. *Opt. Lett.* **31**(16), 2423–2425 (2006).

68. R.J. Zemp, C. Kim, and L.H.V. Wang, Ultrasound-modulated optical tomography with intense acoustic bursts. *Appl. Opt.* **46**(10), 1615–1623 (2007).

69. E. Bossy, A.R. Funke, K. Daoudi, A.C. Boccara, M. Tanter, and M. Fink, Transient optoelastography in optically diffusive media. *Appl. Phys. Lett.* **90**(17), 174111 (2007).

70. K. Daoudi, A.C. Boccara, and E. Bossy, Detection and discrimination of optical absorption and shear stiffness at depth in tissue-mimicking phantoms by transient optoelastography. *Appl. Phys. Lett.* **94**(15), 154103 (2009).

71. H.J. Vanstaveren, C.J.M. Moes, J. Vanmarle, S.A. Prahl, and M.J.C. Vangemert, Light-scattering in intralipid-10-percent in the wavelength range of 400–1100 nm. *Appl. Opt.* **30**(31), 4507–4514 (1991).

72. J. Bercoff, M. Tanter, M. Muller, and M. Fink, The role of viscosity in the impulse diffraction field of elastic waves induced by the acoustic radiation force. *IEEE Trans. Ultrason. Ferroelectr. Freq. Control* **51**(11), 1523–1536 (2004).

73. R. Li, L.P. Song, D.S. Elson, and M.X. Tang, Parallel detection of amplitude-modulated, ultrasound-modulated optical signals. *Opt. Lett.* **35**(15), 2633–2635 (2010).

74. J. Honeysett, E. Stride, T. Leung, and University College London Group, Monte Carlo simulations of acousto-optics with microbubbles, in *Photons Plus Ultrasound: Imaging and Sensing 2010*, A.A. Oraevsky and L.V. Wang, eds., *Proc. SPIE* **7564** (2010).

75. Z. Yaqoob, D. Psaltis, M.S. Feld, and C. Yang, Optical phase conjugation for turbidity suppression in biological samples. *Nat. Photonics* **2**(2), 110–115 (2008).

76. I.M. Vellekoop and A.P. Mosk, Focusing coherent light through opaque strongly scattering media. *Opt. Lett.* **32**, 2309–2311 (2007).

77. X. Xu, H. Liu, and L.V. Wang, Time-reversed ultrasonically encoded optical focusing into scattering media. *Nat. Photonics* **5**, 154–157 (2011).

78. S.M. Popoff, G. Lerosey, M. Fink, A.C. Boccara, and S. Gigan, Image transmission through an opaque material. *Nat. Commun.* **1**, Art. No. 81 (2010).

79. S.M. Popoff, G. Lerosey, R. Carminati, M. Fink, A.C. Boccara, and S. Gigan, Measuring the transmission matrix in optics: An approach to the study and control of light propagation in disordered media. *Phys. Rev. Lett.* **104**(10), Art. No. 100601 (2010).

21

Optoacoustic Tomography: From Fundamentals to Diagnostic Imaging of Breast Cancer

Alexander A. Oraevsky
TomoWave Laboratories, Inc.

21.1 Definition of Optoacoustic Tomography

Optoacoustic tomography (OAT) is a method of image acquisition and reconstruction based on time-resolved detection of acoustic pressure profiles induced in the tissue through absorption of optical pulses under irradiation conditions of temporal pressure confinement during optical energy deposition [1,2]. The phrase "irradiation conditions of temporal pressure confinement" means that optical energy (or other heat-generating energy) must be delivered to the tissue faster than resulting acoustic wave can propagate the distance in the tissue equal to the desirable spatial resolution, δ. For example, having a desirable resolution of optoacoustic images of $\delta = 15$ μm and the speed of sound propagation in the tissue of $v_s = 1.5$ μm/ns, one needs optical pulses shorter than $\tau_L < 10$ ns. Thus, utilization of short (nanosecond) optical pulses represents necessary (but not sufficient) condition to achieve desirable spatial (axial) resolution of OAT [3,4]. The sufficient conditions to obtain desirable spatial resolution also include requirement for the detectors of acoustic waves (transducers) to possess fast temporal response function of not worse than $t \leq \delta/v_s$. Satisfaction of irradiation conditions of temporal pressure confinement is also required for the optoacoustic signals to accurately resemble profiles of absorbed optical energy in the tissue [5,6]. Distribution of absorbed optical energy can be used to visualize and characterize quantitatively various tissue structures and their physiological functions based on variations in tissue optical properties. In order to reproduce tissue structure on optoacoustic images, the acoustic detectors must be capable of resolving not only rapid changes in optoacoustic signals associated with sharp edges and boundaries in tissues but also reproduce slow changes associated with smooth variation in optical properties within one type of tissue. In other words, acoustic detectors must be capable of detecting both high and low ultrasonic frequencies of acoustic pressure signals. These types of acoustic detectors are called ultrawideband acoustic transducers [7,8]. These transducers have relatively equal detection sensitivity over the entire ultrasonic range from 20 kHz to 20 MHz (and in some cases even higher up to 100 MHz) [5,8,9]. The ultrasonic detection bandwidth of acoustic transducers defines the limits of axial resolution. The lateral resolution of OAT, on the other hand, is defined by dimensions of each acoustic transducer, pitch between two neighboring transducers in the array (or distance between two measurement points in the scanning mode), and the total aperture and geometry of the transducer array (measurement surface) [9,10]. In order to acquire an accurate tomographic image, the object of interest should be surrounded by transducers, so that all detector positions form a closed surface. Otherwise, reconstruction will be made using incomplete set of data measurements, which is not quantitatively accurate [11]. Complete sets of temporary resolved optoacoustic data can be acquired using either 2D arrays of transducers or by 1D scanning of linear array of transducers or by 2D scanning of a single transducer [12–14].

In the following sections of this chapter, we will expand on every aspect given in the definition of OAT, including explanation of optoacoustic profiles, ultrawideband acoustic transducers, algorithms of optoacoustic image reconstruction, and medical applications of OAT. This chapter provides introductory and background information for students, scientists, engineers, and medical professionals interested in imaging methods employing light and ultrasound. OAT has been the fastest-growing field of biomedical imaging in the past decade. Limited volume of this chapter, however, does not allow for comprehensive theoretical treatment of optoacoustic phenomena in biological tissue or detailed description of all existing optoacoustic imaging systems. Therefore, while citing the most important works of others, technological examples of the optoacoustic imaging systems in this chapter will be limited to the systems developed in our group, and biomedical applications will be demonstrated based on our own research and the works of our collaborators.

21.2 History of Development

Theoretical and experimental optoacoustic studies of the 1970s and the early 1980s performed with nonbiological media created theoretical and experimental background for the development of biomedical optoacoustics [15]. The initial idea driving the progress in laser optoacoustics was the well-known exceptional sensitivity of piezoelectric detection [16]. Optoacoustic signal profiles were first studied with temporal resolution after the successful development of acoustic transducers with fast (nanosecond) response time [17]. The first proposed optoacoustic applications aimed at sensitive detection of lesions in biological tissue based on measurements of arrival time of acoustic signals with no attention to the information contained in the profile of optoacoustic signals [18]. Later it was realized that the optoacoustic method with temporal resolution could be applied for monitoring of the laser energy deposition in optically absorbing media during the ablation process [19,20]. The lack of theoretical basis, however, did not allow the researchers to get quantitative results at that time. It was a challenge to develop an opto-acoustic method suitable for applications in biological tissue due to its complex heterogeneous structure and optical properties determined by three parameters: absorption coefficient, scattering coefficient, and scattering anisotropy. A rapid progress in the area of biomedical optoacoustics was associated with understanding that under irradiation conditions of temporal pressure confinement, the profile of the laser-induced pressure transients accurately replicates the distribution of absorbed optical energy in the irradiated volume of the tissue [3,4]. In other words, under experimental conditions when laser energy is being deposited faster than propagation of acoustic wave through the volume of the tissue with character-istic dimensions of desirable spatial resolution, one can obtain quantitative information on tissue optical properties from time-resolved profiles of laser-induced pressure. It was then realized that time-resolved optoacoustic profile allows visualization of the distribution of absorbed optical energy in one, two, and three dimensions inside clear [21] and opaque highly scattering media, such as biological tissue [2–4].

The first patented thermoacoustic imaging technology was described by Bowen, but never practi-cally materialized and, therefore, was obscured for more than 15 years [22]. In the last decade of the twentieth century, the first imaging systems based on optical generation of acoustic waves in biological tissues were practically implemented [23–26]. With understanding that red and near-infrared (NIR) wavelength range represents the most optimal energy of optical photons for generation of high image contrast and simultaneously deep penetration of the optical illumination into biological tissue, the hybrid system that combined the most compelling features of optical and acoustic imaging was called laser optoacoustic imaging system (LOIS) [2,23–26]. Simultaneously, the term photoacoustic tomog-raphy was introduced, which broadens the term OAT from optical photons to photons with higher or lower electromagnetic energy [27,28]. Thermal pulses of microwave radiation have also been used for generation of acoustic transients in breast tissue as an alternative to optical energy [28]. This type of imaging technology called thermoacoustic computed tomography has advantage of deeper penetration of excitation energy in the tissue at the price of lower tissue contrast [29–31].

In the late 1990s, optoacoustic imaging experiments were performed in live biological (and human) tissues in vivo with high resolution [25,28,32–38], which stimulated substantial interest to this technol-ogy from the international communities of biomedical optics and ultrasonics. After the turn of the twenty-first century, optoacoustic/photoacoustic imaging grew exponentially and emerged as a new method of biomedical imaging being successfully utilized for tomographic visualization of deep tissue with submillimeter resolution [13,39,40] and for scanning of superficial tissue layers and lesions with microscopic resolution [41–43]. The most useful niche for biomedical optoacoustic imaging is to provide physician with distributions of functional and molecular constituents in the depth of live tissue. The short-term goal of the present development is to achieve high-resolution visualization of human tis-sue enabling high-contrast differentiation of normal and abnormal functional conditions. This chapter reviews contributions of our group to this goal using the systems of OAT, which allow real-time 2D and rapid 3D visualization of large tissue volumes. Due to the limited volume of this chapter, we only give references to the most important works of other groups toward the same goal. The long-term aim is to achieve quantitative optoacoustic imaging of the optical absorption coefficient in the volume of the tissue and apply laser spectroscopy methods to identify and measure concentrations of molecular con-stituents associated with specific health condition or disease. The works toward this challenging long-term goal are ongoing [43–50], but it may take another decade to develop commercially viable solutions.

21.3 Optoacoustic Transducers

A distinct feature of optoacoustic signals is their wide spectral band of ultrasonic frequencies [51]. A typical transient pulse of acoustic pressure, generated in the tissue by a 5–10 ns pulse from a Q-switched laser, contains a wide frequency band of 0–100 MHz. While very low frequencies are typically filtered for the purpose of better visualization of smaller objects and very high frequencies are strongly attenuated by tissues, the optoacoustic signals detected at the tissue surface have the ultrasonic frequency spectrum from about 100 kHz to about 10 MHz. An ultrasonic transducer with equally high sensitivity within such an ultrawideband can enable quantitatively accurate detection of optoacoustic signals. However, the majority of commercial ultrasonic transducers and array developed for medical ultrasound possess relatively narrow band (50%–80% of the central frequency) as a compromise between their capabilities to transmit and simultaneously detect ultrasonic pulses [52]; the ultimate optoacoustic transducer with the bandwidth of close to 200% of the central frequency is yet to be developed.

Optical detectors utilizing interferometric techniques [43,53–55], oblique-incidence reflectance [56], microring resonators [57], fiber-optic lines [58,59], and laser beam deflection [60,61] can also be applied to detect ultrawideband optoacoustic signals. In addition to ultrawideband sensitivity, there are three main advantages of optical detection: (1) possibility for remote (noncontact) optoacoustic detection; (2) small finite size of the virtual detectors enabled by the tightly focused laser beam, which in turn yields high lateral resolution; and (3) possibility of avoiding acoustic diffraction and wavefront distortion in the handheld probes operating in the backward mode [62]. On the other hand, selection of the optoacoustic detection method for deep tissue imaging is dominated by one major parameter—sensitivity or noise-effective pressure (NEP). The NEP of the most sensitive modern optical methods is ~100 Pa by the order of magnitude, and the noise level increases significantly in the range of acoustic frequencies greater than 1 MHz [8]. Therefore, piezoelectric transducers represent ultrasonic detectors of choice especially when low thermal noise and sensitive detection is required [8]. Low acoustic impedance closely matching that of the tissue and ability to operate in wide ultrasonic frequency band are the advantages of optoacoustic detectors made from polyvinylidene difluoride (PVDF) polymers and copolymers [8]. On the other hand, piezoelectric transducers have their own trade-offs and limitations. One major issue with piezoelectric materials is associated with significant reduction of their electrical capacitance with decrease of density, so that materials with acoustic impedance matching that of water and biological tissue have very low electrical capacitance when made small [63]. In spite of this difficulty, we have the capability to design optoacoustic imaging systems with NEP ~ 1 Pa and achieve the highest-contrast optoacoustic imaging at maximum depths ≥ 60 mm [8,26,64]. Piezoelectric polymers (such as PVDF homopolymer and a wide range of copolymers) are the materials of choice for ultrasonic transducers with a large area of elements (>0.25 cm^2), 1–3 composite materials based on single-crystal piezoelectric relaxors are the materials of choice for transducer elements with the active area of >1 mm^2, and design of endoscopic and intravascular systems with very small elements requires pure piezoceramics or composites with high density of piezoceramics. Piezoelectric composite transducers optimized as detectors can be made sufficiently sensitive within an ultrawideband approaching 150%–180%, especially using multilayer assembly techniques [65]. Industrial fabrication of such transducers is not available yet but remains critically important for the development of clinical OAT systems for applications that require quantitative measurement of the optical absorption coefficient throughout the volume of diagnostic interest.

21.4 Laser Generation of Optoacoustic Transients

The generation of acoustic waves by the consecutive transformation of optical energy into heat and then to mechanical stress is referred to as the optothermal mechanism of pressure generation [15]. Short laser pulses allow for the most efficient generation of the thermal pressure [3,4]. Absorption of laser radiation in a medium followed by a fast nonradiative relaxation of the excited states converts the laser energy into heat. Subsequently, thermal expansion of the tissue heated instantly (or more precisely, under conditions of temporal pressure confinement within the voxel to be resolved in the optically illuminated tissue) causes a pressure rise, ΔP [3,4,51]:

$$\Delta P = \frac{1}{\gamma}\frac{\Delta V}{V} = \frac{1}{\gamma}\beta\Delta T = \frac{1}{\gamma}\frac{\beta E_a}{\rho C_V} = \frac{\beta c_0^2}{C_p}\mu_a\,F = \Gamma(z)\,\mu_a(z)\,F(z), \tag{21.1}$$

where γ (Pa^{-1}) is the thermodynamic coefficient of isothermal compressibility (4.59×10^{-5} bar^{-1} for water)

$$\gamma = \frac{1}{\rho c_0^2} \frac{C_p}{C_V}, \qquad (21.2)$$

where

c_0 (m/s) is the sound velocity in the tissue

ΔV (cm³) is the volume increase caused by the thermal expansion

V is the laser-irradiated volume initially at room temperature

ρ (g/cm³) is the density of a medium

C_p (J/gK) is the heat capacity at constant pressure

C_V is the heat capacity at constant volume

The pressure increase is proportional to the thermal coefficient of volume expansion, β (K⁻¹), of the given medium, and the absorbed energy density, E_a (J/cm³), which in turn equals the product of the laser fluence, $F(z)$ (J/cm²), and the absorption coefficient of the tissue, μ_a (cm⁻¹). Pressure measured in (J/cm³) can be equally expressed in MPa or decabar (see SI and CGS units).

Equation 21.1 is strictly valid only in the case when the heating process is much faster than the medium expansion to dimensions of desirable resolution and conditions of temporal pressure confinement are satisfied. In cases where laser pulse does not satisfy the conditions of temporal pressure confinement, optoacoustic imaging will lose both sensitivity and resolution.

The expression $(\beta c_0^2 / C_p)$ in Equation 21.1 represents thermoacoustic efficiency, often called as the Grüneisen parameter, Γ, which equals 0.1 for water and aqueous solutions at room temperature, $T = 20°C$. The Grüneisen parameter is a dimensionless, temperature-dependent factor proportional to the fraction of thermal energy converted into mechanical stress. For liquid water with temperature range between 4°C and 100°C, Γ can be expressed with the following empirical formula [51]:

$$\beta(T) = -0.033 + 0.007T - 0.0000236T^2, \qquad (21.3)$$

where temperature, T, is measured in degrees Celsius.

For blood at room temperature, physiological temperature, Γ, is about 10%–30% higher than that in water and dependent on blood physiological properties [66]. To compare, $\Gamma = 0.25$–0.4 for fats, lipids, and oils, the most efficient biological media for generation of optoacoustic pressure (data from Refs. [67–69]).

21.5 Optoacoustic Profiles and Detection Geometry

21.5.1 Modes of Optoacoustic Detection

In contrast to majority of scanning optoacoustic imaging techniques where the image information is obtained through direct measurements of the signal amplitude from a given voxel, OAT is based on time-resolved measurements and analysis of the optoacoustic signal profiles. The optoacoustic profiles generated under irradiation conditions of temporal pressure confinement replicate axial profiles of the absorbed optical energy (where the axis extends into the depth of the tissue orthogonally from the center of the optoacoustic transducer). Usually irradiation of the tissue in OAT is performed through an optically and acoustically transparent medium (optoacoustic coupling medium) designed to provide effective coupling of the incident light from the laser source into the tissue and the resulting ultrasonic waves from the tissue into the acoustic detector.

The pulsed laser heating of the absorbing tissue with a wide beam of optical energy results in generation of an ultrasonic transient wave being launched in all directions: forward, into the volume of irradiated medium; backward, into the transparent medium; and orthogonally to the laser beam.

The amplitude and the temporal profile of the optoacoustic signals depends on the position of ultrasonic transducers relative to the irradiated tissue surface, area of the surface visible by the transducer, and also the ratio of acoustic impedances of the absorbing and transparent media [4,10,51]. There are three possible modes of the optoacoustic imaging as depicted schematically in Figure 21.1a, b, and c. Depending on the location of the laser illumination relative to ultrasonic detection, the three optoacoustic modes are known as *forward* [4,70], *backward* [62], and *orthogonal* [63]. These three imaging modes allow certain flexibility for in vivo and in vitro measurements with OAT. Each detection mode has its advantages and drawbacks. In the backward mode, the optoacoustic transient, propagated backward in the direction opposite to incident laser beam, is detected at the site of laser irradiation (Figure 21.1a). This is the most convenient and frequently used mode of imaging, since typically only one surface of skin or hollow organ is available for measurements. Different designs of optoacoustic imaging systems operating in the backward mode permit tissue illumination either through a hole in the single focused transducer [5,36], through a prism transparent to light but 100% reflecting for acoustic waves [37,71], or through delivering light on the side (around) ultrasonic transducer or array [40,41,50]. The main concern of the backward mode is that significant optical fluence and acoustic energy generated in the skin enter back the array of detectors overwhelming useful optoacoustic signals. In the forward detection mode, the optoacoustic signal propagated forward along the laser beam into the depth of absorbing medium is detected at the rear surface of the irradiated medium (Figure 21.1b). This would be a desirable geometry if two skin surfaces opposite each other are available at the volume of the tissue under examination. The detection of laser-induced transient pressure at the

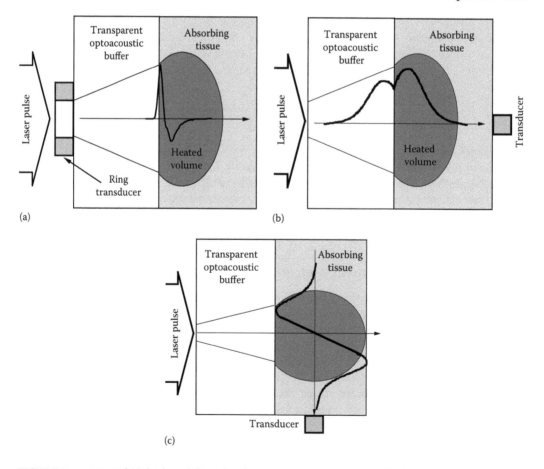

FIGURE 21.1   Forward (a), backward (b), and orthogonal (c) modes of optoacoustic signal detection.

opposite side from the irradiated surface makes the design of the ultrasonic detector much simpler. The third mode of optoacoustic imaging utilizes optical illumination orthogonally to the direction of the optoacoustic signal detection (Figure 21.1c). The mode is free of artifacts associated with the illuminated surface, and thus, it is the most desirable mode for volumetric imaging. The forward and backward modes enable measurements of both optical and acoustic absorption and scattering coefficients of the tissue over a wide range of optical and ultrasonic wavelength/frequency ranges. The orthogonal mode is the most appropriate to image tissue structures based on variations of the optical absorption and minimize influence of the spatial distribution of the optical fluence [72].

21.5.2 One-Dimensional Optoacoustic Profiles

21.5.2.1 Depth Profiles in Plane-Wave Geometry

The optoacoustic profile generated in absorbing tissue, propagated through this tissue to the acoustic detector, and detected with temporal resolution is well established and quantitatively investigated theoretically and experimentally [51]. Figure 21.2a and b shows typical optoacoustic profiles detected in forward (a) and backward (b) mode geometries. The temporal profiles of the detected optoacoustic (pressure) signals can be presented as a solution

$$p^{tr}\left(\tau^{tr}=t+\frac{z}{c_0^{tr}}\right)=T_{ac}\frac{c_0^2\beta}{2c_p}\int_0^{+\infty}\left(\tau^{tr}-\theta\right)Q\left(c_0\theta\right)d\theta \tag{21.4}$$

$$p'\left(\tau=t-\frac{z}{c_0}\right)=T_{ac}\frac{c_0^2\beta}{2c_p}\int_0^{+\infty}\left(\tau^{tr}-\theta\right)Q^{tr}\left(-c_0\theta\right)d\theta \tag{21.5}$$

of the nonstationary thermal wave equation [15]:

$$\frac{\partial^2\rho'}{\partial t^2}-c_0^2\,\Delta p'=\rho c_0^2\beta\frac{\partial^2 T'}{\partial t^2}. \tag{21.6}$$

Here, we used the following terms: c_0, c_0^{tr} is the speed of sound in the tissue and in transparent optoacoustic buffer, β is the thermal expansion coefficient for the tissue, and $Q(z)$ and $Q^{tr}(z)$ represent distributions of absorbed optical (thermal) energy in the tissue and in the zone of negative z that also accounts for reflection of acoustic waves from the boundary:

$$Q=\mu_a F(z), \quad Q^{tr}\left(z\right)=\begin{cases}Q(z), & z>0;\\ R_{ac}Q(-z), & z<0.\end{cases} \tag{21.7}$$

Coefficients of acoustic transmission and reflection from the boundary are defined by the acoustic impedances of the transparent buffer, $z_b = \rho^b c_0^b$, and the absorbing tissue, $z_t = \rho^t c_0^t$, as follows:

$$T_{ac}=\frac{2z_b}{z_b+z_t}, \quad R_{ac}=\frac{z_b-z_t}{z_b+z_t}, \tag{21.8}$$

where
  ρ^b, ρ^t (g/m³) are the densities
  c_0^b, c_0^t (m/s) are the velocities of ultrasound waves of the buffer and the tissue

Therefore, the reflected profile can either be in phase with the original profile ($z_b > z_t$, as at quartz–tissue boundary) or in contraphase with the original profile ($z_b < z_t$, as at air–tissue boundary). The optoacoustic

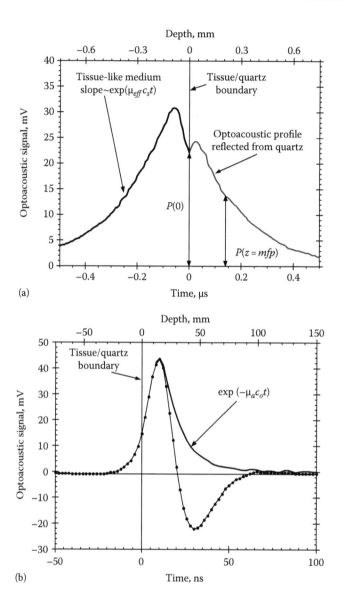

FIGURE 21.2 Optoacoustic profile generated in optically absorbing and scattering medium tissue-like medium covered by an optically transparent window with significantly higher acoustic impedance (quartz). (a) Optoacoustic profile detected in the forward mode and (b) optoacoustic profile detected in the backward mode and the same profile corrected for acoustic diffraction. The detection bandwidth of acoustic transducer was approximately 80 MHz.

profile in the forward mode is described by convolution of the spatial distribution of laser-induced acoustic sources and the temporal shape of the laser pulse [15,51]. Therefore, for sufficiently short laser pulses, $\mu_{eff} c_0 \tau_L \ll 1$ (where μ_{eff} is the effective optical attenuation in the tissue and $\tau_L = \int_{-\infty}^{+\infty} f(t)dt$ is the laser pulse duration), the optoacoustic profiles replicate the distribution profile of the absorbed laser energy:

$$p^{tr}\left(\tau^{tr} = t + \frac{z}{c_0^{tr}}\right) = \begin{cases} 0, & \tau^{tr} < 0; \\ \\ T_{ac} \dfrac{c_0^2 \beta \tau_L}{2c_p} Q\left(c_0 \tau^{tr}\right), & \tau^{tr} > 0; \end{cases} \tag{21.9}$$

$$p\left(\tau = t - \frac{z}{c_0}\right) = \begin{cases} \dfrac{c_0^2 \beta \tau_L}{2 c_p} Q(-c_0 \tau), & \tau < 0; \\[3mm] R_{ac} \dfrac{c_0^2 \beta \tau_L}{2 c_p} Q(c_0 \tau), & \tau > 0. \end{cases} \tag{21.10}$$

The temporal profile of optoacoustic transients generated under irradiation conditions of temporal pressure confinement and detected in the forward mode without signal distortion replicates the profile of spatial distribution of absorbed optical energy (Figure 21.2a). The signals from acoustic sources generated by laser pulses in the depth of the tissue are the first to arrive to a transducer (detector) placed at the rear surface of the tissue. These signals from the depth of the tissue are followed by signals from sources located closer to the irradiated surface. A plane-wave optoacoustic profile generated in the tissue by a wide laser beam propagates in two opposite directions. Therefore, the temporal profile consists of two components moving with the speed of sound: the rising (original) spatial profile followed by a falling profile that corresponds to the reflection from the tissue/quartz boundary with acoustic reflection coefficient, *Rac*. Depending on the sign of *Rac*, the falling slope could be either compressive ($z_b > z_t$, as in the case of rigid quartz/tissue) or tensile ($z_b < z_t$, as in the case of free air/tissue) boundary. The transition zone at the boundary has duration equal to that of the laser pulse.

In case of backward detection mode (see Figure 21.2b), the profile consists of a sharp rising front at $\tau_{tr} = 0$ with the duration of the integrated laser pulse, followed by an exponential trailing slope. The trailing slope resembles the profile of absorbed optical energy in the tissue, which is determined by the optical attenuation coefficient and the speed of sound. This optoacoustic profile can be represented either by a compression transient wave (when $\beta > 0$, like in the tissue at room temperature) or by a tensile transient wave (when $\beta < 0$, like in water in the temperature range of 0°C–4°C). However, due to acoustic diffraction in the quartz optoacoustic buffer, the signal detected in the backward mode is described by the bipolar derivative of the original laser-induced optoacoustic profile, as shown in Figure 21.2b.

Finite duration of laser pulses leads to widening of all components of the optoacoustic profile. Initially, the pulse duration extends central transition zone of the optoacoustic transients detected in the forward mode and the front of the optoacoustic profile detected in the backward mode. Further increase in the pulse duration results in optoacoustic profile that does not resemble the distribution of laser-induced acoustic sources and, instead, replicated the shape of the laser pulse in most cases. The optoacoustic profile detected in the forward mode from the tissue having free irradiated surface (free acoustic boundary produced between tissue and air) represents the exception, when the optoacoustic profile follows derivative of the laser pulse [15,51].

21.5.2.2 Optoacoustic Profile from Absorbing Sphere

Spherical objects in tissues irradiated with NIR light may be considered optically semitransparent, which means that the effective optical penetration depth in tissues is greater than the linear dimensions (radius, *a*) of the absorbing objects (such as tumors). Furthermore, when $\mu_{eff} \ll 1/a$, distribution of optical energy inside spherical objects may be considered homogeneous.

For the sake of simplicity, let us consider a spherical object in tissues with optical properties dominated by the optical absorption (scattering is apparent but may be neglected). In the spherical coordinates with the center coinciding with the center of the object, the radial distribution of thermal energy in this object and around could be approximated with the following function:

$$Q(r) = \begin{cases} \mu_\alpha F_0\, ch(\mu_\alpha r)/ch(\mu_\alpha r), & 0 \le r \le a; \\[2mm] 0, & a < r, \end{cases} \tag{21.11}$$

where F_0 is the laser fluence at the surface of the absorbing sphere, which depends on the effective optical attenuation by absorption and scattering in tissues:

$$F_o = F_0 \exp(-\mu_{eff} z). \tag{21.12}$$

The transient acoustic wave resulting from laser heating of the spherical object will have spherical symmetry and can be given by the following equation:

$$\frac{\partial^2 (rp')}{\partial t^2} - c_0^2 \frac{\partial^2 (rp')}{\partial r^2} = \frac{c_0^2 \beta}{c_p} r Q(r) \frac{df}{dt} \tag{21.13}$$

with the boundary condition associated with the finite pressure in the center of the sphere:

$$\left. (rp') \right|_{r=0} = 0. \tag{21.14}$$

The reflection of the acoustic wave from the center of the sphere occurs in the contraphase. The system of Equations 21.13 and 21.14 is similar to the planar case with free (air/tissue) boundary, Equation 21.6. Therefore, solution (21.5) with reflection coefficient, $R_{ac} = -1$, can be employed for the following case:

$$p'\left(\tau = t - \frac{r}{c_0}\right) = \frac{\mu_\alpha F_0 c_0^2 \beta}{2rC_p} \int_{-a/c_0}^{+a/c_0} f(\tau-\theta)(-c_0\theta)\frac{ch(\mu_\alpha c_0\theta)}{ch(\mu_\alpha a)} d\theta. \tag{21.15}$$

Like in the case of planar acoustic waves, the optoacoustic profile of a spherical acoustic wave can be expressed as the convolution of the temporal profile of laser pulse with the depth profile of the absorbed optical energy modified for contraphase reflection of acoustic wave from the center of the sphere. Under irradiation conditions of temporal pressure confinement (short laser pulses) so that $\mu_\alpha c_0 \tau_L \ll 1$ and for relatively large dimensions of the absorbing sphere, $c_0 \tau_L \ll a$, the optoacoustic profile replicates that of the absorbed (thermal) energy distribution:

$$p'\left(\tau = t - \frac{r}{c_0}\right) = \frac{\mu_\alpha F_0 c_0^2 \beta}{2rc_p} \begin{cases} (-c_0\tau)ch(\mu_\alpha c_0\tau)/ch(\mu_\alpha c_0\tau), & |\tau| < a/c_0; \\ 0, & |\tau| > a/c_0. \end{cases} \tag{21.16}$$

The optoacoustic profile for relatively weakly absorbing objects, $\mu_\alpha a < 1$, possesses the so-called N-shape with duration, $\tau_N = 2a/c_0$, associated with sound propagation through the object. The optoacoustic profile detected from a strongly absorbing object, $\mu_\alpha a \gg 1$, can be described with two short pulses, where a tensile pulse follows the leading compression pulse with a delay equal to the time of sound propagation through the object.

Figure 21.3 shows a typical experimentally measured optoacoustic profile detected in the forward mode from absorbing spheres inside bulk tissue-like phantom irradiated with NIR laser pulses. A wide laser beam was used for illumination of this phantom, which resulted in planar acoustic wave with profile resembling depth (axial) distribution of the absorbed optical energy. On the background of the main exponential trend due to the effective optical attenuation, this optoacoustic profile contains two N-shaped wavelets resulted from spherical acoustic waves from the two absorbing spheres. Since both spheres were positioned on one axis with the irradiation–detection system, the pressure profile in Figure 21.3 includes signals simultaneously recorded from both spheres. These phantom studies demonstrated that the accuracy of localization and the accuracy of *tumor* dimension measurements could be better than 0.5 mm.

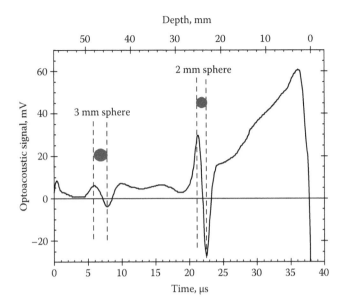

FIGURE 21.3 Laser-induced optoacoustic profile measured with a wideband acoustic transducer along the axis with two gel spheres of 2 and 3 mm in diameter colored with hemoglobin of blood. Two N-shaped signals are shown. The signal at $t = 0$ representing the transducer response to direct illumination was used for calibration of the timescale. Optical attenuation of the bulk phantom was $\mu_{eff} = 1.4$ cm^{-1}.

In case of microscopic absorbing objects in the tissue $(c_0\tau_L \gg a)$, one can transform Equation 21.15 into the following expression for the optoacoustic profile that replicates the derivative of the laser pulse:

$$p'\left(\tau = t - \frac{r}{c_0}\right) = \frac{\beta F_0 4\pi a^2}{4\pi r c_p}\left[th(\mu_\alpha a) - \frac{2(\mu_\alpha a - th(\mu_\alpha a))}{(\mu_\alpha a)^2}\right]\frac{df}{d\tau}. \tag{21.17}$$

If small (microscopic) structures in the tissue also possess relatively small optical absorbance, that is, $\mu_a a \ll 1$, then optoacoustic amplitude linearly increases with the absorption coefficient:

$$p'\left(\tau = t - \frac{r}{c_0}\right) = \frac{\beta I_s 4\pi a^2}{4\pi r c_p}\frac{\mu_\alpha a}{3}\frac{df}{d\tau}. \tag{21.18}$$

If those microspheres possess strong absorption, then the optoacoustic amplitude saturates:

$$p'\left(\tau = t - \frac{r}{c_0}\right) = \frac{\beta I_s 4\pi a^2}{4\pi r c_p}\frac{df}{d\tau}. \tag{21.19}$$

This type of behavior is explained by the fact that optoacoustic signal amplitude is determined by the total absorbed optical energy.

21.5.3 Signal Distortion upon Propagation

The optoacoustic profile can be altered in the course of propagation to the transducer through the tissue, coupling medium, and optoacoustic buffers. The two major phenomena that contribute to the distortion of the optoacoustic profile are acoustic attenuation and diffraction [5,15]. Roughness of the irradiated tissue surface also distorts propagating signals, especially their high-frequency components [8,9]; however, acoustic coupling medium may alleviate those distortions.

The expressions for planar (Equations 21.3 and 21.4) and spherical (Equation 21.15) optoacoustic profiles did not include the acoustic diffraction. On the other hand, acoustic diffraction is the most prominent phenomenon in deep tissue OAT, even when ideal detectors are used and the medium under investigation decreases the amplitude but does not noticeably distort the signal profile due to acoustic attenuation (such is true for ultrasonic frequencies below 10 MHz).

Based on expression 21.18, one can describe the optoacoustic profile, in cases which include the acoustic diffraction:

$$p'(t,\mathbf{r}) = \frac{\beta}{4\pi c_p} \frac{\partial}{\partial t} \int \frac{Q(\mathbf{r}')}{|\mathbf{r}-\mathbf{r}'|} f\left(t - c_0^{-1}|\mathbf{r}-\mathbf{r}'|\right) dV', \tag{21.20}$$

which considers the divergent acoustic wave only outside the volume occupied with laser-induced acoustic sources, $Q(r)$. Solution 21.20 represents the main expression for OAT. The goal of OAT is to invert expression 21.20 in order to image the spatial distribution of the acoustic sources, $Q(r)$.

The acoustic diffraction of the optoacoustic profiles can be described with the following parabolic equation [15,76]:

$$\frac{\partial^2 p'}{\partial \tau \partial z} = \frac{c_0}{2} \Delta_\perp p', \tag{21.21}$$

where
$\Delta_\perp$ is the Laplacian in the transversal coordinates $\{x,y\}$
z is the depth coordinate

The boundary conditions for Equation 21.21 in case of wide laser beams (commonly used in OAT) can be taken in the form of solutions (21.4) and (21.5) obtained upon consideration of planar acoustic waves.

Since optical illumination usually has Gaussian cross-sectional profile, the first approximation for the distribution of laser-induced acoustic sources in the plane perpendicular to the axis of optical illumination may also be taken as Gaussian:

$$p'(z = 0, \tau, \mathbf{r}_\perp) = p_0(\tau) \exp\left(\frac{-\mathbf{r}_\perp^2}{a_0^2}\right), \tag{21.22}$$

where $p_0(\tau)$ is the temporal profile of the optoacoustic signal at the irradiated tissue surface.

It is specific for optoacoustic signals to contain an ultrawide range of ultrasonic frequencies. The effective length, L_D, of the acoustic diffraction depends on the ultrasonic frequency (acoustic wavelength). The acoustic beam cross section, πa_0^2, doubles after propagation of a distance equal to the effective diffraction length:

$$L_D = \frac{\pi a_0^2}{\lambda_{ac}} = \frac{a_0^2 \omega_{ac}}{c_0}, \tag{21.23}$$

where λ_{ac} is the wavelength of the acoustic wave with ultrasonic frequency, ω_{ac} [76,77]. Therefore, different spectral components of the optoacoustic profiles undergo different degrees of acoustic diffraction;

the lower ultrasonic frequencies contribute the most alteration in the optoacoustic profile. The higher frequencies undergo minimal acoustic diffraction, thus propagating mainly along the axis perpendicular to the acoustic front. Considering the importance of the effective diffraction length as a function of ultrasound frequency, the solution for the system of Equations 21.21 and 21.22 can be found in the spectral domain:

$$p'\left(z,\tau=t-\frac{z}{c_0},\mathbf{r}_\perp\right)=\int_{-\infty}^{\infty}\exp\left(-i\omega(\tau-t)-\frac{\mathbf{r}_\perp^2}{a_0^2}\frac{\omega}{\omega+i(2c_0z/a_0^2)}\right)\left(\omega+i\frac{2c_0z}{a_0^2}\right)^{-1}\omega d\omega.\qquad(21.24)$$

Since high ultrasonic frequencies concentrate near the axis of the acoustic beam, the highest resolution in OAT can be obtained by detecting optoacoustic profiles propagating along the axis of the laser beam. The optoacoustic profile at the axis $r_\perp=0$ can be obtained from Equation 21.24 and expressed as

$$p'(z,\tau,\mathbf{r}_\perp=0)=p_0(\tau)-\int_{-\infty}^{\tau}\omega_D\exp(-\omega_D(\tau-t))p_0(t)dt,\qquad(21.25)$$

where $\omega_D=2c_0z/a_0^2$ is the characteristic frequency of acoustic diffraction defined as the frequency for which the characteristic diffraction length is equal to the length of propagation, z. The first item in expression (21.24) replicates the optoacoustic profile at the irradiated tissue surface, and the second item describes the influence of the limited radial dimensions of the acoustic wave. In the far diffraction zone ($z \to \infty$), solution (21.24) can be simplified as

$$p'(z,\tau,\mathbf{r}_\perp=0)=\frac{a_0^2}{2c_0z}\frac{dp_0}{d\tau}.\qquad(21.26)$$

The effect of the acoustic diffraction is to produce derivative of the original optoacoustic profile in the far zone. The task of OAT is to employ optoacoustic profiles at the irradiated surface for image reconstruction. Thus, for the purposes of OAT, one needs to invert expression (21.25), which yields the following result:

$$p'(\tau,z=0,\mathbf{r}_\perp=0)=p'(\tau,z,\mathbf{r}_\perp=0)+\omega_D\int_{-\infty}^{\tau}p'(\vartheta,z,\mathbf{r}_\perp=0)d\vartheta.\qquad(21.27)$$

The acoustic diffraction is the most prominent in the backward detection mode where quartz acoustic buffer (with high acoustic impedance) is placed between the tissue and the transducer. The influence of acoustic diffraction can be compensated, and the original laser-induced profile can be reconstructed with a procedure that convolves detected optoacoustic profile and the reference profile detected from a highly absorbing medium (with $\mu_{eff}> \Delta f_{at}/c_0$, where Δf_{at} is the ultrasonic detection bandwidth of the acoustic transducer) [62]. The detected reference signal replicates the profile of the laser pulse, with Fourier spectrum altered by the signal transmission path and the detection system, which include all distortion factors including the acoustic diffraction, the acoustic attenuation, and the sensitivity response of the acoustic transducer.

21.5.4 Signal Distortion by the Detection System

Properties of the detection system (including pressure-sensitive transducer and electronics) contribute substantially to the distortion of the optoacoustic signals [73–75]. The ultrasonic transducer properties can be characterized in terms of their impulse response [76]. The impulse response of ultrasonic transducers depends on their electromechanical properties and geometrical dimensions [74,77]. The electromechanical impulse response (EIR) can be measured by placing the transducer surface orthogonally to the incident delta-pulse acoustic wave with well-characterized ultrawide ultrasonic frequency spectrum. Figure 21.4 shows EIR for a narrowband commercial ultrasound transducer (Figure 21.4a), an ultrawideband PVDF transducer (Figure 21.4b), and corresponding ultrasonic frequency spectra obtained by fast Fourier transform (FFT) of the temporal profiles (Figure 21.4c). While the narrowband transducer distorts the incident delta pulse resulting in long ringing reverberations, the ultrawideband transducer having approximately constant sensitivity for a wide range of ultrasonic frequencies from 0 to about 15 MHz accurately reproduces the incident delta pulse. The spatial impulse response (SIR) can be measured by varying the angle of incidence of the acoustic wave to the transducer aperture [74]. SIR can be expressed as a function $h(r_0,t)$ describing the transducer response to a delta pressure pulse radiated from the point source, M, at position, r_0 (see diagram Figure 21.4d):

$$h(r_0,t) = \int_\sigma \frac{\delta(t - t' - |r_0 - r'|/c_0)}{2\pi|r_0 - r'|} dS'. \tag{21.28}$$

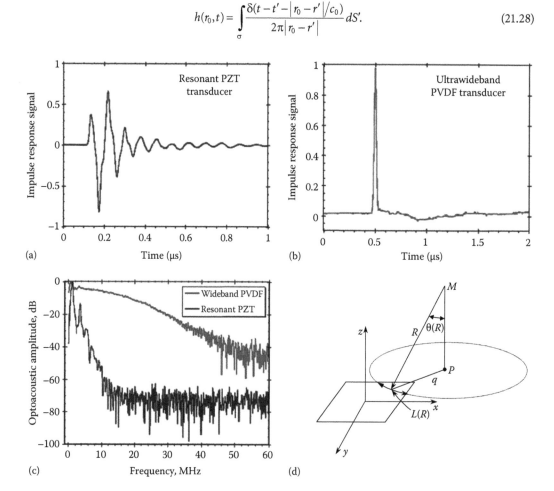

(a)

(b)

(c)

(d)

FIGURE 21.4 Temporal profiles of the EIRs of resonant (a) and ultrawideband (b) ultrasonic transducers and corresponding ultrasonic frequency spectra (c) calculated using Fourier transfer. Geometry for determining the SIR for the rectangular receiving transducer (d), where the point source is located at the position, M, having coordinate (x, y, z).

Transducers with finite dimensions can integrate optoacoustic signals incident at an angle significantly deviating from orthogonal and thereby reduce maximum resolution achievable with these detected signals. It is desirable, therefore, to use small point-like transducers in order to avoid filtering out high ultrasonic frequencies and to widen aperture (directivity) of detection for a more accurate tomography. Deconvolution of EIR and SIR from the measured signals should be incorporated either into signal processing or into the image reconstruction algorithm to obtain OAT images of greater mathematical and physical accuracy [75].

21.6 Raster Scan Optoacoustic Imaging vs. Optoacoustic Tomography

Two-dimensional optoacoustic images can be acquired either by using a stationary linear array of acoustic transducers or by scanning a single transducer along the tissue surface. Figure 21.5 depicts schematic diagrams of the two image acquisition modes. One or the other mode may have advantages of faster image acquisition, sensitivity, and resolution for specific tissue geometry in biomedical applications. Stationary arrays of acoustic transducers allow real-time imaging deep inside the tissue within a large field of view and simplicity of no mechanical translation and/or rotation. On the other hand, any array has limited field of view equally accessed by all transducers. Therefore, transducer arrays yield their maximum lateral resolution when imaging large tissue volumes in the far zone of the detector, especially in human organs than can be surrounded by the array (such as breast). A single focused transducer (or a group of transducers) focused into a point (or a line) can directly detect signals from a single voxel (or a limited number of voxels) with efficiency equal to all voxels available through the scanning. This is an advantage of the scanning mode relative to tomography, which comes with a price of slower rate of image acquisition.

Figure 21.5a shows scanning of a single focused ultrasonic transducer along the skin surface for acquisition of 2D images of subsurface layers. Laser pulses illuminate the tissue through a fiber-optic light delivery system. When the optical beam can be focused in the optically clear media and thin layers of biological tissue, the optoacoustic images can be obtained with optical resolution equal to the waist diameter of the focused laser beam [78]. Due to strong optical scattering in biological tissues, deep tissue imaging can only be obtained with acoustic resolution [79]. Confocal optoacoustic imaging where optical and acoustic focal points are designed to match within the tissue produces higher contrast compared with optoacoustic imaging with wide beam optical illumination [36,37]. Scanning a focused transducer or focused array is the most frequently used in the backward mode of optoacoustic imaging, that is, with acoustic detection at the site of optical illumination. An acoustic detector can be focused within a bright optical field produced by a wide optical beam illuminating the tissue right under the transducer (see Figure 21.5a), or the acoustic detector can be focused within a dark optical field in the middle of the ring-shaped optical illumination or between two optical beams [80]. The former method provides better sensitivity for weakly absorbing objects with bright wide beam illumination; however, the optical fluence gradient into the depth of the tissue has to be compensated to normalize the contrast along the depth axis. The latter method provides better contrast to the dark background illuminated only by diffused light and relatively homogeneous scattered illumination throughout the depth of about 10 mm; however, low optical fluence of diffused light may be insufficient to image objects with lower optical absorption coefficient. In order to obtain 3D images in the scanning mode, focused transducers have to be translated in both horizontal and vertical directions, a scan taking typically a long time. The scanning time may be significantly reduced using ultrasonic transducers with very narrow directivity (i.e., sensitive to acoustic waves incident only orthogonally to the transducer). A very narrow angle of optoacoustic signal acceptance in these transducers permits utilization of the entire duration of the time-resolved signal for obtaining depth information without loss of lateral resolution [81].

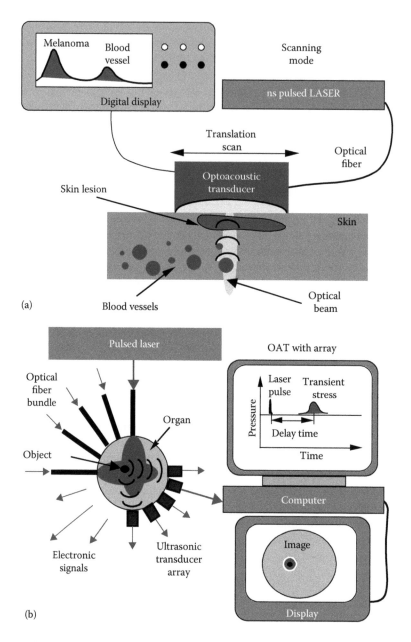

FIGURE 21.5 Schematic diagram of optoacoustic scanning mode (a) and tomography mode (b).

Figure 21.5b shows an array of acoustic transducers employed for deep tissue imaging in the forward mode. Optical pulses can be delivered to the tissue surface with one or more optical fibers as shown on the drawing of an organ (such as breast, arm, leg, or neck). As an alternative, a wide laser beam can be used to illuminate the entire surface skin opposite to the ultrasonic transducers. Objects of interest (such as tumors and blood vessels) having stronger optical absorption compared with surrounding tissue produce optoacoustic signals with amplitude detectable at significant depths of 5–7 cm. The optically generated acoustic waves propagate in the tissue in all directions as expanding spheres and can be detected with an array of ultrasonic transducers. The product of temporal width of the optoacoustic signal produced in an object and the speed of sound yields the object dimension in the direction of the axis between the object and the transducer (detector). The product of the speed of sound in the tissue and the delay time between the laser pulse and the transient pressure wave arrival at the transducer is equal to the distance between the object and the transducer. Linear or arc-shaped arrays of acoustic transducers can be used for 2D tomography. Flat linear probes have advantage of the better compliance with the skin surface, while arc-shaped probes provide better lateral resolution due to the larger angular aperture within the same physical dimensions as the flat linear probe.

21.7 Laser Optoacoustic Imaging System

21.7.1 System Components

LOIS was developed for OAT of deep tissue structures of large organs. LOIS combines the most compelling features of optical and ultrasound imaging systems, pronounced optical contrast, and high resolution of ultrawideband ultrasound detection, yielding a more sensitive imaging modality with excellent resolution throughout the large volume of the tissue. The hybrid of optical and acoustic technologies permit to overcome the problems of pure optical imaging associated with the loss of resolution and sensitivity due to strong light scattering and problems of pure ultrasound imaging associated with low-acoustic-impedance contrast in soft tissues and incapability to provide functional and molecular information.

The heart of LOIS is an array of ultrawideband acoustic transducers. One of the first LOIS prototypes developed in 1998 had only 12 relatively wide piezoelectric elements in a short linear array, which provided a very limited spatial resolution [32]. Advances in OAT over the period of the past 15 years resulted in the design and development of more sophisticated 1D and 2D arrays with a larger number of piezoelectric transducers of smaller dimensions and shaped as an arc to improve spatial resolution [39,64,72,82]. Figure 21.6 shows photographs of the first prototypes of the ultrawideband ultrasonic arrays based on PVDF. From flat array with flat elements (Figure 21.6a) to arc-shaped arrays with flat elements (Figure 21.6b and c) to bifocal array with arc-shaped elements (Figure 21.6d), this was the progress that permitted gradual increase of the spatial resolution in LOIS systems. Artifact-free optoacoustic imaging requires that the piezoelectric element does not vibrate at its thickness-related resonance frequency after detecting an optoacoustic signal and the frequency band of ultrasonic detection in an ideal design should match the wide spectral band of ultrasonic frequencies present in the typical optoacoustic signals emitted by biological tissue structures (about 0.1–10 MHz). To achieve such ultrawideband matching in the ultrasonic transducer, PVDF films with thickness of 25–100 micron were optimal when combined with backing resin material having acoustic impedance similar to that of PVDF. This design was quite effective for mechanical matching and complete damping of reverberations even without front acoustic impedance matching layer. Being supersensitive, these arrays required good grounding for electromagnetic shielding. The front surface of the transducer arrays was covered by a thin aluminum film with its thickness optimized for the optimum compromise between ultrasound penetration and electric noise reduction. The entire housing was made from hypoechoic materials and optically reflective materials with low thermal expansion that allowed us to avoid artifacts associated with laser illumination of the transducer housing.

21.7.2 Sensitivity

Piezoelectric polymer materials, such a PVDF and especially copolymers, such as polyvinylidene fluoride trifluoroethylene (PVDF-TrFE), possess high sensitivity within a wide band of ultrasonic frequencies:

$$S = g_{33}d = (0.14 \div 0.38)\,\text{Vm/N} \times (52 \div 110)\,\mu\text{m} = (7.8 \div 41.8)\,\mu\text{V/Pa}, \tag{21.29}$$

where
   g_{33} is the piezoelectric voltage constant in the thickness direction for copolymer
   d is the thickness of the piezoelement

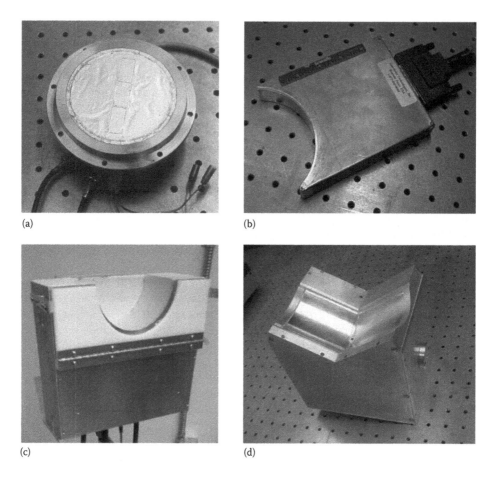

FIGURE 21.6 Photographs of arc-array transducers made of PVDF for OAT: flat array with 16 flat elements (a), arc-shaped arrays with 32 and 64 flat elements (b, c), and (d) bifocal array with 64 arc-shaped elements.

However, this theoretically maximum sensitivity is rarely achieved in practical implementations due to (1) the contribution of the electromechanical coupling coefficient and (2) the defects of bonding between the metal ground electrode of the piezoelectric film and front acoustic impedance matching layer, which give rise to acoustic energy losses at the boundary of the ultrasonic transducer. Furthermore, for satisfactory electromagnetic shielding of the transducer, the metal ground electrode must be relatively thick, resulting in additional losses of the optoacoustic signal at higher ultrasonic frequencies. When optimized for detection mode (without the need of emitter capability), these polymer transducers having relatively low acoustic impedance, ρc_s, can be effectively mechanically coupled to soft tissues for minimal signal losses. For example, for ultrasonic transducers made of PVDF, $\rho c_s = 1780 \text{ kg/m}^3 \times 2200 \text{ m/s} = 3.916 \times 10^6 \text{ kg/m}^2\text{s}$, which is only twice larger than that of soft tissue, $\rho c_s = 1.1 \text{ kg/m}^3 \times 1.5 \text{ km/s} = 1.65 \times 10^6 \text{ kg/m}^2\text{s}$.

Proper detection of the optoacoustic signal requires a wideband ultrasound transducer with a spectral band of sensitivity matching that of the detected signal. An optimum balance between ultrasonic frequency bandwidth (which decreases with increasing thickness of the piezoelement) and sensitivity (which increases with increasing thickness) was found for transducers made of PVDF copolymer having the thickness of the piezoelectric layer, $d = 52$–110 μm. Polymer films with smaller thickness (down to 9 μm) would be preferred for smaller-size transducers for OAT and higher-frequency transducers for optoacoustic microscopy.

Detection of the optoacoustic signal incident obliquely on a piezoelectric transducer with finite dimensions can alter its profile [9,74]. Therefore, an ideal piezoelectric element would have dimensions significantly smaller than the shortest detected acoustic wavelength, λ_{ac}. However, small dimensions yield a small value of electrical capacitance of the transducer piezoelement, C_{pe}, which can be found from the following formula:

$$C_{pe} = \frac{\varepsilon \varepsilon_0 A}{d}, \tag{21.30}$$

where

A is the surface area of the piezoelement
ε is the dielectric constant or permittivity of the transducer material
ε_0 is the electric constant of the vacuum ($\varepsilon_0 \approx 8.854 \times 10^{-12}$ F/m)

In order to avoid shunting effect of electronic circuitry, the capacitance of each transducer element should not be lowered to a level comparable with the stray capacitance of connecting wires and input capacitance of electronic preamplifier. The shunting effect can potentially be the source of significant loses of sensitivity in the detection system. Piezoceramic materials possess much higher relative dielectric permittivity ($\varepsilon/\varepsilon_0 \sim 1000 - 5000$) compared with PVDF type polymers ($\varepsilon/\varepsilon_0 \sim 7 - 13$). On the other hand, piezoceramics have very high mechanical resonance quality ($Q_m \sim 100 - 1000$), which makes it impossible to fabricate wideband ultrasonic transducers from pure ceramics. Therefore, for the optoacoustic system designs that require small-area ultrasonic transducers, one may prefer one to three composite materials made of a matrix of piezoelectric ceramic microcolumns filled with resin. It is the volume fraction ratio of ceramics to resin in the composite material that allows one to trade sensitivity and electrical capacitance for bandwidth and coupling efficiency. The integral under the curve of sensitivity as a function of ultrasonic frequency is constant for transducers made of a specific piezoelectric material. In order to compare performance of various piezoelectric materials in the design of ultrasonic and optoacoustic transducers, we introduce the term bandwidth-effective sensitivity [8]. Table 21.1 presents properties of piezoelectric polymer and ceramic materials, which can be used to construct composite optoacoustic transducers.

The signal-to-noise ratio (SNR) defines the detection efficiency of the acoustic transducer, which can be calculated as the absolute signal amplitude in volts divided to the NEP. NEP depends on the thermal noise in the piezoelectric element and can be found from the following expression [8]:

$$NEP = \frac{M f_{max}}{g_{33} c_l} \sqrt{\frac{kT_0}{C_{pe}}}, \tag{21.31}$$

where

f_{max} is the upper ultrasonic frequency of the transducer detection band
c_l is the longitudinal speed of sound in the piezoelectric element
kT_0 is the product of Boltzmann constant (1.38×10^{-23} J/K) and the ambient temperature (300 K)

The numerical coefficient, M, in the numerator depends on whether the transducer operates in open ($M = 4.6$) or short ($M = 6.5$) electrical circuit [8].

TABLE 21.1 Properties of Piezoelectric Materials Compiled from Technical Specification Sheets of Commercially Available Materials Most Suitable for Optoacoustic Imaging Systems

Material	c_0 (km/s)	ρ (kg/m³)	$\varepsilon/\varepsilon_0$	d_{33} (pC/N)	g_{33} (Vm/N)	k_t	Q_m
PVDF	1.4–2.2	1.5–1.8	6–12	13–22	0.14–0.33	0.14–0.2	10
P(VDF-TrFE)	2.4	1.88	7	32	0.38	0.3	3–15
PZT-5H	3.97	7.45	3400	595	0.02	0.55	65
PMN-PT [010] single crystal	3.1	8.2	3650	2000	0.043	0.6	33

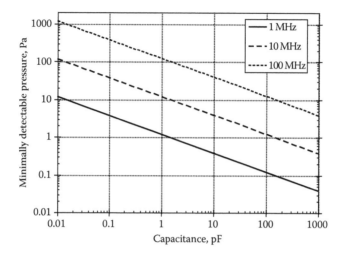

FIGURE 21.7 Acoustic pressure generated by thermal noise as a function of capacitance of acoustic transducer made of PVDF film and operating in the open circuit mode. Three curves for three values of upper ultrasonic frequency (1, 10, and 100 MHz) of the transducer detection band are shown.

Minimally detectable pressure is presented in Figure 21.7 as a function of the transducer capacitance, the main variable parameter for PVDF material of the piezoelectric element operating in the open circuit. This plot demonstrates that pressures in the range of 1 Pa can be detected with LOIS. The minimally detectable pressure of the ultrawideband ultrasonic transducer also depends on the electrical signal coupling into the electronic preamplifier. It is difficult to calculate all possible losses of acoustic energy and electromagnetic noises. Therefore, direct measurement of sensitivity for all transducers in array is of great importance. The experimental variability on the sensitivity between array elements is usually about 10%–15% and needs to be taken into account in the process of image reconstruction.

21.7.3 Spatial Resolution

The axial (depth) resolution, δ_{ax}, of the pulsed optoacoustic system operating under optical energy deposition conditions of temporal pressure confinement is directly defined by the detection bandwidth of ultrasonic transducers. The temporal response time of an ultrawideband acoustic transducer is defined as $1.5/f_{max}$, where f_{max} is the upper frequency limit of the piezoelectric element. The coefficient 1.5 accounts for the fact that for resolved detection of a sphere with diameter $2a_{min}$, one needs to record at least three data samples. According to the Sparrow criterion, two coherently emitting identical spherical acoustic sources with radius, a_{min}, will be detected as separate objects if the space between their centers equals or is greater than $\delta_{ax} = 2a_{min}$ [9,77]. Using this transducer for imaging in the tissue having speed of sound, c_0, one can obtain spatial resolution of

$$\delta_{ax} = 2a_{min} = 3\frac{c_0}{f_{max}}. \tag{21.32}$$

The upper frequency limit of ultrasonic detection band $f_{max}=c_l/2d$ is defined by the transducer thickness and the frequency bandwidth of the preamplifier employed. In LOIS design employing 110 μm thick PVDF film, the upper frequency limit was 4 MHz, which provided 1.1 mm axial (depth) resolution. Later designs of LOIS were fabricated using the PVDF copolymer with a thickness of 52 mm, and LOIS-3D for preclinical research in small animals employed ultrasonic transducers made of 1–3 composite of calcium-modified lead titanate (PTCa) in the poly(ether–ether–ketone) (PEEK) polymer matrix, giving a wider bandwidth of 8.5 MHz while preserving low frequencies. The resolution estimated using the Sparrow criterion is 0.5 mm. While the Sparrow criterion provided a very conservative estimate of the spatial resolution, experimental measurement of the full-width half-maximum (FWHM) cross section of a 100 mm thin hair on optoacoustic images showed 280 mm resolution for LOIS-3D (see Section 21.5 for details).

The lateral resolution of the optoacoustic system is determined by geometry of the array of ultrasonic transducers. The greater the aperture of the array (defined by its shape and the distance between the end elements) and the smaller the pitch between centers of individual elements, the better spatial resolution could be achieved [76,77]. The arc-shaped geometry of the transducer array provides enhanced lateral resolution, especially in the area near the focal center of the arc curvature. This geometry of the array is the most beneficial for imaging within circular field of view. In this area, the lateral resolution can be estimated as the width of synthetic directivity pattern produced by the entire aperture of the array of (see diagram in Figure 21.8)

$$\delta_l = \frac{1.22\lambda_{ac}}{2\,NA} = \frac{0.61\lambda_{ac}}{\sin\theta} \sim \frac{c_0\tau_{ac}}{r/R}, \tag{21.33}$$

where
  $\theta = \arcsin(r/R)$ is the angular aperture of the array
  R is the radius of the arc curvature
  r is the aperture radius
  $\tau_{ac} = 2a_{min}/c_0$ is the duration of acoustic pulse from the minimally detectable sphere

In case of detection of optoacoustic transients, the spatial pulse duration, $c_0\tau_{ac}$, should be employed as equivalent of the shortest detectable acoustic wavelength, λ_{ac}. Expression 21.33 is equivalent to the expression for a size of the waist of the focused transducer with the same configuration, obtained for the radiation of harmonic waves [9]. This formula works well as long as all transducers in the array make equal contributions to the formation of the synthetic aperture. Diffraction can reduce the sensitivity of some transducers when they receive the acoustic transients from the points located outside the central zone. The acoustic diffraction can, therefore, reduce the lateral resolution. The resolution depends on the position of the acoustic sources relative to the array. With the multielement arc-shaped arrays depicted in Figure 21.6b and c, lateral resolution of 0.25 mm can be obtained close to the focal area of the array. In the vicinity of the ultrasonic

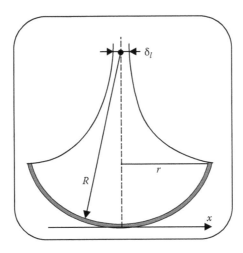

FIGURE 21.8 Schematic diagram of directivity of acoustic detection for an arc-shaped array of piezoelectric transducers.

transducers, the lateral resolution is $\delta_l \sim 1$ mm. For the arc-shaped transducer array described earlier, the ratio r/R equals approximately 0.87; therefore, expression 21.32 can be simplified as $\delta_l \approx 0.7\lambda_{ac}$. This estimation is valid for the monofrequency acoustic waves. In case of ultrawideband detection, it is necessary to take into account the detection frequency spectrum and to choose the value of the effective λ_{ac} correctly.

21.7.4 Signal Processing

Signal processing algorithm realized for LOIS operating in the forward mode is shown schematically in Figure 21.9a. Each signal detected by acoustic transducers in the array consists of the following three components: (1) useful component represented by an N-shaped pulse generated by an absorbing object (such as a blood vessel or a tumor), (2) thermoelectrical noise component represented by a high-frequency fluctuation, and (3) acoustic component represented by a sharp peak produced at the illuminated surface followed by a low-frequency smoothly ascending exponential slope produced by the attenuation of optical intensity inside the tissue. For demonstration purposes, we assumed that the cross section of the object of interest has a spherical shape with radius, a. The duration of the N-shaped pulse is defined by the time of sound propagation through the sphere. The delay in time of signal arrival depends on the object location relative to transducer. Therefore, position of the object and its dimensions can be determined from the optoacoustic signals detected on a surface surrounding the object of interest.

Before the signal could be used for image reconstruction, it is necessary to eliminate its high-frequency noise and low-frequency slope associated with the effective optical attenuation inside the tissue. The high-frequency thermal noise can be removed with a low-pass filter, which typically does not represent a challenge (thus not shown in Figure 21.9a). The removal of the smooth exponential trend in the optoacoustic profile is more difficult but could be achieved either (i) with wavelet filtering [83,84]; (ii) with band-pass numeric hyper-Gaussian filter, which performed better than other

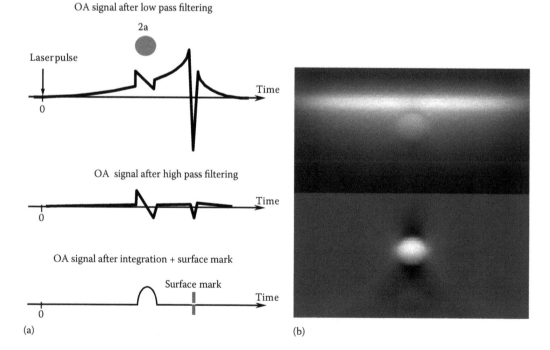

(a)   (b)

FIGURE 21.9 (a) Depiction of 3 steps of signal processing in LOIS, (b) 2D optoacoustic image of a sphere embedded in tissue showing low contrast due to optical fluence gradient (top image) and a filtered image showing enhanced contrast of the sphere after processing using principal component analysis (bottom image).

band-pass filtering of fast Fourier transformed signals [35]; or (iii) through the principal component analysis [85]. The cutoff frequency and the slope of the transfer function of filters (i) and (ii) could be varied conveniently by the imaging operator, so that the high-frequency thermoelectrical noise can be removed with the same filters as the low-frequency component. Removal of the optoacoustic slope associated with the effective optical attenuation in the tissue significantly increases contrast of the object of interest (see Figure 21.9b).

The portion of an optoacoustic signal generated by laser pulses in the skin typical has the highest amplitude compared with any other portion of the entire detected optoacoustic profile. Therefore, the signal gradient has its maximum at the tissue surface, which yields high ultrasound frequencies. High ultrasound frequencies that fall near the resonance frequency, f_{max}, of piezoelements can induce significant reverberation in the transducer. The transducers employed in LOIS are designed to damp resonance frequencies and widen the range of detectable frequencies. Nevertheless, a strong reverberation takes place after the arrival of the signal from the surface of the tissue. These reverberations, however, do not affect the useful part of the optoacoustic profile in the forward mode. It is convenient to employ the sharp peak with high gradient (derivative) for automatic determination of the tissue surface. The sharp surface mark, generated for each transducer position relative to the illuminated volume of the tissue, is quite useful for displaying skin outline of the organ being imaged, so that the location of internal tissue structures could be correlated to the illuminated surface of the tissue. In the backward mode, the skin reverberation represents significant problem for the signal processing. Furthermore, in the backward mode, the signal profile is more complex compared with the forward mode, which requires deconvolution of the system transfer function for restoration of the absorbed energy distribution [62]. In the orthogonal mode, the illuminated surface is not visible, making the first and the most challenging signal processing step unnecessary [72].

21.7.5 Algorithms of Image Reconstruction

Based on the optoacoustic signals received at multiple detector positions, the distribution of the absorbed optical energy in the illuminated volume can be reconstructed using tomography methods. A number of analytical filtered back-projection algorithms have been developed for OAT [33,86–92]. The inverse problem solutions employed in these analytical algorithms have rigorous solution for complete data sets and 3D reconstruction [89]; however, back-projection algorithms yield significant artifacts and only approximate distribution of image brightness from incomplete data sets acquired using optoacoustic detector arrays with limited view. On the other hand, analytical methods are more practical for real-time imaging, especially in clinical applications.

The basic concept of the filtered back projection for OAT is presented schematically in Figure 21.10. The image represents spatial distribution of a product of thermoacoustic efficiency, optical absorption coefficient, and effective optical fluence in the tissue. As a reasonable first approximation, one may consider biological tissues as an acoustically lossless homogeneous medium. It is convenient to consider optoacoustic wave equation in terms of the velocity potential, $\phi(\vec{r},t)$:

$$\left(\nabla^2 - \frac{1}{c_0^2}\frac{\partial^2}{\partial t^2}\right)\phi(\vec{r},t) = \frac{\beta}{\rho C_p}H(\vec{r},t), \tag{21.34}$$

where $\phi(\vec{r},t)$ is related to the optoacoustic pressure through $p(\vec{r},t) = -\rho[\partial\phi(\vec{r},t)/\partial t]$, $H(r,t)$ $a(r)F(r,t)$ is the thermal energy deposited through pulsed laser illumination of tissue with the optical absorption coefficient, $\mu a(r)$. When the object of interest is part of acoustically, thermally, and mechanically homogeneous medium, one can assume constant speed of sound, c_0; constant density, ρ; and constant thermoacoustic efficiency, Γ. The velocity potential for convenience can be replaced in Equation 21.34 with

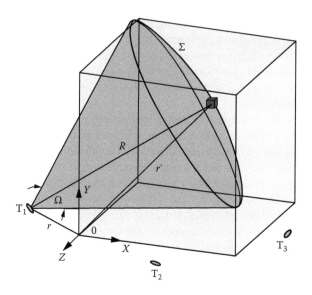

FIGURE 21.10 Geometry of the inverse problem in OAT.

temporal integral of acoustic pressure, $u(\vec{r},t)$, detected by transducer located in the point, $\vec{r}$, which can be expressed in the following form [33]:

$$u(\vec{r},t) = \int_{-\infty}^{t} p(\vec{r},t')dt' = \frac{\beta}{4\pi C_p} \int_V \frac{\mu_a(\vec{r}')I(\vec{r}')L\left(t - (|\vec{r} - \vec{r}'|/c_0)\right)}{|\vec{r} - \vec{r}'|}d\vec{r}', \tag{21.35}$$

where $L(t)$ is the laser pulse temporal profile. All other notations used in formula 21.35 are either defined under Equation 21.1 or explicitly shown in Figure 21.10.

The integral in Equation 21.35 is calculated over the entire space, V. It means that the acoustic pressure $p(\vec{r},t)$ measured at the time t and the point $\vec{r}$ is determined by the acoustic sources located on the spherical shell with radius $|\vec{r} - \vec{r}'|$ and thickness $d\vec{r}'$. Acoustic waves arrive to the measurement point $\vec{r}$ with time delay $|\vec{r} - \vec{r}'|/c_0$. If the laser (illuminating) pulses are sufficiently shorter than the time of thermal expansion of each voxel (conditions of acoustic stress confinement are satisfied), then generation of thermal sources may be considered instantaneous and the laser pulse waveform function can be expressed in the form $L(t) = \tau_L \delta(t)$, where τ_L is the laser pulse duration and $\delta(t)$ is Dirac's delta function. After these simplifications, Equation 21.35 can be rewritten for the pressure, $p(\vec{r},t)$, recorded at transducer location, $\vec{r}$, which can be expressed as a solution of Equation 21.34 subject to initial $p(\vec{r},0) = \Gamma Q(\vec{r})$ and boundary $\partial p(\vec{r},t)/\partial t\big|_{t=0} = 0$ conditions:

$$p(\vec{r},t')dt' = \frac{\beta}{4\pi C_p} \int_V d^3\vec{r}' Q(\vec{r}) \frac{d}{dt} \frac{\delta\left(t - (\vec{r} - \vec{r}'/c_0)\right)}{|\vec{r} - \vec{r}'|}, \tag{21.36}$$

where $F(\vec{r})$ is the distribution of the laser fluence and the nonnegative function $Q(\vec{r}) = \mu_a(\vec{r})F(\vec{r})$ describes the spatial distribution of the absorbed optical energy in the acoustic sources.

Equation 21.36 can be considered fundamental for OAT. The optoacoustic pressure amplitude detected by transducer at the time, t, is the superposition of the laser-induced acoustic sources located on the sphere of radius, $R = c_0 t$. The inverse problem in OAT is to determine an estimate of $Q(\vec{r})$ from knowledge of $p(\vec{r},t)$, that is, the measured optoacoustic signal.

When a complete set of optoacoustic signal data can be acquired through the entire 4π solid angle, the universal back-projection algorithm offers exact reconstruction of pressure $p_0(\vec{r})$ in the acoustic sources for the planar, spherical, and cylindrical geometries [89]:

$$p_0(\vec{r}) = \Gamma(\vec{r})\mu_a(\vec{r})F(\vec{r}) = \frac{2}{\Omega_0}\int_S d\Omega\left[p(\vec{r},t) - t\frac{\partial p(\vec{r},t)}{\partial t}\right]\Bigg|_{t=|\vec{r}-\vec{r}'|/c_0} \tag{21.37}$$

where

Ω_0 is the solid angle of the entire detection surface S with respect to a given source point at $\vec{r}'$

$p(\vec{r},t)$ is the pressure received at detecting position $\vec{r}$ and time t

Equation 21.37 indicates that $p_0(\vec{r})$ can be obtained by back-projecting the filtered data function $[p(\vec{r},t) - t(\partial p(\vec{r},t)/\partial t)]$ onto concentric spherical surfaces centered at each ultrasonic transducer (see Figure 21.10). The magnitude of each data sample is then normalized to the factor, $Rd\Omega/\Omega_0$, which applies proper weight to voxels located at a distance, R, from the ultrasonic transducers and visible within element aperture $d\Omega$ of each transducer relative to the total aperture of the array Ω_0.

Analytical reconstruction algorithms for OAT assume ideal ultrasonic transducers with full 2π wide directivity (ideal SIR) and delta function-type EIR (equal sensitivity over entire range of ultrasonic frequencies). In the real world, however, the pressure waveform can be significantly distorted by the finite dimensions and the finite bandwidth of the ultrasonic transducers, causing artifacts on optoacoustic images. To compensate for transducer physical dimensions and electromechanical properties, iterative image reconstruction algorithms have been developed based on the transducer characteristics, which are described by time-invariant linear systems with the transducer SIR and EIR as convolution kernels [91]. Based on these imaging models, optoacoustic images can be reconstructed much more accurately, especially for geometries when only incomplete set of tomography data can be acquired (such as for handheld probes operating in the backward mode) [75,90–92]. The iterative numerical methods provide quantitatively much more accurate images at the expense of time required for image reconstruction. This quantitative information is invaluable for functional biomedical imaging and measurements of tissue molecular composition [42]. A comprehensive discussion of the state of the art in the optoacoustic image reconstruction can be found in Ref. [93].

21.8 Two-Dimensional vs. Three-Dimensional Optoacoustic Tomography

One of the merits of OAT is the possibility to acquire a sequence of images in real time or at the video frame rate. All necessary data for a 2D image can be measured from a single laser pulse illumination, so that making 2D optoacoustic slices through the tissue has become a common technology in the past decade. On the other hand, 2D images have their limitations. The major drawback of 2D optoacoustic images is that these images are typically obtained with a handheld probe having limited aperture (field of view), which limits accuracy of quantitative information and capability to display complex shapes of objects. Three-dimensional optoacoustic images are free of these limitations. Three-dimensional images rigorously reconstructed from complete sets of data (full 4π view) contain quantitatively accurate distribution of the absorbed optical energy, which may be beneficial for a number of clinical and preclinical applications [13,72,94]. Real-time 3D full-view optoacoustic imaging seems possible using a 2D array of ultrasonic transducers with a large number of elements. However, it is unreasonably expensive with the present cost of detectors and electronics. Partial-view 3D images (3D resolved thick slices) can be obtained in real time with 2D transducer arrays having an affordable number of 256–512 parallel channels [95]. Full-field-of-view 3D images can be reconstructed by stacking thick slices or by rotational scanning of a 1D array.

21.9 LOIS for Preclinical Research

Optoacoustic imaging systems designed for small laboratory animals offer possibility to model human disease in mice and rats and perform preclinical research visualizing tissue structures and physiological processes with excellent resolution through the whole body of the animal. There are four different designs of the system presently available to researchers [72,96–98]. Here, we describe LOIS-3D, the system that rapidly generates optoacoustic images of the whole body and head with high contrast attainable not only in small tissue structures and microvasculature but also in large mouse organs such as kidneys, liver, and spleen and resolution of 0.3–0.5 mm depending on the high-ultrasonic-frequency cutoff (6 or 3 MHz) in the array of ultrawideband transducers. The optoacoustic mouse imaging system consists of four main components: fiber-optic light delivery, mouse holder with translation and rotation, an array of ultrasonic transducers (detectors), and data acquisition and imaging electronics. Various pulsed lasers operating in the NIR spectral range can be used as sources of optical illumination: Nd:YAG, alexandrite, OPO, and Ti:sapphire. The Nd:YAG-pumped Ti:sapphire laser (SpectraWave, Quanta System, Italy) is the most robust, stable, and easy-to-operate system tunable from 730 to 850 nm and also generating pulses at the wavelengths of 1064 and 532 nm, 10 or 20 Hz pulse repetition rate, ~120 mJ energy per pulse, and pulse duration of ~6 ns. Light delivery in LOIS-3D is performed orthogonally to the array of acoustic transducers by a bifurcated, randomized fiber bundle (Figure 21.11a). Imaging is performed in a water tank, which can be customized for specific applications, but typically is a cylinder with a diameter of ~20 cm. The temperature in the water-like optoacoustic coupling medium is maintained in the imaging module at 36°C by heating elements and measured with precision of 0.1 C. The tight control of the temperature ensures stable speed of sound in water surrounding the mouse, which is necessary for accurate reconstruction of the 3D mouse volumes. During the image acquisition, either an animal, placed in the special holder, can be rotated about its central vertical axis or the ultrasonic transducer array can be rotated around the animal. The rotation is performed by a dc motor with an optical encoder, while the initial alignment of the probe position relative to the animal is controlled by linear translation stages. The optoacoustic signals are acquired with a 64-element (3 MHz) or 128-element (6 MHz) arc-shaped piezocomposite ultrasound transducer array. The frequency bandwidth of the ultrasonic transducers

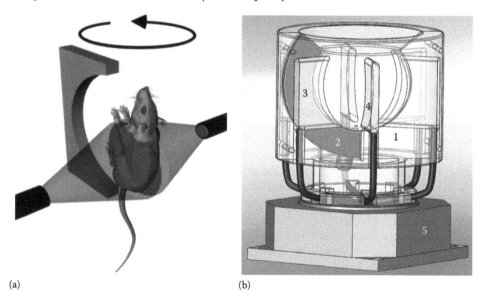

(a)							(b)

FIGURE 21.11	(a) Schematic diagram of the optical illumination in LOIS-3D, (b) imaging module, 1; containing an array of ultrawideband ultrasonic transducers, 2; fiber-optic bundles for NIR laser illumination of the animal, 3, 4; and computer-controlled rotational step motor, 5.

was about 80%–100% at the −6 dB point, when measured in the transmit–receive mode, and expanded to ~160%–180% when optimized for receive-only mode with proper electrical matching to the input of the analog amplifier. The piezocomposite elements had a square dimension of 1 mm^2 and were spaced 0.35 mm apart. The focal length of the array is 65 mm and the overall angular aperture of the array is 150°. The step size for the rotation is set to ensure even detector spacing in equatorial and meridian directions. The data acquisition system consists of a set of two or four low-noise 32-channel analog amplifier boards featuring high input impedance, a variable gain between 0 and 70 dB, a bandwidth of 100 kHz to 13 MHz at the −3 dB point, and an input noise of level of 12 μV. Data digitalization was performed with two or four in-house-designed 32-channel boards containing analog-to-digital converters with a sampling rate of up to 40 MHz, field-programmable gate array (FPGA, Stratix, Altera) for signal processing, and data transfer to personal computer through the Ethernet protocol. A standard dual-core personal computer running LOIS software is used to capture the data and rapidly reconstruct optoacoustic images (<30 s/10 million voxels) using multicore GPU in a CUDA-enabled NVIDIA video card [99].

21.10 Functional and Molecular Optoacoustic Imaging

21.10.1 Tissue Chromophores in the Near Infrared

Optoacoustic imaging may be called hemato imaging, since blood plays the dominant role in the optoacoustic image contrast. The optical absorption coefficient values for hemoglobin ($\mu_a^{[Hb]} = 1 \div 10$ cm^{-1}) and oxyhemoglobin ($\mu_a^{[HbO2]} = 1 \div 10$ cm^{-1}) are the highest among all possible tissue chromophores in the NIR spectral range [100]. Since delivery of blood loaded with oxygen and removal of blood loaded with carbon dioxide and other products of metabolic reactions are pivotal for all tissues in every animal (human) body, all tissues, soft and hard, contain blood and thus can be visualized based on the optical absorption of blood. Distribution of water in soft tissues creates a relatively homogeneous background and becomes significant only for wavelengths longer than 970 nm [101]. Lipids (fats) absorb noticeably only within the bands peaking at 930 and 1200 nm and create low background outside of these two bands, which is important mostly for intravascular imaging of atherosclerotic plaques [102–104]. Melanin with its smooth featureless optical absorption spectrum, contained within a very thin layer of epidermis, plays a minor role of a weak neutral density filter in the skin but becomes an important tissue chromophore for applications of optoacoustic imaging associated with detection of the melanoma cancer [105] and the retinal pigmented epithelium [106].

21.10.2 Functional Optoacoustic Imaging

Supply of blood carrying oxygen and nutrients to tissues is important for normal functioning of the tissues. Any deviation from normal blood supply causes immediate health problems: hypoxia, anemia, hypoglycemia (due to decreased blood concentration), or hematoma (due to increased blood concentration in the interstitial space). That is why imaging of vasculature, blood circulation, and blood distribution in tissues and measurements of [Hb] and [HbO$_2$] concentrations are included in the so-called functional imaging. Important biomedical applications of functional imaging are in angiography (studies of blood hemodynamics in the body) and angiogenesis (studies of microvascular network of aggressively growing cancerous tumors).

When spatial distribution of the optical fluence, $F(\vec{r})$, is known and the Gruneisen parameter, $\Gamma(\vec{r})$, of the thermoacoustic efficiency may be considered constant through the object of interest, one can obtain spatial distribution of the optical absorption coefficient, $\mu_a(\vec{r})$, from the optoacoustic images. Since the optical absorption spectra for the molecular extinction coefficients of oxygenated hemoglobin, $\varepsilon_{HbO2}^{\lambda}$, and deoxygenated hemoglobin, $\varepsilon_{Hb}^{\lambda}$, are well known [100], one can potentially determine concentrations of these molecules [HbO$_2$] and [Hb] in the body. For purposes of functional biomedical diagnostics, parameters of the total hemoglobin, THb, and blood oxygen saturation, SO$_2$, can be determined from optoacoustic images acquired at multiple wavelengths, λ_i, of the optical illumination. In the simplest case when other tissue chromophores do not make noticeable contribution to the overall optical absorption, the functional parameters THb and SO_2 can be measured from optoacoustic images acquired at two wavelengths, λ_1, λ_2, as follows [107]:

$$\text{THb}(\vec{r}) = [\text{Hb}](\vec{r}) + [\text{HbO}_2](\vec{r}) = \frac{\mu_a^{\lambda_1}\left(\varepsilon_{HbO_2}^{\lambda_2} - \varepsilon_{Hb}^{\lambda_2}\right) - \mu_a^{\lambda_2}\left(\varepsilon_{HbO_2}^{\lambda_1} - \varepsilon_{Hb}^{\lambda_1}\right)}{\varepsilon_{Hb}^{\lambda_1}\varepsilon_{HbO_2}^{\lambda_2} - \varepsilon_{Hb}^{\lambda_2}\varepsilon_{HbO_2}^{\lambda_1}};$$ (21.38)

$$SO_2(\vec{r}) = \frac{[\text{HbO}_2]}{[\text{Hb}](\vec{r}) + [\text{HbO}_2](\vec{r})} = \frac{\mu_a^{\lambda_2}\varepsilon_{Hb}^{\lambda_1} - \mu_a^{\lambda_1}\varepsilon_{Hb}^{\lambda_2}}{\mu_a^{\lambda_1}\left(\varepsilon_{HbO_2}^{\lambda_2} - \varepsilon_{Hb}^{\lambda_2}\right) - \mu_a^{\lambda_2}\left(\varepsilon_{HbO_2}^{\lambda_1} - \varepsilon_{Hb}^{\lambda_1}\right)}.$$ (21.39)

It is desirable to select the two wavelengths close to each other, so that changes in the optical scattering as a function of wavelength can be neglected and the distribution of the optical fluence, $F(\vec{r})$, can be considered similar at both wavelengths, and therefore the optical absorption coefficient, $\mu_a(\vec{r})$, can be determined from the reconstructed absorbed energy density, $Q(\vec{r})$, using Equation 21.37.

In the past decade, there were a number of impressive studies that generated functional images in vivo, however in the limited volume or at a limited depth in the tissue [41]. An experimental demonstration of functional optoacoustic imaging in the mouse body using LOIS-3D is depicted in Figure 21.12 [108]. In the course of this experiment, oxygen supply to the mouse was abruptly reduced, which resulted in dramatic reduction of the oxyhemoglobin concentration and visualized as changes in the optical absorption coefficient on optoacoustic images acquired at the wavelength of 760 nm, while the optical fluence distribution remained unchanged between the three measurements, Figure 21.12a, b, and c. Estimates of $SO_2(r)$ and $HbT(r)$ were not computed, since a method of accurate measurement of the optical fluence distribution through the whole body of a mouse is not yet developed.

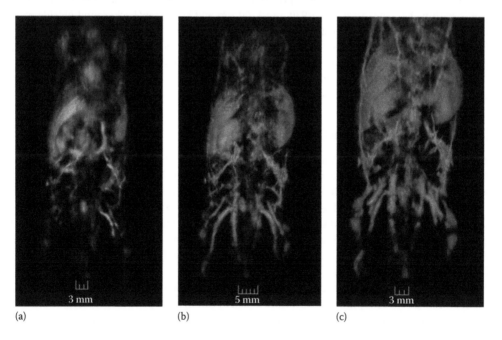

(a)   (b)   (c)

FIGURE 21.12 Laser illumination wavelength of 760 nm matches peak of the optical absorption in deoxyhemoglobin. (a) Normal oxygen saturation, (b) decreased oxygen saturation immediately after death, (c) totally hypoxic blood postmortem.

21.10.3 Molecular Optoacoustic Imaging

Optoacoustic imaging possesses molecular specificity to optically absorbing molecules. Based on optical absorption of endogenous molecular chromophores, such as hemoglobin and oxyhemoglobin, one can acquire functional images of entire small animal body or a human organ. On the other hand, there are a large number of physiologically important molecules, such as cellular protein receptors and nucleic acids of the cell nuclei that do not possess optical absorption in the red and NIR spectral ranges. These biological targets can be imaged with OAT enhanced with exogenous contrast agents.

Organic dyes, nanoparticles, and chromophore molecules resulting from reporter gene activity can be excellent optoacoustic contrast agents. The contrast agents may be especially effective when targeted to specific molecular receptors and/or accumulated in abnormal tissues of interest, such as cancer metastases. The main advantage of dyes is that these typically small molecules have short lifetime in the living body, being either excreted or biodegraded, and thus relatively nontoxic. A number of dyes (such as indocyanine green and methylene blue) absorbing in the NIR have been approved for human use. On the other hand, it is difficult or impossible to accumulate these dyes in the specific molecular target areas.

The advantage of nanoparticles is in their inherent large dimensions compared with dyes, which permits generation of much stronger signal per specific molecular target (the signal is proportional to the nanoparticle volume). The optoacoustic signal amplitude is further enhanced by an exceptionally large optical absorption cross section ($\sigma_a > 10-10$ cm^2) for certain types of metal nanoparticles (such as hollow gold nanospheres, gold and silver nanorods, gold nanocages) that possess strong plasmon resonance in the NIR spectral range [109]. The peak plasmon resonance wavelength in these nanoparticles can be conveniently tuned to a desirable wavelength in the NIR spectral range to minimize the background signal and maximize SNR for the useful optoacoustic signal. Furthermore, the nanoparticles can be covalently bioconjugated to various targeting ligands, such as monoclonal antibodies, nanobodies, short peptides, aptamers, and other specific ligands. The selective targeting of nanoparticles enables their effective accumulation in the cells of interest and high-contrast optoacoustic imaging with molecular specificity. There is a great interest in the biomedical community in the development of diagnostic contrast agents for optoacoustic imaging based on nanoparticles. These works have been recently reviewed [110]. Here, we give just one example of molecular optoacoustic imaging performed at TomoWave Laboratories. In the experiment depicted in Figure 21.13, a 10-week-old immunodeficient athymic nude mouse was inoculated with a xenograft tumor made of breast cancer cells, BT474, that overexpress HER2/neu receptors in concentrations over 1 million/cell. Gold nanorods (GNR) with aspect ratio of 3.4 were bioconjugated with monoclonal antibody raised against HER2/neu antigens. As the tumor grew to about 4 mm in size, the gold nanorods were administered through a tail vein into the mouse in concentration of 7×10^8 GNR/µL and the total volume of 400 µL (two consecutive injections of 200 µL each within the interval of about 10 min). The mouse was imaged with LOIS-3D described in Section 21.7. The imaging was performed prior to GNR bioconjugate injection and 24 h after the injection. Figure 21.13 shows dramatic enhancement of the optoacoustic contrast in the tumor following administration of the GNR-based targeted contrast agent. While prior to administration of exogenous contrast agent the tumor was visible on the optoacoustic image due to the network of microvasculature supporting growth of this tumor, after administration of GNR bioconjugates the optoacoustic contrast was dominated by gold nanorods accumulated in the tumor cells. This was documented by measuring the optoacoustic image brightness within the tumor at a number of wavelengths around 760 nm and matching it to the plasmon resonance absorption band of the gold nanorods.

The products of reporter gene activity can be also imaged with OAT. This genetic molecular imaging was first demonstrated in Ref. [111]. Gliosarcoma cells transfected with LacZ genes were inoculated into a Sprague–Dawley rat. As the tumor grew, LacZ genes were expressed to produce β-galactosidase enzyme, which metabolized the locally injected lactose-like substrate into highly absorbing blue products, thereby providing optoacoustic contrast. Since the early works in this field, the authors expanded the range of reporter genes and demonstrated genetic imaging at the depth of 50 mm in the tissue where conventional optical fluorescence imaging loses its sensitivity and resolution [112].

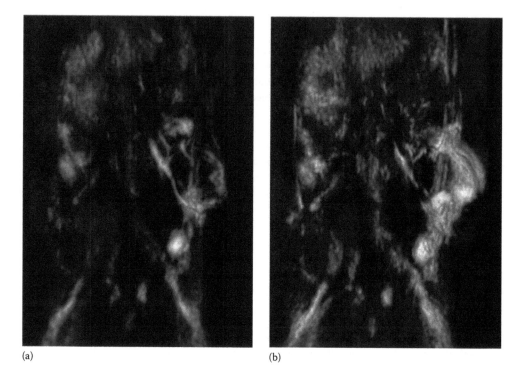

(a)   (b)

FIGURE 21.13 2D projections of 3D optoacoustic images of a live athymic nude mouse bearing xenograft tumor grown from BT474 breast cancer cells. HER2/neu protein receptors are visualized using targeted contrast agent based on gold nanorods conjugated with monoclonal antibody Herceptin. (a) Image acquired prior to administration of the contrast agent. (b) Image acquired 24 h after intravenous injection.

21.11 Application of LOIS for Diagnostic Imaging of Breast Cancer

The only clinical imaging modality officially approved for breast cancer detection has serious limitations. X-ray-based mammography, the current gold standard for breast cancer screening, uses ionizing radiation and generates images with relatively low contrast between diseased and normal tissue in radiologically dense breasts of younger women. And even in elderly women about 10%–20% of cancerous lesions are missed, while 70%–80% of the results are false positive leading to excessive biopsies [113]. Conventional B-mode ultrasonography is often used as an adjunct modality to determine which breast lesions should be biopsied, but the rate of negative biopsies remains high. Numerous publications that report sensitivity and specificity of the digital mammography followed by either diagnostic mammography (higher dose of x-rays) or breast ultrasound, may disagree in specific numbers characterizing tumor detection and differentiation utility and woman's age at which mammography is justified. However, all of them agree in one conclusion that a new imaging modality capable of more sensitive tumor detection and more accurate differentiation between suspicious but not malignant masses and cancerous lesions will significantly improve breast cancer survival rate and reduce the total cost of breast cancer care. All agree in one conclusion that new imaging modality capable of more sensitive detection and more accurate differentiation between suspicious but not malignant masses and cancerous tumors will significantly improve breast cancer survival rate.

The opportunity to detect and diagnose breast cancer noninvasively differentiating malignant carcinomas from benign adenomas has been the main driving force for developments in the field of OAT since the early pioneering works [23,25,32]. After more than a decade of active development, diagnostic imaging of breast cancer is emerging as the first commercial clinical application for the LOIS [50]. LOIS combines advantages of pronounced optical contrast and sensitive, high-resolution ultrasonic detection resulting in a more advanced imaging system for breast cancer [33,35,64,85].

21.11.1 Optoacoustic Contrast in Breast Tumors

Rapidly growing cancer cells need additional blood supply and gradually develop a dense microvascular network inside or around tumors required for tumor growth and proliferation [114,115]. Even though there is little functional difference between low-grade invasive tumors and benign tumors, dense tumor-associated neovascularization is associated with aggressive tumor growth, bleeding, and metastases. It was demonstrated that malignant breast tumors (carcinoma) have not only enhanced blood content but also contain noticeably hypoxic blood [116–118]. In contrast, benign tumors have relatively normal level of blood oxygenation. Considering prior achievements of diffuse optical imaging using several optical wavelengths, spectroscopic OAT may allow the noninvasive, in vivo imaging and quantification of oxygenated and deoxygenated hemoglobin that reflects physiological functions of breast tumors [119]. Stronger absorption of NIR light in malignant tumors with developed angiogenesis leads to a greater than twofold average optoacoustic contrast in tumors compared with normal tissue [33,35,64,84]. In contrast to pure optical tomography, where the tumor contrast is significantly diminished through integration of the signal over the entire optical path, the optoacoustic imaging permits direct reconstruction of the absorbed optical energy in tumors from the optoacoustic pressure profiles measured on the surface surrounding the breast. Tumors with dimensions of 5–10 mm illuminated with short laser pulses present themselves as sources of ultrasonic pressure waves with dominating ultrasonic frequencies ranging from 150 to 300 kHz. For desirable spatial resolution of ~0.5 mm, one does not need to detect ultrasonic frequencies higher than 3–5 MHz. Such ultrasonic waves can propagate in tissues with insignificant attenuation and deliver spatially resolved information to the surface of the tissues [23,120]. In order to achieve similar resolution in B-mode ultrasound imaging, one has to transmit and detect ultrasonic reverberations at 10–15 MHz, which can be substantially attenuated in the breast. Therefore, LOIS utilizing sensitive detection of optoacoustic waves instead of the detection of optical waves or scattered ultrasound waves can alleviate limitations associated with the pure optical and pure ultrasound technologies.

21.11.2 Optoacoustic Sensitivity to Small Tumors and Blood Vessels

One of the important parameters of LOIS is its potential capability to detect small breast tumors (in situ) [26,85]. OAT systems, having high optical contrast and the ultrasonic detection bandwidth of 0.1–10 MHz, are well suited for detection of small objects such as blood vessels and small tumors. The low-frequency cutoff corresponds to a dimension $a_T \sim c_s/f_{ac} = \dfrac{1.5 \text{ mm/μs}}{0.1 \text{μs}^{-1}} = 15$ mm. Therefore, only boundaries and heterogeneous distribution of microvasculature can be visualized for tumors larger than 15 mm. Also, the lateral resolution of the optoacoustic imaging systems with limited field of view (such as handheld probes) is reduced for larger objects (see Section 21.7.3).

Let us consider small breast tumor as a sphere with diameter, $2a_T$, and optical absorption coefficient, μ_a^T. Let this tumor be located at such a depth, d, where the energy of laser pulses exponentially attenuated in the normal breast tissue can generate optoacoustic signals with the SNR = 1. The maximum depth of the tumor detection can be estimated as [26]

$$d_{max} = -\frac{1}{\mu_{eff}} \ln\left(\frac{2R\,\text{NEP}}{\Gamma \mu_a^T a_T F_0}\right),$$ (21.40)

where
   μ_{eff} is the effective optical attenuation coefficient in breast tissue
   R is the distance between the tumor and transducer

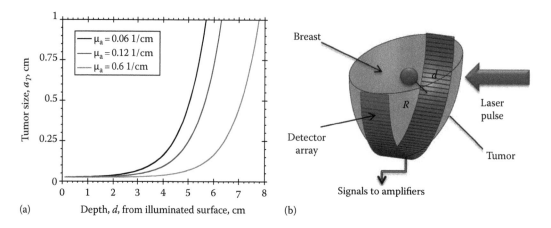

(a)   Depth, *d*, from illuminated surface, cm   (b)

FIGURE 21.14 (a) Minimally detectable dimensions, a_T, of a model tumor calculated as a function of depth, d, from the illuminated surface of surrounding normal tissue. Optical absorption coefficient of 0.6 cm⁻¹ corresponds to the average relative blood content of 10% in the tumor. (b) Schematic diagram of the model showing variable depth d and fixed radius of the arc-shaped array of ultrasonic transducers (distance, R, from the tumor to the transducers is fixed at 65 mm).

Fluence, F_0, of laser pulses at the breast surface must be lower than 20 mJ/cm², as defined by the safety requirement for medical laser procedures with low repetition rate of NIR laser pulses [121]. Gruneisen parameter, Γ, which characterizes the thermoacoustic efficiency in the breast tissues at 37°C, varies in the range of 0.2–0.5 reaching maximum in fatty tissues. The NEP in Equation 21.40 is calculated according to Equation 21.31 for SNR = 1. The root-mean-square of noise voltage, U_{RMS}, produced by the transducer is defined by the thermoelectrical noise of transducer–capacitor and input noise of preamplifiers. For LOIS, the anticipated value of U_{RMS} is about ~10 μV. The noise voltage is reduced $\sqrt{N}$ times if the signal averaging by N pulses is employed. The optimal number of acquisitions for the optoacoustic signal averaging equals $N = 16$, which should allow to get value of effective noise pressure less than 1 Pa.

Using the experimental data of tumor optical properties obtained in the course of clinical studies, we could calculate minimal diameter of spherical tumors with various blood contents, which can be detected inside the breast with the 64-channel LOIS system described in Ref. [64]. The radius of the minimal detectable spherical tumor is plotted in Figure 21.14a as a function of depth from the irradiated surface for optical absorption coefficients $\mu_a = 0.06$, 0.12, and 0.6 cm⁻¹ (at $\lambda = 757$ nm) corresponding to average blood content in tumors of about 1%, 2%, and 10%. Figure 21.14a depicts calculations based on Equation 21.40. Substituting NEP, the characteristic of LOIS in formula (21.40) yields the maximum depth of tumor detection of about 6 cm, assuming the tumor to be a sphere of 4 mm diameter with $\mu_a = 0.6$ cm⁻¹ or, respectively, greater or smaller depths for tumors with higher and lower absorption coefficients. Figure 21.14b shows geometry of the model used for calculations presented in Figure 21.14a.

21.11.3 Detection of Breast Cancer

Every feasibility study usually begins with the demonstration of safety for a new imaging technology. The first prototype of LOIS system designed for detection of breast cancer was tested for safety in the Radiology Department at the University of Texas Medical Branch. In this phase, 15 patients have been studied in the surgery suite prior to radical mastectomy. The pathology studies performed on breasts surgically excised after LOIS imaging demonstrated safety of laser illumination and absence of thermo-mechanical damage to tissues after the LOIS procedures [35]. The next phase was the demonstration of feasibility of breast cancer detection. Results of clinical testing in 27 patients with tumors or areas of the breast suspected for malignancy helped to gradually improve the system hardware and software. Biopsy was performed on each patient after examination with LOIS to make the final pathological determination of the type of tumors found in the breast. These pilot studies tested the hypothesis that LOIS with its high resolution and contrast based on blood in the tumor angiogenesis can improve detection sensitivity of the current gold standard modality, x-ray mammography followed by the ultrasound B-scan.

Although statistically significant conclusions regarding the false-positive and false-negative rates and sensitivity and specificity of LOIS modality could not be made due to the fact that LOIS components were continuously modified, the following examples demonstrate clinical utility of OAT as an imaging modality for breast cancer. Figure 21.15a, b, and c depicts an x-ray mammography image and corresponding ultrasound and optoacoustic images of a breast with poorly differentiated infiltrating ductal carcinoma grade 3/3. While the tumor could not be readily detected on x-ray mammogram due to high radiologic density of the breast (Figure 21.15a), it is seen clearly on the ultrasonic and optoacoustic images (Figure 21.15b and c). The dimensions of this tumor were about 23×15 mm and its center was located at a depth of about 21 mm from the laser-illuminated surface. The optoacoustic contrast measured as the ratio of the average tumor brightness and the average background brightness in proximity of the tumor was higher than that on ultrasound image. The high optoacoustic contrast of this tumor obtained with laser illumination at the wavelength of 757 nm (Figure 21.15c) indicates the presence of advanced angiogenesis with hypoxic blood. The same tumor was not visualized well when imaged at the wavelength of 1064 nm. This example gives evidence that OAT may significantly exceed the sensitivity of x-ray mammography while examining breast of younger women. Two main conclusions may be drawn from clinical experiments with LOIS on breast cancer patients: The first is that sufficient optoacoustic

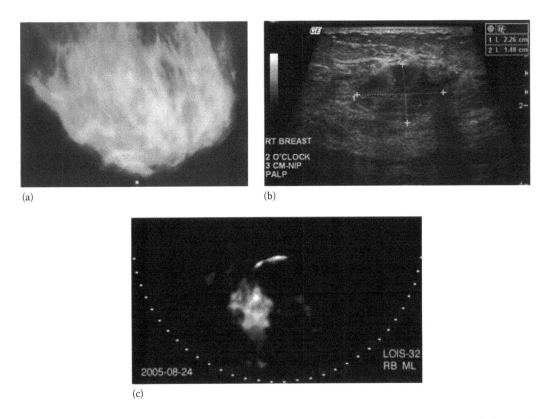

(a)   (b)

(c)

FIGURE 21.15 X-ray mammogram (a), ultrasound image (b), and optoacoustic image (c) of the right breast of a female patient. The x-ray results are inconclusive due to high breast density, but the presence of a tumor is confirmed by the ultrasound showing enhanced tissue density and by the optoacoustic image showing high concentration of hypoxic blood in the tumor angiogenesis.

contrast exists between normal and cancerous breast tissues and most breast tumors can be reliably visualized (18 out of 20 breast carcinomas were detected, while failure to detect tumors was likely associated with their incorrect positioning in the probe during the imaging procedure). The second conclusion is that the wavelength of 757 nm provides better optoacoustic contrast in cancerous tumors compared with 1064 nm, which correlates with the decreased level of oxygen saturation of hemoglobin in the tumors. The tissue optoacoustic contrast was greatly variable due to natural variation of tissue optical properties in such heterogeneous disease as breast cancer. However, no advanced malignant tumors examined had contrast less than twofold relative to background in normal glandular or fatty tissue. Optoacoustic contrast in the breast tumors being angiogenesis dependent can serve as means for accurate detection of aggressively growing and metastatic malignancies. Similar conclusions have been made by the research groups at the University of Twente [122] and Kyoto University [123], developing optoacoustic/photo-acoustic imaging systems for diagnostic imaging of breast cancer in parallel to our own efforts.

21.11.4 Diagnostic Imaging of Breast Cancer

Diagnostic imaging of breast cancer has been a field of rapid advances, especially with the novel modalities of ultrasound elasticity imaging (UEI), Doppler ultrasound imaging (DUSI), positron emission tomography (PET), functional nuclear magnetic resonance (fMRI), and bioelectric and optical/spectroscopic cancer visualization strategies [113]. All of these technologies, however, are not completely satisfactory for breast radiologists, indicating the need for a safer, more accurate, and easy-to-use technology. A combined ultrasonic plus optoacoustic imaging system Imagio™ based on a handheld probe and operating with video rate is being developed by Seno Medical Instruments to meet the challenges of more accurate diagnostics and demand for an advanced yet simple-to-use modality [50]. Optoacoustic imaging is inherently based on ultrasonic detection, which makes the combination of ultrasound and optoacoustics in one modality both natural and logical. The combined system provides fully coregistered structural information of breast tumor morphology and functional information of blood oxygenation and its concentration in the tumors relative to the background of normal tissue. Because the optoacoustic functional imaging system is combined with the widely used anatomical imaging of B-mode ultrasound, Imagio should be readily accepted by radiologists and ultrasonographers, who are very familiar with diagnostic ultrasound procedures using handheld probes.

The enabling feature of Imagio was the design of a handheld probe that combined laser illumination beams delivered to the probe through a fiber bundle with a linear array of 128 wideband ultrasonic transducers. The design of the light delivery system permitted bright-field illumination from the lower dermis down to the depth of breast tissues. Variation of the illumination wavelength permits imaging of the tissue with the image brightness determined by the relative concentration of the total hemoglobin and the level of blood oxygen saturation (see Section 21.10.2). To measure these two functional parameters from the optoacoustic images, the optical illumination is performed sequentially at two wavelengths: 757 nm (which is predominantly absorbed by hypoxic blood) and 1064 nm (which is absorbed predominantly by oxygenated blood). The ultrasonic transducer array was designed from one to three composites of single-crystal piezoelectric material to obtain maximum possible sensitivity within a wide band of ultrasonic frequencies from 0.1 to 10 MHz. Mechanical matching of the transducer to the tissue and optically protected acoustic lens permitted imaging not affected by reverberations. Electrical matching of the transducer to the input of low-noise wideband preamplifier permitted to extend the detection band into the lower frequency range, which was essential for functional optoacoustic imaging.

The system displays in real-time panels of three 2D images: (1) tissue morphology based on grayscale ultrasound, (2) normalized distribution of the total hemoglobin using yellow palette superimposed with ultrasound, and (3) blood oxygen saturation displayed in red-green color map superimposed with ultrasound. Figure 21.15 shows two panels of exemplary functional–anatomical maps (FAMs) of volunteer women present with breast tumors detected with digital x-ray mammography. The dynamic range of the images was fixed, so that brightness of functional colored images (such as Figure 21.16a and b) can be

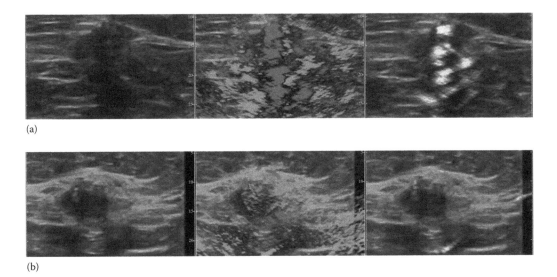

(a)

(b)

FIGURE 21.16 Images obtained using combined optoacoustic–ultrasonic system Imagio of patients with breast tumors: (a) malignant tumor of invasive ductal carcinoma and (b) benign tumor of fibroadenoma. Left, ultrasonic anatomical image; center, optoacoustic functional image of blood oxygen saturation coregistered and superimposed with ultrasonic image; right, optoacoustic functional image of the relative total hemoglobin coregistered and superimposed with ultrasonic image.

compared. In order to make tissue morphology visible through the functional images of the total hemoglobin, the yellow color map was selected and the lower bits of the images were made transparent. The threshold selection was based on statistical analysis of THb images of the background breast tissues. For the same purposes, SO_2 images were displayed using a color map with red colors representing low levels of oxygenation and green colors representing high level of blood oxygen saturation, while total transparency was assigned to SO_2 range representing statistically average background. Figure 21.16a shows a breast tumor with rough boundaries and heterogeneous functional map with significantly elevated THb and reduced SO_2. In contrast, Figure 21.16b shows a breast tumor with smooth boundaries, homogeneous functional map with low-to-average THb, and slight increased-to-average SO_2. The breast tumor biopsy was performed after Imagio procedure to compare conclusion of noninvasive diagnosis with histology for differentiation of breast tumors. Biopsy established that the images of Figure 21.16a represent malignant tumor of invasive ductal carcinoma and the images of Figure 21.16b represent benign tumor of fibroadenoma. Figure 21.16a and b demonstrates that coregistration and correlation of a structural image based on ultrasonic contrast and a functional image based on optical contrast may be used in clinic to visualize and differentiate breast lesions.

The combination of high-contrast functional color maps and better-defined boundaries of ultrasound images makes the superimposed images from Imagio more specific to the type of tissue than ultrasound alone. The statistical analysis performed independently of the system manufacturer, based on a pilot study of 79 patients, with images interpreted by five independent blinded readers revealed that sensitivity of tumor detection was improved and specificity of noninvasive diagnosis using Imagio was significantly greater than S&S of ultrasound alone [124]. The most significant findings were that (1) Imagio helps to diagnose the most ambiguous cases of BIRADS-4B with >30% greater accuracy and (2) the difference in the probability of malignancy (POM) estimated using Imagio was >42% even at the maximum level of sensitivity, which is quite large considering all varieties of breast tumors.

While breast tumors typically occur at the depth of 10–40 mm from the skin, it was important to estimate maximum depth of tumor detection. For this purpose, we used a breast tissue–mimicking phantom made of milk diluted to match average optical properties of the breast at the wavelength of 757 nm

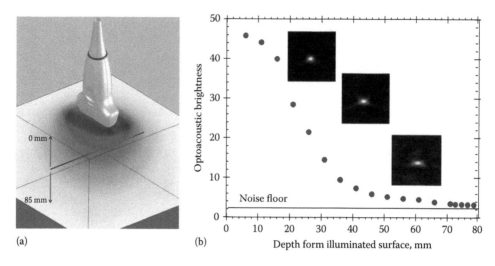

(a)   (b)

FIGURE 21.17 Optoacoustic image brightness of a blood vessel as a function of depth in a breast tissue–mimicking phantom. Cross-sectional optoacoustic images of the blood vessel are depicted at the depth of 30, 45, and 60 mm.

($\mu_a = 0.05\,\text{cm}^{-1}$, $\mu_s = 180\,\text{cm}^{-1}$; $g = 0.95$). A blood vessel with lumen diameter of 0.98 mm filled with blood was placed inside the phantom and was imaged using handheld optoacoustic–ultrasonic probe (see Figure 21.17a) while changing the distance between the probe and the vessel. In Figure 21.17b, the observed opto-acoustic brightness for the blood vessel cross section is shown as a function of the depth of the blood vessel in the phantom. As the depth of the object becomes greater, its contrast decreases as the optoacoustic signals approach the noise floor of the system ($0.7\,\text{nV} \times \sqrt{10}\,\text{MHz} \times 80\,\text{dB} = 2.2\,\mu\text{V} \times 10^4 = 22\,\text{mV}$). Simultaneously, one can observe gradual loss of the lateral resolution due to the limited aperture of the handheld probe. On the other hand, the blood vessel was still visible and resolved at the depth of 65 mm from the probe. Since the average blood content in cancerous tumors is about 10%, one may expect to detect breast tumors at the depth of about 45–50 mm. This conclusion made for optoacoustic imaging in the backward mode (Figure 21.17) corresponds well to our prediction presented in Figure 21.14 for the orthogonal mode.

Thus, by combining two types of image contrast, Imagio has the potential to provide radiologists with additional information helping to increase sensitivity and specificity of the diagnostic imaging procedure. Through correlation of the two types of tissue contrasts, (1) molecular contrast of deoxygen-ated hemoglobin associated with the function of aggressive malignancy to develop angiogenesis and consume oxygen, and (2) structural contrast based on increased density of tumors, breast cancer will be detected and localized more accurately. Also, unnecessary biopsies may be minimized through the tumor characterization based on noninvasive diagnostics. As recently demonstrated at the University of Washington in St. Louis, similar system can also be used for noninvasive detection of sentinel lymph nodes, guiding needle biopsies [125]. One more potential clinical application is the monitoring of the effects of cancer therapy, especially chemotherapy directed against angiogenesis [126].

Although 2D system will have utility for clinical diagnostic imaging, it cannot be used for screen-ing. The main limitation of the current design of Imagio is associated with its limited aperture dic-tated by the need for compact, light, and convenient handheld probe. The reconstruction algorithms for optoacoustic images based on incomplete data obtained within limited field of view provide only an approximation of the absorbed optical energy. The measurement accuracy for the optical absorp-tion coefficient is further reduced due to estimates of the effective optical fluence within the tissues based on average optical properties of the breast tissues. On the other hand, this design matches present regulatory requirements for qualitative imaging and diagnostics based on radiologist perception of the breast images. Computer-assisted diagnostics may be adopted by the regulatory agencies in the future, when 3D full-view imaging modalities will become the standard of breast cancer care. Specifically, 3D laser optoacoustic–ultrasonic imaging system, which visualizes the entire volume of the breast with details unattainable for 2D imaging, can be used for both screening and diagnostics. Provided rigorously reconstructed quantitative images and multispectral image analysis, such system has the potential to become a new safe and effective standard of care for breast cancer patients. This type of system is presently in the early stage of development and feasibility testing [94,127,128].

21.12 Summary and Future Directions

About two decades ago, our group began basic research and development of LOISs for cancer detection in various organs. Presently, 3D optoacoustic/photoacoustic systems are actively used in preclinical research on small laboratory animal models. Combined optoacoustic and ultrasonic imaging systems are expected to find a wide range of applications in biology and medicine. Major preclinical applications include imaging of angiogenesis-related microcirculation of tumors, response of tumors to therapeutic interventions, angiography, visualization and characterization of brain functions, molecular markers of diseases, and gene activity.

Initial clinical applications will include diagnostic imaging of cancer and monitoring of cancer therapy, intravascular imaging of atherosclerotic plaques, assessment of vascular circulation in human extremities, and neonatal brain imaging. A 2D laser optoacoustic–ultrasonic system is being presently evaluated in multicenter clinical trials under FDA guidance as a diagnostic modality for breast cancer. Active development of clinical 3D imaging systems is underway. LOIS is uniquely capable of *in vivo* imaging based only on endogenous contrast of blood. On the other hand, the development of biodegradable and effective optoacoustic contrast agents will expand capabilities of LOIS to molecular medicine. While the main merit of OAT is its capability of deep tissue imaging and molecular specificity defined by optical spectroscopy, the scalability of OAT to microscopy provides a unique opportunity to study the same biomedical system at multiple scales using one and the same optical absorption contrast.

Future advancements of LOIS and various similar systems are envisioned in the direction of developing quantitative imaging capability and improved imaging parameters (sensitivity and resolution), accommodating the needs of continuous real-time monitoring of rapid physiological processes, and in producing displays that intelligently combine structural, molecular, and functional information. The emphasis continues to be on maximizing accuracy of quantitative information, minimizing image acquisition and processing time and costs, and improving easiness of image interpretation through computer-assisted analysis. Recent breakthroughs in all-solid-state laser technology and miniaturization and integration of multifunctional electronic components allow a portable and compact design of future commercial laser optoacoustic–ultrasonic imaging systems.

Acknowledgments

The author would like to express his deep gratitude to his collaborator of many years, Dr. Alexander Karabutov, and to all colleagues at TomoWave Laboratories and Seno Medical Instruments for their invaluable contributions to the development of OAT systems described in this chapter. Financial support for research grants R43ES021629, R01CA167446, R43EB015287, R44CA110137, and R44CA128196 from the National Cancer Institute is also acknowledged.

References

1. Oraevsky, A.A., Jacques, S.L., Esenaliev, R.O., Tittel, F.K., Direct measurement of laser fluence distribution and optoacoustic imaging in heterogeneous tissues, *Proc. SPIE* **2323**, 250, 1994.
2. Oraevsky, A.A., Jacques, S.L., Esenaliev, R.O., Laser optoacoustic imaging for medical diagnostics, USPTO Serial # 05,840,023, 31 January 1996.

3. Oraevsky, A.A., Jacques, S.L., Tittel, F.K., Determination of tissue optical properties by time-resolved detection of laser-induced stress waves, *Proc. SPIE* **1882**, 86, 1993.

4. Oraevsky, A.A., Jacques, S.L., Tittel, F.K., Measurement of tissue optical properties by time-resolved detection of laser-induced transient stress, *Appl. Opt.* **36**, 402, 1997.

5. Oraevsky, A.A., A nanosecond acoustic transducer with applications in laser medicine, *LEOS Newslett.* **8**(1), 6, 1994.

6. Oraevsky, A.A., Jacques, S.L., Esenaliev, R.O., Tittel, F.K., Time-resolved optoacoustic imaging in layered biological tissues, in: *Advances in Optical Imaging and Photon Migration*, edited by Robert R. Alfano, Academic Press, New York, vol. 21, pp. 161–165, 1994.

7. Oraevsky, A.A., Andreev, V.G., Karabutov, A.A., Esenaliev, R.O., Two-dimensional optoacoustic tomography, transducer array and image reconstruction algorithm, *Proc. SPIE* **3601**, 256, 1999.

8. Karabutov, A.A., Oraevsky, A.A., Ultimate sensitivity of wide-band detection for laser-induced ultrasonic transients, *Proc. SPIE* **3916**, 228, 2000.

9. Andreev, V.G., Karabutov, A.A., Oraevsky, A.A., Detection of ultrawide-band ultrasound pulses in optoacoustic tomography, *IEEE Trans. UFFC* **50**(10), 1383–1391, 2003.

10. Oraevsky, A.A., Esenaliev, R.O., Jacques, S.L., Thomsen, S.L., Tittel F.K., Lateral and z-axial resolution in laser optoacoustic imaging with ultrasonic transducers, *Proc. SPIE* **2389**, 198, 1995.

11. Xu, Y, Wang, L.V., Ambartsoumian, G., Kuchment, P., Reconstructions in limited-view thermoacoustic tomography. *Med. Phys.* **31**(4), 724–733, 2004.

12. Wang, Y., Erpelding, T.N., Jankovic, L., Guo, Z., Robert, J.L., David, G., Wang, L.V., In vivo three-dimensional photoacoustic imaging based on a clinical matrix array ultrasound probe, *J. Biomed. Opt.* **17**(6), 061208, 2012.

13. Kruger, R.A., Kiser, W.L., Reinecke, D.R., Kruger, G.A., Miller K.D., Thermoacoustic molecular imaging of small animals, *Mol. Imaging* **2**(2), 113–123, 2003.

14. Song, K.H., Stoica, G., Wang L.V., In vivo three-dimensional photoacoustic tomography of a whole mouse head, *Opt. Lett.* **31**(16), 2453–2455, 2006.

15. Gusev, V.E., Karabutov, A.A., *Laser Optoacoustics*, AIP, New York, 1993.

16. Tam, A.C., Applications of photoacoustic sensing techniques, *Rev. Modern Phys.* **58**(2), 381, 1986.

17. Sigrist, M.W., Laser generated acoustic waves in liquids and solids, *J. Appl. Phys.* **60**, R83, 1986.

18. Wolbarsht, M.L., A proposal to localize an intraocular melanoma by photoacoustic spectroscopy, *Sov. J. Quant. Electron.* **11**(12), 1623, 1981.

19. Cross, F.W., Al-Dhahir, R.K., Dyer, P.E., MacRobert, A.J., Time-resolved photoacoustic studies of vascular tissue ablation at three laser wavelengths, *Appl. Phys. Lett.* **50**(15), 1019, 1987.

20. Oraevsky, A.A., Esenaliev, R.O., Letokhov, V.S., Temporal characteristics and mechanism of atherosclerotic tissue ablation by picosecond and nanosecond laser pulses, *Lasers Life Sci.* **5**(1–2), 75, 1992.

21. Diebold, G.J., Photoacoustic monopole radiation: Waves from objects with symmetry in one, two, and three dimensions, in: *Photoacoustic Imaging and Spectroscopy*, edited by L.V. Wang, CRC Press, Boca Raton, FL, vol. 144, pp. 3–17, 2009.

22. Bowen, T., Radiation-induced thermoacoustic soft tissue imaging, in: *IEEE Proceedings of Ultrasonics Symposium*, edited by B.R. McAvoy, Chicago, IL, vol. 1, pp. 817–822, October 14–16, 1981.

23. Oraevsky, A.A., Esenaliev, R.O., Jacques, S.L., Tittel, F.K., Medina, D., Breast cancer diagnostics by laser optoacoustic tomography, in: *Trends in Optics and Photonics*, edited by R.R. Alfano and J.G. Fujimoto, OSA Publishing House, Washington, DC, vol. II, pp. 316–321, 1996.

24. Esenaliev, R.O., Oraevsky, A.A., Jacques, S.L., Tittel, F.K., Laser optoacoustic tomography for medical diagnostics: Experiments with biological tissues, *Proc. SPIE* **2676**, 84–90, 1996.

25. Esenaliev, R.O., Tittel, F.K., Thomsen, S.L., Fornage, B., Stelling, C., Karabutov, A.A., and Oraevsky, A.A., Laser optoacoustic imaging for breast cancer diagnostics, limit of detection and comparison with x-ray and ultrasound imaging, *Proc. SPIE* **2979**, 71–82, 1997.

26. Esenaliev, R.O., Karabutov, A.A., Oraevsky, A.A., Sensitivity of laser optoacoustic imaging in detection of small deeply embedded tumors, *IEEE J. Sel. Top. Quant. Electron.* **5**(4), 981–988, 1999.

27. Kruger, R.A., Pingyu, L., Fang, Y., Appledorn, C.R., Photoacoustic ultrasound—Reconstruction tomography, *Med. Phys.* **22**(10), 1605, 1995.

28. Hoelen, C.G.A., de Mul, F.F.M., Pongers, R., Dekker, A., Three dimensional photoacoustic imaging of blood vessels in tissue, *Opt. Lett.* **28**(3), 648, 1998.

29. Kruger, R.A., Kopecky, K.K., Aisen, A.M., Reinecke, D.R., Kruger, G.A., Kiser Jr., W.L., Thermoacoustic CT with radio waves, a medical imaging paradigm, *Radiology* **211**(1), 275, 1999.

30. Kruger, R.A., Miller, K.D., Reynolds, H.E., Kiser Jr., W.L., Reinecke, D.R., Kruger, G.A., Breast cancer in vivo: Contrast enhancement with thermoacoustic CT at 434 MHz-feasibility study, *Radiology* **216**(1), 279–283, 2000.

31. Ku, G., Wang, L.V., Scanning thermoacoustic tomography in biological tissue, *Med. Phys.* **27**(5), 1195–1202, 2000.

32. Oraevsky, A.A., Andreev, V.G., Karabutov, A.A., Fleming, R.Y.D., Gatalica, Z., Sindh, H., Esenaliev, R.O., Laser optoacoustic imaging of the breast: Detection of cancer angiogenesis, *Proc. SPIE* **3601**, 352, 1999.

33. Andreev, V.G., Karabutov, A.A., Solomatin, V.S., Savateeva, E.V., Aleynikov, V., Julina, Y.V., Fleming, R.Y.D., Oraevsky, A.A., Optoacoustic tomography of breast cancer with arc-array-transducer, *Proc. SPIE* **3916**, 36, 2000.

34. Karabutov, A.A., Savateeva, E.V., Oraevsky, A.A., Imaging vascular and layered structure of skin in vivo with optoacoustic (front surface) transducer, *Proc. SPIE* **3601**, 284, 1999.

35. Oraevsky, A.A., Karabutov, A.A., Solomatin, V.S., Savateeva, E.V., Andreev, V.G., Gatalica, Z., Singh, H., Fleming, R.Y.D., Laser optoacoustic imaging of breast cancer *in vivo*, *Proc. SPIE* **4256**, 12, 2001.

36. Oraevsky, A.A., Savateeva, E.V., Karabutov, A.A., Bell, B., Johnigan, R., Pasricha, J.P., Motamedi, M., Application of confocal opto-acoustic tomography in detection of squamous epithelial carcinoma at early stages, in: *In Vivo Optical Imaging, Workshop at National Institutes of Health*, 15 September 1999, edited by A. Gandjbakhche, Optical Society of America Press, Washington, DC, p. 153, 2000.

37. Savateeva, E.V., Karabutov, A.A., Bell, B., Johnigan, R., Motamedi, M., Oraevsky, A.A., Noninvasive detection and staging of oral cancer in vivo with confocal optoacoustic tomography, *Proc. SPIE* **3916**, 55, 2000.

38. Karabutov, A.A., Savateeva, E.V., Andreev, V.G., Solomatin, S.V., Fleming, R.D.Y., Gatalica, Z., Singh, H., Henrichs, P.M., Oraevsky, A.A., Optoacoustic images of early cancer in forward and backward modes, European conference on biomedical optics, *Proc. SPIE* **4443**, 21, 2001.

39. Karabutov, A.A., Savateeva, E.V., Oraevsky, A.A., Optoacoustic tomography: New modality of laser diagnostic systems, *Laser Phys.* **13**(5), 711–723, 2003.

40. Niederhauser, J.J., Jaeger, M., Lemor, R., Weber, P., Frenz, M., Combined ultrasound and optoacoustic system for real-time high-contrast vascular imaging in vivo, *IEEE Trans. Med. Imaging* **24**(4), 436–440, 2005.

41. Wang, X., Pang, Y., Ku, G., Xie, X., Stoica, G., Wang, L.V., Noninvasive laser-induced photoacoustic tomography for structural and functional in vivo imaging of the brain, *Nat. Biotechnol.* **21**(7), 803–806, 2003.

42. Zhang, H.F., Maslov, K., Stoica, G., Wang L.V., Functional photoacoustic microscopy for high-resolution and noninvasive in vivo imaging, *Nat. Biotechnol.* **24**(7), 848–851, 2006.

43. Zhang, E., Laufer, J., Beard, P., Backward-mode multiwavelength photoacoustic scanner using a planar Fabry–Perot polymer film ultrasound sensor for high-resolution three-dimensional imaging of biological tissues, *Appl. Opt.* **47**(4), 561–577, 2008.

44. Yuan, Z., Jiang, H., Quantitative photoacoustic tomography: Recovery of optical absorption coefficient maps of heterogeneous media, *Appl. Phys. Lett.* **88**, 231101, 2006.

45. Cox, B., Laufer, J.G., Arridge, S.R., Beard, P.C., Quantitative spectroscopic photoacoustic imaging: A review. *J. Biomed. Opt.* **17**(6), 061202, 2012.

46. Shao, P., Cox, B., Zemp, R.J., Estimating optical absorption, scattering and Gruneisen distributions with multiple-illumination photoacoustic tomography, *Appl. Opt.* **50**(19), 3145–3154, 2011.

47. Ripoll, J., Ntziachristos, V. Quantitative point source photoacoustic inversion formulas for scattering and absorbing media, *Phys. Rev. E* **71**, 031912, 2005.

48. Sivaramakrishnan, M., Maslov, K., Zhang, H.F., Stoica, G., Wang, L.V., Limitations of quantitative photoacoustic measurements of blood oxygenation in small vessels, *Phys. Med. Biol.* **52**, 1349, 2007.

49. Tsyboulski, D., Liopo, A., Su, R., Ermilov, S., Bachilo, S., Weisman, R.B., Oraevsky, A.A., Enabling in vivo measurements of nanoparticle concentrations with three-dimensional optoacoustic tomography, *J. Biophotonics* 2013.

50. Zalev, J., Clingman, B., Smith, R., Herzog, D., Miller, T., Stavros, A.T., Ermilov, S.A. et al., Clinical feasibility study of combined opto-acoustic and ultrasonic imaging modality providing coregistered functional and anatomical maps of breast tumors, *Proc. SPIE* **8581**, 858103, 2013.

51. Oraevsky, A.A., Karabutov, A.A., Time-resolved detection of optoacoustic profiles for measurement of optical energy distribution in tissues, in: *Handbook of Optical Biomedical Diagnostics*, edited by V.V. Tuchin, SPIE Press, Bellingham, WA, Chapter 10, pp. 585–646, 2002.

52. Shung, K.K., *Diagnostic Ultrasound: Imaging and Blood Flow Measurements*, CRC Press, Boca Raton, FL, 2006.

53. Beard, P.C., Mills, T.N., An optical detection system for biomedical photoacoustic imaging, *Proc. SPIE* **3916**, 100, 2000.

54. Nuster, R., Holotta, M., Kremser, C., Grossauer, H., Burgholzer, P., Paltauf, G., Photoacoustic microtomography using optical interferometric detection, *J. Biomed. Opt.* **15**(2), 021307, 2010.

55. Speirs, R.W., Bishop, A.I., Photoacoustic tomography using a Michelson interferometer with quadrature phase detection, *Appl. Phys. Lett.* **103**(5), 053501, 2013.

56. Paltauf, G., Schmidt-Kloiber, H., Measurement of laser-induced acoustic waves with a calibrated optical transducer, *J. Appl. Phys.* **82**(4), 1525–1531, 1997.

57. Chen, S.L., Huang, S.W., Ling, T., Ashkenazi, S., Guo, L.J., Wideband photoacoustic tomography using polymer microring resonators, *Proc. SPIE* **7177**, Photons Plus Ultrasound: Imaging and Sensing, 71772B, 2009.

58. Berer, T., Veres, I.A., Grün, H., Bauer-Marschallinger, J., Felbermayer, K., Burgholzer, P., Characterization of broadband fiber optic line detectors for photoacoustic tomography, *J. Biophotonics* **5**(7), 518–528, 2012.

59. Lamela, H., Gallego, D., Gutierrez, R., Oraevsky, A., Interferometric fiber optic sensors for biomedical applications of optoacoustic imaging, *J. Biophotonics* **4**(3), 184–192, 2011.

60. Davidsoni, G.P., Emmony, D.C., A schlieren probe method for the measurement of the refractive index profile of a shock wave in a fluid, *J. Phys. E: Sci. Instrum.* **13**, 92–97, 1980.

61. Conjusteau, A., Maswadi, S., Ermilov, S., Brecht, H.-P., Barsalou, N., Glickman, R., Oraevsky, A., Detection of gold-nanorod targeted pathogens using optical and piezoelectric optoacoustic sensors: Comparative study, *Proc. SPIE* **7177**, 71771P (pp. 1–10), 2009.

62. Karabutov, A.A., Savateeva, E.V., Podymova, N.B., Oraevsky, A.A., Backward mode detection of laser-induced wide-band ultrasonic transients with optoacoustic transducer, *J. Appl. Phys.* **87**(4), 2003, 2000.

63. Xia, W., Piras, D., van Hespen, J.C., van Veldhoven, S., Prins, C., van Leeuwen, T.G., Steenbergen, W., Manohar, S., An optimized ultrasound detector for photoacoustic breast tomography, *Med. Phys.* **40**(3), 032901, 2013.

64. Ermilov, S.A., Khamapirad, T., Conjusteau, A., Lacewell, R., Mehta, K., Miller, T., Leonard, M.H., Oraevsky, A.A., Laser optoacoustic imaging system for detection of breast cancer, *J Biomed. Opt.* **14**(2), 024007 (pp. 1–14), 2009.

65. Cochran, A., Multilayer piezoelectric and polymer ultrawideband ultrasonic transducer, *J. Acoust. Soc. Am.* **130**(1), 629–630, 2011.

66. Savateeva, E.V., Karabutov, A.A., Solomatin, S.V., Oraevsky, A.A., Optical properties of blood at various levels of oxygenation and sedimentation rate studied by time-resolved detection of laser-induced thermoelastic stress, *Proc. SPIE* **4619**, 63–75, 2002.

67. Kikoin, I.K., *Tables of Physical Parameters*, Atomizdat, Moscow, Russia, 1976 and *Handbook of Chemistry and Physics*, 54th edition, 1974.

68. Goss, S.A., Johnston, R.L., Dunn, F., Comprehensive compilation of empirical ultrasonic properties of mammalian tissues, *J. Acoust. Soc. Am.* **64**(2), 423–457, 1978.

69. Duck, F.A., *Physical Properties of Tissue*, Academic Press, London, U.K., 1990.

70. Manohar, S., Kharine, A., van Hespen, J.C.G., Steenbergen, W. van Leeuwen, T.G., Photoacoustic mammography laboratory prototype: Imaging of breast tissue phantom, *J. Biomed. Opt.* **9**(6), 1172–1181, 2008.

71. Yao, J., Maslov, K.I., Puckett, E.R., Rowland, K.J., Warner, B.W., Wang, L.V., Double-illumination photoacoustic microscopy, *Opt. Lett.* **37**(4), 659–661, 2012.

72. Brecht, H.-P., Su, R., Fronheiser, M., Ermilov, S.A., Conjusteau, A., Oraevsky, A.A., Whole body three-dimensional optoacoustic tomography system for small animals, *J. Biomed. Opt.* **14**(6), 0129061–0129068, 2009.

73. Conjusteau, A., Ermilov, S.A., Su, R., Brecht, H.-P., Fronheiser, M.P., Oraevsky, A.A., Measurement of the spectral directivity of optoacoustic and ultrasonic transducers with a laser ultrasonic source, *Rev. Sci. Instrum.* **80**, 093708 (1–5), 2009.

74. Andreev, V.G., Ponomarev, A.E., Karabutov, A.A., Oraevsky, A.A., Detection of optoacoustic transients with rectangular transducer of finite dimensions, *Proc. SPIE* **4619**, 153–162, 2002.

75. Wang, K., Ermilov, S.A., Su, R., Brecht, H.-P., Anastasio, M.A., Oraevsky, A.A., An imaging model incorporating ultrasonic transducer properties for three-dimensional optoacoustic tomography, *IEEE Trans. Med. Imaging* **30**(2), 203–214, 2011.

76. Morse, P.M., Ingard, K.U., *Theoretical Acoustics*, McGraw-Hill, New York, 1968.

77. Kino, G.S., *Acoustic Waves, Devices, Imaging and Analog Signal Processing*, Prentice-Hall, Englewood Cliffs, NJ, 1987.

78. Maslov, K., Zhang, H.F., Hu, S., Wang, L.V., Optical-resolution photoacoustic microscopy for in vivo imaging of single capillaries, *Opt. Lett.* **33**(9), 929–931, 2008.

79. Favazza, C.P., Jassim, O., Cornelius, L.A., Wang, L.V., In vivo photoacoustic microscopy of human cutaneous microvasculature and a nevus. *J. Biomed. Opt.* **16**(1), 016015, 2011.

80. Maslov, K., Stoica, G., Wang, L.V., In vivo dark-field reflection-mode photoacoustic microscopy, *Opt. Lett.* **30**(6), 625–627, 2005.

81. Maswadi, S., Optoacoustic imaging system using probe beam deflection, US Patent App. 20130041247A1, Filed December 10, 2009.

82. Kozhushko, V., Khokhlova, T., Zharinov, A., Pelivanov, I., Solomatin, V., Karabutov, A., Focused array transducer for two-dimensional optoacoustic tomography, *J. Acoust. Soc. Am.* **116**(3), 1498–1506, 2004.

83. Oraevsky, A.A., Esenaliev, R.O., Karabutov, A.A., Laser optoacoustic tomography of layered tissues: Signal processing, *Proc. SPIE* **2979**, 59–70, 1997.

84. Ermilov, S.A., Stein, A., Conjusteau, A., Gharieb, R., Lacewell, R., Miller, T., Thompson, S. et al., Detection and noninvasive diagnostics of breast cancer with two-color laser optoacoustic imaging system, *Proc. SPIE* **6437**, 6437031–6437037, 2007.

85. Ermilov, S., Fronheiser, M., Brecht, H.-P., Su, R., Conjusteau, A., Mehta, K., Otto, P., Oraevsky, A., Development of laser optoacoustic and ultrasonic imaging system for breast cancer utilizing handheld array probes, *Proc. SPIE* **7177**, 717703, 2009.

86. Kruger, R., Liu, P., Fang R., Photoacoustic ultrasound (PAUS)—Reconstruction tomography, *Med. Phys.* **22**(10), 1605–1609, 1995.

87. Andreev, V.G., Popov, D.A., Sushko, D.V., Karabutov, A.A., Oraevsky, A.A., Inverse radon transform for optoacoustic imaging, *Proc. SPIE* **4256**, 119–129, 2001.

88. Cox, B.T., Beard, P.C., Fast calculation of pulsed photoacoustic fields in fluids using k-space methods, *J. Acoust. Soc. Am.* **117**, 3616–3627, 2005.

89. Xu, M., Wang, L.V., Universal back-projection algorithm for photoacoustic computed tomography, *Phys. Rev. E* **71**, 016706, 2005.

90. Burgholzer, P., Matt, G.J., Haltmeier, M., Paltauf, G., Exact and approximate imaging methods for photoacoustic tomography using an arbitrary detection surface, *Phys. Rev. E* **75**, 046706, 2007.

91. Rosenthal, A., Ntziachristos, V., Razansky, D., Model-based optoacoustic inversion with arbitrary-shape detectors, *Med. Phys.* **38**, 4285–4295, 2011.

92. Wang, K., Su, R., Oraevsky, A.A., Anastasio, M.A., Investigation of iterative image reconstruction in three-dimensional optoacoustic tomography, *Phys. Med. Biol.*, **57**(17), 5399–5423, 2012.

93. Wang, K., Anastasio, M.A., Photoacoustic and thermoacoustic tomography: Image formation principles, in: *Handbook of Mathematical Methods in Imaging*, edited by O. Scherzer, Springer, New York/Heidelberg, Germany, pp. 781–815, 2011.

94. Kruger, R.A., Richard, B., Lam, R.B., Reinecke, D.R., Del Rio, S.P., Doyle, R.P., Photoacoustic angiography of the breast, *Med. Phys.* **37**(11), 6095–6098, 2010.

95. Buehler, A., Deán-Ben, X.L., Claussen, J., Ntziachristos, V., Razansky, D., Three-dimensional optoacoustic tomography at video rate, *Opt. Express* **20**(20), 171986, 2012.

96. Xia, J., Chatni, M., Maslov, K., Guo, Z., Wang, K., Anastasio, M., Wang, L.V., Whole-body ring-shaped confocal photoacoustic computed tomography of small animals in vivo, *J. Biomed. Opt.* **17**, 050506, 2012.

97. Lam, R.B., Kruger, R.A., Reinecke, D.R., DelRio, S.P., Thornton, M.M., Picot, P.A., Morgan, T.G., Dynamic optical angiography of mouse anatomy using radial projections, *Proc. SPIE* **7564**, 756405, 2010.

98. Razansky, D., Buehler, A., Ntziachristos, V., Volumetric real-time multispectral optoacoustic tomography of biomarkers, *Nat. Protoc.* **6**(8), 1121–1129, 2011.

99. Wang, K., Huang, C., Kao, Y.-J., Chou, C.-Y., Oraevsky, A.A., Anastasio, M.A., Accelerating image reconstruction in three-dimensional optoacoustic tomography on graphics processing units, *Med. Phys.* **40**, 023301, 2013.

100. Roggan, A., Friebel, M., Doerschel, K., Hahn, A., Mueller, G., Optical properties of circulating human blood in the wavelength range 400–2500 nm, *J. Biomed. Opt.* **4**(1), 36–46, 1999.

101. Hale, G.M., Querry, M.R., Optical constants of water in the 200 nm to 200 µm wavelength region, *Appl. Opt.* **12**, 555–563, 1973.

102. Henrichs, P.M., Meador, J., Fuqua, J., Oraevsky, A.A., Atherosclerotic plaque characterization with optoacoustic imaging, *Proc. SPIE* **5697**, 217–223, 2005.

103. Wang, B., Su, J.L., Amirian, J., Litovsky, S.H., Smalling, R., Emelianov, S., Detection of lipid in atherosclerotic vessels using ultrasound-guided spectroscopic intravascular photoacoustic imaging, *Opt. Express* **18**(5), 4889–4897, 2010.

104. Allen, T.J., Beard, P.C., Photoacoustic characterisation of vascular tissue at NIR wavelengths, Photons plus ultrasound: Imaging and sensing. *Proc. SPIE* **7177**, 71770A, 2009.

105. Oh, J.T., Li, M.L., Zhang, H.F., Maslov, K., Stoica, G., Wang, L.V., Three-dimensional imaging of skin melanoma in vivo by dual-wavelength photoacoustic microscopy, *J. Biomed. Opt.* **11**(3), 34032, 2006.

106. Jiao, S., Jiang, M., Hu, J., Fawzi, A., Zhou, Q., Shung, K.K., Puliafito, C.A., Zhang, H.F., Photoacoustic ophthalmoscopy for in vivo retinal imaging, *Opt. Express* **18**(4), 3967–3972, 2010.

107. Villringer, A., Chance, B., Non-invasive optical spectroscopy and imaging of human brain function, *Trends Neurosci.* **20**, 435–442, 1997.

108. Su, R., Ermilov, S.A., Liopo, A.V., Oraevsky, A.A., Optoacoustic 3D visualization of changes in physiological properties of mouse tissues from live to postmortem, *Proc. SPIE* **8223**, 82230K, 2012.

109. Oraevsky, A.A., Gold and silver nanoparticles as contrast agents for optoacoustic imaging, in: *Photoacoustic Imaging and Spectroscopy*, edited by L. Wang, CRC Press, Boca Raton, FL, 2009.

110. Liopo, A.V., Oraevsky, A.A., Nanoparticles as contrast agents for optoacoustic imaging, in: *Nanotechnology for Biomedical Imaging and Diagnostics*, edited by M. Berezin, Chapter 5, John Wiley & Sons, Hoboken, NJ, 2014, 550p.

111. Li, L., Zemp, R.J., Lungu, G., Stoica, G., Wang, L.V., Photoacoustic imaging of lacZ gene expression *in vivo*, *J. Biomed. Opt. Lett.* **12**(2), 0205041–0205042, 2007.

112. Cai, X., Li, L., Krumholz, A., Guo, Z., Erpelding, T.N., Zhang, C., Zhang, Y., Xia, Y., Wang, L.V., Multi-scale molecular photoacoustic tomography of gene expression, *PLoS ONE* 7(8), e43999, 2012.

113. Kopans, D.B., *Breast Imaging*, Wolters Kluwer Health, Philadelphia, PA, 1114pp., 2007.

114. Folkman, J., Clinical applications of research on angiogenesis, *N. Engl. J. Med.* **333**, 1757–1763, 1995.

115. Weidner, N., Semple, J.P., Welch, W.R., Folkman, J., Tumor angiogenesis and metastasis—Correlation in invasive breast carcinoma, *N. Engl. J. Med.* **324**, 1–7, 1991.

116. Alacam, B., Yazici, B., Chance, B., Nioka, S., Characterization of breast tumors with NIR methods using optical indices, *Proceedings of the 29th Annual International Conference of the IEEE EMBS*, Lyon, France, pp. 5186–5189, August 23–26, 2007.

117. Glunde, K., Gillies, R.G., Neeman, M., Bhujwalla, Z.M., Molecular and functional imaging of tumor microenvironment, in: *Molecular Imaging: Principles and Practice*, edited by R. Weissleder, B.D. Ross, A. Rehemtulla, S.S. Gambhir, Peoples Medical Publishing House, Shelton, CT, Chapter 50, p. 846, 2010.

118. Grosenick, D., Wabnitz, H., Moesta, K.T., Mucke, J., Schlag, P.M., Rinneberg, H., Time-domain scanning optical mammography: Optical properties and tissue parameters of 87 carcinomas, *Phys. Med. Biol.* **50**, 2451–2468, 2005.

119. Ntziachristos, V., Chance, B., Probing physiology and molecular function using optical imaging: Applications to breast cancer, *Breast Cancer Res.* 3(1), 41–46, 2001.

120. D'Astous, F.T., Foster, F.S., Frequency dependence of ultrasound attenuation and backscatter in breast tissue, *Ultrasound Med. Biol.* **12**(10), 795–808, 1986.

121. American National Standard for Safe Use of Lasers, ANSI Z136.1, American Laser Institute, New York, 2007.

122. Heijblom, M., Piras, D., Xia, W., van Hespen, J.C.G., Klaase, J.M., van den Engh, F.M., van Leeuwen, T.G., Steenbergen, W., Manohar, S., Visualizing breast cancer using the Twente photoacoustic mammoscope: What do we learn from twelve new patient measurements? *Opt. Express* **20**(11), 11582–11597, 2012.

123. Kitai, T., Torii, M., Sugie, T., Kanao, S., Mikami, Y., Shiina, T., Toi, M., Photoacoustic mammography: Initial clinical results, *Breast Cancer* **4**, 1–8, 2012.

124. Otto, P.M., Kist, K., Stavros, A.T., Lavin, P.T., Clingman, B.A., Zalev, J., Ermilov, S.A., Oraevsky, A.A., Coregistered molecular and morphological imaging: Clinical feasibility for improved noninvasive diagnosis of breast cancer, *Translational & Clinical Oncology—SS29, Abstracts of World Molecular Imaging Congress*, Dublin, Ireland, September 6, 2012.

125. Kim, C., Erpelding, T.N., Maslov, K.I., Jankovic, L., Akers, W.J., Song, L., Achilefu, S., Margenthaler, J.A., Pashley, M.D., Wang, L.V., Handheld array-based photoacoustic probe for guiding needle biopsy of sentinel lymph nodes, *J. Biomed. Opt.* **15**(04), 046010, 2010.

126. Siphanto, R.I., Thumma, K.K., Kolkman, R.G.M., Leeuwen, T.G., de Mul, F.F.M., van Neck, J.W., van Adrichem, L.N.A., Steenbergen, W., Serial noninvasive photoacoustic imaging of neovascularization in tumor angiogenesis, *Opt. Express* 13(1), 88–95, 2005.

127. Ermilov, S.A., Conjusteau, A., Hernandez, T., Su, R., Nadvoretskiy, V.V., Tsyboulski, D., Anis, F., Anastasio, M.A., Oraevsky, A.A., 3D laser optoacoustic ultrasonic imaging system for preclinical research, *Proc. SPIE* **8581**, 85810N, 2013.

128. Wenfeng Xia, W., Piras, D., Singh, M.K.A., van Hespen, J.C.G., van Leeuwen, T.J., Steenbergen, W., Manohar, S., Design and evaluation of a laboratory prototype system for 3D photoacoustic full breast tomography, *Biomed. Opt. Express* **4**(11), 2555, 2013.

22

Raman Spectroscopy: From Benchtop to Bedside

Anita Mahadevan-Jansen
Vanderbilt University

Chetan A. Patil
Vanderbilt University

Isaac J. Pence
Vanderbilt University

22.1 Introduction

Light can interact with tissue in different ways and probing this interaction can yield information about the state of tissue with respect to its physiology as well as pathology. The use of fiber optics allows applications of optical techniques in tissue to be performed remotely and with minimal damage. Since tissue response is virtually instantaneous, the results are obtained in real time, and the use of data processing techniques allows for automated detection of disease. These properties have resulted in a variety of applications where optical techniques have been used for tissue diagnosis.

When a photon is incident on a molecule, it may be transmitted, absorbed, or scattered. Different spectroscopic techniques arise from these different light–tissue interactions. These techniques include

- Absorption spectroscopy
- Reflectance spectroscopy
- Fluorescence spectroscopy
- Raman spectroscopy

Each of these techniques has been studied for the purpose of tissue diagnosis with varying degrees of success. Of these, fluorescence spectroscopy is perhaps the most investigated technique for tissue diagnosis.

There is much evidence to indicate that fluorescence spectroscopy of both exogenous (see, e.g., Ref. [1]) and endogenous chromophores can be used to identify neoplastic transformations in cells, precancerous tissue, and cancer in breast [2], lung [3], bronchus [4], oral cavity [5], cervix [6], and gastrointestinal (GI) tract [7,8]. Despite the success of this technique, results indicate that the specificity of fluorescence is limited and benign abnormalities such as inflammation and metaplasia are similar in many patients [6–8]. This suggests that the use of fluorescence diagnosis in situations where incidence is expected to be low may result in an unacceptably high false-positive rate. Vibrational spectroscopy has been considered as a viable approach to enhance diagnostic accuracy due to its inherent biochemical specificity. The focus of this chapter then is the application of Raman spectroscopy in biomedicine, especially as it pertains to disease detection.

Raman spectroscopy has been used for many years to probe into the biochemistry of various biological molecules [9,10]. In recent years, there has been interest in using this technique in diagnostics [11–14], particularly in vivo. These include a wide range of applications from the detection of (pre)malignant lesions in various organ sites to quantitative detection of blood analytes such as glucose, from measurement of skin hydration to the study of aging. The focus of each of the various applications is toward quantitative, in vivo, nonintrusive, automated detection in real-time.

The chapter is laid out to describe the concept, instrumentation, and application of Raman spectroscopy as it applies to biomedicine. It starts with a description of the basic concepts behind Raman spectroscopy and Raman signatures of materials. This is followed by a review of past, present, and future directions of the instrumentation that facilitates the use of this technique for detection of disease. Finally, some sample applications of Raman spectroscopy for disease diagnosis are reviewed, with reference to work at the molecular and microscopic levels. The chapter concludes with a presentation of the future perspectives as they pertain to clinical applications.

22.2 Principles of Raman Spectroscopy

The basis of Raman spectroscopy arises from the Raman effect by which energy can be exchanged between incident photons and scattering molecules. The Raman effect was discovered by Dr. C.V. Raman in 1928 when he experimented with the scattering of light through various liquids and observed "a modified scattered radiation of degraded frequency," later referred to as *Raman lines* from these liquids [15]. Classically speaking, when the energy of the incident photon is unaltered after collision with a molecule, the scattered photon has the same frequency as the incident photon. This is Rayleigh or elastic scattering [16,17]. During the collision, when energy is transferred either from the molecule to the photon or vice versa, the scattered photon then has a different frequency than the incident photon. This is inelastic or Raman scattering (Figure 22.1). Quantum mechanically, Raman scattering is the result

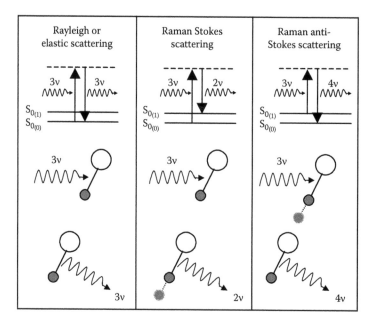

FIGURE 22.1   Schematic illustration of classical and quantum mechanical explanation of scattering.

of an energy transition of the scattering molecule to a virtual excited state and its return to a higher (or lower) vibrational state with the emission of an altered incident photon (Figure 22.1). Since energy can be transferred from the photon to the molecule or from the molecule to the photon, the scattered photon can have less or more energy as compared to the incident photon. When the scattered photon has less energy than the incident photons, the process is referred to as Raman Stokes scattering. When the scattered photon has more energy than the incident photons, the process is referred to as Raman anti-Stokes scattering.

A Raman spectrum is a plot of scattered intensity as a function of the frequency shift (which is proportional to the energy difference) between the incident and scattered photons (Figure 22.2). Together, the frequency shifts are characteristic of the molecule with which the photon collided. The resultant spectrum is characterized by a series of Raman lines or bands that individually correspond to the various vibrational modes of that molecule. The locations of the Raman bands are typically presented in terms of relative wavenumbers (or Raman shift) defined as shifts in wavenumbers (inverse of wavelength in cm^{-1}) from the incident frequency, which is set to zero. This is because the location of Raman bands for a given molecule in relative wavenumbers remains constant regardless of the incident frequency (within the physical constraints of the light–tissue interaction).

Raman signals are usually weak (one in a million scattered photons) and require powerful sources and sensitive detectors. Typically, Raman peaks are spectrally narrow (a few wavenumbers) and in many cases can be associated with the vibration of a particular chemical bond (or normal mode dominated by the vibration of a single functional group) in a molecule. Consider a complex molecule such as glucose (Figure 22.2). Each of the stretching and bending modes of vibration of this molecule has a characteristic frequency. When a photon is incident on this molecule, each mode of vibration results in a characteristic shift in frequency that is indicated in the Raman spectrum. Since each type of bond has characteristic modes of vibration, each type of molecule has its own spectral *fingerprint*. Thus, in a complex mixture of molecules such as in tissue, the presence of the unique bands of glucose can be traced resulting in the quantitative evaluation of the sample's chemical composition, which can then be related to the tissue pathology for diagnosis.

Raman spectroscopy probes different characteristics of materials than fluorescence [16]. The energy transitions of molecules are solely between the vibrational levels. Fluorescence arises from the emission of absorbed energy between electronic transitions. Only a limited number of biological molecules such as flavins, porphyrins, and structural proteins (collagen and elastin) contribute to intrinsic tissue

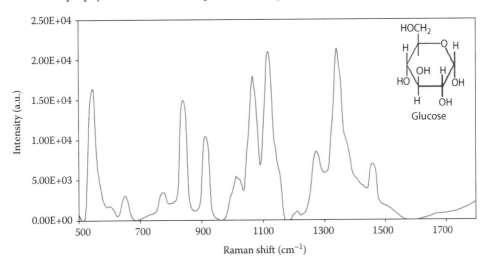

FIGURE 22.2 Raman spectrum of glucose in powdered form obtained with dispersive Raman spectroscopy at 785 nm excitation.

fluorescence, most with spectrally overlapping, broadband emission. In contrast, most biological molecules are Raman active with fingerprint spectral characteristics. In principle, this can be used to overcome some of the limitations of fluorescence diagnosis of precancers and cancers.

Several different modalities based on Raman scattering have been used to analyze the structure of various biological molecules [18,19]. Some of these techniques include near-infrared (NIR) dispersive Raman, Fourier transform Raman (FT-Raman), surface-enhanced Raman (SERS), and ultraviolet resonance Raman (UVR) spectroscopy [16,17]. More recently developed techniques include stimulation Raman, tip-enhanced Raman, and coherent anti-Stokes Raman scattering [20–22]. Pursued extensively as a viable technique for in vivo human application, NIR dispersive Raman scattering is typically excited in the range of 780–1100 nm where minimal fluorescence is produced making detection of the weak Raman signal easier, particularly in biological materials. Early adoption of Raman spectroscopy for biological applications with minimal interference from fluorescence relied on FT-Raman spectroscopy, where the Fourier transform of the scattered signal is detected and then inversely transformed to give the actual Raman signature. This technique yields improved signal-to-noise ratio (SNR) of hard to detect events but requires long collection times [11] that is not practical for in vivo human implementation. With the recent developments in laser and detector technology, FT-Raman methods have become more or less obsolete at least as it pertains to tissue diagnosis. Thus, while some early results from FT-Raman studies are referenced, the focus of the chapter will be on dispersive Raman spectroscopy.

SERS is used to investigate the vibrational properties of single adsorbed molecules [16,17,23]. It was discovered that the rather weak Raman effect can be greatly strengthened (by a factor of up to 14 orders of magnitude) if single molecules are attached to nanometer-sized metal structures that are highly reflective and of a suitable roughness. Many groups have used SERS to detect single molecules attached to colloidal silver particles either adhered to a glass slide or even in an aqueous solution. The advantages of these methods are that they are fast, they can supply some structural information about the molecules, and they do not bleach the molecules as in fluorescence. Single-molecule detection is of great practical interest in chemistry, biology, medicine, and pollution monitoring; examples include DNA sequencing and the tracing of interesting molecules such as those used in bioterrorism. Combining atomic force microscopy (AFM) with SERS by coating the AFM tip with SERS-active metal or metal nanoparticles can yield Raman information on the scale of 100 nm. This combined approach—tip-enhanced Raman spectroscopy—has been applied to a range of samples; however, the practical implantation of TERS is complex and cannot be applied in vivo at this time.

The discovery of nanoparticles and the increasing research effort dedicated to their development has allowed SERS to become possible in an in vivo setting. Researchers have developed biocompatible and nontoxic nanoparticles that can be functionalized and introduced in to mouse models [24–28]. This approach has been applied to such applications as the detection of cancer, inflammation, and glucose sensing. The disadvantage of SERS for clinical use is that nanoparticles and their functionalization are still predominantly in the research phase, and therefore not yet ready or approved for human applications. Furthermore, tracking the trace amounts of functionalized nanoparticles in the human body remains a significant challenge.

When the excitation frequency approaches or enters the region of electronic absorption of a molecule, a resonance Raman spectrum of that molecule is obtained [29]. By choosing appropriate excitation frequencies, a sample is selectively excited at the maximum absorption frequency of a characteristic molecule to detect that feature above all else. Resonance excitation increases the scattering intensity by several orders of magnitude. Typical absorption frequencies of biological molecules such as proteins and nucleic acids are in the UV portion of the spectrum where the Raman and fluorescence signatures may be spectrally resolved. However, high intensities of UV light may cause photolysis of the sample and destroy it over time. Besides, this signal may be attenuated by simultaneous intensified absorption and fluorescence emission [29]. In addition to these factors, the mutagenicity of UV radiation limits the application of this technique for clinical in vivo use [30,31].

Other methods of Raman spectroscopy include nonlinear Raman techniques such as coherent anti-Stokes Raman spectroscopy (CARS) and stimulated Raman scattering that take advantage of nonlinear processes for increased signal levels. However, these techniques are constrained by the need for complex ultrafast laser systems, which can make clinical in vivo human use impractical. Since the focus of this chapter is the application of Raman spectroscopy from bench to bedside, we will therefore concentrate the rest of this chapter on the implementation of dispersive Raman methods for clinical applications. Based on the success of Raman spectroscopy in biology, many groups have recognized its potential in the study and diagnosis of disease. However, early attempts to measure Raman spectra of cells and tissues were hindered by two factors: (1) the highly fluorescent nature of these samples and (2) instrument limitations, which necessitated long integration times and high power densities to collect spectra with good SNRs. Improvements in instrumentation in the last 20 years, particularly in the NIR region of the spectrum, where fluorescence is reduced, have engendered a dramatic increase in biomedical applications of dispersive Raman spectroscopy. Recent reviews of this field [32–34] illustrate the diversity of potential applications, ranging from monitoring of cataract formation in vivo [35] to the precise molecular diagnosis of atherosclerotic lesions in coronary arteries [36,37]. Many researchers have shown that Raman spectroscopy has the potential to diagnose disease in human tissues in vivo [38,39].

22.3 Instrumentation Considerations

Early applications of Raman spectroscopy for tissues used visible laser excitation, such as argon laser lines (see, e.g., Refs. [40,41]). FT-Raman spectroscopy was an advancement that improved the fidelity of tissue Raman spectra, typically using 1064 nm (Nd:YAG) for excitation with germanium detectors [10]. The development of diode lasers and cooled silicon CCD cameras with enhanced NIR sensitivity has enabled the use of Raman spectroscopy in a wide range of applications beyond the laboratory. Diode lasers can provide excitation in the region of 750–850 nm, which allows the use of silicon detectors (sensitive only to 1100 nm). The advantage of NIR *dispersive* Raman spectroscopy is that the fluorescence emission is reduced and spectra with acceptable SNR can be achieved with relatively short integration times of the order of a few seconds or less [42]. Thus, NIR Raman spectroscopy is now commonly used in environmental monitoring and manufacturing. Advances in Raman instrumentation realized by the commercial sector that supplies the aforementioned industries has positively impacted the application of Raman spectroscopy in biomedicine, making the future of Raman spectroscopy for clinical use a viable one.

22.3.1 Basic Instrumentation

The basic instrument capable of measuring Raman spectra is similar to any spectroscopic system in that it consists of a light source, which is typically a laser, light delivery and collection, and a detection system. Figure 22.3 represents the schematic of a typical clinical Raman system used today.

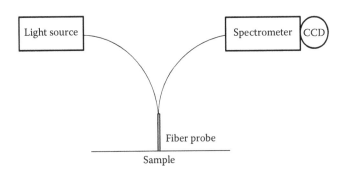

FIGURE 22.3 Schematic of a typical NIR dispersive Raman spectrometer used for tissue diagnosis today.

The weak nature of the Raman phenomenon is largely responsible for the design specifications that must be considered to successfully perform tissue measurements with this basic system. While the three basic components are coupled in terms of the overall system performance, as a first approximation, they can be looked at as individual components contributing to the system. Significant technological advances have been made in each of these areas resulting in Raman instruments that are superior to like systems from the previous decade. We will thus address these components individually, although their ultimate selection will be dependent on the intended use of the system. For example, a system capable of confocality will require a single-mode laser and appropriate optics. A clinical fiber-based Raman system can use a multimode diode laser and will require a rugged design that facilitates portability.

22.3.2 Light Sources

Traditional Raman systems used the argon ion laser for visible excitation, ND:YAG laser for FT-Raman applications, and the Ti:sapphire laser for NIR excitation due to their high output powers, single spatial and longitudinal mode operation, and Gaussian beam profile, which allows for near-diffraction-limited optical performance [43]. However, the size of these lasers and their electronic and cooling requirements make their utility in a portable clinical system impractical. Some current Raman instruments, especially those with confocal capabilities, still use the Ti:sapphire laser. However, advances in diode laser technology have completely changed the footprint of a typical Raman system. Diode lasers utilize electro-optical components (diodes), which emit light as a function of applied current and operating temperature. The laser diodes themselves are small (<1 mm^3) and require precision electronic controls to obtain a stable output. Laser diodes require highly stabilized temperature controllers to minimize thermoelastic effects on the laser cavity length (and thus output frequency) and highly stabilized current sources to minimize output power fluctuations. Laser diodes are also characterized by their elliptical beam output (due to the rectangular shape of the output facet) and astigmatism (due to unequal beam divergence from each dimension of the rectangular facet). These issues make free beam coupling of diode lasers non-trivial and beam-shaping optics are typically necessary for efficient fiber coupling. Nevertheless, most commercial diode lasers are available with a pigtail option where a fiber is coupled directly to the laser diode thus minimizing the losses due to astigmatism and elliptical nature of the beam.

In recent years, external cavity diode lasers (ECDLs) have emerged as robust and cost-effective light sources for Raman applications. By extending the length of the resonant cavity of a laser diode, the distance between the diode's longitudinal modes can be extended, thereby minimizing the effect of small thermoelastic changes on the output frequency. As compared to a bare laser diode, the ECDL nearly eliminates mode hops, minimizes spectral bandwidth of the output light, allows substantial wavelength tunability, and markedly decreases frequency dependence on temperature stabilization. The ability of ECDLs to provide laser linewidths of <0.001 nm (at 785 nm) with mode locking is vital for medical applications where measurement repeatability and spectral resolution are important performance parameters. ECDLs are commercially available in tunable Littman–Metcalf or Littrow configurations, as well as at tailored wavelengths using a distributed Bragg reflector configuration [44,45]. While tunable ECDLs have their advantages, ECDLs based on distributed Bragg reflectors are currently more reliable and rugged, which is an important design consideration when developing bedside Raman systems. Diode lasers that are mode stabilized with powers in the order of 300 mW, in single mode as well as multimode configurations are now commercially available. Some vendors specifically design sources for Raman spectroscopy, which eases the system development burden for researchers.

22.3.3 Detectors and Spectrometers

A typical dispersive Raman detection system consists of a short focal length imaging spectrograph attached to a cooled charge-coupled device (CCD) camera. Clinical implementation of the Raman system requires spectral acquisition in the order of a few seconds. This fast acquisition in turn needs a fast spectrograph and a highly sensitive detector especially given the weak nature of the Raman signal. A typical CCD camera used in spectroscopy consists of a rectangular chip wherein light is dispersed as a function of wavelength on the horizontal axis and the vertical axis is used to stack multiple collection fibers in an effort to optimize collection efficiency. The CCD output is then typically binned in the vertical direction to improve signal-to noise. Technological advances have led to CCD chips with quantum efficiencies on the order of 90% in the NIR. While different types of chips are commercially available for different applications, a back-illuminated, deep-depletion CCD is highly recommended for NIR Raman spectroscopy. These chips are known to be susceptible to the so-called etaloning effect wherein the thin silicon chip acts as an etalon resulting in the introduction of sharp peaks in the sample signal that are difficult to differentiate from the narrow Raman lines. However, commercial cameras are now available that incorporates technology that effectively eliminates this etaloning effect. Most laboratory-grade systems currently utilize CCDs actively cooled to at least −80°C in order to realize excellent dark noise performance. Liquid-nitrogen cooling was previously common; however, the development of thermoelectric (TE) multistage Peltier cooling systems with similar performance is far more advantageous for clinical applications because they require less maintenance. Although liquid nitrogen is still capable of deeper cooling with lower dark current, the short integrations times of current Raman measurements from biological systems make them obsolete. Currently, most researchers prefer TE cooling for most biomedical applications where the detected signal is primarily limited by shot noise.

Dispersive Raman spectroscopy is limited by tissue fluorescence which manifests as a background signal that must be removed so that Raman bands can be discerned. Most tissue fluorophores are primarily excited at UV and visible (UV/VIS) wavelengths below 600 nm. Therefore, NIR sources at wavelengths such as 633, 785, and 830 nm are preferred over those in the UV/VIS due to the less intense fluorescent background. Selection of appropriate NIR wavelengths for excitation is often governed by competing factors. The longer the wavelength, the lower the fluorescence background; however, the Raman scattering also decreases and is generally proportional to $1/\lambda^4$. In addition to minimizing background autofluorescence, acquisition of high SNR spectra also requires efficient detection of the scattered photons. Although the CCD detectors previously mentioned are capable of excellent performance over most of the NIR, the quantum efficiency decreases rapidly with increasing wavelength, falling below 15% at 1000 nm. The competing parameters of Raman scattering intensity, tissue autofluorescence, and detector efficiency all warrant careful consideration. For example, the use of an 830 nm source to acquire spectra from the high-wavenumber region ($v = 2400$–3800 cm^{-1}, $\lambda = 1036$–1212 nm) can be quite inefficient when using silicon-based detectors. For longer wavelengths, other types of detectors such as indium gallium arsenide (InGaAs), germanium, and indium phosphide (InP) detectors can suffer from either lower quantum efficiency and/or increased noise in comparison to silicon detectors. Nevertheless, instrument configurations utilizing Nd:YAG sources and multichannel InP/InGaAsP detectors have recently reported the feasibility of Raman spectroscopy of tissues such as the lung and gastric tissue at 1064 nm with acquisition times on the order of hundreds of seconds [46,47].

A Raman-sensitive detection system requires an appropriate imaging spectrograph that couples to the sample interface (such as a fiber probe) on one end and the CCD of choice at the other end. In order to resolve details of the Raman bands, the Raman detection system should have a spectral resolution of at most 8 cm^{-1}. Compact, rugged, spectrographs optimized for Raman use are now commercially available with *f*-number matching for standard fiber optics and high throughput for rapid acquisition. Since the Raman phenomenon is weak, high throughput is a critical performance feature. Spectrometers based on holographic transmissive gratings are most commonly used; however, there has recently been renewed interest in reflective and prism-based approaches for dispersion [48,49]. Recent interest in the high-wavenumber band has also resulted in the commercial availability of spectrometers with extended spectral coverage at the expense of either resolution or overall size. All of these spectrographs are compact in design and rugged for portable use. Additional components of the detection system include rejection filters that remove any laser light as well as the elastically scattered light from the detected signal. Holographic notch filters can block the laser wavelength with an optical density of six with steep edges and provide 90% transmission elsewhere with a relatively flat curve.

Most Raman measurements acquired for medical applications today are taken using state-of-the-art, high-cost, high-performance Raman systems [50,51]. One example of such a device would consist of a Kaiser Optical Systems imaging spectrograph with a Princeton Instruments or Andor TE-cooled, deep-depletion, back-illuminated CCD detector, a 300 mW Innovative Photonics Solutions diode laser, and a custom fiber probe. Typical integration times are on the order of 1–3 s for this type of system.

22.3.4 Light Delivery and Collection (Fiber Optics)

A critical aspect of translating Raman spectroscopy from the benchtop to bedside is an appropriate light delivery and collection. Raman scattering is a weak phenomenon but most materials are Raman active, which allows for molecular specific study of samples. On the other hand, since most molecules are Raman active, the optics used in the Raman system themselves can interfere with the detection of sample signal. With the development and availability of diode lasers, imaging spectrographs, and cooled CCD cameras, it is now possible to build compact NIR Raman systems that acquire spectra with short integration times. However, the limiting factor remains the signal generated in the delivery systems (luminescence and Raman) used for remote sensing [52]. Light is typically delivered using optical fibers made of silica in a remote sensing spectroscopic system. However, silica itself has a strong Raman signal, which overrides sample signal. The signal generated is proportional to the fiber length and limits the detection capability of the technique [53]. Figure 22.4 shows the Raman spectra of fused silica fibers (Diaguide fiber from Mitsubishi Cable) used to design a probe. Raman signal was observed to be generated from the core as well as the cladding and buffer of the fiber [53,54]. This signal can have magnitudes equal to and sometimes greater than that of the sample under study and thus needs careful consideration [52]. Fiber signal is generated in the delivery fiber by the excitation light. In addition, background signal is also generated in the collection fibers by the elastically scattered excitation light returning into the collection fiber(s). Mathematical techniques cannot be used to remove this unwanted fiber signal as it depends on the reflective and scattering nature of the sample. A feasible probe design must therefore prevent unwanted signal generated in the delivery fiber from illuminating the sample as well as prevent elastically scattered excitation light from entering the collection fibers and generating unwanted signal.

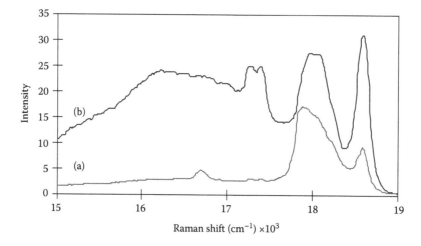

FIGURE 22.4 Raman and luminescence spectra at 488 nm excitation of (a) core in a 200 μm core silica fiber and (b) cladding and buffer of the same optical fiber.

Several different designs have been proposed for potential clinical acquisition of Raman spectra using fiber-optic probes. Early on, Angel et al. developed different dual-fiber probes, which could be used under different conditions with maximum collection efficiency but minimum fiber interference [52]. Most fiber designs since then have been based on similar concepts with modifications. In general, Raman probe designs utilize a band-pass filter placed after the excitation fiber lens, thus allowing only the transmission of the excitation light from the delivery fiber. In addition, the cutoff wavelength of dielectric band-pass filters shifts to the blue with increasing angle of incidence and has therefore been shown to act as a one-way mirror for elastically scattered light [55]. This phenomenon increases the overall efficiency of the probe by preventing multiply scattered incident photons from exiting the tissue and returning into the source fiber. Longpass or notch filters are also placed in front of the collection fibers to block the transmission of Fresnel reflected excitation light as well as to prevent the elastically scattered light from entering the collection fibers. These filters are placed at the tip of the probe for maximum effectiveness and have to be sized on the order of a few millimeters or smaller. There is thus a demand for high-quality optical coatings and micro-optical components that will simplify the design of compact fiber-optic probes for Raman spectroscopy in biomedicine.

Different designs yield different sample geometries and probe diameters, which in turn affect the application under consideration. It is therefore critical to consider the anatomy of the sample to be studied and the physiological/pathological process to be measured. A number of different sampling probes have been developed in order to meet specific design criteria, such as rapid acquisition time, depth selectivity, or the collection of data sets from complementary modalities. Here, we present an overview of the light delivery and collection designs that have been reported with the intent of clinical application.

22.3.4.1 Volumetric Approach

The most common design utilized to measure samples is a conventional, forward-looking design. Consisting of multiple collection fibers bundled with one or more excitation fibers, this design is intended to collect signal from the sample volume directly beneath the tip of the probe. The volume of sample measured is a function of the size, number, and configuration of collection fibers, as well as the optical properties of the sample itself. Using NIR excitation, these designs can measure up to several millimeters in depth depending upon sample extinction values.

Multifiber bundles have been utilized for fluorescence measurements of tissue by several groups [6–8]. Such a bundle commonly consists of a central excitation fiber surrounded by many collection fibers, which are linearly aligned in front of the spectrometer. McCreery et al. used this design and tested it on different samples [56]. Although spectra with good SNR could be obtained from transparent samples, fiber background was still a serious problem in samples with high elastic scattering such as tissue. Feld et al. adapted a design used in solar energy collection for improved signal collection to allow spectral acquisition in a few seconds [57]. A hollow compound parabolic concentrator (CPC) was used at the distal tip of the probe to yield signals with seven times greater collection than a fiber probe without the CPC. Fiber background was reduced by using a dichroic mirror and separate excitation and collection fiber geometries. This probe design was used to acquire Raman spectra for transcutaneous blood glucose measurements. Their design was subsequently modified to use a hyperbolic concentrator with improved results [58]. Both the McCreery probe and the CPC probe were designed for transcutaneous measurements where fiber background could be circumvented using a macroscopic arrangement. In fact, many commercially available probes are designed for remote access of exposed samples where dimensions of the device are not a concern.

However, other applications such as in the colon, cervix, and oral cavity require a more compact configuration and probe design. One of the first designs of a compact fiber probe used clinically in the cervix was reported by the author [59]. As stated before, a feasible probe design must prevent unwanted signal generated in the delivery fiber from illuminating the sample as well as prevent elastically scattered excitation light from entering the collection fibers and generating unwanted signal. Experimental results show

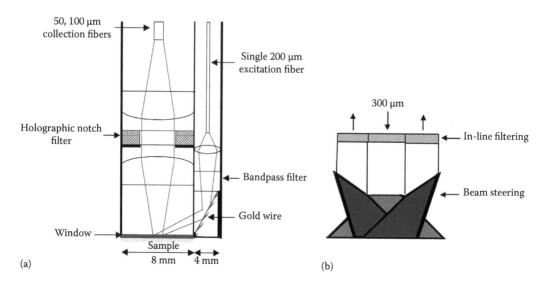

FIGURE 22.5 (a) Transverse section of the clinical Raman probe implemented in the cervix and (b) Enviva beam-steered probe from Visionex, Inc.

that significant proportions of silica signal are generated in the excitation *and* collection fibers, indicating the need for filters in both the excitation and collection legs of the probe. Figure 22.5 shows a transverse section of the design that was implemented as a Raman probe for the cervix [59]. Rather than placing the excitation leg at an angle (as in Ref. [57]), a mirror surface is placed in the excitation path to deflect the beam onto the sample. This probe was designed using the smallest available physical dimensions of both the band-pass and holographic notch filters at that time. An angularly polished gold wire was glued in place such that the deflected excitation and normal collection spots overlap. One of the collection fibers was used to provide an aiming beam during placement of the probe on the sample. A quartz shield was used at the tip of the common end of the probe forming a barrier between the probe optics and the sample. Quartz was selected as the material of choice as its fluorescence and Raman signal were known and any additional background signal from the probe could be identified. The inner surfaces of the metal tubings used to house the probe optics were anodized to reduce the incidence of multiple reflections of light.

This probe was tested in a pilot clinical study approved by the IRB. Raman spectra of the cervix were successfully measured in vivo [59]. Since this initial report, several designs for a Raman probe have been reported. One design that saw widespread use in the 1990s and early twenty-first century is the beam-steered Enviva Raman probe designed by Visionex, Inc. (now Cirrex, Corp.), which incorporated in-line filtering of the laser light and the scattered light at the tip of the probe [60]. The beam steering allowed improved overlap of the excitation and collection volumes thus improving signal collection efficiency (Figure 22.5b). Another unique feature of this probe was its overall dimension, which was on the order of 1–3 mm. No other commercially available fiber Raman probes could be found with such a small over-all diameter. However, these probes are no longer available commercially. Attempts have been made by other companies such as InPhotonics, Inc., to fill the gap. In a survey of currently available probes for biomedical Raman use, it was found that commercially available probes are typically bulky (up to several millimeters in diameter) and expensive (~$3500 or more). Thus, proponents of Raman spectroscopy for tissue diagnosis must rely on custom-designed fiber probes built using commercial vendors.

As a result, new designs have been recently reported. For example, the Feld group proposed a design using ball lens and optical coatings for breast cancer detection [61]. The author's group relies on probes built by Emvision, Inc., whose designs provide dimensions similar to the Enviva probes but without the beam steering [62]. Custom-designed fiber designs also provide the option of customizing depth selectivity, volume of collection, and probe dimensions based on the sample geometry and access.

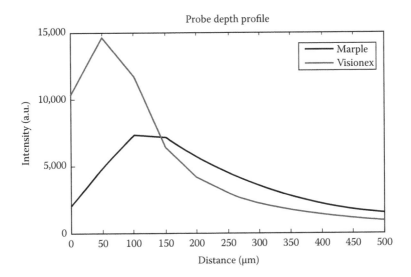

FIGURE 22.6 Spectral intensity of a given Raman band as a function of depth for two different Raman probes: Visionex, beam-steered probe shown in Figure 22.5b, and Marple, 6-around-1 fiber probe with in-line filtering.

Recent developments in the field of microfabrication (MEMs) open a new avenue for compact probe designs such as those presented by Dochow et al. [63].

Although bundled fiber probes can be designed to allow for efficient collection of inelastically scattered light, the sample volume from which signals are collected tend to be on the order of hundreds of microns to millimeters and therefore probe macroscopic volumes of the sample. These probes typically do not provide depth selectivity and resolution. The depth–response profile follows an exponential decay function as per the attenuation of light in tissue (Figure 22.6).

Some of the potentially promising clinical challenges addressable with Raman spectroscopy, such as noninvasive biochemical characterization of bone [64,65] or the detection of skin cancers [66], can benefit from collection of spectral information with a degree of depth sensitivity. While there have been recent attempts to design fiber probes that only collect Raman light from the superficial 100–200 μm of the sample, looking deeper into samples such as tissue require more advanced methods of design. Ultrafast time-gated Raman spectroscopy is an approach that relies on picosecond pulsed excitation sources and ultrafast optical shutters to realize temporal resolutions sufficient to distinguish superficially scattered photons from their more deeply penetrating counterparts [67]. However, much like CARS, this approach requires large, extensive instrumentation along with high peak power sample illumination and therefore may be impractical for routine clinical use. The two most practical methods for acquiring subsurface weighted Raman signals from tissue in vivo include confocal Raman spectroscopy (CRS) and spatially offset Raman spectroscopy (SORS). CRS is capable of optical sectioning with an axial resolution on the scale of microns but provides limited penetration depth. SORS, on the other hand, has the ability to isolate the Raman signature of a specific tissue layer deeper within the tissue, but does not directly acquire light from specific depths. CRS and SORS achieve depth sensitivity through different mechanisms, thus requiring entirely different considerations in the design of a sample interface. Although the two techniques are both capable of collecting spectra that originate below the tissue surface, they may ultimately prove to provide information that is more complementary than it is competing.

22.3.4.2 Confocal Raman Spectroscopy

CRS of living cells [43,68–70] and tissues is a mature approach to interrogating biological specimens due to the fact that it is easily adapted to microscopes and proven commercial systems are available from companies such as Renishaw and Horiba Scientific. In confocal collection, a high numerical aperture (NA) objective lens is used, and scattered light passes through an aperture that rejects out-of-focus light and allows axial resolutions of as small as 1 μm. Since the Raman spectrum is a molecular signature, measurement performed at high resolution with spatial overlay can simplify interpretation of complex biological spectra and provide valuable insight into the compositional as well as microstructural features of cells and tissues. Confocal Raman microscopes have been used extensively in tissues, using Raman maps to evaluate cellular components and processes associated with disease [71–73]. However, most of these studies have been performed in vitro using a benchtop device. The confocal approach can also be implemented using micro-optics into a handheld instrument that can be applied in vivo.

Confocal Raman probes for in vivo measurements were initially developed for analysis of the most easily accessible organ, the skin [74], and utilized an optical design similar to that of a conventional inverted microscope. This design has ultimately been adapted into a specially designed clinical microscope and commercialized by River Diagnostics, International. Lieber et al. developed a handheld confocal Raman microscope that miniaturized the optical design while still utilizing bulk optics and a microscope objective for focusing light onto the sample [66]. The resulting handheld probe (Figure 22.7) could then be easily maneuvered to acquire measurements from various locations across the body. The laser light source and spectrograph were tethered to the probe via fiber optics. The Raman collection fiber also served as the confocal aperture and provided an axial resolution of 14 μm.

In addition to bulk-optic confocal probes, a number of groups have reported fiber-optic probes with focused collection designs that aim to reproduce the depth selectivity of confocal Raman microscopy. Yamamoto et al. reported the development of a fiber-optic probe that incorporated a hollow fiber with a ball lens at the distal tip [75,76]. Although the probe is not confocal, the probe does allow for collection of depth resolved measurements with an axial resolution of 46 μm. Day et al. reported a miniaturized fiber-optic Raman probe for endoscopic use that is capable of being placed in the auxiliary channel of an endoscope [76,77]. This design is based on separate fibers for light delivery and collection and the use of a single 2.4 mm diameter aspheric lens as the objective. Duraipandian et al. [78] have reported a similarly designed probe that uses a sapphire ball lens as the objective. Both probes report axial resolutions of approximately 150 μm. Although the resolutions are much larger than in true confocal probes, they do still allow for isolated

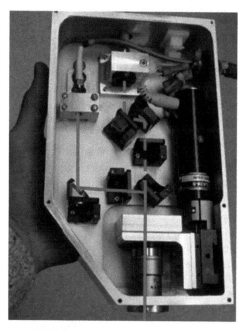

FIGURE 22.7 Handheld probe reported by Lieber et al. Solid line indicates optical path of laser source and dashed line indicates optical path of Raman collection.

measurements of epithelial tissues, as demonstrated by subsequent in vivo studies in the esophagus and cervix. The design of fiber-optic focused probes also requires careful selection of the appropriate filters to eliminate fluorescence in the fibers and minimization of elastic scatter, as in nonfocused probes.

Confocal Raman approaches provide the opportunity for information with high spatial resolution and cellular level detail. However, tissue diagnosis often depends on bulk tissue effects and a multitude of cellular features that may be lost in a system with microlevel resolution. The near confocal probes described earlier are more beneficial in that they yield features of a few cells as opposed to subcellular detail and may be considered to be more amenable to disease detection. One main limitation of confocal probes is the loss of SNR and limited penetration depth that can be achieved. Thus, selection of such an approach should be made based on the sample and condition under study.

22.3.4.3 Spatially Offset Raman Spectroscopy

Early work in photon migration theory performed by Chance et al. detailed the concept of performing optical measurements of elastic scattering at the surface of turbid tissues with improved sensitivity to underlying layers by introducing a spatial offset between the source and detector [79]. This concept has been applied in a variety of techniques including absorption and scattering spectroscopies for deep tissue probing as well as for tomographic applications. SORS introduces depth selectivity in the spectral measurements with a spatial offset between the source and detector elements of the system. Photon migration theory dictates that photons incident on the tissue surface that reemerge after only a few scattering events are likely to undergo minimal transverse shift and travel through the most superficial depths (Figure 22.8). Photons that undergo many scattering events are more likely to undergo a larger transverse shift and also travel deeper within the tissue, due to the fact that the scattering phase function of tissue is primarily in the forward direction. The intensity of the Raman-scattered light at zero spatial

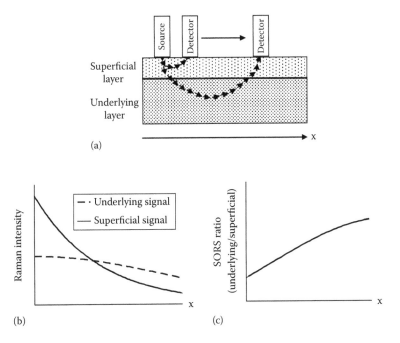

FIGURE 22.8 Illustration of SORS signal as a function of lateral offset in a simplified two-layer sample (a). The measured signal at any given spatial offset contains contributions from both the superficial and underlying layers; however, as the spatial offset increases, the spectral intensity of features arising from the superficial layers falls off faster than the intensity arising from the underlying layers (b). The result is an increase in the relative signal intensity arising from the underlying layer (c).

offset includes contributions from both the superficial and underlying layers. However, as the spatial offset increases, the signal intensity from the superficial layers falls off more rapidly than the intensity of the signal from the underlying layers increasing the relative proportion of signal from the deeper layers. The SORS signal can be collected through a range of spatial offsets, and computational techniques such as band-targeted entropy minimization (BTEM) or partial least-squares regression can be applied to isolate the spectral signature from the individual layers [80,81]. Further, if the structure and optical properties of the sample's layers are known, SORS can be used to determine depth-dependent properties of the sample [82,83]. It is important to note that while SORS can yield Raman spectra from deep within the tissue, it does so in a numerical fashion that is based on the tissue having a layered architecture in which the spectral signatures of the layers are separable. This stands in contrast to confocal RS, which explicitly rejects out-of-focus light and is thus capable of collecting spectra from a well-defined depth. This makes SORS better suited for a more *low-resolution* depth-dependent measurement of features at greater depths than confocal RS.

While a classic Raman system as shown in Figure 22.3 can also be used to make SORS measurements, the challenge is in designing appropriate light delivery and collection interfaces for tissue applications. A number of illumination and collection geometries are possible in the design of a SORS probe. In the simplest configuration, the SORS signal from a single illumination spot is collected from a single spatially offset collection spot (Figure 22.8). This arrangement is possible with either separate optical fibers or through bulk optics with different illumination and collection axes. Bulk-optic designs are possible with an axicon collection lens [84] and have the advantage of allowing a full annular ring to be collected while maintaining flexibility over the exact spatial offset. When the desired spatial offset(s) are generally known, a fiber-optic implementation can be pursued for a more rugged design with increased collection efficiency. Probes have been developed with a ring of collection fibers at a fixed distance from the central illumination fiber [64] or in a fan-shaped array [85] (Figure 22.9). At the distal end of these probes, the detection fibers are arranged vertically for transmission through the slit of the spectrograph. The practical limitation of these configurations is the finite height of the CCD. Inverse SORS represents an alternative approach in which the illumination and collection axes are reversed. The benefit is that illumination over an annular ring can increase the photon flux while maintaining a similar irradiance at the sample surface, thus improving SNR and decreasing integration times. In addition, the number of collection fibers can be reduced, which simplifies spectrograph coupling and detection. However, if the subsurface target tissue is not uniformly illuminated due to its size or shape, it is possible that many of the incident photons can miss their mark, thus reducing overall efficiency.

Matousek first demonstrated SORS in diffusely scattering media using a two-layer phantom in which each layer had a chemical with a distinctive spectrum, and the measured spectra became more similar to the bottom layer with increased separation [86]. The same group provided Monte Carlo simulation results of similar setups [82] and demonstrated the first biological application of this technique in detecting the strong Raman signature of bone through several millimeters of soft tissue [64]. Since that time, Okagbare et al.

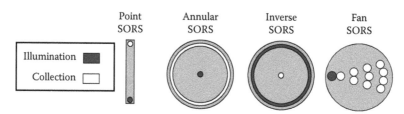

FIGURE 22.9 SORS illumination/collection geometries. From left to right: point SORS where one fiber is connected to the source and one fiber to the detector. Annular SORS uses a multitude of detection fibers at a defined spatial offset. Inverse SORS uses a multitude of source fibers to a single detector fiber at a defined offset. Fan SORS uses a single-source fiber with an increasing number of detector fibers at a series of spatial offset with comparable SNR from each ring.

and Maher et al. have reported valuable developments that will accelerate the application of SORS to the study of bone as it pertains to cancer, aging, and osteoarthritis [87–89]. Matousek and Stone, and Stone et al. have also used SORS to detect the Raman spectral features of hydroxyapatite, a mineral commonly present in breast cancer calcifications, through varying thicknesses of overlying lean chicken breast tissue [90,91]. SORS has also been used to distinguish between layers of soft tissues that have more subtle differences in Raman features as compared to strong scatterers such as bone and calcifications [92]. Soft tissue SORS has also been successfully developed for the ex vivo intraoperative assessment of breast cancer margins in tumor resection surgery using the fan-type SORS probe [85].

An exciting development in the field of SORS is the tomographic reconstruction of Raman spectra via inverse modeling of photon diffusion to yield a 3D Raman tomogram. This approach was initially demonstrated by Schulmerich et al. who reconstructed a section of canine tibia and verified the image using computed tomography (CT) scans [83]. A subsequent report demonstrated the ability to improve the accuracy and contrast of tomographic reconstruction using spatial priors generated from CT [93]. The potential of SORS as a 3D technique for evaluating the compositional properties of bone represents an exciting frontier that may have significant clinical significance in mapping bone quality noninvasively.

22.3.4.4 Multimodal Approaches

Clinically, differential diagnosis of disease is a complex challenge in which physicians typically combine or integrate information from multiple sources to arrive at a conclusion. Raman spectroscopy can provide valuable biochemical information; however, there are a number of powerful optical technologies that offer complementary information to Raman spectra. In an effort to improve the clinical potential of Raman spectroscopy, a number of groups have pursued the development of multimodal optical technologies that include both imaging techniques as well as alternative spectroscopic modalities.

Since creating Raman maps of tissue morphology or structure can be difficult in a clinically relevant time frame, the addition of high-speed imaging techniques such as optical coherence tomography (OCT) and confocal reflectance microscopy, as well as other wide-field imaging modalities has become an area of active interest. One of the primary limitations to clinical implementation of CRS is the fact that epithelial tissues, particularly diseased epithelial tissues, contain significant structural and compositional heterogeneity on the micron scale. As a result, the specific location at which data are collected can dramatically influence the resultant Raman spectra. The combination of confocal reflectance microscopy with Raman spectroscopy can result in collection of image-guided confocal Raman spectra and reduce sampling error. In addition, since confocal reflectance images do not contain molecularly specific contrast, the two techniques can be mutually beneficial. Combined confocal reflectance imaging–CRS instruments have typically used the same laser light source for both modalities and split the optical path of the detection legs using dichroic mirrors [94,95]. Early work in combining confocal reflectance with confocal Raman demonstrated the feasibility of the approach for imaging the skin using a Lucid microscope with Raman spectroscopy [95]. With the benefit of image guidance, localized spectra from glandular structures and capillaries, as well as registered spectral information of natural moisturizing factor in the stratum corneum (topmost layer of skin), could be obtained. More recently, a miniaturized handheld combined confocal reflectance–confocal Raman device has been developed using a MEMS optical scanner to create confocal images [94]. This device offers promise for further work in clinical translation (Figure 22.10).

Interpretation and analysis of Raman spectra on a larger spatial scale can also benefit from the presence of registered images. OCT is a rapidly growing imaging technique with millimeter-scale images at micron-scale resolution. Unlike confocal imaging, which creates en face images, OCT creates cross-sectional images similar to histopathology slides, which can help physicians' interpretation. As in confocal imaging, OCT displays structural features and does not contain any biochemically specific information. The combination of OCT with Raman spectroscopy offers the opportunity for image-guided Raman acquisition to minimize the likelihood of sampling error when targeting underlying microstructural features that may be difficult to visualize. In addition, clinical interpretation of images

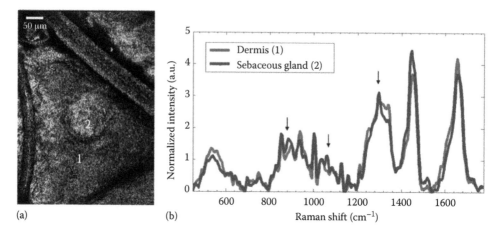

(a)   (b)

FIGURE 22.10 Combined confocal reflectance image (a) and Raman spectra (b) of a sebaceous gland in comparison to adjacent normal dermis. Spectra acquired from within the glandular structure shows characteristic features of sebum and fatty acids at 884, 1157, and 1297 cm^{-1}.

alongside spectra can increase clinician's confidence in spectral classification. A number of groups have reported combined Raman spectroscopy–OCT instruments [96–98], which typically consist of independent Raman and OCT systems that have a common sample arm. The systems are integrated by coaligning the Raman illumination beam with the OCT beam in order to register the images and spectra, and recorded signals are detected by two independent devices. An alternative system design has been reported in which the Raman and OCT systems were integrated to combine both the sample as well detection arms [99]. This technology takes advantage of the spectral domain OCT system architecture to use the same spectrograph and camera for Raman and OCT. Light from the two modalities is offset on the detector chip, which is then binned accordingly to separate Raman from OCT light. By integrating the two detection systems, the sampling volumes are coaligned and each technique can be used to improve on the performance of the other. The value of Raman and OCT to perform morphological and biochemical assessment of tissues has been demonstrated in tissues including skin [98,100], breast [98], bone [98], and the retina [96]. More recent work has seen the development of a clinical Raman–OCT system for assessing skin cancers [100]. This work highlighted challenges related to evaluating skin lesions using either Raman or OCT alone and demonstrated how the combination of the two techniques can be used to thoroughly characterize structural and compositional properties together (Figure 22.11).

Endoscopic assessment of diseases is an area where both optical imaging techniques such as narrowband and autofluorescence imaging have seen measured clinical success in disease diagnosis alongside Raman spectroscopy. However, both narrowband imaging and autofluorescence suffer from low diagnostic specificity, a strength of Raman spectroscopy. The complementary nature of these three modalities motivated the development of a trimodal endoscopic probe that incorporated all three techniques along with traditional white-light imaging [101]. The Raman illumination and detection channels were isolated from the other three but registered in the image frame. The feasibility and value of the device was demonstrated with in vivo images and spectra taken during investigation of the upper GI tract. Similar to the previously mentioned combinations with confocal reflectance and OCT, this type of multimodal instrument has strong potential for further clinical use due to its ability to leverage the unique strengths of each incorporated modality.

In addition to multimodal devices that combine imaging and spectroscopy, multiple spectroscopic approaches have been combined for improved disease detection. The Feld group developed a multimodal spectroscopy device that incorporated intrinsic autofluorescence, Raman, and diffuse reflectance spectroscopy for the evaluation of vascular disease and atherosclerosis [37,102]. Each modality requires

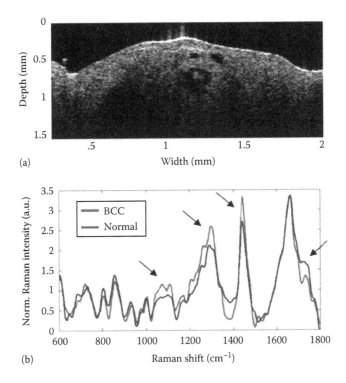

FIGURE 22.11 Clinical Raman–OCT data from BCC. BCC tumor cell nests appear as dark hyporeflective features in OCT image (a); however, hyporeflective features are also observed in noncancerous skin lesions. Spectral analysis of the tumor identifies a spectral lineshape characteristic of BCC, with increased relative intensity in comparison to matched normal skin in the region surrounding 1100, at 1270, 1440, and near 1680 cm^{-1} (b).

its own light source, and the three techniques are integrated into a common multimodal probe. The distinctly different spectral ranges of the illumination sources (UV/VIS for autofluorescence, white light for diffuse reflectance, and IR for Raman) result in each modality probing the tissue over different depth scales, which can be a valuable feature. This is particularly true in atherosclerosis, where the risk of intravascular plaque is dependent on the composition of their cap, superficial regions, and underlying core. The combination of Raman and autofluorescence spectroscopy has also shown potential for improving the assessment of skin lesions [103]. Researchers have combined NIR autofluorescence generated with the Raman light source with the acquired Raman signals to improve the statistical classification of the skin [104]. More recently, a multimodal technique utilizing UV autofluorescence along with NIR Raman has been reported as an alternative over infrared approaches alone [103]. Often, multimodal approaches are developed in an effort to improve the performance of a single modality alone. However, it is important to consider that limitations in performance may be a function of physiological variability and adding more modalities may not add to its success. One must also weigh the potential improvement in diagnosis with reasonable and practical cost of implementing such combined approaches.

22.3.5 Effect of Sample Conditions

The design and construction of a Raman system is clearly a critical part of the process. An often forgotten aspect in the use of a technique deals with the application itself. In developing and applying an approach, the technology must first be tested in a model system before it can be applied in vivo. Subsequently, when it is ready for in vivo use, several factors unique to clinical use must also be considered. These issues are addressed in the following.

22.3.5.1 Tissue Model Selection

There exist two philosophies in the field of spectroscopy on the approach to use in testing the feasibility of a given technique. Some researchers prefer to use an animal model that resembles human tissues in function and structure to simulate the behavior of human tissues, while others prefer in vitro human tissue studies before tackling in vivo studies. Each of these approaches needs to be carefully considered in the context of the human in vivo model.

While an animal model allows in vivo testing, Raman spectra of animal tissues can in some cases differ from that of human tissues resulting in invalid conclusions. One example of this is the use of mouse eye lenses for the study of lens aging [105]. In early studies, Yu suggested that the intensity of Raman bands at 2580 cm^{-1} due to sulfhydryl groups (–SH) and 508 cm^{-1} due to disulfide groups (–S–S) can be used to calculate their relative concentrations, which can then be related to aging and cataract formation. In an extensive study of mouse lenses, a fall in –SH concentration and a corresponding increase in –S–S concentration was observed along the visual axis of mouse lens nucleus from age 1 to 6 months. A tandem increase in protein development with a decrease in sulfhydryl was concluded to accompany the normal aging process. However, on repeating these studies on guinea pig and human lenses, a different phenomenon was observed. Although guinea pig lenses also showed a decrease in sulfhydryl intensity, no corresponding increase in disulfide band was observed. Human eye lenses behaved similar to guinea pig lenses. This study clearly indicates the pitfalls in improper selection of an animal model and indicates that independent verification of the model is needed to ensure that results will be applicable to human conditions.

A primary concern in devising a clinical diagnostic system based on Raman spectroscopy is whether the spectra of excised tissue resemble those of tissue spectra acquired in vivo and whether the information obtained from these in vitro studies can be applied to a clinical setting. It is well known that the spectra acquired from in vitro tissues especially those that have undergone the freeze–thaw process differ from those acquired in vivo [106]. Spectra from intact human stratum corneum were compared to that from excised human stratum corneum [107]. Significant differences in the Raman spectral features were observed. Increased intensity of the C–C stretching vibrational bands at 1030 and 1130 cm^{-1} was observed in vivo. An additional spectral band at 3230 cm^{-1} of unknown origin is observed only in vivo. Fixed tissues specimens typically exhibit Raman bands associated with the fixative as well as other biochemical effects such as protein denaturation and an overall decrease in signal intensity [108]. Thus, spectra acquired from fixed tissues cannot be compared to in vivo conditions and any conclusions drawn must be carefully considered. Thus, it is important to be aware of the potential differences that may occur when moving from in vitro studies to in vivo conditions. Most researchers who follow this approach use the in vitro studies as proof of concept before moving directly into in vivo studies.

22.3.5.2 In Vivo Considerations

In vivo clinical application of the technology is a primary goal for many researchers in this field. However, there are various issues that are specific to working in vivo that need to be considered in the planning of these clinical studies. There are logistic issues such as Institutional Review Board approval and consent forms, which have become challenging processes today. When building a clinical system, some of the practical issues that need to be considered are as follows. The probe needs to be sterilized or disinfected depending on the application, thus, should be designed to withstand the physical and chemical conditions of these processes. The power consumption of the Raman system needs to be such that hospital and/or clinic systems are not overloaded. This can be verified via the engineering department of the hospital. Acquisition times need to be on the order of a few seconds for the sake of patient as well as clinician participation. The system itself needs to be self-contained and nonobtrusive. While some of these considerations appear to be trivial, each of these issues contributes to the smooth running of clinical studies.

Application of any technique that uses lasers must follow certain safety standards to avoid potential hazards. Safety standards for laser exposure of skin and eye have been set by the American National

Standards Institute (ANSI). The power densities used for successful Raman spectral acquisitions can be quite high and warrant consideration of safety hazards. The maximum permissible exposures as set by ANSI are wavelength dependent and can be calculated for a given exposure time following the directions laid out in the ANSI laser safety manual [109].

22.3.5.3 Sources of Variability

Experimentally, there are various sources of variability that can affect spectral measurements made in vivo and should be taken into consideration. These include instrumentation effects, ambient effects, operator variation, pressure effects, and procedural interference. In a recent parametric study, duplicate systems with two similar excitation sources, probe designs, spectrographs, and detectors were compared to determine the influence from each component on the collected Raman signal. While laser source, spectrograph, and detector had only minimal impact on the acquired signal, differences in the fiber probe significantly altered the signal obtained from a sample. Therefore, spectra recorded with a specific probe can be reliably compared regardless of other instrumentation combinations used to obtain the measurements.

Regardless of the short duration of the integration times used for Raman acquisition, ambient effects can significantly influence spectral integrity. Room lights as well as daylight (from the sun) will introduce spectral features that simple mathematical algorithms may not reliably remove. While room lights can be turned off, some patients may not be comfortable in a dark room. Windows can present a greater challenge, since standard window shades do not entirely eliminate background sunlight; therefore, it is important to carefully plan the clinical setting of a Raman spectroscopy study. Other sources of variability include those that arise between different operators or physicians. The effect of varying pressures applied to the probe and angular placement of the probe during acquisition should be considered. Another critical source of variability in the validation of a Raman spectroscopy study is the correlation between measurement site and biopsy site. Since histology continues to be the gold standard against which we must compare this technology, it is critical that the biopsy be obtained from the precise site of spectral measurement using such techniques as marking inks placed appropriately. In addition, it is important to consider intra- and interpatient variability that simply reflects the innate physiological variability of organs and tissues [110]. Certainly, the patient-to-patient variability is the most significant source of uncertainty introduced in any comparative study (Figure 22.12). The high sensitivity of Raman spectroscopy to tissue biochemistry can produce spectral variance that correlates with subtle physiological differences such as those associated with hormonal cycling. In expansive epithelial tissues such as the GI tract and the skin, there is a significant amount of innate variability in the organization and molecular composition of tissue that is important to consider during data analysis. Thus, there exist various sources of variability beyond those related to the instrument that need to be accounted for when acquiring and analyzing Raman spectra from human patients in vivo.

Prior work to assess these sources of variability indicates that when properly used, contact pressure, probe angle, and probe replacement have no significant contribution to spectral variability [110]. Thorough analysis of the potential sources of measurement error should be conducted with any system to understand the obtained results, ideally prior to initiation of the study. To limit the user-induced and physiological variability detected, several steps should be taken during the design and execution of in vivo Raman measurements. These steps include the following: (1) Standardized tissue cleaning protocols, such as cleaning with alcohol or saline, should be used to minimize error contribution (such as from cosmetics and lotions in skin, mucus from the cervix); (2) measurements with the probe should use low but consistent pressure during collection, keeping the probe approximately normal to the surface (user should be trained); (3) for normal control measurements, studies show that intrapatient variability is negligible and therefore a single collection per location is sufficient (Figure 22.12); (4) paired measurements could provide normalization of a spectrum to the inherent signal based on anatomical location and person-specific signals; and (5) the selection of the location for a normal paired measurement should be carefully determined, avoiding confounding signatures such as those arising from hair follicles and major superficial blood vessels in skin measurements. Furthermore, adjacent and contralateral

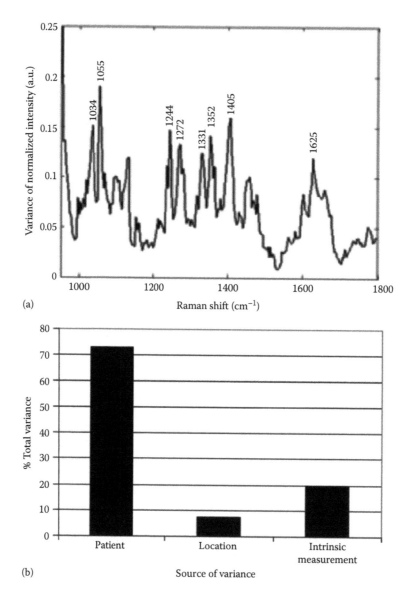

(a)

(b)

FIGURE 22.12 Components of variance. A total of 180 spectra of normal ectocervix from 29 patients were used for the analysis. (a) Total variance at each wavenumber, (b) percent of total variance due to interpatient (between patients), intrapatient (between locations), and intrinsic measurement variability.

normal measurements at a single location should be investigated for consistency. Thus, there exist various sources of variability beyond those related to the instrument that need to be accounted for when acquiring and analyzing Raman spectra from human patients in vivo.

22.3.6 Data Processing

Once a Raman spectrum is acquired, the spectrum needs to be processed for various reasons before interpretation. These include source variation, detector response, noise smoothing, fluorescence elimination, and binning to name a few. Other processing methods may need to be applied depending on the needs of the analysis tools and the variability in the data.

22.3.6.1 Calibration

Since different researchers have different approaches to the development of a given application for Raman spectroscopy, a standard needs to be set to allow transferability of data across systems and methods. Thus, calibration for system response is a key component to data processing immediately following data acquisition. Some of the calibration needs to occur at the time of acquisition, while others may be implemented later. Source compensation is a standard process that is applied to control for variability in the source from measurement to measurement. Instrument response variations require two types of calibration: spectral calibration and intensity calibration. Spectral calibration is used to convert the horizontal measurement axis from pixel numbers to relative wavenumbers. The spectrum of a known calibrated source such as a neon lamp is typically used to calibrate the horizontal axis into absolute wavenumbers (cm^{-1}). Relative wavenumber calibration is performed using the spectrum of the laser line and then validated through the acquisition of substances with well-characterized Raman features and strong Raman scatter, such as naphthalene and acetaminophen. In addition, spectral standards such as the fluorophore rhodamine 6G and a weak Raman scatterer such as methylene blue can be used as intensity standards to account for day-to-day variations in the spectral intensity.

Calibration of the intensity axis is necessary to account for the wavelength-dependent response of the various components in the detection leg of the system such as the grating, the filters, optics, and quantum efficiency of the CCD chip. This is typically performed using a NIST-calibrated source such as a tungsten lamp to generate intensity correction factors for variations in instrument throughput [54]. Such calibration is essential for comparison of the measured and process spectra to those measured using other instruments for the same sample. Perturbation of any of the optical components such as that caused by moving the system from the laboratory to the clinic can affect the calibration and therefore a method for day-to-day calibration of the system performance must be developed. Collection of a tungsten lamp intensity spectrum can often be impractical in a clinical situation due to the experimental controls necessary to ensure that the bright, diffuse emission of the lamp traverses only its intended path through the Raman instrument to the detector, along with the safety concerns that correspond to the spectral intensity in the UV portion of the spectrum. More recently, spectral intensity standards consisting of green-colored Schott glass have been explored by NIST and other groups [111] as more practical alternatives, but no consensus has been reached yet on their applicability. Thus, as calibrated Raman spectra are acquired by the various researchers, a library of tissue Raman spectra can be created that can be used to study cross-links in the chemical compositions and correlation in tissue pathologies as well as to strengthen and standardize the use of Raman spectroscopy for tissue diagnosis.

22.3.6.2 Fluorescence Elimination

Recent years have seen an explosion in the use of Raman spectroscopy for biological purposes such as tissue diagnosis, blood analyte detection, and cellular examination. The greatest benefit of this technique is its high sensitivity to subtle molecular (biochemical) change, as well as its capability for nonintrusive application. But biological applications of Raman spectroscopy involve turbid, chemically complex, and widely varying target sites. Thus, much of the challenge in using Raman spectroscopy for biological purposes is not only the acquisition of viable Raman signatures but also the suppression of inherent noise sources present in the target media. Perhaps the greatest contributor of *noise* to biological Raman spectra is the intrinsic fluorescence of many organic molecules in biological materials. This fluorescence is often several orders of magnitude more intense than the weak chemical transitions probed by Raman spectroscopy and, if left untreated, can dominate the Raman spectra and render analysis of tissue biochemistry as probed by the technique impractical. Therefore, in order to extract Raman signal from the raw spectra acquired, it is necessary to process the spectrum to remove this fluorescence. Even though most biological fluorescence occurs in the UV/VIS, sufficient fluorescence is observed in the NIR to interfere with the collected Raman spectrum and therefore must be removed before spectral analysis.

A number of techniques, implemented both in hardware and software, have been proposed for fluorescence subtraction from raw Raman signals. Hardware methods such as wavelength shifting and time gating have been shown to effectively minimize fluorescence interference in Raman spectra but require modification of the spectroscopic system to achieve their results [112,113]. Mathematical methods implemented in software require no such system modifications and have thus become the norm for fluorescence removal. These methods include first- and second-order differentiation [114,115], frequency-domain filtering [112], wavelet transformation [116,117], and manual polynomial fitting [54,118]. Though each of these methods has been shown to be useful in certain situations, they are not without limitations.

Differentiation can be implemented in various ways. One way is by measuring the spectra at two slightly shifted excitation wavelengths and taking their difference [119]. The fluorescence remains unchanged at both excitation wavelengths whereas the Raman peaks are shifted. The difference of the two spectra is comparable to the first derivative of the Raman spectrum; integrating the difference spectrum yields the original Raman signal. A similar result can be obtained by measuring the spectrum at a single excitation wavelength and taking the first derivative of the spectrum (Figure 22.10). The Raman spectrum can be obtained by integrating the noise-smoothed derivative spectrum following baseline correction [112,115]. The derivative method is entirely unbiased and very efficient in fluorescence subtraction, yet it severely distorts Raman lineshapes and relies on complex mathematical fitting algorithms to reproduce a traditional spectral form [112]. While many of these methods were developed and tested in the early 1990s, shifted excitation methods for removing this undesirable fluorescent signal, coined as modulated wavelength Raman spectroscopy, are coming back into vogue, utilizing multiple closely spaced excitation sources and signal processing algorithms to remove fluorescence signal [120]. While newer sources allow the use of multiple excitation wavelengths to improve the accuracy of the method, issues related to a DC offset remain.

Frequency filtering can be achieved by using the fast Fourier transform (FFT). In this technique, the measured spectrum is Fourier transformed to the frequency domain by taking the FFT of the signal. The FFT signal can then be multiplied with a linear digital filter to eliminate the fluorescence (Figure 22.10). The inverse FFT then yields the Raman spectrum free of fluorescence [112]. This method can cause artifacts to be generated in the processed spectra if the frequency elements of the Raman and noise features are not well separated.

A more elegant method to subtract fluorescence that is both simple and accurate is to fit the measured spectrum containing both Raman and fluorescence information to a polynomial of high-enough order to describe the fluorescence lineshape but not the higher-frequency Raman lineshape. Polynomial curve fitting has a distinct advantage over other fluorescence reduction techniques in its ability to retain the spectral contours and intensities of the input Raman spectra. However, simply fitting a polynomial curve to the raw Raman spectrum in a least-squares manner will not efficiently reproduce the fluorescence background, as the fit will be based on minimizing the differences between the fit and the measured spectra, which includes both the fluorescence background and the Raman peaks. Thus, subsequent subtraction of this fit polynomial, then, will result in a spectrum that varies about the zero baseline. This technique then traditionally relies on user-selected spectral locations on which to base the fit from regions that do not include the more intense Raman bands. Unfortunately, this intervention has several drawbacks. It is time consuming, as the user must process each spectrum individually to identify non-Raman-active spectral regions to be used in the fit. In addition, identification of non-Raman-active frequencies is not always trivial, as biological Raman spectra sometimes contain several adjacent peaks or peaks that are not immediately obvious. The end effect is a method that is highly subjective and prone to variability. In order to address the limitations of existing methods of fluorescence subtraction, various methods to automate polynomial curve fitting have been developed, which retain the benefits of manual curve fitting, without the need for user intervention.

In one implementation of this automation, the basis is a simple sliding-window mean filter, in which the center pixel intensity in the window is set equal to the mean of all the intensities within the window [121]. The modification involved in this method is that any filtered pixels that have an intensity value higher than the original are automatically reassigned to the original intensity. Therefore, the smoothing only eliminates high-frequency Raman peaks while retaining the underlying shape of the baseline fluorescence. This smoothing is repeated over the entire spectrum until a specified coefficient of determination (R^2) of the processed spectrum with an nth-order polynomial (typically fifth) is obtained. The smoothed spectrum is then subtracted from the raw spectrum to yield the Raman bands on a near-null baseline. This algorithm can be implemented easily in MATLAB®, thus automating the entire procedure.

Figure 22.13 shows the Raman spectrum of a rhodamine 6G, as well as the processed Raman spectrum using derivative, FFT, and automated polynomial fluorescence subtraction techniques for direct comparison of the methods. The figure shows the effectiveness of the automated polynomial method to remove the slow varying fluorescence baseline while retaining the Raman features of rhodamine especially in comparison to the other methods.

Each of the different techniques has advantages and disadvantages and the method used should be selected based on the specific application and measurement technique used. Mosier-Boss et al. tested the use of the shifted excitation, first derivative, and FFT techniques for fluorescence subtraction and a preference for using the FFT was indicated due to its ability to filter out random noise from the spectrum [112]. In an analysis of the different techniques by the author for in vivo tissue applications, the use of a polynomial fit was found to be the simplest technique from experimental as well as computational points of view. More recently, a modified polynomial fitting algorithm that accounts for noise levels has been proposed [122]. This technique has been shown to minimize the presence of artificial peaks in low SNR spectra, which can be common in measurements of tissue with high autofluorescence.

Other methods have utilized advanced signal processing techniques to separate underlying autofluorescence from the desired Raman signal. Wavelet detection and penalized least-squares fitting techniques [123] and principal component analysis (PCA) have been described for suppression of the confounding signal components [124]. Wavelet transformation is highly dependent on the decomposition method used and the shape of the fluorescence background, whereas PCA assumes that the highest

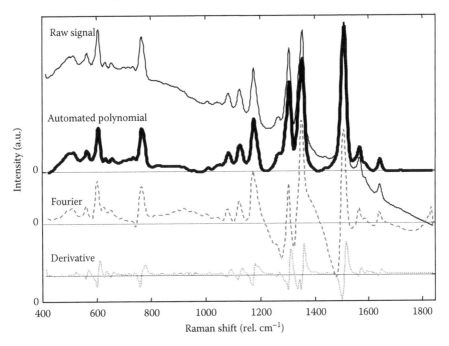

FIGURE 22.13 Raman spectra of rhodamine 6G processed using the derivative, manual curve fitting, and the modified mean methods.

signal variance is due to the fluorescence background, which may not be valid in certain applications. Thus, there are pros and cons to each methods and the choice may be governed by the application at hand and the preference of the investigator.

22.3.6.3 Noise Smoothing and Binning

Since Raman scattering is such a weak phenomenon, the SNRs of most measured Raman spectra are such that noise smoothing needs to be applied as part of the processing procedure. Various types of filters have been effectively used. These include the median filter, the moving average window filter, the Gaussian filter whose full width at half maximum is typically set equal to half the spectral resolution of the system, and the Savitzky–Golay filter of various orders [51]. In using any of these or other methods of noise smoothing, care should be taken to retain the integrity of the spectral lineshape especially in case of multiple peaks that are close to each other. Validating the method using spectra from weak Raman samples should be an essential step in the development process.

Other preprocessing methods include binning of the spectral data set due to a large number of variables for computational ease. Depending on the variability in the acquired data and the needs of the analysis methods used, various normalization methods may also be applied to allow comparison of the spectra. Such methods include normalization to intensity standards, normalization to its own maximum intensity or area under the curve, and mean scaling to the average spectrum acquired from a given patient. Some researchers prefer to use difference spectra to achieve the same normalization effect to account for intra- and interpatient variability observed.

22.3.7 Analysis

One of the advantages of spectroscopic diagnosis is automation, which allows objective and real-time diagnosis of pathologies. Differences in spectral features can be incorporated into diagnostic algorithms that can in turn be implemented in real time to yield classification using multivariate statistical methods; several statistical approaches have been identified and applied to feature extraction and classification of tissues toward automated, clinical diagnosis. Since Raman spectroscopy is a molecular specific technique, the contribution of the various participating chromophores can also be extracted from the measured spectra. These can then in turn be used in diagnostic algorithms as well as in understanding of the spectral signature as it pertains to the disease process. Additionally, concentration of specific components such as glucose can be obtained for diagnostic use as well.

22.3.7.1 Automated Diagnosis

During the 1980s, as the first papers on the application of Raman spectroscopy for disease detection was reported, Raman spectra were analyzed for differences in intensity, shape, and location of the various Raman bands between normal and nonnormal materials such as tissues. Based on consistent differences observed between the various tissue categories, diagnostic algorithms were developed using empirical methods. These algorithms may be based on changes in intensity or ratios of intensities or number and location of peaks. For example, the intensity ratio of the CH_2 bending vibrational mode at 1450 cm^{-1} to the amide I vibrational mode at 1655 cm^{-1} has been observed to vary with disease in several applications including breast cancers and gynecologic cancers and precancers [125,126]. These empirical algorithms indicate the specific changes that occur in the spectra acquired and provide an indication about the biochemical processes that result in these spectral differences.

This empirical analysis, however, has two important limitations. First, clinically useful diagnostic information is typically contained in more than just the few wavenumbers surrounding peaks or valleys observed in tissue; a method of analysis and classification that includes all the available spectral information can potentially improve the accuracy of detection. Second, empirical algorithms are optimized for the spectra within the study. Hence, the estimates of algorithm performances will be biased toward that tissue population. An unbiased estimate of the performance of the algorithms is required for an accurate evaluation of the performance of Raman spectroscopy for tissue diagnosis. To address these limitations, multivariate statistical techniques have become standardized practice in order to develop and evaluate algorithms that differentiate between normal and nonnormal tissues.

In recent years, the potential for using multivariate techniques for spectroscopic data analysis in disease detection has been exploited with great success [54]. Discrimination techniques like linear regression as well as classification techniques such as neural networks have been used [54,127]. Data compression tools such as PCA are used to account for the variability in the data [128]. Linear and nonlinear methods have been used for feature extraction. Subsequently, methods including heirarchical cluster analysis (HCA) [12] and linear discriminant analysis (LDA) [127] have been used to yield classification algorithms for disease differentiation. Partial least squares, a regression-based technique, as well as hybrid linear analysis, has been used to extract accurate concentrations of analytes such as glucose using NIR Raman spectra for transcutaneous blood analysis [129]. More complex multivariate and machine learning methods have also been utilized, including support vector machines, logistic regression models, genetic algorithms, and generalized linear models [38,62]. These methods allow the integration of non-Gaussian constraints and variable weights to optimize classification performance. In small sample sets, one often relies on the leave-one-out or K-fold methods of cross validation. Rigorous, unbiased estimates may be obtained by developing robust discrimination algorithms using a test set and its performance quantified in a validation set; the two sets formed ideally by random distribution of the subject population into two equal data sets. The true measure of success of Raman spectroscopy for tissue diagnosis requires validation of the tested algorithm given earlier in an extensive unbiased (and independent) validation set [130].

22.3.7.2 Component Extraction

Analyzing the Raman spectra for the purpose of disease classification may be sufficient when the goal of the study is to achieve tissue diagnosis alone. However, most researchers not only want to know if they can diagnose disease but also why they can do so. In the case of Raman spectroscopy, the wealth of information provided in these spectra especially with respect to biochemical composition allows us to study the question of *why* in detail that can subsequently be used to enhance diagnostic performance.

Puppels et al. have utilized skin Raman spectra to obtain quantitative information about skin hydration [11]. Feld et al. have developed comprehensive models for biochemical component extraction that have subsequently been used for disease classification [131]. More recently, Huang et al. have performed semiquantitative biomolecular least-squares modeling based on representative basis spectra in order to distinguish spectral sources for neoplastic lesions in multiple patients [132]. Each of these methods is based on the acquisition of Raman spectra from individually identified chromophores either as morphological tissue components or as extracted biochemical constituents. Pixelated Raman microspectroscopy is typically used (with or without confocality) to measure Raman spectra from individual morphologic tissue components using tissue sections. A Raman spectrometer is coupled to a microscope and is scanned across the tissue section to obtain Raman images that can then be correlated with serial hematoxylin- and eosin-stained sections to identify relevant morphologic components and their Raman signature. Alternatively, tissue chromophores can be extracted from biochemical assays and Raman spectra can be acquired from each of these extracted chromophores. Using mathematical models such as those developed by the Feld group, contributions of each of the extracted or morphologic components to intact tissue spectra can then be extracted.

Thus, a portable, clinically viable instrument with a fiber-optic probe can be used to acquire Raman spectra in vivo. The ability of Raman spectroscopy in a particular tissue can be tested in animals in vivo or in vitro and subsequently applied for in vivo human detection. The acquired spectra can then be processed and analyzed and information extracted about the performance of the technique as well as information about the biochemical components that contribute to the ability of the method to separate samples.

22.4 Clinical Application of Raman Spectroscopy

In order to fully evaluate the potential of Raman spectroscopy for clinical diagnosis, in vivo studies are required. Several groups have initiated this process with varying degrees of success. This progression has been made possible by the development of sensitive instrumentation, use of fiber optics, and development of automated algorithms. There has been an increase in the reports of Raman spectroscopy in vivo over the last decade although these are limited to select research groups who have successfully translated the technique from in vitro to clinical studies. Nevertheless, these are critical studies that set the road map for the future of Raman spectroscopy in biomedicine.

Several biological molecules such as nucleic acids, proteins, and lipids have distinctive Raman features that yield structural and environmental information. These molecules have been studied in solutions as well as in their natural microscopic environment [54]. The molecular and cellular changes that occur with disease result in distinct Raman spectra that can be used for diagnosis. The transitional changes in precancerous tissues as well as in benign abnormalities such as inflammation can also yield characteristic Raman features that allow their differentiation. Several groups have indicated the potential of vibrational spectroscopy for disease diagnosis in various organ sites. These groups have shown that features of the vibrational spectrum can be related to molecular and structural changes associated with disease. Raman spectroscopy has been studied extensively for tissue diagnosis in many organ sites. Here, we report summaries of its application in four select organ sites: breast, GI tract, cervix, and skin.

22.4.1 Breast

Perhaps one of the most widely investigated areas in the area of Raman spectroscopy for cancer detection has been for breast cancers. This is the most common type of cancer among women, accounting for 18% of all cancer deaths among women [133]. The breast consists of mammary glands arranged in lobes separated by fibrous connective tissue and a considerable amount of fatty tissue [134]. Pathologies in the breast may be benign or malignant, and current methods of noninvasive diagnosis are limited in their specificity in distinguishing between these two. Fibrocystic changes are benign proliferative processes that vary from the innocuous to those associated with increased risk of carcinomas. These benign changes may exist in three forms—cyst formation and fibrosis, hyperplasia, and adenosis—in most afflicted breasts, all forms occur simultaneously in fibroadipose stroma. Breast tumors may arise from the ductal and lobular epithelium or connective tissue. These tumors vary from benign adenomas and malignant adenocarcinomas to benign fibromas and malignant fibrosarcomas. Infiltrating ductal carcinoma (IDC), the most frequent invasive form of breast cancer, has been studied using Raman spectroscopy. IDCs typically show an increase in dense fibrous stromal tissue as well as malignant proliferation of ductal epithelium [135]. Although routine screening using mammography can aid in early detection of malignancy, lesions identified with this method must be biopsied and evaluated histopathologically to determine the presence of malignancy. A number of spectroscopic techniques have been attempted for breast cancer diagnosis [2,136–138]. Although fluorescence spectroscopy has shown some promise as a diagnostic tool, Raman spectroscopy has shown the ability to provide more definitive characteristics of disease that allow for differential diagnosis of benign and malignant tumors in a direct, side-by-side comparison [139].

Several groups have studied the potential of Raman spectroscopy for pathologies of the breast from detection of breast cancers to study of capsules from breast implants [140]. Alfano et al. obtained the first Raman spectra from excised normal human breast tissues, benign and malignant breast tumors, using an FT-Raman system and discussed the feasibility of using FT-Raman spectroscopy for differentiating normal and malignant breast tissues [136]. The vibrational spectra of benign breast tissues (which include normal tissues) showed four characteristic bands at 1078, 1300, 1445, and 1651 cm^{-1}. The spectra of benign tumors showed bands at 1240, 1445, and 1659 cm^{-1} and malignant tumors displayed only two Raman bands at 1445 and 1651 cm^{-1}. The intensity ratio of 1445–1651 cm^{-1} was found to be larger in benign tissues in comparison to benign tumors and the same ratio was found to be even lower in malignant tumors.

Raman spectroscopy using visible excitation was used to study excised human breast tissues, by Redd et al. [137,141]. Spectra were also obtained from pure compounds, and the features observed in tissue spectra were determined to be primarily due to carotenoids, myoglobin, and lipids. The Raman spectra of normal breast tissues showed peaks that were assigned to carotenoids at 1005, 1157, and 1523 cm^{-1} (not observed with IR excitation); peaks that were assigned to lipids, primarily oleic acid derivatives, at 1302, 1442, and 1653 cm^{-1}; a peak at 1370 cm^{-1} due to myoglobin; and several other smaller unassigned peaks. In a subsequent study by McCreery et al., the feasibility of using NIR Raman spectroscopy for breast cancer detection was assessed. Chromophore contributions differed as excitation was shifted from the visible (yielding carotenoid and lipid bands) to the NIR (yielding only lipids bands) in normal tissues. However, NIR Raman spectroscopy yielded signals with lower fluorescence interference and higher SNR, validating this approach.

NIR Raman spectra were measured from excised normal human breast tissues, tissues with fibrocystic change and IDC at 784 nm excitation by Frank et al. [137]. The ratio of the areas under the peaks at 1654 and 1439 cm^{-1} were found to increase in malignant breast tissues as compared to normal breast tissues. This increase is consistent with the changes reported by Alfano et al. The intensity of the 1654 cm^{-1} C=C stretching band varies with the degree of fatty acid unsaturation and the CH_2 scissoring band at 1439 cm^{-1} depends on the lipid to protein ratio. The spectra from IDC tissues showed an overall decrease in intensity with respect to normal tissue. Several differences were also observed when IDC tissues were compared with benign abnormal tissue. In benign tissue, the intensities of the bands at 1656 and 1259 cm^{-1} were smaller than the band at 1449 cm^{-1} and this band is further shifted to 1446 cm^{-1}. The region of 850–950 cm^{-1} showed only two bands in benign tissue as compared to four in IDC samples. The peaks observed in normal tissues were primarily attributed to oleic acid methyl ester, a lipid, and the peaks observed in IDC and benign tissues were primarily attributed to collagen I. This is consistent with histopathology where IDC and benign tissues show an increase in interstitial tissues microscopically. These spectral differences were found to be significant, and subsequently, this group reported the development of a clinical probe and system for in vivo testing. Preliminary testing of the probe was reported on in vitro samples but no other reports were subsequently published.

More recently, several groups have investigated the potential of Raman spectroscopy for both the diagnosis of primary breast tumors [38,91,142,143] as well as surgical guidance [85,144]. Haka et al. reported the ability of Raman spectroscopy to classify malignant from benign calcified breast lesions using principal components based primarily on spectral signatures arising from calcium hydroxyapatite with elevated calcium carbonate and reduced protein spectral signatures [145]. Subsequent ex vivo work by the same group developed a linear model for reconstruction of bulk tissue breast spectra based on confocal spectral signatures obtained from the cell cytoplasm, cell nucleus, fat, β-carotene, collagen, calcium hydroxylapatite, calcium oxalate dihydrate, cholesterol-like lipid deposits from breast tissue, as well as water [146]. This model was then used to characterize spectra acquired from bulk breast tissue specimens and produce a classification algorithm, which was able to diagnose normal from benign tissue with 94% sensitivity and 96% specificity [147]. More recently, a 21-patient prospective study by the same group reported a sensitivity of 83% and a specificity of 93% when separating normal tissue from cancerous [143]. Ex vivo Raman studies conducted by Chowdary et al. confirmed earlier work by Feld that Raman spectra of normal, benign, and malignant breast tissue could be separated through direct PCA of measured spectra [148], and spectral deconvolution of peaks corresponding to lipids, proteins, collagen, and DNA could also facilitate separation of normal, benign, and malignant breast tissues [149]. The ability to classify normal from cancerous tissue is valuable; however, specifically identifying histopathological classes of ductal carcinoma in situ (DCIS), invasive ductal carcinoma, fibroadenoma, and normal breast tissue has more clinical significance in the context of aiding in physician's decision-making process. Reports by different groups have shown Raman's ability to classify histopathological groups with 99% overall accuracy [139], as well as indicated strong potential for segmenting subtypes of DCIS [150].

In other works, fiber-optic-probe-based measurements of fresh biopsy specimens was able to identify the presence of microcalcifications, which are believed to be an early mammographic sign of breast cancer [38,151]. These studies reflect the potential of Raman spectroscopies use in a hierarchical diagnosis paradigm in which questionable mammography findings can be investigated with increased specificity using Raman measurements conducted via needle biopsy probe. Finally, recent work by Matousek and Stone describes the development of transmission Raman spectroscopy, an approach that seeks to detect spectral signatures of calcified tissue through large thickness (>20 mm) of breast tissue [90,152]. Although promising, this work is currently under development and has only been demonstrated in tissue phantoms to date.

The in vivo potential of Raman spectroscopy for the breast was demonstrated in a study that was performed during partial mastectomy procedures [153]. The study reported 93% overall accuracy in spectral classification of normal, fibrocystic change, and cancerous spectra and also indicated the potential of intraoperative margin assessment with Raman spectroscopy. While there are numerous reports in the literature on the application of Raman spectroscopy for breast cancer diagnosis, this is the only report published on Raman measurements performed in the breast in vivo although the focus of the report was not for breast cancer diagnosis but for margin assessment. Current surgical standards for margin assessment in breast cancer resection require establishing margins at least 2 mm clear of residual tumor, as opposed to sampling the surgical cavity for residual tumor. The Haka paper presents a volumetric approach to breast margin assessment [153] without the 2 mm depth selectivity. A study by Keller et al. reported that it was possible to assess margin status from surgically resected lumpectomy specimens using SORS. The developed SORS probe was used to scan up to 2 mm of the resected breast specimen intraoperatively to determine margin status with 95% sensitivity and 100% specificity [85]. Further studies to scan the entire lump are reported to be in progress.

Raman spectroscopy in the breast has therefore been used by a number of researchers for applications ranging from cancer diagnosis to detection of calcifications to assessing margins during surgical resection. Interestingly, only one group has reported in vivo results. Regardless, the clinical potential of this technique for the breast has been evaluated by many researchers with varying degrees of success and portents the potential of Raman spectroscopy (Figure 22.14).

22.4.2 Cervix

The various gynecologic tissues differ structurally as well as functionally [135,154]. The cervix with its well-characterized disease process has been under much study for the development of spectroscopic detection. The cervix is the most inferior portion of the uterus, which typically measures 2.5–3.0 cm in diameter in the human adult. The cervix is covered by two types of epithelia: The multilayered squamous epithelium covers most of the ectocervix and is separated from the stroma by the basal layer. The glandular epithelium consists of a single layer of columnar cells and covers the surface of the endocervical canal. The interface of the two epithelia is called the squamocolumnar (SQ) junction. Over time, the glandular epithelium is replaced by squamous epithelium, which causes the SQ junction to move towards the os. This transitional epithelium is termed as *squamous metaplasia* [154]. Virtually all squamous cervical neoplasias (new growth) begin at the functional SQ junction and the extent and limit of their precursors coincide with the distribution of the transformation zone [154]. Cervical intraepithelial neoplasia (CIN) refers to the precancerous stages of cervical carcinoma and is often also referred to as cervical dysplasia. Other pathologies that are known to affect the cervix include cervicitis or inflammation, which is usually a tissue response to injury [154], and the human papilloma viral infection. Similarities observed in the morphological changes of the epithelial cells between those induced by HPV and precancer have led to recent research that shows that certain high-risk strains of HPV are

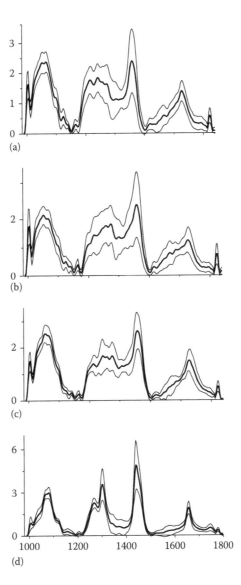

FIGURE 22.14 Mean Raman spectra (thick solid lines) of (a) invasive ductal carcinoma ($n = 86$), (b) DCIS ($n = 18$), (c) fibroadenoma ($n = 55$), and (d) normal ($n = 134$) breast tissue samples.

involved in the incipient stages of cervical precancer and other strains aid in the progression of the disease. Persistent infection of high-risk HPV has been shown to catalyze the higher grades of CIN (grade 2–3) and invasive cervical cancers [155]. Thus, the presence of HPV strains 16 and 18 (in the United States) is indicative of a CIN that will most likely progress and is treated as opposed to those CIN I cases without HPV that are more likely to regress. Thus, current care requires HPV testing as part of routine patient screening and is an important indicator of cervical cancer. Endocervical cancers are typically adenocarcinomas, arising within the endocervix as opposed to cervical epithelial lesions, which arise in the SQ junction.

Cervical cancer is the second most common malignancy among women worldwide. It is estimated that in 2013, 4,030 deaths will occur in the United States from this disease and 12,340 new cases of cervical cancer will be diagnosed [156]. Although early detection of cervical precancer has played a central role in reducing the mortality associated with this disease over the last 50 years, the incidence of preinvasive squamous carcinoma of the cervix has risen dramatically, especially among women under the age of 50. The primary screening tools for cervical precancer are the Papanicolaou (Pap) smear, where scrapings from the walls of the ecto- as well as endocervix that contain a variable number of cells are examined for diagnosis and HPV testing [154]. Although the widespread application of the Pap smear as a screening tool has greatly decreased the incidence of cervical cancer [157], sampling and reading errors lead to high false-positive and false-negative rates. HPV testing requires several days and is an expensive process at this time. Thus, treatment ultimately relies on directed biopsies and subsequent pathological findings.

Alfano et al. were the first to report on the feasibility of using FT-Raman spectroscopy for detecting cancers from various gynecologic tissues [126]. Characteristic features of normal tissues and malignant tumors from the cervix, uterus, endometrium, and ovary were described. Three significant peaks were noted to differ in the Raman spectra of normal and benign cervix compared to cancerous lesions. In cancerous tissues, the intensity of the amide I stretching vibration band at 1657 cm^{-1} is less than the intensity of the C—H bending vibrational band at 1445 cm^{-1}. The amide III band at 1262 cm^{-1} is broadened in cancerous lesions. The author has reported in vitro as well as in vivo studies on the application of Raman spectroscopy for the detection of CIN [51,128]. In her early work, Raman spectra of cervical tissues were measured to characterize the spectral signatures of the different tissue types and assess the feasibility of using Raman spectroscopy for cervical precancer diagnosis. Primary tissue Raman peaks are observed at 626, 818, 978, 1070, 1246, 1330, 1454, and 1656 cm^{-1} ($\pm$10 cm^{-1}), present in all samples. Both empirical and multivariate techniques were used to explore the diagnostic capability of NIR Raman spectra from cervical tissues. A multivariate discrimination algorithm developed using the entire Raman spectrum could differentiate cervical precancers from non-precancers with a sensitivity and specificity of 91% and 90% [128].

Raman spectra were measured in vivo from 79 patients using a system similar to that described in Figure 22.3. Raman spectra from the separate diseases show differences at various spectral bands as can be seen in Figure 22.15. Using multivariate statistical methods and the entire spectrum, Raman spectroscopy could distinguish CIN 2–3 from normal ectocervix and squamous metaplasia with a sensitivity of 92% and specificity of 96%. However, when 24 additional patients with CIN I were added to this study, they were misclassified as normal 26% of the time. Further study for the basis of this misclassification demonstrated that Raman spectroscopy is sensitive to the hormonal cycle of the cervix and could separate normal premenopausal patients from postmenopausal patients with 100% accuracy [158]. The performance of Raman spectroscopy in classifying CIN I cases improved from 74% to 96% when considering only premenopausal women. Additional improvement in performance could be achieved when the patients were further stratified based on the body-mass index and parity. Raman spectroscopy was also shown to have 98.5% classification accuracy between HPV-negative and HPV-positive human cervix measurements from 91 enrolled patients [159].

Several other groups have also developed Raman spectroscopy to study the cervix [78,160]. Researchers have applied high-wavenumber Raman spectroscopy as well as confocal microspectroscopy for cervical precancer detection. Response to radiotherapy in patients with cervical cancer was assessed with Raman spectroscopy and results demonstrated that the spectra could be used to differentiate between responders and nonresponders to therapy [161]. In other applications of the cervix, researchers have demonstrated the potential of Raman spectroscopy to track the pregnant cervix and develop an understanding of cervical remodeling that occurs with pregnancy [162]. These studies clearly indicate the in vivo capability of Raman spectroscopy and the sensitivity of the technique to subtle changes in tissue biochemistry that can be used to enhance its performance.

22.4.3 Skin

The skin is the largest organ of the body and has many different functions. It is divided into two main regions: the epidermis and the dermis. The epidermis primarily consists of keratinocytes and varies in thickness throughout the body. Melanocytes, the pigment-producing cells of the skin, are found

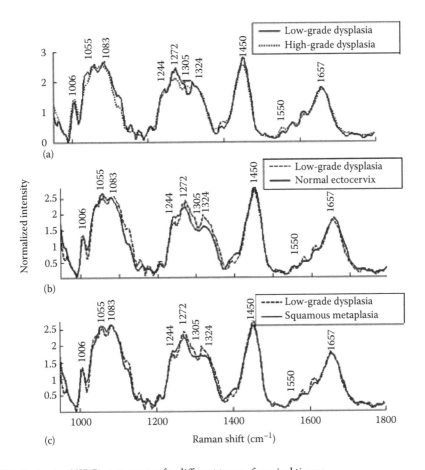

FIGURE 22.15 In vivo NIR Raman spectra for different types of cervical tissues.

throughout the epidermis [134]. The dermis consists mostly of fibroblasts, which are responsible for secreting collagen and elastin giving support and elasticity to the skin. There are two major groups of skin cancers: malignant melanoma and nonmelanoma skin cancers. Cancers that develop from melanocytes are called melanoma. Nonmelanoma skin cancers are the most common cancers of the skin. Among these, two of the most common nonmelanoma types are basal cell carcinoma (BCC) and squamous cell carcinoma (SCC). About 75% of all skin cancers are BCCs. It has a high likelihood of recurrence after treatment either at the same site or elsewhere [133]. SCCs account for about 20% of all skin cancers. SCCs are more likely to invade tissues beneath the skin and to distant parts of the body than are BCCs.

While most people believe they are not at risk for skin cancer, cancers of the skin (including melanoma and nonmelanoma skin cancers) are the most common of all cancers and accounts for about half of all cases in the United States [133]. American Cancer Society predicts 12,650 deaths this year, 9,480 from melanoma and 3,170 from other skin cancers. Melanomas account for about 4% of skin cancer cases but causes about 77% of skin cancer deaths. The number of new cases of melanoma found in this country is on the rise. The American Cancer Society predicts that in the year 2013, there will be 76,690 new cases of melanoma in the United States. For most skin cancer patients (including melanoma and nonmelanoma skin cancers), early diagnosis and thorough treatment (i.e., complete resection) are the keys to gaining a favorable prognosis. Current diagnostic methods for skin cancers rely on physical examination of the lesion in conjunction with skin biopsy. Suspicious areas are selected upon visual inspection by the clinician, after which those lesions are partially or wholly biopsied for complete histological evaluation [133]. The biopsy is then sectioned and stained for pathological investigation and diagnosis. This protocol for skin lesion diagnosis is accepted as the gold standard; however, it is subjective, invasive, and time consuming. Hence, there is considerable interest in developing a noninvasive diagnostic tool, which can accurately detect skin lesions noninvasively in real time especially in its early stages.

Early studies on skin cancer detection using optical spectroscopy were primarily limited to fluorescence and diffuse reflectance spectroscopy and produced limited success [157]. The major limitation has been the interference of skin pigment and external agents such as creams and soaps that limit the success of these techniques. Despite the ease of studying the skin, the first published reports of skin Raman spectra appeared only in the early 1990s. These early studies were, however, focused on characterizing skin components. Research was conducted to study skin hydration, skin aging, and effect of UV radiation, among others [51]. Williams et al. utilized FT-Raman spectroscopy to examine a number of skin features and correlate the Raman spectra with the biochemical agents responsible [163,164]. Gniadecka et al. utilized FT-Raman spectroscopy to successfully differentiate BCC from normal, healthy skin in vitro in 16 patients [165]. Early attempts to use Raman spectroscopy to diagnose skin lesions relied on FT-Raman spectroscopy, a technique that has limitations that preclude clinical applications [165,166]. While promising results were reported, FT-Raman spectroscopy is not a feasible technique for clinical diagnosis. Later, Caspers et al. utilized confocal Raman microspectroscopy to ascertain the in vivo Raman signal characteristics emanating from each layer of normal human skin and showed that each layer of the human skin contained Raman features that can be highly correlated with the protein and chemical content of each respective layer [167]. Additional studies have shown that it is possible to extract carotenoid contribution from Raman spectra in vivo of various skin tissues [168].

In vitro studies have demonstrated the sensitivity of confocal RS to features of skin cancer, such as pilomatrixoma, a benign tumor of the hair follicles [169], as well as the ability of confocal RS to differentiate normal, BCC, and SCC [170]. Figure 22.16 shows the Raman spectra of normal skin, BCC, SCC, and melanoma tissues at a depth where optimal differences between the various tissue types were observed.

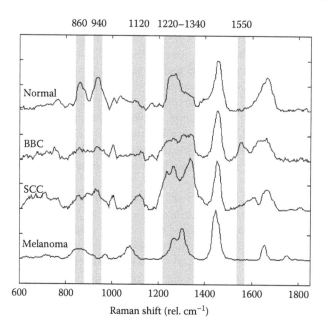

FIGURE 22.16 NIR Raman spectra of normal and cancerous skin lesions acquired in vitro using a confocal Raman microspectrometer.

Key differences in the spectra are observed at several Raman bands including those seen at 860, 940, 1120, 1220–1340, and 1550 cm^{-1}. In addition to the fingerprint region, spectral features from the high-wavenumber region (2800–3125 cm^{-1}) have shown potential for accurately classifying BCC from uninvolved perilesional skin [171].

In vivo studies of Raman spectroscopy's potential for disease diagnosis have been equally promising. An early study conducted using a handheld confocal Raman probe was able to identify differences between BCC, SCC, inflammation, and normal skin [66]. The study enrolled 21 patients and collected Raman spectra with a 30 s integration time. The authors observed qualitative differences in confocal Raman spectra acquired from 40 μm below the tissue surface indicate spectral differences between pathological samples at 920–940, 1000–1010, 1060–1070, 1250–1330, 1445, and 1650 cm^{-1}. The data were classified with an algorithm using a nonlinear machine learning algorithm to perform classification of tissue types with a 95% overall accuracy.

While the skin is a layered tissue with an accepted depth range for initial cancer presentation, several research groups have investigated diagnosis with Raman instruments that are not inherently depth selective. Many groups have investigated various structural and biochemical aspects of skin disease [172–174]. Researchers have used Raman spectra in combination with fluorescence or advanced multivariate statistical techniques to improve performance of discriminating between normal and cancerous tissues [104,175–177]. Recent reports have focused on clinical implementation of conventional fiber-optic-probe-based Raman spectroscopy and reported distinctive spectra obtained from a large patient population and the development of efficient, real-time software tools for processing and analysis of Raman spectra [173,177]. One such study was performed using a 53-around-1 fiber-optic probe capable of 1 s acquisition times and also reported promising findings over a far greater enrollment. The study evaluated 453 patients with lesions that included melanomas, BCCs, SCCs, actinic keratoses, atypical nevi, melanocytic nevi, blue nevi, and seborrheic keratosis [177]. Lesion classification was performed using a principal component with general discriminant analysis as well as partial least-squares discrimination. The authors reported the ability to differentiate cancerous and precancerous lesions from benign with a specificity of 64% and a positive predictive value of 67% when the sensitivity as set at 90%. This technology has been commercialized by Verisante and represents a promising tool to help clinicians and guide screening and diagnosis.

Skin is the most easily accessible as well as the most difficult organ to work with. The variability of the organ across the body and from patient to patient as well as the highly scattering and absorbing nature of the tissue makes it particularly challenging from an optical perspective. However, the critical nature of the disease and the capability of Raman spectroscopy to detect even subtle changes in tissue presents a unique opportunity for the successful clinical application of the technique.

22.4.4 Gastrointestinal Tract

The GI tract is a functionally diverse set of organs that extend from the mouth to the anus. The general anatomy for these organs, including the esophagus, stomach, and bowel, consists of four concentric layers in the following order: mucosa, submucosa, *muscularis externa*, and serosa. The surface exposed to the lumen is an epithelial layer of columnar cells that can be accessed with relative ease via endoscopic techniques. However, routine white-light endoscopy is insensitive in detecting micromorphological and/or biochemical changes involving the mucosal lining of the GI tract. For instance, the detection of mucosal dysplasia (neoplastic epithelium) in patients with Barrett's esophagus (BE) or the differentiation of hyperplastic from neoplastic colon polyps routinely requires taking multiple biopsies for histopathological analysis. For many of these organs, patients suffering from GI cancers have poor survival rates due primarily to the advanced stage at the time of the initial diagnosis. This limit to detection and subsequent medical intervention indicates the need for accurate, sensitive, and noninvasive techniques that can detect cancerous lesions at an early stage.

All accessible with standard endoscopic techniques, the esophagus, stomach, and colon are major organs associated with cancer entities. The pathogenesis of the diverse cancers in the GI tract is not fully understood, but increasing levels of variability and subtypes of disease class are complicating factors for histological evaluation, which is the *gold standard* for diagnosis. An estimated 103,170 cases of colon and 40,290 cases of rectal cancer were expected to occur in the United States in 2012. Colorectal cancer is the third most common cancer in both men and women and was estimated to account for 9% of all US cancer deaths. Gastric and oral cancers, while less prevalent in the United States, are among the most common cancers globally, especially in developing countries [178]. Optical and imaging techniques have been explored in the GI tract for identifying cancerous growths, and more recently, Raman techniques have demonstrated the sensitivity needed for minimally invasive diagnostics when coupled with endoscopy procedures. Demonstrated initially by Shim et al., endoscopic applications of Raman spectroscopy have been utilized for cancer detection in the mouth [178–180], esophagus [132,181–183], stomach [47,132,184–186], and colon [183,187–190] with high sensitivities and specificities.

Raman techniques have been successfully used in cancer and precancer detection, based on differences between normal and adenocarcinoma corresponding to nucleic acid changes [191,192]. Raman has also been used in classifying colon polyps and obtained an accuracy of 95%–99% in distinguishing between adenomatous and hyperplastic polyps both in vitro and in vivo [187] as well as ex vivo studies [189,190]. A database cataloging the intrinsic Raman signatures of various GI cancers including the colon is available [183], and the work showed that colon tissues can be classified with near 90% efficiency [183]. Oral cancers, BE, and other esophageal cancers have been investigated in vivo with recently developed and optimized endoscopic tools. Huang et al. investigated spectral variability of normal anatomical sites in normal tissue of the oral cavity in vivo [179]. Oral cancers have been measured in vivo, classified with multivariate techniques, and reported sensitivities >90% [180]. Cancers of the esophagus have been studied by several groups. Huang et al. reported a study of 107 patients undergoing endoscopy, with a 93.9% sensitivity to cancerous tissues in the esophagus [132], while Kendall et al. reported an 86% sensitivity to high-grade dysplasia and adenocarcinoma during ex vivo Raman spectroscopy measurements [181].

While cancer is the primary research focus for Raman spectroscopy in the GI tract, groups have begun to investigate other pathologies such as inflammatory bowel disease. In vitro studies have demonstrated the biochemical sensitivity of Raman spectroscopy for detecting disease-related changes specific to Crohn's disease and ulcerative colitis through both fiber-optic-probe-based [193] and microspectroscopy [72] detection schemes. Both reports utilized multivariate statistical methods to achieve classification performance with >95% accuracies between diseases. Future in vivo studies applied to this and other disease entities of the colon and GI tract are expected, based on the demonstrated sensitivity of Raman techniques to biochemical changes associated with multiple distinct disease processes.

As observed in the other applications described here, the endoscopic accessibility of the GI tract has allowed the in vivo application of Raman spectroscopy for GI cancers, as well as other noncancer applications. Successful implementation in vivo and the availability of direct organ access, provided during procedures including routine screening colonoscopy, present an avenue for clinical use of Raman spectroscopy with improved diagnostic utility and therefore an opportunity for clinical translation of this technique.

22.4.5 Other Applications

The aforementioned examples show the various stages of development in the implementation of Raman spectroscopy for disease detection in vivo. There are many more applications of this versatile technique that are not specifically reported here. Some of these include the application of Raman spectroscopy for the detection of various pathologies in the brain [80], ovary [58], eye [194], bone [195], and lung [196], among others. The technique has been used to study such diverse conditions as Alzheimer's disease [197], arthritis [198], aging [199], and infections [200]. Besides tissue studies, Raman spectroscopy has also been used for the determination of various analytes such as glucose [201], cholesterol [202], carotenoids [203], and fibrinogen [204]. For example, there are studies reported on the determination of glucose concentration in diabetes patients [205,206]. A recent study reported the transdermal measurement of blood glucose using tissue modulation for signal extraction [207]. There have been extensive studies on the application of Raman spectroscopy for the detection of atherosclerotic plaques [208] and other cardiovascular disease [209]. Thus, there exists a vast variety of applications where researchers in the field are developing the use of Raman spectroscopy in a clinical setting. Interesting applications may be found in the analysis of biological fluids for forensic science and biological warfare. Results in all of these appear promising and poises Raman spectroscopy to the next level of implementation.

22.5 Perspectives on the Future

Technology has come far in the last decade to make clinical implementation of Raman spectroscopy feasible. Advances in diode laser technology and CCD detector technology alone have contributed tremendously to this process. However, there still exists a need for compact Raman probes and integrated systems that would make this technology even more versatile. Currently, several integrated systems are available for the application of Raman spectroscopy in environmental and manufacturing processes. A similar move is required in the field of biomedicine as well. The introduction of micro-optics and microfabrication can further fulfill the need for compact small-diameter probes.

This chapter presents a review of concepts, instrumentation, and sample applications of Raman spectroscopy for disease detection in vivo. The success of the technique has led to the development of feasible clinical systems that can measure Raman signals from tissue with short collection times [136,137]. Many of these systems have already undergone preliminary testing and several others are currently in the process of being tested. These studies clearly indicate that clinical application of Raman spectroscopy is imminent and may be expected to change the face of disease detection in the near future. While extensive studies are required to form a true assessment of the capability of Raman spectroscopy for disease detection, results thus far are extremely encouraging. What makes this technique so invaluable is that not only can it be used for disease classification but the acquired spectra can also be evaluated for biochemical composition making this a viable clinical as well as research tool furthering the technology of patient care as well the understanding of the disease process.

References

1. Stummer, W. et al., Fluorescence-guided resection of glioblastoma multiforme by using 5-aminolevulinic acid-induced porphyrins: A prospective study in 52 consecutive patients. *Journal of Neurosurgery*, 2000. **93**(6): 1003–1013.
2. Alfano, R.R. et al., Optical spectroscopic diagnosis of cancer and normal breast tissues. *Journal of the Optical Society of America B-Optical Physics*, 1989. **6**(5): 1015–1023.
3. Kennedy, T.C., S. Lam, and F.R. Hirsch, Review of recent advances in fluorescence bronchoscopy in early localization of central airway lung cancer. *The Oncologist*, 2001. **6**(3): 257–262.
4. Hung, J. et al., Autofluorescence of normal and malignant bronchial tissue. *Lasers in Surgery and Medicine*, 1991. **11**(2): 99–105.
5. Gillenwater, A. et al., Noninvasive diagnosis of oral neoplasia based on fluorescence spectroscopy and native tissue autofluorescence. *Archives of Otolaryngology: Head & Neck Surgery*, 1998. **124**(11): 1251.
6. Ramanujam, N. et al., Spectroscopic diagnosis of cervical intraepithelial neoplasia (CIN) in vivo using laser-induced fluorescence spectra at multiple excitation wavelengths. *Lasers in Surgery and Medicine*, 1996. **19**(1): 63–74.

7. Cothren, R.M. et al., Gastrointestinal tissue diagnosis by laser-induced fluorescence spectroscopy at endoscopy. *Gastrointestinal Endoscopy*, 1990. **36**(2): 105–111.

8. Schomacker, K.T. et al., Ultraviolet laser-induced fluorescence of colonic tissue: Basic biology and diagnostic potential. *Lasers in Surgery and Medicine*, 1992. **12**(1): 63–78.

9. Johnson, C.R. et al., UV resonance Raman spectroscopy of the aromatic amino acids and myoglobin. *Journal of the American Chemical Society*, 1984. **106**(17): 5008–5010.

10. Nie, S. et al., Applications of near-infrared Fourier transform Raman spectroscopy in biology and medicine. *Spectroscopy*, 1990. **5**(7): 24.

11. Caspers, P. et al., Automated depth-scanning confocal Raman microspectrometer for rapid in vivo determination of water concentration profiles in human skin. *Journal of Raman Spectroscopy*, 2000. **31**(8–9): 813–818.

12. Choo-Smith, L.P. et al., Medical applications of Raman spectroscopy: From proof of principle to clinical implementation. *Biopolymers*, 2002. **67**(1): 1–9.

13. Gellermann, W. et al., *In vivo* resonant Raman measurement of macular carotenoid pigments in the young and the aging human retina. *Journal of the Optical Society of America. A, Optics, Image Science, and Vision*, 2002. **19**(6): 1172–1186.

14. Pilotto, S. et al., Analysis of near-infrared Raman spectroscopy as a new technique for a transcutaneous non-invasive diagnosis of blood components. *Lasers in Medical Science*, 2001. **16**(1): 2–9.

15. Raman, C. and K. Krishnan, A new type of secondary radiation. *Nature*, 1928. **121**(3048): 501–502.

16. Colthup, N.B., L.H. Daly, and S.E. Wiberley, *Introduction to Infrared and Raman Spectroscopy*, 1990. New York, NY: Academic Press.

17. Ferraro, J.R. and K. Nakamoto, *Introductory Raman Spectroscopy*, 1994. San Diego, CA: Academic Press.

18. Carey, P., Biochemical applications of Raman and resonance Raman spectroscopies. *Journal of Molecular Structure*, 1984. **112**: 337.

19. Twardowski, J. and P. Anzenbacher, *Raman and IR Spectroscopy in Biology and Biochemistry*, 1994. Ellis Horwood: New York.

20. Bailo, E. and V. Deckert, Tip-enhanced Raman scattering. *Chemical Society Reviews*, 2008. **37**(5): 921–930.

21. Masihzadeh, O. et al., Coherent anti-Stokes Raman scattering (CARS) microscopy: A novel technique for imaging the retina. *Investigative Ophthalmology & Visual Science*, 2013. **54**(5): 3094–3101.

22. Saar, B.G. et al., Video-rate molecular imaging *in vivo* with stimulated Raman scattering. *Science*, 2010. **330**(6009): 1368–1370.

23. Cialla, D. et al., Surface-enhanced Raman spectroscopy (SERS): Progress and trends. *Analytical and Bioanalytical Chemistry*, 2012. **403**(1): 27–54.

24. Ma, K. et al., In vivo, transcutaneous glucose sensing using surface-enhanced spatially offset Raman spectroscopy: Multiple rats, improved hypoglycemic accuracy, low incident power, and continuous monitoring for greater than 17 days. *Analytical Chemistry*, 2011. **83**(23): 9146–9152.

25. Maiti, K.K. et al., Multiplex targeted *in vivo* cancer detection using sensitive near-infrared SERS nanotags. *Nano Today*, 2012. **7**(2): 85–93.

26. McQueenie, R. et al., Detection of inflammation in vivo by surface-enhanced Raman scattering provides higher sensitivity than conventional fluorescence imaging. *Analytical Chemistry*, 2012. **84**(14): 5968–5975.

27. Qian, X. et al., In vivo tumor targeting and spectroscopic detection with surface-enhanced Raman nanoparticle tags. *Nature Biotechnology*, 2007. **26**(1): 83–90.

28. Zavaleta, C.L. et al., Multiplexed imaging of surface enhanced Raman scattering nanotags in living mice using noninvasive Raman spectroscopy. *Proceedings of the National Academy of Sciences*, 2009. **106**(32): 13511–13516.

29. Szymanski, H.A., *Raman Spectroscopy: Theory and Practice*, 1967. Plenum Publishing Corporation, New York.

30. Asher, S.A., UV resonance Raman spectroscopy for analytical, physical, and biophysical chemistry. *Analytical Chemistry*, 1993. **65**(4): 201A–210A.

31. Feld, M.S. and J.R. Kramer, Mutagenicity and the XeCl excimer laser: A relationship of consequence? *American Heart Journal*, 1991. **122**(6): 1803–1805.

32. Ellis, D.I. et al., Illuminating disease and enlightening biomedicine: Raman spectroscopy as a diagnostic tool. *Analyst*, 2013. **138**(14): 3871–3884.

33. Krafft, C. et al., Diagnosis and screening of cancer tissues by fiber-optic probe Raman spectroscopy. *Biomedical Spectroscopy and Imaging*, 2012. **1**(1): 39–55.

34. Tu, Q. and C. Chang, Diagnostic applications of Raman spectroscopy. *Nanomedicine: Nanotechnology, Biology and Medicine*, 2012. **8**(5): 545–558.

35. Zhuang, Z. et al., Study of molecule variation in various grades of human nuclear cataracts by confocal micro-Raman spectroscopy. *Applied Physics Letters*, 2012. **101**(17): 173701–173701-3.

36. Peres, M.B. et al., Classification model based on Raman spectra of selected morphological and biochemical tissue constituents for identification of atherosclerosis in human coronary arteries. *Lasers in Medical Science*, 2011. **26**(5): 645–655.

37. Šćepanović, O.R. et al., Multimodal spectroscopy detects features of vulnerable atherosclerotic plaque. *Journal of Biomedical Optics*, 2011. **16**(1): 011009-1–011009-10.

38. Barman, I. et al., Application of Raman spectroscopy to identify microcalcifications and underlying breast lesions at stereotactic core needle biopsy. *Cancer Research*, 2013. **73**(11): 3206–3215.

39. Short, M.A. et al., Using high frequency Raman spectra for colonic neoplasia detection. *Optics Express*, 2013. **21**(4): 5025–5034.

40. Clarke, R.H. et al., Laser Raman spectroscopy of calcified atherosclerotic lesions in cardiovascular tissue. *Applied Optics*, 1987. **26**(16): 3175–3177.

41. Yu, N.-T. and E.J. East, Laser Raman spectroscopic studies of ocular lens and its isolated protein fractions. *Journal of Biological Chemistry*, 1975. **250**(6): 2196–2202.

42. Manoharan, R. et al., Raman spectroscopy for cancer detection: Instrument development and tissue diagnosis. *International Symposium on Biomedical Optics Europe'94*, 1994. Universite de Lille, Faculte de Medecine Lille, France, International Society for Optics and Photonics.

43. Puppels, G. et al., Studying single living cells and chromosomes by confocal Raman microspectroscopy. *Nature*, 1990. **347**(6290): 301–303.

44. Rudder, S.L., J.C. Connolly, and G.J. Steckman, Hybrid ECL/DBR wavelength and spectrum stabilized lasers demonstrate high power and narrow spectral linewidth. *Proceedings of SPIE*, 2006. **6101**: 61010I-1–61010I-8.

45. Wang, W., A. Major, and J. Paliwal, Grating-stabilized external cavity diode lasers for Raman spectroscopy—A review. *Applied Spectroscopy Reviews*, 2011. **47**(2): 116–143.

46. Min, Y.K. et al., 1064 nm near-infrared multichannel Raman spectroscopy of fresh human lung tissues. *Journal of Raman Spectroscopy*, 2005. **36**(1): 73–76.

47. Kawabata, T. et al., Optical diagnosis of gastric cancer using near-infrared multichannel Raman spectroscopy with a 1064-nm excitation wavelength. *Journal of Gastroenterology*, 2008. **43**(4): 283–290.

48. Keltner, Z. et al., Prism-based infrared spectrographs using modern-day detectors. *Applied Spectroscopy*, 2007. **61**(9): 909–915.

49. Lieber, C.A., E.M. Kanter, and A. Mahadevan-Jansen, Comparison of Raman spectrograph throughput using two commercial systems: Transmissive versus reflective. *Applied Spectroscopy*, 2008. **62**(5): 575–582.

50. Stone, N. et al., Raman spectroscopy for early detection of laryngeal malignancy: Preliminary results. *Laryngoscope*, 2000. **110**(10 Pt 1): 1756–1763.

51. Utzinger, U. et al., Near-infrared Raman spectroscopy for in vivo detection of cervical precancers. *Applied Spectroscopy*, 2001. **55**(8): 955–959.

52. Myrick, M. and S. Angel, Elimination of background in fiber-optic Raman measurements. *Applied Spectroscopy*, 1990. **44**(4): 565–570.

53. Myrick, M.L., S.M. Angel, and R. Desiderio, Comparison of some fiber optic configurations for measurement of luminescence and Raman scattering. *Applied Optics*, 1990. **29**(9): 1333–1344.

54. Mahadevan-Jansen, A. and R. Richards-Kortum, Raman spectroscopy for the detection of cancers and precancers. *Journal of Biomedical Optics*, 1996. **1**(1): 31–70.

55. Matousek, P., Raman signal enhancement in deep spectroscopy of turbid media. *Applied Spectroscopy*, 2007. **61**(8): 845–854.

56. Schwab, S.D. and R.L. McCreery, Versatile, efficient Raman sampling with fiber optics. *Analytical Chemistry*, 1984. **56**(12): 2199–2204.

57. Tanaka, K. et al., Compound parabolic concentrator probe for efficient light collection in spectroscopy of biological tissue. *Applied Optics*, 1996. **35**(4): 758–763.

58. Kong, C.-R. et al., A novel non-imaging optics based Raman spectroscopy device for transdermal blood analyte measurement. *AIP Advances*, 2011. **1**(3): 032175.

59. Mahadevan-Jansen, A. et al., Development of a fiber optic probe to measure NIR Raman spectra of cervical tissue in vivo. *Photochemistry and Photobiology*, 1998. **68**(3): 427–431.

60. Shim, M.G. et al., Study of fiber-optic probes for in vivo medical Raman spectroscopy. *Applied Spectroscopy*, 1999. **53**(6): 619–627.

61. Motz, J.T. et al., Optical fiber probe for biomedical Raman spectroscopy. *Applied Optics*, 2004. **43**(3): 542–554.

62. Vargis, E. et al., Effect of normal variations on disease classification of Raman spectra from cervical tissue. *Analyst*, 2011. **136**(14): 2981–2987.

63. Dochow, S. et al., Multicore fiber with integrated fiber Bragg gratings for background-free Raman sensing. *Optics Express*, 2012. **20**(18): 20156–20169.

64. Matousek, P. et al., Noninvasive Raman spectroscopy of human tissue in vivo. *Applied Spectroscopy*, 2006. **60**(7): 758–763.

65. Matousek, P. and N. Stone, Recent advances in the development of Raman spectroscopy for deep non-invasive medical diagnosis. *Journal of Biophotonics*, 2013. **6**(1): 7–19.

66. Lieber, C.A. et al., In vivo nonmelanoma skin cancer diagnosis using Raman microspectroscopy. *Lasers in Surgery and Medicine*, 2008. **40**(7): 461–467.

67. Everall, N. et al., Picosecond time-resolved Raman spectroscopy of solids: Capabilities and limitations for fluorescence rejection and the influence of diffuse reflectance. *Applied Spectroscopy*, 2001. **55**(12): 1701–1708.

68. Chan, J.W. et al., Micro-Raman spectroscopy detects individual neoplastic and normal hematopoietic cells. *Biophysical Journal*, 2006. **90**(2): 648–656.

69. Xie, C. et al., Real-time Raman spectroscopy of optically trapped living cells and organelles. *Optics Express*, 2004. **12**(25): 6208–6214.

70. Notingher, I. et al., *In situ* characterisation of living cells by Raman spectroscopy. *Spectroscopy: An International Journal*, 2002. **16**(2): 43–51.

71. Minamikawa, T. et al., Label-free detection of peripheral nerve tissues against adjacent tissues by spontaneous Raman microspectroscopy. *Histochemistry and Cell Biology*, 2013. **139**(1): 181–193.

72. Bielecki, C. et al., Classification of inflammatory bowel diseases by means of Raman spectroscopic imaging of epithelium cells. *Journal of Biomedical Optics*, 2012. **17**(7): 076030.

73. Cals, F.L.J. et al., Method development: Raman spectroscopy-based histopathology of oral mucosa. *Journal of Raman Spectroscopy*, 2013. **44**(7): 963–972.

74. Caspers, P.J. et al., In vitro and in vivo Raman spectroscopy of human skin. *Biospectroscopy*, 1998. **4**(5 Suppl): S31–S39.

75. Yamamoto, Y.S. et al., Subsurface sensing of biomedical tissues using a miniaturized Raman probe: Study of thin-layered model samples. *Analytica Chimica Acta*, 2008. **619**(1): 8–13.

76. Day, J.C.C. et al., A miniature confocal Raman probe for endoscopic use. *Physics in Medicine and Biology*, 2009. **54**(23): 7077.

77. Kendall, C. et al., Evaluation of Raman probe for oesophageal cancer diagnostics. *Analyst*, 2010. **135**(12): 3038–3041.

78. Duraipandian, S. et al., Simultaneous fingerprint and high-wavenumber confocal Raman spectroscopy enhances early detection of cervical precancer in vivo. *Analytical Chemistry*, 2012. **84**(14): 5913–5919.

79. Cui, W., C. Kumar, and B. Chance, Experimental study of migration depth for the photons measured at sample surface. *Proceedings of SPIE*, 1991. **1431**: 180–191.

80. Schulmerich, M.V. et al., Subsurface Raman spectroscopy and mapping using a globally illuminated non-confocal fiber-optic array probe in the presence of Raman photon migration. *Applied Spectroscopy*, 2006. **60**(2): 109–114.

81. Eliasson, C. and P. Matousek, Noninvasive authentication of pharmaceutical products through packaging using spatially offset Raman spectroscopy. *Analytical Chemistry*, 2007. **79**(4): 1696–1701.

82. Matousek, P. et al., Numerical simulations of subsurface probing in diffusely scattering media using spatially offset Raman spectroscopy. *Applied Spectroscopy*, 2005. **59**(12): 1485–1492.

83. Schulmerich, M.V. et al., Noninvasive Raman tomographic imaging of canine bone tissue. *Journal of Biomedical Optics*, 2008. **13**(2): 020506-1–020506-3.

84. Matousek, P., Inverse spatially offset Raman spectroscopy for deep noninvasive probing of turbid media. *Applied Spectroscopy*, 2006. **60**(11): 1341–1347.

85. Keller, M.D. et al., Development of a spatially offset Raman spectroscopy probe for breast tumor surgical margin evaluation. *Journal of Biomedical Optics*, 2011. **16**(7): 077006.

86. Matousek, P. et al., Subsurface probing in diffusely scattering media using spatially offset Raman spectroscopy. *Applied Spectroscopy*, 2005. **59**(4): 393–400.

87. Okagbare, P.I. et al., Noninvasive Raman spectroscopy of rat tibiae: Approach to in vivo assessment of bone quality. *Journal of Biomedical Optics*, 2012. **17**(9): 090502-1.

88. Maher, J.R. et al., Overconstrained library-based fitting method reveals age- and disease-related differences in transcutaneous Raman spectra of murine bones. *Journal of Biomedical Optics*, 2013. **18**(7): 077001.

89. Okagbare, P.I. et al., Development of non-invasive Raman spectroscopy for in vivo evaluation of bone graft osseointegration in a rat model. *Analyst*, 2010. **135**(12): 3142–3146.

90. Matousek, P. and N. Stone, Prospects for the diagnosis of breast cancer by noninvasive probing of calcifications using transmission Raman spectroscopy. *Journal of Biomedical Optics*, 2007. **12**(2): 024008.

91. Stone, N. et al., Subsurface probing of calcifications with spatially offset Raman spectroscopy (SORS): Future possibilities for the diagnosis of breast cancer. *Analyst*, 2007. **132**(9): 899–905.

92. Keller, M.D., S.K. Majumder, and A. Mahadevan-Jansen, Spatially offset Raman spectroscopy of layered soft tissues. *Optics Letters*, 2009. **34**(7): 926–928.

93. Srinivasan, S. et al., Image-guided Raman spectroscopic recovery of canine cortical bone contrast in situ. *Optics Express*, 2008. **16**(16): 12190.

94. Patil, C.A. et al., A handheld laser scanning confocal reflectance imaging-confocal Raman microspectroscopy system. *Biomedical Optics Express*, 2012. **3**(3): 488–502.

95. Caspers, P.J., G.W. Lucassen, and G.J. Puppels, Combined in vivo confocal Raman spectroscopy and confocal microscopy of human skin. *Biophysical Journal*, 2003. **85**(1): 572–580.

96. Evans, J.W. et al., Optical coherence tomography and Raman spectroscopy of the ex-vivo retina. *Journal of Biophotonics*, 2009. **2**(6–7): 398–406.

97. Khan, K.M. et al., Depth-sensitive Raman spectroscopy combined with optical coherence tomography for layered tissue analysis. *Journal of Biophotonics*, 2013. **7**: 77–85.

98. Patil, C.A. et al., Combined Raman spectroscopy and optical coherence tomography device for tissue characterization. *Optics Letters*, 2008. **33**(10): 1135–1137.

99. Patil, C.A. et al., Integrated system for combined Raman spectroscopy-spectral domain optical coherence tomography. *Journal of Biomedical Optics*, 2011. **16**(1): 011007.

100. Patil, C.A. et al., A clinical instrument for combined Raman spectroscopy-optical coherence tomography of skin cancers. *Lasers in Surgery and Medicine*, 2011. **43**(2): 143–151.
101. Huang, Z. et al., Integrated Raman spectroscopy and trimodal wide-field imaging techniques for real-time in vivo tissue Raman measurements at endoscopy. *Optics Letters*, 2009. **34**(6): 758–760.
102. Šćepanović, O.R. et al., A multimodal spectroscopy system for real-time disease diagnosis. *Review of Scientific Instruments*, 2009. **80**: 043103.
103. Cicchi, R. et al., Combined fluorescence-Raman spectroscopic setup for the diagnosis of melanocytic lesions. *Journal of Biophotonics*, 2013. **7**: 86–95.
104. Huang, Z. et al., Raman spectroscopy in combination with background near-infrared autofluorescence enhances the in vivo assessment of malignant tissues. *Photochemistry and Photobiology*, 2005. **81**(5): 1219–1226.
105. Yu, N.-T. et al., Disulfide bond formation in the eye lens. *Proceedings of the National Academy of Sciences*, 1985. **82**(23): 7965–7968.
106. Palmer, G.M. et al., Optimal methods for fluorescence and diffuse reflectance measurements of tissue biopsy samples. *Lasers in Surgery and Medicine*, 2002. **30**(3): 191–200.
107. Williams, A.C. et al., A critical comparison of some Raman spectroscopic techniques for studies of human stratum corneum. *Pharmaceutical Research*, 1993. **10**(11): 1642–1647.
108. Huang, Z. et al., Effect of formalin fixation on the near-infrared Raman spectroscopy of normal and cancerous human bronchial tissues. *International Journal of Oncology*, 2003. **23**(3): 649–656.
109. Institute, A.N.S., *Safe Use of Lasers in Research, Development, or Testing*, 2012. Orlando, FL: Laser Institute of America.
110. Pence, I.J., E. Vargis, and A. Mahadevan-Jansen, Assessing variability of in vivo tissue Raman spectra. *Applied Spectroscopy*, 2013. **67**(7): 789–800.
111. Krishnamoorthi, H. and A. Mahadevan-Jansen, Calibration of Raman systems for biomedical and clinical applications. *SPIE Photonics West*, San Francisco, CA, 2010.
112. Mosier-Boss, P.A., S. Lieberman, and R. Newbery, Fluorescence rejection in Raman spectroscopy by shifted-spectra, edge detection, and FFT filtering techniques. *Applied Spectroscopy*, 1995. **49**(5): 630–638.
113. Van Duyne, R.P., D.L. Jeanmaire, and D. Shriver, Mode-locked laser Raman spectroscopy. New technique for the rejection of interfering background luminescence signals. *Analytical Chemistry*, 1974. **46**(2): 213–222.
114. O'Grady, A. et al., Quantitative Raman spectroscopy of highly fluorescent samples using pseudosecond derivatives and multivariate analysis. *Analytical Chemistry*, 2001. **73**(9): 2058–2065.
115. Zhang, D. and D. Ben-Amotz, Enhanced chemical classification of Raman images in the presence of strong fluorescence interference. *Applied Spectroscopy*, 2000. **54**(9): 1379–1383.
116. Barclay, V., R. Bonner, and I. Hamilton, Application of wavelet transforms to experimental spectra: Smoothing, denoising, and data set compression. *Analytical Chemistry*, 1997. **69**(1): 78–90.
117. Cai, T.T., D. Zhang, and D. Ben-Amotz, Enhanced chemical classification of Raman images using multiresolution wavelet transformation. *Applied Spectroscopy*, 2001. **55**(9): 1124–1130.
118. Vickers, T.J., R.E. Wambles, and C.K. Mann, Curve fitting and linearity: Data processing in Raman spectroscopy. *Applied Spectroscopy*, 2001. **55**(4): 389–393.
119. Baraga, J.J., M.S. Feld, and R.P. Rava, Rapid near-infrared Raman-spectroscopy of human tissue with a spectrograph and CCD detector. *Applied Spectroscopy*, 1992. **46**(2): 187–190.
120. De Luca, A.C. et al., Online fluorescence suppression in modulated Raman spectroscopy. *Analytical Chemistry*, 2009. **82**(2): 738–745.
121. Lieber, C.A. et al., Diagnostic tool for early detection of ovarian cancers using Raman spectroscopy. *BiOS 2000 the International Symposium on Biomedical Optics*, 2000. San Jose, CA, International Society for Optics and Photonics.
122. Zhao, J. et al., Automated autofluorescence background subtraction algorithm for biomedical Raman spectroscopy. *Applied Spectroscopy*, 2007. **61**(11): 1225–1232.

123. Cadusch, P.J., M.M. Hlaing, S.A. Wade, S.L. McArthur, and P.R. Stoddart, Improved methods for fluorescence background subtraction from Raman spectra. *Journal of Raman Spectroscopy*, 2013. **44**: 1587–1595.

124. Zhang, Z.M. et al., An intelligent background-correction algorithm for highly fluorescent samples in Raman spectroscopy. *Journal of Raman Spectroscopy*, 2010. **41**(6): 659–669.

125. Liu, C. et al., Near-IR Fourier transform Raman spectroscopy of normal and atherosclerotic human aorta. *Lasers in the Life Sciences*, 1992. **4**(4): 257–264.

126. Liu, C.H. et al., Raman, fluorescence, and time-resolved light scattering as optical diagnostic techniques to separate diseased and normal biomedical media. *Journal of Photochemistry and Photobiology B*, 1992. **16**(2): 187–209.

127. Petrich, W., Mid-infrared and Raman spectroscopy for medical diagnostics. *Applied Spectroscopy Reviews*, 2001. **36**(2–3): 181–237.

128. Mahadevan-Jansen, A. et al., Near-infrared Raman spectroscopy for in vitro detection of cervical precancers. *Photochemistry and Photobiology*, 1998. **68**(1): 123–132.

129. Berger, A.J. et al., Multicomponent blood analysis by near-infrared Raman spectroscopy. *Applied Optics*, 1999. **38**(13): 2916–2926.

130. Mahadevan-Jansen, A. et al., *Biomedical Vibrational Spectroscopy II: 19–20 January, 2002, San Jose [California] USA. Progress in Biomedical Optics and Imaging*, 2002. Bellingham, WA: SPIE, p. vii, 172pp.

131. Shafer-Peltier, K.E., A.S. Haka, M. Fitzmaurice, J. Crowe, J. Myles, R.R. Dasari, and M.S. Feld, Raman microspectroscopic model of human breast tissue: Implications for breast cancer diagnosis in vivo. *Journal of Raman Spectroscopy*, 2002. **33**: 552–563.

132. Bergholt, M.S. et al., Characterizing variability in in vivo Raman spectra of different anatomical locations in the upper gastrointestinal tract toward cancer detection. *Journal of Biomedical Optics*, 2011. **16**(3): 037003.

133. *Cancer Facts and Figures*, 2012. Atlanta, GA: American Cancer Society.

134. Pearce, E.C., *Anatomy and Physiology for Nurses*, 14th edn., 1966. London, U.K.: Faber, 383pp.

135. Robbins, S.L., R.S. Cotran, and V. Kumar, *Pathologic Basis of Disease*, 3rd edn., 1984. Philadelphia, PA: Saunders, p. x, 1467pp.

136. Alfano, R. et al., Human breast tissues studied by IR Fourier transform Raman spectroscopy. *Lasers in the Life Sciences*, 1991. **4**(1): 23–28.

137. Frank, C.J., R.L. McCreery, and D.C. Redd, Raman spectroscopy of normal and diseased human breast tissues. *Analytical Chemistry*, 1995. **67**(5): 777–783.

138. Manoharan, R. et al., Raman spectroscopy and fluorescence photon migration for breast cancer diagnosis and imaging. *Photochemistry and Photobiology*, 1998. **67**(1): 15–22.

139. Majumder, S.K. et al., Comparison of autofluorescence, diffuse reflectance, and Raman spectroscopy for breast tissue discrimination. *Journal of Biomedical Optics*, 2008. **13**(5): 054009.

140. Centeno, J.A. et al., Laser-Raman microprobe identification of inclusions in capsules associated with silicone gel breast implants. *Modern Pathology*, 1999. **12**(7): 714–721.

141. Redd, D.C. et al., Raman spectroscopic characterization of human breast tissues: Implications for breast cancer diagnosis. *Applied Spectroscopy*, 1993. **47**(6): 787–791.

142. García-Flores, A. et al., High-wavenumber FT-Raman spectroscopy for in vivo and ex vivo measurements of breast cancer. *Theoretical Chemistry Accounts*, 2011. **130**(4–6): 1231–1238.

143. Haka, A.S. et al., Diagnosing breast cancer using Raman spectroscopy: Prospective analysis. *Journal of Biomedical Optics*, 2009. **14**(5): 054023-1–054023-8.

144. Horsnell, J. et al., Raman spectroscopy—A new method for the intra-operative assessment of axillary lymph nodes. *Analyst*, 2010. **135**(12): 3042–3047.

145. Haka, A.S. et al., Identifying microcalcifications in benign and malignant breast lesions by probing differences in their chemical composition using Raman spectroscopy. *Cancer Research*, 2002. **62**(18): 5375–5380.

146. Shafer-Peltier, K.E. et al., Raman microspectroscopic model of human breast tissue: Implications for breast cancer diagnosis in vivo. *Journal of Raman Spectroscopy*, 2002. **33**(7): 552–563.

147. Haka, A.S. et al., Diagnosing breast cancer by using Raman spectroscopy. *Proceedings of the National Academy of Sciences of the United States of America*, 2005. **102**(35): 12371–12376.

148. Chowdary, M.V.P. et al., Discrimination of normal, benign, and malignant breast tissues by Raman spectroscopy. *Biopolymers*, 2006. **83**(5): 556–569.

149. Chowdary, M.V.P. et al., Biochemical correlation of Raman spectra of normal, benign and malignant breast tissues: A spectral deconvolution study. *Biopolymers*, 2009. **91**(7): 539–546.

150. Rehman, S. et al., Raman spectroscopic analysis of breast cancer tissues: Identifying differences between normal, invasive ductal carcinoma and ductal carcinoma in situ of the breast tissue. *Journal of Raman Spectroscopy*, 2007. **38**(10): 1345–1351.

151. Saha, A. et al., Precision of Raman spectroscopy measurements in detection of microcalcifications in breast needle biopsies. *Analytical Chemistry*, 2012. **84**(15): 6715–6722.

152. Stone, N. and P. Matousek, Advanced transmission Raman spectroscopy: A promising tool for breast disease diagnosis. *Cancer Research*, 2008. **68**(11): 4424–4430.

153. Haka, A.S. et al., In vivo margin assessment during partial mastectomy breast surgery using Raman spectroscopy. *Cancer Research*, 2006. **66**(6): 3317–3322.

154. Ferenczy, A. and B. Winkler, Cervical intraepithelial neoplasia and condyloma. In: *Blaustein's Pathology of the Female Genital Tract*, Kurman, R.J., ed., 3rd edn., 1987. New York: Springer-Verlag, pp. 184–191.

155. Walboomers, J.M. et al., Human papillomavirus is a necessary cause of invasive cervical cancer worldwide. *The Journal of Pathology*, 1999. **189**(1): 12–19.

156. Siegel, R., D. Naishadham, and A. Jemal, Cancer statistics, 2013. *CA: A Cancer Journal for Clinicians*, 2013. **63**(1): 11–30.

157. Myers, E.R. et al., Setting the target for a better cervical screening test: Characteristics of a cost-effective test for cervical neoplasia screening. *Obstetrics & Gynecology*, 2000. **96**(5, Part 1): 645–652.

158. Vargis, E. et al., Sensitivity of Raman spectroscopy to normal patient variability. *Journal of Biomedical Optics*, 2011. **16**(11): 117004.

159. Vargis, E. et al., Near-infrared Raman microspectroscopy detects high-risk human papillomaviruses. *Translational Oncology*, 2012. **5**(3): 172.

160. Kamemoto, L.E. et al., Near-infrared micro-Raman spectroscopy for *in vitro* detection of cervical cancer. *Applied Spectroscopy*, 2010. **64**(3): 255–261.

161. Vidyasagar, M. et al., Prediction of radiotherapy response in cervix cancer by Raman spectroscopy: A pilot study. *Biopolymers*, 2008. **89**(6): 530–537.

162. Vargis, E. et al., Detecting biochemical changes in the rodent cervix during pregnancy using Raman spectroscopy. *Annals of Biomedical Engineering*, 2012. **40**(8): 1814–1824.

163. Williams, A.C., H.G.M. Edwards, and B.W. Barry, Fourier-transform Raman-spectroscopy—A novel application for examining human stratum-corneum. *International Journal of Pharmaceutics*, 1992. **81**(2–3): R11–R14.

164. Williams, A.C., H.G.M. Edwards, and B.W. Barry, Raman-spectra of human keratotic biopolymers—Skin, callus, hair and nail. *Journal of Raman Spectroscopy*, 1994. **25**(1): 95–98.

165. Gniadecka, M., H.C. Wulf, N.N. Mortensen, O.F. Nielsen, and D.H. Christensen, Diagnosis of basal cell carcinoma by Raman spectroscopy. *Journal of Raman Spectroscopy*, 1997. **28**(2-3): 125–129.

166. Sterenborg, H. et al., In vivo fluorescence spectroscopy and imaging of human skin tumours. *Lasers in Medical Science*, 1994. **9**(3): 191–201.

167. Caspers, P.J., G.W. Lucassen, E.A. Carter, H.A. Bruining, and G.J. Puppels, In vivo confocal Raman microspectroscopy of the skin: Noninvasive determination of molecular concentration profiles. *Journal of Investigative Dermatology*, 2001. **116**(3): 434–442.

168. Hata, T.R. et al., Non-invasive Raman spectroscopic detection of carotenoids in human skin. *Journal of Investigative Dermatology*, 2000. **115**(3): 441–448.

169. Cheng, W.T. et al., Micro-Raman spectroscopy used to identify and grade human skin pilomatrix-oma. *Microscopy Research and Technique*, 2005. **68**(2): 75–79.

170. Lieber, C.A. et al., Raman microspectroscopy for skin cancer detection in vitro. *Journal of Biomedical Optics*, 2008. **13**(2): 024013.

171. Nijssen, A. et al., Discriminating basal cell carcinoma from perilesional skin using high wave-number Raman spectroscopy. *Journal of Biomedical Optics*, 2007. **12**(3): 034004.

172. Huang, Z. et al., Raman spectroscopy of in vivo cutaneous melanin. *Journal of Biomedical Optics*, 2004. **9**(6): 1198–1205.

173. Zhao, J. et al., Real-time Raman spectroscopy for non-invasive skin cancer detection—Preliminary results. *Conference Proceedings: Annual International Conference of the IEEE Engineering in Medicine and Biology Society*, 2008. **2008**: 3107–3109.

174. Huang, Z. et al., Rapid near-infrared Raman spectroscopy system for real-time in vivo skin measurements. *Optics Letters*, 2001. **26**(22): 1782–1784.

175. Gniadecka, M. et al., Melanoma diagnosis by Raman spectroscopy and neural networks: Structure alterations in proteins and lipids in intact cancer tissue. *The Journal of Investigative Dermatology*, 2004. **122**(2): 443–449.

176. Sigurdsson, S. et al., Detection of skin cancer by classification of Raman spectra. *IEEE Transactions on Bio-medical Engineering*, 2004. **51**(10): 1784–1793.

177. Lui, H. et al., Real-time Raman spectroscopy for in vivo skin cancer diagnosis. *Cancer Research*, 2012. **72**(10): 2491–2500.

178. Malini, R. et al., Discrimination of normal, inflammatory, premalignant, and malignant oral tissue: A Raman spectroscopy study. *Biopolymers*, 2006. **81**(3): 179–193.

179. Bergholt, M.S., W. Zheng, and Z.W. Huang, Characterizing variability in in vivo Raman spectroscopic properties of different anatomical sites of normal tissue in the oral cavity. *Journal of Raman Spectroscopy*, 2012. **43**(2): 255–262.

180. de Carvalho, L.F. et al., Spectral region optimization for Raman-based optical biopsy of inflammatory lesions. *Photomedicine and Laser Surgery*, 2010. **28**(S1): S-111–S-117.

181. Almond, L.M. et al., Endoscopic Raman spectroscopy enables objective diagnosis of dysplasia in Barrett's esophagus. *Gastrointestinal Endoscopy*, 2014. **79**(1): 37–45.

182. Shetty, G. et al., Raman spectroscopy: Elucidation of biochemical changes in carcinogenesis of oesophagus. *British Journal of Cancer*, 2006. **94**(10): 1460–1464.

183. Stone, N. et al., Raman spectroscopy for identification of epithelial cancers. *Faraday Discussions*, 2004. **126**: 141–157; discussion 169–183.

184. Huang, Z. et al., In vivo early diagnosis of gastric dysplasia using narrow-band image-guided Raman endoscopy. *Journal of Biomedical Optics*, 2010. **15**(3): 037017.

185. Stone, N. et al., Near-infrared Raman spectroscopy for the classification of epithelial pre-cancers and cancers. *Journal of Raman Spectroscopy*, 2002. **33**(7): 564–573.

186. Teh, S.K. et al., Diagnosis of gastric cancer using near-infrared Raman spectroscopy and classification and regression tree techniques. *Journal of Biomedical Optics*, 2008. **13**(3): 034013.

187. Molckovsky, A. et al., Diagnostic potential of near-infrared Raman spectroscopy in the colon: Differentiating adenomatous from hyperplastic polyps. *Gastrointestinal Endoscopy*, 2003. **57**(3): 396–402.

188. Shim, M.G. et al., In vivo near-infrared Raman spectroscopy: Demonstration of feasibility during clinical gastrointestinal endoscopy. *Photochemistry and Photobiology*, 2000. **72**(1): 146–150.

189. Chowdary, M.V. et al., Discrimination of normal and malignant mucosal tissues of the colon by Raman spectroscopy. *Photomedicine and Laser Surgery*, 2007. **25**(4): 269–274.

190. Widjaja, E., W. Zheng, and Z.W. Huang, Classification of colonic tissues using near-infrared Raman spectroscopy and support vector machines. *International Journal of Oncology*, 2008. **32**(3): 653–662.

191. Feld, M.S.M., R. Manoharan, J. Salenius, J. Orenstein-Carndona, T.J. Romer, J.F. Brennan, R.R. Dasari, and. Y. Wang, Detection and characterization of human tissue lesions with near infrared Raman spectroscopy. In: *Advances in Fluorescence Sensing Technology*, Lakowicz, J.R., ed., 1995. Bellingham, WA: SPIE.

192. Lakowicz, J.R., Advances in fluorescence sensing technology II. *Proceedings of SPIE*, 1995. **2388**, 56–66.

193. Bi, X. et al., Development of spectral markers for the discrimination of ulcerative colitis and Crohn's disease using Raman spectroscopy. *Diseases of the Colon and Rectum*, 2010. **54**(1): 48–53.

194. Gosselin, M.-È. et al., Raman spectroscopic evidence for nuclear disulfide in isolated lenses of hyperbaric oxygen-treated guinea pigs. *Experimental Eye Research*, 2007. **84**(3): 493–499.

195. Morris, M.D. and G.S. Mandair, Raman assessment of bone quality. *Clinical Orthopaedics and Related Research*, 2011. **469**: 2160–2169.

196. Short, M.A. et al., Using laser Raman spectroscopy to reduce false positives of autofluorescence bronchoscopies: A pilot study. *Journal of Thoracic Oncology*, 2011. **6**(7): 1206–1214.

197. Chen, P. et al., Raman signature from brain hippocampus could aid Alzheimer's disease diagnosis. *Applied Optics*, 2009. **48**(24): 4743–4748.

198. Esmonde-White, K.A. et al., Raman spectroscopy of synovial fluid as a tool for diagnosing osteoarthritis. *Journal of Biomedical Optics*, 2009. **14**(3): 034013.

199. Tfayli, A. et al., Raman spectroscopy: Feasibility of in vivo survey of stratum corneum lipids, effect of natural aging. *European Journal of Dermatology*, 2012. **22**(1): 36–41.

200. Saleem, M. et al., Optical diagnosis of dengue virus infection in human blood serum using Raman spectroscopy. *Laser Physics Letters*, 2013. **10**(3): 035602.

201. Shao, J. et al., In vivo blood glucose quantification using Raman spectroscopy. *PLoS ONE*, 2012. **7**(10): e48127.

202. Zhang, L.-F. et al., Feasibility research on using Raman spectroscopy with PLS for the quantitative detection of cholesterol content in serum. *Spectroscopy and Spectral Analysis*, 2013. **33**(5): 1253–1256.

203. Chan, G.M. et al., Resonance Raman spectroscopy and the preterm infant carotenoid status. *Journal of Pediatric Gastroenterology and Nutrition*, 2013. **56**(5): 556–559.

204. Poon, K.W. et al., Quantitative reagent-free detection of fibrinogen levels in human blood plasma using Raman spectroscopy. *Analyst*, 2012. **137**(8): 1807–1814.

205. Koljenovi, S. et al., Discriminating vital tumor from necrotic tissue in human glioblastoma tissue samples by Raman spectroscopy. *Laboratory Investigation*, 2002. **82**(10): 1265–1277.

206. Motz, J.T. et al. Development of optical fiber probes for biological Raman spectroscopy. In: *Biomedical Optical Spectroscopy and Diagnostics. OSA Biomedical Topical Meetings, Technical Digest*. Optical Society of America, Washington, DC, 2002.

207. Peterson, C.M. et al., Non-invasive monitoring of blood glucose using Raman spectroscopy. *Diabetes*, 2000. **49**(S1): 490.

208. Motz, J.T., Development of in vivo Raman spectroscopy of atherosclerosis. Thesis, 2003. Cambridge, MA: Massachusetts Institute of Technology.

209. Luneva, O. et al., Ion transport, membrane fluidity and haemoglobin conformation in erythrocyte from patients with cardiovascular diseases: Role of augmented plasma cholesterol. *Pathophysiology*, 2007. **14**(1): 41–46.

23

Recent Developments in Fourier Transform Infrared (FTIR) Microspectroscopic Methods for Biomedical Analyses: From Single-Point Detection to Two-Dimensional Imaging

Rohit Bhargava
*National Institutes
of Health*

Ira W. Levin
*National Institutes
of Health*

23.1 Introduction

Since both biological structures and systems of interest within the materials research community are chemically heterogeneous at the microscopic level, the spatial distribution of the underlying chemical species defining the molecular complex often determines the function and properties of the macroscopic assembly. As a corollary, changes in the microscopic molecular heterogeneity may alter significantly the chemical and physical attributes of a substance. While optical microscopy techniques may be employed to survey molecular heterogeneity, they provide little information on, for example, the chemical composition, molecular structure, or local packing characteristics. In contrast, microspectroscopic techniques, such as those involving vibrational spectroscopy, afford potentially powerful complementary approaches for addressing these questions. Thus, a combination of microscopy methodologies and infrared spectroscopy, in particular, retains the spectroscopic advantages of experimental versatility and the availability of extensive databases, while introducing the spatial selectivity inherent in microscopic techniques. In particular, the mid-infrared spectral region (4000 to 400 cm^{-1}), which has been the focus of microspectroscopic examinations for many decades, has proved to be an invaluable source of compositional and structural information for a wide variety of materials. In this brief survey, we first review the instrumentation required for conducting mid-infrared microspectroscopy and then describe several examples illustrating recent developments in this area.

Infrared microspectroscopy involves the measurement of a vibrational spectral response from a prescribed, small region of an appropriately derived sample. Historically, attempts to harness infrared spectroscopy for microscopic measurements have been successful in various forms for more than 50 years.[1,2] In the last 20 years, a number of approaches have become commonly accepted, and numerous commercial instruments are now either available or being developed. Simultaneously, the growth in the number and variety of studies involving infrared microspectroscopy has been explosive. Although spectral specificity for this technique may be achieved in various ways, the most widely employed current methods involve infrared interferometry. In general, the three basic instrumental approaches for obtaining infrared microspectroscopic measurements are to (1) provide incident infrared radiation to a small area of the sample, (2) restrict detection of the signal from the sample to only a small spatial area, and (3) detect wide field signal radiation through the use of multichannel detectors. Based on integration of a single element or multichannel detector to an interferometer and microscope assembly, we divide our discussion into two parts: (1) single-element microscopy and (2) imaging using multichannel detectors.

23.2 Single-Element Detector FTIR Microspectroscopy

Fourier transform infrared (FTIR) spectroscopy became commercially viable approximately three decades ago, and within 10 years attempts were made to use interferometers for microscopic measurements. Specifically, the advantages of radiation throughput, spectral reproducibility, and time averaging afforded by FTIR spectroscopy were particularly conducive to examining small spatial regions. In addition, the development of stable, sensitive, fast-response cryogenic detectors allowed high-fidelity measurements of spectral intensities.[3] Infrared interferometers coupled to infrared microscopes incorporating these sensitive detectors were introduced in the 1980s.[4] Today, these systems and their advanced versions are used in microscopic infrared analyses in thousands of laboratory locations.

23.2.1 Instrumentation

In single-element microspectroscopic instrumentation,[5] modulated radiation from an interferometer is diverted to a set of optics that condense light to a prescribed spatial area, allowing spectral information to be obtained from small samples. Using opaque apertures of controlled size, smaller and better-defined spatial areas can be imaged by restricting the region illuminated by the infrared beam. Subsequently, the radiation is collected by another set of optical components and focused onto a detector. In this manner, infrared spectra may be obtained from highly specified microscopic locations. To uniquely identify the sample area to be spectroscopically examined, a corresponding white light optical image is also acquired. Clearly, focusing the infrared beam for maximal throughput and minimal dispersion in the sample plane requires the optical and infrared paths to be parfocal and collinear. Hence, an optical microscope is integrated into the infrared microscope assembly. A schematic drawing of the system is shown in Figure 23.1.

Important differences exist between a microscope used for infrared spectroscopy and one used for optical microscopy. While optical microscopy is performed by employing high-quality refractive optics made of glass, infrared microscopes usually consist of all-reflective optics. Glass cannot be employed because it does not transmit radiation wavelengths in the mid-infrared spectrum longer than ~5 µm. Further, spectral fidelity is of paramount concern in the infrared spectral domain, where optical

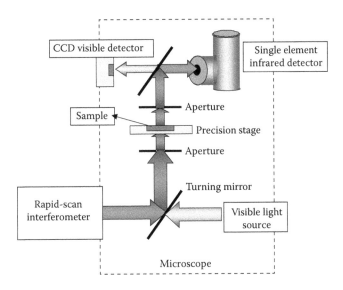

FIGURE 23.1 Schematic diagram of a mapping spectrometer incorporating a single element detector.

aberrations resulting in spectral nonlinearities must be minimized. The source of modulated radiation in the infrared spectral region is derived from an attached rapid-scan interferometer. In principle, any type of modulator may be employed (e.g., step-scan interferometers); rapid-scan interferometers are generally used because they offer cost advantages. Radiation corresponding to small spatial areas is governed by carbon-black-coated metal apertures. In some later designs, specialty infrared absorbing glasses were used, allowing visible imaging while providing restricted infrared imaging.

The instrumentation described above permits the examination of either microscopic samples or narrowly defined regions within larger sample areas and is capable of routinely examining samples in the microgram range. This approach is appropriate particularly for studying small impurities or defects in samples but is of limited utility in obtaining quantitative information from large, heterogeneous materials for which information on the presence and distribution of specific chemical species is desired. By moving the sample, which is easier than moving the optics, different sample locations may be spectroscopically examined. Thus, the sequential movement of the sample in a predetermined manner allows a large sample area to be mapped point by point.[6] Hence, this single-element infrared microspectroscopy using apertures is also referred to as "point mapping" or "point scanning" infrared spectroscopy. Clearly, a sample holder capable of precise microscopic movements must be employed, and for every spatial point a registration of the sample movement to the spectrum corresponding to each spatial index must be maintained. This is accomplished by an automated, programmable microscope stage and an attached computer, which can also be used to control the instrument and to synchronize the various events that are required to map large sample areas.

23.2.2 Capabilities and Limitations

While apertures permit infrared microspectroscopy, they also result in loss of light due to diffraction effects when the aperture is small. In practice, radiation transmitted through an aperture results in the formation of a diffraction pattern and can lead to the detector sampling light from outside the apertured region due to the secondary lobes of the diffraction pattern. The effects of this stray light may compromise the spectral content as far as 40 μm away from the points of interest in the sample.[7] This problem may be circumvented by employing a second aperture in tandem to reject radiation even further. However, this also results in loss of signal from the desired sample area under study, thus degrading the spectral signal-to-noise ratio (SNR) and necessitating larger data-acquisition times to improve data quality. Alternately, large apertures are required for permitting greater radiation throughput, which then incurs a tradeoff between the time required for accumulating data and the achieved spatial resolution. Thus, spatial fidelity and spectral quality are intimately linked in single-element systems incorporating apertures; a balance between the two is required to maximize the efficacy of the sampling protocol.

The design of infrared microscopes that employ apertures for mapping considers the largest aperture that may be employed during the course of experiments. Typically, the largest apertures are approximately on the order of 100×100 μm.[2] Thus, the spot size at the sample plane allowed by the optics is fixed at a larger spot size (hundreds of micrometers in diameter) to account for all aperture sizes that a user might utilize. The effective area available for light throughput is determined, however, by the area of the aperture opening. Thus, the flexibility to employ large aperture sizes implies that the efficiency of light utilization is anywhere from 0.25% to 100%.

23.2.3 Data Processing

Once the spectral response from a sample area is obtained, the absorbance magnitude of a specific vibrational mode is plotted to obtain a map of the distribution of that chemical species. Maps of the relative abundance of chemical species are variously termed "chemical maps" or "functional group maps." Clearly, both the large amount of time required to record data and the optical configuration of a single element detector are not suited either for high spatial resolution or for high spectral resolution mapping over large sample areas. Hence, the acquired data sets usually contain less than 1000 spectral resolution elements and hundreds of spatial resolution elements. Sophisticated spectral data processing may, however, be carried out readily in short time periods. Spatial data processing is of little use because small spatial features are usually below the resolution limit of the technique, and the small number of recorded spatial elements renders the results of many spatial processing routines meaningless. Thus, most data-processing strategies are usually extensions of those developed for a single spectrum acquired by conventional infrared spectrometers.

The usual baseline corrections, normalizations for thickness, and other such steps taken prior to plotting the data for a chemical map are routinely applied. Complex multivariate analyses may be implemented, and library matching of the entire data set is usually feasible. In general, even the most complex data-processing protocols are rapid due to the small data sizes and can be accomplished in a matter of minutes. Computation speeds and power requirements are moderate because less than 1000 spectra are usually processed. One common strategy for use in the spatial domain is to apply deconvolution methods after the point data are acquired, with the points of observation being separated by a distance smaller than the aperture dimension along the direction of separation. Since the collected spectra are often few in number, it is usually more effective to collect data for a longer time than to apply sophisticated techniques for improving the SNR ratio in order to extract molecular information.

23.3 FTIR Raster Imaging Using Multichannel Detectors

While single-element microspectroscopy provides the capability for obtaining spectra from small spatial regions, poor SNR characteristics, diffraction effects, and stray light issues resulting from the use of apertures limits the applicability of these methods. Further, the point-by-point mapping approach results in large collection times and poor utilization of the hundreds of focal plane spot sizes whose diameters measure in the micrometers. An approach to resolve some of these issues has recently been implemented[8] in which, as an improvement over single element detectors, a linear array detector is employed to image an area corresponding to a rectangular spatial area on the sample. Unfortunately, the imaged area may not be sufficiently representative of the distribution of chemical species in the sample, and, hence, a technique to image larger areas is required. To compensate for this the linear array is moved precisely to sequentially image a selected, relatively large spatial region of the sample. This is referred to as "push-broom" mapping or "raster scanning." The process is conceptually similar to point mapping but takes advantage of the multiple channels of detection. Imaging a large sample area is faster by a factor of m for a linear array containing m detector elements.

While detectors for point-by-point mapping are typically 100–250 µm in size, modern array detector pixels are sized in the tens of micrometers. Employment of a linear array thus eliminates the need for apertures because small array detectors directly image different spatial regions. The spatial resolution is determined by the optics; in one commercial implementation,[8] the detectors are 25 µm in size, and the instrument can be operated at either a 1:1 magnification or 4:1 magnification to provide a 25- or 6.25-µm spatial resolution. Such magnification ratios can be readily achieved by employing available infrared optics that are expected to be relatively aberration-free. However, the optical and infrared paths must be collinear, and the visible image must be referenced to acquire infrared data. Further, a precision stage that reproducibly steps in small spatial increments is required for any mapping larger than that achieved by one row of detectors. Since a precision stage is an integral part of the instrument and a record of the visible image is required, the instrument does not require any visual observation accessories. Once the sample is manually positioned a visual image can be constructed by using the visible-light camera and by moving the sample stage. The sample area from which infrared spectroscopic data are to be determined is therefore delineated, and acquisition may then be initiated.

23.3.1 Instrumentation

The schematic diagram of the instrumentation, shown in Figure 23.2, is similar to that required for single-element infrared microscopy but incorporates several important changes. First, no apertures are required; consequently, the unavoidable deficiency in utilizing radiation in point mapping systems is mitigated. Second, the requirements for high-quality optics are simpler and not as stringent as those for the single-element microscope. Third, the spot size can be smaller and matched to the size of the detector array. Since the infrared radiation is more effectively utilized, a reduced intensity source can be employed. Further, the small number of detectors allows fast readout times, and, with the interferometer being operated in a continuous scan mode, instrumental costs decrease. By combining a small multichannel detector with rapid-scan spectroscopy to allow mirror scanning in a favorable Fourier frequency regime, and by utilizing frequency domain filtering, higher SNR data can be obtained. Compared to single element detector systems, the removal of apertures allows for higher radiation

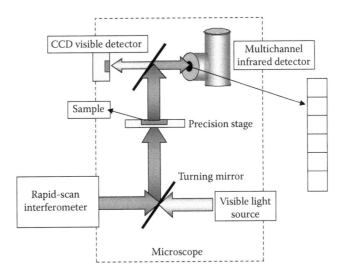

FIGURE 23.2 Schematic diagram of raster-scanning instrumentation for FTIR microspectroscopy.

throughput and provides additional increases in the SNR of data obtained. Hence, with respect to point mapping procedures, the performance of raster-scanning systems is enhanced for both the spatial and spectral domains.

23.3.2 Data and Data Processing

A data set from a raster-scanning system can be quite large compared to a single element detector system. For the same data-acquisition time the data set increases by at least the number of channels present in the detector. Further, as discussed above, the SNR per measurement time is higher; hence, in a given time, larger data sets are obtained. The spatial resolution of raster-scanning systems is essentially diffraction-limited, resulting in chemical concentration plots over the field of view being comparable to the visualization afforded by optical microscopy methods. Many data-processing techniques for enhancing visible images can be effectively applied to the infrared spectroscopic data. In addition, since large numbers of spectra are accumulated in each data set, multivariate methods allow statistically rigorous conclusions to be determined.

23.4 Global FTIR Spectroscopic Imaging

The state of the art in FTIR microspectroscopic instrumentation is the combination of a focal plane array (FPA) detector and an interferometer.[9,10] FPA detectors consist of thousands of individual detectors placed in a two-dimensional grid pattern. Compared to a linear array, the increase in the number of detectors increases the multichannel advantage; for example, a $p \times p$ pixel focal plane array detector provides a p^2 time savings compared to a single-element detector and a p^2/m time saving compared to a linear array detector, where m is the number of detector elements in the linear array detector. For a 256×256 element detector compared to the single-element case, the advantage is a factor of 65,536; in comparison to the 16-element detector, the multichannel advantage is a factor of 4096. Further, the two-dimensional detectors are capable of imaging large spatial areas. An FPA matched to the characteristics of the optical system is capable of imaging the entire field of view afforded by the optics and of utilizing a large fraction of the infrared radiation spot size at the plane of the sample. Among the available various infrared microspectroscopic methods, FPA-based global imaging represents the most versatile approach toward viewing large sample areas and in recording spectral intensities.

Since the methodology of microspectroscopy employing FPA detectors is similar to the acquisition of images from an optical microscope, the technique has been termed "infrared spectroscopic imaging." FTIR coupled with an FPA detector provides spatially resolved images across a wide field of view in data-collection times comparable to the time required to record a single spectrum at a single spatial location using a single element detector. This enormous advantage in acquisition time allows both spatially and spectrally specific analyses. For example, a single spectrum from a small sample region, comparable to a single FPA pixel, may be examined or a spectroscopic signal from a spectral feature representative of the entire field of view can be imaged. Due to the considerable reduction in experimental recording times both the imaging of large areas of static samples[11] and the examination of dynamic processes are feasible and rapid.

23.4.1 Instrumentation

The schematic of a typical FTIR microimaging system shown in Figure 23.3 interfaces an interferometer to an infrared microscope, yielding a specified spot size at the sample plane. This spot, which is typically hundreds of micrometers in size, is magnified by the optical train and imaged onto a focal plane array that is tens of millimeters in diameter. The spatial resolution is thus determined both by the optics that determine magnification and the size of an individual detector element on the focal

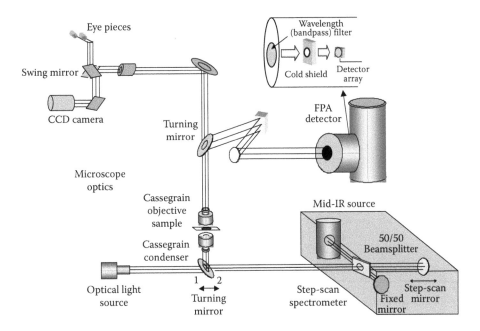

FIGURE 23.3   Schematic diagram of an FTIR imaging spectrometer incorporating a focal plane array detector.

plane array. Even though the nominal spatial resolution is determined by the optics and the detector, the actual resolution limit usually depends upon the diffraction limit of the wavelengths of interest incident upon the sample.

The first and, to date, most popular approach to FTIR microimaging spectrometers incorporates a step-scan interferometer, which provides a means for maintaining constant optical retardations for desired (often large) time periods. A constant retardation over extended time periods is employed both for signal averaging purposes and for computer storage of the acquired data. An initial small time delay prior to data acquisition allows for mirror stabilization at each interferometer step. The data-acquisition and readout formats may be spatially sequential (rolling mode) or simultaneous (snapshot) across the array. In either case, the signal is integrated for only a fraction of the time required for the collection of each frame. The integration time, number of frames coadded, and number of interferometer retardation steps, which is determined by the desired spectral resolution, determine the time required for the experiment. Since signal integration governs the data quality, efforts are made to increase the ratio of the integration time to the total data-acquisition time.

Imaging configurations utilizing a continuous scan[12] or rapid-scan[13] interferometer have been proposed for small detector arrays. Since a large number of detector elements generally precludes regular rapid scanning velocities due to slow readout rates, many instrumental configurations employ a continuously-scanning interferometer at slow speeds. Some manufacturers employ fast step-scan modes where the mirror is partially stabilized to achieve the same retardation error as in continuous-scan spectroscopy; this approach is termed "slow-scan." While slow-scan approaches appear to be similar to rapid-scan methods, they do not have the advantage afforded by the coupled Fourier frequencies as in rapid scanning and merely delay FPA nonlinearity corrections until after the completion of the interferometer scan. We believe that the utility of these slow-scan methods is limited and of little consequence in acquiring high SNR data. A generalized data-acquisition scheme that permits true rapid-scan data acquisition for large arrays or higher mirror speed acquisitions from small arrays has been proposed.[13] The integration time for individual frames collected by the FPA detector is small enough to be considered negligible on the time scale of interferogram collection. For most FPA detectors available today, however, the motion of the moving mirror in a continuous-scan mode does not allow the coaddition of frames per interferometer retardation step. Compared to step-scan approaches, rapid-scan data collection allows fast interferogram acquisition because there is no requirement for mirror stabilization; however, the image stored per resolution element is noisier. Although random FPA noise is dominant, the error arising from the deviation in mirror position during frame collection is considered the next largest contributor. The advantage of continuous-scan interferometry lies in reduced instrumentation costs compared to step-scan units and more efficient data collection because mirror-stabilization times are eliminated.

23.4.2 Post-Collection Operations

The major difference between all other forms of FTIR spectroscopy and FTIR spectroscopic imaging is the extremely large volumes of data handled in the latter mode of operation. For a 256 × 256 element FPA, a user may acquire tens of gigabytes of data per hour. Further, the human comprehension of such a large volume of data in its entirety is not only impossible but also undesirable. Hence, the most common operation is to reduce the data in some manner to allow compact visualization of desired features. A number of analytical approaches have been suggested with the data presented in a variety of forms. Since the information content of the data decreases as the complexity of the representation decreases, the best data-extraction methods cannot be determined *a priori* but are implemented on a case-by-case basis. For example, the most common representations either visualize the two-dimensional distribution of the intensity of a specific vibrational mode over the field of view, project a limited number of spectra from any desired sample region or microdomain, or present statistical distributions of a chemical species. Often, several data-analysis approaches are employed in tandem to provide an effective visualization of the distribution of chemical species.

Another facet of data processing not commonly encountered in conventional infrared spectroscopy is the need to reduce noise in the data set. The low SNR in FTIR images arises both from the characteristics of the FPA and from data-acquisition schemes. While efforts to improve FPAs for spectroscopic imaging have been suggested and advances are constantly being made, the modification of data-acquisition methods is an area of considerable attention. A common data-acquisition approach has been to coadd as many frames as possible during the available experimental time. While this approach results in significant gains, as expected, the SNR, as a function of coadded frames, achieves a plateau.[14] Thus, after the coaddition of a limited number of frames, the benefits are relatively minor compared to the large increase in experimental time expenditures. The coaddition of complete image data sets was shown to be effective in increasing the fidelity of the data, with an optimum sampling strategy being derived by combining both frame and image data-set coaddition. While image coaddition results in improved SNR characteristics, the process involves a $2n^2$ increase in collection time for an SNR improvement factor of n. This rules out image coaddition as a technique to increase the SNR for either real-time imaging of rapidly changing systems or for the expeditious examination of large numbers of samples.

A low-noise, single-beam background ratioed to a single-sample, single-beam image was shown to exhibit lower noise characteristics, allowing for imaging measurements of dynamic systems.[15] This method, termed "pseudo coaddition," is also limited in achievable benefits because noise from the sample's single beam tends to dominate the resultant spectra. Spectra from sample areas with the same true absorbances can be coadded in a similar statistical manner to yield low-noise-average spectra.[15] Mathematical noise reduction, using, for example, the minimum noise fraction (MNF) transform, is an alternate pathway toward obtaining higher-fidelity images after data acquisition.[16] The transformation and inverse transformation after eliminating components due to noise is computationally intensive but does not result in loss of image content or affect image-collection times. The gain in the SNR depends on the SNR characteristics of the original data. Noise is reduced by a factor greater than five if the noise in the initial data is sufficiently low.

23.5 Applications

A recent survey of FTIR techniques, including microspectroscopy, extended to biological materials has been compiled.[17] Although examples of global FTIR imaging applied to biological systems have been discussed elsewhere,[18] we include here several specific studies to illustrate the range of applications and to outline potential future directions. Since FTIR imaging is a noninvasive, nondestructive technique, analyses of intact cells or biopsied tissues are not only a relatively straightforward process but are also of enormous contemporary interest. Conventional cell and tissue examinations are conducted using visible microscopy at various magnification levels. To assist in discrimination between different constituent morphological features of the specimen, samples are stained with reagents responsive to specific chemical components. Although staining methods are generally useful for visualizing tissue structure, they are relatively nonspecific for obtaining detailed chemical information. Moreover, the choice of a specific staining protocol or application of other immunohistochemical techniques often depends on a preliminary biochemical knowledge of the system or disease under scrutiny. FTIR imaging presents, however, an opportunity to directly visualize detailed chemical and morphological characteristics without concern for sample history or disease etiology. As inherent chemical properties of the molecular composition dictate contrast between various components, no sample staining is required. In contrast to conventional IR microscopic methods, the large numbers of spectral data that are obtained through global imaging allow quantitative analyses based on statistical techniques. From the simple demonstration of imaging a lipid [C(16)-lysophosphatidylcholine] distribution in a KBr disk,[19] FTIR imaging applications have grown to include, for example, various tissue sections, single cells, pharmaceutical devices, and food grains.

23.5.1 Human and Animal Tissue Sections

23.5.1.1 Brain

Concentration distributions of various components in thin monkey brain sections[20] revealed specific lipid/protein distributions corresponding to morphological features. Concentration abundance images constructed from spectral data indicated that a greater proportion of lipids occurred in white-matter regions relative to the lipid proportion in gray-matter areas. Since visualization of the entire data set is difficult, a number of statistical methodologies, including scatter plots, histograms, and profile matching, were suggested for data analysis to extract the desired information. These techniques, based on a statistically significant number of observations (spectra), can then be employed to characterize different regions of the tissue. Once the characteristic spectral features of specific regions of a tissue and their inherent variations are known, significant deviations from these may be used to characterize biochemical imbalances, even in cases where morphological changes may be small or nonexistent. This is the fundamental philosophy of employing imaging for biomedical analyses.

Neurotoxic effects of an antineoplastic drug (cytarabine [Ara-C]) on Purkinje cells, which are cells in rat cerebella that have been shown to strongly influence motor coordination and memory processes, were visualized using FTIR imaging.[21,22] Based on the total absorbance inherent in the IR brightfield images, it was observed that the IR images contained more contrast compared to the visible microscopy images. The packing properties of the tissue influenced the refractive index in the infrared spectral region, resulting in better contrast. An analysis of the spectroscopic image from rat cerebella revealed a chemical basis for contrast between different parts of the tissue. This contrast was characterized by a ratio of the lipid-to-protein concentration. The relative lipid concentration exhibited significant differences among sample regions and could be employed as an index to characterize subtle structural changes. The higher protein-packing density of the Purkinje layer was shown to possess increased fractions of disordered lipid acyl chains. Hence, spatially resolved structural changes are determinable based on the molecular information contained in the vibrational spectra.

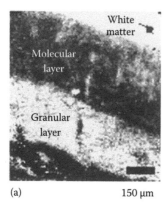
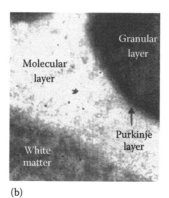
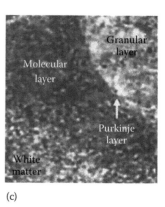

(a)   150 μm   (b)   (c)

FIGURE 23.4 Infrared spectroscopic images of thin cerebellar sections from a control and Ara-C-treated animal. Spectroscopic image showing the spatial distribution of lipid/protein ratios in a rat treated with (a) saline and (b) cytarabine rat. (c) Spectroscopic image depicting the distribution of phosphatidylcholine in a cerebellar section from a cytarabine treated animal. The image is derived from the intensity of a vibrational absorption band centered at approximately 3060 cm⁻¹, assigned to the methyl (CH_3) stretching vibration of the lipid choline headgroup. (From Lester, D.S. et al., *Cell. Mol. Biol.*, 44, 29, 1998. With permission.)

Changes in these measures can be employed to detect and to quantify effects that result from diseases and the effects of drugs or foreign agents. The infrared spectroscopic images reflecting various tissue regions are shown in Figure 23.4.

Neuropathologic effects of a genetic lipid storage disease, Niemann–Pick type C, were investigated by examining sections of control and affected mice cerebella in an effort to understand the chemical basis of the observed morphological changes and to relate these changes to disease pathology.[23] By employing infrared imaging, various cellular layers were readily identified, and the diseased and control samples were distinguished without external, histological staining on the basis of spectral features characteristic of each layer. Lipid depletion was found in diseased samples in comparison to control tissue sections; other molecular differences were discerned in the granular-layer region of the tissue. The observed chemical changes were consistent with demyelination within the cerebellum of the diseased animal. In this manner, morphology and underlying chemical changes are readily correlated. Of particular interest is that separate analyses for each constituent chemical are not required. Instead, a single spectroscopic experiment yields information on the many types of chemical species that are present and their relative concentrations.

23.5.1.2 Bone

As opposed to grinding bone for average spectroscopic analyses, which destroys local structure and may introduce artificial changes, spatially resolved measurements have been carried out on bone-related systems since the 1980s using point mapping. Spatially resolved FTIR imaging[24] has recently allowed the examination of bone in a nondestructive manner, where the advent of imaging allows the rapid characterization of different structures.[25] The spatial variations of chemical components representing the main structural ingredients in bone formation can be easily monitored. For example, hydroxyapatite and protein distributions, as shown in Figure 23.5, illustrate the morphological distributions of these chemicals. Not only can the two-dimensional structure of a thin section be observed, but FTIR imaging also allows the three-dimensional structure of bone, as shown in Figure 23.5, to be visualized in terms of the distribution of its chemical constituents.[26]

The nondestructive nature of the two-dimensional infrared imaging technique also allows the determination of molecular orientation in addition to simple concentration analyses.[24] Chemical-composition data from FTIR imaging and morphology were correlated for human iliac crest biopsies.[27]

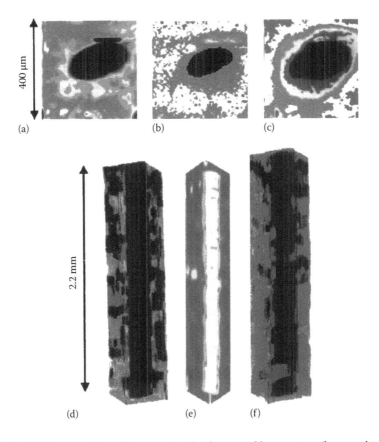

FIGURE 23.5   (a–c) 2D images of three IR parameters for the cortical bone section (human tibia) shown as follows: (a) nonreducible/reducible collagen crosslinks, measured by the 1660/1690 peak height ratio in the amide I spectral region; (b) hydroxyapatite crystallinity index, measured by shape changes in PO_4^{3-} v_1, v_3 mode and quantitated by the 1030/1020 peak height ratio; (c) mineral-to-matrix ratio, measured by the phosphate v_1, v_3/amide I area ratio. Black and blue indicate low numerical values while green, yellow, and red indicate progressively increasing numerical values of the particular parameter. The dimensions of each image are 400 × 400 µm. (d–f) 3D reconstructed views of three IR parameters for the cortical bone section (human tibia), as follows: (d) view of the collagen crosslink parameter measured as the 1660/1690 height ratio in the amide I spectral region; (e) PMMA distribution in a cortical bone section. The relative concentration of PMMA is determined from the integrated intensity of the C=O stretching mode; (f) 3D reconstructed oblique view of the relative amounts of mineral-to-matrix as measured by the phosphate v_1, v_3/amide I area ratio. The dimensions represented in each image are 400 µm × 400 µm × 2.2 mm. (From Ou-Yang, H. et al., *Appl. Spectrosc.*, 56, 419, 2002. With permission.)

The known developmental processes in bone were related to observed gradients in mineral levels by examining spatial profiles from the middle of the osteon to the periphery. The observations were found to be consistent with the models for structure development in the Haversian model of bone development. Protein content, which could be readily monitored using the Amide I contour (1620–1680 cm^{-1}), revealed nonmineralized, high-protein-content regions, namely, the osteoid. A measure of crystallinity and bone maturity was determined using the phosphate v_1, v_3 contour and was found to increase away from the osteonal center. Due to the design of experiments, sample-selection limitations, and the myriad approaches for characterizing extracted chemicals, the available databases are often contradictory and often lead researchers to accept the historical understanding of osteoporosis as a mass deficiency of otherwise healthy bone materials. Using imaging techniques investigators have shown from their examination of spectral data from known, localized sites of mineralized tissue that the conventional view of the disease is not entirely correct. When imaging data from normal and osteoporotic human iliac crest biopsies were compared,[28] two spectral parameters were found useful in characterizing the biochemical changes. The first, which is indicative of the extent of mineral (hydroxyapatite) formation in the tissue, was obtained using a ratio of the integrated areas of the phosphate contour and the amide I peak. This parameter also served to normalize any thickness variations arising from the sample preparation process. The second parameter, indicative of the size and perfection of the crystals, was obtained by taking a ratio of absorbance at 1030 cm^{-1} to the absorbance at 1020 cm^{-1}. It was shown that the average mineral levels in osteoporotic samples are considerably reduced compared to normal bone and that the crystal size and crystal perfection were substantially degraded.

The analysis protocol was applied to examine the effects of estrogen therapy on fracture healing in rat femurs. The mineral content per unit matrix in the estrogen-treated samples was found to be higher, demonstrating the effectiveness of the treatment. Similarly, the crystal sizes and perfection ratios were also found to be elevated in the treated samples. When healing bone was monitored, it was found that several sites along the fracture contained a disproportionately large protein content, indicating that these were sites for the formation of new mineral. In addition, cellular activity was detected at the fracture sites by signals corresponding to cellular-membrane fatty acids. It is clear that FTIR imaging may be employed to detect and monitor normal structure, structure development, and pathological changes in bone through the chemical alterations reflected by localized spectral changes.[24-28]

23.5.1.3 Prostate

Prostate cancer, specifically prostatic adenocarcinoma originating in the epithelial regions of the prostate gland, is prevalent in the western world. In the United States, almost 180,000 men are diagnosed with prostate cancer each year. Similarly, cancer of the prostate is the most common male cancer affecting British men, with the average lifetime risk of development approximately 1 in 13, with nearly 21,000 men diagnosed with prostate cancer every year in the U.K. Early detection and correct diagnoses may increase considerably the number of treatment options available for this disease. We have attempted to discern chemical markers of the onset of prostatic adenocarcinoma before it becomes apparent in morphological changes, which are typically profound for late-stage cancers but extremely subtle and often difficult to discern in the early phases of the disease. The chemical specificity of FTIR spectroscopy is particularly useful in the study of this disease because it can be combined with the spatial selectivity afforded by imaging when analyzing tissue. For prostatic adenocarcinoma, it is particularly important to assess spectral changes in small (5–20 μm wide), localized regions around prostatic ducts, or lumens. A comparison of a stained visible image, as employed for conventional morphological analyses, and an infrared spectroscopic image of the distribution of chemical components is shown in Figure 23.6. Preliminary studies indicate that the analysis of localized spectral changes is an attractive means for characterizing spectral changes for disease diagnosis and for monitoring its progression. Since the spectral changes involved are subtle, large numbers of samples must be examined, and FTIR imaging techniques that provide superior data quality, as indicated in Figure 23.6,[29] must be employed.

23.5.1.4 Breast

Silicone breast implants, consisting of an elastomeric shell filled with silicone gel material, are used extensively for breast enhancement procedures. The silicone gel may leak from the implant due either to material failure as a consequence of aging or to a rupture in the casing. Among the complications arising from this leakage are capsular contracture, calcification, and connective tissue disorders. To reliably assess any histopathological changes it is first necessary to confirm the presence of implant material in the breast tissue. Since silicone gel differs in chemical composition from surrounding tissue,

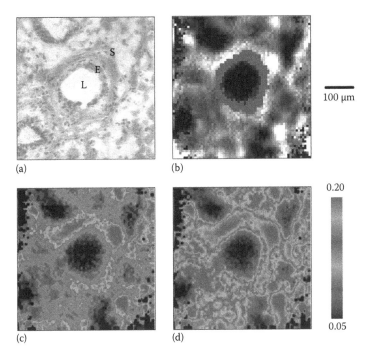

FIGURE 23.6 (a) H&E stained section corresponding to the unstained section used to obtain spectroscopic images. The circular lumen (L) of prostatic gland in the center is lined by a double layer of epithelial cells (E) and supported by a smooth muscular and fibrocollagenous stroma (S). (b) Unstained section with the epithelial regions highlighted in red. Images of the distribution of absorbance obtained by applying (c) no gain ranging at a gain setting of one and (d) gain ranging for gains 1 and 10 with a gain ranging radius of 10 points. The images represent a sample area of 500 μm × 500 μm as indicated by the size bar. The color-coded images show the distribution of the absorbance at 1245 cm^{-1} between the indicated limits. (From Bhargava, R. et al., *Appl. Spectrosc.*, 55, 1580, 2001. With permission.)

it is easily detected in tissue sections using FTIR spectroscopic imaging.[30] The presence of an inclusion was revealed by monitoring the Si-CH$_3$ characteristic stretching vibrations, which are normally absent in human tissue. Silicone gel contaminations in regions as small as ~10 μm could be observed even for inclusions where conventional optical microscopy contrast was poor and chemical specificity was lacking. Dacron, a commercial name for poly(ethylene terepthalate), threads due to fixative patches were also distinguished. In particular, the rapid analysis and minimal sample preparation allowed the detection of contamination within minutes of sectioning the tissue.[30] These advantages imply that FTIR imaging may potentially be useful in settings requiring real-time analysis, for example, in surgical facilities.

23.5.2 Single Cells

The high spatial resolution of infrared imaging, which has allowed the examination of small morphological features in tissues, may also be employed to image single biological cells.[31] An example of single-cell imaging and the associated spectral data that are collected are shown in Figure 23.7. It is expected that in the future the spatial-resolution limits and spectral SNR that can be obtained will allow relatively complete chemical characterizations of single cells and their intracellular components. In particular, the monitoring of biochemical changes within single cellular assemblies that have either been modified in a specific manner or harvested from specific types of tissue will make more detailed approaches to biomedical analyses achievable.

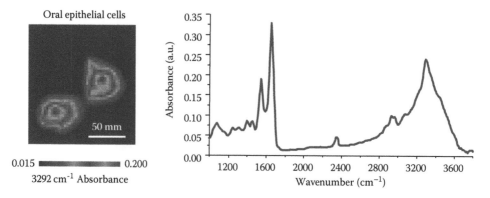

FIGURE 23.7 IR spectroscopic image of single oral epithelial cells (left) and the corresponding spectrum from a part of the cell. The high signal-to-noise ratio of the data allows for detailed analysis of subtle chemical changes.

23.6 Summary

FTIR spectroscopic imaging employing an infrared interferometer and infrared-sensitive multichannel detectors have considerably enhanced the ability to rapidly acquire high-fidelity, spatially resolved data at unprecedented levels of spatial resolution and chemical detectivity. These approaches are particularly suited to detailed biochemical and biological studies in which localized chemical signatures combined with large numbers of recorded data points lead to robust characterization protocols for biomedical analyses. An increase in the number and sophistication of available chemometric tools coupled to this powerful technique undoubtedly will contribute to an explosive growth in the acceptance and use of FTIR spectroscopic imaging in biomedical venues. Significant efforts in the authors' laboratory are under way to demonstrate fully the utility of infrared vibrational spectroscopic imaging for disease detection and diagnosis.

References

1. Barer, R., Cole, A.R.H., and Thompson, H.W., Infra-red spectroscopy with the reflecting microscope in physics, chemistry and biology, *Nature*, 163, 198, 1949.
2. Gore, R.C., Infrared spectrometry of small samples with the reflecting microscope, *Science*, 110, 710, 1949.
3. Reffner, J.A., Instrumental factors in infrared microscopy, *Cell. Mol. Biol.*, 44, 1, 1998.
4. Kwiatkoski, J.M. and Reffner, J.A., FT-IR microscopy advances, *Nature*, 328, 837, 1987.
5. Messerschmidt, R.G., Minimizing optical nonlinearities in infrared microspectroscopy. In: *Practical Guide to Infrared Microspectroscopy*, Humecki, H.J., Ed., Marcel Dekker, New York, 1995, pp. 3–39.
6. Reffner, J.A., Molecular microspectral mapping with the FT-IR microscope, *Inst. Phys. Conf. Ser.*, 98, 559, 1989.
7. Sommer, A.J. and Katon, J.E., Diffraction-induced stray light in infrared microspectroscopy and its effect on spatial resolution, *Appl. Spectrosc.*, 45, 1663, 1991.
8. Spotlight FT-IR Imaging system by Perkin-Elmer Company.
9. Colarusso, P., Kidder, L.H., Levin, I.W., Fraser, J.C., Arens, J.F., and Lewis, E.N., Intrared spectroscopic imaging: From planetary to cellular systems, *Appl. Spectrosc.*, 52, 106A, 1998.
10. Lewis, E.N., Treado, P.J., Reeder, R.C., Story, G.M., Dowrey, A.E., Marcott, C., and Levin, I.W., Fourier-transform spectroscopic imaging using an ingrared focal-plane array detector, *Anal. Chem.*, 67, 3377, 1995.

11. Koenig, J.L. and Snively, C.M., Fast FT-IT imaging: Theory and applications, *Spectroscopy*, 13, 22, 1998.

12. Snively, C.M., Katzenberger, S., Oskarsdottir, G., and Lauterbach, J., Fourier-transform infrared imaging using a rapid-scan spectrometer, *Appl. Opt.*, 24, 1841, 1999.

13. Huffman, S.W., Bhargava, R., and Levin, I.W., A generalized implementation of rapid-scan Fourier transform infrared spectroscopic imaging, *Appl. Spectrosc.*, 56, 965, 2002.

14. Snively, C.M. and Koenig, J.L., Characterizing the performance of a fast FT-IR imaging spectrometer, *Appl. Spectrosc.*, 53, 17, 1999.

15. Bhargava, R., Ribar, T., and Koenig, J.L., Towards faster FT-IR imaging by reducing noise, *Appl. Spectrosc.*, 53, 1313, 1999.

16. Bhargava, R., Wang, S.-Q., and Koenig, J.L., Processing FT-IR imaging data for morphology visualization, *Appl. Spectrosc.*, 54, 1690, 2000.

17. Gremlich, H.-U. and Yan, B., *Infrared and Raman Spectroscopy of Biological Materials*, Marcel Dekker, New York, 2000.

18. Bhargava, R. and Levin, I.W., Fourier transform infrared imaging: A new spectroscopic tool for microscropic analysis of biological tissue, *Trends Appl. Spectrosc.*, 3, 57, 2001.

19. Lewis, E.N. and Levin, I.W., Advances in vibrational imaging microscopy, *J. Microsc. Soc. Am.*, 1, 35, 1995.

20. Lewis, E.N., Gorbach, A.M., Marcott, C., and Levin, I.W., High-fidelity Fourier transform infrared spectroscopic imaging of primate brain tissue, microscopy in neurotoxicity, *Appl. Spectrosc.*, 50, 263, 1996.

21. Lewis, E.N., Kidder, L.H., Levin, I.W., Kalasinsky, V.F., Hanig, J.P., and Lester, D.S., High-fidelity Fourier transform infrared imaging microscopy in neurotoxicity, *Ann. N. Y. Acad. Sci.*, 820, 234, 1997.

22. Lester, D.S., Kidder, L.H., Levin, I.W., and Lewis, E.N., Infrared microspectroscopic imaging of the cerebellum of normal and cytarabine treated rats, *Cell. Mol. Biol.*, 44, 29, 1998.

23. Kidder, L.H., Colarusso, P., Stewart, S.A., Levin, I.W., Appel, N.M., Lester, D.S., Pentchev, P.G., and Lewis, E.N., Infrared spectroscopic imaging of the biochemical modifications induced in the cerebellum of the Niemann–Pick type C mouse, *J. Biomed. Opt.*, 4, 7, 1999.

24. Paschalis, E.P., DiCarlo, E., Betts, F., Sherman, P., Mendelsohn, R., and Boskey, A.L., FTIR microspectroscopic analysis of human osteonal bone, *Calcif. Tissue Int.*, 59, 480, 1996.

25. Marcott, C., Reeder, R.C., Paschalis, E.P., Boskey, A.L., and Mendelsohn, R., Infrared microspectroscopic imaging of biomineralized tissues using a mercury-cadmium-telluride focal-plane array detector, *Phosphorus Sulfur*, 146, 417, 1999.

26. Ou-Yang, H., Paschalis, E.P., Boskey, A.L., and Mendelsohn, R., Chemical structure-based three-dimensional reconstruction of human cortical bone from two-dimensional infrared images, *Appl. Spectrosc.*, 56, 419, 2002.

27. Mendelsohn, R., Paschalis, E.P., and Boskey, A.L., Infrared spectroscopy, microscopy, and microscopic imaging of mineralizing tissues: Spectra-structure correlations from human iliac crest biopsies, *J. Biomed. Opt.*, 4, 14, 1999.

28. Mendelsohn, R., Paschalis, E.P., Sherman, P.J., and Boskey, A.L., IR microscopic imaging of pathological states and fracture healing of bone, *Appl. Spectrosc.*, 54, 1183, 2000.

29. Bhargava, R., Schaeberle, M.D., Fernandez, D.C., and Levin, I.W., Novel route to faster Fourier transform infrared spectroscopic imaging, *Appl. Spectrosc.*, 55, 1580, 2001.

30. Kidder, L.H., Kalasinsky, V.F., Luke, J.L., Levin, I.W., and Lewis, E.N., Visualization of silicone gel in human breast tissue using new infrared imaging spectroscopy, *Nat. Med.*, 3, 235, 1997.

31. Bhargava, R., Fernandez, D.C., and Levin, I.W., FTIR imaging of biological tissue for histopathological analyses, Presentation at *Pittcon 02*, New Orleans, LA, 2002.

24

Diffuse Optical Spectroscopy: Frequency-Domain Techniques

Albert E. Cerussi
*University of
California, Irvine*

Bruce J. Tromberg
*University of
California, Irvine*

24.1 Diffuse Optical Spectroscopy

24.1.1 What Is Diffuse Optical Spectroscopy?

Diffuse optical spectroscopy (DOS) is a technique that combines experimental measurements and model-based data analysis to measure the bulk absorption and scattering properties of highly scattering media. DOS typically uses red and near-infrared (NIR) light, especially from 600 to 1000 nm, where light propagation in tissue is heavily dominated by scattering [1]. DOS measurements of tissue optical properties (i.e., absorption and scattering) are assumed to contain information about tissue structure and function. The term diffuse optics refers to photons that propagate randomly throughout the tissue. DOS utilizes the photons that conventional optical techniques discard; instead of collimated or coherent photons, DOS measures incoherent, multiply scattered photons that are spread out over space and time. Diffusive photons probe a large sample volume, providing *macroscopically averaged* absorption and scattering properties at depths up to *a few centimeters* in tissues.

In the red and NIR spectral regions, the dominant molecular absorbers in tissue are oxygenated (Hb-O$_2$) and reduced hemoglobin (Hb-R), water, and lipids [2,3]. Myoglobin (which is indistinguishable from hemoglobin in the NIR), cytochrome aa$_3$, and other hemoglobin states also absorb in the NIR but are found in small concentrations.*

The frequency-domain DOS techniques featured in this article measure absorption independently from scattering; not all NIR diffusive measurements do this. Such distinction is important because NIR photon attenuation is chiefly due to scattering. Traditional absorption spectroscopy assumes negligible scattering. With the help of DOS techniques, one can recover undistorted absorption spectra from within tissues and ultimately quantify absorber concentrations. Scattering spectra also can provide useful information about tissue structure and composition.

24.1.2 Historical Development

The dramatic growth of clinical laser applications during the 1990s has stimulated intense research into the fundamental nature of light-tissue interactions. Although studies in highly scattering biological materials were performed in the 1930s [4], significant advances in the quantitative characterization of tissue optical properties in vivo were not made until the early 1990s. Bonner et al. introduced *photon migration* in tissue by proposing a random-walk theory to infer bulk tissue scattering, absorption, and photon path lengths [5]. Delpy [6] and Chance [7] employed time-resolved spectroscopy to measure photon path lengths and thereby determine hemoglobin concentration in tissue. Transport theory models had been developed earlier [8] but did not become widely accepted for modeling in tissue optics until the late 1980s [9,10], Patterson et al. measured absorption independently from scattering using analytic time- and frequency-domain models [11,12].

Fishkin and Gratton first applied frequency-domain methods to turbid media and described the propagation of intensity-modulated light in terms of photon density waves (PDWs) [13]. Svaasand and Tromberg characterized the frequency dependence of PDWs and employed measurements of PDW dispersion to quantify absorption and scattering in turbid media [14]. Rapid and inexpensive means for measuring absorption and scattering in turbid media soon followed [15]. There are several advantages to the frequency-domain method in terms of information content, measurement speed, and cost [16].

Tissue physiology can be inferred from reliable measurements of tissue absorption [2]. DOS systems typically feature two wavelengths, the bare minimum needed to recover [Hb-O$_2$] and [Hb-R].† Restricting systems to only two or three wavelengths can lead to significant errors, even for relative parameters such as the hemoglobin saturation, S$_t$O$_2$ [17].‡ Increased spectral bandwidth adds more information content and improves accuracy [18].

Recent reviews suggest that diffuse optical methods can provide unique information and will play an important role in medicine [19–21]. As of this writing, there are several commercial devices based upon the technology described in this chapter. Although many possibilities exist, the most important general application of DOS lies in quantifying thick tissue hemodynamics. Because the DOS signal represents a volume average of tissue, the diffusively measured S$_t$O$_2$ is primarily representative of the tissue microvasculature [22]. This exquisite sensitivity to microvasculature suggests many broad applications in medicine (see Section 24.5 of this chapter for examples).

---

* The validity of this statement depends upon both tissue site and physiological condition.
† The brackets "[ ]" will be used to denote concentration.
‡ The hemoglobin saturation is defined as S$_t$O$_2$ = [Hb-O$_2$]/THC, with THC = [Hb-R] + [Hb-O$_2$].

24.2 Working in the Frequency Domain

24.2.1 Basics of the Frequency-Domain Method

The time- and frequency-domain methods are general tools used to study light propagation in tissues. Time-domain spectroscopy measures the *temporal broadening* of an initial narrow pulse of light as it interacts with a sample (Figure 24.1). Typical mechanisms behind these propagation delays include photon scattering and fluorescence lifetimes. The broadened pulse shape contains quantitative information about the decay mechanisms involved.

Frequency-domain spectroscopy measures the propagation of harmonic signals (Figure 24.2). We start with an *intensity-modulated* light source, characterized by an average intensity (DC), an oscillating intensity (AC), and a phase (ϕ), which has the form

$$I_s = DC_s + AC_s \cos(\phi - \omega t). \tag{24.1}$$

In the previous expression, I is the total intensity, ω is the angular frequency (such that $\omega = 2\pi f$, where f is the *modulation frequency*), and the subscript "s" denotes the source. The modulation frequency is the on–off rate of source and is not related to the photon energy. The source need not be modulated at a single frequency; any waveform may be described as a sum of the terms of Equation 24.1. The detected wave and source wave repeat at the same frequency.

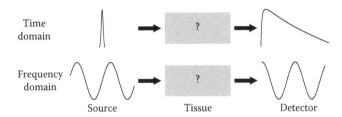

FIGURE 24.1 Time-domain spectroscopy measures the temporal broadening in an incident pulse. Frequency-domain spectroscopy measures changes in wave characteristics relative to the incident wave.

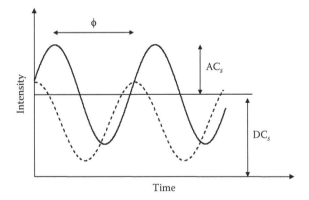

FIGURE 24.2 The measured frequency-domain parameters are a phase shift (ϕ) and a modulation decrease (i.e., ratio of AC to DC components) of the detected wave with respect to the source. Both source and detected waves oscillate at the same frequency f.

Figure 24.2 demonstrates the measured frequency-domain parameters. The detected response (dotted wave) is *shifted* in phase (ϕ) and *reduced* in modulation (M) with respect to the source (solid wave). The term *modulation*, or *modulation depth*, refers to AC_s/DC_s at f and ideally is equal to unity. In frequency-domain spectroscopy, there is no carrier wave; we do not modulate the frequency (frequency modulation, or FM), the AC amplitude (amplitude modulation, or AM), or the phase (phase modulation, or PM) of the optical wave.

An important point is that ϕ and M denote *relative quantities* that describe *absolute values*. Such relative measurements are insensitive to artifacts that can complicate absolute intensity measurements. Modulated signals can be discriminated against background signals at different frequencies (such as unwanted room light). Measurements in both time and frequency domains are equivalent, being related by temporal Fourier transforms. Since it is possible to obtain enough information for DOS using a single frequency, frequency-domain measurements can be very rapid and cost-effective [15].

24.2.2 Need for the Frequency Domain

The richer frequency-domain information content (or equivalent time domain) is usually needed to perform quantitative absorption and scattering spectroscopy in thick tissues. The intensity of light transmitted through a purely absorbing medium (i.e., negligible scattering) is related to the incident intensity I_0 via the Beer–Lambert law:

$$AB = \log\left(I_0/I\right) = \varepsilon[C]L,\tag{24.2}$$

where
  AB is the absorbance
  L is the photon path length (cm)
  $[C]$ is the absorber concentration
  ε is the molar extinction coefficient (mol/L cm^{-1}, or cm^2/mol)*

In terms of μ_a, the Beer–Lambert law is $I = I_0 \exp(-\mu_a L)$, so that μ_a is proportional to the absorber concentration:

$$\mu_a \approx 2.303\varepsilon[C].\tag{24.3}$$

In purely absorbing media, it is relatively simple to measure μ_a (or $[C]$ if ε is known) since L is equal to the width of the sample. However, in the case of multiple scattering, L is not known a priori. Scattering *increases the photon path length* beyond the geometrical path of the light (Figure 24.3). L must be known in order to accurately determine $[C]$. Frequency-domain spectroscopy provides a method that effectively measures L so that $[C]$ may be determined.

There is another way to view this dilemma. In the infinite medium geometry, diffusion theory predicts DC intensity at a detector placed a distance r from the source with the form

$$DC_d \propto \frac{1}{r}\exp\left[-r\sqrt{\mu_a\mu_s'}\,\right],\tag{24.4}$$

where the subscript "d" refers to the detected intensity. It is not possible to separate analytically the effects of μ_a from μ_s' using a single measurement because of the product between μ_a and μ_s'. Under certain conditions,

---

* This ε is based upon a base 10-logarithm scale.

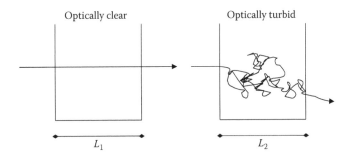

Optically clear   Optically turbid

L_1 L_2

FIGURE 24.3 Multiple scattering increases the photon path length. Although both samples have the same thickness, $L_2 \gg L_1$ due to intense multiple scattering. The absorber concentration cannot be determined unless L is known.

it is possible to separate μ_a from μ_s' while performing steady-state multiple-distance measurements on a tissue surface (i.e., spatially resolved reflectance), although the method involves source–detector separations that are too small for characterizing tissue optical properties at depths beyond several millimeters [17].

24.3 Frequency-Domain Solution to the Diffusion Equation

24.3.1 General Transport of Light in Turbid Media

Transport theory is a statistical bookkeeping scheme that treats photons as noninteracting point particles undergoing elastic interactions. The quantity of interest is the photon density (photons mm^{-3}).* The transport equation is easy to assemble, but difficult to solve analytically, even in simple cases [23]. DOS can use numerical solutions, but important physical insight has come from simple analytic models. The general P_n approximation allows tractable analytic solutions. The P_1 approximation keeps only first-order spherical harmonic expansion terms of the transport equation [23]. Forcing the photon density to discard its true angular dependence introduces limitations that must be carefully understood. The P_1 approximation is sometimes referred to as the *diffusion approximation*, but there are some important differences between these approximations [24]. Excellent reviews exist on this topic [25,26].

24.3.2 P_1 Approximation: Infinite Medium Solution

24.3.2.1 Formal Theory

Assuming an isotropic point source, keeping terms to first order reveals the P_1 *equation*, expressing the photon density, $U(\mathbf{r},t)$, in terms of the optical properties of the tissue [24,27]:

$$vD\left[\frac{3}{v^2}\frac{\partial^2 U(\mathbf{r},t)}{\partial t^2} - \nabla^2 U(\mathbf{r},t)\right] + (1+3\mu_a D)\frac{\partial U(\mathbf{r},t)}{\partial t} + v\mu_a U(\mathbf{r},t) = Q(\mathbf{r},t) + \frac{3D}{v}\frac{\partial Q(\mathbf{r},t)}{\partial t}, \quad (24.5)$$

where
v is the speed of light inside the medium
$Q(\mathbf{r},t)$ is the photon density per unit time injected by the source
$vD \equiv v(3\mu_s'+3\mu_a)^{-1} \equiv v(3\mu_{tr})^{-1}$ is the optical diffusion coefficient (mm^2 s^{-1})†

---

* Some texts use the radiance as the fundamental quantity, which is the power per unit area per solid angle. The magnitude of this vector, averaged over the solid angle, divided by the photon energy, gives the photon density.
† μ_s' represents a scattering length where the direction of the photon has been randomized. Actual scattering events occur on a much smaller length scale.

The variables $|\mathbf{r}|$ and t represent distance from the source and time, respectively. Three important assumptions make this expansion possible: (1) The medium is assumed to be *macroscopically homogeneous*, (2) we must be *far* from sources and boundaries (i.e., more than one transport mean-free-path, *mfp*), and (3) the medium must be *strongly scattering* (i.e., $\mu_s \gg \mu_a$). These limitations stem from restricting the angular dependence of U; thus, Equation 24.5 is only valid in regions where anisotropy is low.

The P_1 equation is simple to solve in the frequency domain. Noting that $i^2 = -1$, a frequency-domain point source has the form

$$Q(\mathbf{r}, \omega, t) = S(\omega) \exp\left[-i\left(\omega t - \phi_0(\omega)\right)\right] \delta(\mathbf{r}). \tag{24.6}$$

We have not broken the source into AC and DC components as in Equation 24.1 since the DC component results from setting $\omega = 0$. The terms $S(\omega)$ and $\phi_0(\omega)$ are frequency-dependent instrumental factors, called the source strength (photons $mm^{-3}\ s^{-1}$) and source phase (degrees), respectively. The delta function represents a point source centered at $\mathbf{r} = 0$. In the frequency domain, all time-dependent factors become $\exp(-i\omega t)$, as in Equation 24.6. If we substitute $U(\mathbf{r}, \omega)\exp(-i\omega t)$ for $U(\mathbf{r}, t)$ and so on, we arrive at the following expression for Equation 24.5:

$$\left[\nabla^2 - k^2(\omega)\right] U(\mathbf{r}, \omega) = -\frac{S(\omega)}{vD} \exp\left[-i\phi_o(\omega)\right] \delta(\mathbf{r}). \tag{24.7}$$

$$k^2(\omega) \equiv \frac{\mu_a}{D}\left[1 - i\frac{\omega}{v\mu_a}(1 + 3\mu_a D)\right]. \tag{24.8}$$

Equation 24.7 is a *Helmholtz equation*, whose solutions are known to be *waves*. Within this framework, ik is a wave vector (mm^{-1}). It is critical to note that k depends upon μ_a, μ_s', and ω. Using infinite medium boundary conditions (i.e., $U(r, \omega) \to 0$ as $r \to \infty$), we can write down a 1D solution to Equation 24.7:

$$U(r, \omega) = \frac{S(\omega)\exp\left[-i\phi_0(\omega)\right]}{4\pi vD} \frac{1}{r} \exp\left[-k(\omega) r\right]. \tag{24.9}$$

The frequency-domain solution emerges as a *damped-spherical-photon-density wave*. These PDWs exhibit classical wave phenomena such as diffraction, reflection, and refraction [13,28]. The phase and amplitude of the PDW described by Equation 24.7 are

$$\Theta_{\text{inf}}(r, \omega) = k_{imag}(\omega) r + \phi_0 \qquad A_{\text{inf}}(r, \omega) = \frac{S(\omega)}{4\pi vD\ r} \exp\left[-k_{real}(\omega)\ r\right]. \tag{24.10}$$

The subscript "inf" reminds us these equations are valid in infinite media. k_{real} and k_{imag} represent the real and imaginary parts of k, respectively. We have written Equation 24.10 as functions of r and ω since measurements of μ_a and μ_s' depend upon changing r and/or ω.

24.3.2.2 Frequency Dependence

Figure 24.4 demonstrates the dispersion of the components of k for a medium with optical properties of $\mu_a = 0.006\ mm^{-1}$ and $\mu_s' = 1.0\ mm^{-1}$. k_{real} is representative of the wave attenuation; higher-frequency components have higher k_{real} and higher attenuation. The sensitivity of k to the optical properties changes with f. Intuitively, we may rewrite absorption and transport coefficients (μ_{tr}) as relaxation frequencies ($f_a \equiv v\mu_a$ and $f_{tr} \equiv v\mu_{tr} = v(\mu_a + \mu_s')$, respectively) or as relaxation times ($\tau_a = 1/f_a$ and $\tau_{tr} = 1/f_{tr}$). In the DC case ($\omega = 0$), the wave vector values become

$$k_{real}(0) = \sqrt{3\mu_a\mu_s'} \quad \text{and} \quad k_{imag}(0) = 0. \tag{24.11}$$

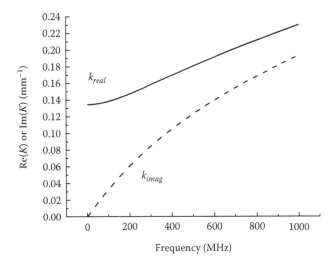

FIGURE 24.4 PDW characteristics are determined by the real (solid line) and imaginary (dashed line) parts of the wave vector, k. The plot uses $\mu_a = 0.006$ mm^{-1} and $\mu'_s = 1.0$ mm^{-1}. The sensitivity of k to μ_a and μ'_s depends upon f (i.e., wave dispersion).

In the DC regime, the product $\mu_a\mu'_s$ determines the attenuation and there is no phase information. k_{real} is very sensitive to changes in μ_a and μ'_s, but changes in μ_a cannot be distinguished from changes in μ'_s. If we increase f with a low-frequency expansion (i.e., $\omega \gg v\mu_a$) of Equation 24.8,

$$k_{real}(\omega) \approx \sqrt{3\mu_a\mu'_s}\left\{1 + \frac{1}{8}(\omega\tau_a)^2\right\} \quad k_{imag}(\omega) \approx \sqrt{3\mu_a\mu'_s}\,\frac{\omega\tau_a}{2}, \tag{24.12}$$

where we have made the assumption $\mu_a \ll \mu'_s$ for diffusive media. The term *low frequency* implies frequencies well below f_a, where most frequency-domain measurements have been performed. In most tissues, μ_a ranges from 0.002 to 0.02 mm^{-1}, and thus, f_a ranges from 60 to 680 MHz. Within this low-frequency approximation, ϕ is linear in f (see Equation 24.10).

As f increases above f_a, the character of the k changes considerably. A higher-frequency expansion of the real and imaginary parts of Equation 24.8 reveals ($\omega \gg f_a$ but $\omega^2 \ll f_a f_{tr}$) [29]:

$$k_{real}(\omega) = k_{imag}(\omega) = \sqrt{\frac{3}{2}\frac{\omega}{v}\mu'_s}. \tag{24.13}$$

In this limit, the wave vector loses dependence upon μ_a. Eventually, this behavior changes; in the limit where $\omega^2 \gg f_a f_{tr}$, transport theory breaks down, leaving us with

$$k_{real}(\omega \to \infty) = 0 \quad \text{and} \quad k_{imag}(\omega \to \infty) = 3\frac{\omega}{v}. \tag{24.14}$$

Photons described by this behavior are ballistic in nature and are not scattered. These expressions also describe the leading edge of the time-domain pulse [24].

24.3.2.3 Diffusion Wavelength

The diffusion wavelength, or $\lambda_{PDW} \equiv 2\pi/k_{imag}(\omega)$, has nothing to do with the photon energy. λ_{PDW} depends upon the optical properties of the medium. Given a modulation frequency of 200 MHz, $\mu_a = 0.006$ mm^{-1}, and $\mu'_s = 1.0$ mm^{-1}, and λ_{PDW} is about 105 mm. The wave-front speed is given by $v_{PDW} = \lambda_{PDW}\,f$, setting

$v_{PDW} \sim 2.1 \times 10^{10}$ mm s^{-1}. The diffusive wave-front speed proceeds at approximately one order of magnitude slower than the speed of an individual photon. λ_{PDW} is generally much greater than our typical sampling distances of a few centimeters so that in general, we record PDW phase and amplitude in a *near-field* region. Higher modulation frequencies reduce λ_{PDW}, signifying greater attenuation and lower penetration.

24.3.3 P_1 Approximation: Semi-Infinite Medium Solution

24.3.3.1 Changes in the Theory

There are two types of discontinuities that impose important boundaries for light propagation in tissues: (1) index of refraction and (2) optical property. For example, the abrupt index of refraction mismatch at the air–tissue interface can lead to total-internal reflection. Encounters with this boundary will alter the spatial distribution of the PDW. In order to accurately quantify average tissue optical properties, it is essential to modify the light transport model to account for this interface. In practical terms, this permits the use of measurement geometries that place the source and detector outside the tissue (i.e., in a nonscattering medium). Our approach uses the method of images to place an image source at the same point above the boundary as the actual source below the boundary forces. This configuration forces U to vanish along any plane perpendicular to the surface normal. Moving the condition of $U = 0$ to a plane *external* to the medium forces a sort of quasi-isotropic condition at the boundary by using the reflected flux at the boundary [31]. The location of the extrapolated boundary, z_b, is given by

$$z_b = \frac{2}{3}\frac{1+R_{eff}}{1-R_{eff}}l_{tr},$$ (24.15)

where R_{eff} represents an effective Fresnel coefficient for the tissue-outside medium interface. Typical values for z_b are about 2 mm beyond the physical boundary. Groenhuis et al. have provided an empirical expression for R_{eff}, whereas Haskell et al. have calculated this coefficient to be 0.493 and 0.431 when the air–tissue interfaces are $n = 1.4$ and 1.33, respectively [30,31].

Using the subscript "si" to denote semi-infinite, solutions to the extrapolated boundary problem take the form of $U_{SI}(r,\omega,t) = U_{INF}(r_a,\omega,t) - U_{INF}(r_i,\omega,t)$. Solving this equation with a modified extrapolated boundary condition yields the phase shift and amplitude of a PDW in a semi-infinite medium [31]:

$$\Theta_{si}(\rho,\omega) = k_{imag}(\omega)r_0 - \arctan\left(\frac{\eta}{\xi}\right) + \phi_0(\omega)$$ (24.16)

$$A_{si}(\rho,\omega) = \frac{S(\omega)}{4\pi vD}\sqrt{\xi^2 + \eta^2},$$ (24.17)

where

$$\xi = \frac{1}{r_0}\exp\left[-k_{real}(\omega)r_0\right] - \cos\left[k_{imag}(\omega)(r_{0b} - r_0)\right]\frac{1}{r_{0b}}\exp\left[-k_{real}(\omega)r_{0b}\right]$$

$$\eta = \sin\left[k_{imag}(\omega)(r_{0b} - r_0)\right]\frac{1}{r_{0b}}\exp\left[-k_{real}(\omega)r_{0b}\right]$$ (24.18)

and

$$r_a = \sqrt{\rho^2 + \left(l_{tr}\right)^2} \qquad r_a = \sqrt{\rho^2 + \left(2z_bl_{tr}\right)^2}.$$ (24.19)

24.3.3.2 Sensitivity to the Optical Properties

Figures 24.5 and 24.6 present the photon density as functions of the experimental variables r and f, respectively. For the sake of comparison, each line style represents the same set of optical coefficients: solid line ($\mu_a = 0.01$ mm^{-1}, $\mu_s' = 1$ mm^{-1}), dotted line ($\mu_a = 0.01$ mm^{-1}, $\mu_s' = 0.5$ mm^{-1}), and dashed line ($\mu_a = 0.002$ mm^{-1}, $\mu_s' = 1$ mm^{-1}). In each graph, Equations 24.16 and 24.17 provide (a) the AC intensity and (b) the phase. In Figure 24.5, intensities and phases have been normalized to the $r = 10$ mm value.

Changes in μ_s' and in μ_a have different effects upon A and Θ. For example, assume μ_s' increases while keeping μ_a constant (dotted line vs. solid line). Increasing μ_s' results in greater attenuation (i.e., lower A). This same increased μ_s' allows longer-path-length photons to be detected

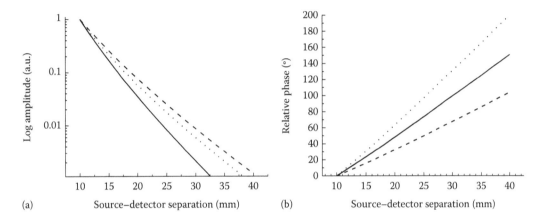

(a)   Source–detector separation (mm)   (b)   Source–detector separation (mm)

FIGURE 24.5 Calculated changes in PDW amplitude (a) and phase (b) as a function of r for three sets of optical properties: solid line ($\mu_a = 0.01$ mm^{-1}, $\mu_s' = 1$ mm^{-1}), dotted line ($\mu_a = 0.01$ mm^{-1}, $\mu_s' = 0.5$ mm^{-1}), and dashed line ($\mu_a = 0.002$ mm^{-1}, $\mu_s' = 1$ mm^{-1}). Intensities and phases have been normalized to the $r = 10$ mm value. Note the linearity of the phase and log (amplitude).

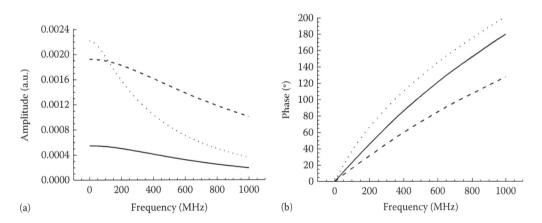

(a)   Frequency (MHz)   (b)   Frequency (MHz)

FIGURE 24.6 Calculated changes in PDW amplitude (a) and phase (b) as a function of f. See Figure 24.5 for line definitions. Note that the curvature changes vary with changes in μ_a and μ_s'.

(i.e., higher Θ). These longer-path-length photons increase the overall phase of the detected signal. However, if we increase μ_a and keep μ'_s constant (dashed line vs. solid line), the attenuation increases as before, but the longer-path-length photons will be deleted and hence decrease the phase. Thus, A and Θ have *different sensitivities* to μ_a and μ'_s, allowing them to be *measured independently* from each other.

24.3.4 Standard Diffusion Equation

In the standard diffusion equation (SDE), a few more approximations simplify the mathematics: (1) the scattering mfp must be *much smaller* than the absorption mfp, or $\mu'_s \gg \mu_a$, and (2) $3\omega Dv^{-1} \ll 1$. The physical meaning of the term $3\omega Dv^{-1}$ is an isotropic collision period ($\tau_{coll} = 1/v\mu'_s$). The source has its own period too: $\tau_{mod} = 1/f = 2\pi/\omega$. The condition $3\omega Dv^{-1} \ll 1$ is another way of saying that there must be many collisions within a single modulation period [24]. Tissues on average possess $\mu'_s \sim 1$ mm^{-1}, so that τ_{coll} is typically about 5 ps, limiting $f < 1$ GHz. It has been shown conclusively that the diffusion approximation breaks down at higher frequencies [24].

The approximations earlier simply change the layout of our previous Helmholtz equation. The solutions (infinite and semi-infinite) remain the same, but the wave vector simplifies to

$$k^2(\omega) \equiv \frac{\mu_a}{D}\left(1 - i\frac{\omega}{v\,\mu_a}\right). \tag{24.20}$$

In many cases, there is little difference between the P_1 and diffusion approximations. The slight edge in frequency response and range of μ'_s makes P_1 the more rigorous choice.

24.3.5 Measurements of PDW

Changing r and f have different effects upon the PDW intensity and phase (Figures 24.5 and 24.6). In each case, it is possible to infer the optical properties of the medium by monitoring the response of the intensity and phase to changes in r and/or f.

Tromberg et al. measured the optical properties of turbid media by changing the modulation frequency [29]. Sweeping f assures the sampling of regions where A and Θ are sensitive to μ_a and μ'_s. For example, measurements of Θ versus f can recover μ_a and μ'_s, but only when a sufficient frequency range is used that samples PDW dispersion [14,24]. Fitting A and Θ *simultaneously* produces the best results [33]. Frequency-swept methods also allow measurements at a single r, limiting depth-sampling errors (Figure 24.7). However, instrumentation artifacts S and ϕ_0 must be removed by a calibration measurement performed on a phantom of known optical properties. Simultaneous fitting of A and Θ must be performed with multiple initial guesses to ensure that nonlinear global fits converge upon a true global minimum.

Fantini et al. demonstrated that the diffusion equation in both the infinite [15] and semi-infinite geometries [32] possesses a linear relationship between Θ and r (Figure 24.5). In addition, $\ln(A\,r)$ is linear in r in the infinite medium geometry; a function related to $\ln(A\,r^2)$ is linear with r in the semi-infinite geometry. The optical properties are related to the *slopes* of the measured frequency-domain parameters versus r. All source term information (i.e., S and ϕ) is constrained to the intercepts. Thus, simple linear fits of the intensity and phase slopes yield a *direct* calculation of μ_a and μ'_s. Measurements can be performed at a single modulation frequency, greatly simplifying the instrumentation. However, one must be careful to not use f in a region of low sensitivity to μ_a or μ'_s [29]. If multiple light sources are used for each r, then the intensities and phases of each must be calibrated, again on a phantom of known optical properties. Changing r probes different tissue volumes (Figure 24.7), while changing f over frequencies around f_a changes the probed volume to a lesser extent.

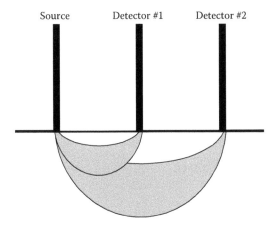

FIGURE 24.7 Different source–detector separations sample different depths of tissue. The shaded areas represent the average volume probed by the light for a given source–detector separation. Differences in probed volume can cause problems in some layered (such as in the brain) or inhomogeneous (such as in a tumor) media. Note that changes in modulation frequency also change the probing depth but to a lesser extent.

24.4 Frequency-Domain Instrumentation

24.4.1 Frequency-Domain Instrument

Figure 24.8 shows the essential elements of a frequency-domain instrument. There have been several detailed descriptions of frequency-domain photon migration (FDPM) devices [16,33–35]. An intensity-modulated light source (at frequency f) excites a sample. Diffusely reflected light is collected from the sample at frequency f and guided to an optical detector. Typically, the detector is modulated at $f + \Delta f$ to process the high-frequency signal. The detected signal is then digitized and processed. Special consider-ations are required since some components must respond to $f > 100$ MHz.*

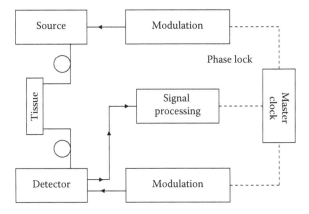

FIGURE 24.8 Simple schematic for a frequency-domain instrument. The key element is that the modulation of source and detector must be synchronized (i.e., phase locked).

---

* We will use the designation RF to describe the MHz regime.

In order to detect modulated optical signals, both source and detector clocks must be *phase-locked* together. A phase shift between two unsynchronized waves is random, obscuring any physical meaning of the phase. Locking together the clocks of these waves synchronizes them. Most frequency-domain systems use a 10 MHz master clock signal as a phase lock. One notable *exception* is the system developed by Tromberg, which uses a commercial network analyzer as both radio-frequency (RF) source and RF detector, eliminating the need for external phase locking [33]. Typically, the light source is referenced to account for drifts in the source phase and intensity. When it is not possible or practical to employ this optical reference, an electronic reference may be used instead.

24.4.2 Frequency-Domain Source

24.4.2.1 Internal Modulation

Light sources can be modulated internally by directly modulating their supply power. The modulation of the supply current of laser diodes (LDs) and light-emitting diodes (LEDs) alters the optical output. Conventional lamps can also be modulated internally, but at frequencies far too low for use in DOS. Some lasers are modulated internally by *mode locking* or coordinating the phases between different longitudinal modes within the laser cavity. A typical titanium–sapphire laser, such as the Coherent Mira system, is mode locked with 150 fs pulses firing at approximately 80 MHz.

Semiconductor technology has substantially advanced biomedical optics by providing inexpensive and portable light sources. A DC bias current turns on the LD by marginally exceeding the threshold current I_{th}. A small RF current on top of the DC bias current drives the diode above and below I_{th}, switching the diode on and off (Figure 24.9). This condition yields the maximum modulation depth of the source (100%). One may trade modulation depth for increased optical power. Increasing the DC bias and RF currents results in more optical power, but to maintain the same modulation depth, more RF current is needed. Solid-state devices can only handle so much RF current and will typically fail if the current drives negative. In general, NIR LEDs can be modulated in the 100 MHz range and LDs up to and beyond 1 GHz.

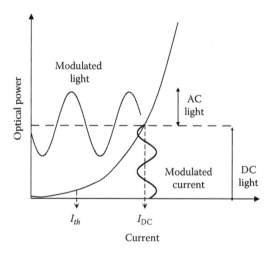

FIGURE 24.9 Modulation of solid-state devices consists of exceeding the threshold current with a modulated current. For a given amount of RF power, the modulation depth decreases as the optical power increases; thus, a balance must be made between modulation depth and total output power. Note that this same general principle applies to modulating a solid-state detector such as an APD.

24.4.2.2 External Modulation

External modulation occurs outside the light source. Mechanical choppers can achieve modulation, but not at frequencies high enough to be useful in DOS. External devices, such the acousto-optic modulator (AOM) and the Pockels cell, may be used on either laser beams or lamps, although modulation efficiency is highly sensitive to input beam quality.

By inducing birefringence in a crystal from the application of an oscillating applied voltage, the Pockels cell is essentially a fast-switching polarizer [36]. Required voltages range from 0.1 to over 1 kV, depending upon the cell material and configuration. Pockels cells made from ammonium dihydrogen phosphate (ADP), for example, modulate light in the 0.3–1.2 µM spectral range up to about 500 MHz. Higher-index materials such as lithium niobate can modulate light well above 1 GHz. The ability of the power source to produce voltages of adequate amplitude and frequency also limits the bandwidth of the Pockels cell. High FM is achievable only with collimated light.

The AOM uses an applied voltage to induce ultrasonic standing waves inside a crystal to diffract light. The diffracted spots are modulated, whereas the center beam is unmodulated [37]. Two AOMs in series can be used to beat signals together, thereby increasing the frequency range [38]. Materials such as gallium phosphide can achieve bandwidth up to 1 GHz in the NIR, although a rather large supply voltage is required. Tellurium dioxide AOMs offer lower bandwidths of 300 MHz over a broader spectral region and with a considerable reduction in supply power. Compared to Pockels cells, AOMs have lower overall bandwidth and more modest voltage requirements [36]. The AOM working distance is large since the diffraction angles are small.

24.4.3 Frequency-Domain Detector

24.4.3.1 Signal Detection

Accurately sampling a 100 MHz wave requires a clock running well into the GHz range. One method that allows accurate phase and amplitude measurements of 100 MHz signals is known as *heterodyning*, which is the same process used by AM radio receivers. Consider two signals, a source wave $A_1\sin(\omega t + \phi_1)$ and a detected wave $A_2\sin([\omega + \Delta\omega]t + \phi_2)$. In mixing these waves together (i.e., multiply them), the product becomes

$$\frac{1}{2}A_1A_2\big(\cos(\Delta\omega t + \Delta\phi) - \cos(2\omega t + \Delta\omega t + \phi_1 + \phi_2)\big), \tag{24.21}$$

where $\Delta\phi \equiv \phi_2 - \phi_1$. Equation 24.21 expresses the sum and difference of the frequencies of two waves (i.e., a beat). f is typically 100 MHz or greater, and Δf is in the range of 1 kHz. Under these conditions, the first term of Equation 24.21 can be easily filtered from the second term. The usefulness of heterodyning is that the $\Delta\omega$ term is proportional to A_2 and depends upon $\Delta\phi$. Heterodyning *translates* a high-frequency signal into a low-frequency signal while *retaining* the amplitude and phase information of the detected wave. This low-frequency signal may now be easily processed by standard electronic digitization methods.

Two additional configurations require comment. In the configuration devised by Tromberg, a network analyzer performs all heterodyning operations internally [33]. One can use any detector without concern for additional RF electronics. Secondly, lock-in detection can be used in principle, but in practice can be difficult since (1) both reference and detected signals must be carefully matched in power and (2) most lock-ins are not meant to work in the 100 MHz regime.

24.4.3.2 Photoemissive Detectors

Photomultiplier tubes (PMTs) have been the most commonly used detector in DOS. PMT's are highly inefficient in the NIR, resulting in quantum efficiencies well below 10% out to 800 nm.* A commonly used PMT is the Hamamatsu R928, which has an effective NIR spectral range of 600–840 nm. Advantages of this PMT are its high gain of 10^7 and low dark current (3 nA, with typical signal currents in the 30 μA range). The R928 also has a rise time of 2.2 ns, allowing in principle the detection of signals up to 400 MHz for well-focused light. Additional concerns for using any PMT are their high voltage considerations (the R928 requires about 1200 V).

Shutting off a dynode early in the chain and stopping the avalanche of electrons from reaching the anode modulates a PMT. Applying a sinusoidal voltage at frequency f to the first dynode will turn the PMT on and off at the frequency f [39]. Microchannel plate (MCP) detectors have also been used in DOS [24]. The MCP offers immensely increased bandwidth, often exceeding several GHz. However, the dramatically lower signal currents require high-precision microwave electronics.

24.4.3.3 Solid-State Detectors

The most useful solid-state detector for FDPM is the avalanche photodiode (APD). Photodiodes in general have excellent NIR sensitivity (Si and InGaAs), reaching quantum efficiencies near 100% at 800 nm. Conventional photodiodes have no gain mechanism, while the APD has internal gains that can reach 10^2–10^3 with a low-noise figure. Photodiodes in general are very good frequency-domain detectors capable of processing optical signals in excess of 1 GHz. An APD can be modulated via its supply voltage, as with the PMT (see Figure 24.9). APDs used in DOS are usually reverse biased, with bias voltages below 300 V. One major drawback of the APD is the small active area. An active area of 1 mm² translates into about a 600 MHz bandwidth for the Hamamatsu model S2383 APD; higher active areas generally decrease the frequency response. The APD has adequate sensitivity over the entire NIR range.

24.5 Current Clinical Examples

In the following, we provide a sample of frequency-domain DOS applied to medical problems. This list is not exhaustive, but only representative of frequency-domain DOS in tissues. Space does not permit mention of important works by other authors. Of course, frequency-domain DOS has not been the only method to investigate the examples we describe. The common thread in these emerging applications is that all measurements are quantitative and noninvasive and reveal important aspects of tissue function that were not observed by other methods.

24.5.1 Breast Spectroscopy

24.5.1.1 Past Efforts

Optical transillumination was applied to breast in 1929 as a tool to visualize the shadows cast by breast lesions. Attempts at spectroscopy started in the early 1980s by dividing images into red and NIR bands. Throughout the 1980s, many clinical trials compared transillumination with mammography as a screening tool; a potpourri of conflicting clinical conclusions was the result. By 1990, transillumination sensitivity and specificity were found inferior to mammography [18].

Classical transillumination (sometimes called diaphanography) made no attempt to distinguish between absorption and scattering and could not provide measures of tissue chromophore concentrations. Although direct visualization of lesion anatomy is difficult, if not impossible with visible/NIR optics, *spectroscopic* visualization of tissue function is an entirely different matter. Early studies have shown that red and NIR light absorption in breast is highly sensitive to hemoglobin. However, the

---

* See, for example, the PMT catalog of Hamamatsu (Japan).

presence of blood alone is not sufficient criteria for the diagnosis of cancer, a weakness that probably contributed to the high false-positive rate of transillumination. Neglecting scattering diminishes contrast even further. Additional information about water and lipid content may help improve sensitivity and specificity.

24.5.1.2 New Contributions

Frequency-domain DOS measurements of breast tumors have shown increased absorption by hemoglobin and water, as well as lower S_tO_2 compared to normal tissue [40]. The sources of NIR contrast in healthy breast tissue have been quantified; studies have demonstrated that NIR-derived breast tissue composition and metabolism correlates with known histological changes that occur from long-term and short-term hormonal use [41,42]. These measurements demonstrate clearly that DOS has the sensitivity to detect small functional changes in breast that may prove useful in detecting cancer and monitoring the effectiveness of cancer therapies. The use of endogenous contrast (i.e., hemoglobin) alleviates concerns for any unknown dynamics and undesirable toxicity of exogenous contrast agents.

Pogue et al. have constructed a frequency-domain imager that combines spectral information from 650 to 850 nm [34]. Pilot study results have shown that tumor hemoglobin concentrations correlate with tumor vascularity [43]. This finding indicates that DOS techniques could be used to monitor the progression of anti-angiogenesis drugs in the breast. It is important to note that this work uses model-based reconstructions of tissue optical properties and does not rely upon nonspectroscopic images of shadows. Wideband tissue spectroscopy coupled with this fast image capability may provide an important new approach for imaging tumor angiogenesis.

24.5.2 Functional Brain Monitoring

Rapid frequency-domain techniques have proved useful in probing human brain function. There have been numerous attempts to measure changes in brain hemoglobin concentrations using NIR spectroscopy (see Chapter 9 for greater detail about NIR functional imaging). Activation events, or the so-called *slow* brain signals, are hemodynamic in nature, occurring on a 2–10 s timescale. Relatively simple optical instruments can monitor these hemodynamic changes via absorption. However, it has been observed that changes in brain optical properties are also due to changes in scattering, the so-called *fast* events (50–500 ms). Classic NIR methods that cannot separate absorption from scattering will not quantify these events.

E. Gratton, an early pioneer in the application of frequency-domain methods, used frequency-domain DOS to measure absorption and scattering changes in the brain in vivo [44]. Gratton and colleagues have reported fast (i.e., <1 s) brain optical signal changes that are apparently the result of scattering fluctuations occurring during localized neural tissue activation. Using a commercial two-wavelength, multidistance device with a measurement time of 160 ms (ISS, Urbana, IL), Gratton et al. measured both fast and slow changes in brain optical properties that correlate with brain activity in response to periodic stimuli. In addition, they have shown that these optical changes correlate with electrical changes in the brain. Further work has also centered around measuring correlations in phase and amplitude as a means of quantifying brain optical property changes [45].

24.5.3 Measurements of Tissue Physiology

24.5.3.1 Deep-Tissue Arterial and Venous Oximetry

Pulse oximetry provides the hemoglobin saturation in arterial blood (S_aO_2) by monitoring pulsatile changes in NIR attenuation. The technique is generally limited to thin sections of tissue, such as the fingertip or earlobe. Frequency-domain DOS provides the S_tO_2, which is more representative of the tissue capillary bed (i.e., mixed arterial and venous). Franceschini and coworkers have used a multidistance frequency-domain technique to measure independently the arterial [46] and venous saturations (S_vO_2) [47] in thick tissues. The frequency-domain technique is required to provide the photon path length, which standard NIR techniques cannot do. The discrimination between S_vO_2 and S_aO_2 is accomplished by locking onto the harmonic content of changes in μ_a. Changes in μ_a at the heartbeat frequency correspond to arterial signals, whereas changes in μ_a at the respiratory frequency correspond to venous signals. This technique could be important in both brain and muscle physiology, since there is no way to measure S_vO_2 noninvasively. The technique can be performed in real time.

24.5.3.2 Monitor of Photodynamic Therapy Response

Photodynamic therapy (PDT) drugs provide new treatment options in the management of cancer. A photosensitizing drug in the presence of oxygen will cause tissue necrosis after absorbing an appropriate amount of optical radiation. Without knowledge of the optical properties of the tissue, the exact amount of light dosage required for treatment remains an unknown variable, limiting the effectiveness of the treatment.

Pham et al. used a frequency-domain multifrequency approach to measure changes in tumor physiology in response to a photosensitizer in a rat ovarian cancer model [48]. DOS revealed significant decreases in *THC* and S_tO_2 after the application and subsequent optical activation of the photosensitizer. Histologic inspection of the tumors revealed that the long-term efficacy of the treatment highly correlated with the measured changes in *THC* and S_tO_2. As PDT use increases in clinical practice, DOS could provide rapid feedback about the effectiveness of the delivered photosensitizer dose.

Acknowledgments

We wish to thank many people who have worked with us in contributing to the basic development of DOS: Tuan Pham, Joshua Fishkin, Olivier Coqouz, Eric Anderson, Steen Madsen, and Lars Svaasand. We would like to thank many organizations for their generous support during the development of the ideas in this chapter: National Institutes of Health (NIH) Laser Microbeam and Medical Program (P41RR01192 and P41EB015890), NIH (#R29-GM50958), Department of Energy (DOE #DE-FG03-91ER61227), Air Force Office of Scientific Research (#F49620-00-1-0371), and the Beckman, Whitaker, and Hewitt Foundations. A.E.C. cheerfully acknowledges support from the U.S. Army Medical Research and Materiel Command (DAMD17-98-1-8186).

References

1. Wilson, B. C. et al. Tissue optical properties in relation to light propagation models and in vivo dosimetry, in *Photon Migration in Tissues*, Chance, B., Ed. Plenum, New York, 1988, p. 25.
2. Sevick, E. M. et al. Quantitation of time-resolved and frequency-resolved optical spectra for the determination of tissue oxygenation. *Anal. Biochem.* 195: 330, 1991.
3. Ertefai, S. and Profio, A. E. Spectral transmittance and contrast in breast diaphanography. *Med. Phys.* 12: 393, 1985.
4. Chance, B. et al. Photon migration in muscle and brain, in *Photon Migration in Tissues*, Chance, B., Ed. Plenum, New York, 1990, p. 121.
5. Bonner, R. F. et al. Model for photon migration in turbid biological media. *J. Opt. Soc. Am. A* 4: 423, 1987.
6. Delpy, D. T. et al. Estimation of optical pathlength through tissue from direct time of flight measurement. *Phys. Med. Biol.* 33: 1433, 1988.
7. Chance, B. et al. Comparison of time-resolved and time-unresolved measurements of deoxyhemoglobin in brain. *Proc. Natl. Acad. Sci. USA.* 85: 4971, 1988.
8. Ishimaru, A. *Wave Propagation and Scattering in Random Media*, 1st edn. Academic Press, New York, 1978, p. 572.

9. Star, W. M., Marijnissen, J. P. A., and van Gemert, M. J. C. Light dosimetry in optical phantoms and in tissues. I. Multiple flux and transport theory. *Phys. Med. Biol.* 33: 435, 1988.

10. Profio, A. E. and Doiron, D. R. Transport of light in tissue in photodynamic therapy. *Photochem. Photobiol.* 46: 591, 1987.

11. Patterson, M. S., Chance, B., and Wilson, B. C. Time resolved reflectance and transmittance for the non-invasive measurement of tissue optical properties. *Appl. Opt.* 28: 2331, 1989.

12. Patterson, M. S. et al. Frequency-domain reflectance for the determination of the scattering and absorption properties of tissue. *Appl. Opt.* 30: 4474, 1991.

13. Fishkin, J. B. and Gratton, E. Propagation of photon-density waves in strongly scattering media containing an absorbing semi-infinite plane bounded by a straight edge. *J. Opt. Soc. Am. A* 10: 127, 1993.

14. Svaasand, L. O. and Tromberg, B. J. On the properties of optical waves in turbid media, in *Future Trends in Biomedical Applications of Lasers*. Proc. SPIE 1525, Svaasand, L. Ed, Bellingham, WA, p.41, 1991.

15. Fantini, S. et al. Quantitative determination of the absorption spectra of chromophores in strongly scattering media: A light-emitting-diode based technique. *Appl. Opt.* 33: 5204, 1994.

16. Chance, B. et al. Phase measurement of light absorption and scatter in human tissue. *Rev. Sci. Instrum.* 69: 3457, 1998.

17. Hull, E. L., Nichols, M. G., and Foster, T. H. Quantitative broadband near-infrared spectroscopy of tissue-simulating phantoms containing erythrocytes. *Phys. Med. Biol.* 43: 3381, 1998.

18. Cerussi, A. E. et al. Spectroscopy enhances the information content of optical mammography. *J. Biomed. Opt.* 7: 60, 2002.

19. See *Journal of Biomedical Optics*, 5, 2000 and *Applied Optics*, 36, 1997 special issues.

20. Muller, G. et al. *Medical Optical Tomography: Functional Imaging and Monitoring*. SPIE, Bellingham, WA, 1993.

21. Chance, B. *Photon Migration in Tissues*. Plenum, New York, 1990.

22. Liu, H. et al. Influence of blood vessels on the measurement of hemoglobin oxygenation as determined by time-resolved reflectance spectroscopy. *Med. Phys.* 22: 1209, 1995.

23. Duderstadt, J. J. and Hamilton, L. J. *Nuclear Reactor Analysis*. John Wiley & Sons, New York, 1976, p. 143.

24. Fishkin, J. B. et al. Gigahertz photon density waves in a turbid medium: Theory and experiments. *Phys. Rev. E* 53: 2307, 1996.

25. Starr, W. M. Diffusion theory of light transport, in *Optical-Thermal Response of Laser Irradiated Tissue*, van Gemert, M. J. C., Ed. Plenum Press, New York, 1995, p. 131.

26. Yodh, A. and Chance, B. Spectroscopy and imaging with diffusing light. *Phys. Today* 48: 34, 1996.

27. Kaltenbach, J. M. and Kaschke, M. Frequency- and time-domain modeling of light transport in random media, in *Medical Optical Tomography: Functional Imaging and Monitoring*, Müller, G. et al., Eds., SPIE, Bellingham, WA, 1993, p. 65.

28. Boas, D. A. et al. Scattering and wavelength transduction of diffuse photon density waves. *Phys. Rev. E* 47: R2999, 1993.

29. Tromberg, B. J. et al. Properties of photon density waves in multiple-scattering media. *Appl. Opt.* 32: 607, 1993.

30. Groenhuis, R. A. J., Ferwerda, H. A., and Ten Bosch, J. J. Scattering and absorption of turbid materials determined from reflection measurements. I. Theory. *Appl. Opt.* 22: 2456, 1983.

31. Haskell, R. C. et al. Boundary conditions for the diffusion equation in radiative transfer. *J. Opt. Soc. Am. A* 11, 2727, 1994.

32. Fantini, S., Franceschini, M. A., and Gratton, E. Semi-infinite-geometry boundary problem for light migration in highly scattering media: A frequency-domain study in the diffusion approximation. *J. Opt. Soc. Am. B* 11: 2128, 1994.

33. Pham, T. et al. A Broad bandwidth frequency domain instrument for quantitative tissue optical spectroscopy. *Rev. Sci. Instrum.* 71: 1, 2000.

34. McBride, T. O. et al. A parallel-detection frequency-domain near-infrared tomography system for hemoglobin imaging of the breast in vivo. *Rev. Sci. Instrum.* 72: 1817, 2001.

35. Franceschini, M. A. et al. Optical study of the skeletal muscle during exercise with a second generation frequency-domain tissue oximeter, in *Optical Tomography and Spectroscopy of Tissue*, Proc. SPIE 2979, Chance, B. and Alfano, R.R. Eds., Bellingham, WA, p.807, 1997.

36. http://www.rp-photonics.com/pockels_cells.html (accessed March 28, 2014).

37. Saleh, B. E. A. and Teich, M. C. *Fundamentals of Photonics*. John Wiley & Sons, New York, 1991, p. 800.

38. Piston, D. W. et al. Wide-band acousto-optic light modulator for frequency domain fluorometry and phosphorimetry. *Rev. Sci. Instrum.* 60: 2596, 1989.

39. Gratton, E. and Limkeman, M. A continuously variable frequency cross-correlation phase fluorometer with picosecond resolution. *Biophys. J.* 44: 315, 1983.

40. Tromberg, B. J. et al. Non-invasive in vivo characterization of breast tumors using photon migration spectroscopy. *Neoplasia* 2: 1, 2000.

41. Cerussi, A. E. et al. Sources of absorption and scattering contrast for non-invasive optical mammography. *Acad. Radiol.* 8: 211, 2001.

42. Shah, N. et al. Non-invasive functional optical spectroscopy of human breast tissue. *Proc. Natl. Acad. Sci. U. S. A.* 98: 4420, 2001.

43. Pogue, B. W. et al. Quantitative hemoglobin tomography with diffuse near-infrared spectroscopy: Pilot results in the breast. *Radiology* 218: 261, 2001.

44. Gratton, E. et al. Measurements of scattering and absorption changes in muscle and brain. *Philos. Trans. R. Soc. Lond. B* 352: 727, 1997.

45. Cheung, C. et al. In vivo cerebrovascular measurement combining diffuse near-infrared absorption and correlation spectroscopies. *Phys. Med. Biol.* 46: 2053, 2001.

46. Franceschini, M. A., Gratton, E., and Fantini, S. Noninvasive optical method of measuring tissue and arterial saturation: An application to absolute pulse oximetry of the brain. *Opt. Lett.* 24: 829, 1999.

47. Franceschini, M. A. et al. Near-infrared spiroximetry: Non-invasive measurements of venous saturation in piglets and human subjects. *J. Appl. Physiol.* 92: 372, 2002.

48. Pham, T. H. et al. Monitoring tumor response during photodynamic therapy using near-infrared photon-migration spectroscopy. *Photochem. Photobiol.* 73: 669, 2001.

Index

Milton Keynes UK
Ingram Content Group UK Ltd.
UKHW050309111024
449327UK00049B/435